PEDIATRIC PRACTICE

Infectious Disease

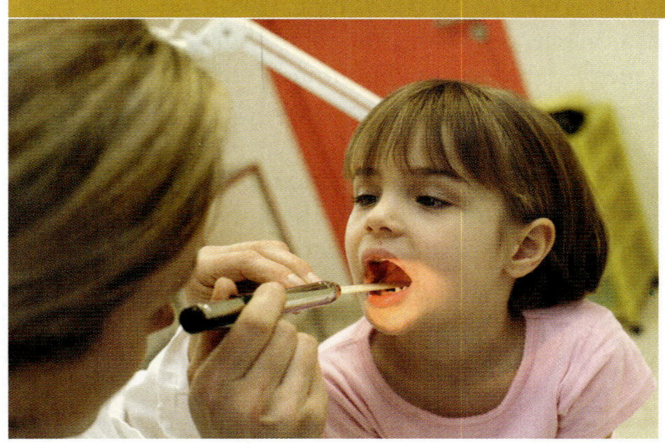

NOTICE

PEDIATRIC PRACTICE

Infectious Disease

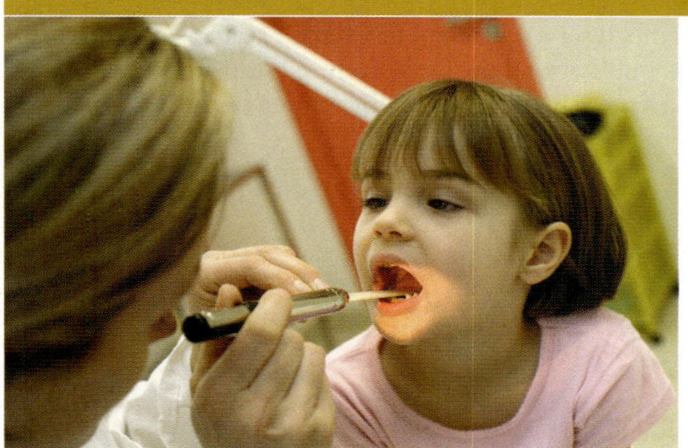

EDITOR

Samir S. Shah, MD, MSCE
Assistant Professor
Departments of Pediatrics and Epidemiology
Senior Scholar
Center for Clinical Epidemiology and Biostatistics
University of Pennsylvania School of Medicine
Attending Physician
Divisions of Infectious Diseases and General
Pediatrics
The Children's Hospital of Philadelphia
Philadelphia, Pennsylvania

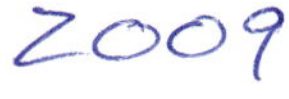

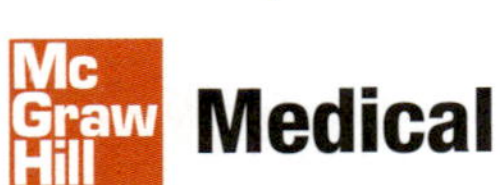

New York Chicago San Francisco Lisbon London Madrid Mexico City
Milan New Delhi San Juan Seoul Singapore Sydney Toronto

The McGraw-Hill Companies

Pediatric Practice: Infectious Disease

1 2 3 4 5 6 7 8 9 0 CTP/CTP 12 11 10 9 8

ISBN 978-0-07-148924-9
MHID 0-07-148924-X

This book was set in Minion by Aptara®, Inc.
The editors were Anne Sydor and Alyssa Fried.
The production supervisor was Phil Galea.
Project management was provided by Sandhya Joshi, Aptara®, Inc.
The designer was Janice Bielawa; the cover designer was David Dell'Accio.
The indexer was Sudeshna Maiti.
China Translation & Printing Services, Ltd. was printer and binder.

This book is printed on acid-free paper.

Photo Credits:
Cover: Credit: Ian Hooton/Photo Researchers, Inc. Caption: Throat examination.
Part 3 opener. Credit: LADA/Hop Americain, Photo Researchers, Inc.
Part 5 opener: Credit: Phanie/Photo Researchers, Inc.
Part 7 opener: Credit: Lea Paterson/Photo Researchers, Inc.
Part 9 opener: Credit: Publiphoto/Photo Researchers, Inc.
Part 11 opener: Credit: Dr P. Marazzi/Photo Researchers, Inc.
Part 13 opener: Credit: BSIP/Photo Researchers, Inc.
Part 14 opener: Credit: Andy Crump, TDR, WHO/Photo Researchers, Inc.
Part 15 opener: Credit: Ian Hooton/Photo Researchers, Inc.
Part 16 opener: Credit; Chris Priest/Photo Researchers, Inc.
Part 17 opener: Credit: Blair Seitz/Photo Researchers, Inc.
Part 18 opener: Credit: Guy Gillette/Photo Researchers, Inc.
Part 19 opener: Credit: Michelle Del Guercio/Photo Researchers, Inc.

Library of Congress Cataloging-in-Publication Data
Pediatric practice. Infectious disease / editor, Samir S. Shah.
p. ; cm.
Includes bibliographical references and index.
ISBN-13: 978-0-07-148924-9 (alk. paper)
ISBN-10: 0-07-148924-X (alk. paper)
1. Communicable diseases in children—Handbooks, manuals, etc. I. Shah, Samir S. II. Title: Infectious disease.
[DNLM: 1. Communicable Diseases. 2. Adolescent. 3. Bacterial Infections. 4. Child. 5. Infant. 6. Mycoses. 7. Parasitic Diseases. 8. Virus Diseases. WC 100 P3727 2009]
RJ401.P435 2009
618.92'9—dc22

2008046422

This book is dedicated to my wife, Kara, and my children, Avani and Siddharth.
Their love and support inspire me.

Contents

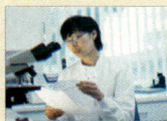

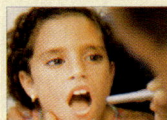

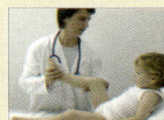

Section 4: Ophthalmologic Infections / 173

Section 5: Oral Cavity and Neck Infections / 205

Section 6: Upper Respiratory Infections / 239

Section 7: Lower Respiratory Infections / 283

Section 8: Cardiac Infections / 349

Section 9: Gastrointestinal Infections / 379

Section 10: Genitourinary Infections / 407

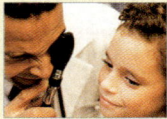

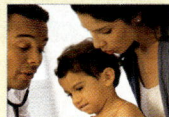

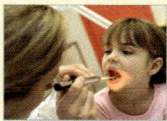

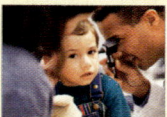

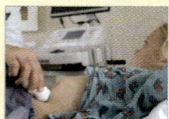

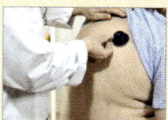

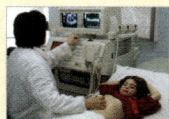

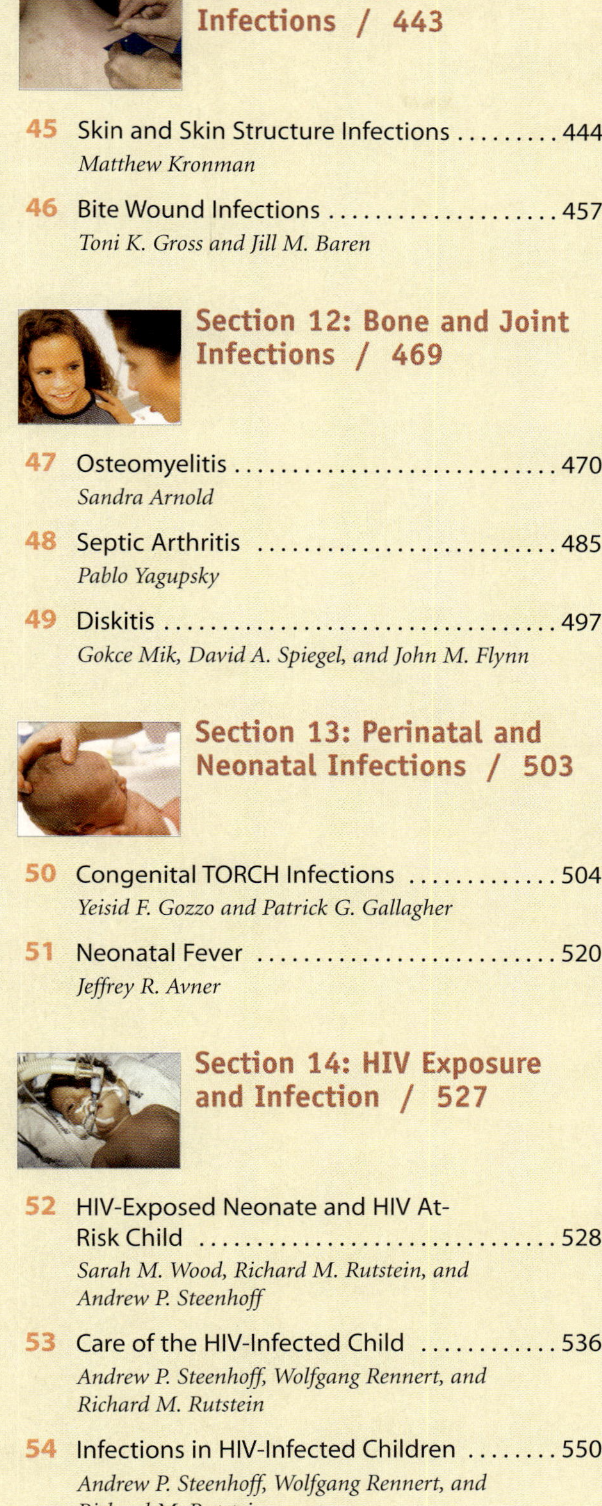

Section 11: Skin Infections / 443

Section 12: Bone and Joint Infections / 469

Section 13: Perinatal and Neonatal Infections / 503

Section 14: HIV Exposure and Infection / 527

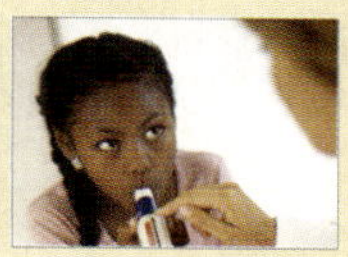

Section 15: Infections Complicating Chronic Diseases / 577

Section 16: Congenital Immunodeficiency Syndromes / 609

Section 17: Fever Syndromes / 623

Section 18: Travel-Related Infections / 665

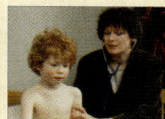

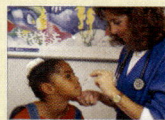

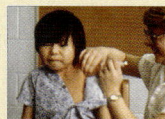

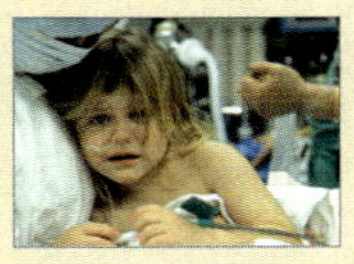

Section 19: Health-Care Acquired Infections / 737

Contributors

Brian K. Alverson, MD
Assistant Professor of Pediatrics
Department of Pediatrics
Brown University School of Medicine
Hospitalist
Department of Pediatrics
Hasbro Children's Hospital/Rhode Island Hospital
Providence, Rhode Island

Donald H. Arnold, MD, MPH
Assistant Professor
Emergency Medicine and Pediatrics
Vanderbilt University School of Medicine
Nashville, Tennessee

Sandra Arnold, MD
Associate Professor
Department of Pediatrics
University of Tennessee
Memphis, Tennessee

Erika F. Augustine, MD
Clinical Fellow in Neurology
Department of Neurology
Harvard Medical School
Resident in Neurology
Department of Neurology
Children's Hospital Boston
Boston, Massachusetts

Robert Avery, DO
Division of Neurology
The Children's Hospital of Philadelphia
Philadelphia, Pennsylvania

Jeffrey R. Avner, MD
Professor of Clinical Pediatrics
Albert Einstein College of Medicine
Chief
Division of Pediatric Emergency Services
Children's Hospital at Montefiore
Bronx, New York

Megan Aylor, MD
Assistant Professor
Department of Pediatrics
Oregon Health and Science University
Portland, Oregon

Jill M. Baren, MD, MBE, FACEP, FAAP
Associate Professor of Emergency Medicine and Pediatrics
Department of Emergency Medicine
University of Pennsylvania School of Medicine
Attending Physician
Division of Emergency Medicine
The Children's Hospital of Philadelphia
Philadelphia, Pennsylvania

Yodit Belew, MD
Adjunct Instructor in Pediatrics
The George Washington University
Washington, District of Columbia

Jay Berry, MD, MPH
Instructor of Pediatrics
Harvard Medical School
Associate in Medicine
Complex Care Service
Children's Hospital Boston
Boston, Massachusetts

Mercedes M. Blackstone, MD
Fellow
Emergency Medicine
The Children's Hospital of Philadelphia
Clinical Instructor
Pediatrics
University of Pennsylvania School of Medicine
Philadelphia, Pennsylvania

Evelien J. Bodar, MD
Department of General Internal Medicine
Radboud University Nijmegen Medical Center
Nijmegen, The Netherlands

Kristina Bryant, MD
Assistant Professor
Department of Pediatrics
Division of Pediatric Infectious Diseases
University of Louisville
Hospital Epidemiologist
Kosair Children's Hospital
Louisville, Kentucky

Jon M. Burnham, MD, MSCE
Attending Physician
Division of Rheumatology
The Children's Hospital of Philadelphia
Assistant Professor of Pediatrics
University of Pennsylvania School of Medicine
Philadelphia, Pennsylvania

Jane C. Burns, MD
Professor and Chief
Division of Allergy, Immunology, and Rheumatology
Rady Children's Hospital and Department of Pediatrics
University of California at San Diego School of Medicine
San Diego, California

Michael G. Camitta, MD
Assistant Professor of Pediatrics
Division of Pediatric Cardiology
Medical Director
Pediatric Echocardiography Laboratory
Duke University Medical Center
Durham, North Carolina

Cynthia J. Campen, MD
Division of Child Neurology
The Children's Hospital of Philadelphia
Philadelphia, Pennsylvania

Michael Cappello, MD
Professor of Pediatrics, Microbial Pathogenesis, and Epidemiology & Public Health
Director
Program in International Child Health
Yale University School of Medicine
New Haven, Connecticut

John C. Christenson, MD
Professor of Clinical Pediatrics
Indiana University School of Medicine
Director, Pediatric Travel Medicine Clinic
Center for International Adoption and Geographic Medicine
Ryan White Center for Infectious Diseases
Riley Hospital for Children
Indianapolis, Indiana

Peter Clement, MD, PhD
Professor of Otorhinolaryngology
Chairman
ENT Department
University Hospital (V.U.B)
Free University Brussels
Brussels, Belgium

Kevin James Downes, MD
Pediatrics Resident
Cincinnati Children's Hospital Medical Center
Cincinnati, Ohio

Joost P.H. Drenth, MD, PhD
Professor of Molecular Gastroenterology & Hepatology
Department of Gastroenterology and Hepatology
Radboud University Nijmegen Medical Center
Nijmegen, The Netherlands

Orooj Fasiuddin, MD
Assistant Professor of Pediatrics
Paul C. Gaffney Diagnostic Referral Service
Children's Hospital of Pittsburgh
Pittsburgh, Pennsylvania

Kristen Feemster, MD, MPH, MSHPR
Fellow
Division of Infectious Diseases
The Children's Hospital of Philadelphia
Philadelphia, Pennsylvania

Evan Fieldston, MD, MBA
Robert Wood Johnson Clinical Scholar
University of Pennsylvania School of Medicine
The Children's Hospital of Philadelphia
Philadelphia, Pennsylvania

Elizabeth K. Fiorino, MD
Fellow
Division of Pulmonary Medicine
The Children's Hospital of Philadelphia
Philadelphia, Pennsylvania

Brian T. Fisher, DO, MPH
Assistant Professor
Department of Pediatrics
University of Pennsylvania School of Medicine
Attending Physician
Division of Infectious Diseases
The Children's Hospital of Philadelphia
Philadelphia, Pennsylvania

John M. Flynn, MD
Associate Chief of Orthopaedic Surgery
The Children's Hospital of Philadelphia
Associate Professor of Orthopaedic Surgery
University of Pennsylvania School of Medicine
Philadelphia, Pennsylvania

Gary Frank, MD
Pediatric Hospitalist
Scottish Rite Pediatric and Adolescent Consultant
Clinical Assistant Professor
Emory University School of Medicine
Atlanta, Georgia

Joel A. Friedlander, DO, MBe
Fellow
Division of Gastroenterology, Hepatology and Nutrition
The Children's Hospital of Philadelphia
Instructor
Department of Pediatrics
University of Pennsylvania School of Medicine
Philadelphia, Pennsylvania

Patrick G. Gallagher, MD, FAAP
Professor
Department of Pediatrics
Yale University School of Medicine
New Haven, Connecticut

Johanna Goldfarb, MD
Head
Pediatric Infectious Diseases
Children's Hospital Cleveland Clinic
Professor of Pediatrics
Cleveland Clinic Lerner College of Medicine at Case Western Reserve University
Cleveland, Ohio

Mark P. Gorman, MD
Clinical Fellow
Neurology
Children's Hospital Boston
Boston, Massachusetts

Yeisid F. Gozzo, MD
Fellow
Division of Neonatal/Perinatal Medicine
Department of Pediatrics
Yale University School of Medicine
New Haven, Connecticut

Toni K. Gross, MD, MPH
Assistant Professor
Department of Pediatrics
University of Pennsylvania School of Medicine
Attending Physician
Division of Emergency Medicine
The Children's Hospital of Philadelphia
Philadelphia, Pennsylvania

Barbara A. Haber, MD
Associate Professor
Department of Pediatrics
University of Pennsylvania School of Medicine
Attending Physician
Division of Gastroenterology,
Hepatology and Nutrition
The Children's Hospital of Philadelphia
Philadelphia, Pennsylvania

Margaret R. Hammerschlag, MD
Professor of Pediatrics and Medicine
Department of Pediatrics
State Univesity of New York
Downstate Medical Center
Brooklyn, New York

Laura Hammitt, MD
Clinical Epidemiologist
Centre for Tropical Medicine
University of Oxford
Kilifi, Kenya

Marvin B. Harper, MD
Assistant Professor of Pediatrics
Harvard Medical School
Attending Physician
Infectious Diseases and Emergency Medicine
Children's Hospital Boston
Boston, Massachusetts

Harry R. Hill, MD
Professor
Departments of Pathology, Pediatrics and Medicine
University of Utah School of Medicine
Salt Lake City, Utah

Richard L. Hodinka, PhD
Director, Clinical Virology Laboratory
Department of Pathology and Laboratory Medicine
The Children's Hospital of Philadelphia
Associate Professor
Department of Pediatrics
University of Pennsylvania School of Medicine
Philadelphia, Pennsylvania

Julia Hutter, MD
Fellow
Pediatric Infectious Diseases and Tropical Pediatrics
Center for Vaccine Development
School of Medicine
University of Maryland
Baltimore, Maryland

Mary Anne Jackson, MD
Chief
Section of Pediatric Infectious Diseases
Children's Mercy Hospital & Clinics
Professor of Pediatrics
University of Missouri-Kansas City
School of Medicine
Kansas City, Missouri

Emma Jacobs, MD
International Adoption Clinic
Floating Hospital for Children
Tufts Medical Center
Boston, Massachusetts

Samay Jain, MD
Assistant Professor of Neurology
Clinical Director
Movement Disorders Division
Department of Neurology
University of Pittsburgh
Pittsburgh, Pennsylvania

Chandy C. John, MD, MS
Associate Professor
Departments of Pediatrics and Medicine
Director
Center for Global Pediatrics
University of Minnesota Medical School
Minneapolis, Minnesota

Jessica K. Hart, MD
Resident in Pediatrics
The Children's Hospital of Philadelphia
Philadelphia, Pennsylvania

Binita M. Kamath, MBBChir
Assistant Professor
Department of Pediatrics
University of Pennsylvania School of Medicine
Attending Physician
Division of Gastroenterology,
Hepatology and Nutrition
The Children's Hospital of Philadelphia
Philadelphia, Pennsylvania

Nadeem Karimbux, DMD, MMSC
Associate Professor
Department of Oral Medicine, Infection and Immunity
Harvard School of Dental Medicine
Boston, Massachusetts

David Kim, DDS, DMSc
Assistant Professor
Director of Oral Medicine, Infection and Immunity
Harvard School of Dental Medicine
Boston, Massachusetts

Terry Klassen, MD
Professor and Chair
Department of Pediatrics
University of Alberta
Regional Clinic Program Director
Child Health
Stollery Children's Hospital
Capital Health
Edmonton, Alberta, Canada

William C. Koch, MD
Associate Professor
Department of Pediatrics
Division of Infectious Diseases
Virginia Commonwealth University School of Medicine
Richmond, Virginia

Sarah Kranick, MD
Department of Neurology
Hospital of the University of Pennsylvania
Philadelphia, Pennsylvania

Matthew Kronman, MD
Fellow
Division of Infectious Diseases
The Children's Hospital of Philadelphia
Philadelphia, Pennsylvania

Timothy R. La Pine, MD
Associate Professor of Pediatrics and Pathology
University of Utah School of Medicine
Salt Lake City, Utah

Miriam K. Laufer, MD
Assistant Professor of Pediatrics
Center for Vaccine Development
University of Maryland School of Medicine
Baltimore, Maryland

Matthew B. Laurens, MD, MPH
Fellow
Pediatric Infectious Diseases and Tropical Pediatrics
Department of Pediatrics
University of Maryland School of Medicine
Baltimore, Maryland

Melissa A. Lerman, MD, PhD
Fellow
Division of Rheumatology
The Children's Hospital of Philadelphia
Philadelphia, Pennsylvania

Leonard J. Levine, MD
Assistant Professor
Department of Pediatrics
Division of Adolescent Medicine
St. Christopher's Hospital for Children
Drexel University College of Medicine
Philadelphia, Pennsylvania

Rebecca E. Levorson, MD
Pediatric Infectious Disease Fellow
Division of Infectious Disease
Children's National Medical Center
Pediatric Infectious Disease Fellow
George Washington University School of Medicine
Washington, District of Columbia

Jennifer S. Li, MD
Professor of Pediatrics
Division of Pediatric Cardiology
Duke University Medical Center
Duke Clinical Research Institute
Durham, North Carolina

Daniel J. Licht, MD
Assistant Professor of Neurology and Pediatrics
Division of Child Neurology
The Children's Hospital of Philadelphia
Philadelphia, Pennsylvania

Scott M. Lieberman, MD, PhD
Fellow
Division of Rheumatology
The Children's Hospital of Philadelphia
Instructor in Pediatrics
University of Pennsylvania School of Medicine
Philadelphia, Pennsylvania

Latania K. Logan, MD
Pediatric Infectious Diseases Fellow
Department of Pediatrics
Children's Memorial Hospital
Northwestern University
Feinberg School of Medicine
Chicago, Illinois

Nisha Manickam, DO
Fellow
Division of Infectious Diseases
Department of Pediatrics and Department of Internal Medicine
Yale University School of Medicine
New Haven, Connecticut

Shannon Manzi, Pharm D
ED Clinical Pharmacist
Children's Hospital Boston
Clincial Assistant Professor
Bouve College of Pharmacy
Northeastern University
Boston, Massachusetts

Ben J. Marais, MD
Associate Professor
Department of Paediatrics and Child Health
Tygerberg Children's Hospital
Stellenbosch University
Cape Town, South Africa

Beth C. Marshall, MD
Assistant Professor
Department of Pediatrics
Division of Infectious Diseases
Virginia Commonwealth University School of Medicine
Richmond, Virginia

Peter Mattei, MD
Assistant Professor
Department of Surgery
University of Pennsylvania School of Medicine
General, Thoracic and Fetal Surgery
The Children's Hospital of Philadelphia
Philadelphia, Pennsylvania

Randolph P. Matthews, MD, PhD
Assistant Professor of Pediatrics
University of Pennsylvania School of Medicine
Division of Gastroenterology, Hepatology, and Nutrition
The Children's Hospital of Philadelphia
Philadelphia, Pennsylvania

Alexander J. McAdams, MD, PhD
Medical Director of Infectious Diseases Division
Department of Laboratory Medicine
Children's Hospital Boston
Assistant Professor
Department of Pathology
Harvard Medical School
Boston, Massachusetts

Sarah C. McBride, MD
Staff Physician
Department of Medicine
Children's Hospital
Instructor in Pediatrics
Harvard Medical School
Boston, Massachusetts

Gokce Mik, MD
Division of Orthopedic Surgery
The Children's Hospital of Philadelphia
Philadelphia, Pennsylvania

Laurie C. Miller, MD
Associate Professor of Pediatrics
Director
International Adoption Clinic
Tufts University School of Medicine
Boston, Massachusetts

Jason G. Newland, MD
Section of Pediatric Infectious Diseases
Children's Mercy Hospital & Clinics
Assistant Professor of Pediatrics
Department of Pediatrics
University of Missouri-Kansas City
Kansas City, Missouri

Howard B. Panitch, MD
Professor of Pediatrics
University of Pennsylvania School of Medicine
Director of Clinical Programs
Division of Pulmonary Medicine
The Children's Hospital of Philadelphia
Philadelphia, Pennsylvania

Mark S. Pasternack, MD
Chief
Pediatric Infectious Disease Unit
Massachusetts General Hospital
Associate Professor of Pediatrics
Harvard Medical School
Boston, Massachusetts

Jacques Pepin, MD, FRCPC, MSC
Department of Microbiology and Infectious Diseases
University of Sherbrooke School of Medicine
Sherbrooke, Canada

Nadja G. Peter, MD
Clinical Assistant Professor
Pediatrics
Craig Dalsimer Division of Adolescent Medicine
University of Pennsylvania
The Children's Hospital of Philadelphia
Philadelphia, Pennsylvania

Annapurna Poduri, MD, MPH
Instructor
Department of Neurology
Harvard Medical School
Assistant
Department of Neurology
Children's Hospital Boston
Boston, Massachusetts

Scott L. Pomeroy, MD, PhD
Neurologist-in-Chief
Children's Hospital Boston
Bronson Crothers Professor of Neurology
Harvard Medical School
Boston, Massachusetts

Adam J. Ratner, MD, MPH
Assistant Professor
Pediatrics and Microbiology
Columbia University
New York, New York

Wolfgang Rennert, MD, DMSc, DTMTH, FAAP
Residency Program Director
Department of Pediatrics
Georgetown University Hospital
Washington, District of Columbia

Richard M. Rutstein, MD
Associate Professor
University of Pennsylvania School of Medicine
Medical Director
Special Immunology Service and Family Care Center
The Children's Hospital of Philadelphia
Philadelphia, Pennsylvania

Daniel J. Salchow, MD
Assistant Professor of Ophthalmology and Visual Science
Director
Pediatric Ophthalmology and Strabismus Section
Department of Ophthalmology & Visual Science
Yale University School of Medicine
New Haven, Connecticut

Joshua W. Salvin, MD, MPH
Assistant in Cardiology
Department of Cardiology
Division of Cardiac Intensive Care
Children's Hospital Boston
Instructor in Pediatrics
Harvard Medical School
Boston, Massachusetts

Nadia Sam-Agudu, MD
Fellow
Division of Infectious Diseases and Global Pediatrics Program
University of Minnesota Medical School
Minneapolis, Minnesota

Thomas J. Sandora, MD
Hospital Epidemiologist
Medical Director of Infection Control
Division of Infectious Diseases
Children's Hospital Boston
Harvard Medical School
Boston, Massachusetts

Robert Seese, MD
Hospitalist
Department of Pediatrics
Licking Memorial Hospital
Newark, Ohio

Kara N. Shah, MD, PhD
Assistant Professor of Pediatrics and Dermatology
University of Pennsylvania School of Medicine
Attending Physician
Section of Pediatric Dermatology
The Children's Hospital of Philadelphia
Philadelphia, Pennsylvania

Samir S. Shah, MD, MSCE
Assistant Professor
Departments of Pediatrics and Epidemiology
Senior Scholar
Center for Clinical Epidemiology and Biostatistics
University of Pennsylvania School of Medicine
Attending Physician
Divisions of Infectious Diseases and General Pediatrics
The Children's Hospital of Philadelphia
Philadelphia, Pennsylvania

Rahul K. Shah, MD, FAAP
Assistant Professor of Otolaryngology and Pediatrics
Children's National Medical Center
George Washington University School of Medicine
Washington, District of Columbia

Udayan K. Shah, MD, FACS, FAAP
Director
Fellow and Resident Education in Pediatric Otolaryngology
Nemours-Alfred I duPont Hospital for Children
Wilmington, Delaware
Associate Professor
Otolaryngology-Head & Neck Surgery
Jefferson Medical College
Thomas Jefferson University
Philadelphia, Pennsylvania

Anna Simon, MD, PhD
Department of General Internal Medicine
Radboud University Nijmegen Medical Center
Nijmegen, The Netherlands

Joseph Sleiman, MD
Clinical Assistant Instructor
Department of Pediatric Infectious Diseases
Children's Hospital at SUNY Downstate Medical Center
Brooklyn, New York

Michael J. Smith, MD
Division of Infectious Diseases
The Children's Hospital of Philadelphia
Philadelphia, Pennsylvania

Philip R. Spandorfer, MD, MSCE
Attending Physician
Emergency Medicine
Children's Healthcare of Atlanta at Scottish Rite
Atlanta, Georgia

David A. Spiegel, MD
Assistant Professor of Orthopedic Surgery
University of Pennsylvania School of Medicine
Division of Orthopedic Surgery
The Children's Hospital of Philadelphia
Philadelphia, Pennsylvania

David M. Spiro MD, MPH
Associate Professor of Emergency Medicine and Pediatrics
Section Chief
Pediatric Emergency Medicine
Doernbecher Children's Hospital
Oregon Health and Science University
Portland, Oregon

Joseph W. St. Geme III, MD
Professor
Department of Pediatrics
Department of Molecular Genetic & Microbiology
Duke University Medical Center
Durham, North Carolina

Andrew P. Steenhoff, MBBCH, DCH(UK), FCPaed(SA)
Instructor, Department of Pediatrics
Center for AIDs Research
University of Pennsylvania School of Medicine
Attending Physician
Division of Infectious Diseases
The Children's Hospital of Philadelphia
Philadelphia, Pennsylvania

Sanjeev Swami, MD
Fellow
Division of Infectious Diseases
Department of Pediatrics
The Children's Hospital of Philadelphia
Philadelphia, Pennsylvania

Tina Q. Tan, MD
Associate Professor of Pediatrics
Department of Pediatrics
Feinberg School of Medicine
Northwestern University
Pediatric Infectious Diseases Physician
Department of Pediatrics
Children's Memorial Hospital
Chicago, Illinois

Sarah M. Taub, MD
Attending Physician
Advocare Haddon Pediatrics
Haddonfield, New Jersey

Oana Tomescu, MD
Fellow
Craig Dalsimer Division of Adolescent Medicine
The Children's Hospital of Philadelphia
Philadelphia, Pennsylvania

Adriana H. Tremoulet, MD
Adjunct Assistant Professor
Division of Pharmacology and Drug Discovery
Rady Children's Hospital
Department of Pediatrics
University of California
San Diego, California

Adriana Tremoulet, MD
Adjunct Assistant Professor
Division of Pharmacology and Drug Discovery
Rady Children's Hospital
Department of Pediatrics
University of California, San Diego
San Diego, California

Louis Valiquette, MD
Associate Professor
Department of Microbiology and Infectious Diseases
Faculté de médecine, Université de Sherbrooke
Sherbrooke, Québec, Canada

Kishore Vellody, MD
Assistant Professor of Pediatrics
University of Pittsburgh School of Medicine
The Paul C. Gaffney Diagnostic Referral Service
Children's Hospital of Pittsburgh
Pittsburgh, Pennsylvania

Sarah M. Wood, MD
Resident Physician
General Pediatrics
The Children's Hospital of Philadelphia
Philadelphia, Pennsylvania

Robert Bruce Wright, MD, FRCPC, FAAP
Assistant Director
Division of Pediatric Emergency Medicine
Assistant Professor
Department of Pediatrics
University of Alberta
Edmonton, Alberta, Canada

Pablo Yagupsky, MD
Director
Clinical Microbiology Laboratory
Soroka University Medical Center
Ben-Gurion University of the Negev
Beer-Sheeva, Israel

Catherine Yen, MD, MPH
Pediatric Infectious Diseases
Columbia University Medical Center
New York, New York

Matt Zahn, MD
Medical Director
Louisville Metro Department of Public Health and Wellness
Assistant Professor
Division of Pediatric Infectious Disease
University of Louisville School of Medicine
Louisville, Kentucky

Basil J. Zitelli, MD
Professor of Pediatrics
University of Pittsburgh School of Medicine
Chief
The Paul C. Gaffney Diagnostic Referral Service
Children's Hospital of Pittsburgh
Pittsburgh, Pennsylvania

Joseph J. Zorc, MD, MSCE
Associate Professor of Pediatrics
Department of Pediatrics
The University of Pennsylvania School of Medicine
Attending Physician
Emergency Medicine
The Children's Hospital of Philadelphia
Philadelphia, Pennsylvania

Preface

Our understanding of infectious diseases has increased exponentially over the past few decades. We have new diagnostic tests, new diseases, and new pathogens. We also have the recognition of new syndromes caused by well-known pathogens and the resurgence of "old" diseases, once thought conquered. Consequently, the amount of knowledge required to manage even common childhood infections is mind boggling. This book was written in order to provide the generalist pediatrician, both office- and hospital-based, a practical, reliable, and evidence-based resource to diagnose and treat commonly encountered pediatric infections.

The book is divided into four parts. The first part addresses practical aspects such as basics of the clinical microbiology and virology laboratories, vaccine safety, infection control and prevention, and important concepts in infectious diseases epidemiology. The second part covers common signs and symptoms where infections are often part of the differential diagnosis. The third part reviews infections by anatomic site. The fourth part discusses special situations that fall outside the scope of organ systems such as perinatally acquired infections and the care of children with human immunodeficiency virus infection. This last section also includes topics such as infections in children with atopic dermatitis and infections in internationally adopted children that sometimes fall outside the scope of textbooks aimed at the pediatric generalist.

The challenge in organizing this book was to ensure that chapters were sufficiently detailed and thoroughly referenced while adhering to our philosophy of providing practical management strategies. The authors, despite the many demands on their time, succeeded in reaching this objective in a timely manner. I hope this book will serve as a daily infectious diseases reference to the practicing pediatrician.

Samir S. Shah
Philadephia, Pennsylvania

SECTION 1

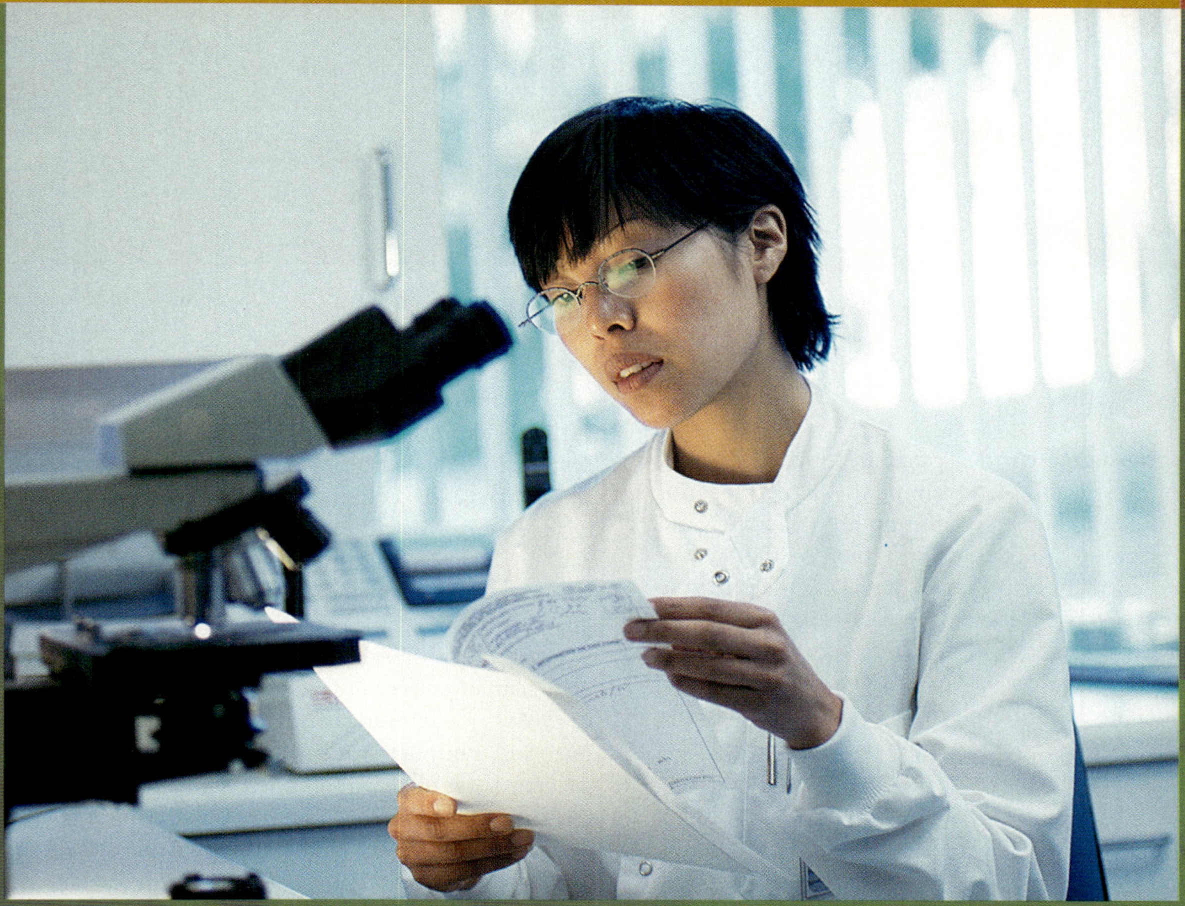

Practical Aspects

1. Laboratory Diagnosis of Bacterial, Parasitic and Fungal Diseases
2. Laboratory Diagnosis of Viral Diseases
3. Vaccines and Vaccine Safety
4. Office Infection Control
5. Infection Control in the Hospital
6. Infectious Diseases Epidemiology

CHAPTER 1

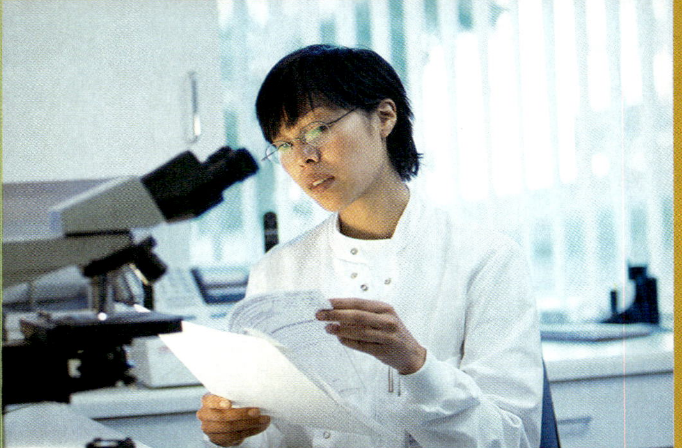

Laboratory Diagnosis of Bacterial, Parasitic and Fungal Diseases

Alexander J. McAdam

INTRODUCTION

The appropriate use of tests for infectious diseases of children is critical to determining the correct diagnosis. The keys to successful testing are collection and transport of an appropriate specimen to the laboratory and correct performance of the right test in the laboratory. Communication between the clinician and laboratory staff is important in diagnostic testing, particularly if a rare or fastidious organism is suspected. General guidelines for specimen collection and transport are included in this chapter, but it is important to seek guidance from the laboratory which will be performing the test, as practice varies between laboratories.

SPECIMEN COLLECTION AND TRANSPORT FOR BACTERIA AND FUNGI

Because bacteria and fungi are living organisms, they can proliferate or die during transportation of the specimen to the laboratory. Survival of the pathogen is required for culture, however, growth of organisms during transport is undesirable, if the quantity of bacteria is important in making a diagnosis (e.g., in urine culture) or if overgrowth by flora makes detection of a pathogen less likely (e.g., in stool culture). The time for transport to the laboratory should be minimized to reduce death or excessive growth of organisms. When transport time exceeds 1–2 hours, as in the outpatient office where transport times of up to 24 hours are sometimes required, use of specialized transport media is essential for most specimens.

If it is practical to obtain them, body fluids, tissues, and purulent material are generally preferred to specimens collected on a swab. The quantity of material, which can be collected on a swab, is small and bacteria may remain trapped on the swab, where they cannot be detected. Throat and genital specimens for bacterial culture are an exception to this rule and adequate specimens can be collected from these sites using swabs. If swabs must be submitted, submit one swab for each stain or culture ordered.

Many commercial transport systems include a swab and transport media in a tube. These systems work well for most medically important bacteria and fungi. Organisms, which do not survive well during transport (even with transport media), include *Neisseria* spp., *Streptococcus pneumoniae*, *Haemophilus influenzae*, *Campylobacter* spp., and obligate anaerobic bacteria. If these organisms are suspected, transport time to the laboratory should be minimized (<6–12 h) or media should be inoculated and incubated immediately after specimen collection or nonculture methods of detection should be used. Submission of swabs without transport media to the microbiology laboratory should be avoided, except for throat cultures for group A streptococci (*Streptococcus pyogenes*), which survives well for 24 hours on either dry swabs or in commercial transport media.

Obligate anaerobic bacteria are killed by the presence of oxygen, so special transport systems are used for specimens from infections that are likely to include these organisms. These include deep abscesses, fasciitis, and infections which have spread from sites heavily colonized by anaerobic bacteria, such as the oropharynx and intestine. Specimens from the oropharynx, intestine, and vagina, which are normally colonized by obligate anaerobic bacteria, generally should not be submitted for anaerobic culture, because the growth of these organisms is expected and susceptibility testing is not typically performed on anaerobic bacteria. In addition, superficial skin and wound infections are unlikely to include obligate anaerobic bacteria and so anaerobic culture is generally not useful for these infections. Unless the specimen will reach the laboratory very quickly (minutes for small specimens and up to 2 hours for larger specimens), a commercial anaerobic transport tube, jar or bag should be used to protect the viability of the bacteria. Fluids, which must be transported without an anaerobic transport system, should be sent in a capped syringe from which all the air has been purged.

Specimens for yeast culture can be transported as described for bacterial culture. The following comments apply to specimens in which a hyphael fungus (i.e., mold) is suspected, although if yeast cells are present, they will also remain viable. Tissue, fluids (respiratory, urine, sterile body fluids), hair, or nail specimens for fungal culture can generally be transported in a clean, dry container without transport media. If the specimen will not reach the laboratory within 2 hours, specimens from normally sterile sites can be kept at 37°C, while those from body sites with bacterial flora can be kept at 4°C.

TESTS FOR BACTERIAL INFECTIONS

Laboratory Methods for Detection and Identification of Bacteria

Detection and identification of bacteria can be performed by several methods, including microscopic examination of stained specimens, culture, antigen detection, and nucleic acid amplification tests (NAAT), which include polymerase chain reaction (PCR) and transcription mediated amplification.

The Gram stain remains a valuable tool for rapid detection and preliminary identification of bacteria. Gram-positive bacteria appear dark blue or purple because they have a thick cell wall composed of peptidoglycan, which retains crystal violet and iodine during destaining with alcohol. In contrast, Gram-negative bacteria have a thin layer of peptidoglycan surrounded by an outer membrane, and the alcohol rinse removes the crystal violet and iodine. After a counter stain with safranin, gram-negative bacteria appear pink. The Gram stain also reveals the shape and arrangement of bacteria. The morphology of commonly isolated bacteria is summarized in Table 1–1. Yeast usually stain Gram-positive and they are easily differentiated from bacteria by their greater size.

Stains for mycobacteria include stains with carbol fuchsin and auromine-O. These stains can be routinely performed on respiratory specimens and tissue, and might be performed on other specimens at the discretion of the physician and laboratory. The modified acid-fast stain is a less stringent stain than the acid-fast stain and is useful in detection and identification of *Nocardia*, *Rhodococcus*, *Tsukamurella*, and *Gordona*, all of which are positive by modified acid-fast stain, but negative by regular acid-fast stain.

Culture and biochemical tests are the mainstay of detection and identification of most bacteria. Most aerobic and facultative anaerobic bacterial pathogens will grow rapidly in routine culture, however, some species require the use of special media and so the laboratory should be informed if these are suspected. Infections with some organisms, which require special culture, are better detected by serology, NAAT or antigen tests and these are noted in the tables later in this chapter.

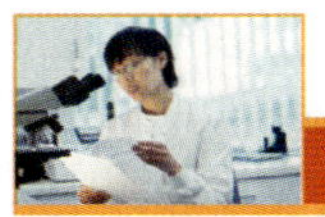

Table 1–1.

Morphology of Organisms Frequently Detected by Gram Stain

Morphology	Likely Organisms
Gram-positive cocci in pairs and short chains	*Streptococcus pneumoniae*, *Enterococcus* species
Gram-positive cocci in chains	*Streptococcus* species other than *S. pneumoniae*
Gram-positive cocci in clusters	*Staphylococcus* species
Gram-positive bacilli	*Listeria monocytogenes* (small, regular rods)
	Corynebacterium species (small, irregular rods)
	Bacillus and *Clostridium* species (large, regular rods, may have spores)
Gram-negative cocci in pairs	*Neisseria* species
	Moraxella catarrhalis
Gram-negative bacilli	Many enteric bacteria, including *Escherichia coli*, *Yersinia enterocolitica*, *Salmonella* species, *Shigella* species
	Pseudomonas aeruginosa

Detection of mycobacteria in culture usually requires specific media, although rapid-growing mycobacteria (e.g., *Mycobacterium fortuitum, Mycobacterium chelonae, Mycobacterium abscessus)* may be detected in routine bacterial culture. *Mycobacterium tuberculosis* often takes several weeks to grow in culture, although the time for growth is significantly reduced by using liquid culture media. Identification of mycobacteria is also time consuming, although nucleic acid probes can now be used to identify most mycobacteria from culture quickly and accurately.

Antigen detection assays use antibodies specific for bacterial proteins or carbohydrates to test for bacteria. Rapid antigen tests for *S. pyogenes* (group A *Streptococcus*) are highly specific (>95%). These tests have sensitivities of approximately 70–85%, though the sensitivity is considerably lower (approximately 50%) when performed by nonlaboratory personnel.[1,2] Because of the moderate sensitivities of these tests, specimens with negative results by antigen tests for *S. pyogenes* should be submitted for culture.[1] The Binax NOW® test for *S. pneumoniae* antigen in urine is very sensitive (100%) for pneumococcal disease in children, however, it is also positive in asymptomatic children colonized with *S. pneumoniae* and so it has a specificity of only 50–60%.[3] Antigen tests performed on CSF are discussed below, in the section on meningitis.

NAAT, such as PCR, are very sensitive because they amplify nucleic acid from the pathogen in logarithmic fashion, doubling the number of DNA or RNA molecules several times. As a result, NAAT can be more sensitive than culture, particularly for fastidious organisms. The number of U.S. Food and Drug Administration (FDA)-approved NAAT is still small, however, many large laboratories have validated non-FDA-approved tests using either commercial kits or "home-brew" assays. NAAT for *Chlamydia trachomatis, Neisseria gonorrhoeae, Bordetella pertussis*, and *M. tuberculosis* are discussed later in this chapter.

There are FDA-approved PCR tests for *S. agalactiae* (group B *Streptococcus*) in vaginal/rectal samples for screening pregnant women[4] and for methicillin-resistant *S. aureus* in nasal swabs, for infection control screens.[5] The results of these assays compare well to those obtained with conventional culture and PCR results may be available more quickly.

Antibiotic Susceptibility Testing

Several methods are used for determination of antibiotic susceptibility. The minimum inhibitory concentration (MIC) is the concentration of antibiotic, which inhibits visible growth of bacteria. The MIC can be determined by several methods, including culturing bacteria in a titration of antibiotics in agar or broth, or by using automated devices. The minimum bactericidal concentration (MBC) is the concentration of an antibiotic, which kills 99.9% of bacteria. In practice, the MIC is easily determined and predicts the susceptibility of bacteria to antibiotics, while determination of the MBC is technically cumbersome and rarely adds information beyond that from the MIC or disk-diffusion testing, and so MBC testing is seldom done. One circumstance in which determining the MBC may be useful is in selection of an aminoglycoside for treatment of endocarditis with enterobacteriaceae (enteric gram-negative rods).[6]

Disk-diffusion susceptibility testing is performed by coating an agar plate with a known concentration of bacteria, and then placing paper disks impregnated with antibiotics onto the plate. The antibiotic diffuses out of the paper disk and a gradient of antibiotic forms around the disk. After 16–24 hours of incubation, the diameter of the zone of growth inhibition around the disk is measured. The zone of growth inhibition around the disk is inversely proportional to the MIC, and the relationship between these values is the basis for interpretation of disk-diffusion testing results.

The interpretation of MIC values or disk diffusion zones as "susceptible," "intermediate," or "resistant" is performed according to guidelines which are published by the Clinical and Laboratory Standards Institute (CLSI) in the United States.[7] An organism is considered susceptible, if it is inhibited by concentrations of antibiotic which will be achieved at the relevant body site with the recommended dosage, and it is considered resistant if it is not. An interpretation of intermediate means that failure of antibiotic therapy is more likely than if the organism is susceptible, but that drugs which are normally concentrated at the site of infection (e.g., penicillin in urine) or drugs given at higher doses than usual (e.g., penicillin for intermediate *S. pneumoniae* in meningitis) may be effective. The intermediate range also includes a buffer zone for technical variation in the test. The absorption, metabolism, and excretion of an antibiotic determine whether it will reach an effective concentration at the site of infection and so laboratories selectively report susceptibility testing based on the body site from which bacteria are isolated. For example, susceptibility results with nitrofurantoin are only reported for bacteria isolated from urine, because nitrofurantoin is concentrated in urine while reaching only subtherapeutic levels in serum and tissue. Furthermore, the interpretation of antibiotic susceptibility may vary depending upon the site infected. For example, interpretation of the MICs of *S. pneumoniae* with cefotaxime and ceftriaxone depends on whether the patient has meningitis or infection only outside the central nervous system because the levels of these drugs in the central nervous system and the rest of the body differ.[8]

Laboratory testing can, in a few cases, be used to predict that there is a significant risk that an organism, which is apparently susceptible to an antibiotic, is likely to develop resistance to that antibiotic. An increased MIC to naladixic acid in *Salmonella* indicates that the bacterium has mutations which make it more likely to become fully resistant to fluoroquinolones, and so treatment of these organisms with fluoroquinolones in extra-intestinal infections may be ineffective.[9] An increased chance of developing resistance to clindamycin in *Staphylococcus* and β-hemolytic *Streptococci* can be detected by testing for erythromycin-inducible clindamycin resistance.[10] This is done by placing clindamycin and erythromycin disks close together in disk-diffusion susceptibility testing and looking for a flattening of the zone of growth inhibition around the clindamycin disk (the "D-test"). Organisms with a positive D-test are reported as clindamycin resistant, although the laboratory may report that clindamycin may still be effective in some patients.

The only test for antibiotic synergy, which is routinely performed, is a screen for synergy of the aminoglycosides gentamicin and streptomycin with the cell wall synthesis inhibitors penicillin, ampicillin and vancomycin against *Enterococcus.* This is done by simply testing the growth of the *Enterococcus* isolate with a high level of the aminoglycoside alone. Although synergy testing is available for antibiotic resistant gram-negative organisms from patients with cystic fibrosis, there is no evidence that use of these results leads to improved patient outcomes.[11]

TESTS FOR FUNGAL INFECTIONS

Laboratory Methods for Detection and Identification of Fungi

"Fungi" include both molds and yeasts. The distinction between molds and yeasts is based on their shape, rather than true biological relationships between the fungi. Molds grow primarily as hyphae (elongated structures that form a colony which looks fuzzy) and spore-forming structures. *Aspergillus*, the Zygomycetes (e.g., *Mucor* and *Rhizopus*) and the dermatophytes (e.g., *Trichphyton*) are all molds. Yeast grow predominantly as round or oval forms and divide by budding. Colonies of yeast can look smooth or rough, but not fuzzy. Yeast include *Candida* spp. and *Cryptococcus neoformans.* Dimorphic fungi grow as yeast at body temperature (including in tissue), but as molds at 25–30°C and these include *Histoplasma capsulatum, Coccidiodes immitis, Blastomyces dermatitidis, Sporothrix schenkii, Paracoccidioides brasiliensis,* and *Penicillium marneffei.*

Microscopic examination of specimens for fungi requires specific stains because Gram stain may stain these organisms poorly. Treatment of specimens with KOH makes most host tissues clear, but fungi remain visible. Calcofluor white stain, which can be combined with KOH, binds to fungal cell walls and fluoresces under ultraviolet light, making it easy to detect fungal structures. Geimsa or Wright's stains are useful for detecting *H. capsulatum* in blood or bone marrow smears. Gomori methenamine silver stain is used to stain fungi such as *Pneumocystis jiroveci* (formerly *P. carinii*) in fixed tissue

Several different media are available for fungal culture and the choice of appropriate media depends on the specimen type and suspected fungus. It is therefore important that the specimen type (body site) be specified. *Malassezia* require addition of lipids to the media to grow, and so it is also important to tell the laboratory if *Malassezia* is suspected. *Malassezia* cause catheter-related infections in children receiving lipid-rich parenteral nutrition and also cause tinea versicolor, and less commonly, folliculitis, seborrheic dermatitis, and intravascular catheter-associated sepsis.[12]

Identification of fungi, particularly molds and dimorphic fungi, is primarily based on the macroscopic and microscopic morphology of the organism. It may take several days to weeks for a mold to develop the distinctive morphology required for identification. Yeast can usually be identified more quickly. The germ-tube assay is a test for identification of *Candida albicans,* which can be completed within a few hours after isolation of the organism in culture. Biochemical and morphological identification of other yeast can usually be accomplished in less than a week.

Several antigen tests for fungal infections are available. The galactomannan assay detects a cell wall structure from *Aspergillus* and *Penicillium.* Studies in children, although large, include only small numbers of patients with invasive *Aspergillus.* The test has been very sensitive (100%) in the small number of children with confirmed or probable invasive *Aspergillus.*[13] In adults, the sensitivity of the galactomannan test for invasive *Aspergillus* ranges from 29% to 100%, with higher values generally occurring in profoundly immunocompromised patients.[14] The specificity of galactomannan in children at risk of invasive *Aspergillus* as a result of hematological disease is 89.9–97.5%.[13,15] The specificity of the assay is lower in neonates and children than in adults, perhaps because of translocation of the antigen across the pediatric gut.[14] False-positive results with galactomannan occur in patients treated with piperacillin-tazobactam and the assay may be positive due to infection with other fungi, including *C. neoformans* and *Geotrichum capitatum.*[15,16]

The β-1, 3-D glucan assay detects an antigen produced by many fungi, including *Candida, Aspergillus, Fusarium, Trichosporon,* and others. Infections with

Cryptococcus neoformans and the Zygomycetes (*Rhizopus*, *Mucor*, *Rhizomucor*, *Cunninghamella* and *Absidia*) cannot be detected by the (1,3)-β-D-glucan tests. In the United States, a (1,3)-β-D-glucan test is marketed as Fungitell (Associates of Cape Cod). There are not adequate studies of the use of the Fungitell assay for detection of invasive fungal infections in children. The reference range for adults may not be appropriate for children, in whom the normal levels are (1,3)-β-D-glucan are slightly higher.[17] In adults, the (1,3)-β-D-glucan assay is 64.4% sensitive and 81.1% specific for invasive fungal disease when a single specimen is used.[18] If specimens are collected twice weekly in neutropenic adults with acute myelogenous leukemia or myelodysplastic syndrome, the sensitivity of the test is 100% in those with proven or probable invasive fungal infection if a single abnormally high value is counted as positive, and a positive value occurs a median of 10 days before a clinical diagnosis.[19] (1,3)-β-D-glucan is common in the environment and in medical devices or solutions, and positive results have been reported as a result of dialysis, administration of immunoglobulin or surgical gauze and bandages.[20]

Antifungal Susceptibility Testing

Susceptibility testing for fungi is still advancing and only limited tests are available. The CLSI guideline for yeast includes *Candida* and *C. neoformans*. Interpretations of susceptibility tests are available for fluconazole, itraconazole and flucytosine.[21] There are no guidelines for interpretation of testing amphotericin B susceptibility, although organisms with an MIC greater than 1 μg/mL are probably resistant. The guidelines for molds include methods for testing the MIC with amphotericin, flucytosine, fluconazole, ketoconazole, and itraconazole; however, there are no interpretive standards for determining whether an isolate is susceptible.

SPECIMEN COLLECTION AND TRANSPORT FOR PARASITES

It is important to use one or more preservatives for transport of stool for parasite examination because some parasites rapidly become undetectable. Many laboratories request that the stool be sent in two separate preservatives: 10% buffered formalin for preparation of a stool concentrate and a preservative with polyvinyl alcohol for preparation of a permanent stained slide. Commercial kits with these preservatives are available and these have convenient tight-fitting screw caps and "fill to" lines. Preservatives, which can be used for both the concentrate and permanent stained slide, are available but the laboratory should be consulted before these are used.

Pinworms (*Enterobius vermicularis*) and their eggs are not readily found in stool because the female worms exit the anus and lay their eggs on the adjacent skin. To collect the eggs for diagnosis, the sticky side of cellulose (clear) tape can be applied repeatedly to different areas of the peri anal skin, preferably first thing in the morning (before passing stool). The tape is then applied to a microscope slide, with the sticky side against the glass and submitted to the laboratory. Opaque or frosted tape should not be used. Commercial collection kits with sticky transparent paddles are available and simpler to use than tape.

If blood-borne parasites are suspected, blood anticoagulated with EDTA (purple top tube) should be submitted for preparation of blood smears.

TESTS FOR PARASITIC INFECTIONS

Routine testing for intestinal parasites includes microscopic examination of a wet concentrate and a permanent stained slide of stool or, for *E. vermicularis*, tape-preparation specimens. Routine examination of stool includes a concentrated wet preparation for detection of helminths, protozoan cysts, coccidia and microsporidia, and a permanent stain-smear for protozoa. A few intestinal parasites require special stains to be detected. If these parasites are suspected, it is important to tell the microbiology laboratory so that the right methods will be used. These parasites, along with the method used for detection and the recommended specimen, are listed in Table 1–2.

Blood-borne parasites include *Plasmodium* (malaria), *Babesia*, *Trypanosoma*, and several species of filaria. These pathogens can be detected by microscopic examination of Giemsa-stained blood smears. The use of thick blood films increases the sensitivity for *Plasmodium* and *Babesia*, however, thin smears should also be made because the morphology of the parasites is better preserved in this preparation so that species identification can be made. The Binax NOW® ICT malaria test is an FDA-approved rapid immunochromatographic test which differentiates *P. falciparum* from the other species of Plasmodium. It is sensitive for *P. falciparum* (96%) and *P. vivax* (87%), but less sensitive for *P. ovale* and *P. malariae* (both 62%) and has an overall specificity of 99%.[22]

SPECIMEN COLLECTION AND TESTING FOR SELECTED BODY SITES

Blood

Blood culture bottles specifically intended for pediatric use may provide some advantage over use of adult blood culture bottles in children, although the data

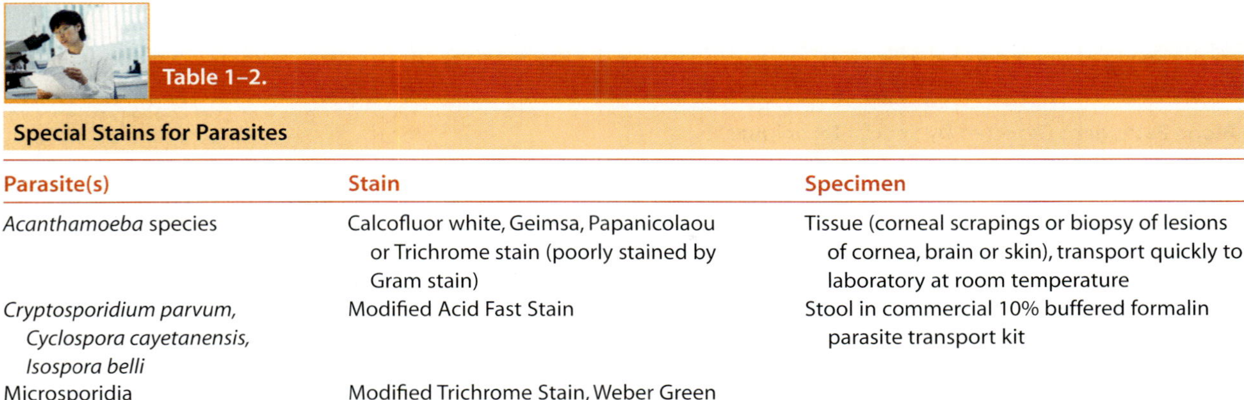

Table 1–2.

Special Stains for Parasites

Parasite(s)	Stain	Specimen
Acanthamoeba species	Calcofluor white, Geimsa, Papanicolaou or Trichrome stain (poorly stained by Gram stain)	Tissue (corneal scrapings or biopsy of lesions of cornea, brain or skin), transport quickly to laboratory at room temperature
Cryptosporidium parvum, Cyclospora cayetanensis, Isospora belli	Modified Acid Fast Stain	Stool in commercial 10% buffered formalin parasite transport kit
Microsporidia	Modified Trichrome Stain, Weber Green Stain, Ryan Blue Stain	

supporting this are limited.[23] Pediatric blood culture bottles contain a smaller volume of media than those intended for use in adults and also have a lower concentration of sodium polyanethol sulfonate (SPS), which is an anticoagulant also inhibits the antibacterial effects of blood. SPS has been suggested to inhibit growth of some bacteria (e.g., *Neisseria meningitidis*), however, the antibacterial effect of SPS does not appear to be significant in practice.[24]

The concentration of bacteria in the blood of a septic child can be quite low, so the chance of detecting a bacterial pathogen is significantly increased by culturing a larger volume of blood. The concentration of bacteria in blood is less than 1 colony-forming units (viable bacteria) per mL of blood in 23.1% of children, and less than 10 colony-forming units per mL of blood in 60.3% of children with culture-confirmed bacteremia.[25] The sensitivity of blood culture in children increases when higher volumes of blood are cultured (e.g., sensitivity increases by approximately 20% when the volume is increased from 2 to 6 mL.)[26]

Because limited blood volume is available from children and because the yield of aerobic culture is greater than of anaerobic culture from children, anaerobic culture should be performed only in children with risk factors for sepsis with obligate anaerobes.[27,28] Widely used automated continuous-monitoring pediatric blood culture systems reliably detect facultative but not obligate anaerobes. Although data are limited, risk factors for sepsis with obligate anaerobic bacteria in children may include decubitis ulcers, abdominal processes (pain, breakdown of the anatomic barrier of the intestinal tract), and neutropenia.[27,28] Obligate anaerobic bacteria are also associated with deep abscesses and infections of the head and neck which extend from the oropharynx, and so anaerobic culture may also be useful in children with such infections.

Several bacteria and fungi in blood require special culture conditions or alternative methods of detection (Table 1–3).[29,30] Yeast, including *Candida*, can be detected in conventional blood culture bottles.

Cerebrospinal Fluid

Cerebrospinal fluid (CSF) culture and Gram stain and blood culture should be routinely sent if bacterial meningitis is suspected. CSF should be transported to the microbiology laboratory at room temperature within 1 hour of specimen collection. Routine Gram stain and culture will detect most common and uncommon causes of meningitis in children. Gram stain will detect approximately half of cases of bacterial meningitis, and false-positive CSF Gram stain results, although uncommon, may be caused by observer misinterpretation, reagent contamination, or the use of an occluded lumbar needle which leads to contamination of the specimen with skin flora. Tests for bacterial antigens in CSF should not be performed as these are insensitive and nonspecific and do not add information to that from Gram stain and culture results.[31] Even when bacterial antigens are detected in CSF, the result rarely affects patient care because the Gram stain is nearly always positive in these patients as well.[32,33] Obligate anaerobic bacteria are an uncommon cause of meningitis in children. Anaerobic culture of CSF should be considered when there are other infections which may give anaerobes access to the meninges or blood (e.g., sinusitis, chronic ear infections, or gastrointestinal disease) or when the anatomic protection of the meninges is compromised (e.g., owing to ventricular shunt or skull fractures).[34]

Tests for fungi in CSF should be sent in selected patients. Immunocompromised patients, particularly those with HIV infection or prolonged corticosteroid treatment, are at risk for meningitis caused by *C. neoformans*. Tests for cryptococcal antigen in CSF and blood can be done quickly and are sensitive and specific.[35] In adults, tests for cryptococcal antigen on CSF

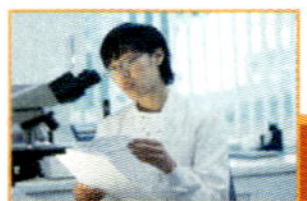

Table 1–3.

Blood Pathogens Detected by Special Techniques

Pathogen	Culture	Comments
Bartonella species	Collect blood in Isolator tube* Culture takes up to 5 wk	Serology or NAAT recommended
Borrielia species (relapsing fever)	Seldom available (research use)	Collect blood during fever, submit for microscopic examination Serology recommended
Brucella species	Conventional blood culture bottles require extended incubation and blind subculture	Notify laboratory, as *Brucella* is a potential hazard to laboratory staff Consider bone marrow culture Serology recommended
Ehrlichia and *Anaplasma* species	Seldom available (research use)	Microscopic examination of blood for inclusions may be helpful, but is insensitive Serology and NAAT recommended
H. capsulatum	Collect blood in Isolator tube* for fungal culture or collect blood in Myco/F lytic bottle†	Specimen collected in Isolator tube will yield growth faster Contact laboratory for preferred bottle
Leptospira interrogans	Inoculate oleic acid-albumin media with 1–2 drops of blood at bedside (preferred) or collect blood with sodium polyamethol sulfonate and submit to laboratory	Contact laboratory so that media will be available Multiple cultures may be needed to detect Serology recommended
Malasezia species (catheter infections)	Innoculate fungal media with blood, overlay with olive oil	Contact laboratory so that media will be available Also submit blood from port for Gram stain
Mycobacterium species	Use an Isolator tube* or culture bottles specific for mycobacteria (Myco/F lytic bottle†, Bactec 13 A‡ or BacT/Alert MB§)	Contact laboratory for preferred bottle Specimen collected in Isolator tube will yield growth slower
Streptobacillus moniliformis (rat-bite fever)	Collect blood in citrate anticoagulant, culture with serum-supplemented media	Contact laboratory so that media will be available

**Isolator system from Wampole Laboratories.*
†Myco/F lytic bottle from Becton Dickinson and Company.
‡Bactec 13 A bottle from Becton Dickinson and Company.
§BacT/Alert MB from BioMerieux Incorporated.

are more than 95% sensitive for cryptococcal meningitis regardless of HIV status.[36] Serum tests for cryptococcal antigen to diagnose cryptococcal meningitis are approximately 75% sensitive in adults without HIV and 95% sensitive in adults with HIV.[36] False-negative tests for cryptococcal antigen can be avoided by pronase treatment of serum specimens and by titration of serum and CSF specimens to overcome the inhibitory prozone effect of high levels of antigen.[35,37] India ink stains will detect less than half of cases of cryptococcal meningitis and should not be done unless cryptococcal antigen tests are not available.[38] *H. capsulatum* and *C. immitis* may also be detected by antigen tests and these results will often be available more quickly than culture results. It is reasonable to do fungal culture in addition to antigen assays if fungi are suspected, but it is important to note that fungi often take weeks to grow in culture.

Stool

Routine stool culture usually includes *Salmonella*, *Shigella*, and *Campylobacter*. If other pathogens, such as enterohemorrhagic *E. coli* (EHEC or *E. coli* O157:H7), *Y. enterocolitica* or *Vibrio* are suspected, culture for these organisms should be specifically requested. Excreted stool is preferable to swab specimens; swab specimens should only be collected from infants or patients who are unable to produce a specimen. If a stool specimen cannot be transported to the laboratory in less than an

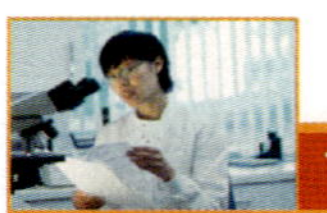

Table 1–4.

Gastrointestinal Pathogens Detected by Special Techniques

Pathogen	Culture	Comments
C. difficile (colitis)	Common flora in children, so presence in culture may be normal If culture needed, anaerobic transport is required	Immunoassays or tissue-culture cytotoxicity assays for *C. difficile* toxins are recommended
Enterohemmorhagic *E. coli* (including O157:H7)	Transport media (modified Cary-Blair) needed if transport time >1 h Culture on sorbitol-MacConkey's agar for *E. coli* O157	Stool preferred to swabs Other (non-O157) enterohemmorhagic *E. coli* can be detected by immunoassay for shiga-like toxin
Helicobacter pylori	Gastric antral biopsy (not stool) should be transported to laboratory as soon as possible in culture broth (e.g., tryptic soy broth) If transport time >1 h, transport at 4°C Grows on 5% sheep blood-agar or modified Thayer-Martin in humidified microaerobic environment (5% O_2)	Serology or stool antigen tests are recommended
Vibrio species	Transport media (e.g., modified Cary-Blair) needed if transport time >1 h Grow on MacConkey's or 5% sheep's blood media, but selective alkaline broth and thiosulfate citrate bile sucrose media enhance recovery	Stool preferred to swabs Contact laboratory to determine availability of selective broth and media
Y. enterocolitica	Transport media (e.g., modified Cary-Blair) needed if transport time >1 h Grow on MacConkey's agar at 37°C, but culture at 25°C enhances recovery	Stool preferred to swabs Cold enrichment (4°C) enhances recovery from stool, but takes weeks and so is of limited utility

hour, it should either be transported at 4°C, or with transport media to preserve the bacteria. Enteric pathogens, which require special culture conditions, are shown in Table 1–4.

EHEC is among the most common bacterial causes of diarrhea in children.[39] EHEC can be detected either by culture or by immunoassay for the shiga-like toxin which they produce. Some laboratories only test for EHEC if the stool is visibly bloody, so it is important to communicate with the laboratory if EHEC is suspected. Approximately half of EHEC are of the serotype O157:H7, and these can be detected using MacConkey's agar containing sorbitol, which these organisms do not ferment.[40] Most laboratories in the United States use sorbitol containing media for detection of EHEC. Assays for shiga-like toxin, which is produced by all serotypes of EHEC, will detect significantly more cases of EHEC infection, however, this test is used in relatively few laboratories.[39,40]

Clostridium difficile-associated diarrhea is best diagnosed by assays for the toxins produced by *C. difficile* because culture has poor specificity for symptomatic infection. Diagnosis of *C. difficile* associated diarrhea in young children is difficult because up to 30% of asymptomatic children younger than age 1 year are colonized by *C. difficile* which can lead to positive toxin assays in asymptomatic children or those with another likely cause of diarrhea.[39,41] Positive toxin results in younger children should be interpreted carefully in the context of the patient's history and complete testing for other pathogens.

Respiratory Specimens

If a patient is old enough to produce a sputum sample (typically older than 5 years), sputum should be submitted for Gram stain and bacterial culture. Bacteria that commonly cause pneumonia, including streptococci, staphylococci and *H. influenzae*, can be grown in routine respiratory culture. In children too young or too ill to produce an adequate sputum sample, a sample collection by more invasive means such as tracheal aspiration or bronchoalveolar lavage may be necessary in some circumstances (e.g., child with chronic

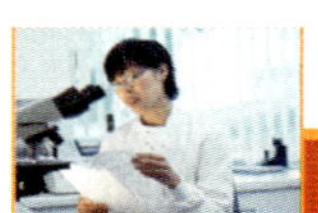

Table 1–5.

Respiratory Pathogens Detected by Special Techniques

Pathogen	Culture	Comments
Bordetella pertussis	Requires enriched media, Regan-Lowe Transport media with charcoal (Aimes with charcoal or Regan-Lowe transport media) will enhance survival	Consider serology or NAAT (more sensitive than culture) Direct fluorescent antibody tests are not adequately sensitive or specific if used alone
Burkholderia cepacia complex	Requires selective media, B. cepacia selective agar (BCSA) or oxidation-fermentation with polymyxin B, bacitracin and lactose (OFPBL)	Consider in patients with cystic fibrosis Difficult to identify and so may require reference laboratory
Corynebacterium diptheriae	Use commercial swab and transport media to swab beneath membrane, if possible Requires selective media, cystine tellurite blood agar or tinsdayle agar	Contact laboratory to determine availability of media or need for send-out to reference laboratory
Legionella pneumophila	Requires enriched media, buffered charcoal-yeast extract (BCYE) If specimen must be transported before culture, transport at 4°C	Consider urine antigen tests
Mycobacterium species	Collect sputum if possible, or bronchoalveolar lavage or three gastric aspirates (see text) for culture Agarose media (e.g., Middlebrook agars) and broth media (MGIT system, MB/BacT, Bactec Myco/F lytic bottles) both inoculated for fastest recovery Takes up to 8 wk	Stain for acid-fast organisms recommended (carbol fuchsin or auromine-O stain) on sputum or BAL NAAT recommended
Mycoplasma pneumoniae	If culture needed, use Mycoplasma transport media (2 SP) or culture media (SP-4) Requires selective media, SP-4, methylene blue-glucose or others Takes up to 4 wk	Serology (IgM) or NAAT are recommended Contact laboratory to determine availability of transport media and culture

granulomatous disease). Regardless of whether a sputum sample is submitted, blood culture should be obtained in patients suspected of having bacterial pneumonia. As discussed above, the Binax NOW® test for *S. pneumoniae* antigen is sensitive, but not specific for invasive pneumococcal disease in children.

There are few studies on interpretation of respiratory Gram stains in children. In adults, a high number of polymorphonuclear leukocytes and low number of epithelial cells on Gram stain suggests that a respiratory specimen is from the lower respiratory tract and that bacterial growth is likely to be significant. A study which evaluated the utility of Gram stain in endotracheal aspirates from mechanically ventilated children found that the absence of bacteria on Gram stain suggests that culture is unlikely to detect a pathogen.[42]

Respiratory pathogens, which are not detected by routine culture, are listed in Table 1–5 and comments on some of these follow.

The appropriate specimen for diagnosis of pulmonary tuberculosis depends on the child's age and ability to produce sputum. If sputum can be produced, three sputum samples collected on separate days should be submitted for stain and culture for acid-fast bacteria. If sputum cannot be obtained, gastric aspirate specimens should be collected. The sensitivity of gastric aspirate culture can be increased by collecting the specimen first thing in the morning (before the patient eats), neutralization of the stomach acid by adding sodium bicarbonate or sodium carbonate to the specimen, and collection of three specimens on separate days before the initiation of therapy.[43] Even with these steps, the sensitivity of culture of gastric aspirates for *M. tuberculosis* is, at best, approximately 50%.[43,44] It is controversial whether gastric aspirate specimens should be stained for acid-fast bacilli, because oral acid-fast organisms can be detected in aspirates from patients who do not have pulmonary tuberculosis. In populations with a high prevalence of pulmonary tuberculosis, staining of gastric aspirates works well, but positive results should be interpreted with caution in patients at a low risk of pulmonary tuberculosis.[44]

Two NAATs have been approved by the FDA, for detection of *M. tuberculosis* in respiratory specimens. These tests are sensitive and specific on respiratory specimens in which acid-fast bacilli are detectable on stain (i.e., "smear-positive" specimens).[45] If acid-fast bacilli are not detectable by stain, these tests are specific, but not very sensitive and so a positive result is highly predictive of tuberculosis, but a negative result should not be used to rule out tuberculosis.[46] NAAT for *M. tuberculosis* should not be used alone, but they are a useful addition to stains for acid-fast bacilli and culture.

B. pertussis can be detected by culture, PCR or serology. Direct immunofluorescent assays for *B. pertussis* are not sensitive or specific and should not be used if other tests are available. If the patient has been symptomatic less than 2 weeks, culture or PCR of a nasopharyngeal swab, aspirate or wash specimen is very sensitive and typically detects two-fold to three-fold more infections than does culture.[47,48] Dacron or rayon swabs with synthetic shafts are preferred because calcium alginate swabs and wooden shafts inhibit PCR. Most PCR tests detect a *B. pertussis* genetic sequence (IS481) that is also present in *Bordetella holmseii,* which is occasionally found in human samples and can lead to false-positive PCR for *B. pertussis.* The high sensitivity of PCR must be weighed against the potential for false-positive results, which have led to costly pseudo-outbreaks of pertussis.[49] PCR for pertussis can be made more sensitive by amplifying other DNA sequences, such as the pertussis toxin gene promoter.[47] There is no FDA approved serology test for antibodies to *B. pertussis*, however, some public health laboratories offer this test.

Infection with *Mycoplasma pneumoniae* is best detected by NAAT of respiratory specimens or by serological testing. There are no FDA-approved NAAT for *M. pneumoniae*, however, many assays have been validated by reference laboratories and have sensitivity of approximately 60% and specificity of more than 95%.[50–52] The sensitivity of paired IgM samples for *M. pneumoniae* ranges widely, from 32% to 84% and specificity is typically approximately 90%, but also varies between assays.[53] Culture is difficult and slower than NAAT or serology.

Sexually Transmitted Infections (Including Perinatal Transmission)

Diagnosis of sexually transmitted infections in adolescents can be done by the same methods used in adults. In younger children, bacteria associated with sexually transmitted infection can be acquired from the mother during delivery or as a result of sexual abuse. The body sites affected and the diagnostic tests can therefore differ in children and adults, because of the routes of transmission and social, legal and psychological consequences of the diagnosis. The collection of genital specimens from a prepubertal girl should be done only by experienced practitioners, as it can be painful when performed incorrectly.

Neisseria gonorrhoeae can be detected by Gram stain, culture or NAAT. Gram stain of a urethral specimen in a symptomatic adolescent male is a sensitive and specific test for *N. gonorrhoeae* infection, however, it should not be used in females or asymptomatic males. Culture for *N. gonorrhoeae* can be performed using urethral, cervical, vaginal, anal/rectal, conjuctival or pharyngeal swabs. The organism is labile and every effort should be made to culture specimens correctly. Culture conditions and alternative tests for genital pathogens are in Table 1–6. Culture is a reasonably sensitive test for *N. gonorrhoeae* (80–86%) and it is the gold standard for specificity. Molecular tests, including NAAT, for *N. gonorrhoeae* and *Chlamydia trachomatis* are discussed together below, as these are usually performed together on a single specimen.

C. trachomatis can be detected by immunoassays (ELISA or immunofluorescent staining), culture, and molecular tests. Immunoassays can give same day results, but the poor sensitivity and specificity of these tests has made them less popular than NAAT. *C. trachomatis* culture is performed by incubating the specimen with mammalian cells, which support replication of the bacteria, and then staining the cells by immunofluorescence with antibodies specific for *C. trachomatis* 2 or 3 days later. The advantages of culture are the high (gold-standard) specificity of the test and acceptability of multiple specimen sources, including urethral, cervical, vaginal, anal/rectal, conjuctival or pharyngeal swabs. Unfortunately, the sensitivity of culture for genital infection with *C. trachomatis* is only 52.3% (female) to 58.9% (male), which is significantly lower than that of NAAT.[54] As a result, culture is used primarily for conjunctival and pharyngeal sites, from which NAAT usually cannot be done, and when sexual abuse is suspected, since the very high specificity makes a false-positive result unlikely.

There are several molecular assays for *C. trachomatis* and *N. gonorrhoeae*. PACE-2 (Gen-Probe Incorporated) is a nonamplified molecular probe test

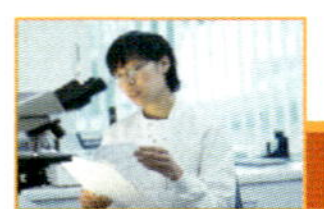

Table 1–6.

Genital Pathogens Detected by Special Techniques

Pathogen	Culture	Comments
C. trachomatis	Requires cell culture If culture needed (e.g., suspected sexual abuse), use Chlamydia transport media (2 SP or SPG)	NAAT are recommended
Haemophilus ducreyi	Immediately inoculate conventional chocolate (5% lysed sheep blood) agar and, if available, chocolate agar supplemented with vancomycin and fetal bovine serum If specimen must be transported before culture, transport at 4°C	Culture is insensitive Contact laboratory to determine availability of media
Neisseria gonorrhoeae	Innoculate room-temperature selective media (Modified Thayer-Martin, Martin-Lewis, or NYC medium) and incubate at 35°C with 5% CO_2 immediately if possible If plates are transported, systems which generate CO_2 should be used (JEMBEC, Gono-Pak, InTray GC)	Consider NAAT Swabs should be cultured within 6 h
Klebsiella (Calymmatobacterium) granulomatis	Seldom available (research use)	Collect scraping or biopsy of edge of lesion, submit for Wright's or Giemsa stain

for *C. trachomatis* and *N. gonorrhoeae*. The sensitivity of PACE-2 is approximately 70% for *C. trachomatis* and 80% for *N. gonorrhoeae* and it is highly specific (>98%) for both organisms.[55–57] Three NAAT are available for *C. trachomatis* and *N. gonorrhoeae*: AMPLICOR (Roche Diagnostic Systems), BDProbeTec (Becton, Dickinson and Company) and APTIMA Combo 2 Assay (Gen-Probe Incorporated). An advantage of NAAT over other tests for *C. trachomatis* and *N. gonorrhoeae* is that urine can be tested, in addition to urethral and cervical specimens. Other specimens (e.g., conjunctival and pharyngeal) are not usually acceptable for NAAT. Most studies of NAAT for diagnosis of these infections are performed in adults and adolescents and data in prepubertal children are quite limited. It is difficult to compare the performance of the available NAAT because of the use of different and problematic gold-standards, but it is clear that NAAT are the most sensitive tests for both *C. trachomatis* and *N. gonorrhoeae*.[57] Most studies of adults find that the NAAT are more than 90% sensitive for both organisms and that the specificities are more than 97%.[58,59] Use of urine from females may be somewhat less sensitive for both organisms (approximately 80–85%) than other acceptable specimens.[58,59]

The selection of tests for diagnosis of *C. trachomatis* and *N. gonorrhoeae* in children who may have been sexually abused is complex. Detection of these bacteria requires a sensitive test (e.g., the NAATs) while the significant legal, social and psychological consequences of a false-positive test requires a very specific test (e.g., culture). See Table 1–7 for a summary of the tests for bacteria and parasites recommended by the Centers for Disease Control and Prevention at initial visit and 2 weeks later for children in cases of suspected sexual abuse.[60] The Centers for Disease Control and Prevention does not recommend use of NAAT for *C. trachomatis* or *N. gonorrhoeae* if culture is available, however, this is an area of controversy.[60–62] Results of a NAAT might not be considered evidence of infection in legal proceedings as a result of the imperfect specificity of these tests, and this can affect the decision to use a NAAT in suspected sexual abuse.[60]

Syphilis can be diagnosed by microscopic detection of *Treponema pallidum* or by serology.[60] If lesions (e.g., chancre) are present, treponemes can be detected by dark-field microscopy or immunofluorescent stain. More commonly, the diagnosis is made by serology in the absence of primary lesions. Nontreponemal serological tests (RPR and VDRL) detect antibodies against a lipid antigen, cardiolipin, rather than against the bacteria. The treponemal serological tests (FTA-ABS and TP-PA) detect antibodies specific for *T. pallidum*. Nontreponemal tests are used as screening tests for syphilis (e.g., in sexually active adolescents)

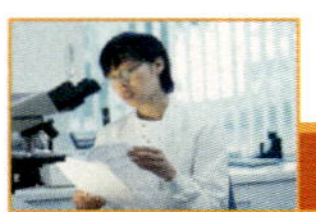

Table 1–7.

Tests for Sexually Transmitted Organisms in Suspected Sexual Abuse

Pathogen	Specimen(s)	Test(s)
Niesseria gonorrhoeae	Pharynx and anus in both boys and girls Vagina (not cervix) in girls and urethra in boys	Culture Request that specimen and isolates be preserved in laboratory
C. trachomatis	Anus in both boys and girls Vagina (not cervix) in girls Meatal swab if urethral discharge present in boys	Culture Request that specimen and isolates be preserved in laboratory If culture is not available, NAAT with confirmation by amplification of separate target if positive
T. vaginalis and bacterial vaginosis	Vagina (not cervix) in girls	Wet-mount for *T. vaginalis* and bacterial vaginosis Culture for *T. vaginalis*

and for following the course of disease, as the titers of the nontreponemal tests fall with successful treatment. Treponemal tests are used to confirm the nontreponemal results, but the treponemal tests usually stay positive for the life of the individual even after successful treatment.

The risk of congenital syphilis should be determined by a nontreponemal antibody test of the pregnant woman in the first trimester of pregnancy and, if the risk of syphilis is high, at delivery.[60] Testing the mother is preferred to testing the child, as a low level of maternal antibody may not be detectable in the newborn. However, once the diagnosis of syphilis is made in the mother, follow-up testing in the newborn should include the same quantitative nontreponemal test as was used in the mother. A higher titer in the newborn (four-fold or greater than the titer in the mother) is highly suggestive of congenital syphilis.[60] Physical manifestations of congenital syphilis and anatomic pathology of the placenta and newborn are also important in determining the risk of congenital syphilis and current guidelines should be consulted.[60]

Trichomonas vaginalis can be detected by wet-mount of vaginal secretions in adolescents, although this test is only 50–70% sensitive.[60] More sensitive tests include culture (the current gold standard) as well as a DNA probe test, Affirm VP (Becton, Dickinson and Company), which is 90.5% sensitive and 99.8% specific for *T. vaginalis* and also separately detects *Candida* and *Gardenerella vaginalis*.[63] A rapid antigen detection test, OSOM Trichomonas Rapid Test (Genzyme Diagnostics) is also available, and is 82% sensitive.[64] Infection with *T. vaginalis* in suspected sexual abuse should be diagnosed by culture because the performance of the nonculture tests has not been adequately assessed in prepubertal children.[60]

Urine

Urine culture is the gold standard for diagnosis of urinary tract infection (UTI), but culture results require a minimum of 24 hours and so rapid screening tests are also valuable. Screening tests for UTI include biochemical tests by rapid dipstick methods (nitrite and leukocyte esterase) and microscopic examination of the urine for bacteria and leukocytes. A meta-analysis of studies of screening tests for UTI in children found that detection of any bacteria by Gram stain was the best screening test for UTI, with an estimated sensitivity of 93% and specificity of 95%.[65] Dipstick assays, which are less technically demanding than Gram stain, also performed well as a screen for UTI. If either leukocyte esterase or nitrite is positive (trace or greater), the dipstick has an estimated sensitivity of 88% and if both results are negative, the dipstick has an estimated specificity of 96%. In the meta-analysis, microscopic examination of urine for leukocytes was inferior to other tests as a screening assay for UTI. But microscopy for urine leukocytes may have some value, as the number of leukocytes in the urine is the best predictor of sepsis associated with UTI in children younger than 90 days.[66] When tested by dipstick methods, urine collected by bag has sensitivity comparable to that of urine collected by catheter, however, the specificity of urine collected by bag is significantly lower than that collected by catheter.[67]

Culture of urine is important because use of the screening tests alone will miss a significant number of

UTI. Collection of specimens from children who are not toilet trained is very important to make an accurate diagnosis. Bag urine specimens are not acceptable for culture as they are frequently contaminated with normal skin and genital flora.[68] Specimens properly collected by suprapubic aspiration should be sterile and growth of any number of gram-negative rods or a few thousand gram-positive cocci per mL very likely indicates a UTI.[69] Pure growth of more than 10,000 pure colonies of a uropathogen collected by transurethral catheterization is likely to indicate true infection and more than 100,000 pure colonies of a uropathogen from midstream urine is also likely to indicate true infection. The presence of small numbers of urogenital flora (e.g., *Lactobacillus*) will usually be ignored by the laboratory, but if urogenital flora are present in quantities roughly equal to a uropathogen, the laboratory will report the culture as mixed and collection of a new culture is needed.

REFERENCES

1. Mirza A, Wludyka P, Chiu TT, Rathore MH. Throat culture is necessary after negative rapid antigen detection tests. *Clin Pediatr (Phila)*. 2007;46(3):241-246.
2. Fox JW, Cohen DM, Marcon MJ, Cotton WH, Bonsu BK. Performance of rapid streptococcal antigen testing varies by personnel. *J Clin Microbiol.* 2006;44(11):3918-3922.
3. Charkaluk ML, Kalach N, Mvogo H, et al. Assessment of a rapid urinary antigen detection by an immunochromatographic test for diagnosis of pneumococcal infection in children. *Diagn Microbiol Infect Dis.* 2006;55(2):89-94.
4. Davies HD, Miller MA, Faro S, Gregson D, Kehl SC, Jordan JA. Multicenter study of a rapid molecular-based assay for the diagnosis of group B Streptococcus colonization in pregnant women. *Clin Infect Dis.* 2004;39(8):1129-1135.
5. Warren DK, Liao RS, Merz LR, Eveland M, Dunne WM, Jr. Detection of methicillin-resistant *Staphylococcus aureus* directly from nasal swab specimens by a real-time PCR assay. *J Clin Microbiol.* 2004;42(12):5578-5581.
6. Baddour LM, Wilson WR, Bayer AS, et al. Infective endocarditis: diagnosis, antimicrobial therapy, and management of complications: a statement for healthcare professionals from the Committee on Rheumatic Fever, Endocarditis, and Kawasaki Disease, Council on Cardiovascular Disease in the Young, and the Councils on Clinical Cardiology, Stroke, and Cardiovascular Surgery and Anesthesia, American Heart Association: endorsed by the Infectious Diseases Society of America. *Circulation.* 2005;111(23):e394-e434.
7. Winkler MA, Cockerill FR, Craig WA, et al. *Performance Standard for Antimicrobial Susceptibility Testing; Seventeenth Informational Supplement.* Wayne: Clinical and Laboratory Standards Institute; 2007.
8. Musher DM, Bartlett JG, Doern GV. A fresh look at the definition of susceptibility of *Streptococcus pneumoniae* to β-lactam antibiotics. *Arch Intern Med.* 2001;161(21):2538-2544.
9. Turner AK, Nair S, Wain J. The acquisition of full fluoroquinolone resistance in Salmonella Typhi by accumulation of point mutations in the topoisomerase targets. *J Antimicrob Chemother.* 2006;58(4):733-740.
10. Patel M, Waites KB, Moser SA, Cloud GA, Hoesley CJ. Prevalence of inducible clindamycin resistance among community- and hospital-associated *Staphylococcus aureus* isolates. *J Clin Microbiol.* 2006;44(7):2481-2484.
11. Aaron SD, Vandemheen KL, Ferris W, et al. Combination antibiotic susceptibility testing to treat exacerbations of cystic fibrosis associated with multiresistant bacteria: a randomised, double-blind, controlled clinical trial. *Lancet.* 2005;366(9484):463-471.
12. Devlin RK. Invasive fungal infections caused by Candida and Malassezia species in the neonatal intensive care unit. *Adv Neonatal Care.* 2006;6(2):68-77; quiz 8-9.
13. Sulahian A, Boutboul F, Ribaud P, Leblanc T, Lacroix C, Derouin F. Value of antigen detection using an enzyme immunoassay in the diagnosis and prediction of invasive aspergillosis in two adult and pediatric hematology units during a 4-year prospective study. *Cancer.* 2001;91(2):311-318.
14. Hope WW, Walsh TJ, Denning DW. Laboratory diagnosis of invasive aspergillosis. *Lancet Infect Dis.* 2005;5(10):609-622.
15. Steinbach WJ, Addison RM, McLaughlin L, et al. Prospective aspergillus galactomannan antigen testing in pediatric hematopoietic stem cell transplant recipients. *Pediatr Infect Dis J.* 2007;26(7):558-564.
16. Giacchino M, Chiapello N, Bezzio S, et al. Aspergillus galactomannan enzyme-linked immunosorbent assay cross-reactivity caused by invasive *Geotrichum capitatum. J Clin Microbiol.* 2006;44(9):3432-3434.
17. Smith PB, Benjamin DK, Jr., Alexander BD, Johnson MD, Finkelman MA, Steinbach WJ. Quantification of 1,3 β-D-glucan levels in children: preliminary data for diagnostic use of the β-glucan assay in a pediatric setting. *Clin Vaccine Immunol.* 2007;14(7):924-925.
18. Ostrosky-Zeichner L, Alexander BD, Kett DH, et al. Multicenter clinical evaluation of the (1->3) β-D-glucan assay as an aid to diagnosis of fungal infections in humans. *Clin Infect Dis.* 2005;41(5):654-659.
19. Odabasi Z, Mattiuzzi G, Estey E, et al. β-D-glucan as a diagnostic adjunct for invasive fungal infections: validation, cutoff development, and performance in patients with acute myelogenous leukemia and myelodysplastic syndrome. *Clin Infect Dis.* 2004;39(2):199-205.
20. Kedzierska A, Kochan P, Pietrzyk A, Kedzierska J. Current status of fungal cell wall components in the immunodiagnostics of invasive fungal infections in humans: galactomannan, mannan and (1->3) β-D-glucan antigens. *Eur J Clin Microbiol Infect Dis.* 2007;26:755-766.
21. Pfaller MA, Chaturvedi V, Espinel-Ingroff A, et al. *Reference Method for Broth Dilution Antifungal Susceptibility Testing of Yeasts; Approved Standard.* Wayne: Clinical and Laboratory Standards Institute; 2002.
22. Farcas GA, Zhong KJ, Lovegrove FE, Graham CM, Kain KC. Evaluation of the Binax NOW ICT test versus polymerase chain reaction and microscopy for the detection of malaria in returned travelers. *Am J Trop Med Hyg.* 2003;69(6):589-592.

23. Lee CS, Tang RB, Chung RL, Chen SJ. Evaluation of different blood culture media in neonatal sepsis. *J Microbiol Immunol Infect.* 2000;33(3):165-168.
24. McDonald JC, Knowles K, Sorger S. Assessment of gelatin supplementation of PEDS Plus BACTEC blood culture medium. *Diagn Microbiol Infect Dis.* 1993;17(3):193-196.
25. Kellogg JA, Manzella JP, Bankert DA. Frequency of low-level bacteremia in children from birth to 15 years of age. *J Clin Microbiol.* 2000;38(6):2181-2185.
26. Isaacman DJ, Karasic RB, Reynolds EA, Kost SI. Effect of number of blood cultures and volume of blood on detection of bacteremia in children. *J Pediatr.* 1996;128(2):190-195.
27. Lee CS, Hwang B, Chung RL, Tang RB. The assessment of anaerobic blood culture in children. *J Microbiol Immunol Infect.* 2000;33(1):49-52.
28. Zaidi AK, Knaut AL, Mirrett S, Reller LB. Value of routine anaerobic blood cultures for pediatric patients. *J Pediatr.* 1995;127(2):263-268.
29. Crump JA, Tanner DC, Mirrett S, McKnight CM, Reller LB. Controlled comparison of BACTEC 13 A, MYCO/F LYTIC, BacT/ALERT MB, and ISOLATOR 10 systems for detection of mycobacteremia. *J Clin Microbiol.* 2003;41(5):1987-1990.
30. Fuller DD, Davis TE, Jr., Denys GA, York MK. Evaluation of BACTEC MYCO/F Lytic medium for recovery of mycobacteria, fungi, and bacteria from blood. *J Clin Microbiol.* 2001;39(8):2933-2936.
31. Nigrovic LE, Kuppermann N, McAdam AJ, Malley R. Cerebrospinal latex agglutination fails to contribute to the microbiologic diagnosis of pretreated children with meningitis. *Pediatr Infect Dis J.* 2004;23(8):786-788.
32. Maxson S, Lewno MJ, Schutze GE. Clinical usefulness of cerebrospinal fluid bacterial antigen studies. *J Pediatr.* 1994;125(2):235-238.
33. Perkins MD, Mirrett S, Reller LB. Rapid bacterial antigen detection is not clinically useful. *J Clin Microbiol.* 1995;33(6):1486-1491.
34. Brook I. Meningitis and shunt infection caused by anaerobic bacteria in children. *Pediatr Neurol.* 2002;26(2):99-105.
35. Tanner DC, Weinstein MP, Fedorciw B, Joho KL, Thorpe JJ, Reller L. Comparison of commercial kits for detection of cryptococcal antigen. *J Clin Microbiol.* 1994;32(7):1680-1684.
36. Dromer F, Mathoulin-Pelissier S, Launay O, Lortholary O. Determinants of disease presentation and outcome during cryptococcosis: the CryptoA/D Study. *PLoS Med.* 2007;4(2):e21.
37. Hamilton JR, Noble A, Denning DW, Stevens DA. Performance of cryptococcus antigen latex agglutination kits on serum and cerebrospinal fluid specimens of AIDS patients before and after pronase treatment. *J Clin Microbiol.* 1991;29(2):333-339.
38. Sato Y, Osabe S, Kuno H, Kaji M, Oizumi K. Rapid diagnosis of cryptococcal meningitis by microscopic examination of centrifuged cerebrospinal fluid sediment. *J Neurol Sci.* 1999;164(1):72-75.
39. Klein EJ, Boster DR, Stapp JR, et al. Diarrhea etiology in a Children's Hospital Emergency Department: a prospective cohort study. *Clin Infect Dis.* 2006;43(7):807-813.
40. Fey PD, Wickert RS, Rupp ME, Safranek TJ, Hinrichs SH. Prevalence of non-O157:H7 shiga toxin-producing *Escherichia coli* in diarrheal stool samples from Nebraska. *Emerg Infect Dis.* 2000;6(5):530-533.
41. Cerquetti M, Luzzi I, Caprioli A, Sebastianelli A, Mastrantonio P. Role of *Clostridium difficile* in childhood diarrhea. *Pediatr Infect Dis J.* 1995;14(7):598-603.
42. Zaidi AK, Reller LB. Rejection criteria for endotracheal aspirates from pediatric patients. *J Clin Microbiol.* 1996;34(2):352-354.
43. Pomputius WF, III, Rost J, Dennehy PH, Carter EJ. Standardization of gastric aspirate technique improves yield in the diagnosis of tuberculosis in children. *Pediatr Infect Dis J.* 1997;16(2):222-226.
44. Berggren Palme I, Gudetta B, Bruchfeld J, Eriksson M, Giesecke J. Detection of Mycobacterium tuberculosis in gastric aspirate and sputum collected from Ethiopian HIV-positive and HIV-negative children in a mixed in- and outpatient setting. *Acta Paediatr.* 2004;93(3):311-315.
45. Nahid P, Pai M, Hopewell PC. Advances in the diagnosis and treatment of tuberculosis. *Proc Am Thorac Soc.* 2006;3(1):103-110.
46. Sarmiento OL, Weigle KA, Alexander J, Weber DJ, Miller WC. Assessment by meta-analysis of PCR for diagnosis of smear-negative pulmonary tuberculosis. *J Clin Microbiol.* 2003;41(7):3233-3240.
47. Qin X, Galanakis E, Martin ET, Englund JA. Multitarget PCR for diagnosis of pertussis and its clinical implications. *J Clin Microbiol.* 2007;45(2):506-511.
48. Knorr L, Fox JD, Tilley PA, Ahmed-Bentley J. Evaluation of real-time PCR for diagnosis of *Bordetella pertussis* infection. *BMC Infect Dis.* 2006;6:62.
49. Kirkland KB, Talbot EA, Lasky RA, et al. Outbreaks of respiratory illness mistakenly attributed to pertussis - New Hampshire, Massachusetts, and Tennessee, 2004-2006. *MMWR.* 2007;56(33):387-842.
50. Daxboeck F, Krause R, Wenisch C. Laboratory diagnosis of *Mycoplasma pneumoniae* infection. *Clin Microbiol Infect.* 2003;9(4):263-273.
51. Michelow IC, Olsen K, Lozano J, Duffy LB, McCracken GH, Hardy RD. Diagnostic utility and clinical significance of naso- and oropharyngeal samples used in a PCR assay to diagnose *Mycoplasma pneumoniae* infection in children with community-acquired pneumonia. *J Clin Microbiol.* 2004;42(7):3339-3341.
52. Pitcher D, Chalker VJ, Sheppard C, George RC, Harrison TG. Real-time detection of *Mycoplasma pneumoniae* in respiratory samples with an internal processing control. *J Med Microbiol.* 2006;55(pt 2):149-155.
53. Beersma MF, Dirven K, van Dam AP, Templeton KE, Claas EC, Goossens H. Evaluation of 12 commercial tests and the complement fixation test for *Mycoplasma pneumoniae*-specific immunoglobulin G (IgG) and IgM antibodies, with PCR used as the "gold standard". *J Clin Microbiol.* 2005;43(5):2277-2285.
54. Crotchfelt KA, Pare B, Gaydos C, Quinn TC. Detection of *Chlamydia trachomatis* by the Gen-Probe AMPLIFIED *Chlamydia Trachomatis* Assay (AMP CT) in urine specimens from men and women and endocervical specimens from women. *J Clin Microbiol.* 1998;36(2):391-394.

55. Wylie JL, Moses S, Babcock R, Jolly A, Giercke S, Hammond G. Comparative evaluation of chlamydiazyme, PACE 2, and AMP-CT assays for detection of *Chlamydia trachomatis* in endocervical specimens. *J Clin Microbiol.* 1998;36(12):3488-3491.
56. Darwin LH, Cullen AP, Crowe SR, Modarress KJ, Willis DE, Payne WJ. Evaluation of the Hybrid Capture 2 CT/GC DNA tests and the GenProbe PACE 2 tests from the same male urethral swab specimens. *Sex Transm Dis.* 2002;29(10):576-580.
57. Olshen E, Shrier LA. Diagnostic tests for chlamydial and gonorrheal infections. *Semin Pediatr Infect Dis.* 2005;16(3):192-198.
58. van Doornum GJ, Schouls LM, Pijl A, Cairo I, Buimer M, Bruisten S. Comparison between the LCx Probe system and the COBAS AMPLICOR system for detection of *Chlamydia trachomatis* and *Neisseria gonorrhoeae* infections in patients attending a clinic for treatment of sexually transmitted diseases in Amsterdam, The Netherlands. *J Clin Microbiol.* 2001;39(3):829-835.
59. Van Der Pol B, Ferrero DV, Buck-Barrington L, et al. Multicenter evaluation of the BDProbeTec ET System for detection of *Chlamydia trachomatis* and *Neisseria gonorrhoeae* in urine specimens, female endocervical swabs, and male urethral swabs. *J Clin Microbiol.* 2001;39(3):1008-1016.
60. Workowski K, Berman S. Sexually Transmitted Diseases Treatment Guidelines, 2006. *MMWR.* 2006;55(RR-11):1-94.
61. Palusci VJ, Reeves MJ. Testing for genital gonorrhea infections in prepubertal girls with suspected sexual abuse. *Pediatr Infect Dis J.* 2003;22(7):618-623.
62. Kellogg ND, Baillargeon J, Lukefahr JL, Lawless K, Menard SW. Comparison of nucleic acid amplification tests and culture techniques in the detection of *Neisseria gonorrhoeae* and *Chlamydia trachomatis* in victims of suspected child sexual abuse. *J Pediatr Adolesc Gynecol.* 2004;17(5):331-339.
63. DeMeo LR, Draper DL, McGregor JA, et al. Evaluation of a deoxyribonucleic acid probe for the detection of *Trichomonas vaginalis* in vaginal secretions. *Am J Obstet Gynecol.* 1996;174(4):1339-1342.
64. Huppert JS, Mortensen JE, Reed JL, et al. Rapid antigen testing compares favorably with transcription-mediated amplification assay for the detection of *Trichomonas vaginalis* in young women. *Clin Infect Dis.* 2007;45(2):194-198.
65. Gorelick MH, Shaw KN. Screening tests for urinary tract infection in children: a meta-analysis. *Pediatrics.* 1999;104(5):e54.
66. Bonsu BK, Harper MB. Leukocyte counts in urine reflect the risk of concomitant sepsis in bacteriuric infants: a retrospective cohort study. *BMC Pediatr.* 2007;7:24.
67. McGillivray D, Mok E, Mulrooney E, Kramer MS. A head-to-head comparison: "Clean-void" bag versus catheter urinalysis in the diagnosis of urinary tract infection in young children. *J Pediatr.* 2005;147(4):451-456.
68. Al-Orifi F, McGillivray D, Tange S, Kramer MS. Urine culture from bag specimens in young children: are the risks too high? *J Pediatr.* 2000;137(2):221-226.
69. American Academy of Pediatrics, Committee on Quality Improvement, Subcommittee on Urinary Tract Infection. Practice parameter: the diagnosis, treatment, and evaluation of the initial urinary tract infection in febrile infants and young children. *Pediatrics.* 1999;103(4 pt 1):843-852.

CHAPTER 2

Laboratory Diagnosis of Viral Diseases

Richard L. Hodinka

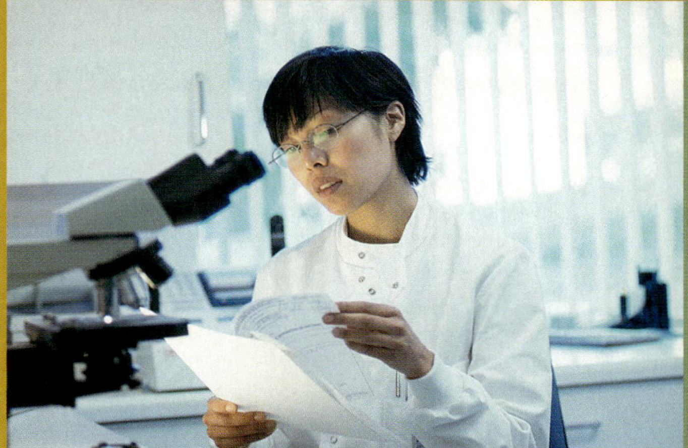

INTRODUCTION

Viruses remain a continuing threat to humankind regardless of age, gender, ethnicity, and socioeconomic status. They are a leading cause of morbidity and mortality worldwide, and severe illness commonly occurs in infants, the elderly, the chronically ill, the malnourished, and the immunocompromised.

The clinical diagnosis of viral diseases can be difficult, and laboratory confirmation is required in patients with serious illnesses since signs and symptoms are often overlapping and not always specific for any one viral agent. This is particularly true in children. Early detection of viral diseases can have a prompt and significant impact on patient care by increasing clinical awareness and providing for more informed decision making for better patient management.[1–8] A rapid and specific diagnosis can help in decreasing the use of unwarranted laboratory tests, hospital procedures, and antimicrobial drugs, resulting in reduced costs related to supportive care and a reduction in hospital stay.[1,3,4,8–13] In some cases where antiviral therapy is available, rapid and accurate viral detection can provide the opportunity for prophylaxis against certain viral infections or early treatment that may limit the extent of disease and reduce associated sequelae.[1,14] Finally, timely laboratory surveillance for viruses can provide for rapid outbreak identification and assist in the prevention of community and hospital spread.[15–18]

Many methods are available for the diagnosis and management of viral diseases (Table 2–1).[19,20] These include (1) cell culture systems for the isolation of viruses in human or animal cells, (2) rapid immunologic and molecular assays for the direct detection and/or quantification of viral proteins or nucleic acids, (3) serologic tests to detect virus-specific IgG and/or IgM antibody responses, (4) electron microscopy to identify viruses based on size and shape of viral particles, (5) histologic and cytologic techniques for detection of viral-induced morphological changes within tissues and exfoliated cells, and (6) genotypic and phenotypic assays to detect antiviral drug resistance and to identify genetic variants that may not respond to therapy. There are notable differences in the use and clinical performance of these methods and the relative importance of certain tests has changed over the years. Therefore, the selection of which assays to perform and the choice of specimens to collect for testing should be made judiciously and in consultation with appropriate laboratory personnel and will depend on the patient population and clinical situation, the intended use of the individual tests, and the capabilities and resources of individual laboratories.

SPECIMEN COLLECTION AND HANDLING

Appropriate specimen collection and handling is absolutely critical to the success of laboratory testing for diagnosis of viral infections.[21] Irrespective of the location of testing or techniques used, specimens that are poorly collected, ill timed, or incorrectly handled between the time of collection and testing are more likely to yield false test results. A comprehensive listing of the selection of viral specimens based on clinical infections, the suspected viral agents, and the tests to be performed are listed in Tables 2–2 to 2–11.

In general, specimens should be collected as close to clinical onset as possible (e.g., within the first 1–3 days). Viral shedding is at its maximum at this time and

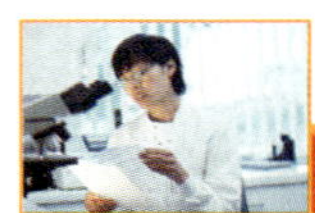

Table 2–1.

Methods Used in Diagnostic Virology Laboratory

Methods	Primary Applications
Cell culture systems	
Conventional tube	Any virus that will grow in defined cell culture system.
Shell vial or multiwell plate	CMV, HSV, VZV, respiratory viruses (e.g., RSV, influenza virus types A and B, parainfluenza virus types 1, 2, 3, adenovirus, metapneumovirus), enterovirus, and others (e.g., measles and rubella viruses).
Direct immunologic tests	
Immunofluorescence	CMV, EBV, HSV, VZV, respiratory viruses (e.g., RSV, influenza virus types A and B, parainfluenza virus types 1, 2, 3, 4, adenovirus, metapneumovirus), measles, mumps, rubella and rabies viruses. For CMV, antigenemia assay can be used to quantify the levels of virus in blood from immunocompromised patients.
Immunoassays	RSV, influenza virus types A and B, metapneumovirus, HBV, rotavirus, adenovirus types 40/41, and norovirus.
Molecular amplification assays	Any virus for which conserved gene sequences are known. Quantitative molecular assays are often used to monitor viral loads of HIV, CMV, EBV, HBV, HCV, HHV-6, BKV, and adenovirus in defined patient populations.
Electron microscopy	Enteric viruses and poxviruses.
Cytology	CMV, HSV, VZV, adenovirus, BK and JC viruses, measles virus, rabies virus, and HPV.
Histology	Any virus for which immunohistochemistry can be done. Primarily CMV, EBV, HSV, BKV, HBV, HPV, parvovirus B19, and adenovirus.
Serology	Any virus.
Genotypic and phenotypic assays	Detection of drug-resistant strains of HIV, CMV, HSV, VZV and influenza virus, and genetic variants of HBV and HCV that may not respond to therapy.

increases the likelihood of virus detection. Most acute viral infections are self-limiting and last for approximately 5–10 days, so delays in specimen collection may adversely affect laboratory testing. The amount of virus present and the duration of viral shedding will vary, however, and depends on the age of the patient, the virus, a competent immune system, the anatomical site chosen for specimen collection, and whether the infection is localized or systemic. Young infants and immunosuppressed children may shed virus for more extended times. The specimen site should be determined by the clinical presentation and the pathogenic potential of the suspected virus (Tables 2–2 to 2–11). Recovery of a given virus may be enhanced by collecting the same specimen type over the course of several days or by collecting various specimens from different body sites. Specimens should be transported to the laboratory as quickly as possible after collection. This is especially true when attempting to grow viruses from clinical specimens since some viruses, particularly those with envelopes, are quite labile outside their natural host and do not survive well under adverse environmental conditions. When immediate transport is not possible, refrigerate the specimens or keep them on wet ice. For delays of more than 24–48 hours, specimens should be processed as needed and rapidly frozen to −70°C and then transported to the laboratory on dry ice. Specimens to be used for the direct detection of viruses (e.g., culture, antigen assays, or molecular methods) should never be stored at room temperature or frozen at −20°C; it is acceptable to freeze serum or plasma at −20°C for transport to and extended storage in the laboratory when being used for detection of viral-specific antibodies. It is recommended that all specimens for molecular testing be stored at 4°C immediately after collection and then promptly sent to the laboratory for appropriate processing and storage for testing. This is critical to ensure the stability and amplification of nucleic acids, particularly for the detection of RNA viruses since RNA is unstable and easily degraded by RNases from the surrounding environment.

Collection Instructions for Selected Specimen Types

Blood for plasma or white blood cells

Approximately 4–7 mL of whole blood should be collected in a suitable anticoagulant such as ethylenediamminetriaminoacetic acid (EDTA), sodium heparin,

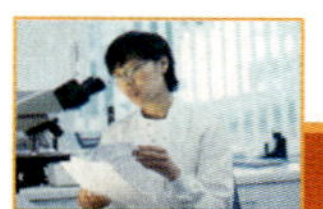

Table 2–2.

Common Specimens and Laboratory Tests for Diagnosis of Viral Respiratory Disease

General Disease Category	Possible Virus	Preferred Methods for Diagnosis: Culture	Antigen Detection	NAAT	Cytology/ Histology	EM	Serology	Suggested Specimens
Respiratory	RSV	X	X	X				NPA or NPW preferred; NPS, OS, BAL, TA, lung tissue acceptable
	Influenza virus	X	X	X				
	Parainfluenza virus	X	X	X				
	Adenovirus	X	X	X				
	Rhinovirus	X	X	X				
	Coronavirus			X				
	Metapneumo virus	X	X	X				
	CMV	X	X	X				BAL, lung tissue, blood
	HSV	X	X	X				BAL, lung tissue
	VZV	X	X	X				BAL, lung tissue
	EBV			X			X	Blood for serology; OS for PCR
	Enteroviruses	X		X				NPA, NPW, NPS, OS
	SARS-Coronavirus*			X			X	Blood for serology; NPA, NPW, NPS, OS, BAL, TA, stool acceptable for PCR
	Hantavirus*			X	X		X	Blood for serology; lung tissue for PCR, histology
	Influenza H5N1		X	X			X	Blood for serology; OS, BAL, TA preferred; NPA, NPW or NPS acceptable for PCR

**Testing is primarily done in State/Reference Laboratories or the Centers for Disease Control and Prevention (CDC).*
NAAT, nucleic acid amplification tests (e.g., PCR, other target and signal molecular amplification technologies); EM, electron microscopy; NPA, nasopharyngeal aspirate; NPW, nasopharyngeal wash; NPS, nasopharyngeal swab; OS, oropharyngeal swab; BAL, bronchoalveolar lavage; TA, tracheal aspirate.

sodium citrate, or acid citrate dextrose. EDTA is currently the preferred anticoagulant for most viral studies that require plasma or white blood cells and is considered to be the best stabilizer of nucleic acids for molecular testing.

Blood for serum

Serum is the preferred specimen for most serological assays. Approximately 1–2 mL of blood should be collected for every two to three tests ordered; collection tubes should not contain anticoagulants or preservatives. A single serum specimen is sufficient to determine the immune status of an individual or for the detection of virus-specific IgM antibody. For the diagnosis of current or recent viral infections, paired serum specimens collected 10–14 days apart are needed when testing for virus-specific IgG antibody. There are exceptions to this general rule and only a single serum for IgG is required for viruses such as Epstein–Barr virus (EBV), hepatitis B virus (HBV), and parvovirus B19. The acute-phase serum should be collected as early as possible in the course of the illness, and the acute and convalescent sera should be tested simultaneously to obtain the most meaningful results. Serum specimens from mother, fetus, and newborn can be submitted for the evaluation of IgG and IgM antibodies for the detection of prenatal, natal, and postnatal viral infections with cytomegalovirus (CMV), rubella virus, herpes simplex virus (HSV), varicella-zoster virus (VZV), parvovirus B19, human immunodeficiency virus (HIV), HBV, hepatitis C virus (HCV), and others. Plasma can be used as an acceptable alternative to serum for serological diagnosis of HIV and hepatitis viruses. Oral mucosal transudates rich in gingival crevicular fluid,[22,24] urine,[23] and dried blood spots[24,25] can be used as noninvasive alternatives to the collection of blood for the detection of HIV-specific antibodies. Cerebrospinal fluid

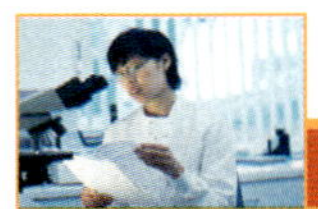

Table 2–3.

Common Specimens and Laboratory Tests for Diagnosis of Viral Infections of Skin and Mucous Membranes

General Disease Category	Possible Virus	Preferred Methods for Diagnosis: Culture	Antigen Detection	NAAT	Cytology/ Histology	EM	Serology	Suggested Specimens
Skin and mucous membranes	HSV	X	X	X				Lesion swab
	VZV	X	X	X				Lesion swab
	EBV			X			X	Blood
	CMV	X	X	X			X	Blood for serology, PCR, antigen; urine, respiratory for culture, PCR
	HHV-6			X			X	Blood
	HHV-7			X			X	Blood
	HHV-8			X			X	Blood for serology and PCR; tissue for PCR
	Parvovirus B19						X	Blood
	Papillomaviruses			X	X			Lesion scrapings, tissue
	Poxviruses				X	X		Lesion scrapings, tissue
	Enterovirus	X		X				Lesion swab, respiratory, stool, urine, blood, CSF
	Measles virus	X	X				X	Respiratory, eye swab for culture and antigen; urine for culture; blood for serology
	Rubella virus	X					X	Respiratory, urine, blood for culture; blood for serology
	HIV	X*		X			X	Blood
	Dengue virus			X			X	Blood
	West Nile Virus			X			X	Blood

**HIV culture requires specialized facilities and expertise and is not available in most diagnostic virology laboratories.*

(CSF) may be collected and paired with a serum specimen from the same date to be tested for viral-specific antibody in patients with viral neurological diseases.[26] However, the yield of such testing is low for most viruses and limited by delays in intrathecal production of antibody, and many hospital laboratories no longer perform antibody testing on CSF samples. Testing for viral-specific antibodies in CSF may be beneficial for certain viruses, including the arboviruses, measles, mumps, and rabies viruses, herpes B virus, and lymphocytic choriomeningitis virus (LCMV).

Respiratory specimens

Traditionally, nasopharyngeal aspirates or nasopharyngeal washes have been the preferred specimens for the detection of respiratory viruses, and are felt to be superior to swabs for the adequate collection of respiratory epithelial cells. Aspirates are particularly useful for infants and young children who produce copious amounts of mucus during their viral respiratory illness, but are not as practical in older children and adults with less respiratory secretions to aspirate. In the latter populations, swabs are far more convenient for medical personnel to use and patients are more willing to allow collection of this specimen type. For optimum recovery of viruses from the respiratory tract when using swabs, collection of combined throat and nasopharyngeal swabs is recommended since recovery of certain viruses can vary depending on the amount of virus present in either the throat or nose. For instance, nasopharyngeal swabs are better than throat swabs for the recovery of seasonal human influenza virus strains, while throat swabs are preferred in humans with respiratory disease caused by avian H5N1 influenza virus since the throat contains higher titers of this virus. Tracheal or transtracheal aspirates or bronchoalveolar lavage specimens are superior for the indication of lower respiratory tract infections. Sputum has been used for the detection of respiratory viruses, but normally contains less than the optimum amount of viruses required for testing and is not

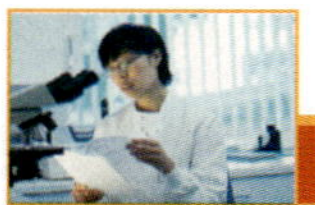

Table 2–4.

Common Specimens and Laboratory Tests for Diagnosis of Viral Encephalitis and Meningitis

General Disease Category	Possible Virus	Preferred Methods for Diagnosis: Culture	Antigen Detection	NAAT	Cytology/ Histology	EM	Serology	Suggested Specimens
Encephalitis/ meningitis	HSV			X				CSF
	CMV			X				CSF (quantifying level of CMV in CSF can be useful)
	EBV			X			X	Blood for serology; CSF for PCR
	VZV			X				CSF
	HHV-6			X				Blood, CSF
	Herpes B virus*	X		X			X	Lesions at bite site, CSF for culture and PCR; blood, CSF for serology
	Enterovirus	X		X				CSF, urine, blood, respira tory, stool for PCR (preferred) or culture (acceptable)
	Arboviruses*			X			X	Blood, CSF for PCR and serology
	Rabies*	X	X	X			X	Neck biopsy for antigen; saliva for culture; saliva, neck biopsy for PCR; blood, CSF for serology
	Measles virus						X	Blood, CSF for IgG
	Mumps virus	X		X			X	CSF, respiratory, urine for culture or PCR; blood, CSF for IgM
	Rubella virus	X						CSF
	Influenza virus	X		X				CSF
	Parainfluenza virus	X		X				CSF
	Adenovirus	X		X				CSF
	HIV			X				CSF
	JC virus			X				CSF
	LCMV						X	Blood

Testing is primarily done in State/Reference Laboratories or the Centers for Disease Control and Prevention (CDC).

recommended. Regardless of the respiratory specimen chosen for collection, children generally shed respiratory viruses at higher titers for longer periods than adults. Excess dilution of respiratory specimens during collection may decrease test performance in the laboratory and should be avoided.

Nasopharyngeal aspirate Obtain a mucus trap, a sterile French gauge suction catheter, and a vacuum aspiration pump. The length and diameter of the catheter and suction pressure to be used will vary with the age of the patient and should be appropriate for an infant, child, or adult. Attach the catheter to the trap and then connect the trap to the vacuum aspiration pump. Insert the catheter into the nose, directed posteriorly and toward the opening of the external ear. The depth of the catheter insertion necessary to reach the posterior pharynx is equivalent to the distance between the anterior nares and external opening of the ear. Apply vacuum aspiration. Using a rotating movement, collect as much of the secretions as possible and then slowly withdraw the catheter. The catheter should remain in the nasopharynx for no longer than 10 seconds. Hold the trap upright to prevent the secretions from going into the pump. Rinse the catheter (if necessary) with approximately 2 mL of viral transport

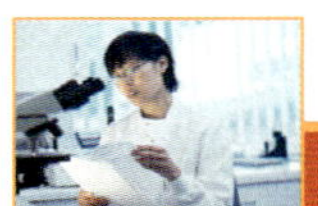

Table 2–5.

Common Specimens and Laboratory Tests for Diagnosis of Viral Congenital and Perinatal Diseases

General Disease Category	Possible Virus	Preferred Methods for Diagnosis: Culture	Antigen Detection	NAAT	Cytology/ Histology	EM	Serology	Suggested Specimens
Congenital/ perinatal	CMV	X		X			X	*In utero*: Amniotic fluid for PCR *Postpartum*: Urine for PCR or culture; serum for IgM
	Rubella virus	X		X			X	*In utero*: Amniotic fluid for PCR *Postpartum*: Throat swab, urine, blood, CSF for PCR or culture; serum for IgM
	HSV	X	X	X				*Postpartum*: Lesions for antigen, culture or PCR; respiratory, ocular, skin, urine, blood, rectal swab, CSF for PCR or culture
	Enterovirus	X		X				*In utero*: Amniotic fluid for PCR *Postpartum*: CSF, blood, urine, stool, respiratory for PCR or culture
	VZV	X	X	X				*In utero*: Amniotic fluid for PCR *Postpartum*: Lesions, throat swab, blood for culture or PCR; lesions for antigen
	Parvovirus B19			X			X	*In utero*: Amniotic fluid for PCR *Postpartum*: Blood for IgM and PCR
	HIV	X*		X			X	*Postpartum*: Blood on mom for serology; blood on baby for PCR and/or culture
	HBV						X	*Postpartum*: Blood
	HCV			X			X	*Postpartum*: Blood

**HIV culture requires specialized facilities and expertise and is not available in most diagnostic virology laboratories.*

medium if the secretions do not move freely through the tubing into the trap; disconnect the suction catheter and vacuum pump and close off the trap for transport to the laboratory.

Nasal wash: Syringe method Obtain a 3–5-cc syringe and fill the syringe with sterile saline. Attach an appropriately sized French gauge catheter to the syringe, and, as above, insert the tubing into the nose to reach the posterior nasopharynx. Quickly instill the saline into the nasopharynx and immediately withdraw the fluid back into the syringe to recover the specimen material. Inject the aspirated specimen from the syringe into a suitable dry, sterile container or one containing a specified volume of viral transport medium.

Nasal wash: Bulb method Suction 3–5 mL of saline into a clean sterile 1–2 oz. tapered rubber bulb. Insert the bulb into one nostril until the nostril is occluded. Instill the saline into the nostril with one squeeze of the

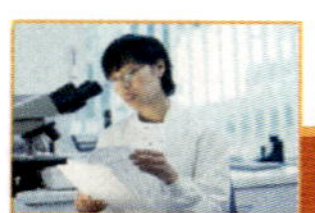

Table 2–6.

Common Specimens and Laboratory Tests for Diagnosis of Viral Ocular Disease

General Disease Category	Possible Virus	Preferred Methods for Diagnosis: Culture	Antigen Detection	NAAT	Cytology/ Histology	EM	Serology	Suggested Specimens
Ocular	Adenovirus	X	X	X				Conjunctival swab; collection of other specimens depends on associated systemic features
	Enterovirus	X		X				
	Measles	X	X					
	HSV	X	X	X				Conjunctival/corneal swabs, tear sample, lesion swab/scraping, aqueous humor, vitreous humor, corneal biopsy, retinal biopsy
	VZV	X	X	X				
	CMV	X		X				Aqueous humor, vitreous humor, subretinal fluid, retinal biopsy
	EBV						X	Blood
	Papillomavirus			X	X			Lesion scrapings, tissue biopsy
	Poxvirus	X			X	X		

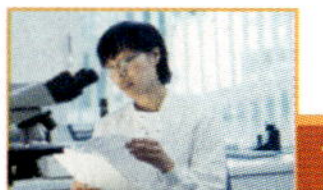

Table 2–7.

Common Specimens and Laboratory Tests for Diagnosis of Viral Gastrointestinal Disease

General Disease Category	Possible Virus	Preferred Methods for Diagnosis: Culture	Antigen Detection	NAAT	Cytology/ Histology	EM	Serology	Suggested Specimens
Gastroenteritis	Rotavirus		X*	X		X		Stool preferred, rectal swabs acceptable
	Adenovirus types 40/41		X*	X		X		
	Norovirus		X*	X		X		
	Sapovirus			X		X		
	Astrovirus		X	X		X		
Colitis	CMV	X	X	X	X			Lesion biopsy for culture, PCR, antigen, histology; stool for culture or PCR; blood for antigenemia, PCR
Proctitis	HSV	X	X	X				Lesion swab for antigen, culture, or PCR; rectal swab for culture or PCR
	Papillomavirus			X	X			Lesion biopsy

**Conventional EIAs are commercially available for these viruses.*

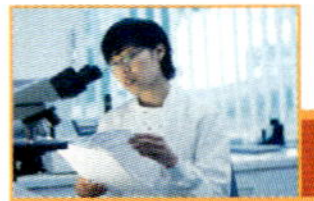

Table 2–8.

Common Specimens and Laboratory Tests for Diagnosis of Viral Diseases in Immunocompromised Hosts

General Disease Category	Possible Virus	Preferred Methods for Diagnosis: Culture	Antigen Detection	NAAT	Cytology/ Histology	EM	Serology	Suggested Specimens
Diseases in immunocompro mised hosts	CMV		X	X	X			*Transplant recipients and AIDS patients*: Blood for quantitative monitoring of antigen or nucleic acid *Pneumonia, colitis*: Tissue for histology/antigen testing, PCR, or culture *CNS disease*: CSF for PCR
	EBV			X	X			*Primary CNS lymphoma*: CSF for PCR *PTLD*: Posttransplant monitoring of blood by quantitative PCR; tissue for PCR and histology
	HSV	X	X	X				*Meningoencephalitis*: CSF for PCR *Lesions*: Swab of lesions for culture, antigen, or PCR
	VZV	X	X	X				*Encephalitis, myelitis*: CSF for PCR *Lesions*: Swab of lesions for culture, antigen, or PCR
	HHV-6			X				*Transplant recipients*: Posttransplant monitoring of blood by quantitative PCR; CSF, bone marrow, lung tissue for PCR
	JC virus			X				*PML in AIDS*: CSF
	BK virus			X				*Hemorrhagic cystitis, nephropathy, ureteral stenosis in transplant recipients*: Blood, urine for quantitative PCR monitoring
	Adenovirus	X		X				*Disseminated disease in transplant or cancer patients*: Blood for PCR monitoring; conjunctival swab, stool, respiratory, urine for PCR and/or culture
	Parvovirus B19			X				*Aplastic crisis, chronic anemia*: Blood

CNS, central nervous system; PTLD, posttransplant lymphoproliferative disease.

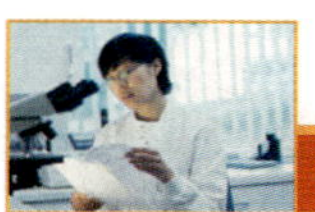

Table 2–9.

Common Specimens and Laboratory Tests for Diagnosis of Viral Hepatitis

General Disease Category	Possible Virus	Preferred Methods for Diagnosis: Culture	Antigen Detection	NAAT	Cytology/ Histology	EM	Serology	Suggested Specimens
Hepatitis	Hepatitis A virus						X	Blood
	Hepatitis B virus			X			X	Blood; can test for HBV DNA in certain cases where antigen negative mutants are likely; can quantify HBV DNA before therapy and for monitoring response
	Hepatitis C virus			X			X	Blood; can test for HCV RNA to detect seronegative infection and to confirm presence of virus in patients that are seropositive; can quantify HCV RNA before therapy and for monitoring response
	Hepatitis D virus						X	Blood
	Hepatitis E virus						X	Blood
	Adenovirus	X	X	X				Liver tissue, blood
	CMV	X	X	X				Liver tissue, blood
	HSV	X	X	X				Liver tissue, blood
	VZV	X	X	X				Liver tissue, blood
	EBV			X			X	Blood
	Enterovirus	X		X				Blood, urine, stool, respiratory, liver tissue
	HIV	X*		X			X	Blood

**HIV culture requires specialized facilities and expertise and is not available in most diagnostic virology laboratories.*

bulb and immediately release the bulb to recover the nasal specimen. Empty the bulb into a suitable dry, sterile container or one containing a specified volume of viral transport medium.

Nasopharyngeal or oropharyngeal swabs (See below for swab specimens.)

Sterile body fluids

Urine, CSF, amniotic, pleural and pericardial fluids, and other sterile body fluid specimens should be submitted to the laboratory in sterile, leak proof containers. Do not dilute these specimens in viral transport medium. All body fluid specimens must be of sufficient quantity, and, as a general rule, should equal a minimum of 0.5 mL per test requested. Shedding of some viruses in urine may be intermittent (e.g., CMV) and collecting two to three urine specimens over time may enhance recovery. Sampling of amniotic fluid should be done after 21–23 weeks of fetal gestation for best testing sensitivity when using either serological or direct detection methods for prenatal diagnosis.

Stool

Stool is the specimen of choice for the detection of enteric viruses. Approximately 2–4 mL of liquid stool or

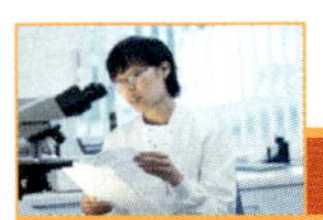

Table 2–10.

Common Specimens and Laboratory Tests for Diagnosis of Viral Myocarditis and Pericarditis

General Disease Category	Possible Virus	Preferred Methods for Diagnosis: Culture	Antigen Detection	NAAT	Cytology/ Histology	EM	Serology	Suggested Specimens
Myocarditis/ pericartitis	Enterovirus	X		X				Biopsy from myocardium, endocardium, or pericardium, pericardial fluid for PCR and/or culture; serum for serology; other sites (blood, urine, stool, respiratory) for culture, antigen, PCR for certain viruses
	CMV	X	X	X				
	EBV			X			X	
	HSV	X		X				
	Adenovirus	X		X				
	Parvovirus B19			X			X	
	Influenza virus types A and B	X		X				
	Paramyxoviruses (measles virus, mumps virus, parainfluenza virus, RSV)	X		X				
	HIV	X*		X			X	

*HIV culture requires specialized facilities and expertise and is not available in most diagnostic virology laboratories.

2–4 g of formed stool should be placed in leak proof containers that do not contain media, preservatives, serum, or detergent, as any of these additives may interfere with specific antigen tests for rotavirus and adenovirus types 40 and 41.

Swab specimens

Swabs are used for collecting specimens from dermal, rectal, respiratory, and ocular sites. Plastic- or metal-shafted swabs with rayon, Dacron, cotton, or polyester tips should be used; calcium alginate or wooden-shafted swabs are inhibitory to some viruses and are not acceptable. To facilitate binding of cellular material to the swab, the swab can be premoistened with sterile saline. The excess liquid should be adequately expressed from the swab before attempting to collect the specimen. All swab specimens should be placed in viral transport medium immediately after collection. Recently, a new type of swab made with flocked nylon has been developed by Copan Diagnostics (Corona, CA). Use of this swab has resulted in enhanced specimen recovery and improved test performance by allowing for increased absorption of cells to the swab during collection and improved release of the cells from the swab during processing and testing in the laboratory.[27,28]

Eye (conjunctivae) Conjunctival swabs should be taken by stroking the lower conjunctival sac of the eye five to six times with a sterile swab.

Dermal lesions Cells and fluid from fresh vesicles are superior to specimens prepared from other lesion types (e.g., vesicles > pustules > ulcers > crusts) for direct antigen detection, polymerase chain reaction (PCR), and viral culture. Unroof the vesicle with a sterile needle or scalpel blade and use a sterile swab to vigorously swab the margins and base of the lesion to obtain infected epithelial cells. For ulcers, use a swab to remove pus without disrupting the lesion base and then use a fresh sterile swab to firmly swab the lesion as described above. Crusted lesions should have the crust removed and discarded before collection of cells from the lesion base and margins. The yield of HSV or VZV from a crusted lesion is low for rapid antigen and culture-based tests and moderate for PCR, so the utility of collecting specimens from this type of lesions should be considered.

Nasopharyngeal Insert a swab into the posterior nasopharynx. Press the swab tip on the mucosal surface of the midinferior portion of the inferior turbinate and rub or rotate the swab tip several times across the mucosal surface to loosen and collect respiratory epithelial cells.

Oropharyngeal Gently open the mouth or ask the patient (if age appropriate) to open the mouth widely and phonate an "ah" to lift the uvula and reduce the gag

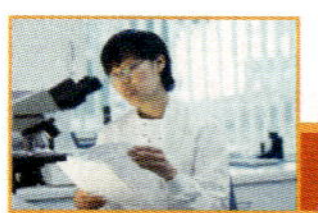

Table 2–11.

Common Specimens and Laboratory Tests for Diagnosis of Miscellaneous Diseases Caused by Viruses

General Disease Category	Possible Virus	Preferred Methods for Diagnosis: Culture	Antigen Detection	NAAT	Cytology/ Histology	EM	Serology	Suggested Specimens
Parotitis	Mumps virus	X	X	X			X	Blood for serology; buccal/throat swabs, urine for culture, PCR; buccal/throat swabs for antigen
Infectious mono-nucleosis	EBV						X	Blood for heterophile antibody in children >4 yrs of age; comprehensive antibody panel in younger children and persons with heterophile-negative IM
	CMV	X	X	X			X	Blood for serology; blood, urine, respiratory for PCR, culture, or antigen
	HIV	X*		X			X	Blood for serology, RNA detection, and/or culture
	Rubella virus	X		X			X	Throat swab, urine, blood for culture or PCR; serum for IgM
Neonatal sepsis	Enterovirus	X		X				Blood, urine, CSF, stool, respiratory
	HSV	X		X				Lesions for antigen, culture or PCR; respiratory, ocular, urine, blood, stool, CSF for PCR or culture
Urinary tract	BK virus			X	X			Urine, blood, tissue
	Adenovirus	X		X				Urine, blood
Genital tract	HSV	X	X	X				Lesion swab
	Papilloma viruses			X	X			Lesion scrapings, tissue biopsy
	Poxvirus				X	X		Lesion scrapings, tissue biopsy

**HIV culture requires specialized facilities and expertise and is not available in most diagnostic virology laboratories.*

reflex. Gently depress the tongue with a tongue blade and guide a swab into the posterior oropharynx. Use a gentle but firm back-and-forth sweeping motion to swab thoroughly behind the uvula and between the tonsillar pillars while avoiding the buccal mucosa, tonsils, tongue, and palate. Collected nasopharyngeal and oropharyngeal swabs should be combined and placed into a single tube of viral transport medium. Doing so usually improves on the number of epithelial cells available for testing and enhances the recovery of viruses from these sources.

Rectal Rectal swabs are normally inferior to stool specimens for the detection of enteric viruses and their collection is discouraged. If it is necessary to collect a rectal swab, a sufficient quantity of fecal material (e.g., at least a pea-sized amount) should be obtained. If fecal material is not clearly visible on the swab, the specimen is most likely inadequate. A swab of the rectal mucosa can be performed if viral proctitis is suspected.

Tissues

Freshly collected tissue specimens should be immediately placed in viral transport medium to prevent drying.

All specimens submitted to the laboratory for diagnostic testing should be labeled with the patient's full name, the medical record number or other unique identifier, date and time of collection, and signature of the collector. Each specimen should be accompanied by a requisition slip containing the same information as on the specimen container as well as the patient's location within the hospital, physician's name, and contact information, specimen site, test(s) requested, virus(es) suspected, and any other relevant clinical data (e.g., clinical diagnosis, current therapy, or factors affecting immune status such as transplantation or malignancy). Specimens must be appropriate for the test(s) requested and/or the clinical situation described. Meaningful communication between health care providers and laboratorians is especially important to determine the appropriateness of specimens for viral diagnosis.

LABORATORY METHODS

See Tables 2–2 to 2–11 for selecting the most appropriate laboratory tests depending on the clinical situation and suspected virus or viruses.

Cell Culture Systems

The isolation and identification of viruses in cell culture remains an important and integral component of most clinical virology laboratories[29–30], and advances in technology over the years have improved the speed and usefulness of cell culture systems for the detection of certain viruses.

Conventional tube cultures

Conventional tube culture systems have long been the cornerstone of diagnostic virology and are the traditional counterpart to growing bacteria in the microbiology laboratory. Unlike bacteria that grow in nutrient broth or on solid agar media, viruses are obligate intracellular parasites and, therefore, require living cells to replicate. Clinical specimens are normally inoculated onto various tissue culture cell lines of animal and human origin grown in 16 × 125-mm glass or plastic tubes and incubated under conditions suitable for isolation of the largest number of viruses. The cultures are examined over a period of time using a standard light microscope, and the presence of viral growth is usually recognized by the development of a virus-induced cytopathic effect (CPE) within infected cells. Each virus that may grow in culture has its characteristic CPE; the rate at which CPE progresses, the type of CPE observed, and the cell line in which the virus replicates are factors in determining the type of virus present. Some viruses, most notably influenza and parainfluenza viruses, often do not produce CPE as primary isolates and their growth in culture is detected by alternative techniques such as measuring hemagglutinin activity and using monoclonal antibodies to visualize specific viral proteins in an immunofluorescence assay. Conventional tube cultures offer the distinct advantage of being able to isolate a wide range of viruses from a given clinical specimen and can detect unknown or unsuspected viral agents. Also, the growth of a virus in a culture is highly specific depending on which cell lines are selected and how the culture system is designed, and low titers of virus present in a specimen can be amplified to sufficient levels for detection and further characterization. Conversely, conventional tube cultures are slow, often taking many days to weeks to obtain a final result and have a limited impact on clinical decision making. They also are time-consuming, labor-intensive, require specialized facilities and expertise, and have a varied sensitivity as many medically relevant viruses are very difficult to grow or cannot be grown at all. Alternatives to conventional tube cultures have been developed and are discussed below. These include shell vial/multiwell plate cultures and the use of genetically engineered and mixed-cell populations.

Shell vial/multiwell plate cultures

Shell vial or multiwell plate cultures were originally designed to decrease the time required for detection of viruses in culture, especially slow-growing viruses like CMV and VZV. With this method, low-speed centrifugation is used to inoculate clinical specimens onto the surface of cell monolayers grown on 12-mm round coverslips in the bottom of 1-dram (3.7 mL) vials or flat-bottomed 24- or 48-well plates to facilitate viral infection of the cells. Following incubation, viral growth is detected prior to the development of CPE using immunofluorescence staining with monoclonal antibodies directed against specific viral proteins. This method has been applied to the rapid detection of CMV, HSV, VZV, enteroviruses, measles and rubella viruses, and respiratory viruses such as respiratory syncytial virus (RSV), influenza virus types A and B, parainfluenza virus types 1, 2, 3, and 4, adenovirus, and more recently, human metapneumovirus.[31] The major advantage of this culture system over conventional tube cultures is that results are available in a much shorter time frame (most in 24–48 hours, but may take up to 5 days for some respiratory viruses). Disadvantages include that only viruses that are being sought can be identified and only one or a few viruses can be detected at a time. Also, this type of culture is normally less sensitive than conventional tube culture systems, and similar to conventional cultures, involves considerable time, labor, and expertise to perform.

Genetically engineered cells

Transgenic cells that have been genetically modified to promote the stable expression of a process or processes required by the virus for entry into or replication within cells have been developed and are being used to facilitate virus detection in culture.[32] An enzyme-linked virus-inducible culture system (ELVIS) has been commercially developed by Diagnostic Hybrids (Athens, OH) for the rapid detection of HSV-1 and HSV-2.[33,34] The system uses genetically engineered baby hamster kidney cells containing the lac Z gene of *Escherichia coli* driven by the ICP6 promoter from the UL39 gene of HSV-1. Clinical specimens are inoculated by centrifugation onto cell monolayers in 24-well plates and incubated for 16–24 hours. Cells infected only with HSV express β-galactosidase and are identified by their blue color following histochemical staining for β-galactosidase activity and examination by light microscopy. The assay is rapid and relatively simple to perform and requires less labor and expertise than the more conventional centrifugation-assisted cultures described above. It has the important advantage of easily detecting a color change that is readily induced following infection with either HSV type. To enhance the recovery of enteroviruses in culture, buffalo green monkey kidney (BGMK) cells have been transfected with the gene for human decay-accelerating factor (hDAF), a receptor that certain enterovirus types interact with during entry into a cell.[35] The developed genetically engineered cell line, BGMK-hDAF, has an expanded host range and increased sensitivity for the detection of various enteroviruses and has been commercialized for use in a mixed-cell culture system like the one described below. A genetically engineered human embryonic kidney 293T cell line with a reporter gene inducible by influenza A virus has also been developed for the rapid detection of multiple strains of influenza A.[36] The major limitations of these transgenic cell lines are that they will detect only the virus for which they were designed and they are available for only a small number of viruses, thereby limiting their diagnostic use.

Mixed-cell populations

A more recent development in cell culture involves the mixing of two cell lines together to form a single monolayer in shell vials or multiwell plates. As above, clinical specimens are inoculated by centrifugation onto the monolayers and viruses that can grow in either or both of the mixed cell lines and are detected by immunofluorescence using viral-specific monoclonal antibodies conjugated with different fluorochromes. The major advantage of using mixed cell populations is that multiple viruses can be detected in a single vial or well-thereby decreasing the need to use multiple single tubes as is done with conventional tube cultures. The mixed-cell culture system also takes advantage of the speed involved in virus detection when using the techniques of centrifugation-assisted inoculation and identification of viruses prior to the development of CPE. Cocultivated cell lines of this type are now commercially available for the detection of HSV and VZV,[37] enteroviruses,[35] and respiratory viruses, which include RSV, influenza virus types A and B, parainfluenza virus types 1, 2, and 3, and adenovirus.[38–40]

In general, the use and relative importance of cell culture systems for viral isolation is declining with the continued development of rapid and accurate immunologic and molecular tests. However, viral isolation is still one of the most practical and convenient methods for many clinical virology laboratories that are attempting to diagnose viral diseases. Also, specific needs for culture-based systems will most likely always remain. For example, laboratory confirmation of antiviral drug resistance may be important in certain clinical situations involving viruses such as CMV, HSV, VZV, HIV, and influenza A and B viruses. To this end, culture-based, phenotypic antiviral susceptibility assays have been developed (see Ref. 41 for a review). Virus replication within cultured cells is measured in the presence or absence of an antiviral drug and the susceptibility of the virus is expressed as the drug concentration required to inhibit viral replication by 50% relative to infected cell cultures containing no drug. The disadvantages of these tests are that they are relatively costly and labor-involved, and usually have turnaround times of 2–6 weeks depending on the virus examined and the assay used. They are also only available in a limited number of reference laboratories. The major advantage is that culture-based, phenotypic assays are a direct measure of the action of an antiviral drug on a live, growing virus.

Direct Detection Tests

Antigen detection assays

Immunologic tests for direct detection of viral antigens in clinical material are now commercially available for many viruses and all or some of the assays are routinely used in most clinical laboratories. The tests are rapid, inexpensive, relatively simple to perform, and, unlike culture-based systems, do not require viable virus for detection. The sensitivity and specificity of these tests are variable and are highly dependent on the virus to be detected, the testing format, and the quality of the specimen. In general, antigen detection assays are usually not as accurate as viral culture or molecular amplification techniques. Also, similar to the centrifugation-assisted cultures described above, direct antigen detection assays can only identify the specific viruses for which the test was designed.

Immunofluorescence Immunofluorescence is used extensively for the direct visualization of antigens of a number of viruses,[42–48] including CMV, EBV, HSV, VZV, RSV, influenza virus types A and B, parainfluenza virus types 1, 2, 3, and 4, adenovirus, metapneumovirus, and measles, mumps, rubella, and rabies viruses. Monoclonal antibodies are now available for these and many other less common viruses, and manufacturers now provide kits that contain all of the necessary reagents for staining. When using immunofluorescence, cells from submitted clinical specimens are fixed to the surface of glass slides and viral antigens within infected cells are detected using virus-specific primary antibodies. A direct or indirect immunofluorescence assay can be used to detect the antigen–antibody complexes. In the direct method, the virus-specific antibody is directly conjugated with a fluorochrome, while in the indirect method, the primary antibody is allowed to react with viral antigen and the specific complexes are detected using an antispecies-specific antibody conjugated with a fluorochrome. The choice of the method to be used depends on the availability and quality of conjugated and unconjugated antibodies and the particular viral antigen to be detected. The assays normally take 1–3 hours to complete and microscopic examination of the slides requires considerable expertise for correct reading and interpretation of the results. By using immunofluorescence, the quality of specimens can be assessed and specimens can be screened for multiple viruses of interest depending on the number of available antibodies. Immunofluorescence is more likely to be performed in larger academic medical centers and public health laboratories rather than in community hospitals because of the need for an immunofluorescence microscope and the requirement for a higher level of expertise to perform these assays. Also, the method is not available for viral infections caused by enteroviruses, rhinoviruses, and viral agents of gastroenteritis because of the limited availability of appropriate reagents. An immunofluorescence test for CMV, called the antigenemia assay, is widely used for the detection and quantification of CMV from blood leukocytes.[49,50] The assay is used for the routine monitoring of patients at high risk for severe CMV disease, including recipients of solid-organ and bone marrow transplants and individuals infected with HIV. The assay can be used to predict and differentiate CMV disease from asymptomatic infection, monitor the efficacy of antiviral therapy and predict drug resistance, and to make decisions regarding the initiation of preemptive therapy.

Solid-phase immunoassays Solid-phase immunoassays also can be used for the detection of viral antigens from clinical specimens.[30,48,51] A number of commercial kits are available and include conventional enzyme-linked immunoassays (EIAs) and the more rapid and less sophisticated immunoassays. In conventional EIAs, specific viral antigens, if present in a clinical specimen, will bind to monoclonal antibodies coated onto the surface of a solid phase (e.g., a well of a microtiter plate or a polystyrene bead). Following a wash step, an enzyme-labeled antiviral monoclonal antibody is added. The antibody–antigen–antibody complex is then detected by the addition of a colorless substrate, which becomes colored in the presence of the enzyme. The assays usually take 1–2 hours to complete and the results are read in a spectrophotometer. This type of assay is normally performed in the laboratory and is primarily used for the detection of viral antigens of HBV, rotavirus, adenoviruses, including types 40 and 41, and norovirus.[52,53]

The more recently developed rapid immunoassays involve self-contained, disposable devices and only a single step or a few simple steps. There are several basic formats, including membrane flow-through devices, lateral-flow immunochromatographic strips, and optical immunoassays. An endogenous enzyme assay also has been commercialized for the direct detection of neuraminidase activity of influenza viruses from clinical specimens. The rapid assays require no specialized equipment and require little technical expertise and can be completed in 15–30 minutes. Kits are designed to be used either in the laboratory or at the site where the specimen was collected (e.g., physician's offices, ambulatory clinics, and emergency departments). Rapid assays are available for RSV, influenza virus types A and B, and rotavirus. Although simple and relatively inexpensive to perform, rapid antigen tests are the least accurate of all direct detection tests offered in a diagnostic virology laboratory. A number of false-negative and false-positive results can be generated from these tests depending on how, when, and where the tests are used. This is particularly true for rapid antigen tests for influenza virus, which may vary in sensitivity and specificity depending on the age of the patient, specimen type and adequacy, virus subtype, prevalence of the virus in the community, and the particular test that is selected for testing.[51]

Molecular methods

There has been enormous enthusiasm for the medical and commercial potential of molecular technologies, and in the past two decades, there has been an explosion of technological innovations in molecular diagnostics. The development of rapid and sensitive molecular amplification methods has resulted in one of the most dynamic and dramatic revolutions in clinical laboratory medicine, particularly in the diagnosis of viral diseases. A large and growing number of viruses can now be detected using such methods as PCR, nucleic acid sequence-based amplification, branched chain signal amplification, transcription-mediated amplification, hybrid capture signal amplification, and strand displacement amplification. The sensitivity and specificity of these assays exceed that of more conventional methods in the diagnostic virology laboratory and the clinical applications of these techniques seem endless. As such, the emphasis of the clinical virology laboratory is changing considerably.

The 1990s saw a new wave of change that is still going on today with the advent of real-time quantitative PCR,[54–58] advancements in microfluidics and microelectronics, and the development of sequencing systems, microarrays, biochips, and biosensors.[59–62] Molecular amplification methods are now rapidly displacing the more traditional culture- and antigen-based procedures that have been used for decades and are becoming the new "gold standard" for detecting most viruses of medical importance. These methods can detect viruses for which existing tests are considerably less accurate or for which no tests exist.[63] The technologies are being used successfully to detect unculturable, fastidious, or slow-growing viruses and for detecting viruses that are new or otherwise too dangerous to grow. Molecular amplification methods are especially well suited for detecting viruses present in small specimen volumes or that are in low numbers or nonviable within clinical specimens. Multiplex procedures have been developed and commercialized for the simultaneous detection of multiple viruses from a single specimen.[64–70] Quantitative molecular amplification assays have become invaluable tools to assess disease progression and prognosis, monitor therapy, predict treatment failure and the emergence of drug resistance, and to facilitate our understanding of the transmission and pathogenesis of certain viruses in chronically infected and immunocompromised hosts. Commercial and user-developed assays are now available for the accurate quantification of viral nucleic acids of HIV-1, CMV, EBV, human herpes virus-6 (HHV-6), HHV-7, HHV-8, BK virus (BKV), HBV, and HCV.[71–76] Lastly, molecular genotyping assays that involve using nucleic acid amplification of specific viral genes and direct sequencing of the amplified products have been developed.[74,77] These methods are primarily being used to identify mutations that confer resistance to antiviral drugs used for the treatment of HIV-1 and CMV and for recognition of genetic variants of HBV and HCV that may be refractile to antiviral drugs. Use of genotypic assays also can provide valuable information about the evolution and phylogenetic relationships among closely related viruses and the epidemiological and pathogenic behavior of viruses.

The continued development of molecular amplification procedures has led to an explosive increase in the availability of high-quality commercial reagents. Nucleic acid amplification methods are now an integral and necessary component of many diagnostic virology laboratories, and continuous improvements, automation, and simplification of the technology have made these procedures easier to use and more accessible to laboratories with even limited experience. More recent advances have resulted in new generations of rapid molecular amplification assays for detection, quantification, and typing of viruses. This has greatly increased our ability to accurately detect and monitor viral infections. With the continued arrival of more cost-effective and automated nucleic acid isolation and amplification systems, the future holds great promise for the widespread use of such methods in every clinical virology laboratory. Ultimately, the acceptance of these tests will depend on their clinical performance, convenience, and relative expense. The technology will continue to advance and have even a greater impact on the care and management of ill patients with viral infections. However, enthusiasm for the use of molecular-based technologies must be tempered by recognition of the need for performing rigorous quality control in the laboratory and providing appropriate interpretation of results. The significance of the results must be evaluated with respect to the virus identified, the specimen site, and the clinical situation. Also, there must be a greater availability of assays licensed by the U.S. Food and Drug Administration (FDA) as there are only a few FDA-cleared commercial molecular test kits in the market for laboratories to use. As such, many laboratories have been forced to develop their own molecular assays, thereby limiting much of the molecular testing to laboratories at academic institutions or large reference laboratories with the expertise, personnel, and resources to enable these technologies.

Cytology/histology

Direct cytological or histological examinations of stained clinical material are some of the fastest and oldest methods of detecting viruses. While relatively simple and cost-effective, the tests are insensitive compared with direct antigen or nucleic acid detection methods. The specificity can also be low; Tzanck smears, for example, are limited by their inability to distinguish HSV from VZV infections. Cytologic examination of exfoliated cells has been applied to specific viruses such as CMV, HSV, VZV, adenovirus, the polyomaviruses BK and JC, measles virus, rabies virus, and human papillomaviruses (HPV). Histological examination of impression smears, frozen sections, or formaldehyde-fixed and paraffin-embedded tissue has been used for various viruses, including CMV, EBV, HSV, BKV, HBV, HPV, parvovirus B19, and adenovirus, and may provide useful information regarding tissue inflammation and damage as the result of viral infection. The sensitivity of histological staining can be increased somewhat by using immunohistochemical or in situ hybridization techniques. Overall, these tests are used sparingly in most laboratories.

Electron microscopy

Electron microscopy can be a useful tool for the rapid identification of viral particles based on characteristic size and morphology.[78,79] It offers the main advantage of speed when doing negative staining of liquid samples and can detect fastidious or uncultivable viruses. The method has been mostly applied to the examination of stools for viral agents of gastroenteritis and has been used successfully as an adjunct to other methods for detecting unidentified viruses suspected of causing disease. The major limitations include the high cost of the instrument, the requirement for specialized facilities and expertise, and moderate to low sensitivity and specificity. This procedure has largely been replaced by alternative methods for viral diagnosis and is seldom available in diagnostic laboratories in the United States.

Serology

A number of sensitive and specific tests are available for the detection of antibodies to a variety of viruses.[80] Enzyme immunoassays, immunofluorescence, or passive latex agglutination tests are commonly used by most laboratories to screen for the presence of viral-specific antibodies in a clinical specimen. Immunoblot techniques are available for HIV-1 and -2, HCV, and human T-cell leukemia virus-I and -II (HTLV-I and -II), and are primarily used as confirmatory or supplemental tests to verify the results of positive screening tests. Serological testing can be useful for the diagnosis of recent or chronic viral infections and to determine the immune status of an individual or group. Antibody detection remains at the forefront of diagnosis of infections with HIV-1 and -2[81] and the hepatitis viruses A–E,[82] as well as EBV, the arboviruses, measles, mumps and rubella viruses, parvovirus B19, and HTLV-I and -II. Defining an individual's immunity to a given virus can be beneficial for (1) prenatal and pretransplanatation screening, (2) testing blood and blood products for donation, (3) postexposure monitoring, (4) preemployment screening in a patient care setting, and (5) verifying an immune response following administration of vaccines. Detection of virus-specific IgM in a single serum sample can be diagnostic of primary viral infection and has been used successfully for many viruses. Viruses for which IgM testing can be useful include CMV, EBV, VZV, HHV-6 and -7, measles, mumps and rubella viruses, hepatitis A virus (HAV), HBV, parvovirus B19, and arthropod- and rodent-borne viruses. Seroconversion from a negative to a positive IgG antibody response between acute and convalescent sera collected 2–3 weeks apart can also be used to diagnose a primary infection, but such testing is no longer routinely performed in most hospital diagnostic laboratories since it is retrospective and has a limited impact on the care and management of patients. Detection of virus-specific IgG in a single serum specimen indicates exposure to a virus at some time in the past or a response to vaccination, while finding no detectable antibodies may exclude viral infection. Results of serological tests must be interpreted with caution, as measurements and interpretations of antibody responses to viral infections can be complicated by numerous factors.[80] For most viral infections in the acute phase of illness, rapid antigen and/or nucleic acid detection methods or viral isolation are also available and may yield results in a more sensitive and timely manner.

Rapid and simple tests for the detection of HIV antibodies have been developed and licensed by the FDA.[83–85] These assays involve no special equipment, require little technical expertise, and are performed using self-contained, disposable devices. Most of the assays use serum or plasma for testing, while whole blood and oral fluids have also been incorporated as acceptable specimens for some assays. The assays have been designed to detect HIV-1 only or both HIV-1 and -2, and can be performed at the point of care or in the laboratory. The sensitivity and specificity of the rapid assays are comparable to laboratory-based screening tests, and like laboratory-based assays, confirmation by Western blot or immunofluorescence is required for specimens that are positive for HIV-specific antibody by rapid testing. Rapid HIV tests have been used widely in developing countries as tools for screening and confirmation of an HIV antibody response. They are the preferred test in this setting since resources and facilities may not be available to perform the more technically demanding laboratory-based immunoassays and Western blots. In the United States, these tests are being advocated for use in emergency departments, hospital clinics, sexually transmitted disease (STD) clinics, family planning clinic, and outreach programs. The intended uses of rapid HIV tests include providing greater access to testing and counseling and same-visit results, screening pregnant women with unknown HIV serostatus at the time of delivery, and assessing the risk of HIV transmission following exposure.

CONCLUSION

More so than any other time in the history of diagnostic virology, a number of rapid and accurate laboratory tests are now available to health care providers faced with children who are acutely or chronically ill with viral diseases. The appropriate selection, use, and interpretation of these methods in combination with clinical assessment of the patient can greatly improve care and have a positive impact on the management of these ill patients.

REFERENCES

1. Henrickson KJ. Cost effective use of rapid diagnostic techniques in the treatment and prevention of viral respiratory infections. *Pediatr Ann.* 2005;34(1):24-31.
2. Templeton KE. Why diagnose respiratory viral infection? *J Clin Virol.* 2007;40(suppl 1):S2-S4.
3. Falsey AR, Murata Y, Walsh EE. Impact of rapid diagnosis on management of adults hospitalized with influenza. *Arch Intern Med.* 2007;167:354-360.
4. Bonner AB, Monroe KW, Talley LI, et al. Impact of the rapid diagnosis of influenza on physician decision-making and patient management in the pediatric emergency department: results of a randomized, prospective, controlled trial. *Pediatrics.* 2003;112:363-367.
5. Abanses, JC, Dowd MD, Simon SD, et al. Impact of rapid influenza testing at triage on management of febrile infants and young children. *Pediatr Emerg Care.* 2006;22(3): 145-149.
6. Peck AJ, Corey L, Boeckh M. Pretransplantation respiratory syncytial virus infection: impact of a strategy to delay transplantation. *Clin Infect Dis.* 2004;(39):673-680.
7. Rocholl C, Gerber K, Daly J, et al. Adenovirus infections in children: the impact of rapid diagnosis. *Pediatrics.* 2004; 113(1):e51-e56.
8. Stellrecht KA, Harding I, Woron AM, et al. The impact of an enteroviral RT-PCR assay on the diagnosis of aseptic meningitis and patient management. *J Clin Virol.* 2002; 25:S19-S26.
9. Langley JM, Wang EEL, Law BJ, et al. Economic evaluation of respiratory syncytial virus infection in Canadian children: a Pediatric Investigators Collaborative Network on Infections in Canada (PICNIC) study. *J Pediatr.* 1997; 131(1, pt 1):113-117.
10. Woo PCY, Chiu SS, Seto W-H, et al. Cost-effectiveness of rapid diagnosis of viral respiratory tract infections in pediatric patients. *J Clin Microbiol.* 1997;35(6):1579-1581.
11. Barenfanger J, Drake C, Leon N, et al. Clinical and financial benefits of rapid detection of respiratory viruses: an outcomes study. *J Clin Microbiol.* 2000;38(8): 2824-2828.
12. Byrington CL, Castillo H, Gerber K, et al. The effect of rapid respiratory virus diagnostic testing on antibiotic use in a children's hospital. *Arch Pediatr Adolesc Med.* 2002; 156(12):1230-1234.
13. King RL, Lorch SA, Cohen DM, et al. Routine cerebrospinal fluid enterovirus polymerase chain reaction testing reduces hospitalization and antibiotic use for infants 90 days of age or younger. *Pediatrics.* 2007;120(3): 489-496.
14. D'Heilly SJ, Janoff EN, Nichol P, et al. Rapid diagnosis of influenza infection in older adults: influence on clinical care in a routine clinical setting. *J Clin Virol.* 2008. doi: 10.1016/j.jcv.2007.12.014.
15. Smith MJ, Clark HF, Lawley D, et al. The clinical and molecular epidemiology of community- and healthcare-acquired rotavirus gastroenteritis. *Pediatr Infect Dis J.* 2008;27(1):54-58.
16. Patel MM, Tate JE, Selvarangan R, et al. Routine laboratory testing data for surveillance of rotavirus hospitalizations to evaluate the impact of vaccination. *Pediatr Infect Dis J.* 2007;26(10):914-919.
17. Halasa NB, Williams JV, Wilson GJ, et al. Medical and economic impact of a respiratory syncytial virus outbreak in a neonatal intensive care unit. *Pediatr Infect Dis J.* 2005;24(12):1040-1044.
18. Macartney KK, Gorelick MH, Manning ML, et al. Nosocomial respiratory syncytial virus infections: the cost-effectiveness and cost-benefit of infection control. *Pediatrics.* 2000;106:520-526.
19. Specter S, Hodinka RL, Wiedbrauk DL, et al. Diagnosis of viral infections. In: Richman DD, Whitley RJ, Hayden FG, eds. *Clinical Virology.* 2nd ed. Washington, DC: ASM Press; 2002:243.
20. Storch GA. Diagnostic virology. *Clin Infect Dis.* 2000;31: 739-751.
21. Forman MS, Valsamakis A. Specimen collection, transport, and processing: Virology. In: Murray PR, Baron EJ, Jorgensen JH, et al. eds. *Manual of Clinical Microbiology.* 9th ed. Washington, DC: ASM Press; 2007:1284.
22. Hodinka RL, Nagashunmugam T, Malamud D. Detection of human immunodeficiency virus antibodies in oral fluids. *Clin Diag Lab Immunol.* 1998;5(4);419-426.
23. Almeda J, Casabona J, Matas L, et al. Evaluation of a commercial enzyme immunoassay for HIV screening in urine. *Eur J Clin Microbiol Infect Dis.* 2004;23(11):831-835.
24. Spielberg F, Critchlow C, Vittinghoff E, et al. Home collection for frequent HIV testing: acceptability of oral fluids, dried blood spots and telephone results. HIV Early Detection Study Group. *AIDS.* 2000;14(12):1819-1828.
25. Sarge-Njie R, Schim van der Loeff M, Ceesay S, et al. Evaluation of the dried blood spot filter paper technology and five testing strategies of HIV-1 and HIV-2 infections in West Africa. *Scand J Infect Dis.* 2006;38(11-12):1050-1056.
26. Andiman WA. Organism-specific antibody indices, the cerebrospinal fluid-immunoglobulin index and other tools: a clinician's guide to the etiologic diagnosis of central nervous system infection. *Pediatr Infect Dis J.* 1991; 10(7):490-495.
27. Daley P, Castriciano S, Chernesky M, Smieja M. Comparison of flocked and rayon swabs for collection of respiratory epithelial cells from uninfected volunteers and symptomatic patients. *J Clin Microbiol.* 2006;44(6):2265-2267.
28. Chan KH, Peiris JSM, Lim W, et al. Comparison of nasopharyngeal flocked swabs and aspirates for rapid diagnosis of respiratory viruses in children. *J Clin Virol.* 2008. doi:10.10161j.jcv.2007.12.003.
29. Landry ML, Hsiung GD. 2000. Primary isolation of viruses. In: Specter S, Hodinka RL, Young SA, eds. *Clinical Virology Manual.* 3rd ed. Washington, DC: ASM Press; 2000:27.

30. Leland DS, Ginocchio CC. Role of cell culture for virus detection in the age of technology. *Clin Microbiol Rev.* 2007;20(1):49-78.
31. Landry ML, Ferguson D, Cohen S, et al. Detection of human metapneumovirus in clinical samples by immunofluorescence staining of shell vial centrifugation cultures prepared from three different cell lines. *J Clin Microbiol.* 2005;43(4):1950-1952.
32. Olivo PD. Transgeneic cell lines for detection of animal viruses. *Clin Microbiol Rev.* 1996;9(3):321-334.
33. Stabell EC, Olivo PD. Isolation of a cell line for rapid and sensitive histochemical assay for the detection of herpes simplex virus. *J Virol Methods.* 1992;38:195-204.
34. Stabell EC, O'Rourke RR, Storch GA, Olivo PD. Evaluation of a genetically engineered cell line and a histochemical β-galactosidase assay to detect herpes simplex virus in clinical specimens. *J Clin Microbiol.* 1993;31(10):2796-2798.
35. Huang YT, Yam P, Yan H, Sun Y. Engineered BGMK cells for sensitive and rapid detection of enteroviruses. *J Clin Microbiol.* 2002;40(2):366-371.
36. Lutz A, Dyall J, Olivo PD, Pekosz A. Virus-inducible reporter genes as a tool for detecting and quantifying influenza A virus replication. *J Virol Methods.* 2005;126: 13-20.
37. Huang YT, Hite S, Duane V, Yan H. CV-1 and MRC-5 mixed cells for simultaneous detection of herpes simplex virus and varicella zoster virus in skin lesions. *J Clin Virol.* 2002;24(1-2):37-43.
38. Fong CK, Lee MK, Grith BP. Evaluation of R-Mix Fresh-Cells in shell vials for detection of respiratory viruses. *J Clin Microbiol.* 2000;38(12):4660-4662.
39. Barenfanger J, Drake C, Mueller T, et al. R-Mix cells are faster, at least as sensitive and marginally more costly than conventional cell lines for the detection of respiratory viruses. *J Clin Virol.* 2001;22(1):101-110.
40. St George K, Patel NM, Hartwig RA, et al. Rapid and sensitive detection of respiratory virus infections for directed antiviral treatment using R-Mix cultures. *J Clin Virol.* 2002;24(1–2):107-115.
41. Arens MQ, Swierkosz EM. Susceptibility test methods: Viruses. In: Murray PR, Baron EJ, Jorgensen JH, et al. eds. *Manual of Clinical Microbiology.* 9th ed. Washington, DC: ASM Press; 2007:1705.
42. Grandien M. Viral diagnosis by antigen detection techniques. *Clin Diag Virol.* 1996;5:81-90.
43. Coffin SE, Hodinka RL. Utility of direct immunofluorescence and virus culture for detection of varicella-zoster virus in skin lesions. *J Clin Microbiol.* 1995;33(10):2792-2795.
44. Landry ML, Ferguson D, Wlochowski J. Detection of herpes simplex virus in clinical specimens by cytospin-enhanced direct immunofluorescence. *J Clin Microbiol.* 1997;35(1):302-304.
45. Shetty AK, Treynor E, Hill DW, et al. Comparison of conventional viral cultures with direct fluorescent antibody stains for diagnosis of community-acquired respiratory virus infections in hospitalized children. *Pediatr Infect Dis J.* 2003;22(9):789-794.
46. Landry ML, Ferguson D. SimulFluor respiratory screen for rapid detection of multiple respiratory viruses in clinical specimens by immunofluorescence staining. *J Clin Microbiol.* 2000;38(2):708-711.
47. Landry ML, Cohen S, Ferguson D. Impact of sample type on rapid detection of influenza virus A by cytospin-enhanced immunofluorescence and membrane enzyme-linked immunosorbent assay. *J Clin Microbiol.* 2000;38(1): 429-430.
48. Henrickson KJ, Hall CB. Diagnostic assays for respiratory syncytial virus disease. *Pediatr Infect Dis J.* 2007;26(11): S36-S40.
49. Mazzulli T, Rubin RH, Ferraro MJ, et al. Cytomegalovirus antigenemia: clinical correlations in transplant recipients and in persons with AIDS. *J Clin Microbiol.* 1993;31(10): 2824-2827.
50. Hodinka RL. Human cytomegalovirus. In: Murray PR, Baron EJ, Jorgensen JH, et al. eds. *Manual of Clinical Microbiology.* 9th ed. Washington, DC: ASM Press; 2007:1549.
51. Storch GA. Rapid diagnostic tests for influenza. *Curr Opin in Pediatr.* 2003;15:77-84.
52. Castriciano S, Luinstra K, Petrich A, et al. Comparison of the RIDASCREEN norovirus enzyme immunoassay to IDEIA NLV Gi/GII by testing stools also assayed by RT-PCR and electron microscopy. *J Virol Methods.* 2007;141(2): 216-219.
53. Wilhelmi de Cal I, Revilla A, del Alamo JM, et al. Evaluation of two commercial enzyme immunoassays for the detection of norovirus in faecal samples from hospitalised children with sporadic acute gastroenteritis. *Clin Microbiol Infect.* 2007;13(3):341-343.
54. Espy MJ, Uhl JR, Sloan LM, et al. Real-time PCR in clinical microbiology: applications for routine laboratory testing. *Clin Microbiol Rev.* 2006;19(1):165-256.
55. Niesters HGM. Molecular and diagnostic clinical virology in real time. *Clin Microbiol Infect.* 2004;10:5-11.
56. Mackay IM. Real-time PCR in the microbiology laboratory. *Clin Microbiol Infect.* 2004;10:190-212.
57. Watzinger F, Ebner K, Lion T. Detection and monitoring of virus infections by real-time PCR. *Mol Asp Med.* 2006;27:254-298.
58. Gunson RN, Collins TC, Carman WF. Practical experience of high throughput real time PCR in the routine diagnostic virology setting. *J Clin Virol.* 2006;35:355-367.
59. Jain KK. Nanotechnology in clinical laboratory diagnostics. *Clin Chim Acta.* 2005;358:37-54.
60. Kricka LJ. Microchips, microarrays, biochips and nanochips: personal laboratories for the 21st century. *Clin Chim Acta.* 2001;307(1–2):219-223.
61. Sampath R, Russell KL, Massire C, et al. Global surveillance of emerging influenza virus genotypes by mass spectrometry. *PLoS One.* 2007;2(5):e489.
62. Blyn LB, Hall TA, Libby B, et al. Rapid detection and molecular serotyping of adenovirus by use of PCR followed by electrospray ionization mass spectrometry. *J Clin Microbiol.* 2008;46(2):644-651.
63. Wiedbrauk DL, Hodinka RL. Applications of the polymerase chain reaction. In: Specter S, et al. eds. *Rapid Detection of Infectious Agents.* New York: Plenum Press; 1998:97.
64. Fan J, Henrickson KJ, Savatski LL. Rapid simultaneous diagnosis of infections with respiratory syncytial viruses A and B, influenza viruses A and B, and human parainfluenza virus types 1, 2, and 3 by multiplex quantitative reverse transcription-polymerase chain reaction-enzyme

hybridization assay (Hexaplex). *Clin Infect Dis.* 1998;26: 1397-1402.

65. Dunbar SA. Applications of Luminex xMAP technology for rapid, high-throughput multiplexed nucleic acid detection. *Clin Chim Acta.* 2006;363:71-82.
66. Schmitt M, Bravo IG, Snijders PJ, et al. Bead-based multiplex genotyping of human papillomaviruses. *J Clin Microbiol.* 2006;44(2):504-512.
67. Mahony J, Chong S, Merante, F, et al. Development of a respiratory virus panel test for detection of twenty human respiratory viruses by use of multiplex PCR and a fluid microbead-based assay. *J Clin Microbiol.* 2007;45(9): 2965-2970.
68. Lee, W-M, Grindle K, Pappas T, et al. High-throughput, sensitive, and accurate multiplex PCR-microsphere flow cytometry system for large-scale comprehensive detection of respiratory viruses. *J Clin Microbiol.* 2007;45(8):2626-2634.
69. Brunstein J, Thomas E. Direct screening of clinical specimens for multiple respiratory pathogens using the Genaco Respiratory Panels 1 and 2. *Diagn Mol Pathol.* 2006;15(3):169-173.
70. Legoff J, Kara R, Moulin F, et al. Evaluation of the one-step multiplex real-time reverse transcription-PCR ProFlu-1 assay for detection of influenza A and influenza B viruses and respiratory syncytial viruses in children. *J Clin Microbiol.* 2008;46(2):789-791.
71. Berger A, Preiser W. Viral genome quantification as a tool for improving patient management: the example of HIV, HBV, HCV and CMV. *J Antimicrob Chemother.* 2002;49: 713-721.
72. Peter JB, Sevall JS. Molecular-based methods for quantifying HIV viral load. *AIDS Patient Care STD.* 2004;18(2): 75-79.
73. Smith TF, Espy MJ, Mandrekar J, et al. Quantitative real-time polymerase chain reaction for evaluating DNAemia due to cytomegalovirus, Epstein–Barr virus, and BK virus in solid organ transplant recipients. *Clin Infect Dis.* 2007;45:1056-1061.
74. Domiati-Saad R, Scheuermann RH. Nucleic acid testing for viral burden and viral genotyping. *Clin Chim Acta.* 2006;363:197-205.
75. Drew LW. Laboratory diagnosis of cytomegalovirus infection and disease in immunocompromised patients. *Curr Opin Infect Dis.* 2007;20:408-411.
76. Hodinka RL. Human herpesviruses 6, 7, and 8. In: Detrick B, Hamilton RG, Folds JD, eds. *Manual of Molecular and Clinical Laboratory Immunology.* 7th ed. Washington, DC: ASM Press; 2006:658.
77. Arens M. Clinically relevant sequence-based genotyping of HBV, HCV, CMV, and HIV. *J Clin Virol.* 2001;22:11-29.
78. Hazelton PR, Gelderblom HR. Electron microscopy for rapid diagnosis of infectious agents in emergent situations. *Emerg Infect Dis.* 2003;9(3):294-303.
79. Curry A, Appleton, H, Dowsett B. Application of transmission electron microscopy to the clinical study of viral and bacterial infections: present and future. *Micron.* 2006;37:91-106.
80. Hodinka RL. Serological tests in clinical virology. In: Lennette EH, Smith TF, eds. *Laboratory Diagnosis of Viral Infections.* 3rd ed. New York: Marcel Dekker; 1999:195.
81. Hodinka RL. Human immunodeficiency virus. In: Truant AL, ed. *Manual of Commercial Methods in Clinical Microbiology.* Washington, DC: ASM Press; 2002:100.
82. Hodinka RL. Laboratory diagnosis of viral hepatitis. In: Specter S, ed. *Viral Hepatitis: Diagnosis, Therapy, and Prevention.* Totowa, NJ: Humana Press; 1999:193.
83. Greenwald JL. Routine rapid HIV testing in hospitals: another opportunity for hospitalists to improve care. *J Hosp Med.* 2006;1:106-112.
84. Greenwald JL, Burstein GR, Pincus J, et al. A rapid review of rapid HIV antibody tests. *Curr Infect Dis Rep.* 2006;8(2):125-131.
85. Roberts KJ, Grusky O, Swanson A-N. Outcomes of blood and oral fluid rapid HIV Testing: a literature review, 2000-2006. *AIDS Patient Care STD.* 2007;21(9):621-637.

CHAPTER 3

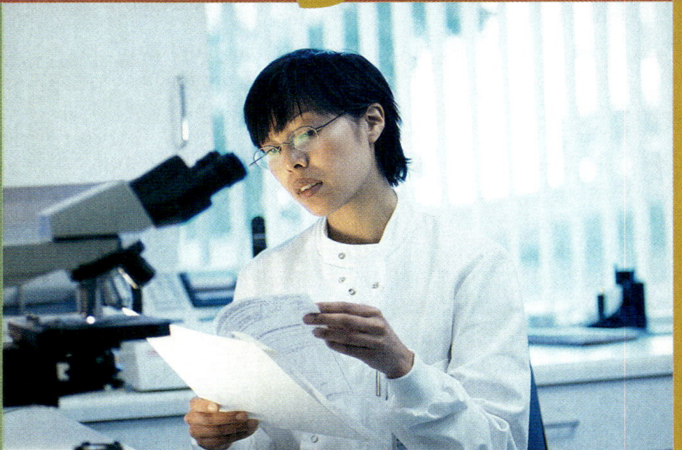

Vaccines and Vaccine Safety

Michael J. Smith

INTRODUCTION

Vaccines represent one of the most successful public health interventions of all time. Diseases that once killed thousands of children each year have been virtually eliminated from the United States (Table 3–1). Because vaccines have been so effective, many parents and younger physicians have little firsthand experience with the infectious diseases they prevent. In this context, attention has shifted away from concerns of vaccine-preventable diseases themselves toward concerns of vaccine safety, both perceived and real.

Figure 3–1 graphically depicts what may occur if the public loses faith in the immunization system. Disease incidence begins to decline when a new vaccine is introduced. If there is loss of confidence in the vaccine among a critical proportion of the population, outbreaks may occur. Continued decrease in disease incidence with potential disease eradication can only occur if public confidence in the vaccine program is restored.

There are several historical examples of what may occur when immunization practices suddenly shift. For instance, the incidence of pertussis was found to be 10–100 times lower in countries that maintained high levels of whole-cell diphtheria–tetanus–pertussis (DTP) vaccination in the 1980s as compared to countries with prominent anti-DTP movements.[1] In Japan during the mid-1990s, immunizations were made optional after the

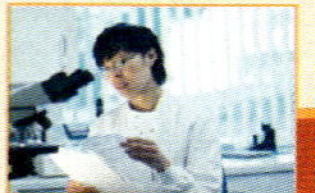

Table 3–1.

Impact of Vaccines in the Twentieth Century

Disease	Twentieth Century Annual Morbidity	2005 Total	% Decrease
Smallpox	48,164	0	100
Diphtheria	175,885	0	100
Pertussis	147,271	25,616	83
Tetanus	1,314	27	98
Polio (paralytic)	16,316	1*	>99.9
Measles	503,282	66	>99.9
Mumps	152,209	314	>99
Rubella	47,745	11	>99.9
Congenital rubella	823	1	99.8
Haemophilus influenzae (<5 years)	20,000 (EST)	226 (Serotype B or unknown serotype)	99

**Imported vaccine-associated paralytic polio.*

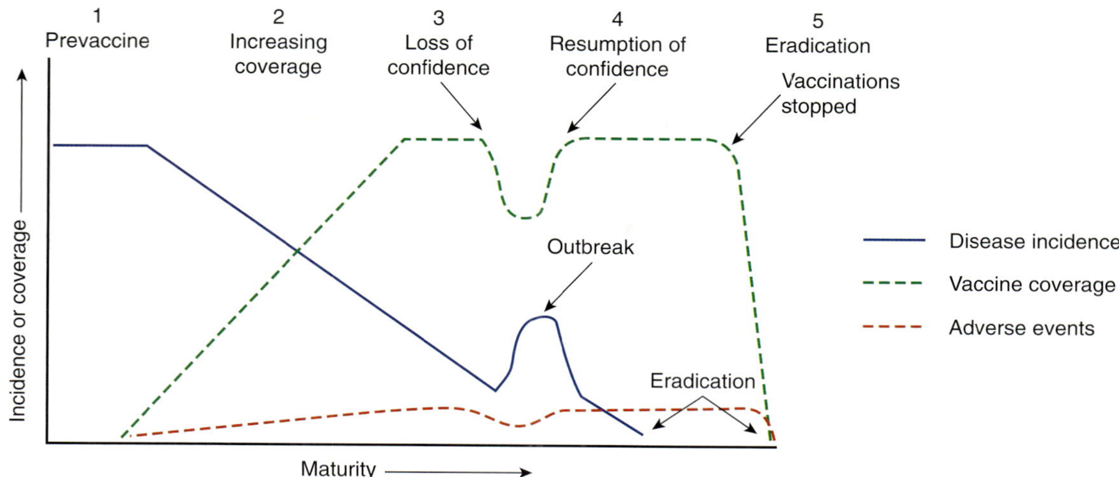

(1) Before vaccines are introduced, the incidence of vaccine-preventable diseases is high.
(2) As vaccine coverage increases, disease incidence decreases.
(3) As more people are vaccinated, adverse events associated with immunization begin to appear. Because disease is no longer common, this results in loss of public confidence in the immunization program. Subsequent decreases in vaccination coverage result in outbreaks of disease.
(4) If public confidence is restored, vaccination rates increase and disease incidence falls again.
(5) Over time, the disease may be completely eradicated and the vaccination program may be terminated. To date, this has happened only for smallpox.

FIGURE 3–1 ■ Life cycle of an immunization program.

occurrence of rare case reports of aseptic meningitis associated with measles–mumps–rubella (MMR) receipt. Consequently, measles made a recurrence, resulting in more than 100,000 cases and 50–100 deaths per year.[2]

Even in the United States, where many parents feel that there is no risk for infectious diseases, outbreaks have occurred when individuals are unvaccinated. These outbreaks are more likely to occur in clusters of vaccine-resistant communities.[3] For example, in Colorado there were 14 measles outbreaks between 1987 and 1998.[4] Children who were exempted from vaccination were 22 times more likely to acquire measles as children who were vaccinated. Another outbreak occurred in Indiana in the summer of 2005 when 34 members of a church acquired measles after an unvaccinated member returned from a missionary trip to Romania. 32 of the 34 affected individuals were unvaccinated, primarily due to concerns of vaccine safety.[5] As the number of unvaccinated individuals increases, the potential for a large-scale outbreak in the United States becomes greater. In 2008, 127 cases of measles in 15 states were reported to the Centers for Disease Control and Prevention (CDC) as of the end of June, mostly in unvaccinated individuals.[58] Although these data are for the first half of the year alone, this already represents the greatest number of cases reported since 1997, when 138 people were diagnosed with measles.

In this chapter, we review the process of assessing vaccine safety. We then review the biologic and epidemiologic data surrounding popular myths about vaccines.

THE CHALLENGES OF VACCINE SAFETY

Vaccines are unique among pharmaceutical agents in that they are given to healthy children to prevent disease in the future. This poses several challenges. First, if parents have even the slightest concern about the safety of a vaccine, the perceived risk of vaccination may outweigh the perceived benefit of protection against a disease that is no longer prevalent. Second, because nearly all children are vaccinated, it is difficult to determine whether adverse events that occur after vaccination are truly as a result of vaccine receipt or mere coincidence. While vaccines are highly efficacious, they can prevent only a small percentage of infectious diseases, and do not prevent other childhood adverse outcomes.[6] This may be confusing when diseases with uncertain etiology such as autism are diagnosed at the same age as most vaccines are given. Finally, most vaccines are given simultaneously with other vaccines and it can be difficult to determine which specific vaccine, if any, is responsible for a given adverse event.

Randomized controlled trials (RCTs) provide the strongest epidemiologic evidence of a causal relationship. However, postlicensure RCTs are not ethically feasible once a vaccine becomes recommended for routine pediatric use. Therefore, vaccine safety has traditionally been studied as part of prelicensure RCTs and further monitored using postlicensure surveillance.

Prelicensure RCTs are usually designed to assess vaccine efficacy and may be underpowered to detect uncommon vaccine adverse effects. A notable exception is the prelicensure trials surrounding the newly approved pentavalent bovine rotavirus vaccine (RotaTeq), which enrolled nearly 70,000 children.[7] This large study was designed because of safety issues with an earlier rotavirus vaccine (Rotashield), which was found to be associated with intussusception in an estimated 1 in 10,000 vaccine recipients.[8] Because the Rotashield prelicensure study included only slightly more than 10,000 children, it was not large enough to detect this adverse effect. Ideally, one would simply increase the size of vaccine prelicensure RCTs. However, some vaccine side effects occur too rarely to be detected in an RCT. For instance, a trial designed to detect a threefold increase in relative risk for an outcome with a background incidence of 0.01 would require a two-arm trial with 175,000 children.[9] Even if it were possible to design a study of this size, it might not be financially feasible.

THE VACCINE ADVERSE EVENT REPORTING SYSTEM

Postlicensure monitoring of vaccine safety uses the Vaccine Adverse Event Reporting System (VAERS). VAERS is a passive postlicensure reporting system, maintained jointly by the Food and Drug Administration (FDA) and the Center for Disease Control (CDC). It allows any individual who believes that a vaccine-associated adverse effect has occurred to report this to the system. The strength of VAERS is that it incorporates data from the entire country and is therefore widely generalizable.[6] However, VAERS also has several limitations. First, simply reporting an adverse effect does not imply causation. In fact, common, acute symptoms such as fever occur in up to 10% of healthy children regardless of vaccination status and so the observed association may be attributed to chance alone.[10] Second, there is no denominator that can be used to calculate the incidence of adverse effects. While the total number of delivered doses can be obtained from pharmaceutical companies, it is difficult to determine how many doses have actually been administered. Furthermore, the distribution of vaccine across age groups, which would be helpful for calculating age-specific incidence rates, is unknown.[6] Finally, there is potential for significant bias in reporting. In one recent analysis it was found that a large percentage of VAERS reports were filed by attorneys involved in lawsuits against vaccine companies.[11] Similarly, parental and physician reports may be influenced by public perception. In another study, parents who reported autism as a vaccine-associated adverse effect to VAERS were much more likely to do so after the publication of a paper that claimed a link between MMR and autism, even though their children were vaccinated several years before.[12] On the other hand, there may be significant underreporting to VAERS. While there are data to suggest that serious adverse events such as intussusception and death are reported,[13] more common and benign events that occur after vaccination may be overlooked by parents and physicians. Despite these limitations, VAERS is able to detect potential vaccine-associated adverse events that may be further evaluated using other epidemiologic methods.

THE VACCINE SAFETY DATALINK

One such method uses the Vaccine Safety Datalink (VSD), which was created in 1990 and is modeled after other pharmacoepidemiologic-linking studies.[14] It is partnered with eight large managed care organizations (MCOs), and prospectively collects data on 5.5 million individuals each year.[15] Vaccinations are entered into the medical record as part of routine medical care, and any subsequent medical history, including adverse events, can be detected. This allows for a true denominator that may be used to calculate the incidence of adverse reactions after vaccination. While this system offers a higher standard of epidemiologic data than VAERS, it is still unable to account for the fact that most children in the United States are vaccinated.[16] Another limitation is that it only includes data on children enrolled in managed care organizations, who may not be representative of the entire population. Despite the lack of unvaccinated children, the VSD can be used to determine the risk of acute vaccine adverse effects using the case-crossover study design, in which cases serve as their own controls.[6] Several of the studies included in this chapter are based on VSD data. In the sections below, we will focus on specific concerns about vaccine safety.

VACCINES AND AUTISM

Measles–Mumps–Rubella Vaccine

In February 1998, researchers in Britain suggested that receipt of the MMR vaccine may cause autism.[17] This was based on a small series of 12 children, all of whom had inflammatory bowel disease and 8 of whom also had autism. This study was significantly flawed. First, case reports do not offer strong proof of causal association. Second, the exposure—MMR vaccination—relied on parental recall. Because these parents believed that MMR was responsible for their children's autism, it is not surprising that they reported a temporal association between MMR vaccination and the development of autistic symptoms. More importantly, the lead author was funded by a group of lawyers who were representing the families of the eight autistic children in a lawsuit against the manufacturer of MMR.[18] Ten of the original 13 authors eventually retracted their statement of causality.[19]

Despite these limitations, this story was widely published in the popular media and on the Internet. In Britain, national MMR immunization rates fell from 92% to 75%, which resulted in several measles outbreaks and the first death caused by measles in a decade.[20] In the United States, immunization rates have remained fairly high because of school-entry requirements, yet pediatricians do report that parents are concerned about the possible association between MMR and autism. These concerns led the Institute of Medicine (IOM) to investigate the potential relationship between MMR and autism.[21,22] In 2001, and again in 2004, the IOM concluded that there was sufficient data to reject the hypothesis that MMR caused autism.

These decisions were based in part on several large epidemiologic studies. The most rigorous study was performed in Denmark in 2002.[23] The investigators incorporated data from 537,303 children born in Denmark from 1991 to 1998, for a total of 2,129,864 person-years. Of these, there were 1,647,504 person-years of follow-up for children who received MMR and 482,360 person-years of follow-up for children who did not receive MMR. After adjusting for age, calendar year, sex, birth weight, gestational age, maternal education, and socioeconomic status, there was no significant difference in rates of autism (relative risk [RR] 0.92; 95% confidence interval [CI], 0.68–1.24) or other autistic-spectrum disorders (RR 0.83; 95% CI, 0.65–1.07) between children who had received MMR and those who had not.

Other research has relied upon ecologic analyses.[24] Two studies compared rates of autism before and after the introduction of national MMR immunization programs, and found that the prevalence[25] and incidence[26] of autism decreased after the introduction of MMR. Other studies employing time-series approaches found that trends in the number of children diagnosed with autism did not parallel trends in MMR coverage.[27–30] If MMR did cause autism, autistic children who received MMR might have developed symptoms at an earlier age than autistic children who were unvaccinated. This does not appear to be the case.[23,26,29]

THIMEROSAL AND AUTISM

Shortly after the MMR–autism controversy began, a new concern about vaccines and autism emerged. In 1999, the FDA released a report suggesting that the levels of ethyl mercury, a metabolite of the preservative thimerosal that is used in some childhood vaccines, exceeded acceptable levels as determined by the Environmental Protection Agency (EPA). Based on preliminary data that suggested an increasing trend in autism at the same time as the emergence of new thimerosal-containing vaccines, the Advisory Committee for Immunization Practices and American Academy of Pediatrics (AAP) issued a statement recommending that thimerosal be removed from all childhood immunizations.[31] At that time, it was felt that the risk of a potential association outweighed the benefit of using thimerosal-containing vaccines. However, the Environmental Protection Agency data are based on data for methyl mercury, a common environmental toxin. In contrast, thimerosal is metabolized to ethyl mercury, which has different pharmacokinetics and is excreted from the body much more quickly.[32] Despite the removal of thimerosal from all childhood vaccines in 2001 (except for the injectable influenza vaccine), rates of autism in the United States continue to increase, making it implausible that thimerosal causes autism. Finally, there have been several large epidemiologic studies that suggest that thimerosal exposure is not associated with autism.

One study based on the VSD-incorporated data from 124,170 children vaccinated at three health maintenance organizations (HMOs).[33] In one HMO, researchers discovered a statistically significant association between cumulative thimerosal exposure and tics at 3 months, but not at 1 or 7 months. This association was not seen at the other HMOs. At the second HMO, there was a statistically significant association with language delay at 3 and 7 months. There were no associations observed between thimerosal exposure and any other developmental conditions, including autism and attention-deficit disorder. In a third HMO, consisting on 16,717 children, no statistically significant associations were noted between thimerosal and any developmental diagnoses. Because there was no consistent relationship between thimerosal exposure and developmental disorders, it was concluded that the two observed statistical associations were attributed to chance alone.

A study performed in Denmark found no association between autism and ethyl mercury exposure.[34] This study took advantage of the fact that Danish children had received thimerosal in vaccines only until 1992. Therefore, the authors were able to compare rates of autism among children who were exposed to significant levels of thimerosal, some thimerosal, and no thimerosal. The authors studied thimerosal exposure in three separate analyses. Comparing any thimerosal receipt to no thimerosal receipt, there was no association with autism. When these results were stratified by dose of thimerosal, there was still no association. Finally, when thimerosal was treated as a continuous variable there was also no association.

Another study performed in Denmark found that the discontinuation of thimerosal-containing vaccines was actually associated with an increase in autism.[35] Finally, a study combining data from California, Sweden, and Denmark found that rates of autism continued to increase after discontinuation of thimerosal-containing vaccines.[36] Based on these data, and others, the IOM concluded in 2004 that there was sufficient evidence to reject the hypothesis that thimerosal is causally associated with autism.[22]

TOO MANY SHOTS

In a nationally representative telephone survey conducted in 1999, 23% of parents reported concern that children receive too many immunizations and 25% of parents believed that their child's immune system could be weakened as a result of too many immunizations.[37] Since the publication of this report, even more vaccines have been added to the immunization schedule.[38] Despite these new vaccines, most childhood infections are not vaccine-preventable.[39] Therefore, vaccines represent only a small proportion of the antigenic burden to the developing immune system. Additionally, while the number of vaccine-preventable childhood diseases has increased from 1 (smallpox) in 1900 to 13 in 2007, the total number of antigens to which children are exposed in current vaccines is significantly less than it had been for most of the twentieth century. This is because of the discontinuation of the whole-cell pertussis vaccine, which contained 3000 proteins; and the smallpox vaccine, which contained 200 proteins.[40] In contrast, the combined antigenic burden of all current childhood vaccines is less than 200 proteins or polysaccharides.[40] Another concern is that receipt of immunizations may actually weaken the immune system. This does not appear to be the case. In fact, children who are vaccinated may actually be protected against infections that are not included in the childhood vaccines.[41,42] Additionally, several studies have shown that vaccine immunogenicity is not altered by giving multiple vaccines at the same time.[40]

VACCINES AND VIRAL ILLNESS

Another common misperception shared by parents and medical providers is that children should not receive vaccinations when they are sick. One study did find decreased serologic evidence of measles immunity in children with upper respiratory illness (URI) at the time of vaccination as compared to asymptomatic children.[43] However, the results from this study have not been replicated. Two subsequent studies[44,45] found no difference in seroconversion rates between children with afebrile URI and asymptomatic children. Finally, a prospective cohort study including 356 children compared seroconversion after MMR vaccination in asymptomatic children with children who had either URI, otitis media, or diarrhea, excluding children with temperature greater than 37.4°C.[46] The authors found no significant difference in seroconversion between these groups. In fact, children with mild illness had slightly higher rates of seroconversion, although this did not reach statistical significance. While it is recommended that immunizations be deferred for children who have severe infections requiring hospitalization, this is not because of concerns about vaccine effectiveness. Instead, vaccine deferral is recommended to decrease the likelihood of an adverse event associated with hospitalization being misattributed to vaccination.[40]

VACCINES AND ASTHMA/ALLERGIES

There is also concern that vaccines may be responsible for allergies and the development of asthma. This theory is rooted in the "hygiene hypothesis," which suggests that children with better hygiene are more likely to develop allergies.[47,48] Vaccines, some argue, prevent natural infection with viruses and bacteria that would normally stimulate the immune system. However, most infections that occur during the first year of life are caused by viruses that are not prevented by vaccines.[39,47] Furthermore, all infants are exposed to environmental antigens such as pollen, cigarette smoke, dust mites, and pet dander that also contribute to immune system development.[39] Finally, several studies have failed to find an association between vaccination status and development of allergies or asthma.

One such study used the Vaccine Safety Datalink (VCD) to assess risk factors for asthma in 167,240 children.[49] In multivariable regression, receipt of MMR, DTP, and OPV were not associated with asthma. *Haemophilus influenza* type B (RR 1.18; 95% CI, 1.02–1.36) and hepatitis B (RR 1.20; 95% CI, 1.13–1.27) vaccines were associated with a small increase in relative risk for asthma. Infants who were enrolled in but did not receive long-term medical care in the managed care organizations would appear to be unvaccinated and would also have no record of asthma. This might artificially decrease the risk of asthma among unvaccinated children. A subanalysis including only those children with two or more health care visits was performed to correct for this bias, and revealed no association between any vaccines and asthma. Another study of allergic responses within a randomized controlled pertussis vaccine trial found no association between vaccine receipt and allergic diagnoses.[50] Finally, a recent ecologic study demonstrated that the increase in asthma seen in the United States during the 1990s occurred before the increase in the number

Box 3–1. Strategies for Vaccine Risk Communication

- Listen carefully and respectfully to parental concerns about vaccine safety.
- Explain the risks of getting vaccinated as compared to the risks of remaining unvaccinated.
- If parents are concerned about pain associated with multiple injections, consider pain reduction strategies or alternative vaccination schedules that minimize the number of injections per visit.
- If parents are concerned about specific vaccines, they may accept other immunizations.
- Discharging families from one's practice because vaccine refusal is not generally recommended.

of recommended vaccines that occurred in the late 1990s.[51] This further suggests that the increasing numbers of vaccines are not responsible for observed increases in asthma during the last decade.

STRATEGIES FOR VACCINE RISK COMMUNICATION

In this chapter, we have described the mechanisms in place for monitoring vaccine safety in the United States and have addressed some of the more common myths surrounding childhood immunizations. This information may be useful during discussions with parents who have concerns about vaccine safety. Additional strategies for discussing immunizations with vaccine-hesitant parents have recently been published by the American Academy of Pediatrics, [52,53] and are summarized in Box 3–1. Despite increasing coverage of vaccine controversies in the media and on the Internet, physicians remain the most influential source of immunization information for parents,[37,54,55] including those who believe that vaccines are unsafe[56] and those who request exemptions.[57] Physician familiarity with vaccine safety issues and vaccine risk communication is important in order to maintain optimal immunization rates.

REFERENCES

1. Gangarosa EJ, Galazka AM, Wolfe CR, et al. Impact of anti-vaccine movements on pertussis control: the untold story. *Lancet.* 1998;351(9099):356-361.
2. Gomi H, Takahashi H. Why is measles still endemic in Japan? *Lancet.* 2004;364(9431):328-329.
3. May T, Silverman RD. Clustering of exemptions as a collective action threat to herd immunity. *Vaccine.* 2003; 21(11–12):1048-1051.
4. Feikin DR, Lezotte DC, Hamman RF, Salmon DA, Chen RT, Hoffman RE. Individual and community risks of measles and pertussis associated with personal exemptions to immunization. *JAMA.* 2000;284(24):3145-3150.
5. Parker AA, Staggs W, Dayan GH, et al. Implications of a 2005 measles outbreak in Indiana for sustained elimination of measles in the United States. *New Engl J Med.* 2006; 355(5):447-455.
6. Ellenberg SS, Braun MM. Monitoring the safety of vaccines: assessing the risks. *Drug Safety.* 2002;25(3):145-152.
7. Vesikari T, Matson DO, Dennehy P, et al. Safety and efficacy of a pentavalent human-bovine (WC3) reassortant rotavirus vaccine. *New Engl J Med.* 2006;354(1):23-33.
8. Peter G, Myers MG. Intussusception, rotavirus, and oral vaccines: summary of a workshop. *Pediatrics.* 2002; 110(6):e67.
9. Ellenberg SS. Safety considerations for new vaccine development. *Pharmacoepidemiol Drug Saf.* 2001;10(5):411-415.
10. Peltola H, Heinonen OP. Frequency of true adverse reactions to measles–mumps–rubella vaccine: a double-blind placebo-controlled trial in twins. *Lancet.* 1986;1(8487): 939-942.
11. Goodman MJ, Nordin J. Vaccine adverse event reporting system reporting source: a possible source of bias in longitudinal studies. *Pediatrics.* 2006;117(2):387-390.
12. Woo EJ, Ball R, Bostrom A, et al. Vaccine risk perception among reporters of autism after vaccination: vaccine adverse event reporting system 1990-2001. *Am J Public Health.* 2004;94(6):990-995.
13. Rosenthal S, Chen R. The reporting sensitivities of two passive surveillance systems for vaccine adverse events. *Am J Public Health.* 1995;85(12):1706-1709.
14. DeStefano F. The vaccine safety datalink project. *Pharmacoepidemiol Drug Saf.* 2001;10(5):403-406.
15. Vaccine Safety Datalink Project (VSD). http://www.cdc.gov/od/science/iso/research_activties/vsdp.htm. Accessed July 10, 2007.
16. Chen RT, Glasser JW, Rhodes PH, et al. Vaccine safety datalink project: a new tool for improving vaccine safety monitoring in the United States. *Pediatrics.* 1997;99(6): 765-773.
17. Wakefield AJ, Murch SH, Anthony A, et al. Ileal-lymphoid-nodular hyperplasia, non-specific colitis, and pervasive developmental disorder in children. *Lancet.* 1998;351 (9103):637-641.
18. Deer B. MMR doctor given legal aid thousands. *London Sunday Times.* December 31, 2006.
19. Murch SH, Anthony A, Casson DH, et al. Ileal-lymphoid-nodular hyperplasia, non-specific colitis, and pervasive developmental disorder in children. *Lancet.* 2004; 363(9411):750.
20. Deer B. Schoolboy, 13, dies as measles makes a comeback. *London Sunday Times.* April 2, 2006.
21. Institute of Medicine. *Measles-Mumps-Rubella Vaccine and Autism.* Washington, DC: The National Academies Press; 2001.
22. Institute of Medicine. *Immunization Safety Review: Vaccines and Autism.* Washington, DC: National Academies Press; 2004.
23. Madsen KM, Hviid A, Vestergaard M, et al. A population-based study of measles, mumps, and rubella vaccination and autism. *New Engl J Med.* 2002;347(19): 1477-1482.
24. Wilson K, Mills E, Ross C, McGowan J, Jadad A. Association of autistic spectrum disorder and the measles,

mumps, and rubella vaccine: a systematic review of current epidemiological evidence. *Arch Pediatr Adoles Med.* 2003;157(7):628-634.

25. Gillberg C HH. MMR and autism. *Autism.* 1998;2(4): 423-424.
26. Fombonne E, Chakrabarti S. No evidence for a new variant of measles-mumps-rubella-induced autism. *Pediatrics.* 2001;108(4):e58.
27. Dales L, Hammer SJ, Smith NJ. Time trends in autism and in MMR immunization coverage in California. *JAMA.* 2001;285(9):1183-1185.
28. Kaye JA, Melero-Montes MD, Jick H. Mumps, measles, and rubella vaccine and the incidence of autism recorded by general practitioners: a time trend analysis. *BMJ.* 2001; 322(7284):460-463.
29. Taylor B, Miller E, Farrington CP, et al. Autism and measles, mumps, and rubella vaccine: no epidemiological evidence for a causal association. *Lancet.* 1999;353(9169): 2026-2029.
30. Taylor B, Miller E, Lingam R, Andrews N, Simmons A, Stowe J. Measles, mumps, and rubella vaccination and bowel problems or developmental regression in children with autism: Population study. *BMJ.* 2002;324(7334):393-396.
31. Thimerosal in vaccines: a joint statement of the American Academy of Pediatrics and the Public Health Service. *MMWR.* 1999;48(26):563-565.
32. Offit PA, Jew RK. Addressing parents' concerns: do vaccines contain harmful preservatives, adjuvants, additives, or residuals? *Pediatrics.* 2003;112(6):1394-1401.
33. Verstraeten T, Davis RL, DeStefano F, et al. Safety of thimerosal-containing vaccines: a two-phased study of computerized health maintenance organization databases. *Pediatrics.* Nov 2003;112(5):1039-1048.
34. Hviid A, Stellfeld M, Wohlfahrt J, Melbye M. Association between thimerosal-containing vaccine and autism. *JAMA.* 2003;290(13):1763-1766.
35. Madsen KM, Lauritsen MB, Pedersen CB, et al. Thimerosal and the occurrence of autism: negative ecological evidence from Danish population-based data. *Pediatrics.* 2003;112(3):604-606.
36. Stehr-Green P, Tull P, Stellfeld M, Mortenson PB, Simpson D. Autism and thimerosal-containing vaccines: lack of consistent evidence for an association. *Am J Prev Med.* 2003;25(2):101-106.
37. Gellin BG, Maibach EW, Marcuse EK. Do parents understand immunizations? A national telephone survey. *Pediatrics.* 2000;106(5):1097-1102.
38. Recommended immunization schedules for children and adolescents—United States, 2007. *Pediatrics.* 2007;119(1): 207-208.
39. Gregson AL, Edelman R. Does antigenic overload exist? The role of multiple immunizations in infants. *Immunol Allergy Clin North Am.* 2003;23(4):649.
40. Offit PA, Quarles J, Gerber MA, et al. Addressing parents' concerns: do multiple vaccines overwhelm or weaken the infant's immune system? *Pediatrics.* Jan 2002;109(1): 124-129.
41. Otto S, Mahner B, Kadow I, Beck JF, Wiersbitzky SKW, Bruns R. General non-specific morbidity is reduced after vaccination within the third month of life: The Greifswald study. *J Infect.* 2000;41(2):172-175.
42. Miller E, Andrews N, Waight P, Taylor B. Bacterial infections, immune overload, and MMR vaccine. *Arch Dis in Child.* 2003;88(3):222-223.
43. Krober MS, Stracener CE, Bass JW. Decreased measles antibody-response after measles-mumps-rubella vaccine in infants with colds. *JAMA.* 1991;265(16):2095-2096.
44. Dennehy PH, Saracen CL, Peter G. Seroconversion rates to combined measles-mumps-rubella-varicella vaccine of children with upper respiratory-tract infection. *Pediatrics.* 1994;94(4):514-516.
45. Ratnam S, West R, Gadag V. Measles and rubella antibody-response after measles mumps rubella vaccination in children with afebrile upper respiratory-tract infection. *J Pediatr.* 1995;127(3):432-434.
46. King GE, Markowitz LE, Heath J, et al. Antibody response to measles mumps rubella vaccine of children with mild illness at the time of vaccination. *JAMA.* 1996;275(9):704-707.
47. Offit PA, Hackett CJ. Addressing parents' concerns: do vaccines cause allergic or autoimmune diseases? *Pediatrics.* 2003;111(3):653-659.
48. Mullooly JP, Schuler R, Barrett M, Maher JE. Vaccines, antibiotics, and atopy. *Pharmacoepidemiol Drug Saf.* 2007;16(3):275-288.
49. Destefano F, Gu D, Kramarz P, et al. Childhood vaccinations and risk of asthma. *Pediatr Infect Dis J.* 2002;21(6):498-504.
50. Nilsson L, Kjellman NIM, Bjorksten B. A randomized controlled trial of the effect of pertussis vaccines on atopic disease. *Arch Pediatr Adolesc Med.* 1998;152(8):734-738.
51. Enriquez R, Hartert T, Persky V. Trends in asthma prevalence and recommended number of childhood immunizations are not parallel. *Pediatrics.* 2007;119(1):222-223.
52. Diekema DS. Responding to parental refusals of immunization of children. *Pediatrics.* 2005;115(5):1428-1431.
53. American Academy of Pediatrics. Parental refusal of immunization. In: Pickering LK, ed. *Red Book: 2006 Report of the Committee on Infectious Diseases.* 27th ed. Elk Grove Village, IL: American Academy of Pediatrics; 2006:7-8.
54. Gust D, Brown C, Sheedy K, Hibbs B, Weaver D, Nowak G. Immunization attitudes and beliefs among parents: beyond a dichotomous perspective. *Am J Health Behav.* 2005;29(1):81-92.
55. Fredrickson DD, Davis TC, Arnold CL, et al. Childhood immunization refusal: provider and parent perceptions. *Fam Med.* 2004;36(6):431-439.
56. Smith PJ, Kennedy AM, Wooten K, Gust DA, Pickering LK. Association between health care providers' influence on parents who have concerns about vaccine safety and vaccination coverage. *Pediatrics.* 2006;118(5):E1287-E1292.
57. Salmon DA, Moulton LH, Omer SB, DeHart MP, Stokley S, Halsey NA. Factors associated with refusal of childhood vaccines among parents of school-aged children: a case-control study. *Arch Pediatr Adolesc Med.* 2005;159(5):470-476.
58. Measles outbreak hits 127 people in 15 states. Available on-line at: http://www.reuters.com/article/healthNews/idUSNO943743120080709?feedType=RSS&feedName=healthNews&rpc=22&sp=true. Accessed July 14, 2008.

CHAPTER 4

Infection Control in the Office

Thomas J. Sandora

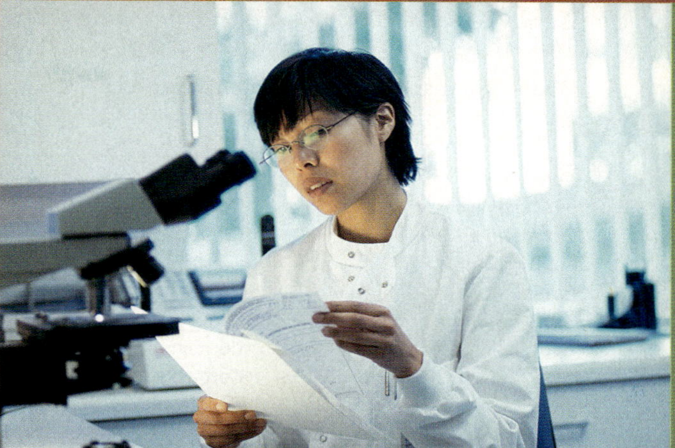

INTRODUCTION

Infection control is a critical component of pediatric practice in the outpatient setting. Children seen in an office for sick visits frequently have infections that may be transmitted to other patients or staff. In addition, as the delivery of complex medical care continues to shift from the hospital to the outpatient setting, careful attention to infection control practices in the office has become increasingly important. Clinicians should understand the epidemiology and modes of transmission of common pediatric infections. In addition, office practitioners must be familiar with regulations that apply to infectious diseases, including requirements for purchasing safety devices for staff, reporting diseases to public health agencies, and cleaning and disinfection in the office environment to prevent the transmission of infections.

ROUTES OF TRANSMISSION OF INFECTIOUS AGENTS

There are three primary modes of transmission by which microorganisms can be spread between patients and health care workers: contact, droplet, and airborne. (Additional routes of transmission, including common vehicle and vector-borne transmission, will not be reviewed here.) The Centers for Disease Control and Prevention (CDC) and the Healthcare Infection Control Practices Advisory Committee issue national guidelines and recommendations for preventing and controlling health-care-associated infections.[1] These guidelines apply to both inpatient and outpatient settings, and they serve as the source for the application of transmission-based precautions in health care settings.

Many common infections encountered in pediatric practice are transmitted by direct or indirect contact. Direct contact refers to person-to-person spread of an organism through direct physical contact. Indirect contact refers to spread that occurs by means of contact with a contaminated intermediate object (often fomites such as stethoscopes, bed linens, etc.), including the hands of health care workers; this route is the most important means of transmission of infections in health care settings.

Transmission via the droplet route occurs when large droplets are generated as an infected person coughs, sneezes, or talks. These droplets are propelled a short distance (generally less than 3 ft), and are deposited on the eyes, nasal mucosa, or mouth of a susceptible host.

Airborne transmission occurs when small droplet nuclei, dust particles, or skin squames containing microorganisms are transmitted to a susceptible host by air currents. Infections that are transmitted by the airborne route may be spread to others who are quite distant in space from the source infection.

Table 4–1 reviews the primary modes of transmission for many common infections that may be encountered in a pediatric practice. Each of these modes of transmission requires a unique strategy to prevent the spread of infection (see "Isolation Precautions in the Outpatient Setting").

HAND HYGIENE

Because contact with contaminated hands of health care workers is the primary means of transmission of infections in the health care setting, hand hygiene is the single most important method of preventing the spread of

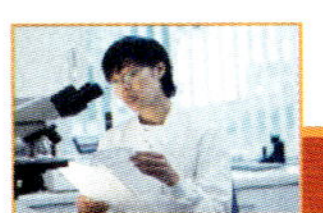

Table 4–1.

Modes of Transmission of Common Infections

Organism	Mode of Transmission
Adenovirus	Droplet and contact
Bordetella pertussis	Droplet
Clostridium difficile	Contact
Enteroviruses	Contact
Giardia	Contact
Group A *Streptococcus*	Droplet
Hepatitis A	Contact
HSV	Contact
Influenza	Droplet
Lice	Contact
Measles	Airborne
MRSA	Contact
Mycobacterium tuberculosis	Airborne
Mycoplasma pneumoniae	Droplet
Neisseria meningitidis	Droplet
Norovirus	Contact
Parainfluenza	Contact
Rotavirus	Contact
RSV	Contact
Salmonella, Shigella, E. coli O157:H7	Contact
Scabies	Contact
Varicella	Airborne and contact
VRE	Contact
Zoster	Contact (may be airborne in immunocompromised patients)

HSV, herpes simplex virus; MRSA, methicillin-resistant Staphylococcus aureus; RSV, respiratory syncytial virus; VRE, vancomycin-resistant enterococcus.

infections. Numerous studies in health care facilities have demonstrated the effectiveness of hand hygiene in reducing health-care-associated infections.[2–8] Several limitations of traditional handwashing with soap and water (including the need for access to sinks and the 15 seconds of vigorous rubbing required for optimal effect) have contributed to poor compliance with hand-hygiene practices in health care settings.[7,9–11] Alcohol-based hand sanitizers have several advantages, including increased killing of many organisms compared with soap and water; no requirement for access to running water; and less time required for proper use. In 2002, CDC endorsed alcohol-based hand sanitizers as the preferred products for decontaminating the hands of health care workers.[12] This recommendation applies to office practice as well; providers should have alcohol-based hand sanitizers available for use in their clinics or office spaces, in addition to sinks (for use when hands are visibly soiled or for particular organisms against which soap and water are more effective, such as *Clostridium difficile*).

DESIGN ISSUES FOR THE PEDIATRIC OFFICE

Several aspects of the design of an ambulatory care facility can impact the transmission of infectious diseases. Detailed information about current recommendations can be found in the most current version of the Guidelines for Design and Construction of Healthcare Facilities from the American Institute of Architects.[13]

Waiting areas should be designed in a fashion that allows for spatial separation of patients with potentially communicable diseases. Contact between healthy children and those with active infections should be minimized to the extent possible.[14] During influenza season, persons in the waiting area (including patients and family members or guardians) should ideally be instructed to practice components of respiratory hygiene and cough etiquette as recommended by CDC.[15] Office providers should post visual alerts containing instructions about how to prevent the spread of infections from coughing, and tissues and hands-free disposal receptacles should be provided. In addition, waiting areas should have easy access to hand-hygiene agents (either alcohol-based sanitizers or sinks with soap and water). Children who present with illnesses that may be transmitted by the airborne route should be immediately placed into an examination room with the door closed. Examination rooms should always contain a sink, and an alcohol-based hand sanitizer should be easily accessible.

BLOODBORNE PATHOGENS

Because of occupational exposures, health care workers are potentially at risk of acquiring several bloodborne viral infections, including human immunodeficiency virus (HIV), hepatitis B, and hepatitis C. The Occupational Safety and Health Administration (OSHA) mandates that health care providers in the outpatient setting adhere to the Bloodborne Pathogen Standard,[16] and the Joint Commission specifies that infection-control policies and procedures be consistent across the inpatient and outpatient arenas within a facility.[17] It is, therefore, incumbent on outpatient providers to understand issues around preventing transmission of these bloodborne pathogens.

The frequency of sharps injuries can be drastically reduced by the use of safety devices. "Safety" versions of needles and other devices are now widely available. These safety devices use technologies such as retractable needles to reduce the likelihood of a sharps injury. OSHA requires that health care facilities use devices with engineered sharps injury protections.[16] Outpatient practices should regularly review their inventory of devices and actively replace products with safety versions where applicable. Devices of particular interest in the outpatient setting include needles used for administration of immunizations, other injectable medications, or phlebotomy; safety versions of all of these devices are currently available.

When needlestick injuries do occur, every outpatient practice needs to have in place a process for managing exposed employees. As a routine, the risk of the particular exposure for transmitting bloodborne pathogens must be assessed, and employees should be counseled about risks and about the decision to take antiretroviral medications as postexposure prophylaxis for HIV. In addition, procedures must be in place to arrange for testing source patients for HIV and hepatitis B and C. Recommendations for management of these scenarios are available from CDC.[18,19] Since most exposed personnel will be adults, many pediatric office providers choose to contract with an adult provider or other resource for assistance in managing exposures.

REPORTING DISEASES TO PUBLIC HEALTH AUTHORITIES

Prompt reporting of communicable diseases is the foundation of public health surveillance and disease control. Information obtained through disease reporting is crucial to alert the public to potential health concerns, monitor disease trends and identify high-risk groups. As of January 2007, there were 63 reportable diseases in the United States at a national level; these diseases are reported weekly in Morbidity and Mortality Weekly Report (www.cdc.gov/mmwr), and are summarized annually by CDC in the "Summary of Notifiable Diseases in the United States." Reporting of these diseases is regulated by individual states. Although the details may differ from state to state, every state has regulations mandating that specified diseases or conditions be reported to local or state public health agencies. All health care providers are responsible for knowing these regulations and for reporting diseases according to their local or state guidelines. In general, certain infections with high mortality or large public health implications (such as meningococcal infections, measles, or smallpox) must be reported immediately; other infections (such as pertussis, varicella, or invasive Group A streptococcal infection) may in some cases be reported in a slightly less emergent fashion (e.g., 1–2 business days). While clinical laboratories have their own reporting requirements, individual providers are also responsible for reporting these conditions. Providers should also be clear about which infections are reported to local boards of health and which are reported directly to the state department of public health. For details about regulations for your own state, refer to your local and state public health agencies.

OFFICE ENVIRONMENT

Many features of the office environment have infection-control implications, and providers should be familiar with requirements pertaining to processes for storage and disposal of regulated products or waste.

Vaccine storage is a key component of an outpatient pediatric practice. While some vaccines (such as varicella) can be stored frozen (5°F or lower), many others including diphtheria/tetanus/acellular pertussis, measles/mumps/rubella, and pneumococcal conjugate vaccine are refrigerated prior to use. Refrigerated vaccines must be stored in the range of 36–46°F to maintain their efficacy. CDC recommends continuously monitoring the temperature of any refrigerator used to store vaccines, since unanticipated failure of cooling could compromise the efficacy of a vaccine if administered to patients.[20] Office practices should keep a log of temperatures on the refrigerator at all times.

Storage of medications and patient specimens must comply with OSHA standards. Medications must be stored in a separate refrigerator from patient specimens (such as urine or other body fluids that could be potentially infectious). Refrigerators used for specimen storage should be clearly marked by the use of a biohazard sticker on the outside of the refrigerator.[16]

OSHA regulations require that sharps and medical waste be disposed of in the appropriate manner.[16] Designated puncture-proof sharps containers must be available as close as is practical to the location where needles or other devices capable of causing injury will be used. The containers must be closable and labeled or color-coded. The containers must not be overfilled with disposed sharps in order to avoid needles sticking out of the opening. Practices frequently choose to contract with a company to empty their sharps containers on a regular basis. Medical waste (sometimes referred to as "infectious waste") is a term used to describe waste that is potentially infectious or hazardous (for instance, linens contaminated with blood). In general, facilities must define which waste is infectious and develop protocols for separating infectious waste from noninfectious waste. Procedures should be in place for proper labeling, storage, and disposal of infectious waste (e.g., red waste containers with a biohazard label). A more complete review of medical waste management is available for providers who are responsible for developing waste management programs for outpatient facilities.[21]

CLEANING AND DISINFECTION

Office providers must be responsible for ensuring that appropriate cleaning and disinfection measures are in place to prevent the transmission of infections within the office. Many different contaminated devices have been implicated in the transmission of infections.[22–24] Following a brief review of disinfection and sterilization principles, several specific items commonly present in outpatient practices will be addressed. Several excellent published reviews of disinfection and sterilization are available for readers who are interested in more details.[25–29]

Sterilization is the complete destruction of all forms of microbial life, including fungal and bacterial spores. Sterilization is accomplished by physical and chemical processes (e.g., steam under pressure, liquid chemicals, etc.). Disinfection eliminates many or all pathogenic organisms, with the exception of spores. Disinfection is usually performed using liquid chemicals or wet pasteurization. The same chemical may act as a sterilant with prolonged exposure time (e.g., 6–10 h), but only as a disinfectant at shorter exposure times (e.g., less than 45 min). Cleaning refers to the removal of all foreign material (e.g., organic matter) from an object, usually through the use of water with detergents or enzymatic products.[27] It is important to note that cleaning of equipment must precede sterilization or disinfection.

Whether a patient care item requires cleaning, disinfection, or sterilization is based on the associated risk of transmission of infection given its intended use. In general, items are divided into three categories: critical, semicritical, or noncritical.[29] Table 4–2 reviews the distinction between these categories and summarizes the appropriate disinfection and sterilization procedures for each group of items.

In the office setting, providers most commonly use noncritical reusable medical equipment, such as stethoscopes and blood pressure cuffs. These items pose little risk of infection to the patient because they only come into contact with intact skin, which functions as a barrier to most microorganisms. The same is true of examination tables and office floors. These items should be disinfected using low-level disinfectants approved by the Environmental Protection Agency, such as quaternary ammonium compounds. Ambulatory facilities should establish a regular schedule for cleaning and disinfection of these items (generally at least daily in addition to when items are soiled). Single-use items such as otoscope specula should be discarded after use; reprocessing of single-use items places the liability on the facility instead of on the manufacturer and, therefore, requires extensive oversight to ensure adequate disinfection and preserved function of equipment.

Multidose vials have been associated with multiple outbreaks in outpatient clinics[30]; if single-dose vials cannot be used because of cost or availability, careful attention must be paid to proper use of multidose vials and appropriate infection-control precautions.

Toys pose a unique challenge in the pediatric ambulatory setting. Toys can serve as fomites in the transmission of infection among patients. Facilities can reduce the risk of transmission by purchasing toys that are easily cleaned or disinfected. Hard, smooth objects made of plastic lend themselves more easily to cleaning procedures than furry stuffed animals or complex games with grooves and ridges that can harbor bacteria or viruses and are difficult to clean. No

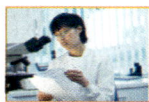

Table 4–2.

Sterilization and Disinfection

Category of Item	Examples	Method
Critical (will enter sterile tissue or vascular system, or blood will flow through it)	Surgical instruments	Sterilization
Semicritical (will come in contact with mucous membranes or nonintact skin)	Respiratory therapy equipment, endoscopes, thermometers	High-level disinfection*
Noncritical (will come in contact with intact skin)	Blood pressure cuffs, stethoscopes, linens, exam tables, floors	Low-level disinfection†

*High-level disinfection refers to killing all microorganisms except spores.

†Low-level disinfection refers to killing most vegetative bacteria, some fungi and some viruses but not spores.

published standards exist to regulate cleaning of toys in health care settings; however, offices should establish cleaning policies that call for toys to be cleaned on a routine basis (often daily in addition to after exposure to secretions or to patients with certain known infections).

ISOLATION PRECAUTIONS IN THE OUTPATIENT SETTING

Isolation precautions for patients with communicable diseases are a critical part of infection control within the hospital setting, and Healthcare Infection Control Practices Advisory Committee guidelines[1] provide recommendations for isolation precautions for specific infections or clinical syndromes. These recommendations also apply to ambulatory health care settings, and providers should be aware of measures to reduce the transmission of infections within the office.

Methicillin-resistant *Staphylococcus aureus* (MRSA) infections have been a part of health care since the 1960s, and their frequency began to rise notably in the 1980s. Initially, most patients with MRSA infections had risk factors for resistant infections, such as frequent contact with health care facilities. Since the mid-1990s, there has been a well-documented rise in the rate of community-acquired MRSA (CA-MRSA) infections in adults and children across the United States[31–33]; at some centers, up to 60–80% of pediatric MRSA infections are now community-acquired. Since these patients are frequently seen in the office setting for concerns such as skin and soft tissue infections, the office practitioner must be cognizant of infection-control measures in the clinic to reduce the likelihood of transmission of MRSA to other patients. Gloves should be worn for contact with any patient with known or suspected MRSA infection. Offices must ensure that an adequate supply of gloves is available at all times, and that they are easily accessible to providers at the point of entry into an examination room. Gowns should be available for encounters in which extensive contact with the patient is anticipated, in order to decrease contamination of clothing. Strict attention to hand hygiene, preferably with an alcohol-based hand sanitizer, is also critical.

C. difficile is another infection that has been seen traditionally in hospitalized patients but has become more prevalent in the community in recent years.[34,35] *C. difficile* is a spore-producing organism that is also transmitted by contact. If a patient with known or suspected *C. difficile* infection is seen in clinic, gloves should be used for contact with the patient. After examining such a patient, hand hygiene should be performed using soap and water rather than an alcohol-based agent, as alcohol has poor activity against spore-forming organisms and therefore is not the preferred method of hand decontamination for this infection.[12,36]

The most common infections seen by pediatricians in the outpatient setting are viral respiratory and gastrointestinal infections, including respiratory syncytial virus (RSV) and rotavirus (among others). These viral infections are also transmitted by contact, and in the hospital setting would require gown and glove use. During the winter and spring when these infections comprise a majority of sick visits to an office, implementing appropriate infection-control measures can seem overwhelming. It is important for practitioners to understand the infectivity of these organisms and their potential for transmission.

Rotavirus is present in high titers in the stool of infected patients, and is shed for an average of 4 days during infection (although the virus may persist for weeks in some cases).[37] The virus can survive on environmental surfaces for several weeks, and contamination of various items (such as toys and patient charts) in the health care setting is well documented.[38]

RSV is also primarily transmitted by contact, as documented in a classic study by Hall and Douglas.[39] Volunteers caring for infants with RSV were divided into three groups: "cuddlers," who held and provided care for the infants; "touchers," who did not touch the infant but had extensive contact with the environment, which had been contaminated with patient secretions; and "sitters," who sat by the crib but did not touch the patient or the environment. RSV infection developed in 5 of 7 cuddlers, 4 of 10 touchers, and 0 of 14 sitters. RSV is usually shed for 3–8 days during infection,[40] and the virus can survive for up to 6 hours on environmental surfaces.[41]

Because of the nature of transmission of these common viral infections, office practitioners should be vigilant about ensuring strict attention to hand hygiene in the office and appropriate cleaning and disinfection of contaminated surfaces. In addition, glove use in the office setting when seeing patients who have infections that are transmitted by contact may help to reduce contamination of the hands with infectious organisms.

MANAGING ILLNESS IN PATIENTS AND STAFF MEMBERS

Clinicians who see patients in an ambulatory setting are asked frequently to answer questions regarding infection-control implications of infectious diseases. Providers should be knowledgeable about potential criteria for excluding children from school or out-of-home child care, as well as methods to prevent infection in staff members and criteria for exclusion from work when staff members become ill.

As of 1999, more than 7.5 million children younger than 5 years of age were enrolled in out-of-home child care.[4] Attendance at child care places children at high risk of acquiring contagious diseases,[42–51] because children readily exchange secretions and staff members face daunting challenges in environmental sanitation.[52,53] The most common infections encountered in the child care setting include viral respiratory and gastrointestinal infections (rotavirus is the most frequent cause of gastroenteritis in child care), enteric bacteria such as *Shigella* and *E. coli* O157:H7, hepatitis A, parasites such as *Giardia* and cryptosporidium, and encapsulated bacteria (such as *Streptococcus pneumoniae*, *Neisseria meningitidis*, and *Haemophilus influenzae*).

In the child care setting, the most common routes of transmission of infections include fecal–oral, droplet, and person-to-person contact. In most situations, common sense hygienic practices will decrease the risk of illness transmission. Mild illness is common among children younger than 5 years, and most children need not be excluded from child care for mild respiratory tract illness. Exclusion is recommended when doing so is likely to decrease the risk of secondary cases. Table 4–3 summarizes some illnesses for which exclusion from child care is reasonable.[54] Examples of illnesses that generally do not require exclusion include rash without fever or behavioral change; parvovirus B19 infection in immunocompetent hosts; cytomegalovirus infection; and HIV or chronic hepatitis B infection in most cases. Each child care center is likely to have its own list of illnesses for which exclusion is required, and written procedures for hand hygiene, environmental sanitation, and managing illness in children and staff members should be in place. Consultation with local and state public health agencies is also recommended when deciding about whether to exclude an ill child from child care, as most states have laws about isolation of persons with specific communicable diseases.

Health care workers who are exposed to or contract selected illnesses should also be restricted from work to decrease the risk of transmission to patients or other staff members. State and local public health regulations should be consulted when creating exclusion policies. Table 4–4 provides a list of illnesses that generally require health care worker exclusion from patient care activities.[55,56] Decisions about work restriction for specific illnesses are made based on the epidemiology of the particular infection and its mode of transmission. Providers should ensure that policies encourage personnel to report their illnesses and that wages are provided during periods of required exclusion even if workmen's compensation laws do not require reimbursement.

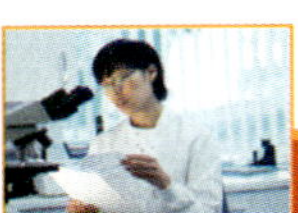

Table 4–3.

Possible Reasons for Exclusion from Child Care*

Illness	Notes
Conjunctivitis	Until resolves
Diarrhea or stools that contain blood or mucus	Until resolves
Head lice	Until after first treatment
Hepatitis A	Until 1 week after onset of symptoms or jaundice
Impetigo	Until 24 hours after therapy instituted
Measles	Until 4 days after onset of rash
Mumps	Until 9 days after onset of parotid swelling
Pertussis	Until 5 days of antimicrobial therapy has been completed
Rash with fever or behavior change	Until determined to be noninfectious
Scabies	Until after treatment
Shigella or E. coli O157:H7	Until diarrhea resolves and 2 stool cultures are negative
Streptococcal pharyngitis	Until 24 hours after therapy instituted
Tuberculosis	Until deemed to be noninfectious by public health authorities or treating physician
Vomiting	If more than twice in prior 24 hours, unless a noninfectious etiology is identified
Varicella	Until all lesions have crusted

**Consult local public health recommendations as well as any rules for a specific child care center.*

Many infections to which health care workers may be exposed can be prevented by vaccination. Office practitioners should be familiar with published recommendations for vaccination of health care workers.[55,57–59] Table 4–5 reviews these recommended vaccines. Review of vaccination status and mandatory immunization of employees should be part of a comprehensive occupational health program for all health care facilities. These activities should occur at the time of hire for new employees and as part of an annual review for current employees, since new vaccines may be added to the list of recommended immunizations and selected vaccines (such as influenza) must be delivered annually.

Tuberculosis (TB) screening for health care workers should also be done based on the risk classification of the facility, according to published CDC guidelines.[60] Outpatient health care settings are

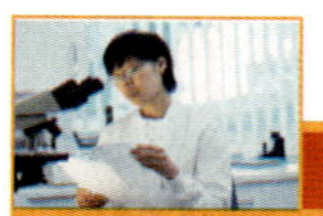

Table 4–4.

Restrictions for Health Care Workers with Infections*

Illness	Work Restriction	Duration
Conjunctivitis	Restrict from patient contact	Until discharge resolves
Gastroenteritis	Restrict from patient contact and food handling	Until symptoms resolve
Hepatitis A	Restrict from patient contact and food handling	Until 7 days after onset of jaundice
Hepatitis B	No restriction; standard precautions should always be observed	
Hepatitis C	No restriction; standard precautions should always be observed	
Herpes simplex virus, orofacial	Restrict from care of high-risk patients, including neonates	Until lesions crust over
Herpes simplex virus, herpetic whitlow	Restrict from patient contact	Until lesions crust over
HIV	No restriction; standard precautions should always be observed	
Measles	Exclude from office	For active disease, until 4 days after rash onset; for exposure in susceptible personnel, from 5th day after first exposure through 21st day after last exposure
Meningococcus	Exclude from office	Until 24 hours after starting effective therapy
Mumps	Exclude from office	Until 9 days after onset of parotitis
Pediculosis (lice)	Restrict from patient contact	Until treated and observed to be free of lice
Pertussis	Exclude from office	Until 5 days after start of effective therapy; personnel who have been exposed but are asymptomatic may work if they are receiving antimicrobial prophylaxis
Respiratory viral infections with fever	Consider excluding from care of high-risk patients during community outbreaks of influenza or RSV	Until symptoms resolve
Rubella	Exclude from office	Until 5 days after rash onset
Scabies	Restrict from patient contact	Until treated
Streptococcal pharyngitis	Restrict from patient contact	Until 24 hours after start of effective therapy
Tuberculosis, active disease	Exclude from office	Until proven noninfectious; personnel with latent TB infection (skin test positive but no active disease) may work without restriction
Varicella	Exclude from office	Until all lesions crust over; exposed susceptible personnel should be excluded from 10th day after first exposure through 21st day after last exposure
Zoster	Cover lesions and restrict from care of high-risk patients, including neonates and immunocompromised persons	Localized zoster–until all lesions crust over; zoster in an immunocompromised health care worker—restrict from patient contact

**State and local public health regulations should always be followed.*
HIV, human immunodeficiency virus; RSV, respiratory syncytial virus.

currently classified as low risk if fewer than three TB patients were seen during the preceding year, and medium risk if more than three TB patients were seen during the preceding year. For low-risk settings, health care workers should undergo TB screening at hire and then only need additional screening if an exposure to TB occurs. In contrast, for medium-risk settings, annual TB screening of health care workers should be performed. Clinics that are part of a larger health care setting might fall under different risk classification criteria based on the types of services provided and frequency of TB visits, and each facility should review the CDC guideline to determine its own risk classification and recommendations for screening.

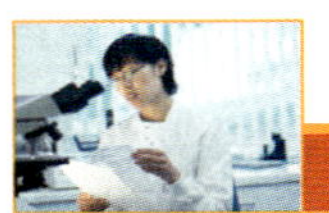

Table 4–5.

Recommended Immunizations for Health Care Workers

Vaccine	Notes
Measles	All employees who do not have proof of immunity, including those born before 1957
Mumps	All employees who do not have proof of immunity, including those born before 1957, can be considered immune
Rubella	All employees who do not have proof of immunity; adults born before 1957, *except* women who can become pregnant, can be considered immune
VZV	All employees who do not have evidence of immunity, defined as: documentation of two doses of vaccine; laboratory evidence of immunity or laboratory confirmation of disease; or health care provider verification of a history or diagnosis of varicella or zoster
Hepatitis B	Recommended for all health care workers, particularly those at risk for exposure to blood or body fluids
Influenza	Should receive vaccine annually prior to onset of flu season
Tdap	Health care workers who have direct patient care contact should receive a single dose as soon as feasible, at an interval as short as 2 years from the last dose of Td; those without direct patient contact should receive a single dose to replace the next scheduled Td (no greater than 10 years since the last Td, but they are encouraged to receive Tdap at an interval as short as 2 years following the last Td)

VZV, varicella-zoster virus (live vaccine); Tdap, tetanus/diphtheria/acellular pertussis; Td, tetanus/diphtheria.

SUMMARY

Infection control in the outpatient setting is complex and requires constant vigilance by providers as well as systematic attention to high-risk activities. Emphasis should be placed on proper hand hygiene, in addition to other fundamental principles to prevent the transmission of infections, including isolation precautions and surface disinfection. Clinicians should be familiar with appropriate regulations and should be aware of relevant literature to guide infection-control practices. Providers who have questions about infection-control issues should consult available resources, including infection-control practitioners at affiliated health care facilities, as well as local and state public health officials.

REFERENCES

1. Siegel JD, Rhinehart E, Jackson M, Chiarello L, and the Healthcare Infection Control Practices Advisory Committee. 2007 guideline for isolation precautions: preventing transmission of infectious agents in healthcare setting. *Am J Infect Control.* 2007;35(10 Suppl 2):S65-S164.
2. Fendler EJ, Ali Y, Hammond BS, Lyons MK, Kelley MB, Vowell NA. The impact of alcohol hand sanitizer use on infection rates in an extended care facility. *Am J Infect Control.* 2002;30(4):226-233.
3. Hilburn J, Hammond BS, Fendler EJ, Groziak PA. Use of alcohol hand sanitizer as an infection control strategy in an acute care facility. *Am J Infect Control.* 2003;31(2):109-116.
4. Doebbeling BN, Stanley GL, Sheetz CT, et al. Comparative efficacy of alternative hand-washing agents in reducing nosocomial infections in intensive care units. *N Engl J Med.* 1992;327(2):88-93.
5. Maki DG. The use of antiseptics for handwashing by medical personnel. *J Chemother.* 1989;(1 suppl 1):3-11.
6. Mortimer EA, Jr., Lipsitz PJ, Wolinsky E, Gonzaga AJ, Rammelkamp CH, Jr. Transmission of staphylococci between newborns. Importance of the hands to personnel. *Am J Dis Child.* 1962;104:289-295.
7. Pittet D, Hugonnet S, Harbarth S, et al. Effectiveness of a hospital-wide programme to improve compliance with hand hygiene. Infection Control Programme. *Lancet.* 2000;356(9238):1307-1312.
8. Webster J, Faoagali JL, Cartwright D. Elimination of methicillin-resistant Staphylococcus aureus from a neonatal intensive care unit after hand washing with triclosan. *J Paediatr Child Health.* 1994;30(1):59-64.
9. Gould D. Nurses' hand decontamination practice: results of a local study. *J Hosp Infect.* 1994;28(1):15-30.
10. Larson E, Kretzer EK. Compliance with handwashing and barrier precautions. *J Hosp Infect.* 1995;30 (suppl):88-106.
11. Watanakunakorn C, Wang C, Hazy J. An observational study of hand washing and infection control practices by healthcare workers. *Infect Control Hosp Epidemiol.* 1998; 19(11):858-860.
12. Boyce JM, Pittet D. Guideline for Hand Hygiene in Health-Care Settings. Recommendations of the Healthcare Infection Control Practices Advisory Committee and the HICPAC/SHEA/APIC/IDSA Hand Hygiene Task Force. Society for Healthcare Epidemiology of America/ Association for Professionals in Infection Control/ Infectious Diseases Society of America. *MMWR Recomm Rep.* 2002;51(RR-16):1-45, quiz CE1-4.
13. The American Institute of Architects & Facilities Guidelines Institute. *Guidelines for Design and Construction of Healthcare Facilities*; 2006.
14. American Academy of Pediatrics. Infection control and prevention in ambulatory settings. In: Pickering LK, ed. *Red Book: 2006 Report of the Committee on Infectious Diseases.* 27th ed. Elk Grove Village, IL: American Academy of Pediatrics; 2006:164-166.
15. Centers for Disease Control and Prevention. Respiratory Hygiene/Cough Etiquette in Healthcare Settings. http://www.cdc.gov/flu/professionals/infectioncontrol/resphygiene.htm. Accessed February 23, 2007.

16. Department of Labor, Occupational Safety and Health Administration. 29 CFR Part 1920.1030, Occupational exopsure to bloodborne pathogens, final rule. *Federal Register December.* 6, 1991;56:64,004-64,182.
17. Joint Commission on Accreditation of Healthcare Organizations. Leadership standard. *Comprehensive Accreditation Manual for Hospital: The Official Handbook.* Oakbrook Terrace, IL: JCAHO;1996:LD-1-LD-52.
18. Panlilio AL, Cardo DM, Grohskopf LA, Heneine W, Ross CS. Updated U.S. Public Health Service guidelines for the management of occupational exposures to HIV and recommendations for postexposure prophylaxis. *MMWR Recomm Rep.* 2005;54(RR-9):1-17.
19. Updated U.S. Public Health Service Guidelines for the Management of Occupational Exposures to HBV, HCV, and HIV and Recommendations for Postexposure Prophylaxis. *MMWR Recomm Rep.* 2001;50(RR-11):1-52.
20. Atkinson WL, Pickering LK, Schwartz B, Weniger BG, Iskander JK, Watson JC. General recommendations on immunization. Recommendations of the Advisory Committee on Immunization Practices (ACIP) and the American Academy of Family Physicians (AAFP). *MMWR Recomm Rep.* 2002;51(RR-2):1-35.
21. Gordon JG, Reinhardt PA, Denys GA. Medical waste management. In: Mayhall CG, ed. *Hospital Epidemiology and Infection Control.* Philadelphia: Lippincott Williams & Wilkins; 2004:1773-1785.
22. Cohen HA, Cohen Z, Kahan E. Bacterial contamination of spacer devices used by children with asthma. *JAMA.* 2003;290(2):195-196.
23. Srinivasan A, Wolfenden LL, Song X, et al. An outbreak of Pseudomonas aeruginosa infections associated with flexible bronchoscopes. *N Engl J Med.* 2003;348(3):221-227.
24. Yardy GW, Cox RA. An outbreak of Pseudomonas aeruginosa infection associated with contaminated urodynamic equipment. *J Hosp Infect.* 2001;47(1):60-63.
25. Rutala WA. APIC guideline for selection and use of disinfectants. 1994, 1995, and 1996 APIC Guidelines Committee. Association for Professionals in Infection Control and Epidemiology, Inc. *Am J Infect Control.* 1996;24(4):313-342.
26. Rutala WA. Disinfection and sterilization of patient-care items. *Infect Control Hosp Epidemiol.* 1996;17(6):377-384.
27. Rutala WA, Weber DJ. Infection control: the role of disinfection and sterilization. *J Hosp Infect.* 1999;43 (suppl): S43-S55.
28. Rutala WA, Weber DJ. New disinfection and sterilization methods. *Emerg Infect Dis.* 2001;7(2):348-353.
29. Rutala WA, Weber DJ. Disinfection and sterilization in health care facilities: what clinicians need to know. *Clin Infect Dis.* 2004;39(5):702-709.
30. Herwaldt LA, Smith SD, Carter CD. Infection control in the outpatient setting. *Infect Control Hosp Epidemiol.* 1998;19(1):41-74.
31. Fergie JE, Purcell K. Community-acquired methicillin-resistant Staphylococcus aureus infections in south Texas children. *Pediatr Infect Dis J.* 2001;20(9):860-863.
32. Buckingham SC, McDougal LK, Cathey LD, et al. Emergence of community-associated methicillin-resistant Staphylococcus aureus at a Memphis, Tennessee Children's Hospital. *Pediatr Infect Dis J.* 2004;23(7): 619-624.
33. Kaplan SL, Hulten KG, Gonzalez BE, et al. Three-year surveillance of community-acquired Staphylococcus aureus infections in children. *Clin Infect Dis.* 2005;40(12): 1785-1791.
34. Centers for Disease Control and Prevention (CDC). Severe Clostridium difficile-associated disease in populations previously at low risk–four states, 2005. *MMWR.* 2005;54(47):1201-1205.
35. Bloomfield SF, Cookson B, Falkiner F, Griffith C, Cleary V. Methicillin-resistant Staphylococcus aureus, Clostridium difficile, and extended-spectrum beta-lactamase-producing Escherichia coli in the community: assessing the problem and controlling the spread. *Am J Infect Control.* 2007; 35(2):86-88.
36. Weber DJ, Sickbert-Bennett E, Gergen MF, Rutala WA. Efficacy of selected hand hygiene agents used to remove Bacillus atrophaeus (a surrogate of Bacillus anthracis) from contaminated hands. *JAMA.* 2003;289(10):1274-1277.
37. American Academy of Pediatrics. Rotavirus infections. In: Pickering LK, ed. *Red Book: 2006 Report of the Committee on Infectious Diseases.* 27th ed. Elk Grove Village, IL: American Academy of Pediatrics; 2006:572-574.
38. Akhter J, al-Hajjar S, Myint S, Qadri SM. Viral contamination of environmental surfaces on a general paediatric ward and playroom in a major referral centre in Riyadh. *Eur J Epidemiol.* 1995;11(5):587-590.
39. Hall CB, Douglas RG, Jr. Modes of transmission of respiratory syncytial virus. *J Pediatr.* 1981;99(1):100-103.
40. American Academy of Pediatrics. Respiratory syncytial virus. In: Pickering LK, ed. *Red Book: 2006 Report of the Committee on Infectious Diseases.* 27th ed. Elk Grove Village, IL: American Academy of Pediatrics; 2006: 560-566.
41. Hall CB, Douglas RG, Jr., Geiman JM. Possible transmission by fomites of respiratory syncytial virus. *J Infect Dis.* 1980;141(1):98-102.
42. Holmes SJ, Morrow AL, Pickering LK. Child-care practices: effects of social change on the epidemiology of infectious diseases and antibiotic resistance. *Epidemiol Rev.* 1996;18(1):10-28.
43. Hurwitz ES, Gunn WJ, Pinsky PF, Schonberger LB. Risk of respiratory illness associated with day-care attendance: a nationwide study. *Pediatrics.* 1991;87(1):62-69.
44. Lemp GF, Woodward WE, Pickering LK, Sullivan PS, DuPont HL. The relationship of staff to the incidence of diarrhea in day-care centers. *Am J Epidemiol.* 1984;120 (5): 750-758.
45. Sullivan P, Woodward WE, Pickering LK, DuPont HL. Longitudinal study of occurrence of diarrheal disease in day care centers. *Am J Public Health.* 1984;74(9): 987-991.
46. Wald ER, Dashefsky B, Byers C, Guerra N, Taylor F. Frequency and severity of infections in day care. *J Pediatr.* 1988;112(4):540-546.
47. Child care and common communicable illnesses: results from the National Institute of Child Health and Human Development Study of Early Child Care. *Arch Pediatr Adolesc Med.* 2001;155(4):481-488.
48. Bartlett AV, Moore M, Gary GW, Starko KM, Erben JJ, Meredith BA. Diarrheal illness among infants and

toddlers in day care centers. II. Comparison with day care homes and households. *J Pediatr.* 1985;107(4):503-509.

49. Fleming DW, Cochi SL, Hightower AW, Broome CV. Childhood upper respiratory tract infections: to what degree is incidence affected by day-care attendance? *Pediatrics.* 1987;79(1):55-60.
50. Louhiala PJ, Jaakkola N, Ruotsalainen R, Jaakkola JJ. Day-care centers and diarrhea: a public health perspective. *J Pediatr.* 1997;131(3):476-479.
51. Osterholm MT, Reves RR, Murph JR, Pickering LK. Infectious diseases and child day care. *Pediatr Infect Dis J.* 1992;11(8 suppl):S31-S41.
52. Goldmann DA. Transmission of infectious diseases in children. *Pediatr Rev.* 1992;13(8):283-293.
53. Goldmann DA. Transmission of viral respiratory infections in the home. *Pediatr Infect Dis J.* 2000;19(10 suppl):S97-S102.
54. American Academy of Pediatrics. Children in out-of-home childcare. In: Pickering LK, ed. *Red Book: 2003 Report of the Committee on Infectious Diseases.* 26th ed. Elk Grove Village, IL: American Academy of Pediatrics; 2003:123-137.
55. Bolyard EA, Tablan OC, Williams WW, Pearson ML, Shapiro CN, Deitchmann SD. Guideline for infection control in healthcare personnel, 1998. Hospital Infection Control Practices Advisory Committee. *Infect Control Hosp Epidemiol.* 1998;19(6):407-463.
56. Shah SS, Zsolway KW. Infection control and office practice management. *Pediatr Ann.* 2002;31(5):299-306.
57. Immunization of health-care workers: recommendations of the Advisory Committee on Immunization Practices (ACIP) and the Hospital Infection Control Practices Advisory Committee (HICPAC). *MMWR Recomm Rep.* 1997;46(RR-18):1-42.
58. Weber DJ, Rutala WA, Weigle K. Selection and use of vaccines for healthcare workers. *Infect Control Hosp Epidemiol.* 1997;18(10):682-687.
59. Kretsinger K, Broder KR, Cortese MM, et al. Preventing tetanus, diphtheria, and pertussis among adults: use of tetanus toxoid, reduced diphtheria toxoid and acellular pertussis vaccine recommendations of the Advisory Committee on Immunization Practices (ACIP) and recommendation of ACIP, supported by the Healthcare Infection Control Practices Advisory Committee (HICPAC), for use of Tdap among health-care personnel. *MMWR Recomm Rep.* 2006;55(RR-17):1-37.
60. Jensen PA, Lambert LA, Iademarco MF, Ridzon R. Guidelines for preventing the transmission of Mycobacterium tuberculosis in health-care settings, 2005. *MMWR Recomm Rep.* 2005;54(17):1-141.

CHAPTER 5

Infection Control in the Hospital

Robert Seese and Johanna Goldfarb

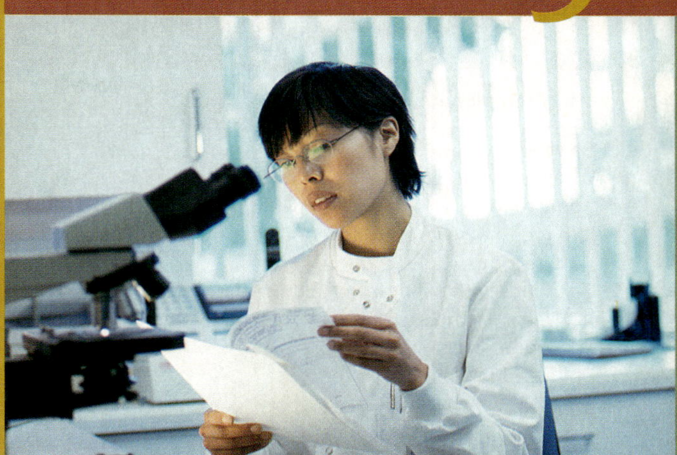

HAND HYGIENE

Hand hygiene is the most important infection-control practice, whether in the hospital, the clinic, or at home. By interrupting the transmission of pathogens, hand hygiene protects not only patients, but also the health care workers (HCWs) who care for them. Monitoring and encouraging compliance with proper hand hygiene is one of the most important goals of every infection control program.

Human skin is naturally colonized with bacteria; our hands have been estimated to have approximately 4 million bacteria/cm^2 of skin, mostly coagulase-negative staphylococci and diptheroids.[1–3] After admission to hospital, patients become colonized with different, more pathogenic organisms, some acquired in hospital, others brought from the community but increasing in number by stress of illness and antibiotic treatment.[4,5] These bacteria can become the source of nosocomial infections. After caring for a hospitalized patient, the hands of a HCW become contaminated with these "transient flora,"[6] which can then be passed onto the next patient cared for, to a chart, phone, or computer, unless removed by hand hygiene.[7] The deeper resident flora remains mostly intact.[8] Viral pathogens such as the respiratory syncytial virus (RSV) and rotavirus are also transmitted to the hands of HCWs during direct patient care,[9] and also by contact with fomites in the room. Hence, hand hygiene is crucial not only after touching a patient but also after entering a hospital room and handling objects in the room.

Gloves are used to decrease the risk of transmission of pathogens to hands of HCWs and have an important role in infection-control guidelines. However, gloves do not completely prevent transmission of organisms to our hands.[10] It is, therefore, necessary to clean hands after removing gloves and to change gloves when going from an infected site to a "clean" site.

Artificial nails can become colonized with gram-negative bacteria,[11,12] and should not be allowed for HCWs involved in direct patient care. In the nursery, rings are removed prior to washing hands on entering the nursery and should remain off until finished with direct patient care.[13] While at least one study has suggested that alcohol-based rubs are not adversely affected by the presence of rings,[14] other studies raise concern about the ability to remove bacteria adequately when rings are left on during hand hygiene.[13]

From Semmelweis' observation that hand hygiene could decrease the risk of puerperal fever and maternal death in an obstetrical ward in 1847, to a recent study showing decreased catheter-related bacteremia with attention to hand hygiene and infection-control guidelines,[15] hand hygiene really does save lives.

How Do We Do Hand Hygiene?

Soaps are detergents that remove organic substances and soiling materials from the hands, removing pathogens mechanically. Plain soaps without any antimicrobial additives reduce the burden of bacteria on the skin. A 15-second handwash can reduce the number of pathogenic bacteria on the skin by 0.6–1.1 $\log_{10}$.[1,16] However, bar soaps can become colonized with gram-negative bacteria and can become a fomite for spread of pathogens.[17] Antimicrobial agents have been added to soaps and most hospitals now use antimicrobial liquid-dispensed soaps to avoid this problem. The most common antimicrobial additives in soaps are triclosan and chlorhexidine, which act to

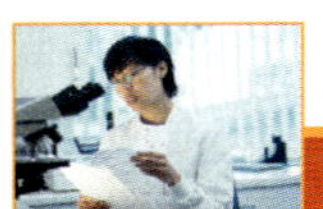

Table 5–1.

Hand Hygiene

Soap and water[45]
Wet hands with warm, not hot water
Apply soap
Rub together vigorously covering all surfaces and fingers for 15 seconds
Dry hands with paper towel and use the towel to turn off the water with the towel to avoid recontaminating hands on hand-operated sink
Estimated time: About 60 seconds

Alcohol-based rubs
Place rub directly in the palm of one hand
Amount is specific to the type and brand
Rub the compound on all surfaces of the hands and fingers
This should take about 15 seconds
Every 5–6 times, washing hands with soap and water will remove residue that may build up with repeated use
Estimated time: 15 seconds

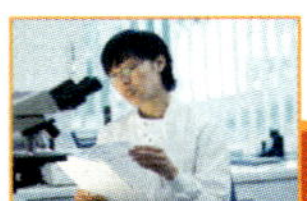

Table 5–2.

CDC 2002 Guide to Hand-Hygiene Recommendations Summarized

Alcohol-based hand rubs can be used:
Before and after each patient contact, before and after leaving a patient's room
Before and after gloving

Wash hands with soap and water:
When hands are visibly soiled
The patient has C. *difficile colitis*
Before eating and after using the rest room
Can be used before and after each patient contact, as you enter and as you leave a patient's room and before and after gloving

Use gloves to help decrease transmission of pathogens:
When touching mucosal surfaces
When touching areas of infection
When handling specimens of bodily fluids such as blood, urine, sputum, etc.
Remember to use hand hygiene after removing gloves and only soap and water if hands are visibly soiled
Remove gloves before examining a new area of the body or after putting down a sample. Clean hands before proceeding to the next part of your examination or going to a chart, phone or computer, or leaving the patient area

destabilize the cytoplasmic membrane of bacteria and yeast. Chlorhexidine also has excellent activity against enveloped viruses like HIV, HSV, RSV, influenza, and hepatitis viruses. Technique is important to be effective (Table 5–1).

In contrast to soaps, alcohol-based hand rubs operate primarily by denaturing proteins contained in microbes. Most commercial rubs contain ethanol, *n*-propanolol, or isopropanolol alcohol at varying concentrations. The most effective concentration of alcohol is between 60% and 95%.[18] At these concentrations, alcohols have activity against gram-positive bacteria, including MRSA and VRE, various gram-negative bacteria, fungi, mycobacteria, HSV, HIV, influenza virus, RSV, hepatitis B virus, hepatitis C virus, and rotavirus. Alcohols are **not** effective in destroying the spores of *Clostridium difficile*, protozoal oocysts and are **not** effective in cleaning visibly soiled hands; mechanical removal by soap and water is therefore recommended after contact with these infections.

Numerous studies, using various methods[19,20] have documented that alcohol-based hand rubs are effective, and many studies suggest increased efficacy compared to soap and water.[21] Newer hand rub products have added emollients and are much better tolerated than earlier products that dried the skin and were not well accepted. Nurses who use an alcohol rub compared to those using soap and water have less drying and cracking of the skin.[22,23] Additionally, studies have shown improved compliance with hand hygiene when hand rubs are made available to HCWs, as they are faster and easier to use effectively, and can be placed in areas where getting to a sink is difficult.[24]

Despite the importance of hand hygiene, many studies continue to show poor compliance with hand hygiene in most hospitals in this country. Important reasons that HCWs fail to comply with hand hygiene include overwork and a sense of not having enough time[25]; lack of role models ("if my attending physician doesn't clean his hands, why should I?"); and lack of understanding the need to use hand hygiene, especially after removing gloves. In response to these considerations and the increasing data that alcohol rubs improve compliance, the CDC in 2002 revised guidelines for hand hygiene and for the first time stressed the use of hand rubs (Table 5–2).[21]

Infection Control and Supporting Hand Hygiene

Methods to support and to promote hand hygiene include education, to be sure that every HCW understands proper hand hygiene; observation of hand hygiene practice with feedback and corrective action, if practice does not improve; placing more hand rubs in places where sinks are difficult to reach; educating patients and families and engaging their support in hand hygiene promotions; institutional role models and a commitment to safety within the institution. (Recommendations are reviewed in detail in reference 21 and at the Institute for Healthcare Improvement (IHI): How-to Guide: Improving Hand Hygiene: www. IHI.org). Hand hygiene is a constant concern and promoting it is necessary as part of each hospital's infection-control and safety programs.

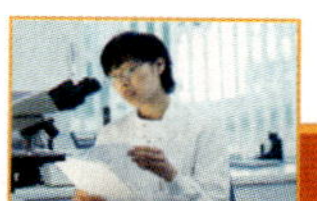

Table 5–3.

Recommendations for Standard Precautions*

Hand hygiene: Before and after each and every patient contact, or after touching blood, body fluids, secretions, excretions or contaminated items, and after removing gloves

Barriers: Personal protective equipment for special situations

Gloves: Put on before touching blood, body fluids, secretions, excretions or contaminated items, and/or touching a mucosal membrane or nonintact skin

Gown: Before doing a procedure or patient care activity when contact of clothing or exposed skin with blood/body fluids, secretions and excretions is anticipated

Mask: Before procedure or patient care likely to cause splashes or sprays of blood, body fluids, secretions, excretions or contaminated items

Eye protection/Face mask: Before a procedure or patient care activity that may cause splashes that could contaminate the eyes or face

Other Recommendations:

Patient Resuscitations: Mouth-to-mouth resuscitation should be avoided; use resuscitation bags and these should be readily available for emergency situations

Used linens and hospital garments should be treated as contaminated and possible sources of infection. They should be transported and processed in a manner that prevents contamination of the clothing, skin, or mucous membranes of HCWs or housekeeping staff

When handling needles and other sharps: Do not recap, bend, or break a sharp; whenever possible, use needle-free safety devices; place sharps in a puncture-resistant container when finished using. If recapping of a needle is necessary, use the single-hand technique **only**

**Standard precautions should be used with every patient encounter.*

TRANSMISSION OF INFECTIONS IN THE HOSPITAL SETTING

Isolation Precautions

All hospitalized patients should be handled with standard precautions, as outlined by the CDC Health Care Infection Control Practices Advisory Committee. These guidelines recognize that not only blood but also other body fluids pose a risk of carrying pathogens and that all patients should be treated in a consistent manner to decrease the risk of transmission of these pathogens between patients and HCWs. Standard precautions are based on the following basic assumptions:

1. Hand hygiene is the most important infection-control practice—the basis of all precautions including standard precautions.
2. Barrier techniques help to avoid contact with any body fluid or mucosal surface to decrease transmission of pathogens and include Gloves, gowns, mask, and eye protection or face shield as appropriate for patient contact.

Standard precautions for pediatrics are summarized in Table 5–3.

Transmission-Based Precautions

More specialized precautions are used to prevent the spread of specific microorganisms when standard precautions are not sufficient. The types of transmission-based precautions are airborne, droplet, and contact precautions (Table 5–4).

Airborne precautions are employed for infectious agents spread primarily by the droplet route, such as *Mycobacterium tuberculosis*, varicella zoster virus, and the measles virus. These organisms are carried on small-particle droplets or dust in the air, remaining suspended for long periods of time, and are subject to spread based on airflow. They can be spread over long distances, and require special ventilation and air handling. Patients should be given a private room with negative air pressure ventilation system that exhausts air externally or filter it through a high-efficiency particulate (HEPA) filter prior to recirculation. If a private room is not possible, patients with the same infectious agent should be cohorted. HCWs susceptible to infection with measles or varicella virus should not care for these patients. If susceptible workers must care for these children, a mask should be worn when in the room. Workers with immunity to measles or varicella do not require masks. N-95 masks, or other sealed respirators should be used in the care of patients with suspected or known cavitary pulmonary tuberculosis. HCWs require "fit" testing, to be sure that the mask selected is properly fit and will be protective, prior to using in the care of patients.

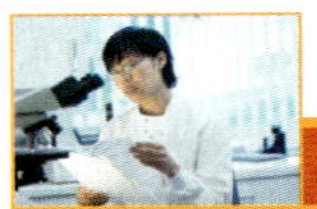

Table 5–4.

Transmission-Based Precautions in the Hospital*

Airborne: Single-patient room with negative air pressure and filtered air and 6–12 air changes per hour
Respirators: N95 mask or Powered Purified Air Respirator (does not require fit testing)
Gowns: No
Gloves: No

Droplet
Single patient room
Masks: Surgical mask put on entry into room
Gowns: No
Gloves: No

Contact
Single-patient room
Mask: No
Gowns: Yes
Gloves: Yes

Droplet precautions are used for organisms with transmission by aerosols from activities such as talking or sneezing. Aerosols deposited on the mucous membranes of another individual transmit infection. These larger droplets spread only over a more limited range of less than 3 ft, compared to airborne organisms. Since these microorganisms are contained in large droplets, they are not readily spread by air currents and therefore do not require negative pressure rooms with high-efficiency particulate filters or outside exhausts. In general, patients with an organism spread by droplet transmission should be given a private room. If a private room is not available, cohorting patients with the same infection is acceptable. If neither of these solutions is possible, then infected patients must be separated from their roommates by a distance of at least 3 ft. HCWs entering the room should wear masks to prevent infection when in close contact with the patient, within 3 ft. Masks should be removed and left in the room or anteroom, with hand hygiene after removing the mask. Organisms that require droplet precautions include adenovirus, diphtheria (pharyngeal), invasive *Haemophilus* type b, Influenza, mumps, *Neisseria meningiditis*, parvovirus prior to rash, pertussis, rubella, streptococcal respiratory infections, and the SARS virus.

Contact precaution is used to prevent both direct and indirect contact transmission. Direct contact transmission occurs when microorganisms are transferred from a patient to a HCW or another patient directly by direct contact (e.g., patient to hand of HCW). In contrast, indirect contact transmission occurs when the spread is via an intermediate object, such as when a HCW touches contaminated linens or bed surfaces and his hands become contaminated. Hand hygiene and barrier methods are particularly important in preventing the spread of these organisms. Patients should be given a private room, or cohorted with other patients with the same infection, and gloves should be worn at all times. If a HCW is likely to have contact with a patient's clothing or with surfaces in the patient's room, gowns should be worn and removed with gloves prior to leaving the room (or in an anteroom) and then hand hygiene. Organisms requiring this isolation include *C. difficile*, conjunctivitis, enteroviruses, *Escherichia coli* O157:H7, hepatitis A, herpes simplex virus: neonatal and cutaneous herpes zoster shingles, parainfluenza virus, RSV, rotavirus, scabies, *Shigella*, and *Staphylococcus aureus* draining wounds.

When the etiology of the infection is unknown, the transmission precautions can be used empirically and can be used in combination. For example, infants who are clinically diagnosed with bronchiolitis should be placed in both droplet and contact precautions if and until their specific pathogen is known. Similarly, pediatric patients with a diarrheal illness that is likely to be infectious should be placed in contact precautions.

Children placed in transmission-based precautions should not be allowed to leave their rooms for visits to the cafeteria or play rooms. Gloves are not required for routine diaper changes unless the child is in contact isolation. A full listing of organisms with isolation recommendations and incubation periods is available at the CDC Web site: www.cdc.gov/ncidod/dhqp/gl_isolation.

INFECTION CONTROL CONSIDERATIONS FOR THE HOSPITAL SETTING

Consoderations for Staff in Children's Units

HCWs should be screened by serology for vaccine-preventable infections and vaccine offered at the time of employment; infections include varicella zoster, measles, rubella, and mumps in addition to hepatitis B. The Tdap vaccine released in 2006 against tetanus, diphtheria, and pertussis should be given to employees 19–65 years of age if they have not received a tetanus booster in the last 2 years or when due for a booster. Yearly vaccination with the influenza virus vaccine should be standard. This vaccine can be given on hospital units, increasing compliance with this important recommendation. HCWs should also be evaluated for tuberculosis yearly, more frequently in high-risk areas. HCWs should be encouraged to stay at home and to avoid direct patient care when they are ill. They should be educated about the devastating effects that mild adult diseases, such as an upper respiratory infection or gastroenteritis, may have on children, especially infants and newborns.

Sibling Visitation

Visitation rules should complement isolation and safety procedures. In pediatric hospitals, family and sibling visits are important to the well-being of patients, but can also be a source of infectious diseases. Siblings should be evaluated outside the ward or intensive care unit by a trained HCW to evaluate each child for symptoms of contagious diseases and history of exposure to a contact with a known contagious disease to which the child is susceptible. Siblings should be excluded from visiting if they have fevers or symptoms of upper respiratory infection, gastroenteritis, or communicable viral exanthema. Some hospitals have utilized a sticker system that notifies the hospital staff that the visiting sibling has been screened and hence is wearing a specified sticker (e.g., green sticker for go).

Pet and Service Animal Visitations

An effective animal visitation policy involving allergic reactions, zoonotic transmission of infection, emotional reactions to the animals must be taken into account.[26] Pets should have documentation of their vaccinations and a certification from the attending veterinarian that the animals are free from disease and appropriate for visiting. Three types of animals are eligible for visits: personal pets, therapeutic animals, and service animals. Only canines and felines are eligible for visitation in the hospital. Children who have indwelling catheters in place should have these devices covered when interacting with the animal. In addition, the animals should be confined to the specific areas and in general, should not be allowed entry into intensive care units or nurseries.

Service animals differ from pets or therapeutic animals in that their presence is necessary to allow the disabled to perform daily tasks.[27] These animals, usually a professionally trained dog, have a role that has been legally defined by the Americans with Disabilities Act. As such, exclusionary rules may not apply as a matter of law. In general, all public facilities must allow service animals to accompany disabled citizens. Service animals may be barred from certain areas of the hospital if their presence would result in a danger to patients or a change in hospital functioning.

Infection Control in the Neonatal Intensive Care Unit

There is no more concerning site for infection control in the hospital than the Neonatal Intensive Care Unit (NICU), the site with the highest rate of nosocomial infections.[28] Neonates, and especially the premature neonate, are immuno-compromised hosts. In the NICU, infants are likely to have underlying medical disease often requiring prolonged hospital stays with invasive procedures and indwelling catheters. The premature infant may also have immature skin, those born before 32-weeks gestation have relatively permeable skin for the first 2 weeks after birth, allowing for the translocation of bacteria across the skin, with resultant transient bacteremias. In a similar manner, the mucosa of the mouth and gastrointestinal tract are underdeveloped and can allow translocation of organisms. The GI tract and upper airway at birth are sterile, becoming colonized with bacteria from the environment, normally that of the mother. If a child is critically ill and is in ICU, the flora is likely to be the more pathogenic flora of the hospital,[4] and even community-acquired flora will be pressured by antibiotic therapy toward more resistant organisms.[29] The immune system of the neonate is immature with decreased neutrophil reserves and neutrophil chemotactic function; immaturity of T-cell function, as well as defects in the complement cascade.[30] Transplacental transmission of immunoglobulin G (IgG) occurs during the last trimester so the immature infant born before 32-weeks gestation is deficient. The newborn has a blunted immunoglobulin response and frequent blood draws in the NICU deplete stores of IgM and IgG, while frequent blood transfusions dilute immunoglobulin levels. Together these factors make the newborn, and especially the very immature infant, at risk for infection.

Outbreaks are a constant concern in the NICU. Hand contamination of the HCW can occur even with routine patient care and allows transmission between infants unless hand hygiene is meticulous between patients.[31,32] A pathogen of increasing concern in the NICU is methicillin-resistant *Staphylococcus aureus* (MRSA).[33] McBryde et al. documented the spread of MRSA from patient clothing and patient beds to the gloved hands of HCWs. [34] Very rarely a HCW is a carrier,[35] but here also, the infection spreads on the hands of a HCW. Some nurseries now routinely screen for MRSA at admission and attempt to contain this organism with isolation of colonized infants. In an outbreak situation, neonates with MRSA should be placed in contact precautions, preferably in a separate room from the rest of the unit and with cohorting of staff, though this may not always be possible.

Resistant gram-negatives and viruses, such as RSV, are other important nosocomial pathogens.[36] While some outbreaks of gram-negatives have been linked to contaminated antibiotics, total parenteral nutrition, or intravenous fluids, most are the result of poor infection-control techniques.[37]

Equipment routinely used should be thoroughly cleaned after use and whenever possible, each neonate should have his own dedicated equipment. The role of hand rubs is evolving in the NICU, but clearly is effective.[38] Parents and staff should avoid the NICU when ill, especially with contagious diseases such as diarrhea, adenoviral conjunctivitis, and herpes simplex infections of the mouth or hands.

Breast milk is often used to feed infants in the nursery, including infants too ill to breastfeed directly. Infection-control policy should address clean methods of collecting, saving, and dispensing fresh and frozen milk to infants. Care should be taken that infants receive only their own mother's milk, or under the guidance of a milk bank, safely stored and screened donor milk.

Infection Control in the Pediatric Intensive Care Unit

After the NICU, the Pediatric Intensive Care Unit (PICU) is the next most important site for nosocomial infections in the children's hospital. Here, as everywhere, hand hygiene and attention to infection-control practice is key for the prevention of nosocomial infections. Meticulous care in starting intravenous lines and following "bundling" recommendations (chlorhexidene skin preparation, full-barrier measures, and meticulous hand hygiene) are crucial.[15] Infection-control issues should be considered for each child at admission to the PICU, and appropriate empiric isolation precautions started.

Each infection control program selects specific infections to monitor as part of hospital surveillance. Catheter-related bloodstream, cerebrospinal fluid and urinary tract infections should be actively monitored in real time to identify outbreaks promptly, especially in the ICU. Catheters should be removed as soon as possible. Catheter-related bloodstream infections are most deadly, especially in the burn unit,[39] septic thrombophlebitis in particular. This life-threatening infection requires prompt recognition and surgical debridement of the vein.

When a multidrug-resistant organism is cultured from a patient in the ICU, a decision about whether to isolate the patient should be made. The more resistant the organism, the more concern about spread of the organism within the ICU. Contact precautions can be used to try to contain the organism. If multiple children are colonized, cohorting will likely be necessary as well.

Ventilator-associated pneumonia is very rare in pediatrics, while nosocomial transmission of respiratory viruses and rotavirus is a more common occurrence. Transmission-based precautions and strict attention to hand hygiene are critical to prevention.

Infection-control programs should maintain surveillance programs to be able to identify outbreaks. Surveillance should reflect particular populations and their specific risks for outbreaks. The program should develop and implement policies to improve safety in the hospital.[40]

Special Situations: Construction

Construction, remodeling, and new additions to a health care facility all carry infection risks that need to be managed and minimized. Infection-control guidelines should be followed in all hospital construction planning and execution. Ceilings, elevator shafts, and insulation have also been found to contain the fungal conidia of *Aspergillus*, a special concern in immunocompromised patients; and they should be removed from areas adjacent to construction,[41] with barriers placed to separate air supply from hospital units.

The hospital water supply is vulnerable to contamination, especially with *Legionella* species.[42] Immunocompromised and transplant patients are especially susceptible. The route of infection is usually via inhalation of contaminated aerosols from environmental sources, including hot water supplied in hospitals. The use of routine surveillance cultures of the water supply is not recommended, but should be used in outbreak situations to identify possible sources.

Disaster Preparedness

Disaster preparedness is an essential role of the infection-control program. Disasters, which include both natural pandemics and acts of biological terrorism, stress the resources and personnel of any health care system. The infection-control program should work with the community to be part of preparedness drills and HCW educational programs. Ideally, personal protective equipment is available and HCWs are trained to use these appropriately. Medications for particular threats may be difficult to stockpile, and should be available from a federal source in the case of a biological attack.[43]

Children are especially vulnerable to disasters and the aftermath. Children with more rapid respiratory rates and increased body/surface areas are at increased risk of exposure and disease, after a toxin or biological weapon attack. Increased body/surface area also makes hypothermia and exposure more serious than for the adult, including during a decontamination procedure. The pediatric population requires different doses of antibiotics and antidote compounds than adult victims, and in an emergency, this information should be readily available. Thus, careful planning and training for possible disasters is essential in maximizing the quality of disaster care children receive in your hospital and local community.[44]

The recently held *Pediatric Preparedness for Disasters and Terrorism: A National Consensus Conference* focused on eight major areas to improve preparedness for disasters like pandemics and terrorism, as well as natural disasters. These areas include emergency and prehospital care, hospital care, emergency preparedness, terrorism preparedness, mental health needs, school preparedness, training and drills, and future research and funding (CDC website: www.CDC.gov).

REFERENCES

1. Price PB. Bacteriology of normal skin: A new quantitative test applied to a study of the bacterial flora and the disinfectant action of mechanical cleansing. *J Infect Dis.* 1938;63: 301-318.
2. Aboelela SW, Stone PW, Larson EL. Effectiveness of bundled behavioural interventions to control healthcare-associated infections: a systematic review of the literature. *J Hosp Infect.* 2007;66(2):101-108.
3. Larson E. Effects of handwashing agent, handwashing frequency, and clinical area on hand flora. *Am J Infect Control.* 1984;12(2):76-82.
4. Goldmann DA, Leclair J, Macone A. Bacterial colonization of neonates admitted to an intensive care environment. *J Pediatr.* 1978;93(2):288-293.
5. Toltzis P, Blumer JL. Problems with resistance in pediatric intensive care. *New Horiz.* 1996;4(3):353-360.
6. Price B. The bacteriology of normal skin: a new quantitative test applied to a study of the bacterial flora and the disinfectant action of mechanical cleansing. *J Infect Dis.* 1938;63:301-318.
7. Sproat LJ, Inglis TJ. A multicentre survey of hand hygiene practice in intensive care units. *J Hosp Infect.* 1994;26(2): 137-148.
8. Pittet D, Allegranzi B, Sax H, et al. Evidence-based model for hand transmission during patient care and the role of improved practices. *Lancet Infect Dis.* 2006;6(10): 641-652.
9. Simon A, Khurana K, Wilkesmann A, et al. Nosocomial respiratory syncytial virus infection: impact of prospective surveillance and targeted infection control. *Int J Hyg Environ Health.* 2006;209(4):317-324.
10. Olsen RJ, Lynch P, Coyle MB, Cummings J, Bokete T, Stamm WE. Examination gloves as barriers to hand contamination in clinical practice. *JAMA.* 1993;270(3): 350-353.
11. Passaro DJ, Waring L, Armstrong R, et al. Postoperative Serratia marcescens wound infections traced to an out-of-hospital source. *J Infect Dis.* 1997;175(4):992-995.
12. Pottinger J, Burns S, Manske C. Bacterial carriage by artificial versus natural nails. *Am J Infect Control.* 1989;17(6): 340-344.
13. Trick WE, Vernon MO, Hayes RA, et al. Impact of ring wearing on hand contamination and comparison of hand hygiene agents in a hospital. *Clin Infect Dis.* 2003;36(11): 1383-1390.
14. Wongworawat MD, Jones SG. Influence of rings on the efficacy of hand sanitization and residual bacterial contamination. *Infect Control Hosp Epidemiol.* 2007;28(3):351-353.
15. Pronovost P, Needham D, Berenholtz S, et al. An intervention to decrease catheter-related bloodstream infections in the ICU. *N Engl J Med.* 2006;355(26):2725-2732.
16. Rotter, ML. In: Mayhall CG. (ed.) *Hand Washing and Hand Disinfection in Hospital Epidemiology and Infection Control.* Philadelphia: Lippincott Williams & Wilkins; 1996:1052-1068.
17. Sartor C, Jacomo V, Duvivier C, Tissot-Dupont H, Sambuc R, Drancourt M. Nosocomial Serratia marcescens infections associated with extrinsic contamination of a liquid nonmedicated soap. *Infect Control Hosp Epidemiol.* 2000;21(3):196-199.
18. Larson EL, Morton HE. *Alcohols.* In: Block SS (ed.). Disinfection, sterilization and preservation, 4th ed. Philadelphia: Lea and Febiger, 1991:642-654.
19. Administration. FaD. Tentative final monograph for healtcare antiseptic drug products; proposed rule. *Federal Register.* 1994;59:31441-31452.
20. Standardization. ECf. Chemical disinfedtants and antiseptics-hygienic hand rub. European Standard EN 1500 1997/Brussels Belgium: Central Secretariat).
21. Boyce JM, Pittet D. Guideline for hand hygiene in health-care settings: recommendations of the healthcare infection control practices advisory committee and the HICPAC/SHEA/APIC/IDSA hand hygiene task force. *Infect Control Hosp Epidemiol.* 2002;23(12 suppl):S3-S40.
22. Boyce JM, Kelliher S, Vallande N. Skin irritation and dryness associated with two hand-hygiene regimens: soap-and-water hand washing versus hand antisepsis with an alcoholic hand gel. *Infect Control Hosp Epidemiol.* 2000; 21(7):442-448.
23. Winnefeld M, Richard MA, Drancourt M, Grob JJ. Skin tolerance and effectiveness of two hand decontamination procedures in everyday hospital use. *Br J Dermatol.* 2000; 143(3):546-550.
24. Bischoff WE, Reynolds TM, Sessler CN, Edmond MB, Wenzel RP. Handwashing compliance by health care workers: the impact of introducing an accessible, alcohol-based hand antiseptic. *Arch Intern Med.* 2000;160(7): 1017-1021.
25. Pittet D. Improving compliance with hand hygiene in hospitals. *Infect Control Hosp Epidemiol.* 2000;21(6): 381-386.
26. DiSalvo H, Haiduven D, Johnson N, et al. Who let the dogs out? Infection control did: utility of dogs in health care settings and infection control aspects. *Am J Infect Control.* 2006;34(5):301-307.
27. Duncan SL. APIC State-of-the-art report: the implications of service animals in health care settings. *Am J Infect Control.* 2000;28(2):170-180.
28. Sohn AH, Garrett DO, Sinkowitz-Cochran RL, et al. Prevalence of nosocomial infections in neonatal intensive care unit patients: results from the first national point-prevalence survey. *J Pediatr.* 2001;139(6):821-827.

29. Toltzis P, Dul MJ, Hoyen C, et al. Molecular epidemiology of antibiotic-resistant gram-negative bacilli in a neonatal intensive care unit during a nonoutbreak period. *Pediatrics.* 2001;108(5):1143-1148.
30. Lewis DB, Wilson CB. *Developmental Immunology and Role of Host Defenses in Fetal and Neonatal Susceptibility to Infection in Infectious Diseases of the Fetus and Newborn.* Philadelphia: WB Saunders Company; 2001: 25-138.
31. Saiman L, Cronquist A, Wu F, et al. An outbreak of methicillin-resistant *Staphylococcus aureus* in a neonatal intensive care unit. *Infect Control Hosp Epidemiol.* 2003;24(5): 317-321.
32. Colodner R, Sakran W, Miron D, Teitler N, Khavalevsky E, Kopelowitz J. Listeria monocytogenes cross-contamination in a nursery [corrected]. *Am J Infect Control.* 2003;31(5): 322-324.
33. James L, Gorwitz RJ, Jones RC, et al. Methicillin-resistant *Staphylococcus aureus* infections among healthy full-term newborns. *Arch Dis Child Fetal Neonatal Ed.* 2008;93: 40-44.
34. McBryde ES, Bradley LC, Whitby M, McElwain DL. An investigation of contact transmission of methicillin-resistant *Staphylococcus aureus. J Hosp Infect.* 2004;58(2): 104-108.
35. Bertin ML, Vinski J, Schmitt S, et al. Outbreak of methicillin-resistant *Staphylococcus aureus* colonization and infection in a neonatal intensive care unit epidemiologically linked to a healthcare worker with chronic otitis. *Infect Control Hosp Epidemiol.* 2006;27(6):581-585.
36. Halasa NB, Williams JV, Wilson GJ, Walsh WF, Schaffner W, Wright PF. Medical and economic impact of a respiratory syncytial virus outbreak in a neonatal intensive care unit. *Pediatr Infect Dis J.* 2005;24(12):1040-1044.
37. Schelonka RL, Scruggs S, Nichols K, Dimmitt RA, Carlo WA. Sustained reductions in neonatal nosocomial infection rates following a comprehensive infection control intervention. *J Perinatol.* 2006;26(3):176-179.
38. Larson E, Silberger M, Jakob K, et al. Assessment of alternative hand hygiene regimens to improve skin health among neonatal intensive care unit nurses. *Heart Lung.* 2000;29(2):136-142.
39. Church D, Elsayed S, Reid O, Winston B, Lindsay R. Burn wound infections. *Clin Microbiol Rev.* 2006;19(2):403-434.
40. Bearman GM, Munro C, Sessler CN, Wenzel RP. Infection control and the prevention of nosocomial infections in the intensive care unit. *Semin Respir Crit Care Med.* 2006;27(3):310-324.
41. Vonberg RP, Gastmeier P. Nosocomial aspergillosis in outbreak settings. *J Hosp Infect.* 2006;63(3):246-254.
42. Berthelot P, Grattard F, Ros A, Lucht F, Pozzetto B. Nosocomial legionellosis outbreak over a three-year period: Investigation and control. *Clin Microbiol Infect.* 1998;4(7): 385-391.
43. Markenson D, Redlener I. Pediatric terrorism preparedness national guidelines and recommendations: Findings of an evidenced-based consensus process. *Biosecur Bioterror.* 2004;2(4):301-319.
44. White SR, Henretig FM, Dukes RG. Medical management of vulnerable populations and co-morbid conditions of victims of bioterrorism. *Emerg Med Clin North Am.* 2002;20(2):365-392, xi.
45. Centers for Disease Control and Prevention. Guidelines for hand hygiene. *Fla Nurse.* 2002;50(4):12.
46. Pediatrics AAo. *Red Book.* 27th ed. 2006;153-166.

CHAPTER 6

Infectious Diseases Epidemiology

Kevin J. Downes and Samir S. Shah

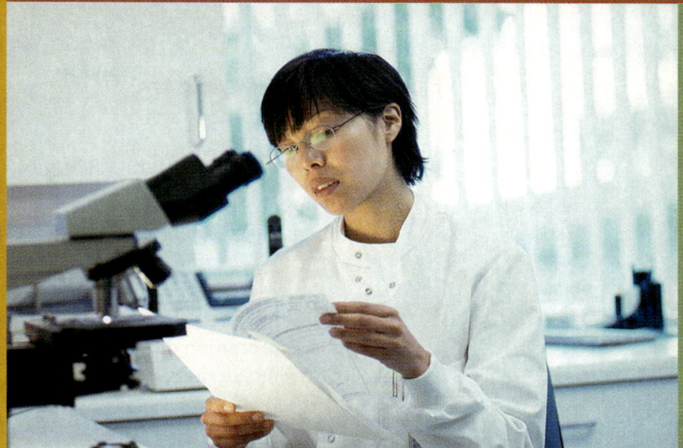

INTRODUCTION

Epidemiology is the study of health and disease in a population. Studying the causes, distribution, risk factors, and treatment of diseases, all of which fall under its scope, provides the cornerstone for research into explaining how and why infectious diseases occur. This chapter is designed to provide a brief introduction to the core principles of clinical research and epidemiology. Our goal is to present clinicians with an overview of the key terms and concepts found throughout published research, and we hope that this chapter will serve as a useful reference for pediatricians seeking to better understand the fundamentals of infectious diseases epidemiology.

In this chapter, we begin with a discussion of study designs, including the strengths and weaknesses of different types of studies. We then explore important concepts used in studies of diagnostic tests: sensitivity, specificity, positive and negative predictive values, and likelihood ratios. Next, we discuss statistical analysis by comparing univariate and multivariate analyses, while explaining terms used to define the magnitude of an effect such as odds ratios (ORs), relative risk (RR), and confidence intervals. Finally, we end the chapter with an examination of relative risk reduction (RRR), absolute risk reduction (ARR), and number needed to treat—measures used to enumerate the benefits of an intervention. We hope that the information presented in this chapter provides a concise overview of the key concepts of epidemiologic and clinical research in infectious diseases.

STUDY DESIGN

A variety of study designs are utilized in clinical research and each allows authors to address different questions. Depending on whether an author would like to determine the prevalence of a disease, the natural course of an infection, or the effectiveness of a treatment, for example, will determine which study design the investigator will use. In general, studies can be broken down into two principle types: descriptive and analytic. *Descriptive studies* include case reports, case series, and survey studies, all of which are used primarily to generate hypotheses.[1–4] As the name implies, these types of study designs allow authors to describe the characteristics of a single patient or group of patients with a common disease. However, since these studies do not use a control or comparison group, they are poorly suited to make causal inferences. Instead, they are more useful for characterizing emerging or rare diseases, such as avian influenza A, where little is known about the natural course of disease.

Analytic studies are hypothesis-testing in nature and are better equipped to explore the relationship between cause and effect. Analytic studies can be further subdivided into observational and experimental studies. *Observational studies* include cross-sectional, case-control, and cohort studies, and provide information about prevalence, incidence, causes, risk factors, and outcomes of disease. *Experimental studies* test the effects of an intervention and include clinical trials, both randomized and nonrandomized. Randomized clinical trials (RCTs) are often considered the most powerful and scientific study designs, and are the gold standard for evaluating the efficacy of therapies and other interventions. While all study designs are subject to varying amounts of *external validity*, or generalizability to other populations or to the population at large, RCTs have the highest *internal validity*, meaning that they are the most capable to conclude that a cause has a specific and real effect. Table 6–1 provides a list of the most common types of study designs and includes information about

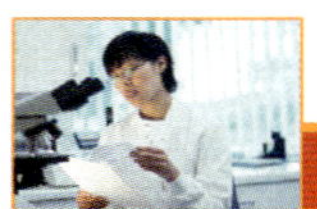

Table 6–1.

Hierarchy of Epidemiologic Study Designs

Study Design	Objective	Strengths	Weaknesses
Descriptive	*Generate hypotheses for future studies*		
Case report	Describes a single instance of a disease in a patient	Emphasizes an important or unique point related to treatment or diagnosis of a disease	No control or comparison group Findings cannot be generalized to any other patients with that disease
Case series	Describes a series of cases that share a common disease, treatment, or outcome	Emphasizes an important point related to treatment or diagnosis of a disease Inexpensive and provides rapid results Useful for providing information about rare diseases	No control group Unable to make causal or temporal inferences Findings cannot be generalized to any other patients with that disease
Survey	Examines relationships among variables across a population	Can be cross-sectional or longitudinal Interviews can be conducted in a variety of formats (in person, over the phone, mail, etc.) Inexpensive	No control group Unable to make causal or temporal inferences Nonresponse leads to questions of validity
Analytic	*Test hypotheses related to causes and outcomes of disease*		
Cross-sectional study	To determine prevalence of exposure, disease, and/or outcome in a population	Can determine associations between exposure and disease or between disease and outcome Data collected at one point in time thus relatively inexpensive and able to provide rapid results	Unable to make causal or temporal inferences Cannot study rare diseases—too few subjects with the disease relative to those without the disease Confounders may not be distributed equally between groups Cannot measure incidence
Case-control study	Retrospective design used to identify factors that are associated with the development of a disease or outcome; compare individuals with a disease or outcome (cases) to those without (controls) and look back to determine presence of an exposure or risk factor	Used to study rare diseases, those with a long period between exposure and outcome, or those with numerous potential risk factors Relatively few cases are needed Less expensive than cohort studies or clinical trials Can express the frequency of an exposure among subjects with a disease relative to those who are disease-free Can assess the impact of numerous risk factors or exposures	Identification of an appropriate control group is difficult Study design is complex and difficult for clinicians to understand Can only assess a single outcome of interest Sampling bias—cases may not be generalizable to all patients with a disease or outcome Recall bias—better recollection of exposure among cases than controls Cannot calculate incidence, relative risk, or attributable risk
Cohort study	Longitudinal study of individuals who share a particular exposure or disease; follow subjects to assess factors related to the development of an outcome of interest among those individuals over time	Prospective or retrospective Can study numerous outcomes among subjects Best studies to assess the natural course of disease Individuals who do not develop an outcome of interest serve as internal controls	Expensive and often requires numerous subjects if outcome of interest is rare, or long follow-up Retrospective cohorts cannot control the selection of subjects or outcomes of interest since data already exist Loss to follow-up can affect results and generalizability

(continued)

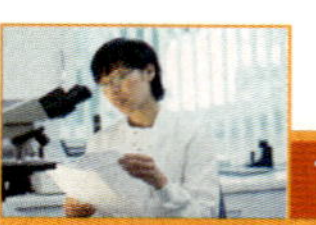

Table 6–1. (Continued)

Hierarchy of Epidemiologic Study Designs

Study Design	Objective	Strengths	Weaknesses
		Useful when randomization to treatment versus placebo is unattainable or unethical Can adequately determine temporality between cause and effect Can calculate incidence, relative risk, and attributable risk	Prospective studies can be very expensive and demand extensive resources Subject to systematic bias, information bias, and recall bias (retrospective cohorts) Confounding may impact the validity of results
Randomized controlled trial	Prospective study used to evaluate treatments or interventions through the use of random assignment of subjects to treatment or control group	Randomization eliminates selection bias and evenly distributes confounders between groups Provides strong evidence for cause and effect Double-blinding minimizes observer bias since researcher does not know if subject is in control or treatment group	Expensive and requires significant time to conduct the study Randomization and blinding may be impossible or unethical May have limited external validity (generalizability to general population)

**Studies listed in order of increasing evidence of causality.*

each design's strengths and limitations.[1–7] In this table, study designs are listed in order of increasing strength of evidence.

One of the primary issues that an investigator must face when designing a study is, "How well can this study design answer the question at hand?" Regardless of design, the main obstacles to the internal validity of any study are bias and confounding. *Bias* is any source of variation that distorts the study findings and creates systematic error, and can only be avoided through careful study design that addresses these issues upfront. Meanwhile, *confounding* is any extrinsic factor that is both associated with the exposure and a cause of the outcome.[5] Unless addressed during the design or statistical analysis phases, confounding variables will alter the association between an exposure and an outcome such that the result is actually an over- or underestimation of the true effect of the exposure on the outcome. Additionally, in any study there is the potential that an investigator's results are false merely owing to random error. This error is unrelated to how the study was designed or conducted, but occurs simply by chance. However, random error will decrease as the sample size increases.

STUDIES OF DIAGNOSTIC TESTS

Many epidemiologic studies examine the utility of diagnostic tests. In infectious diseases, these studies are of particular importance. Clinical decision making relies on an understanding of the reliability of test results and knowledge of how these tests should be used in a clinical context. For example, a child may be admitted to the hospital because of what appears to be a viral syndrome. And, the child's physician suspects that influenza is responsible and would like to send a rapid test for the virus. Before sending the test, there are numerous questions that the physician may ask. What is the probability of influenza in this child (*pretest probability*)? How often will patients with the virus have a positive test result (*sensitivity*)? How often will patients that do not have the virus have a negative test result (*specificity*)? Or, how often will a positive/negative test result mean that the patient actually has/does not have an active viral infection (*positive/negative predictive value*)? Knowledge of these important concepts will affect the ordering of the test, the interpretation of the test results, and the likelihood that the patient does or does not have the disease once the test results are known (*posttest probability*).[8,9]

The utility of diagnostic tests can often be thought of in regard to a 2 × 2 table (Table 6–2) and explained using the following terms:

1. *Sensitivity*—the ability of a test to accurately identify those *with* disease.
   a. Calculated as the proportion of individuals with the disease in whom the test is positive.

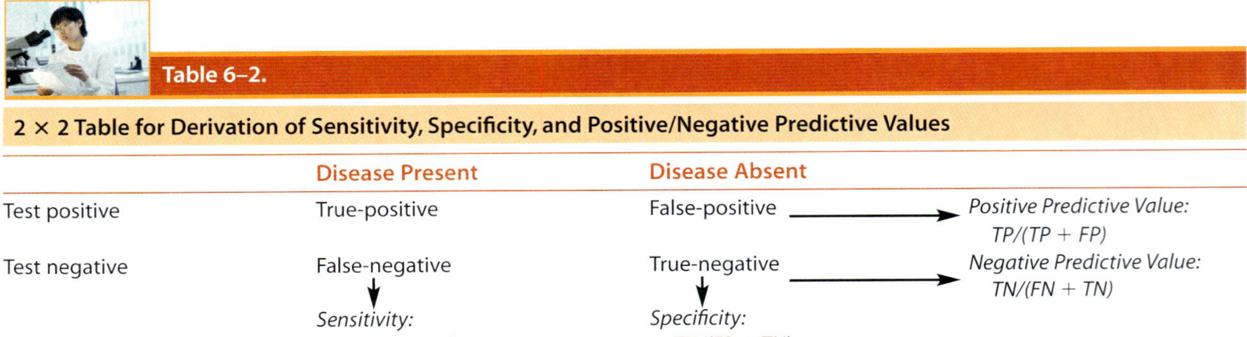

Table 6–2.

2 × 2 Table for Derivation of Sensitivity, Specificity, and Positive/Negative Predictive Values

	Disease Present	Disease Absent	
Test positive	True-positive	False-positive →	*Positive Predictive Value: TP/(TP + FP)*
Test negative	False-negative ↓	True-negative ↓ →	*Negative Predictive Value: TN/(FN + TN)*
	Sensitivity: TP/(TP + FN)	*Specificity: TN/(FP + TN)*	

2. *Specificity*—the ability of a test to accurately identify those *without* disease.
   a. Calculated as the proportion of individuals without the disease in whom the test is negative.
3. *Positive-predictive value (PPV)*—the likelihood that a positive result represents the identification of an individual that actually has the disease.
   a. Calculated as the proportion of individuals that test positive *and* have disease among all individuals that test positive.
4. *Negative-predictive value (NPV)*—the likelihood that a negative result represents the identification of an individual without disease.
   a. Calculated as the proportion of individuals that test negative *and* do not have disease among all individuals that test negative.

There are drawbacks to the use of these test parameters in a clinical setting, however.[8] In general, highly sensitive tests are good screening tests because they will pick up almost all cases of disease. But the increased sensitivity usually comes at the expense of specificity, so highly sensitive tests sometimes have a high false-positive rate. In that setting (high sensitivity but only a modest specificity), a negative test result provides more certainty to the clinician regarding the disease status of the patient. A test that is 100% sensitive, for example, will detect all cases of disease, but if the specificity is only modest (i.e., 85% or less), may also produce numerous false-positives. So, while a negative test result will effectively rule out disease and allow the clinician to reassure the patient, a positive test result will be less helpful, especially if the disease is uncommon (so most positive test results are false-positives), and may warrant further testing to determine true disease status. A good example of such tiered testing is syphilis where a positive nontreponemal antibody test (e.g., rapid plasma regain [RPR]) is typically confirmed with treponemal antibody testing (e.g., FTA-ABS, fluorescent treponemal antibody absorption). On the other hand, a diagnostic test that is highly specific is much more helpful if the test result is positive since high specificity often comes at the expense of decreasing sensitivity. Since tests with high specificity are used to accurately identify those with disease, they are generally regarded as good confirmatory tests because false-positive results are uncommon. Unfortunately, they will likely have numerous false-negatives. Therefore, a positive result can help direct clinical management, while a negative test doesn't necessarily exclude disease in a patient unless the sensitivity is also quite high.

As the above paragraph alludes to the main issue with both specificity and sensitivity is that they do not help clinicians estimate probability of disease in individual patients.[8] They are useful at ruling in or out disease, but cannot be used to determine how likely a patient is to have or not have the disease. Instead, a clinician can use positive and negative predictive values to help predict the likelihood of disease once a test result is known. Both the PPV, which tells the probability of having disease given a positive result, and the NPV, which tells the probability of being disease-free given a negative result, can increase or decrease a clinician's posttest probability. In this manner, test results can be applied to individual patients. However, there is a significant limitation to the use of PPV and NPV: Both are affected by the prevalence of disease. PPV will increase as the prevalence of disease increases, while NPV will decrease, and vice versa when disease prevalence decreases. So, clinicians need to be careful when applying PPV and NPV to test results in their patients, since the prevalence may differ from that of the population used to define the test parameters.

While sensitivity, specificity, PPV, and NPV are useful when interpreting diagnostic test results, they have limitations when assessing the probability of disease in individual patients. Instead, by combining the sensitivity and specificity, *likelihood ratios (LRs)* provide a more clinically useful measure. LRs describe how many times more (or less) likely patients with disease are to have a positive (or negative) test result than those without disease.

1. *Likelihood ratio positive (LR+)* explains the probability of a patient with disease having a positive test result compared to the probability of a patient without disease having a positive test result.
   a. Calculated as the true-positive rate (sensitivity) divided by the false-positive rate (1.0—specificity).
   b. LR+ greater than 1.0 indicates an increased probability of disease.
2. *Likelihood ratio negative (LR–)* explains the probability of a negative result in a patient with disease compared with a negative result in a patient without disease.
   a. Calculated as 1.0—sensitivity of a test divided by the specificity.
   b. LR– less than 1.0 indicates a decreased probability of disease.

Clinical Example

Respiratory syncytial virus (RSV) is a prevalent virus, which is the cause of high levels of morbidity and mortality in infants and young children. Although treatment is largely supportive, rapid detection of RSV may expedite management and prevent the use of additional costly and potentially harmful diagnostic tests. In 2002, Dayan et al. sought to determine the test characteristics of RSV EIA in febrile infants.[10] Using tissue and shell viral cultures as the reference standard, the nasal washings of 174 infants were evaluated using RSV EIA. Table 6–3 demonstrates the comparison of RSV EIA to culture.

Based on these findings, the RSV EIA had a sensitivity of 75%, a specificity of 98%, a PPV of 89%, and a NPV of 95%. The LR+ for this test was found to be 35.5, while the LR– was 0.26. Based on these findings, the RSV EIA is a modest screening test and good confirmatory test for the detection of RSV. It will correctly identify three quarters of febrile infants with RSV (sensitivity), and infants without RSV will be accurately identified as they do not have disease 98% of the time (specificity). Additionally, this study found that a febrile infant with a positive RSV EIA was more than 35 times more likely to have RSV than a febrile infant without RSV (LR+). Based on these results, the RSV EIA has significant clinical utility and the results of testing in a febrile infant can assist clinicians in their management.

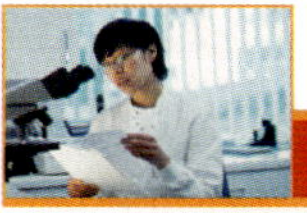

Table 6–3.

2 × 2 Table for the Diagnosis of RSV Using RSV EIA

	RSV Present*	RSV Absent*	Total
RSV EIA positive	24	3	27
RSV EIA negative	8	139	147
Total	32	142	174

**Tissue and shell viral culture used as the reference standard.*

STATISTICAL ANALYSIS

Once data collection has been completed, the next step is statistical analysis. The first step in this process is to conduct *univariate analysis,* which explores the relationship between the dependent variable and each independent variable individually. *Independent variables* are those factors, which may impact the outcome (*dependent variable*) and can take a variety of forms: demographic and historical data, exposures, treatments, interventions, etc. Univariate analysis provides descriptive information about the frequencies and distributions of the independent variables across subjects in a study. Additionally, univariate analysis sets the stage for further analyses. Variables can be summarized across groups of subjects in the study allowing for comparison across exposed and unexposed groups, or across the intervention and nonintervention groups. Thus, through univariate analysis, investigators can determine whether the exposure or intervention group was more or less likely to experience an outcome or event than the unexposed or nonintervention group.

While it is useful to demonstrate that one group was more or less likely to have experienced an event or outcome, it is often necessary to determine how much the groups differed. Two concepts used to quantify the magnitude of an effect are RR or risk ratio, and the OR. Both the OR and RR describe the likelihood of an event between two groups. And, interpretation of OR and RR is somewhat similar: If the RR or OR equals 1.0, the likelihood of an event is comparable between the two groups. If the RR or OR is greater than 1.0, an event is more likely to occur in the exposed or intervention group than in the unexposed or nonintervention group. The opposite is true if the OR or RR is less than 1.0.[11] However, there are important differences between the RR and OR that must be recognized.

The *OR* describes the relative odds of an outcome or event in the exposed group compared to odds of the outcome or event in the unexposed group. On the other hand, the *RR* is the ratio of the probability of an outcome or event in the exposed group to the probability of the outcome or event in the unexposed group. Since the difference between these two concepts is not always clear, it is useful to think in terms of a 2 × 2 table (Table 6–4). The primary difference between OR and RR is the discrepancy between odds and probability. Although both

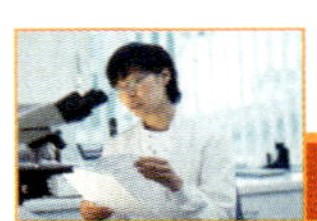

Table 6–4.

Calculating the Odds Ratio* and Relative Risk† Between Groups

		Intervention or Exposure		
		Yes	No	Total
Outcome or	Yes	a	b	a + b
Event	No	c	d	c + d
Total		a + c	b + d	

*Odds ratio = (a/c)/(b/d) = ad/bc.
†Relative risk = (a/a+c)/(b/b+d).

OR and RR are ratios, the concept of RR is more straightforward. RR can be simply understood as the increased or decreased likelihood of an outcome or event in the exposed group versus the unexposed group. And, for most individuals, this is the intuitive way to compare the likelihood of an event between two groups. An RR can be stated as "group A is X times more or less likely to experience Y than group B." However, an OR cannot be understood in this manner. Instead, the OR needs to be interpreted in terms of the prevalence of the event or outcome. As the prevalence of an event or outcome increases, the OR poorly approximates relative risk. In fact, an OR will always overestimate the RR if greater than 1.0 and underestimate a relative risk if less than 1.0. The amount of over- and underestimation will be magnified if the prevalence of the event or outcome is high.[12] Therefore, it is only when the prevalence of a disease or outcome is rare that the OR truly approximates the RR and can be interpreted as such.

So, why would one ever use ORs if their interpretation is difficult? Firstly, the direction of the effect is useful. An OR greater than or less than 1.0 will demonstrate which group is more or less likely to experience an outcome or event. Often, that has as much utility as the magnitude of the effect itself. Secondly, ORs are necessary in case-control studies, since relative risks cannot be calculated in these studies. Because case-control studies are designed to identify risk factors for development of disease, cases and controls are selected based on the presence or absence of disease, respectively. An RR cannot be determined because cases overestimate the likelihood of disease in the population. Therefore, a case-control study cannot estimate the risk of disease and, simply because of the design, cannot calculate the RR of developing disease based on the presence or absence of a risk factor. Instead, an investigator can use ORs to express the relative likelihood of a risk factor in cases and controls. And, since case-control studies study rare diseases, the OR will actually approximate the RR mathematically (*in Table 6–4, cells a and b will be significantly smaller than c and d, and the calculated OR will equate the RR*). Finally, ORs are practical when performing multivariate analyses. It is far easier to adjust the ORs for confounding variables than it is to adjust RRs. Thus, determining ORs will allow for the measurement of the independent effects of variables on the outcome of interest.

Multivariate analysis allows investigators to determine the independent effects of multiple factors on a single event or outcome.[13] When numerous independent variables, or contributing factors, have an effect on a dependent variable, or outcome, multivariate analysis allows investigators to determine the individual contribution of each. As mentioned above, confounding variables are factors associated to the exposure and causally related to the outcome. Multivariate analysis enables researchers to determine the true effect of an exposure on an outcome by adjusting for known or suspected confounders.

There are numerous types of multivariate analysis that are available for researchers: multiple linear regression, multiple logistic regression, and Cox proportional-hazards regression, for example. Linear regression is used when the outcome is a continuous variable (i.e., HIV-viral load), and logistic regression is used when the outcome is a dichotomous, often yes or no, variable (i.e., HIV seroconversion or death). Cox regression is useful when the outcome of interest is a period of time, such as time to positivity for blood cultures.

Once the results of a multivariate model are determined, the adjusted ORs relate to the independent effects of each variable on the outcome of interest. And, while the investigator may have adjusted for all known confounders, there is still the possibility that either random error or unmeasured confounders played a role in the point estimate of the effect between the variable and the outcome. Confidence intervals allow the investigator to present a range of values within which the true value of the effect likely lies. Ninety-five percent confidence intervals, for example, which are most commonly used in clinical research, provide a range of values that contains the true effect with 95% certainty. Wider confidence intervals represent more uncertainty, while more narrow confidence intervals signify greater precision. When the confidence intervals surrounding an OR or an RR include 1.0, the author cannot be certain whether there is actually a difference between the two groups.[11] Therefore, when the confidence intervals include 1.0, a causal relationship between the independent and dependent variables cannot be established.

ADDITIONAL MEASURES OF EFFECT

ORs and RRs are informative when summarizing case-control and cohort studies. However, when an investigator conducts a clinical trial, it is important to enumerate the effects of the intervention being studied. Patients and clinicians alike want to know when the benefits of an intervention outweigh the harms. One way to express the effects of the intervention is in terms of the *RRR*: the relative difference in the rate of an event (i.e., death, hospitalization, etc.) between the intervention and the nonintervention group. RRR is calculated by dividing the difference between rate of an event in the intervention group and nonintervention group by the rate of the event in the nonintervention group. For example, in a hypothetical trial, if an event occurs in 40% of the nonintervention group and in 20% of the intervention group, the RRR from the intervention is 0.50, or 50% (*calculated as 40% minus 20%, divided by 40%*). Another measure of the benefit or harm of an intervention is the *ARR*. This is the absolute difference in the rate of an event between the intervention and nonintervention group. To calculate ARR, the event rate in the intervention group is subtracted from the event rate in the nonintervention group. In the hypothetical trial above, the ARR would be 20%.[11,14,15]

Because the rate of an event in the nonintervention group serves as the denominator for calculating RRR, the RRR will always be greater than the ARR. And, as the event rate becomes smaller, the difference between the relative and ARR will widen, making the RRR appear more dramatic.[14] However, RRR should be interpreted with caution. Because it is a relative measure, it does not take into account the baseline event rate in the control group. Therefore, when the event is very rare or very common, RRR will dramatically overestimate or underestimate, respectively, the true effects of the intervention. Contrarily, ARR does account for the event rate in the nonintervention group at baseline and, thus, provides a more clinically practical measure of the effect of the intervention.[15] Hence, the ARR is often referred to as the attributable risk of an intervention.

Although both RRR and ARR are ways to understand the benefits of an intervention, they are not easily applied to individual patients. Instead, clinicians can employ a measure known as the *number needed to treat* (NNT) to better enumerate these effects in a clinically useful way. The NNT is defined as the number of patients that need to receive a treatment in order to prevent one patient from experiencing an adverse outcome over a specified period of time (the study period).[16] It is calculated as the inverse of the ARR (1/ARR) and the smaller the NNT, the more effective the treatment. In the hypothetical trial above, the ARR was 20%. Therefore the NNT would be five, which is to say that five patients would need to receive the treatment to avoid one adverse outcome. However, the NNT can also be applied to individual patients: In the example, an individual patient has a one in five chance of benefitting from the treatment.[14]

Clinical Example

In January, 2006, Vesikari, et al. published a study examining the safety and efficacy of a live pentavalent human-bovine reassortant vaccine against rotavirus gastroenteritis.[17] This study was a double-blind, placebo-controlled, randomized trial involving more than 69,000 children in 11 countries. Healthy infants between 6 and 12 weeks of age were randomized to receive three doses of oral vaccine or placebo. All subjects were followed for the development of acute gastroenteritis requiring hospitalization or emergency department care, as well as the development of complications such as intussusception.

In this study, 57,134 children were involved in an analysis of health care service use attributed to rotavirus gastroenteritis. For our discussion, we will look simply at the efficacy of the vaccine in reducing hospitalizations resulting from acute rotavirus gastroenteritis. Among the infants who received the vaccine, 6 of 28,646 developed acute rotavirus gastroenteritis requiring hospitalization for 14 days or more following receipt of the last dose of the vaccine. In the placebo group, 138 of 28,488 infants were hospitalized. Children in the vaccine group had an RR of 0.043 for developing rotavirus gastroenteritis requiring hospitalization (*calculated as 6/28,646 divided by 138/28,488*), meaning that vaccinated children had 4.3% of the risk of being hospitalized as a result of rotavirus gastroenteritis compared to unvaccinated children. The RRR from vaccination was 95.7% (*calculated as 138/28,488 minus 6/28,646 divided by 138/28,488*), while because of the low incidence of hospitalization overall, the ARR from vaccination was just 0.46% (*calculated as 138/28,488 minus 6/28,646 times 100*). However, the NNT of 216 (*calculated as 1 divided by the difference of 138/28,488 and 6/28,646, or 0.0046*) means that vaccination of 216 children prevented 1 case of acute rotavirus gastroenteritis requiring hospitalization over the first year of life.

An NNT of 216 may seem high to some readers. However, one needs to take into account the prevalence of disease, as well as the risk-benefit ratio of the intervention. Rotavirus infection affects more than 100 million children annually worldwide and is the leading cause of deaths resulting from acute gastroenteritis.[18] Even in the United States, rotavirus gastroenteritis is responsible for more than 60,000 hospitalizations per year.[19] Therefore, given the cost associated with hospitalization (parental missed days of work, health care costs, etc.), the significant morbidity and mortality associated with severe rotavirus gastroenteritis, the incidence of this disease worldwide, and the relative safety and efficacy of this vaccine, widespread vaccination has a considerable potential benefit.

PEARLS

1. Study designs vary significantly in regard to the strength of evidence. While descriptive studies provide useful anecdotes and often serve as the basis for further investigation, analytic studies have the capacity to have tremendous internal validity and demonstrate true cause and effect.
2. Sensitivity and specificity relate to the ability of a test to identify an individual with and without disease, respectively.
3. The positive and negative predictive values relate to the likelihood that a positive/negative result has accurately identified an individual with or without disease, respectively.
4. LRs describe how many times more (or less) likely patients with disease are to have a positive (or negative) test result than those without disease.
5. ORs and RR are two ways to quantify differences between study groups. An OR or RR greater than 1.0 signifies an increased likelihood of the event in the comparison group, while OR or RR less than 1.0 signifies an increased likelihood of the event in the control group.
6. The NNT, calculated as 1 divided by the ARR, represents the number of individuals that would need to receive the treatment/intervention in order to avoid one adverse outcome.

REFERENCES

1. Nelson KE, Williams CM. *Infectious Disease Epidemiology: Theory and Practice*. 2nd ed. Sudbury, MA: Jones & Bartlett Publishers; 2007.
2. Grimes DA, Schulz KF. An overview of clinical research: the lay of the land. *Lancet*. 2002;359(9300):57-61.
3. Brighton B, Bhandari M, Tornetta P III, Felson DT. Hierarchy of evidence: from case reports to randomized controlled trials. *Clin Orthop Relat Res*. 2003;(413):19-24.
4. Dunn WR, Lyman S, Marx R. Research methodology. *Arthroscopy*. 2003;19(8):870-873.
5. Hulley SB. *Designing Clinical Research: An Epidemiologic Approach*. 2nd ed. Philadelphia: Lippincott Williams & Wilkins; 2001.
6. Mann CJ. Observational research methods. Research design II: cohort, cross sectional, and case-control studies. *Emerg Med J*. 2003;20(1):54-60.
7. Stephenson JM, Babiker A. Overview of study design in clinical epidemiology. *Sex Transm Infect*. 2000;76(4): 244-247.
8. Akobeng AK. Understanding diagnostic tests 1: sensitivity, specificity and predictive values. *Acta Paediatr*. 2007;96(3):338-341.
9. Akobeng AK. Understanding diagnostic tests 2: likelihood ratios, pre- and post-test probabilities and their use in clinical practice. *Acta Paediatr*. 2007;96(4):487-491.
10. Dayan P, Ahmad F, Urtecho J, et al. Test characteristics of the respiratory syncytial virus enzyme-linked immunoabsorbent assay in febrile infants < or = 60 days of age. *Clin Pediatr (Phila)*. 2002;41(6):415-418.
11. Sheldon TA. Biostatistics and study design for evidence-based practice. *AACN Clin Issues*. 2001;12(4):546-559.
12. Davies HT, Crombie IK, Tavakoli M. When can odds ratios mislead? *BMJ*. 1998;316(7136):989-991.
13. Katz MH. Multivariable analysis: a primer for readers of medical research. *Ann Intern Med*. 2003;138(8):644-650.
14. Barratt A, Wyer PC, Hatala R, et al. Tips for learners of evidence-based medicine: 1. Relative risk reduction, absolute risk reduction and number needed to treat. *CMAJ*. 2004;171(4):353-358.
15. Replogle WH, Johnson WD. Interpretation of absolute measures of disease risk in comparative research. *Fam Med*. 2007;39(6):432-435.
16. Sinclair JC, Cook RJ, Guyatt GH, Pauker SG, Cook DJ. When should an effective treatment be used? Derivation of the threshold number needed to treat and the minimum event rate for treatment. *J Clin Epidemiol*. 2001; 54(3):253-262.
17. Vesikari T, Matson DO, Dennehy P, et al. Safety and efficacy of a pentavalent human-bovine (WC3) reassortant rotavirus vaccine. *N Engl J Med*. 2006;354(1):23-33.
18. Parashar UD, Hummelman EG, Bresee JS, Miller MA, Glass RI. Global illness and deaths caused by rotavirus disease in children. *Emerg Infect Dis*. 2003;9(5):565-572.
19. Fischer TK, Viboud C, Parashar U, et al. Hospitalizations and deaths from diarrhea and rotavirus among children <5 years of age in the United States, 1993-2003. *J Infect Dis*. 2007;195(8):1117-1125.

SECTION 2

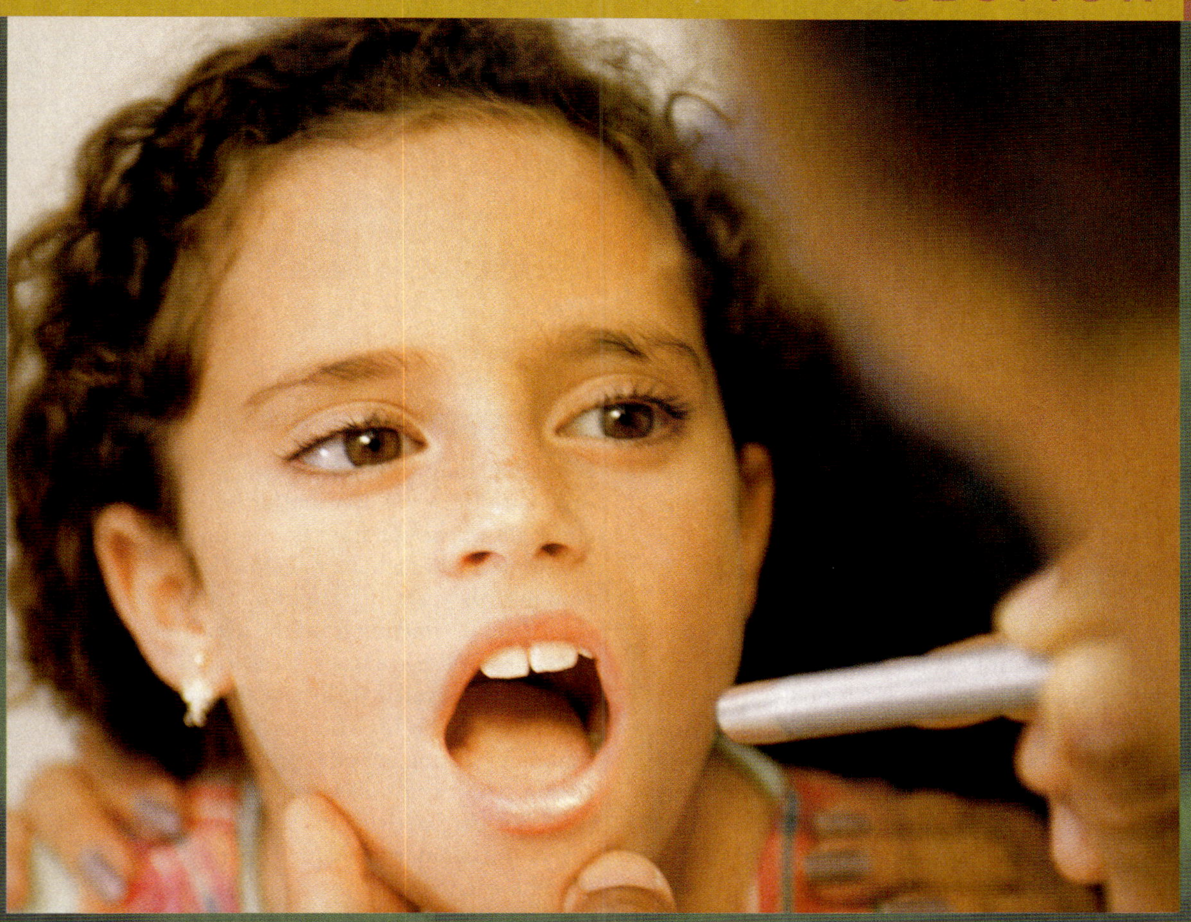

Signs and Symptoms

CHAPTER 7

Chronic Abdominal Pain

Joel Friedlander and Randolph P. Matthews

DEFINITION

Chronic abdominal pain in children is defined as any type of pain localized to the abdomen of at least 2 months duration that inhibits normal activity. It is one of the most common presenting complaints to pediatricians. Up to 17% of high school students experience weekly abdominal pain, and chronic abdominal pain accounts for approximately 4% of pediatric office visits.[1] The vast majority of these children have functional abdominal pain that, while debilitating, cannot be explained by a clear pathophysiologic mechanism. A minority of patients complaining of chronic abdominal pain has a chronic illness, typically of an infectious, inflammatory, anatomic, or biochemical etiology. These conditions, which will be the focus of this chapter, are often treatable and occasionally curable.

DIFFERENTIAL DIAGNOSIS

While the differential diagnosis of chronic abdominal pain is broad, a fairly simple approach can be utilized to help determine the etiology of the pain. The first decision point, as depicted in Figure 7–1, concerns the location of the pain. If the patient defines the location, the differential diagnosis becomes more focused, and the etiology is often discernable from organs in the vicinity of the pain. In general, location alone does not allow for clear differentiation of infectious from noninfectious causes. If the patient cannot define the location, either because the pain is diffuse or the patient is too young or is nonverbal, the clinician must rely on other symptoms to identify the problem. This approach is detailed more fully below.

Right Upper Quadrant

Pain emanating from the right upper quadrant usually originates from the liver and/or biliary tree. Occasionally, right upper quadrant pain is caused by diseases of the stomach, duodenum, or colon (Figure 7–1). Phrenic pain may also present as right upper quadrant pain.

Pain originating from the liver itself is because of stretching of the liver capsule, as that is the only part of the liver innervated with pain fibers. Thus, liver pain occurs when the liver becomes swollen, such as after trauma or during episodes of severe inflammation and edema. This is not likely to cause chronic abdominal pain, but chronic hepatitis may have periods of more severe inflammation, during which the liver may become edematous, causing the capsule to stretch. A more detailed discussion of hepatitis is found elsewhere in this textbook. Perihepatitis, or inflammation of the capsule itself, will lead to right upper quadrant pain. This is occasionally a component of pelvic inflammatory disease (see Chapter 43).

Cholelithiasis refers to the presence of symptomatic gallstones and may present as intermittent severe right upper quadrant pain, or as milder pain following meals. Most children with cholelithiasis have underlying hemolytic disorders such as sickle cell disease, or have a prolonged history of total parenteral nutrition; however, increasing rates of obesity in children have also led to a greater incidence of cholelithiasis.[2] Obstruction of the biliary tree leads to choledocholithiasis, while obstruction of the gallbladder leads to cholecystitis. While these are important causes of acute right upper quadrant pain, cholecystitis in particular may be chronic. Chronic cholecystitis is frequently associated with poor gallbladder emptying (gallbladder dyskinesia) rather than

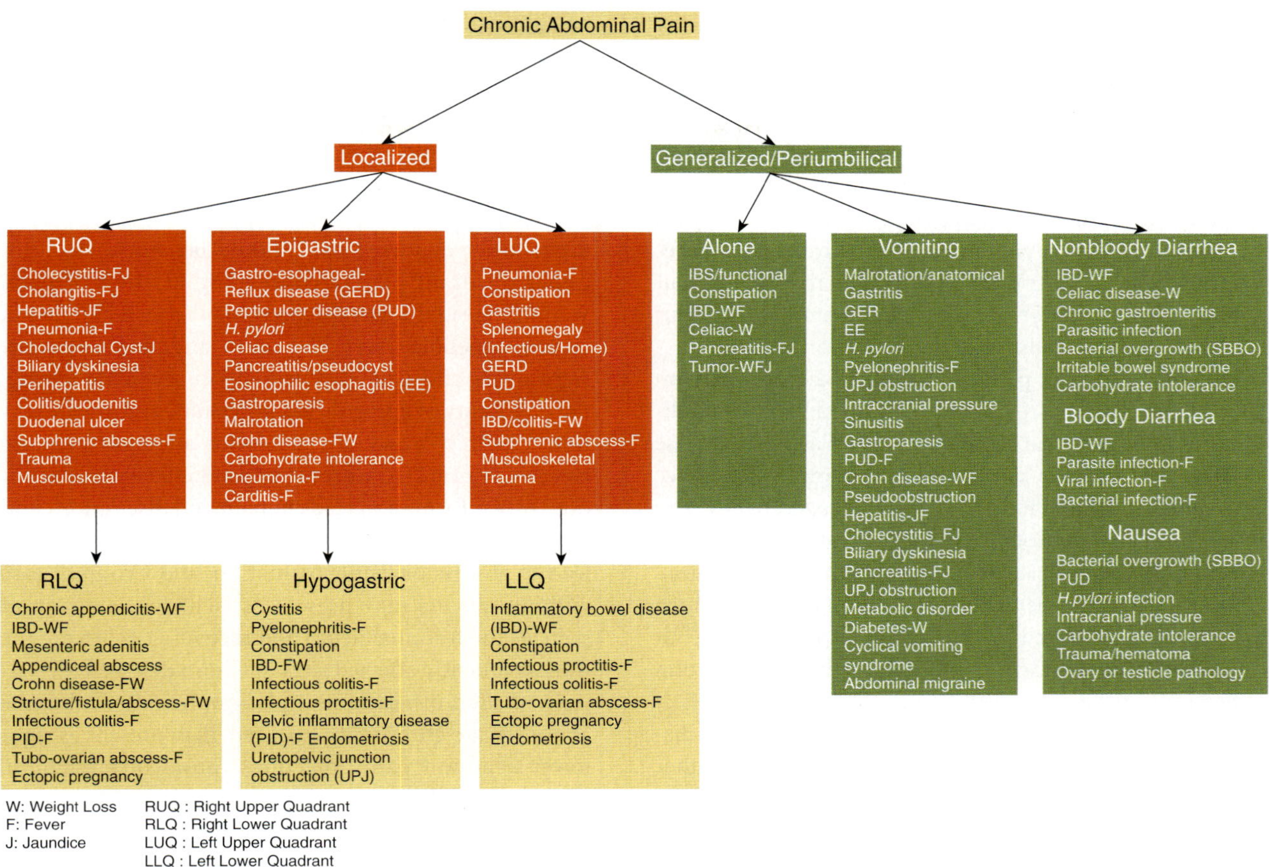

FIGURE 7–1 ■ Differential diagnosis of chronic abdominal pain. Letters W, J and F refer to accompanying symptoms.

obstruction; therefore, jaundice does not typically occur in these patients. Cholangitis refers to inflammation or infection of the intrahepatic biliary tree and rarely causes pain, although it is a risk factor for gallstone formation. Choledochal cysts are congenital malformations of the bile ducts, and typically cause pain when obstructed; as bile flow is generally poor through the cyst, infection and stone formation occur commonly.

Intestinal causes of right upper quadrant pain, such as colitis and bowel ischemia, are discussed more fully below, as they are more frequently causes of lower quadrant pain. Pneumonia and phrenic abscesses lead to right upper quadrant pain because of irritation to the diaphragm, which can be interpreted as right upper quadrant pain.

Epigastric Pain

Pain in this region typically derives from the distal esophagus, stomach, duodenum, or pancreas. Occasionally, functional pain may be epigastric in origin, but other more easily treated entities should be evaluated.

Esophagitis has a multitude of causes. Typically, pain occurs while eating. Esophagitis may be infectious in nature, most commonly in immunocompromised patients where *Candida* spp., herpes simplex virus, and cytomegalovirus are relatively common causes. Retrosternal burning dysphagia and chronic nausea or vomiting should alert the clinician to the possibility of esophageal infection. Gastroesophageal reflux disease may lead to inflammation of the esophagus, but increasingly esophagitis is caused by food or environmental allergies that trigger eosinophilic esophagitis. Pain is not a typical presentation of eosinophilic esophagitis, but given the increasing prevalence of this condition it should be a consideration, particularly in patients with poor response to empiric acid blockade.[3] Gastroesophageal reflux without esophagitis may also lead to epigastric pain, typically associated with heartburn and dyspepsia.

Gastric causes of epigastric pain include gastritis and the related peptic ulcer disease. Gastritis is simply defined as inflammation of the stomach; the most common cause is *Helicobacter pylori.* Less common infectious causes of gastritis include cytomegalovirus, *Mycobacterium tuberculosis, Mycobacterium avium-intracellulare,* and fungi. Chronic nonsteroidal anti-inflammatory drug (NSAID) overuse is also an important cause. Peptic ulcer disease refers to ulcers exacerbated by acid, and in the stomach can be caused by medications such as nonsteroidal anti-inflammatory drugs or glucocorticoids—either exogenous in the form of medication or endogenous from extreme physiologic stress such as burns or trauma. Ulcers from *H. pylori* are more typically found in the duodenum, although gastric ulcers from *H. pylori* do occur. Epigastric pain may also arise from gastroparesis, or delayed gastric emptying. This may be present after either a viral or parasitic gastroenteritis. *H. pylori* may also be associated with this condition.

In addition to peptic ulcers in the duodenum from *H. pylori*, epigastric pain may be caused by chronic illnesses that affect the small bowel, such as celiac disease and Crohn disease. Celiac disease is a chronic intolerance to gluten, a protein found in wheat, rye, and barley; this condition is now recognized as a strikingly common condition, affecting ~1:100 individuals in the United States.[4] Celiac disease can be associated with other features such as diarrhea, constipation, weight loss, or poor growth, but may in fact present with pain as the only feature. Crohn disease is an inflammatory bowel disease that can affect any part of the gastrointestinal tract, and like celiac disease, is frequently, but not always, associated with other features such as diarrhea, vomiting, weight loss, or poor growth. Lactose intolerance is fairly common in select patient populations (persons of Asian, African, and Native American descent[5]) and is often associated with bloating and diarrhea after ingestion of dairy products. Small bowel bacterial overgrowth occurs when there is stasis in the intestinal lumen, such as upstream of strictures, or in individuals with poor intestinal motility; bacteria proliferate in these static regions and lead to symptoms such as pain, nausea, and bloating.

Acute pancreatitis in children most frequently has an infectious cause, although drugs and trauma are also important causes. Infectious causes of acute pancreatitis include multiple viruses (e.g., enteroviruses, adenovirus, cytomegalovirus, Epstein–Barr virus, mumps, measles), bacteria (e.g., *Salmonella* spp., *Campylobacter* spp., *Mycoplasma pneumoniae*, *M. tuberculosis*), and parasites (especially ascariasis).[6] Chronic or recurrent pancreatitis most often is idiopathic and may be triggered by an initial infectious agent, but may also be caused by anatomic anomalies, metabolic disorders, or heritable genetic disorders.[7]

Left Upper Quadrant

Isolated left upper quadrant pain is extraordinarily rare as a complaint. Generally, the etiologies of left upper quadrant are similar to midepigastric pain, as gastric pain may be felt in the left upper quadrant. Phrenic pain may be secondary to pneumonia or a subphrenic abscess. Splenic pain is more frequently associated with hematological conditions such as sickle cell disease or with viral infections such as Epstein–Barr virus. Chronic constipation may occasionally present as left upper quadrant pain, as may colitis.

Right Lower Quadrant

Right lower quadrant pain should be, similar to right upper quadrant pain, a concerning location of pain. Within the right lower quadrant lie the terminal ileum, cecum, appendix, ascending colon, and, in females, the right ovary and adnexa. Certainly in the acute setting, the possibility of appendicitis necessitates prompt attention. Chronic causes of right lower quadrant pain are listed in Figure 7–1. Chronic appendicitis with or without abscess formation leads to pain and discomfort, and may be accompanied by fevers. Crohn disease may also lead to abscess or fistula formation, and Crohn disease without abscess may present as right lower quadrant pain, as the terminal ileum and ascending colon are the most frequently affected sites in Crohn disease.[8] Mesenteric adenitis, in which multiple lymph nodes within the abdomen are chronically enlarged, may present as right lower quadrant pain. Infectious causes of mesenteric adenitis include viruses (e.g., coxsackie viruses, adenovirus, rubeola, human immunodeficiency virus, Epstein–Barr virus), bacteria (most commonly *Yersinia* sp., occasionally nontyphoid *Salmonella*, *M. tuberculosis*, and various *Staphylococcus* and *Streptococcus* spp.), and parasites (commonly *Giardia lamblia*). In female patients, tubo-ovarian abscesses, ectopic pregnancy, and pelvic inflammatory disease may present as right lower quadrant pain. It is possible for constipation or colitis to present as right lower quadrant pain, although this is probably the least likely location for these entities.

Hypogastrum

The hypogastrum, or suprapubic area, covers the bladder, rectum, and the uterus in females. Chronic pain in this region generally derives from inflammation in these structures, with the exception of chronic constipation, which in the absence of other symptoms is the most likely cause. Irritable bowel syndrome may present as chronic hypogastric or infraumbilical pain, and this condition is frequently associated with diarrhea or constipation. Chronic cystitis with or without pyelonephritis may lead to hypogastric pain. Colitis or proctitis may be caused by ulcerative colitis or by an infectious cause. Pelvic inflammatory disease may also lead to hypogastric pain.

Left Lower Quadrant

The left lower quadrant contains the descending and sigmoid colon, as well as the right ovary and adnexa in females. Thus, the causes of chronic left lower quadrant include constipation, colitis (infectious or ulcerative), and pelvic inflammatory disease or tubo-ovarian abscess. Diverticulitis, an important cause of left lower quadrant pain in adults, is rare in children.

Periumbilical/Diffuse

In general, patients with periumbilical or diffuse chronic abdominal pain are less likely to have an organic etiology to their pain. However, when chronic pain is associated with other gastrointestinal symptoms, such as vomiting, diarrhea, or constipation, there is much more likely to be an organic etiology. Thus, it is helpful to subdivide causes of chronic periumbilical pain based on associated symptoms.

Vomiting

Chronic diffuse abdominal pain associated with vomiting may arise from the upper gastrointestinal tract, from intestinal obstruction, or from nongastrointestinal problems. There is considerable overlap between the conditions causing diffuse or periumbilical pain and conditions that can present with localized pain discussed above. Malrotation and associated intermittent volvulus can present with chronic or intermittent abdominal pain and vomiting. The incidence of malrotation in the general pediatric population is estimated at 1/500[9] suggesting that this diagnosis should always be considered in this setting. Chronic intestinal pseudo-obstruction is a debilitating condition in which symptoms are indistinguishable from a true obstruction, but there is no physical obstruction. The etiology of this condition is unclear, and it may result in eventual intestinal failure.[10] A milder version may be seen transiently after gastroenteritis, which is often associated with carbohydrate malabsorption. Parasitic infections, particularly *Giardia* and *Blastocystis hominis*, may lead to chronic abdominal pain with gastroesophageal reflux-like symptoms, and occasional vomiting.

Occasionally, chronic or insidious conditions not within the abdomen lead to abdominal pain, and these conditions may also be associated with vomiting. Increased intracranial pressure, often from a mass, may lead to abdominal pain and vomiting, particularly early in the morning after the patient has been lying down. Various metabolic disorders, in particular fatty acid oxidation disorders and organic acidemias, may present with vomiting and pain, but typically pain is not an important component. If the abdominal pain and vomiting are paroxysmal, the patient may have cyclic vomiting syndrome, a condition associated with a family history of migraine headaches and with potential development of migraines in the patient.[11] Chronic sinusitis may present as abdominal pain and intermittent vomiting because of the persistent postnasal drip. Diabetes may also present as abdominal pain and vomiting, secondary to the ileus that develops from acidosis and severe illness. Patients with eating disorders may also present with chronic abdominal pain, vomiting, and weight loss; these patients almost always have poor body image and have intentional weight loss, in contrast to patients with celiac disease or inflammatory bowel disease.

Constipation

Diffuse abdominal pain is a common complaint of patients with constipation. The vast majority of patients with chronic constipation have functional constipation. There are several potential organic causes of chronic constipation, including Hirschsprung disease, lead toxicity, celiac disease, spina bifida (including occulta) and other spinal cord lesions, hypothyroidism, hypercalcemia and cystic fibrosis. Parasitic infections, particularly pinworm infection, may lead to constipation, but typically not without anal pruritis. Irritable bowel syndrome, a variant of functional abdominal pain, may present with diffuse abdominal pain and episodes of constipation.

Diarrhea

Many of the conditions that cause diarrhea also present with localized pain and thus have been mentioned above. In some cases, the diarrhea is bloody, and that changes the differential diagnosis (Figure 7–1). Patients with nonbloody diarrhea and abdominal pain typically have conditions affecting the small intestine, such as celiac disease, lactose intolerance, or infections such as *Giardia* or *Cryptosporidium*. Crohn disease of the small intestine also may result in nonbloody diarrhea. Crohn disease may be associated with a history of oral ulcers or perianal disease, or with extraintestinal complaints such as fevers, arthralgias or arthritis, and rashes. As stated above, weight loss is also a common feature.

Less commonly, patients may develop a "flat villous lesion," a condition in which intestinal villi have been destroyed following severe gastroenteritis, occasionally requiring parenteral nutrition until the villi have regrown. The lack of intestinal absorption is a common feature of all of these conditions, which results in increased intraluminal water and thus diarrhea. Irritable bowel syndrome may also present as diffuse abdominal pain with intermittent nonbloody diarrhea, although the etiology of this diarrhea is unclear.

As stated above, the presence of bloody diarrhea suggests colitis, whether from an infectious cause or from inflammatory bowel disease, either ulcerative colitis or Crohn disease. *Salmonella, Shigella, E. coli* 0157:H7, and other pathogens most frequently cause acute infectious colitis, as discussed elsewhere. These agents occasionally result in chronic colitis as well, but *Clostridium difficile* infection is more likely to become chronic. While these conditions may produce diffuse abdominal pain, patients with distal colitis or proctitis often will complain of tenesmus, which localizes to the rectum.

No Additional Gastrointestinal Symptoms

Diffuse abdominal pain that is not accompanied by other symptoms is the most common presentation for chronic abdominal pain. While this can certainly be a manifestation of virtually every condition listed above, it most likely represents functional abdominal pain. Functional abdominal pain is defined as debilitating pain for which there is no clear organic etiology. Because organic causes of chronic abdominal pain may present with no other symptoms, though, a thorough evaluation of the patient is usually required prior to diagnosing functional pain.

HISTORY AND PHYSICAL EXAMINATION

The history and physical examination for abdominal pain must focus not only on the abdomen, but on the entire patient. As discussed above, many conditions have extra-abdominal manifestations, and these clues may help determine the diagnosis. The history should begin, as with any, with the onset, location, and the duration of the pain. From there, questions regarding exacerbation and remission are helpful., Once this information is obtained, a careful and complete review of systems is necessary. For example, abdominal pain and vomiting may simply represent infectious gastritis, but with an early morning headache the cause could be an intracranial mass. Alternatively, this presentation with a history of hard and infrequent stools suggests functional constipation. Chronic abdominal pain with vomiting in which the patient also has weight loss, fevers, and arthralgias makes the diagnosis of inflammatory bowel disease more likely. The review of systems assists the clinician in narrowing the differential.

The physical examination must also be thorough to evaluate for associated conditions that have manifestations in the abdomen. Specific findings in other systems may suggest organic causes to chronic abdominal pain, such as jaundice suggesting biliary tract obstruction or liver disease, or mouth ulcers suggesting Crohn disease. An important part of the evaluation of any child is an assessment of growth; in the context of chronic abdominal pain, poor growth or low-weight percentiles suggest celiac disease or inflammatory bowel disease.

Inspection of the abdomen may reveal signs of previous surgery, distention, or a rash. Diminished bowel sounds suggest ileus or pseudo-obstruction, while hyperactive bowel sounds might be heard in a patient with Crohn disease and a partial small bowel obstruction. Palpation of the abdomen will help determine the presence of organomegaly, palpable stool, or tenderness. Localized tenderness in the context of chronic abdominal pain is concerning for an inflammatory or infectious etiology, such as colitis or chronic appendicitis for left or right lower quadrant pain, or for chronic cholecystitis for right upper quadrant tenderness. Palpable stool suggests chronic constipation, while splenomegaly suggests chronic liver disease or an infiltrative process. A rectal examination should always be performed on patients with chronic abdominal pain. Perianal disease is strongly suggestive of Crohn disease, and may be accompanied by signs of a perirectal abscess. Poor anal tone or lack of anal wink in a patient with constipation is concerning for a spinal cord lesion, while increased rectal tone may be consistent with Hirschsprung disease. A large amount of stool or a widened rectal vault suggests functional constipation.

Certain findings on history and physical examination suggest an infectious etiology to chronic abdominal pain (Table 7–1), but it is important to realize that these signs may also be present in chronic inflammatory processes. A history of fever or a fever on presentation, for example, may suggest a chronic infection such as an appendiceal abscess, but may also be present in inflammatory bowel disease. Physical findings consistent with an abscess are important not only for diagnosis of the abscess itself, but for the diagnosis of a possible underlying inflammatory process.

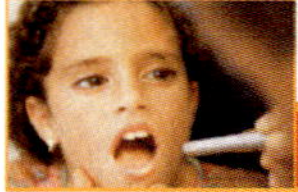

Table 7–1.

History and Physical Findings Suggestive of an Infectious Cause of Chronic Abdominal Pain

History	Physical Examination
Fever	Fever
Rash	Lymphadenopathy
Cough	Abnormal lung examination (crackles, etc.)
Diarrhea	Rash
Dysuria and/or flank pain	
Vaginal or penile discharge	

LABORATORY STUDIES AND EVALUATION

When the history suggests a clear problem such as constipation or gastroesophageal reflux, laboratory studies are typically unnecessary. However, laboratory studies may be helpful to diagnose some specific conditions.

General screening blood tests may include a complete blood count (CBC) with differential, electrolytes with BUN and creatinine, liver function tests, erythrocyte sedimentation rate (ESR), C-reactive protein (CRP), amylase, lipase, and celiac panel. Abnormalities of the above may suggest an organic etiology to chronic abdominal pain, such as an elevated amylase and lipase suggesting chronic pancreatitis. Elevation of the erythrocyte sedimentation rate, C-reactive protein, or white blood cell count, while possibly suggesting an infectious cause, may in fact suggest an inflammatory condition such as Crohn disease or ulcerative colitis. Celiac panels vary by laboratory, but generally the most helpful screening tests are antibodies against tissue transglutaminase (tTG) and anti-endomysial antibodies, with sensitivity and specificity of greater than 95% for both.[12] Other blood tests may be performed as indicated.

General screening studies should also be performed on stool, especially if diarrhea is present. A stool *H. pylori* antigen may be helpful in the absence of diarrhea as an effective screening test for infectious gastritis.[13] If diarrhea is present, then a stool culture, ova and parasite test smear, *C. difficile* toxin assay, and antigen detection for *Cryptosporidium* and *Giardia* should be performed. Urinalysis and urine culture should be obtained if indicated by history, and as a screening test if chronic abdominal pain and vomiting are present, especially in girls. Urine studies or other tests for *Neisseria gonorrhea* or *Chlamydia trachomatis* may also be obtained if indicated (see Chapter 45).

Diagnostic evaluation is generally symptom-oriented, but may be useful as screening as well. An abdominal radiograph will facilitate the diagnosis of constipation and obstruction. All patients with chronic vomiting should have an upper gastrointestinal (UGI) series performed to evaluate for possible intestinal malrotation. Strong suspicion for small intestinal Crohn disease requires that an upper gastrointestinal series with small bowel follow-through be performed. Tests for lactose intolerance such as a breath hydrogen test can be performed; a similar test can be performed to evaluate for small bowel bacterial overgrowth. If an intra-abdominal abscess, mass, or pancreatitis is a potential concern, then either computed tomography (CT) scan or ultrasound may be obtained. Such studies can also help guide aspiration or drainage of any abscesses.

Diagnostic tests suggestive of an infectious cause of chronic abdominal pain are listed in Table 7–1. As with findings on history and physical examination, some findings, such as elevated inflammatory markers, are nonspecific. Clearly, positive cultures are suggestive of an infectious etiology and should be treated appropriately.

INDICATIONS FOR REFERRAL

While consultation with a pediatric gastroenterologist may be initiated at any point in the evaluation of chronic abdominal pain, it may be necessary to obtain such consultation if the cause is unclear despite a thorough history, physical examination, and laboratory testing. Upper and/or lower endoscopy can help diagnose *H. pylori* infection, and is critical in the diagnosis of celiac disease and inflammatory bowel disease. Refractory *H. pylori* infection may require upper endoscopy to obtain gastric cultures to determine an effective antibiotic regimen. Motility studies can be performed, if necessary, to diagnose intestinal pseudo-obstruction. Long-term follow-up with a pediatric gastroenterologist is necessary for many of the conditions described above. Many of these patients, in particular those with functional pain, will benefit from counseling and therapy aimed at restoring some level of function. Some conditions, such as an appendiceal abscess or cholecystitis, should be referred to a surgeon. For those chronic conditions in which a relatively simple treatment can be found, such as antibiotic treatment for chronic giardiasis or small bowel bacterial overgrowth, treatment of the condition and resolution of symptoms can be gratifying for the clinician and a great relief to the patient.

ACKNOWLEDGMENTS

The authors thank Dr. John T. Boyle for critical review of the manuscript.

REFERENCES

1. Chronic abdominal pain in children. *Pediatrics.* 2005; 115(3):e370-e381.
2. Wesdorp I, Bosman D, de Graaff A, Aronson D, van der Blij F, Taminiau J. Clinical presentations and predisposing factors of cholelithiasis and sludge in children. *J Pediatr Gastroenterol Nutr.* 2000;31(4):411-417.
3. Liacouras CA, Ruchelli E. Eosinophilic esophagitis. *Curr Opin Pediatr.* 2004;16(5):560-566.
4. Torres MI, Lopez Casado MA, Rios A. New aspects in celiac disease. *World J Gastroenterol.* 2007;13(8):1156-1161.
5. Sahi T. Genetics and epidemiology of adult-type hypolactasia. *Scand J Gastroenterol Suppl.* 1994;202:7-20.
6. Parenti DM, Steinberg W, Kang P. Infectious causes of acute pancreatitis. *Pancreas.* 1996;13(4):356-371.

7. Lowe ME. Pancreatitis in childhood. *Curr Gastroenterol Rep.* 2004;6(3):240-246.
8. Barton JR, Ferguson A. Clinical features, morbidity and mortality of Scottish children with inflammatory bowel disease. *Q J Med.* 1990;75(277):423-439.
9. Ford EG, Senac MO, Jr., Srikanth MS, Weitzman JJ. Malrotation of the intestine in children. *Ann Surg.* 1992; 215(2):172-178.
10. Connor FL, Di Lorenzo C. Chronic intestinal pseudo-obstruction: assessment and management. *Gastroenterology.* 2006;130(2 suppl 1):S29-S36.
11. Li BU, Misiewicz L. Cyclic vomiting syndrome: a brain-gut disorder. *Gastroenterol Clin North Am.* 2003;32(3): 997-1019.
12. Rostom A, Dubé C, Cranney A, et al. The diagnostic accuracy of serologic tests for celiac disease: a systematic review. *Gastroenterology.* 2005;128(4 suppl 1): S38-S46.
13. Koletzko S, Konstantopoulos N, Bosman D, et al. Evaluation of a novel monoclonal enzyme immunoassay for detection of *Helicobacter pylori* antigen in stool from children. *Gut.* 2003;52(6):804-806.

CHAPTER 8

Ataxia

Erika F. Augustine and Annapurna Poduri

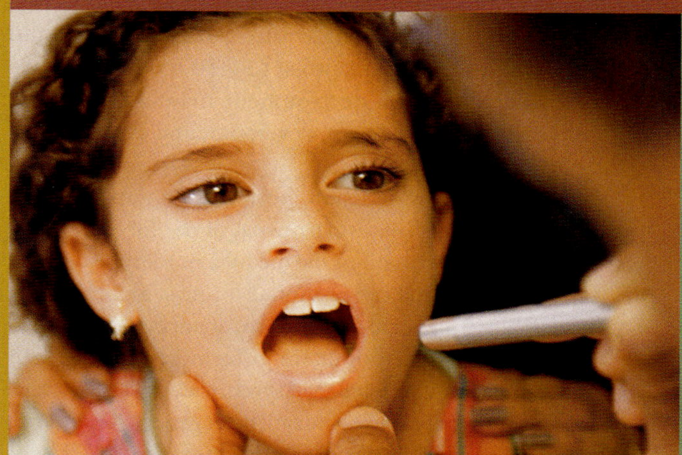

DEFINITION

Ataxia is derived from the Greek word *ataktos*, meaning disorderly, irregular, or unruly. Specifically, ataxia refers to an abnormality of regulation of posture and movement, a disturbance of balance and gait. Although ataxia can be caused by peripheral sensory abnormalities, spinal cord lesions, or injury to cerebellar projections, this chapter will focus on symptoms, signs, and etiologies of cerebellar ataxia with an emphasis on infectious and postinfectious causes.

SIGNS AND SYMPTOMS

Ataxia is characterized by unsteadiness of gait, truncal instability, and incoordination of limb movements. Cerebellar ataxia may be accompanied by other symptoms of cerebellar dysfunction such as dysarthria. Key portions of the history that will guide the differential diagnosis and evaluation include the nature of the onset of symptoms (sudden or gradual), duration of ataxia (hours, days, or months), course of illness (static, episodic, slowly or rapidly progressive), and associated symptoms.

Abnormalities of gait are the most common presenting symptom. Toddlers may present for evaluation of refusal to walk, while older patients may report the sensation of walking on a moving train or boat; adults make comparisons to the sensation of alcohol intoxication. Patients have difficulty ambulating or making sudden turns without assistance; many experience falls due to the instability.

Patients may also present with problems of limb coordination. In particular, difficulties with fine motor skills should be sought on the initial history. Patients may report clumsiness or inability to perform activities of daily living such as eating, writing, or reaching for objects. Difficulties controlling movements or presence of an action tremor may also be described.

Nighttime or early morning awakening with headache, pain that is occipital in location, vomiting, or pain that worsens after lying horizontally, bending, or with cough, sneeze, or Valsalva maneuver suggests increased intracranial pressure.

Lethargy and somnolence are worrisome symptoms, highly suggestive of increased intracranial pressure from cerebral edema, hydrocephalus, or mass. Lesions of the brainstem may also produce alterations in mental status. One should inquire about brainstem localizing symptoms such as diplopia, vertigo, and dysphagia. Fever suggests an infectious etiology, but an infection involving the cerebellum could produce neurological symptoms in the absence of fever.

DIFFERENTIAL DIAGNOSIS

The differential diagnosis of ataxia is quite broad. We will review the differential diagnosis of ataxia according to the time course of presentation—congenital, acute monophasic, episodic or recurrent, and chronic progressive ataxia. Since most in-hospital evaluation for ataxia addresses acute monophasic ataxia, emphasis has been placed on this section.

Congenital

Congenital ataxias are nonprogressive in nature but may become more evident over the course of the first 2 years of life as development progresses. They are typically related to malformations such as congenital cerebellar hypoplasia or dysplasia, or part of broader cerebral malformation syndromes such as Joubert or Dandy–Walker syndrome. Prenatal or perinatal injury, such as trauma or asphyxia, and hydrocephalus should also be considered. In contrast to acquired degenerative cerebellar disorders, development may be delayed in congenital disorders, but developmental regression is not present.

In basilar impression, posterior migration of the odontoid process causes narrowing of the foramen magnum with compression of the medulla or midline cerebellum. Minor trauma can precipitate acute symptoms, such as ataxia, cranial nerve dysfunction, quadriparesis, or sudden death. At-risk populations include patients with Down syndrome, Klippel–Feil syndrome, rickets, Hurler's syndrome, hyperparathyroidism, osteogenesis imperfecta, rheumatoid arthritis, and Paget's disease.

Acute/Subacute Monophasic

During early childhood, in previously healthy patients, drug ingestion (32.5%) and postinfectious acute cerebellar ataxia (35–40%) are the most common causes of acute or subacute ataxia.[1,2]

Particularly in young children and adolescents, it is important to rule out acute intoxication with medications (e.g., barbiturates, benzodiazepines, antiepileptic drugs, and antihistamines), heavy metals, organic chemicals, alcohol, or illicit drugs. Among antiepileptic drugs, phenytoin is the most likely to cause ataxia and nystagmus, although it may occur with other agents as well. Consider psychoactive drugs when alteration in sensorium is present or if seizures occur. Even without these features, toxin exposure should be considered in every patient with new acute onset ataxia.

In postinfectious acute cerebellar ataxia, symptoms are sudden in onset, typically affecting children under the age of 6 years,[1,3] although acute cerebellar ataxia may occur in adulthood.[4] Acute cerebellar ataxia is presumed to be a postinfectious, autoimmune disorder with cerebellar demyelination. Direct viral invasion is an alternate possible mechanism.[2,3] A typical case would be that of a previously well child awakening with dramatic ataxia, maximal at onset. Symptoms often develop within 1–2 weeks of a viral illness, often respiratory or gastrointestinal in nature.[1,4–6] There is a broad spectrum of severity from mild unsteadiness upon standing to complete inability to stand or sit without support. Truncal ataxia, dysmetria, and nystagmus are the most common neurologic findings.[4,6] There is a tendency for the trunk to be more affected than the extremities. Irritability is common, but alertness should remain intact. Depressed mental status may be a sign of malignant cerebellar edema with or without concomitant hydrocephalus. Generally speaking, however, postinfectious cerebellitis is a self-limited illness with an excellent prognosis. Improvement begins within 1–2 weeks of the onset of illness, with full recovery expected over the course of several weeks to months.[5,6] In a series of 60 cases of acute cerebellar ataxia between 1967 and 1989, 91% of patients had complete recovery, with the average duration of cerebellar signs being 2 months.[4] Only five of the 60 patients had sustained learning problems. In another series of 39 cases, all experienced complete recovery within 24 days.[6]

Acute cerebellar ataxia is particularly characteristic of varicella in the postinfectious period, on average 5–6 days after the development of the rash.[7] In one series, 26% of cases of acute cerebellar ataxia were attributed to varicella (in the prevaccination era).[4] Ataxia has been reported preceding the initial skin eruption, with a delay of as long as 2 weeks between ataxia and the development of rash. Thus, varicella should be considered as a potential agent in unvaccinated patients even if the characteristic rash is absent.[8] Acute cerebellar ataxia may also follow varicella vaccination.[9]

Although more commonly postinfectious, acute ataxia may be a presenting sign of viral encephalitis. When fever, altered mental status, symptoms of meningitis or cranial nerve palsies are present, encephalitis should be placed high in the differential diagnosis. Although the potential infectious causes are broad, Epstein–Barr virus (EBV), *Listeria monocytogenes*, human herpes virus 6 (HHV6), varicella, *Mycoplasma pneumoniae*, and enteroviruses have been implicated frequently. See Table 8–1 for further detail.

Ataxia may also be a presenting feature of acute demyelinating encephalomyelitis (ADEM), an immune-mediated multifocal monophasic demyelinating illness. In one series of 84 children with ADEM, 50% of patients demonstrated ataxia among the presenting symptoms.[10] Also postinfectious in nature, the presence of alteration in mental status, multifocal neurologic deficits, and multifocal white matter lesions on magnetic resonance imaging (MRI) are helpful in distinguishing ADEM from postinfectious acute cerebellar ataxia.[10,11]

Multiple sclerosis is largely an illness of young adults, although up to 5% of cases occur in children under the age of 6 years. An episode of cerebellar white matter demyelination could represent a first presentation of multiple sclerosis. When compared to adults with multiple sclerosis, children are more likely to present during a febrile illness with lethargy and nausea or vomiting. History of prior transient focal neurologic symptoms is an important component of making this diagnosis.

In one case series, 12.5% of patients with acute ataxia were diagnosed with Guillain–Barré syndrome (GBS).[1] This included patients with the Miller–Fisher variant of GBS, characterized by ataxia, ophthalmoplegia,

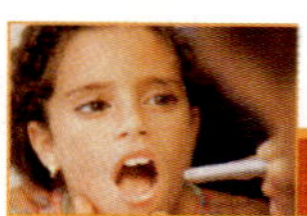

Table 8–1.

Causes of Acute or Recurrent Ataxia[5,12,13,16,17]

Infectious/Postinfectious/Autoimmune
Postinfectious acute cerebellar ataxia
Acute demyelinating encephalomyelitis
Multiple sclerosis
Guillain–Barré syndrome, Miller Fisher variant
Brainstem or cerebellar encephalitis
Bacterial meningitis
Selected infectious agents: Varicella zoster virus, Epstein–Barr virus, HHV6, mycoplasma, listeria, enteroviruses, herpes viruses, HIV, borrelia, Coxsackie, influenza viruses, parvovirus B19, Hepatitis A, malaria, legionella, coxiella, rubeola, typhoid, mumps, pertussis, diphtheria
Cerebellar abscess

Toxin exposure/Drug ingestion
Alcohol intoxication, illicit drug use
Antiepileptic drugs

Neoplasms/Masses/Paraneoplastic
Posterior fossa tumors (see Table 8–2)
Neuroblastoma (opsoclonus-myoclonus-ataxia syndrome)
Cerebellar abscess

Hydrocephalus

Migraine or migraine Equivalents
Basilar migraine
Benign positional vertigo

Trauma
Cerebellar contusion
Cerebellar or posterior fossa hemorrhage
Postconcussive syndrome
Vertebrobasilar occlusion or dissection
Cervical vertebral fracture/dislocation

Epileptic pseudoataxia

Vascular
Cerebellar hemorrhage
Acute infarction, sickle cell anemia, vertebral artery dissection
Vasculitis, Kawasaki disease
Vascular malformations (arteriovenous malformation, aneurysm)

Vestibular disease—may produce balance difficulties though not true ataxia
Otitis media, labyrinthitis
Meniere's disease
Posttraumatic
Perilymphatic fistula
Ototoxicity (antibiotic)

Metabolic/Genetic
Autosomal dominant episodic ataxias
Biotinidase deficiency
Hartnup disease
Hyperammonemia
Hypoglycemia, hyponatremia
Hypothyroidism
Kearns–Sayre syndrome, Leigh's disease, myoclonic epilepsy with ragged red fibers, neuropathy ataxia and retinitis pigmentosa
Maple syrup urine disease
Metachromatic leukodystrophy
Neuronal ceroid-lipofuscinosis
Niemann–Pick disease
Porphyria
Pyruvate dehydrogenase deficiency
Pyruvate carboxylase deficiency
Sialidosis
Vitamin E deficiency
Wernicke encephalopathy
Wilson disease
See Table 8–2 for additional genetic disorders that may present with either recurrent ataxia or chronic progressive ataxia

Conversion reaction

HHV6, human herpes virus 6; HIV, human immunodeficiency virus.

cranial nerve palsies, and areflexia; at times, this can be difficult to distinguish from brainstem encephalitis. Normal mental status and absence of fever are key findings that point toward GBS spectrum disorders rather than encephalitis. Patients present days to weeks after a viral illness or *Campylobacter jejuni* infection in some settings. Recovery is over a period of weeks to months.

If signs of increased intracranial pressure, such as headache, papilledema, vomiting, or lethargy are present, hydrocephalus or posterior fossa mass (e.g., tumor, cyst, or abscess) should be considered. Although gradual onset or chronic symptoms are more common in patients with brain tumors, if rapid tumor growth, hemorrhage, or development of hydrocephalus occurs, patients may present in an acute or subacute manner.

Paraneoplastic ataxic disorders should be considered as well, such as the opsoclonus-myoclonus-ataxia syndrome associated with neuroblastoma. The syndrome is characterized by opsoclonus (chaotic, darting eye movements), myoclonus, ataxia, and often encephalopathy. Symptoms may present prior to the diagnosis of neuroblastoma, with a mean age of onset of 18 months (range 6 months to 3 years). Symptoms evolve gradually over multiple days to weeks, and may wax and wane, in contrast to acute cerebellar ataxia, where symptoms peak within hours and then gradually improve. The encephalopathy most commonly manifests as extreme irritability or personality change.[2]

Ataxia can also occur after head injury as part of a postconcussive syndrome. Associated symptoms include chronic low-grade headaches, lightheadedness, and attention or short-term memory problems. Although the gait may be unsteady, limb dysmetria is not usually present, and the remainder of the neurologic examination is normal. The ataxia typically begins to improve within 1 month from the initial injury and resolves within 6 months.

Although rare in children, neurologic emergencies such as cerebellar hemorrhage and posterior circulation ischemic stroke are also included in the differential diagnosis of acute onset ataxia, and should be evaluated emergently. These diagnoses should be considered in high-risk groups (trauma, those with bleeding diatheses, hypercoagulable states, or congenital heart disease). Trauma to the vertebrobasilar arterial system may occur in high-speed accidents as well as with neck manipulation or sports injuries, causing vertebral artery dissection. Sudden stretch of the vertebral artery system as it travels through the neck may result in thrombosis with subsequent posterior circulation ischemia. Cerebellar hemorrhage can occur spontaneously due to arteriovenous malformation (AVM). Approximately 10% of all intracranial AVMs are located in the cerebellum. Vomiting, headache, neck stiffness, vertigo, cranial nerve signs, weakness, sensory loss, and altered consciousness are seen.

When the gait or balance disturbance is particularly extreme, in the absence of objective signs of cerebellar dysfunction or other neurological signs (e.g., hypotonia, hyporeflexia, weakness, or diminished sensation), conversion or functional gait disorder can be considered but only as a diagnosis of exclusion.

Episodic/Recurrent

There are some notable causes of recurrent episodic ataxia that will likely present with a first episode to a pediatrician or emergency department physician. Evaluation by a neurologist is highly recommended for evaluation of recurrent ataxia. As mentioned above, multiple sclerosis can present with ataxia, and recurrent demyelination of the cerebellum can lead to recurrent episodes of ataxia.

In basilar migraine, patients have recurrent attacks of cerebellar or brainstem dysfunction as a manifestation of migraine headache. The ataxia is followed by throbbing, severe occipital pain, possibly with associated nausea and/or vomiting. The attacks may rarely occur in isolation without headache. Approximately 50% of patients have true ataxia; other neurologic manifestations may include syncope, vertigo, positive visual phenomena (irregular flashes or light or colors), hemiplegia, or paresthesias. Prior history of migraine headache and family history of migraine are helpful. Incidence peaks in adolescence, with girls more likely to be affected compared to boys. Episodes tend to be stereotyped in nature and respond to standard migraine treatments. Over time, a classic migraine picture typically evolves.

In children, transient ischemic attacks are lower on the differential diagnosis, and repeated drug ingestion or metabolic disorder may be more likely unless vascular risk factors are present (Moyamoya disease, vascular anomalies, hypercoagulable states, congenital heart disease, and sickle cell anemia).

In patients with known epilepsy, consider pseudoataxia, an epileptic phenomenon. Patients have episodes of sudden onset ataxia due to generalized 2–3 Hz spike and wave discharges. Ataxia may also be a manifestation of a postictal state.

A number of metabolic disorders can present with ataxia, including urea cycle defects, aminoacidurias, and mitochondrial disorders. Exacerbations may occur in the setting of intercurrent illness and dietary change such as high protein load or other stressors.[12] At the time of first presentation, it may be difficult to separate these disorders from acute cerebellar ataxia. However, family history, developmental delay, cognitive impairment, encephalopathy, organomegaly, and systemic illness provide clues to this group of disorders.

Patients with benign positional vertigo may not display true ataxia on examination, but the vertigo is of a severity that makes standing or position change difficult. Episodes are brief, lasting minutes, and typically occur without headache, alteration in sensorium, or other neurologic symptoms (with the exception of nystagmus).

Chronic/Progressive

Recurrent or progressive ataxias are uncommon in childhood. Most chronic or progressive ataxic disorders are related to inborn errors of metabolism, or genetic disorders, once mass lesions and hydrocephalus have been excluded. The inherited ataxias are a broad group of rare disorders whose range and complexity are beyond the scope of this chapter, but should be considered in conjunction with a neurologist.

Ataxia–telangiectasia (AT) is a rare, progressive, neurodegenerative disorder characterized by ataxia, dysarthria, oculomotor apraxia, movement disorders, and cutaneous telangiectasias. Patients may first present to the primary care physician with recurrent sinopulmonary infections due to immunodeficiency associated with this disorder. Physical examination may reveal telangiectasias of the conjunctivae and exposed skin areas. Patients with AT are also at high risk for development of malignancies, including lymphoma and leukemia, as well as nonlymphoid cancers.[13] See Table 8–2 for other inherited ataxias.

Chronic infections, such as congenital rubella, or Creutzfeldt–Jakob disease may present with a slowly progressive ataxia. In teenagers or adults, consider chronic alcohol use causing cerebellar degeneration.

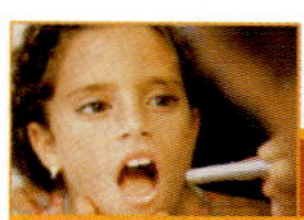

Table 8–2.

Causes of Chronic or Progressive Ataxia[12,13,16,17]

Neoplasms
Cerebellar astrocytoma
Ependymoma
Medulloblastoma
Von-Hippel Lindau disease

Congenital malformations
Cerebellar or vermal aplasias/hypoplasias/dysplasias
Dandy–Walker malformation
Chiari malformation
Basilar impression

Perinatal injury
Cerebellar hemorrhage
Hypoxic ischemic injury

Chronic infection
Creutzfeld–Jacob, Rubella, HIV, measles
Subacute sclerosing panencephalitis

Alcoholic cerebellar degeneration

Hereditary ataxias

Autosomal dominant
Episodic ataxias 1 and 2
Fragile X syndrome
Spinocerebellar ataxias

X-linked
Adrenoleukodystrophy
Leber optic neuropathy

Autosomal recessive
Abetalipoproteinemia
Ataxia–telangiectasia
Ataxia with oculomotor apraxia 1 and 2
Ataxia with episodic dystonia
Ataxia with vitamin E deficiency
Cayman ataxia
Friedreich ataxia
Juvenile GM2 gangliosidosis
Juvenile sulfatide lipidoses
Marinesco–Sjogren syndrome
Olivopontocerebellar ataxias
Ramsay Hunt disease
Refsum diease
Spinocerebellar ataxia with axonal neuropathy

HIV, human immunodeficiency virus infection.

HISTORY/PHYSICAL EXAMINATION

Most young children presenting with acute ataxia have postinfectious acute cerebellar ataxia or have suffered toxin exposure. One goal of the history and physical examination is to exclude serious or emergent causes of ataxia. In addition, the neurologic examination should help to clarify whether ataxia is present or whether other abnormalities of strength or sensation have produced unsteady gait or poor coordination.

History should include review of environmental exposures (cleaning substances, alcohol, illicit drugs, and prescribed and over-the-counter medications) and immunizations. Symptoms of current or recent fever, headache, neck stiffness, vomiting, lethargy, infectious symptoms (respiratory, gastrointestinal systems), infectious exposures, rash, or head/neck trauma are important. Inquiry into signs of cranial nerve dysfunction such as diplopia, head tilt, dysarthria, dysphagia, facial weakness, facial numbness, vertigo, or tinnitus should be sought as well. Elicit whether prior episodes of ataxia or focal neurologic symptoms have occurred, birth history, and preexisting medical conditions (epilepsy, metabolic disorders, migraine). Family history of similar episodes should be identified.

The general physical examination should include careful skin examination for evidence of viral exanthem, vesicles (which suggest varicella), petechiae, or telangiectasias. Furthermore, the ears should be examined to rule out otitis media as a cause of vestibular dysfunction leading to loss of balance. Careful examination should include testing for meningismus. If the ataxia is recurrent, hepatosplenomegaly may provide an insight into a metabolic disorder. Clues to possible drug ingestion may come from pupil examination and vital signs although pupillary abnormalities may occur with increased intracranial pressure, stroke, and mass lesions as well. Macrocephaly or rapidly increasing head circumference in a toddler suggests hydrocephalus or mass lesion.

Children with acute cerebellar ataxia may be irritable, but are typically alert. Alteration in mental status is suggestive of toxin exposure or more acute intracranial pathology, such as hydrocephalus, stroke, encephalitis, or increased intracranial pressure.

Horizontal nystagmus is common, however, vertical nystagmus or additional cranial nerve abnormalities point to a focal brainstem lesion. Papilledema or bilateral sixth nerve palsies, a false localizing sign, indicate increased intracranial pressure until proven otherwise.

Although the child may be most comfortable in a supine position, periods in seated and standing positions should be observed to look for truncal ataxia. Can the child sit without support of the hands or additional assistance? Is there swaying of the trunk? Is head titubation (bobbing) present? Trunk or head involvement is more suggestive of a lesion of the midline cerebellar vermis, while the limbs are predominantly affected in disease of the cerebellar hemispheres.

One may elicit limb ataxia with finger-to-nose or heel-to-shin testing. Rapid movements of the fingers, hands, or feet may be dysrhythmic and uncoordinated as well. If present, cerebellar tremor is most prominent with action or with the upper extremities elevated and outstretched; it is absent at reset. Cerebellar tremor is typically large in amplitude and coarse.

The classic ataxic gait is wide-based and staggering, more prominent with sudden stops or turns. The ataxia is best observed by asking the patient to narrow the base of the gait to perform tandem gait (heel-toe walking). Persistent falls to one side suggest a unilateral cerebellar lesion; falls occur to the same (ipsilateral) side as the lesion. Again, ataxia may be due to lesions outside of the cerebellum as well; a positive Romberg sign suggests sensory pathology, localized to the posterior columns of the spinal cord. In a positive Romberg sign, the ataxia becomes more prominent with loss of visual input (eyes closed). In cerebellar ataxia, findings should be relatively unchanged with eyes open or closed.

In addition to the above described signs/symptoms, key neurologic examination findings may include hypotonia, hyporeflexia, and altered speech. In ataxic disorders, the speech may be dysarthric and has a "scanning" quality. The speech is slow and deliberate with increased separation of words or syllables; the normal variation in intonation is lessened. One should look carefully for opsoclonus, irregular dancing movements of the eyes as seen in the opsoclonus-myoclonus-ataxia syndrome. Cognitive dysfunction, incontinence, dysautonomia, skeletal deformities, organomegaly, or multisystem disease may suggest an inherited metabolic or broader genetic syndrome. Asymmetry in power, tone, or deep tendon reflexes should prompt investigation into disorders other than acute cerebellar ataxia.

LABORATORY STUDIES

History and physical examination are the most important components of the evaluation of acute ataxia. Acute cerebellar ataxia, while one of the most common diagnoses in young patients with acute ataxia, is a clinical diagnosis. Urine and serum toxicology screens may provide the highest yield of all laboratory investigations, even when unsuspected, and thus should be performed in all patients with acute onset of ataxia. Similarly, serum electrolytes, including sodium and glucose should be a standard component of the evaluation of acute ataxia.

Urgent neuroimaging should be considered in patients with cranial nerve palsies, asymmetric neurologic examination, or alteration in mental status to evaluate for mass lesion, stroke, hemorrhage, or hydrocephalus. The head computed tomography (CT) is often normal in acute cerebellar ataxia. MRI of the brain may be normal or show cerebellar edema, bilateral diffuse cerebellar T2 hyperintense lesions (73% of cases in one review[14]), meningeal enhancement around the cerebellum, or obstructive hydrocephalus.[5,14,15] Signal change may be unilateral although this is atypical. For most patients, MRI abnormalities normalize within 10 months, although varying degrees of cerebellar atrophy can be seen.[14] Multifocal asymmetric subcortical enhancing areas of white matter signal abnormality are seen in ADEM. The brain MRI in multiple sclerosis may show multiple small periventricular white matter lesions, while the lesions of ADEM are typically large and subcortical in location. If ischemic infarction is suspected, diffusion-weighted imaging and MR angiography should be included, and ordered emergently.

In acute cerebellar ataxia and ADEM, the peripheral white blood cell count is mildly elevated in approximately one-half of patients, with lymphocytic predominance. Cerebrospinal fluid (CSF) may also display mild lymphocytosis and protein elevation.[4,10] Significant pleocytosis and/or low CSF glucose is more indicative of meningitis, and more specific bacterial or viral studies may be required. Early CSF studies in GBS may show mild pleocytosis but more typically show protein elevation with normal white blood cell (WBC) count; antibodies for the GQ1b protein may be positive. Oligoclonal bands are nonspecific and can be present in multiple sclerosis, ADEM, as well as acute cerebellar ataxia.

If neuroblastoma is suspected due to the presence of the opsoclonus-myoclonus-ataxia syndrome, workup should include measurements of urine homovanillic acid, vanillylmandelic acid, chest and abdomen MRI, and/or metaiodobenzylguanidine (MIBG) scintigraphy to investigate neuroblastoma.

In the absence of positive family history, recurrent episodes, or developmental delay, metabolic workup including lactate, pyruvate, serum amino acids, urine organic acids, and additional studies are unlikely to be of high yield. Further studies, such as electroencephalography (EEG) and/or electromyography (EMG), should be considered in consultation with a neurologist.

EVALUATION

See Table 8–3 for recommendations concerning evaluation of acute ataxia.

INDICATIONS FOR CONSULTATION OR REFERRAL

We feel that all patients with ataxia should be evaluated by a neurologist, especially patients with recurrent episodic and progressive ataxia. In the hospital setting, acute onset ataxia requires immediate emergency department evaluation, laboratory evaluation, neuroimaging, admission to the hospital to establish the course of disease while considering further diagnostic evaluation, and consultation with a neurologist. Any patient with depressed mental status, new onset of seizure, focal cranial nerve palsies, papilledema, or other

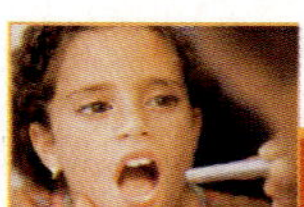

Table 8–3.

Evaluation

Consider strongly in all patients with new presentation of ataxia	Some patients will also need
■ Blood glucose ■ Serum electrolytes, bicarbonate ■ Drug screening (urine), specific serum tests if an exposure is known or suspected ■ Imaging for all children with acute cerebellar ataxia CT if an acute hemorrhage, hydrocephalus, or large stroke is suspected MRI with gadolinium MRI with diffusion weighted imaging and MRA if stroke is suspected	■ Lumbar puncture If fever, lethargy or papilledema are present; first obtain brain imaging Send CSF for viral studies if infection is suspected (VZV, CMV, HSV) ■ Serum viral titers based on common pathogens and specific exposures ■ HVA/VMA, abdominal CT/MRI for opsoclonus-myoclonus-ataxia syndrome ■ Lactate, pyruvate, NH_3, serum amino acids, urine amino/organic acids May be reserved for recurrent episodic ataxia ■ Vitamin E level if sensory neuropathy is suspected ■ ESR, CRP if risk factors for vasculitis are present ■ EEG only if seizures occur or if clinical suspicion for seizure as a cause of ataxia is high

CSF, cerebrospinal fluid; CT, computed tomography; MRI, magnetic resonance imaging; MRA, magnetic resonance angiography; VZV, varicella zoster virus; CMV, cytomegalovirus; HSV, herpes simplex virus; ESR, erythrocyte sedimentation rate; CRP, C-reactive protein; EEG, electroencephalogram; HVA, homovanillic acid; VMA, vanillylmandelic acid.

signs of infection or hydrocephalus should have emergent neuroimaging with CT and lumbar puncture unless the risk for herniation is high. Neurosurgery consultation is indicated for patients with hydrocephalus, hemorrhage, or mass lesions.

REFERENCES

1. Gieron-Korthals MA, Westberry KR, Emmanuel PJ. Acute childhood ataxia: 10-year experience. J Child Neurol. 1994;9(4):381-384.
2. Ryan MM, Engle EC. Acute ataxia in childhood. J Child Neurol. 2003;18(5):309-316.
3. Davis DP, Marino A. Acute cerebellar ataxia in a toddler: case report and literature review. J Emerg Med. 2003; 24(3):281-284.
4. Connolly AM, Dodson WE, Prensky AL, Rust RS. Course and outcome of acute cerebellar ataxia. Ann Neurol. 1994;35(6):673-679.
5. Maggi G, Varone A, Aliberti F. Acute cerebellar ataxia in children. Child Nerv Syst. 1997;13(10):542-545.
6. Nussinovitch M, Prais D, Volovitz B, et al. Post-infectious acute cerebellar ataxia in children. Clin Pediatr. 2003;42(7):581-584.
7. Johnson R, Milbourn PE. Central nervous system manifestations of chickenpox. CMAJ. 1970;102(8):831-834.
8. Liu GT, Urion DK. Pre-eruptive varicella encephalitis and cerebellar ataxia. Pediatr Neurol. 1992;8(1):69-70.
9. Sunaga Y, Hikima A, Ostuka T, et al. Acute cerebellar ataxia with abnormal MRI lesions after varicella vaccination. Pediatr Neurol. 1995;13(4):340-342.
10. Tenembaum S, Chamoles N, Fejerman N. Acute disseminated encephalomyelitis: a long-term follow-up study of 84 pediatric patients. Neurology. 2002;59(8):1224-1231.
11. Apak RA, Kose G, Anlar B, et al. Acute disseminated encephalomyelitis in childhood: report of 10 cases. J Child Neurol. 1999;14(3):198-201.
12. Lyon, G, Kolodny, EH, Pastores, GM, eds. *Neurology of Hereditary Metabolic Diseases of Children.* 3rd ed. New York: McGraw-Hill; 2006.
13. Maricich SM, Zoghbi HY. The cerebellum and the hereditary ataxias. In: Swaiman KF, Ashwal S, Ferriero DM, eds. *Pediatric Neurology: Principles and Practice.* 4th ed. Philadelphia: Mosby Elsevier; 2006.
14. De Bruecker Y, Claus F, Demaerel P, et al. MRI findings in acute cerebellitis. Eur Radiol. 2004;14(8):1478-1483.
15. Bakshi R, Bates VE, Kinkel PR, et al. Magnetic resonance imaging findings in acute cerebellitis. Clin Imag. 1998; 22(2):79-85.
16. Mariotti C, Fancellu R, Di Donato S. An overview of the patient with ataxia. J Neurol. 2005;252(5):511-518.
17. Fenichel, GM. *Clinical Pediatric Neurology: A Signs and Symptoms Approach.* 5th ed. Philadelphia: Elsevier Saunders; 2005.

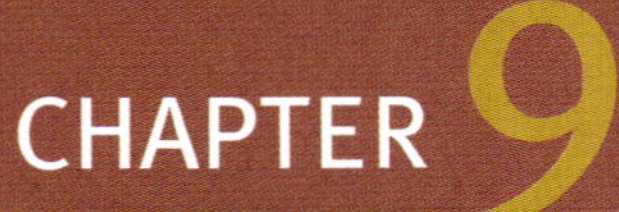

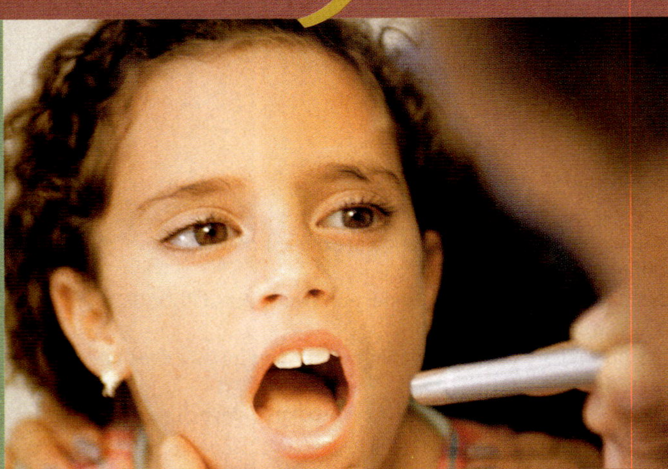

Dysuria

Kristen Feemster

DEFINITION

Dysuria, defined as painful urination, indicates irritation of either the bladder, urethra, or prostate gland.[1] It may be associated with urinary frequency and urgency or may be used to describe the discomfort associated with these symptoms. A complaint of dysuria can be difficult to elicit in younger children who may have difficulty distinguishing between dysuria and perineal or genital irritation.[2]

DIFFERENTIAL DIAGNOSIS

Overall, the most common conditions associated with dysuria are urinary tract infections (UTIs), urethritis, and local irritation. However, there are many other causes to consider (Table 9–1).[2–4] The patient's age and the presence of specific clinical or laboratory findings can help focus the differential diagnosis. Additionally, sexual abuse and pruritis associated with pinworm infestation can mimic dysuria.

Infection

Prepubertal children

A complaint of dysuria can be difficult to ascertain in younger children, but the presence of fever, increased fussiness, decreased appetite, lower abdominal pain, or suprapubic or flank tenderness may signal the presence of a UTI. Among febrile infants and children of age 2 months to 2 years with no other source of fever, the prevalence of a UTI is about 5% with an overall predominance of girls. Male neonates are five to eight times more likely to have a UTI than girls during the neonatal period but after 3 months of age, female infants are two times more likely to be infected and 1–5-year-old girls are 10–20 times more likely to be compared with boys.[5]

A UTI can affect either the upper or lower genitourinary tract. The presence of fever and other signs such as flank pain point to pyelonephritis rather than cystitis. These signs, however, are more reliable in older children. The most common organisms associated with UTI are enterobacteria. *Escherichia coli* is associated with 70–90% of infections.[5,6] Other organisms include *Pseudomonas aeruginosa, Proteus mirabalis,* and *Enterococcus* spp. Viruses, though less common, can also cause cystitis. Adenovirus in particular is a well-described cause of acute hemorrhagic cystitis. Uncommon organisms that cause UTI include *Staphylococcus aureus, Schistosomae* (associated with acute hemorrhagic cystitis), and *Mycobacterium tuberculosis.*[1,5,6] *S. aureus* most commonly causes infection when there is a predisposing condition such as an indwelling catheter or concurrent infection such as a renal abscess.

Other causes of dysuria in the prepubertal child include vaginitis in girls and balanitis in boys. Vaginitis can be caused by group A *Streptococcus, Shigella* spp., or *Candida* spp. Varicella lesions involving the perineum and vagina may also cause dysuria.[4] If there are signs of vaginitis or urethritis and the source is found to be a sexually transmitted organism such as *Chlamydia trachomatis* or *Neisseria gonorrhoeae*, an evaluation for sexual abuse should be initiated.

Postpubertal children

Among adolescents, UTI remains the most common cause of dysuria, particularly in girls. UTIs occur less commonly in postpubertal boys in the absence of an anatomic urinary tract abnormality. Beyond UTI, the most important consideration is sexually transmitted infection causing urethritis, cervicitis, or vaginitis. The

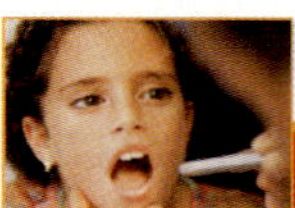

Table 9–1.

Infectious and Noninfectious Causes of Dysuria*

Infectious causes	**Common** –Bacterial cystitis –Pyelonephritis –Urethritis –*N. gonorrhoeae* –*C. trachomatis* –Herpes simplex virus –*Candida* species
	Less common –Viral cystitis[†] –Tuberculosis –Prostatitis –Schistosomiasis —Bulbar urethritis (adolescent males) —Balanitis (prepubertal males)
Noninfectious causes	**Toxic/environmental** –Chemical irritation from bubble bath, detergents, or perfumed soaps –Diaper dermatitis –Systemic drugs (cytoxin) –Contact dermatitis (poison ivy)
	Trauma –Masturbation/Sexual activity –Local injury –Irritation (tight clothing) –Foreign body
	Functional –Dysfunctional elimination –Syndrome/Constipation –Attention-seeking behavior
	Anatomic –Labial adhesions –Urolithiasis –Nephrocalcinosis –Uretheral stricture
	Other –Idiopathic urethritis –Appendicitis –Sarcoma botryoides –Virginal vaginal ulcers
	Systemic causes of urethritis –Stevens–Johnson syndrome –Reiter syndrome –Behcet syndrome –Varicella

**Conditions that predispose to infection, strictures, or urolithiasis include congenital and metabolic causes. Congenital causes include meatal stenosis, posterior urethral diverticula, ureterocele, ectopic ureter, posterior urethral valves, and vesicovaginal fistula. Metabolic causes include hypercalcuria and cystinuria.*
†Adenovirus is the only viral pathogen likely to be found as a cause of urinary tract infection.[6]

symptoms for both urinary tract and sexually transmitted infections overlap such that evaluation for both etiologies is often required in adolescents. One prospective study of adolescent females with dysuria showed that only 17% had a UTI, while 15% had C. *trachomatis* and 29% had urethritis and vaginitis caused by a variety of sexually and nonsexually transmitted agents.[7] UTIs are caused by many of the same pathogens that cause infection in younger children, with the exception of *Staphylococcus saprophyticus*,[7] which occurs more commonly in adolescent girls.

The burden of sexually transmitted infection among adolescents is high. According to the Centers for Disease Control and Prevention (CDC), 40% of all cases of *C. trachomatis* are diagnosed in 15–19-year-old females.[7] Since a history of sexual activity is not always reliable, screening for *N. gonorrhoeae* and *C. trachomatis* should be a routine part of the evaluation of an adolescent with dysuria, particularly if no other cause has been identified. Also, among boys, a complaint of dysuria is much more likely to be due to urethritis rather than UTI.[8] The presence of urethral or vaginal discharge strongly suggests urethritis, most commonly caused by either *N. gonorrhoeae* or *C. trachomatis*. Dysuria can also be associated with genital herpes simplex virus infection or with vaginitis caused by other sexually or nonsexually transmitted agents such as *Candida albicans*, *Trichomonas vaginalis*, and *Gardnerella vaginalis*.[7,9]

In an adolescent with dysuria, fever, and abdominal or flank pain, an upper genitourinary tract infection such as pyelonephritis or pelvic inflammatory disease (PID) should be considered. However, these symptoms can overlap with a wide range of other intra-abdominal conditions such as appendicitis, gastroenteritis, and nephrolithiasis.[7] The presence of flank pain and pyuria helps to distinguish pyelonephritis. Among sexually active adolescent females, assessing for PID is extremely important given the potential long-term sequelae of untreated infection. In addition to dysuria, patients may complain of lower abdominal or pelvic pain, fever, dyspareunia, vaginal discharge, and vaginal bleeding.[9] However, symptoms for PID can be very mild and only include one or two of these findings. In these cases, PID may not be considered in the differential diagnosis and infection can be missed. Minimal criteria defined by the CDC for the diagnosis of PID include cervical motion, uterine, or adnexal tenderness with or without other signs of of lower genitourinary tract infection. These criteria, while not very specific, minimize the frequency of missed infection.

Noninfectious Causes of Dysuria

In younger children, particularly those who present with isolated dysuria, local irritation is a common etiology. Local irritation can be induced by exposure to a variety of products including bubble bath, perfumed soap, or detergents. There may be no apparent signs of irritation on physical examination but symptom resolution will coincide with removal of the offending exposure.

Dysuria is also caused by local trauma associated with genital self-exploration, masturbation, or by direct trauma caused by events such as straddle injuries.[2–4] It is often difficult to elicit a history of trauma. Younger children may not remember an injury event and older children may be reluctant to disclose self-exploration or masturbation.[2–4]

Anatomic abnormalities can also cause dysuria. In young girls, labial adhesions are relatively common. While they are usually asymptomatic, there can be associated dysuria, especially if the urethral meatus is involved. Urinary strictures have also been found to cause dysuria in both younger children and adolescents.[4] Additionally, genitourinary abnormalities can predispose children to infection that results in dysuria. For infants and young children with a first UTI or older children with recurrent infection, evaluation for these abnormalities should be considered.[10]

Dysfunctional elimination syndrome (DES) with associated idiopathic urethritis is a relatively common cause of dysuria in younger children.[11,12] This diagnosis should be strongly considered if there is (1) no evidence of infection, (2) no history of exposure to irritants or trauma, and (3) no anatomic abnormality. Here, dysuria occurs in conjunction with constipation, which causes inadequate bladder emptying and chronic uretheral irritation. Bladder and bowel retraining programs effectively treat the urethritis.[11,12]

If dysuria is accompanied by hematuria and flank or lower abdominal pain with no fever or other signs of infection, urolithiasis should be considered. This is relatively uncommon among children and adolescents unless there is a history of a predisposing metabolic disorder such as hypercalciuria.[13]

When no cause for dysuria is identified, the complaint is isolated or is associated with times of stress, psychogenic dysuria should be considered. It is also important to seek other causes of perineal irritation such as pinworm infestation, which causes discomfort that is misidentified as dysuria.[2,3] If dysuria is associated with multiple symptoms such as rash, fever, conjunctivitis, the systemic causes of dysuria must be ruled out.[2] However, in these cases, dysuria is not usually the presenting complaint.

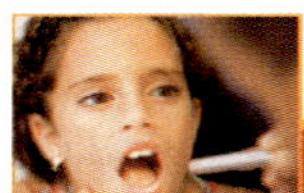

Table 9–2.

Significance of History and Physical Examination Findings in a Child with Dysuria

Finding	Significance
Presence of fever	–Urinary tract infection, pyelonephritis, or pelvic inflammatory disease
Presence of urethral discharge	–Urethritis or vaginitis caused by sexually or nonsexually transmitted infection.
Hematuria	–Nephrolithiasis, genital manipulation, urethral prolapse –Urinary tract infection caused by *S. saprophyticus* –If gross hematuria, hemorrhagic cystitis caused by *Adenovirus* or *Schistosomiasis*
Flank pain	–Pyelonephritis –Nephrolithiasis
Abdominal or pelvic pain	–Cystitis, pelvic inflammatory disease –Appendicitis
Urgency or frequency	–Urinary tract infection –Dysfunctional elimination syndrome
Swelling/redness	–Trauma, local irritation
Lesions	–Herpes simplex –Tumor –Virginal vaginal ulcers
Systemic signs, i.e., rash, conjunctivitis	–Stevens–Johnson syndrome –Reiter syndrome
Abnormal urethra	Presence of an anatomic abnormality, i.e., prolapsed urethra

HISTORY AND PHYSICAL EXAMINATION

The initial history should clarify the presence of dysuria versus perineal irritation and determine whether other accompanying symptoms readily suggest a specific cause (Table 9–2).[3,4,14] While systemic conditions such as Stevens–Johnson syndrome are uncommon, they do require urgent medical attention. The presence of rash, conjunctivitis, or meatal erythema should prompt a more focused evaluation for Stevens–Johnson syndrome. Recurrent dysuria, particularly when associated with oral or genital ulcers suggests Behcet disease. If there is no indication that a systemic condition is present, the clinician should focus on determining the presence of infection. History should assess the following[3]:

1. Is there presence of fever?
2. Is there presence of abdominal or flank pain?
3. Is there any urethral discharge?
4. Is there any blood in the urine?

As discussed earlier, fever and abdominal pain suggest either pyelonephritis or PID, both of which require prompt diagnosis and treatment to prevent late complications associated with these infections. In the absence of these findings, the clinician should attempt to identify other signs of infection such as urinary urgency or frequency. For adolescents, a sexual history should be elicited to assess for the possibility of a sexually transmitted infection. While sexually transmitted infections often present with urethral discharge, they may present with isolated dysuria only.[9] The absence of reported sexual activity does not preclude the possibility of a sexually transmitted infection, as adolescents do not always disclose this history.

Microscopic and gross hematuria may result from a UTI. Some pathogens are more likely to be associated with hematuria. *S. saprophyticus* often causes microscipic hematuria and *Schistosomiasis* and adenovirus often cause gross hematuria.[5,7] While sexually transmitted infections can be associated with abnormal vaginal bleeding, they are usually not associated with hematuria. Therefore, in the context of hematuria, UTI is more likely to be the cause of dysuria rather than sexually transmitted infection unless there is concurrent infection.[7]

If the initial history does not point to infection, the history should then focus upon the common noninfectious causes of dysuria. Exposure to any local irritants or injury should be elicited. Masturbation should also be considered; however, this history may be difficult to elicit

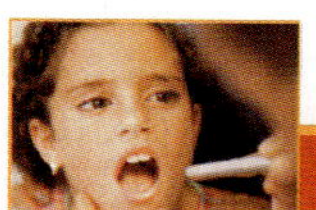

Table 9–3.

Diagnostic Studies to Consider in a Child with Dysuria

Test	Significance
Urinalysis	–Presence of leukocyte esterase and nitrites strongly suggests a urinary tract infection –Presence of WBCs indicates infection. Bacteria may or may not be present –RBCs and/or urine sediment indicates possible urolithiasis. If large number RBCs, consider hemorrhagic cystitis –Presence of crystals suggests nephrolithiasis
Urine bacterial culture[5]	
Clean catch	–$>10^5$ colony forming units per milliliter of a single organism indicates high likelihood of infection –10^4–$<10^5$ is suspicious of infection and should be repeated, especially if symptomatic –$<10^4$ or colony of mixed organisms suggests infection is unlikely
Catheterization	–$<10^4$ suggests highly likely infection –10^3–10^4 suspicious for infection, repeat culture
Suprapubic aspiration	–Any number gram-organisms or >few thousand gram-positive cocci indicates infection
Other urine culture[16]	–Culture for adenovirus can be sent from fresh urine if viral cystitis is suspected. For more rapid diagnosis, can send urine for immunofluoresence or EIA to look for adenovirus antigen. Serum antibody levels of at least 1:32 help confirm diagnosis
Nucelic acid amplification for gonorrhea/chlamydia	–Send in adolescents with history of sexual activity, if presence of discharge or if suspect reliability of sexual history –Urine specimens can be sent in both males and females. Among females, cervical specimens can also be submitted
Wet prep (microscopic examination of vaginal fluid)[9]	–Perform for adolescent females presenting with vaginal discharge. -Clue cells, elevated pH, and a positive Whiff test (odor when drop of KOH is applied to sample) suggest bacterial vaginosis –Budding yeast suggests candidal infection –Presence of motile, flagellated organisms and elevated pH suggest trichomonas
Metabolic studies[13] -Serum electrolytes, creatinine, calcium, phosphorus, uric acid -24-hour urine collection for sodium, calcium, urate, oxalate, citrate, creatinine, and cystine -Parathyroid, thyroid, and adrenocorticoid hormone levels (if hypercalcemia is present)	–Send if suspect nephrolithiasis or if family history metabolic disorder. Most common causes: –Hypercalciuria: Elevated urinary calcium:creatinine ratio, usually normocalcemic. Check parathyroid hormone if hypercalcemic. Usually idiopathic –Hyperoxaluria: Elevated urinary oxalate excretion, exacerbated by malabsorption –Hyperuricosuria: Elevated serum and urinary uric acid. May be associated with disorders of purine metabolism –Cystinuria: Elevated urinary cystine. Associated with disorder of renal tubular transport –In all cases may see signs of renal insufficiency
Imaging studies	–X-ray or ultrasound if suspect nephrolithiasis –Uric acid stones radiolucent and better visualized with ultrasound. Nonenhanced helical CT is most sensitive for detection of stones[13] –Ultrasound if suspect anatomic abnormality –Ultrasound and voiding cysterourethrogram should be performed in girls younger than 3 years with a first UTI, all boys with a first UTI, and all children younger than 5 years with a febrile UTI[17]

from both younger children and adolescents. Flank or abdominal pain and hematuria without fever suggest urolithiasis. Isolated hematuria also suggests either hypercalciuria or nephrolithiasis. A family history of metabolic disorders increases the likelihood of urinary stones. Isolated dysuria with a history of constipation suggests DES.

LABORATORY STUDIES

Evaluation of dysuria begins with a complete history and physical focusing upon the clinical findings detailed above. Unless a systemic condition is suspected as the cause of dysuria, laboratory evaluation should begin with a urinalysis. History, physicial examination, and the results of the urinalysis should direct subsequent testing (Table 9–3).[2–4,8]

Radiologic studies are generally not indicated for the initial evaluation of dysuria unless urolithiasis is suspected, or if there is suspicion of complicated pyelonephritis or a renal abscess. For younger children with a first UTI, imaging should be pursued to diagnose an anatomic abnormality such as posterior urethral valves and to detect the presence of vesicoureteral reflux that predisposes to infection; a voiding cysteurethrogram is the study of choice. A renal ultrasound may be performed to diagnose hydronephrosis or renal scarring. Renal scarring is more likely to occur in younger children after a UTI and identifying any predisposing abnormalities is important to prevent further infection and renal damage.[5]

EVALUATION

An algorithm for the evaluation of dysuria for any age group is described in Figure 9–1.[2,4] After performing the history and physical in all ages, a urinalysis is the first diagnostic test to be performed, even among sexually active adolescents in whom a sexually transmitted infection is suspected since a sexually transmitted infection and UTI can occur concurrently.[7]

In any patient with dysuria older than 6 years of age, while awaiting results of the evaluation, symptomatic relief can be offered with phenazopyridine (Pyridium): 4 mg/kg by mouth three times per day (maximum 12 mg/kg/day) or 100–200 mg three times

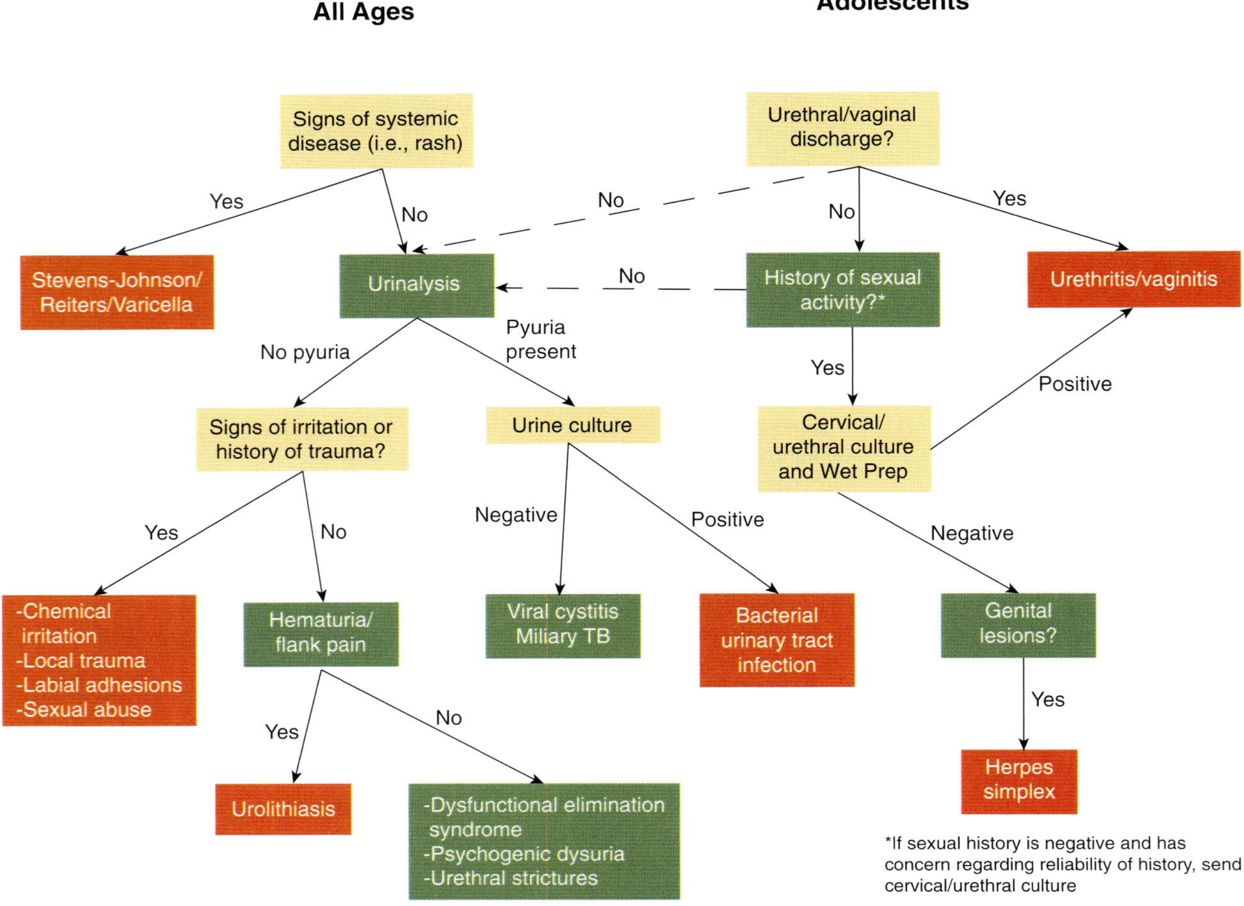

FIGURE 9–1 ■ Algorithm for the evaluation of dysuria.

per day for children older than age 12 years. Treatment should not be given for more than 2 days.[15]

INDICATIONS FOR CONSULTATION OR REFERRAL

Referral to Emergency Department

1. Infants and children with UTI and systemic signs such as high fever or inability to tolerate oral medications should be referred for admission and parenteral antibiotics.[5,10]
2. Any child or adolescent with a UTI who fails oral antibiotic treatment.
3. Any adolescent who fails oral antibiotic treatment for PID.
4. Any child for whom sexual abuse is suspected.

Referral to a Specialist

1. Any child found to have urethral strictures or any other anatomic abnormality should be referred to a pediatric urologist.[3]
2. A child with DES may benefit from a referral to outpatient urology for management if no response to a bowel/bladder retraining program.[11,12]
3. Presence of urinary stones may warrant referral to metabolic or endocrine specialist if the patient appears to have an underlying condition such as hypercalciuria.

REFERENCES

1. McAninch JW. Symptoms of disorders of the genitourinary tract. In: Tangho EA, McAninch JW, eds. *Smith's General Urology*. New York: McGraw-Hill; 2004.
2. Fleisher GR, Ludwig S, Henretig FM. Signs and symptoms: Dysuria. In: Fleisher GR, Ludwig S, Henretig FM, eds. *Textbook of Pediatric Emergency Medicine*. 5th ed. Philadelphia: Lippincott Williams & Wilkins; 2006: 2052.
3. Schwartz C, Schwartz W. Dysuria. In: Schwartz MW, Bell LM, Bingham PM, et al., eds. *5-Minute Pediatric Consult*. Philadelphia: Lippincott Williams & Wilkins; 2005:30-31
4. Fleisher GR. Evaluation of dysuria in children. In: UpToDate, Wiley JP, ed. *UpToDate*. Waltham, MA; 2007.
5. Schlager TA. Urinary tract infections in infants and children. *Infect Dis Clin North Am*. 2003;17:353-365.
6. Lohr JA, Downs SM, Schlager TA. Genitourinary tract infections. In: Long SS, PicKering LK, Prober CG, eds. *Principles and Practices of Pediatric Infectious Diseases*. Philadelphia: Churchill Livingstone; 2003:323-329.
7. Bonny AE, Brouhard BH. Urinary tract infections among adolescents. *Adolesc Med Clin*. 2005;16:149-161.
8. Letterle SJ. Genitourinary emergencies. In: Stone CK, Humphries RL, eds. *Current Emergency Diagnosis and Treatment*. New York: McGraw-Hill; 2004.
9. Holland-Hall C. Sexually transmitted infections: Screening, syndromes and symptoms. *Prim Care*. 2006;33: 433-454.
10. Committee on Quality Improvement. Subcommittee on Urinary Tract Infection. Practice parameter: the diagnosis, treatment and evaluation of the initial urinary tract infection in febrile infants and young children. *Pediatrics*. 1999;103(4):843-852.
11. Herz D, Weiser A, Collette T, Reda E, Levitt S, Franco I. Dysfunctional elimination syndrome as an etiology of idiopathic urethritis in childhood. *J Urol*. 2005;173:2132-2137.
12. Schulman S. Voiding dysfunction in children. *Urol Clin North Am*. 2004;31:481-490.
13. Nicoletta JA, Lande MB. Medical evaluation and treatment of urolithiasis. *Pediatr Clin North Am*. 2006;53:479-491.
14. Gonzales R. Common symptoms. In: McPhee SJ, Papadakis MA, Tierney LM, eds. *Current Medical Diagnosis and Treatment*. New York: McGraw-Hill; 2007.
15. Lee C, Robertson J, Shilkofski N. Drug doses. In: Hospital TJH, Robertson J, Shilkofski N, eds. *The Harriet Lane Handbook*. St. Louis, MO: Elsevier; 2005.
16. Baum SG. Adenoviruses. In: Mandell GL, Bennett JE, Dolin R, eds. *Principles and Practice of Infectious Diseases*. Philadelphia: Churchill Livingstone; 2005.
17. Shaikh N, Hoberman A. Clinical features and diagnosis of urinary tract infection in children. In: UpToDate, Torchi MM, ed. *UpToDate*. Waltham, MA; 2006.

CHAPTER 10

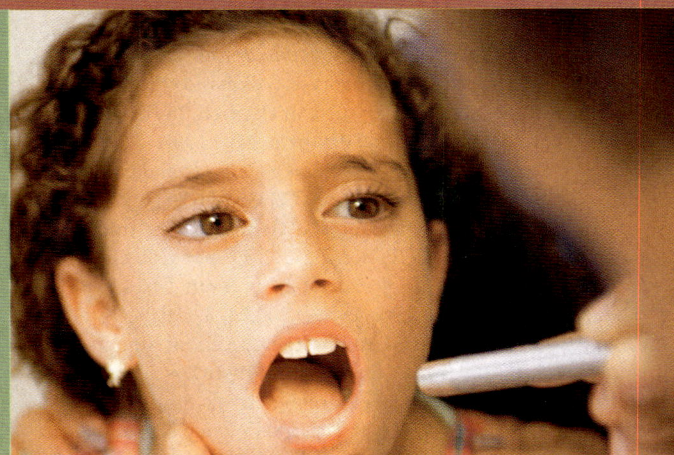

Headache

Robert A. Avery

DEFINITION

Headache is defined as pain located at any part of the head, but not necessarily in a specific nerve distribution. Headaches can be primary or secondary. Primary headaches cannot be attributed to another medical, systemic, or intracranial disorder. A common primary headache is migraine. The criteria for pediatric migraine include at least five attacks lasting between 1 and 72 hours, at least one associated symptom (photophobia, phonophobia, vomiting, nausea) and at least two of the following major criteria: unilateral or bilateral location (i.e., bifrontal or bitemporal as opposed to global); pulsating or throbbing quality; moderate to severe intensity; and worsened headache by physical activity.[1] Secondary headaches are caused by intracranial or medical/systemic disorders.[2] For example, a child with brain tumor and headache has a secondary headache. When fever and headache occur simultaneously, the headache is almost universally a secondary headache.

The ability to classify a headache as primary or secondary may not be readily apparent during the initial evaluation, therefore also categorizing the temporal characteristics of the headache is a useful way to approach pediatric headache. Headaches can be subdivided into acute, acute recurrent, chronic nonprogressive, and chronic progressive. Acute headache occurs without a prior history of similar episodes, whereas acute recurrent headaches have more stereotyped symptoms that return after periods of being symptom free. The headache that increases in severity over time is termed chronic progressive. The severity and frequency of pain may wax and wane in chronic progressive headache, but the overall trend demonstrates progression of symptoms. Chronic nonprogressive headaches occur on a nearly daily basis and do not significantly change in severity, and are typically less severe than chronic progressive headaches.

DIFFERENTIAL DIAGNOSIS

In patients without a prior history of severe headache, the acute headache is concerning to the family and the practitioner. The acute headache occurring concurrently with a systemic (e.g., viral, bacterial, etc.) or localized illness (e.g., sinusitis, otitis media, pharyngitis) is generally due to the accompanying fever or inflammation and represents the most common type of secondary headache presenting to the emergency department.[3–5] However, in a child with fever, any suspicion of central nervous system involvement including a change in mental status, seizure, or meningismus should raise the suspicion of an intracranial infection. Hydrocephalus should be the primary concern in all patients with an indwelling ventricular-peritoneal shunt who present with an acute headache and in patients whose headache is accompanied by double vision or episodes of transient visual loss. Other causative factors to consider in the evaluation of the acute headache include medications, toxins, trauma, seizure, or hypertension. Special consideration should be given to all patients presenting with acute headache that have an active or past significant medical history including leukemia, lymphoma, SLE, sickle cell disease, or HIV. Table 10–1 lists the differential diagnosis of headache based on temporal characteristics.

Acute recurrent headaches typically have similar characteristics that return after a period of being symptom free. Migraine headache is the most common acute recurrent headache. While most adult migraine is unilateral, younger children can have bilateral headache

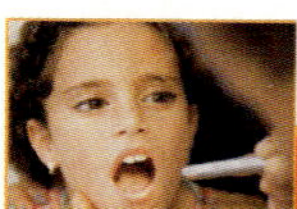

Table 10–1.

Differential Diagnosis of Headache by Temporal Character

Acute
Systemic viral infection
Localized sinus infection
Migraine
Meningitis (bacterial and viral)
Postseizure
Ventricular shunt malfunction/hydrocephalus
Trauma
Dental disease
Brain tumor
Ocular problem
Intracerebral hemorrhage
Cerebral sinovenous thrombosis
Subarachnoid hemorrhage
Toxin (lead poisoning, CO_2 poisoning)
Acute Recurrent
Migraine
Complicated migraine (hemiplegic, opthalmoplegic, basilar, confusional)
Migraine variants
Medications
Seizure disorder
Toxins/Substance abuse
Obstructive sleep apnea
Psychiatric disorders (anxiety, depression)
Chronic Progressive Headache
Medications
Brain tumor
Idiopathic intracranial hypertension (pseudotumor cerebri)
Brain abscess
Cerebral sinovenous thrombosis
Hydrocephalus
Ventricular shunt malfunction/Hydrocephalus
Chronic Nonprogressive
Chronic daily headache
Transformed migraine
Functional headache
Chronic meningitis
Psychiatric disorders

that later in adolescence becomes unilateral. When acute or acute recurrent headaches have accompanying neurologic abnormalities (i.e., weakness, aphasia, or change in mental status), the differential diagnosis should always include stroke, complicated migraine, and seizures. Aura consisting of visual, sensory, or speech disturbances can precede migraine headaches. Positive visual symptoms such as bright spots/lines or colorful scotoma are reassuring, whereas negative symptoms (i.e., visual field cut) are concerning. Children with headache and focal neurologic symptoms should always be examined by a pediatric neurologist.

The chronic progressive headache deserves prompt medical attention, especially in the setting of an abnormal neurologic examination as it most often indicates an elevation in intracranial pressure (ICP) or significant intracranial pathology. Any child with a headache that is increasing in severity and has an abnormal neurologic examination needs emergent imaging. Worsening of headache severity by lying flat should raise the suspicion of increased ICP. Headache is present in half the children presenting with brain tumor, but it is almost always associated with an abnormal neurologic examination.[6] Idiopathic intracranial hypertension (IIH), previously known as pseudotumor cerebri, is another common cause of chronic progressive headache that can also have accompanying abducens (sixth cranial nerve) palsy, decreased visual acuity, visual obscurations, decreased visual fields, or ringing in the ears.[7] Papilledema in the setting of an elevated CSF opening pressure with normal neuroimaging, serum, and CSF studies confirm the diagnosis of intracranial hypertension. When increased ICP is found, a search for contributing factors such as mastoiditis, sinus venous thrombosis, cryptococcus, lyme meningitis, chronic meningitis, or medications (oral contraceptives, tetracycline, Retin-A, chronic steroid use) should be undertaken. Children with cerebral venous thrombosis commonly present with both systemic symptoms and focal neurologic signs.[8] Risk factors for cerebral venous thrombosis include head and neck infections, acute systemic illness, dehydration, iron-deficient anemia, chronic systemic disease (e.g., connective tissue, hematologic, cardiac, or oncologic), or prothrombotic states.[8,9]

The chronic nonprogressive headache is generally milder in severity than acute headaches and less likely represents significant pathology. In the setting of a normal neurologic examination, a history of mild headaches without concerning features suggests chronic daily headache. There is typically a long history of headache that has been refractory to many medical treatments and/or has an emotional component.

HISTORY AND PHYSICAL EXAMINATION

The history and physical examination in pediatric headache is paramount (Figure 10–1). Obtaining a detailed description of the headache can be quite difficult in the uncomfortable child or adolescent. A headache history is particularly difficult in the toddler and young child. As with any medical symptom, the duration, frequency, onset (i.e., gradual versus abrupt), location, quality, severity, and temporal pattern of pain should be obtained. The presence of previous headaches with similar symptoms is

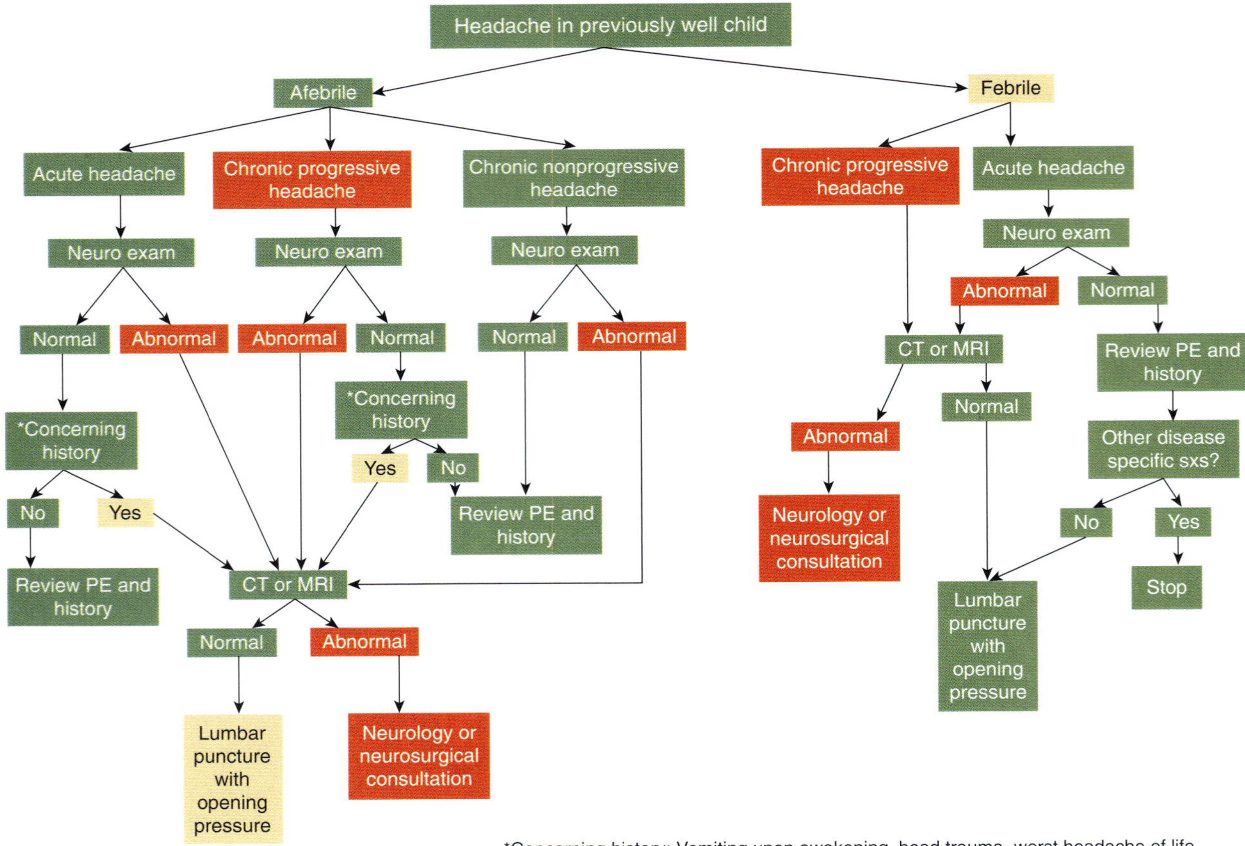

FIGURE 10–1 ■ Evaluation of headache in previously well child. Children with chronic medical conditions presenting with headache should be evaluated with close collaboration of their subspecialty physician and/or a neurologist.

the most useful as discussed in the prior section. Family history of migraine is also very reassuring. Subarachnoid hemorrhage should be considered when children complain of a sudden onset of their worst headache of life.

The headache location can be difficult to pinpoint in some children and may be referred pain from the sinuses, ear, mastoid, neck is but ascribed to the head. Headaches occurring in the occipital region are believed to be suggestive of significant pathology, but this is controversial. Although the quality of the pain (i.e., sharp, dull, pulsing) is a helpful descriptor, its usefulness in ruling out significant disease has not been shown to be helpful. Headaches that awaken a child at night or are present immediately upon awakening are two temporal patterns that should raise concern for intracranial pathology. Special attention to exacerbating factors such as worsening pain when lying flat or performing the valsalva maneuver suggests increased ICP. Headache relief with vomiting or early morning vomiting also suggests increased ICP.

Additional questions in the history should include presence of fever, localized pain, recent infection, trauma, toxin exposure, current medications, and a thorough review of any comorbid medical conditions and their treatment (i.e., congenital heart disease, genetic syndromes associated with vascular anomalies, immunodeficiency, indwelling shunts, oncology patients requiring chemotherapy, postsurgical patients, sickle cell disease, thrombophilia).

Routine vital signs, physical examination, and neurologic examination should be performed in every child presenting with headache. Special attention to the sinusus, nares, dentition, lymph system, mastoid, tympanic membrane, and nuchal rigidity may help elucidate an etiology. A complete neurologic examination should always include a funduscopic examination. If the optic disk and disk margins cannot be adequately visualized, a dilated eye examination by a neurologist or ophthalmologist might be needed in certain clinical situations. Figure 10–2 demonstrates papilledema in a child with 3 weeks of progressive headache who was found to have an elevated opening pressure on lumbar puncture and then diagnosed with idiopathic intracranial hypertension (i.e., pseudotumor cerebri).

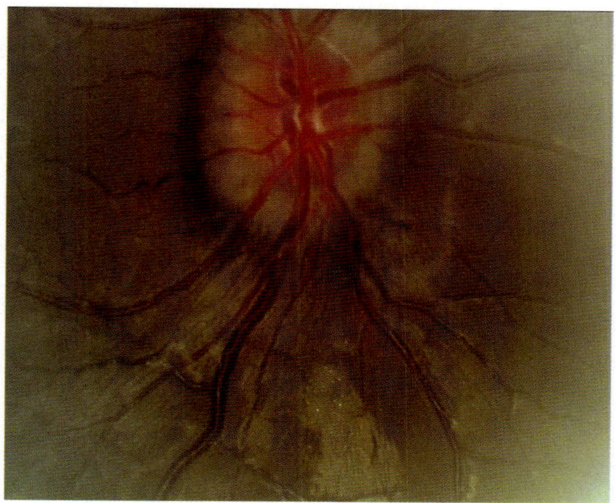

FIGURE 10–2 ■ The photo shows papilledema in a child diagnosed with idiopathic intracranial hypertension (i.e., pseudotumor cerebri). The child had 3 weeks of progressive headache and was found to have an elevated opening pressure on lumbar puncture. Note the elevated optic disk with blurred disk margins. Some, but not all of the vessels are obscured at the disk margins and the overall appearance is hyperemic.

LABORATORY STUDIES

Most laboratory tests are unhelpful in the child presenting with headache and a normal physical and neurologic examination. When indicated, etiology-specific laboratory studies can be sent based on physical examination findings. When meningitis, subarachnoid hemorrhage, or increased ICP are suspected, lumbar puncture is indicated. For cerebral and epidural abscesses, lumbar puncture should be deferred until after neurosurgical consultation. If signs of increased ICP or focal neurologic deficits are present, a noncontrast head CT should be performed prior to lumbar puncture. For suspected infections, routine CSF cultures and viral-specific CSF studies (i.e., enterovirus PCR, HSV PCR) should be sent along with routine cell counts, protein, and glucose. An opening pressure should be a part of every diagnostic lumbar puncture.[10] If there exists a clinical suspicion for subarachnoid or intracerebral hemorrhage, CSF cell counts should be performed on the first and last CSF specimen tubes to evaluate clearing of blood.

Imaging the child with headache can be approached in a systematic manner. Any child with an abnormal neurologic examination or signs of increased ICP requires emergent imaging. In most cases, a noncontrast head CT scan will be sufficient initially. Even when the neurologic examination is normal, if elements of the history are concerning (i.e., vomiting upon awakening, head trauma, worst headache of life, improvement of headache with vomiting, double vision, episodes of transient visual loss, or worsening of headache when lying flat), imaging should be considered. If mastoiditis is present or an epidural abscess is suspected, a noncontrast CT using a temporal bone window is recommended. If cerebral sinovenous thrombosis is suspected, magnetic resonance imaging (MRI) including magnetic resonance venography (MRV) may be warranted. Vertebral artery dissection should be strongly considered in patients with neurologic deficits associated with neck pain or posterior head pain following trauma. Imaging the vasculature of the head and neck using either magnetic resonance angiography (MRA) or CT angiography should be performed in these cases. In children with indwelling ventricular shunts, a shunt series to evaluate the integrity of the shunt as well as a noncontrast head CT should be obtained.

EVALUATION

Many excellent algorithms exist for evaluating the acute pediatric headache.[11] Figure 10–2 lists a simplified algorithm for how to approach headache in a previously healthy child using history and physical examination to guide the laboratory and imaging evaluations. Children with chronic medical conditions presenting with headache should be evaluated with close collaboration of their subspecialty physician and/or a neurologist.

INDICATIONS FOR CONSULTATION OR REFERRAL

Headache with accompanying neurologic deficit requires immediate referral to an emergency department and neurology consultation. Any child with papilledema or other signs of increased ICP needs an urgent neuroimaging study. Neurology consultation is typically warranted in most children with chronic medical conditions presenting with headache. The management of acute recurrent headache suspected to be migraine can initially be managed conservatively with referral to a neurologist on a nonurgent basis. Treatment of complicated migraine (i.e., those with accompanying neurologic symptoms) should be deferred until speaking with a pediatric neurologist.

REFERENCES

1. Hershey AD, Winner P, Kabbouche MA, et al. Use of the ICHD-II criteria in the diagnosis of pediatric migraine. *Headache.* 2005;45(10):1288-1297.
2. The International Classification of Headache Disorders. 2nd ed. *Cephalalgia.* 2004;24(suppl 1):9-160.
3. Burton LJ, Quinn B, Pratt-Cheney JL, Pourani M. Headache etiology in a pediatric emergency department. *Pediatr Emerg Care.* 1997;13(1):1-4.
4. Kan L, Nagelberg J, Maytal J. Headaches in a pediatric emergency department: etiology, imaging, and treatment. *Headache.* 2000;40(1):25-29.

5. Lewis DW, Qureshi F. Acute headache in children and adolescents presenting to the emergency department. *Headache.* 2000;40(3):200-203.
6. The epidemiology of headache among children with brain tumor. Headache in children with brain tumors. The childhood brain tumor consortium. *J Neurooncol.* 1991;10(1):31-46.
7. Liu GT, Volpe NJ, Galetta SL. *Neuro-Ophthalmology: Diagnosis and Management.* Philadelphia: WB Saunders; 2001: 204-214.
8. deVeber G, Andrew M, Adams C, et al. Cerebral sinovenous thrombosis in children. *N Engl J Med.* 2001; 345(6):417-423.
9. Sebire G, Tabarki B, Saunders DE, et al. Cerebral venous sinus thrombosis in children: risk factors, presentation, diagnosis and outcome. *Brain.* 2005;128(pt 3):477-489.
10. Fishman RA. Examination of cerebrospinal fluid: techniques and complications. In: Fishman RA, ed. *Cerebrospinal Fluid and Diseases of the Nervous System.* Philadelphia: WB Saunders; 1992:157-182.
11. Qureshi F, Lewis D. Managing headache in the pediatric emergency department. *Clin Pediatr Emerg Med.* 2003;4:159-170.

CHAPTER 11

Joint Complaints

Scott M. Lieberman, Melissa A. Lerman, and Jon M. Burnham

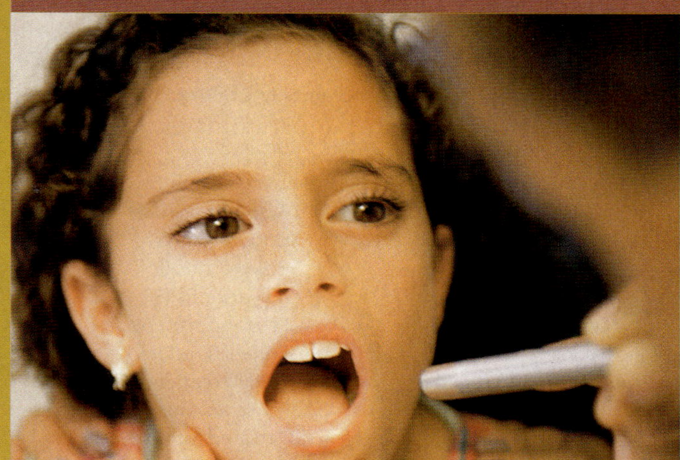

DEFINITIONS

Joint complaints are common in children, and the presentation may vary according to the underlying disease process and the age of the child. An infant may present with a red, swollen joint, decreased use of an extremity, or pain, demonstrated by fussiness with manipulation, such as with diaper changes. A toddler or school aged child may present with a complaint of pain, limp, or swelling noticed by a caregiver or with decreased use of an extremity. An adolescent is more likely to present with a complaint of pain, swelling, or stiffness. Joint complaints may be articular, originating directly from the joint, or nonarticular, arising from surrounding bone, muscles, soft tissue, or organs. This chapter will focus on articular pain.

Arthritis is defined as inflammation of a joint with two of the following: pain, swelling/effusion, limited range of motion, erythema, or warmth. Arthritis may affect a single joint (monoarticular) or multiple joints (oligoarticular if fewer than five; polyarticular if greater than or equal to five) and may be acute, chronic (6 weeks or more), or acute on chronic. Arthralgia is joint pain without other signs of inflammation. Enthesitis represents tenderness and inflammation of the tendon insertion into bone.

DIFFERENTIAL DIAGNOSIS

The causes of joint pain may be classified as infectious, postinfectious, rheumatologic, autoinflammatory, hematologic, oncologic, mechanical/traumatic, and other (including genetic and metabolic) (Table 11–1).

Infectious and Postinfectious

Septic arthritis is an infection of the joint space, usually caused by hematogenous spread rather than direct inoculation or spread from contiguous tissues. Septic arthritis is typically bacterial (e.g., *Staphylococcus aureus*, *Streptococcus pyogenes*, *Neisseria* spp.), although the spirochete *Borrelia burgdorferi* (Lyme disease) may be found in the synovium during acute infection. The presentation is typically acute. Prompt diagnosis and treatment with an appropriate antibiotic is necessary to preserve articular cartilage, which may begin to degrade as early as 8 hours after the onset of a suppurative infection.[1] Of special importance is septic arthritis of the hip, which does not typically present with noticeable joint swelling or redness, making it more difficult to distinguish from less emergent causes of hip pain. In viral arthritides, such as in parvovirus B19, viral particles may be found in the synovium, but the arthritis may be immune complex-mediated.

The peak incidence of septic arthritis is in children younger than 3 years, with boys affected more frequently than girls. Knees and hips are most commonly involved, followed by ankles, elbows, and shoulders, but any joint may be affected. *S. aureus* is by far the most common organism responsible for septic arthritis, with other common organisms varying by age and other risk factors (e.g., *N. gonorrhea* for sexually active adolescents).[1,2] Septic arthritis typically presents with a single exquisitely tender, swollen, erythematous, warm joint with decreased range of motion and pain. The child is often, but not always, febrile and toxic appearing. Although the large majority of cases of septic arthritis affect only one joint, multifocal arthritis is noted in

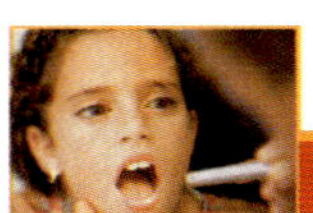

Table 11–1.

Etiologies of Joint Complaints in Children and Adolescents

Infectious	Rheumatologic	Autoinflammatory	Other
Septic arthritis	Juvenile idiopathic arthritis	Familial Mediterranean fever	Glycogen storage disease
Staphylococcus aureus	Systemic arthritis	TRAPS	Cystic fibrosis
Streptococcus pyogenes	Oligoarthritis	Hyper-IgD syndrome	Diabetes mellitus
Neisseria spp.	Polyarthritis (RF−)	CIAS1 Associated Syndromes	Serum sickness
Lyme arthritis	Polyarthritis (RF+)	Neonatal onset multisystem inflammatory disease	Marfan syndrome
Viral Arthritis	Psoriatic arthritis	Muckle-Wells syndrome	Ehlers–Danlos syndrome
Parvovirus B19	Enthesitis related arthritis	Familial cold autoinflammatory syndrome	Hypothyroidism
Hepatitis B and C	Undifferentiated arthritis		
Tuberculosis	Juvenile ankylosing spondylitis		
Osteomyelitis	IBD related arthritis		
Myositis	Systemic lupus erythematosus	**Hematologic and oncologic**	
Cellulitis	Mixed connective tissue disease	Leukemia	
Postinfectious arthritis	Sjögren syndrome	Bone tumors	
Streptococcus pyogenes	Scleroderma	Metastatic disease	
Acute rheumatic fever	Juvenile dermatomyositis	Synovial hemangioma	
Poststreptococcal reactive arthritis	Vasculitis	Pigmented villonodular synovitis	
Enteric infections	Takayasu arteritis	Sickle cell anemia	
Salmonella	Polyarteritis nodosa	Hemarthrosis (often in hemophilia)	
Shigella	Kawasaki disease		
Yersinia	Henoch–Schönlein purpura	**Mechanical**	
Enterobacter	Wegener granulomatosis	Trauma	
Clostridium difficile	Microscopic polyangiitis	Osteochondritis dessicans	
Genitourinary infections	Churg–Strauss syndrome	Foreign body synovitis	
Chlamydia trachomatis	Behçet disease	Slipped capital femoral epiphysis	
Neisseria gonorrheae	Sarcoidosis	Legg–Calvé–Perthes disease	
Mycoplasma pneumoniae		Osgood–Schlatter	
		Benign hypermobility	

5–15% of cases.[1–5] The presence of a known rheumatologic condition, such as juvenile idiopathic arthritis (JIA) or systemic lupus erythematosus (SLE), does not preclude the possibility of developing septic arthritis, especially when being treated with immunosuppressive medications.[6–8] Septic arthritis is discussed in more detail in Chapter 48.

Postinfectious "reactive" arthritis occurs following either bacterial or viral infections. Reactive arthritis presents with an acute onset of severe joint pain and swelling, sometimes with associated erythema, and can occur days to weeks following genitourinary or enteric infections. Poststreptococcal reactive arthritis and acute rheumatic fever occur following untreated group A β-hemolytic streptococcal pharyngitis, most commonly in children 5–15 years old. In acute rheumatic fever, arthralgias may precede a migratory arthritis that usually affects large joints, such as knees, ankles, shoulders, wrists, or elbows. The Jones Criteria for the diagnosis of acute rheumatic fever are presented in Table 11–2.[9] Postinfectious viral processes occur 1–2 months following infection, yet most are transient and resolve within 6 weeks. Toxic synovitis is a mild reactive arthritis

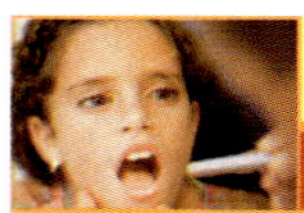

Table 11–2.

Jones Criteria for Diagnosis of Acute Rheumatic Fever* (JAMA 1992)

Major Criteria	Minor Criteria
Joint: migratory polyarthritis	Fever
Carditis: new murmur, (mitral ≥ aortic)	Previous acute rheumatic fever or rheumatic heart disease
Nodules, subcutaneous, and painless	Arthralgia
Erythema marginatum	Elevated inflammatory markers (ESR or CRP)
Sydenham's chorea	Prolonged PR interval on ECG

**Diagnosis requires two major or one major and two minor criteria PLUS evidence of preceding group A Streptococcal infection (positive rapid test or throat culture, elevated or rising ASO or anti-DNase B titer. The presence of Sydenham's chorea may be the only major criterion present and may occur late in the disease.*

of the hip. It commonly occurs following a viral upper respiratory tract infection.

Rheumatologic and Autoinflammatory

Previously referred to as juvenile rheumatoid arthritis (JRA), JIA affects approximately 0.1% of children.[10] By definition, JIA begins before the 16th birthday and symptoms must be present for a minimum of 6 weeks. JIA is divided into seven subsets: systemic arthritis, oligoarthritis, polyarthritis (rheumatoid factor negative), polyarthritis (rheumatoid factor positive), psoriatic arthritis, enthesitis related arthritis, and undifferentiated arthritis.[11] A key distinction is between systemic arthritis and other forms of JIA. Systemic arthritis is defined as arthritis in one or more joints associated with high fevers for at least 2 weeks and "quotidian" for at least 3 days, accompanied by one or more of the following characteristics: (1) evanescent, nonfixed, erythematous rash, (2) generalized lymph node enlargement, (3) hepatomegaly and/or splenomegaly, or (4) serositis. Children are often ill-appearing, particularly during fever spikes, when the rash may be more prominent. Arthritis may be present at initial diagnosis or may become evident later in the disease course, consisting of oligoarthritis or polyarthritis with involvement of any joint.

Other forms of JIA typically present with mild or no constitutional symptoms and variable degrees of pain. Approximately 25% of children with these forms of JIA will have no pain associated with their arthritis. The oligoarthritis subtype most commonly affects the knees or ankles. It typically occurs in young girls and is associated with antinuclear antibody (ANA) positivity and asymptomatic anterior uveitis. Polyarthritis often involves both large and small joints, sometimes in a symmetric pattern. It may be more debilitating, especially if rheumatoid factor is present. Enthesitis-related arthritis may be a harbinger of juvenile ankylosing spondylitis, which is more common in males, involves the sacroiliac joints and spine, and is strongly associated with the presence of HLA-B27. In psoriatic arthritis, the joint symptoms may precede the onset of rash. There is often a family history of psoriasis, prominent nail pits, and painful dactylitis, which has the appearance of a "sausage digit." Arthritis in association with growth delay, weight loss, microcytic anemia, and hypoalbuminemia should alert the clinician to the possibility of inflammatory bowel disease, even in the absence of specific gastrointestinal complaints.

SLE is a multisystem disorder often presenting with fever, fatigue, arthritis, and rashes, including the typical malar "butterfly" rash. Approximately 15% of all cases of SLE present during childhood, most commonly after 8 years of age, with a greater prevalence in females.[12] At presentation, arthritis and rash are present in 70% of children, and nephritis is observed in 50%.

Juvenile dermatomyositis is an autoimmune disorder that presents with rash and progressive proximal muscle weakness. The common "heliotrope" rash is a violet discoloration of the upper eyelids, which are often puffy. A malar rash may be seen. Gottron papules are erythematous lesions seen on the dorsum of the hand, particularly over the metacarpophalangeal as well as proximal and distal interphalangeal joints. Erythematous discoloration of the extensor surfaces of the elbows and knees are common. Up to 60% of children develop nondeforming oligoarthritis or polyarthritis during the course of their disease, but fewer (6–35%) have evidence of arthritis on initial presentation.[13,14]

The two most common vasculitides of childhood are both associated with joint symptoms.[15] Henoch–Schönlein purpura is a small vessel vasculitis that presents with palpable purpura in dependent areas (usually lower extremities), acute arthritis of the lower extremities (usually knees and/or ankles), and abdominal pain, with or without renal involvement. Kawasaki disease is diagnosed by the constellation of fever (5 days or more) and four of the following: nonsuppurative conjunctivitis, changes of the lips and oral cavity (red cracked lips, strawberry tongue), polymorphous rash, cervical lymphadenitis (nonsuppurative lymph node enlargement greater than 1.5 cm), and swelling of the hands and feet. The incidence of arthritis in Kawasaki disease is as high as 45%.[16] Two forms of arthritis have been described, and resolve without sequelae. Arthritis or arthralgia found in the acute stage is characterized by polyarticular involvement of large and small joints. Arthritis in the subacute phase of Kawasaki disease tends to involve the hips, knees, and ankles. Timely treatment decreases risk for long-term coronary artery aneurysms.[16] Arthritis is a common feature of other less common vasculitides, such as polyarteritis nodosa and the antineutrophil cytoplasmic antibody (ANCA) associated vasculitides (Wegener granulomatosis, microscopic polyangiitis, Churg–Strauss syndrome).

Sarcoidosis is a chronic systemic granulomatous disease that can affect almost any organ system. A common presentation during childhood consists of arthritis, rash, and uveitis, particularly in the inherited form associated with mutations in CARD15.[17] The majority of patients will have constitutional symptoms, such as malaise, fevers, and weight loss. Hilar, mesenteric, and peripheral lymphadenopathy are common findings.

Arthritis may be a prominent feature of autoinflammatory syndromes. Acute attacks of arthritis are seen in conditions such as familial Mediterranean fever, tumor necrosis factor receptor-associated periodic syndrome, hyper-IgD syndrome, Muckle–Wells syndrome, and familial cold autoinflammatory syndrome (see Chapter XXX for more detail).[18] In neonatal-onset multisystem inflammatory disease, arthritis may be transient, but a typical severe, deforming arthropathy is usually observed.

Neoplastic

Neoplasms that may present with joint complaints include primary liquid tumors (leukemia), metastatic disease, benign synovial tumors, and osteoid osteoma. Distinguishing malignancies from rheumatologic illnesses in a child presenting with arthritis and systemic symptoms is challenging. For example, in 15–30% of acute lymphoblastic leukemia cases, fever and joint pathology may be seen.[19] Leukemia and neuroblastoma are the most common malignancies that present with joint symptoms. However, other malignancies (such as lymphoma and Ewing's sarcoma) have also been initially misdiagnosed as rheumatologic illnesses delaying appropriate treatment.[20,21] Some features that are atypical for rheumatologic diseases and warrant further workup include: bone pain or tenderness, back pain, night sweats, focal neurologic abnormalities, and bruising.[21] Marrow replacement often causes pain that is worse at night, involves the back and long bones, and may be out of proportion to physical examination findings.[20]

Mechanical/Traumatic

Trauma is a common cause of musculoskeletal complaints in children and adolescents. Prior to maturation of the skeletal system, fractures are more common than ligament or tendon injury. Thus, it is important to image sites of trauma to ensure proper stabilization (surgical vs. nonsurgical) and suggest orthopedic referral. Nonaccidental trauma should always be considered, especially in the case of a neonate, an infant, or a chronically ill child, and in the case of an injury not explained by the proposed mechanism. In a child with multiple fractures or deformities, genetic or metabolic predisposition to such injuries should also be considered. A history of trauma does not preclude the presence of infectious, neoplastic, or rheumatologic condition. In fact, parents often mistakenly attribute the chronic joint swelling of JIA to a minor episode of trauma.

Consider Legg–Calvé–Perthes, or idiopathic osteonecrosis of the proximal femoral epiphysis, especially in a boy 4–8 years old, who presents with painless limp. Pain may develop in the hip, knee, or thigh.[22] This pain is usually worse at the end of the day and may wake a child from sleep. Slipped capital femoral epiphysis is seen in older children and adolescents. Slipped capital femoral epiphysis causes acute or subacute knee, thigh, or hip pain and is especially prevalent in overweight or obese individuals. Bilateral disease is observed in 20–30% of cases and urgent orthopedic referral is indicated.[22,23]

HISTORY AND PHYSICAL EXAMINATION

Characterization of joint complaints should focus on historical information and physical examination findings to determine if the problem is acute or chronic, and to distinguish between etiologies noted above (Table 11–3). Physical examination should focus not only on the most severe area of pain but the entire musculoskeletal system and neurologic system looking for asymptomatic arthritis, muscle weakness, or nerve dysfunction. Examine the area of interest last to allow for a less apprehensive child. A key goal of the physical examination is to determine if the complaint is because of true joint pathology or, rather, to pathology of surrounding tissues. Also pay specific attention to signs of systemic illness or multisystem involvement suggesting rheumatologic, autoinflammatory or neoplastic etiologies.

When examining the affected area, first inspect for color change and visible swelling. Evidence of asymmetric growth, such as limb length discrepancies or muscle

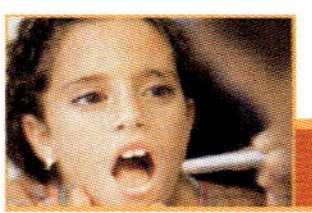

Table 11–3.

Significance of History and Physical Examination Findings in Children with Joint Complaints

Finding	Potential Etiologies
Toxic appearing	Septic arthritis, rheumatologic (SLE, vasculitis), autoinflammatory, neoplastic
Systemic signs/symptoms (fever, rash, fatigue)	Septic arthritis, rheumatologic, autoinflammatory, neoplastic
Morning stiffness or pain worse after inactivity	Inflammatory arthritis
Pain worse with activity	Mechanical/injury or enthesitis
Multiple joint involvement in additive pattern	Inflammatory polyarthritis
Multiple joint involvement with new joints after previous joints resolve (migratory)	Postinfectious (especially ARF), Lyme, leukemia
Preceding illness	Postinfectious, ARF, Lyme
Back pain, weight loss, or night pain	Neoplastic
Limb length discrepancy or atrophy/asymmetry of muscles	Chronic arthritis
Painful acute uveitis	Reactive arthritis, ankylosing spondylitis, enthesitis-related arthritis, psoriatic arthritis, inflammatory bowel disease, Behçet disease, vasculitis
Asymptomatic painless uveitis	Oligoarticular JIA, polyarticular JIA, psoriatic arthritis

atrophy, often indicate a chronic condition, as does the presence of deformities (flexion contracture, boutonniere deformity, swan neck deformity). Next, palpate the joint to assess for warmth and swelling by comparing it with the contralateral joint. Warmth is often best appreciated using the dorsal surface of the hand. Assess for fluid in the joint space, and then examine the muscles and bones above and below for point tenderness and deformity. If the child is old enough to cooperate, ask him/her to move the joint on his/her own. Even if its active range of motion is limited, it is important to also assess passive range of motion of the joint. Mild hypermobility may cause significant pain in children, particularly with and after activities. Extreme hypermobility should alert the clinician to the possibility of a connective tissue disorder, such as Marfan or Ehlers–Danlos syndrome.

Without visible signs of redness and swelling, localizing pain to the hip is more difficult than with other joints. In addition, pathology of the hip may present as thigh or knee pain. Examination of the hip, surrounding joints, bones, muscles, lymph nodes, and testes becomes very important in distinguishing hip pain from pain at other sites that may be referred to the hip. Typically, limited range of motion or pain on log roll of the leg indicates hip pathology. The joint space of the hip has maximal volume when the hip is flexed, externally rotated, and abducted. Pain on movements compressing this maximal joint space suggests the presence of effusion or other space-occupying lesion.[1]

LABORATORY AND IMAGING STUDIES

The differential diagnosis should first be narrowed based on the history and physical examination, and tests should be ordered to specifically distinguish between likely etiologies. In a well-appearing child with an isolated joint complaint and no evidence of arthritis, routine laboratory tests are not generally warranted. However, depending on the degree of clinical suspicion, imaging may be appropriate. In any child with arthritis and systemic signs or symptoms, especially if ill-appearing, a complete blood count with differential, inflammatory markers (erythrocyte sedimentation rate and C-reactive protein concentration), and a blood culture are appropriate. An elevated white blood cell count with a predominance of segmented neutrophils and elevated bands suggests a bacterial infection or in the appropriate clinical context, systemic arthritis or vasculitis (e.g., Kawasaki disease). A normocytic or microcytic anemia and thrombocytosis are common in the presence of chronic inflammation. A decrease in two or more cell lines may be indicative of bone marrow infiltration, suggesting malignancy. There are no specific diagnostic laboratory tests for rheumatic disease as a general category; symptoms and signs must be considered in conjunction with laboratory results. Obtaining an ANA and rheumatoid factor is a common but inaccurate method to "rule out" a rheumatologic disease. A positive ANA is commonly observed in healthy children and many children with rheumatologic disorders (e.g., vasculitis) are ANA negative.[24]

Evaluation of a child suspected to have septic arthritis requires aspiration of the joint fluid for analysis (cell count, Gram stain) and culture (aerobic and anaerobic). Identification of specific organisms occurs in approximately 50–60% of cases from joint fluid cultures and 30–40% of cases from blood cultures.[2] Numerous studies have attempted to define criteria to distinguish postinfectious from septic arthritis of the hip.[25–27] In one prospective study, five diagnostic criteria were used: oral temperature greater than 38.5°C, refusal to bear weight, serum white blood cell count greater than 12,000/mm^3, erythrocyte sedimentation rate greater than 40 mm/h, and C-reactive protein greater than 2 mg/dL.[28] Children with all five factors had a 98% chance of having septic arthritis. If there is a concern for septic arthritis, an arthrocentesis should be performed and empiric antibiotic therapy considered.

The three strongest predictive factors distinguishing leukemia from systemic onset JIA include low white blood cell count, a low or low–normal platelet count, and a history of night pain.[19] An elevated serum lactate dehydrogenase and uric acid suggest high cell turnover. A dissociation of inflammatory markers and the platelet count is suggestive of marrow infiltration in the appropriate clinical setting.[21] If peripheral blasts are seen in a blood smear, an oncologic evaluation should be sought immediately. However, in 75% of cases of acute lymphoblastic leukemia, blast forms were not evident in peripheral blood at presentation.[19] Bone marrow aspiration is often required to differentiate malignancy from rheumatologic illness.

Imaging modalities include conventional radiography, ultrasound, computed tomography, magnetic resonance imaging (MRI), and triple-phase bone scan. X-rays are appropriate for most initial evaluations and may detect effusions (usually noted as joint space widening or displacement of a fat pad) or the presence of bone pathology (e.g., metaphyseal lucencies in leukemia). Similarly, computed tomography scans are most useful for evaluating bone structure and subtle lesions, such as osteoid osteoma. Ultrasound is a noninvasive, nonirradiating modality for detecting effusions; however, it is user-dependent and often less accessible than X-rays. Bone scans are especially useful when multiple foci of bone inflammation are suspected, or to rule out osteomyelitis. MRI is a sensitive tool for the evaluation of the joints, muscles, and bones. In the evaluation of malignancies, MRI can detect bone marrow infiltration. In an individual with arthritis, MRI can distinguish between JIA, pigmented villonodular synovitis, and rare entities such as synovial hemangiomas.

EVALUATION

The approach to a child presenting with joint complaints requires a detailed history, a thorough physical examination, and judicious use of laboratory and imaging modalities. The key first step is determining the true anatomic location of the presenting complaint. Once arthritis or joint involvement has been established, it is imperative to evaluate for the possibility of septic arthritis, a diagnosis for which treatment must begin immediately in order to preserve the joint structure and to prevent joint destruction. Once the clinician has ruled out septic arthritis, evaluation for myriad etiologies of arthritis may begin. Figure 11–1 provides an algorithm to be used in conjunction with the laboratory and radiologic studies discussed above, when appropriate.

INDICATIONS FOR CONSULTATION OR REFERRAL

Consultation with orthopedists, rheumatologists, oncologists, infectious disease specialists, and geneticists should be sought based on the history, physical examination, imaging studies, and laboratory evaluation. These consultants may help focus the diagnostic workup and institute appropriate medical or surgical therapy.

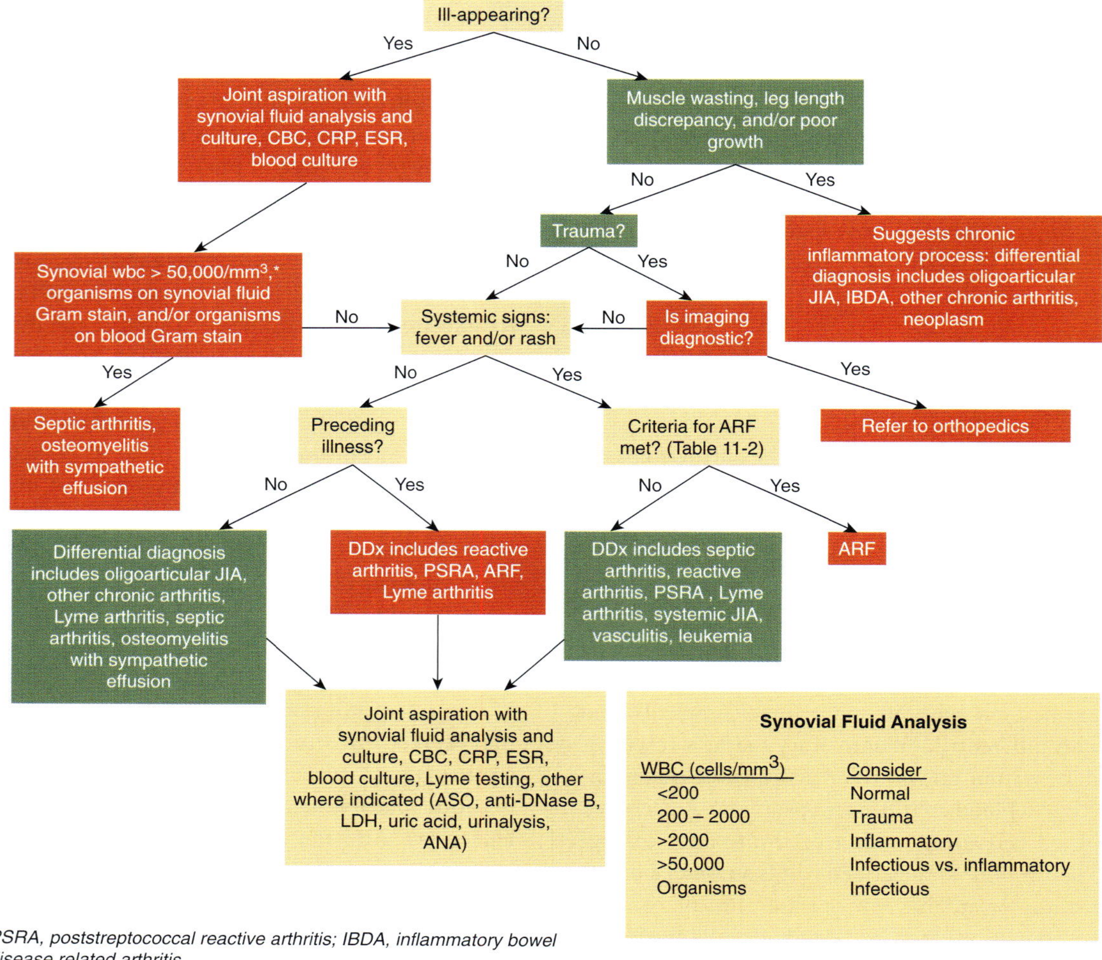

FIGURE 11–1 ■ Evaluation of a child with acute monoarthritis. (Note that bacterial infection may occasionally occur with $\leq$50,000 wbc/mm^3 in joint fluid aspirate.)

REFERENCES

1. Gutierrez K. Bone and joint infections in children. *Pediatr Clin North Am.* 2005;52(3):779-794, vi.
2. Shetty AK, Gedalia A. Septic arthritis in children. *Rheum Dis Clin North Am.* 1998;24(2):287-304.
3. Chang WS, Chiu NC, Chi H, Li WC, Huang FY. Comparison of the characteristics of culture-negative versus culture-positive septic arthritis in children. *J Microbiol Immunol Infect.* 2005;38(3):189-193.
4. Caksen H, Ozturk MK, Uzum K, Yuksel S, Ustunbas HB, Per H. Septic arthritis in childhood. *Pediatr Int.* 2000; 42(5):534-540.
5. Eder L, Zisman D, Rozenbaum M, Rosner I. Clinical features and aetiology of septic arthritis in northern Israel. *Rheumatology (Oxford).* 2005;44(12):1559-1563.
6. Elwood RL, Pelszynski MM, Corman LI. Multifocal septic arthritis and osteomyelitis caused by group A *Streptococcus* in a patient receiving immunomodulating therapy with etanercept. *Pediatr Infect Dis J.* 2003;22(3):286-288.
7. Huang JL, Hung JJ, Wu KC, Lee WI, Chan CK, Ou LS. Septic arthritis in patients with systemic lupus erythematosus: salmonella and nonsalmonella infections compared. *Semin Arthritis Rheum.* 2006;36(1):61-67.
8. Sauer ST, Farrell E, Geller E, Pizzutillo PD. Septic arthritis in a patient with juvenile rheumatoid arthritis. *Clin Orthop Relat Res.* 2004;(418):219-221.
9. Guidelines for the diagnosis of rheumatic fever. Jones Criteria, 1992 update. Special Writing Group of the Committee on Rheumatic Fever, Endocarditis, and Kawasaki Disease of the Council on Cardiovascular Disease in the Young of the American Heart Association. *JAMA.* 1992; 268(15):2069-2073.
10. Manners PJ, Bower C. Worldwide prevalence of juvenile arthritis why does it vary so much? *J Rheumatol.* 2002; 29(7):1520-1530.
11. Petty RE, Southwood TR, Manners P, et al. International League of Associations for Rheumatology classification of juvenile idiopathic arthritis: second revision, Edmonton, 2001. *J Rheumatol.* 2004;31(2):390-392.
12. Bader-Meunier B, Armengaud JB, Haddad E, et al. Initial presentation of childhood-onset systemic lupus erythematosus: a French multicenter study. *J Pediatr.* 2005; 146(5):648-653.
13. Ramanan AV, Feldman BM. Clinical features and outcomes of juvenile dermatomyositis and other childhood onset myositis syndromes. *Rheum Dis Clin North Am.* 2002;28(4):833-857.
14. Pachman LM, Hayford JR, Chung A, et al. Juvenile dermatomyositis at diagnosis: clinical characteristics of 79 children. *J Rheumatol.* 1998;25(6):1198-1204.
15. Dedeoglu F, Sundel RP. Vasculitis in children. *Pediatr Clin North Am.* 2005;52(2):547-575, vii.
16. Newburger JW, Takahashi M, Gerber MA, et al. Diagnosis, treatment, and long-term management of Kawasaki disease: a statement for health professionals from the Committee on Rheumatic Fever, Endocarditis and Kawasaki Disease, Council on Cardiovascular Disease in the Young, American Heart Association. *Circulation.* 2004;110(17): 2747-2771.
17. Rose CD, Wouters CH, Meiorin S, et al. Pediatric granulomatous arthritis: an international registry. *Arthritis Rheum.* 2006;54(10):3337-3344.
18. Padeh S. Periodic fever syndromes. *Pediatr Clin North Am.* 2005;52(2):577-609, vii.
19. Jones OY, Spencer CH, Bowyer SL, Dent PB, Gottlieb BS, Rabinovich CE. A multicenter case-control study on predictive factors distinguishing childhood leukemia from juvenile rheumatoid arthritis. *Pediatrics.* 2006;117(5):e840-e844.
20. Trapani S, Grisolia F, Simonini G, Calabri GB, Falcini F. Incidence of occult cancer in children presenting with musculoskeletal symptoms: a 10-year survey in a pediatric rheumatology unit. *Semin Arthritis Rheum.* 2000; 29(6):348-359.
21. Cabral DA, Tucker LB. Malignancies in children who initially present with rheumatic complaints. *J Pediatr.* 1999; 134(1):53-57.
22. Frick SL. Evaluation of the child who has hip pain. *Orthop Clin North Am.* 2006;37(2):133-140, v.
23. Tse SM, Laxer RM. Approach to acute limb pain in childhood. *Pediatr Rev.* 2006;27(5):170-179; quiz 80.
24. Hilario MO, Len CA, Roja SC, Terreri MT, Almeida G, Andrade LE. Frequency of antinuclear antibodies in healthy children and adolescents. *Clin Pediatr (Phila).* 2004;43(7):637-642.
25. Luhmann SJ, Jones A, Schootman M, Gordon JE, Schoenecker PL, Luhmann JD. Differentiation between septic arthritis and transient synovitis of the hip in children with clinical prediction algorithms. *J Bone Joint Surg Am.* 2004;86-A(5):956-962.
26. Jung ST, Rowe SM, Moon ES, Song EK, Yoon TR, Seo HY. Significance of laboratory and radiologic findings for differentiating between septic arthritis and transient synovitis of the hip. *J Pediatr Orthop.* 2003;23(3):368-372.
27. Kocher MS, Zurakowski D, Kasser JR. Differentiating between septic arthritis and transient synovitis of the hip in children: an evidence-based clinical prediction algorithm. *J Bone Joint Surg Am.* 1999;81(12):1662-1670.
28. Caird MS, Flynn JM, Leung YL, Millman JE, D'Italia JG, Dormans JP. Factors distinguishing septic arthritis from transient synovitis of the hip in children. A prospective study. *J Bone Joint Surg Am.* 2006;88(6):1251-1257.

CHAPTER 12

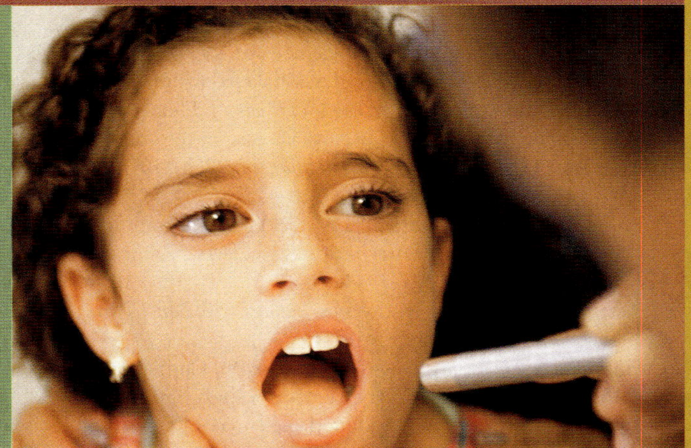

Neck Pain

Orooj Fasiuddin, Kishore Vellody, and Basil J. Zitelli

DEFINITION

Neck stiffness is defined as limited cervical range of motion caused by muscle spasm. This limitation can occur with flexion, extension, rotation, or lateral bending and may or may not be associated with pain. *Nuchal rigidity*, on the other hand, is pain with limitation through all ranges and is typically caused by significant meningeal irritation in the same manner peritonitis causes abdominal rigidity. *Meningismus* describes signs of meningeal irritation, typically pain with limited cervical flexion, in the absence of true meningitis.[1]

DIFFERENTIAL DIAGNOSIS

The differential diagnosis is extensive (Table 12–1). Nearly all infectious causes of neck pain and/or stiffness present acutely (≤7 days) and with fever. The most common infectious causes of neck pain and stiffness are cervical lymphadenitis, meningitis, deep neck space infections, and cervical osteomyelitis.

It is important to note that up to 20% of children with meningitis have no cervical signs of meningeal irritation.[2] Index of suspicion should be high, however, in the febrile, ill-appearing child who also has one or more associated signs or symptoms of meningitis. In the infant, these can be nonspecific and include irritability, inconsolable crying, and lethargy. The older child may complain of headache and photophobia and display altered mental status. Vomiting, seizures, and upper respiratory tract symptoms are also common.[3]

The child with a deep neck space infection can also present with fever, stiff neck, and toxic appearance. However, they may also have torticollis, neck mass, drooling, trismus, or stridor along with intraoral findings, such as tonsillitis and uvular deviation. Superficial neck infections, such as adenitis and cellulitis, less commonly cause toxic appearance, stiffness, and drooling. The presence of these should prompt an evaluation for a deep neck space infection.[4,5]

Children with cervical osteomyelitis are not toxic appearing and typically present with neck pain and stiffness. Fever may be present. Diskitis is rare in the cervical area, almost exclusively occurring in the lumbar area. When cervical diskitis is present, fever is often absent and neck pain is the presenting complaint. In both conditions, duration of symptoms can range from 1 day to 1 month. Examination often reveals point tenderness along the cervical spine and neck stiffness.[6]

Chronic forms of neck stiffness in the absence of fever can be caused by congenital malformations, tumor, fibromatosis colli, and several other conditions (Table 12–1).[1,7,8]

HISTORY

Several key questions can guide the evaluation and focus the differential diagnosis (Table 12–2).

PHYSICAL EXAMINATION

In addition to the distinguishing features mentioned above, several other findings on examination may point toward or away from an infectious etiology (Table 12–3). Unusual neck posturing, such as cervical hyperflexion or guarding the neck with hands, may be associated with space occupying lesions, such as tumors.[7] Conditions causing significant meningeal irritation, such as meningitis and subarachnoid hemorrhage, typically cause

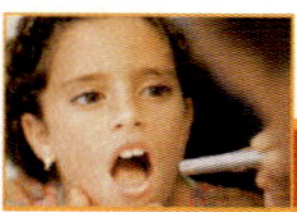

Table 12–1.

Differential Diagnosis of Neck Stiffness and/or Pain

Acute (≤7 days)		Chronic	
Infectious	**Noninfectious**	**Infectious**	**Noninfectious**
Meningitis	Cervical fracture, dislocation, or subluxation	Cervical osteomyelitis	Cervical or paracervical tumor
Encephalitis	SCIOWRA*	Cervical diskitis	Musculoskeletal pain
Cervical osteomyelitis	SCM		Spastic cerebral palsy
Abscess	hematoma, tear or sprain		Fibromatous colli of SCM
Retropharyngeal	Juvenile rheumatoid arthritis		Congenital vertebral anomaly
Brain	Cervical or paracervical tumor		Klippel–Feil syndrome
Epidural	Neuroblastoma		Sprengel deformity
Parapharyngeal	Medulloblastoma		Arnold Chiari malformation
Peritonsillar	Subarachnoid hemorrhage		Juvenile Rheumatoid arthritis
Dental	Arteriovenous malformation		Lead encephalopathy
Postinfectious encephalomyelitis	Extradural hematoma or mass		Sandifer syndrome
Cervical adenitis	Epidural hematoma		Intervertebral disc calcification
Diskitis	Foreign body		Psychogenic
Thyroiditis	Polyarteritis nodosa		Wilson disease
Viral myositis	Dystonic reaction		Huntington disease
Tonsillitis	Black widow spider or scorpion bite		
Epiglottitis	Paroxysmal torticollis		
Parotitis	Increased intracranial pressure		
Tetanus	Cervical fracture, dislocation, or subluxation		
Pneumonia			
Viral myositis			
Myeloradiculopathy			
Poliomyelitis			
Acute cerebellar ataxia			
Jugular thrombophlebitis			
Ludwig's angina			

**SCIOWRA, spinal cord injury without radiographic abnormality; SCM-sternocleidomastoid muscle.*

nuchal rigidity or pain upon cervical flexion. Fracture, subluxation or tumor should be suspected if the child is able to flex, but has limited rotation, extension, or lateral bending.[7,9,10] Meningismus in the absence of fever is seen with subarachnoid hemorrhage and tumors.[7,11]

If neck stiffness (in the absence of fever and altered mental status) is associated with abnormal neurological findings, such as focal muscle weakness, parasthesias, or gait abnormalities, the etiology is unlikely infectious.[6–12]

EVALUATION AND MANAGEMENT

In the child who presents with neck pain, early diagnosis of an infectious process is crucial to prevent spread and progression of the disease. Several laboratory and radiologic studies are useful to definitively diagnose the cause of the symptoms (Table 12–4). A management algorithm is provided in Figure 12–1.

In bacterial meningitis, early diagnosis and treatment is crucial to prevent neurologic sequelae or death.[13] The organisms responsible for bacterial meningitis change with age. In neonates, group B streptococci, gram-negative enteric bacilli, and *Listeria* are most common. Parenteral antibiotic therapy with broad-spectrum coverage (ampicillin and either a third-generation cephalosporin or aminoglycoside) is appropriate initially with more specific therapy once definitive identification and antibiotic susceptibilities are known. In older children, *Streptococcus pneumoniae* and *Neisseria meningitidis* are the most commonly identified organisms and vancomycin with a third-generation cephalosporin should be initiated until resistant *S. pneumoniae* have been excluded.[14]

Deep neck space abscesses have the potential to rupture into the retropharyngeal or parapharyngeal

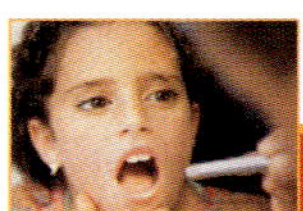

Table 12–2.

History

Acute or chronic	An acute onset of symptoms may be consistent with infection or recent injury. Infections uncommonly produce chronic pain
Age	A younger age (≤4 years) is more consistent with a retropharyngeal abscess since the retropharyngeal lymph nodes have not yet involuted. An older age is more consistent with a peritonsillar abscess
Fever or systemically ill	Fever and/or systemic illness is more likely associated with infectious causes rather than anatomic or congenital disorders. A presentation with rash, seizure, or mental status changes suggests meningitis. Patients with retropharyngeal abscesses may not appear "toxic" early on
Headache	Headache is common in meningitis, retropharyngeal abscess, migraine, or increased intracranial pressure
Oral Intake	Dysphagia from deep neck space infection is likely to limit oral intake
Neck Movement	Pain with neck extension suggests a retropharyngeal abscess. If neck flexion elicits pain, meningitis is more likely. Rotational neck pain may represent a cervical tumor
Recent trauma	A neck injury can result in musculoskeletal pain. A penetrating injury may directly inoculate the CSF or deep neck space resulting in infection
Neck Swelling	A swollen neck is consistent with trauma, retropharyngeal abscess, adenitis, retropharyngeal abscess, Lemierre syndrome, or Ludwig's angina
Illness, immunization status	The presence of intracranial hardware (i.e., ventriculoperitoneal shunt, cochlear implant), incomplete immunizations, or immune deficiencies increase the risk of infection

spaces. Following rupture, the infection may then spread freely from the skull base to mediastinum as well as laterally into the vascular sheath containing the carotid artery and internal jugular vein. This vascular involvement may then result in septic emboli and vastly increase the risk of morbidity and mortality.[15,17] Deep neck space infections are generally caused by *Staphylococcus aureus*, group A streptococci, and anaerobes.

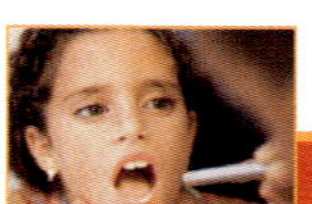

Table 12–3.

Significance of Examination Findings in the Child with Neck Pain and/or Stiffness

Finding	Clinical Significance
Fever and toxic appearance	Meningitis, deep neck space infection
Bulging fontanelle	Meningitis, CNS tumor, CNS hemorrhage
Altered mental status	Encephalitis, meningitis, CNS hemorrhage
Papilledema	Meningitis, CNS tumor, CNS hemorrhage
Dental caries	Dental abscess, Ludwig's angina
Trismus	Deep neck space infection
Drooling	Epiglottitis, foreign body, retropharyngeal, parapharyngeal or peritonsillar abscess
Peritonsillar bulge, uvular deviation	Peritonsillar abscess
Torticollis	Fibromatosis colli, deep neck space infection, ocular torticollis, atlantoaxial subluxation, cervical and paracervical tumors
Nuchal rigidity	Meningitis, subarachnoid hemorrhage, cervical tumor
Midline cervical point tenderness	Diskitis, osteomyelitis, JRA
Paraspinous tenderness without limited range of motion	Musculoskeletal pain
Guarding	Fracture, subluxation, tumor
Cervical adenopathy	Adenitis, deep neck space infection
Stridor	Epiglottitis, retropharyngeal abscess, foreign body
Focal weakness	Tumor, CNS hemorrhage
Abnormal gait	Tumor
Generalized dystonia	Drug-induced, tetanus, acute lead poisoning, black-widow spider and scorpion bite
Sternocleidomastoid muscle mass	Fibromatosis colli

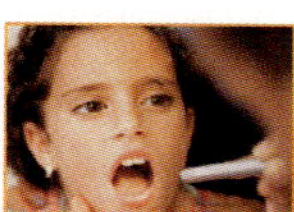

Table 12–4.

Laboratory/Radiologic Studies

Throat culture	A throat culture may isolate the causative organism in peritonsillar or pharyngeal infection.
Complete blood count	Elevation of the WBC count (especially with immature forms) is suggestive of infectious process.
Blood culture	A blood culture could isolate an organism if the infection has spread hematogenously. This is more likely in some disease processes (i.e. epiglottitis, Lemierre syndrome) than in others (i.e., adenitis, deep neck abscess).
ESR/CRP	These are general markers of inflammation. They are not specific, but they can be helpful to determine the treatment course in diskitis/osteomyelitis.
Lumbar puncture	Pleocytosis, visualized bacteria on the Gram stain, low CSF glucose, high CSF protein, or bacterial growth on culture indicates a bacterial meningitis. Viral meningitis can be differentiated from bacterial meningitis based on lack of CSF culture growth, normal CSF glucose, and a normal to high CSF protein.
Neck X-ray	Good technique is essential as artifactual widening of the prevertebral tissue may occur from respiration or swallowing. Fullness of the retropharyngeal space ($\geq 1/2$ the width of the corresponding vertebral body) suggests retropharyngeal abscess or cellulitis. Edema of the submental/submandibular soft tissues suggests Ludwig's angina. X-ray may also uncover vertebral fracture, spondylolysis, spondylolisthesis, or suggest osteomyelitis or diskitis.
Fluoroscopy	This modality may be useful to differentiate true retropharyngeal space thickness from artifact. If the clinician is not very suspicious of a retropharyngeal abscess, this may be helpful to avoid the need for computed tomography.
Neck ultrasound	The main advantages are less expense, less radiation, and no need for sedation. However, ultrasound alone is not sufficient to evaluate for extension deep neck space infection beyond the abscess cavity.
Computed tomography (CT) with contrast	This is essential to define a deep neck space infection location/extension. It has a high false negative and false positive rate in differentiating retropharyngeal cellulitis from abscess. The CT images should include the upper chest to evaluate for mediastinal extension. CT can identify diskitis or osteomyelitis before any X-ray changes occur.
Magnetic resonance imaging (MRI)	MRI has a limited use in the acute setting due to need for staffing, sedation, and expense. It may help define the extent of vascular involvement or spread of a deep neck space infection. MRI is useful in delineating neck anatomy or in diagnosing diskitis or osteomyelitis.

A trial of parenteral antibiotics (clindamycin with or without a third-generation cephalosporin or ampicillin/sulbactam alone) may be successful in preventing the need for surgery.[5,15,16] If surgery is required, intraoral incision and drainage may allow isolation of the causative organism(s) and provide symptomatic relief to the patient.[16]

Osteomyelitis and diskitis are most often caused by *Staph. aureus* or group A streptococci. Penicillinase-resistant penicillins (oxacillin or nafcillin) or first- or second-generation cephalosporins are appropriate. Consideration should be given for clindamycin or vancomycin given the growing number of methicillin-resistant staphylococcal organisms. An initial course of 3–6 weeks of antibiotics should be planned with ultimate length of therapy based on clinical response and improved inflammatory markers.[6,18,19]

CONSULTATION/REFERRAL

Otolaryngology consultation may be needed for patients with deep neck space infection for possible drainage. If abscess rupture and extension has occurred, cardiothoracic surgery and infectious disease consultation is indicated.

In the era of immunizations, bacterial meningitis occurs far less frequently than previously. Infectious disease consultation can be helpful in acute management and long-term follow-up. In cases with residual deficits, long-term follow-up with physical and occupational therapy, audiology, or neurology may be needed.

In cases of osteomyelitis or diskitis, orthopedic surgery and infectious diseases consultants are advisable.

REFERENCES

1. Stein MT, Trauner D. The child with a stiff neck. *Clin Pediatr.* 1982;21(9):559-563.
2. Oostenbrink R, Moons KG, Theunissen CC, et al. Signs of meningeal irritation at the emergency department: how often bacterial meningitis? *Pediatr Emerg Care.* 2001;17(3):161-164.
3. Long SS, Pickering LK, ProberCG. *Principles and Practice of Pediatric Infectious Diseases.* Philadelphia: Elsevier Science; 2003:265.

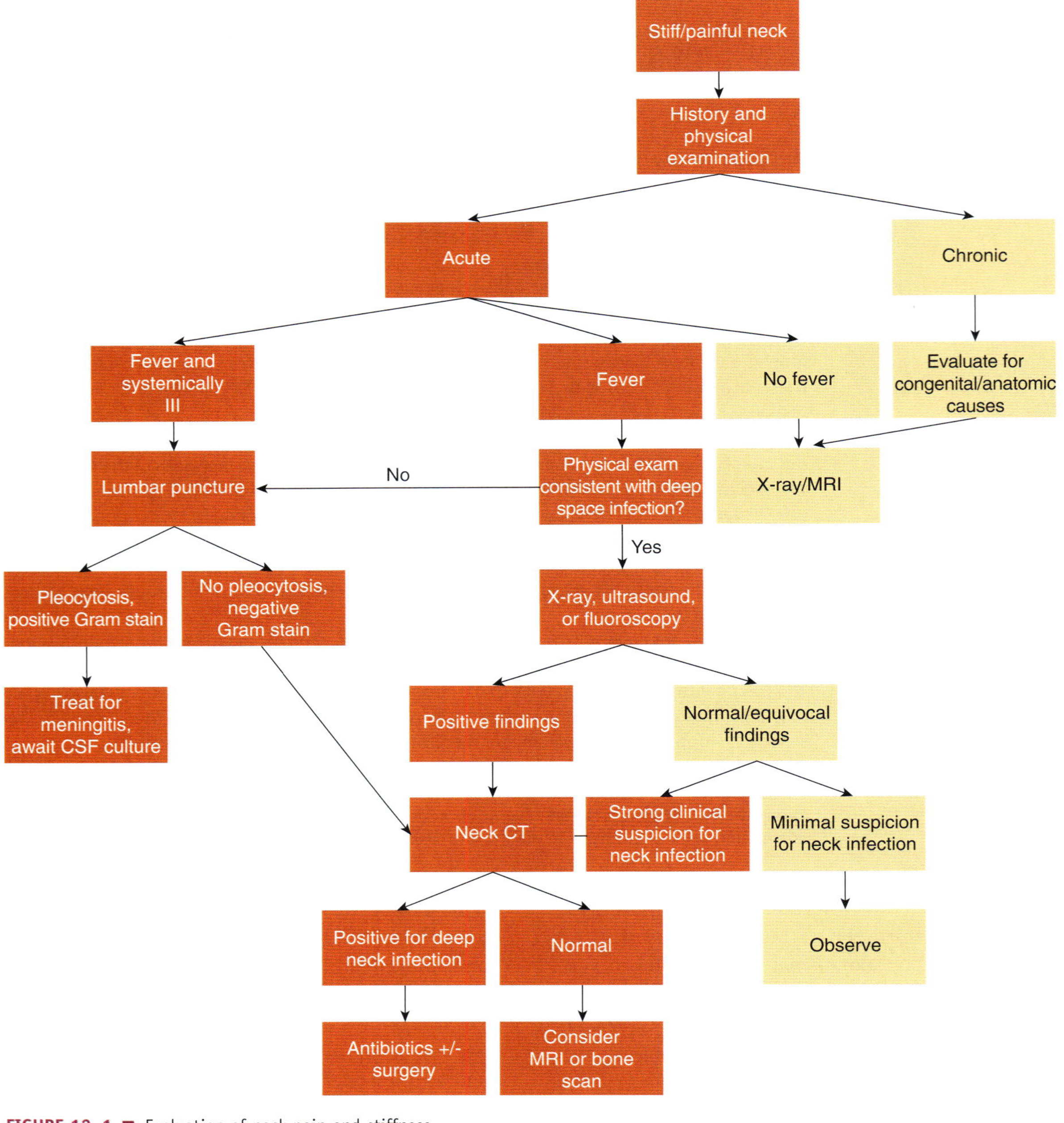

FIGURE 12–1 ■ Evaluation of neck pain and stiffness.

4. Coticchia JM, Getnick GS, Yun RD, et al. Age, site, and time-specific differences in pediatric deep neck abscesses. *Arch Otol Head Neck Surg.* 2004;130:201-207.
5. Craig FW, Schunk JE. Retropharyngeal abscess in children: clinical presentation: clinical presentation, utility of imaging, and current management. *Pediatrics.* 2003;111(6):1394-1398.
6. Fernandez M, Carrol CL, Baker CJ. Discitis and vertebral osteomyelitis in children: an 18-year review. *Pediatrics.* 2000;105:1299-1304.
7. Natarajan A, Yassa JG, Burke DP, et al. Not all cases of neck pain with/without torticollis are benign: unusual presentations in a paediatric accident and emergency department. *Emerg Med J.* 2005;22:646-649.
8. Levine AM, Boriani S, Donati D, et al. Benign tumors of the cervical spine. *Spine.* 1992;17(10 S):S399-S406.
9. Thakar C, Harish S, Saifuddin A, et al. Displaced fracture through the anterior atlantal synchondrosis. *Skeletal Radiol.* 2005;34(9):547-549.
10. Ranjith RK, Mullett H, Burke TE. Hangman's fracture caused by suspected child abuse, a case report. *J Pediatr Orthop.* 2002;11(4):329-332.
11. Seet CM. Clinical presentation of patients with subarachnoid haemorrhage at a local emergency department. *Singapore Med J.* 1999;40(6):383-385.

12. Vallee B, Besson G, Gaudin J, et al. Spontaneous spinal epidural hematoma in a 22-month old girl. *J Neurosurg.* 1982;56(1):135-138.
13. Chavez-Bueno S, McCracken Jr., GH. Bacterial Meningitis in Children. *Pediatr Clin N Am.* 2005;52:795-810.
14. Yogev R, Guzman-Cottrill J. Bacterial meningitis in children: critical review of current concepts. *Drugs.* 2005; 65(8):1097-1112.
15. Roberson DW. Pediatric retropharyngeal abscesses. *Clin Pediatr Emerg Med.* 2005
16. Dudas R. Retropharyngeal abscess. *Pediatr Rev.* 2006; 27(6):e45-e46.
17. Venglarcik J. Lemierre's syndrome. *Pediatr Infect Dis J.* 2003;22(10):921-923.
18. Vazquez M. Osteomyelitis in children. *Curr Opin Pediatr.* 2002;14(1):112-115.
19. Sharif I. Current treatment of osteomyelitis. *Pediatr Rev.* 2006;26(1):38-39.

CHAPTER 13

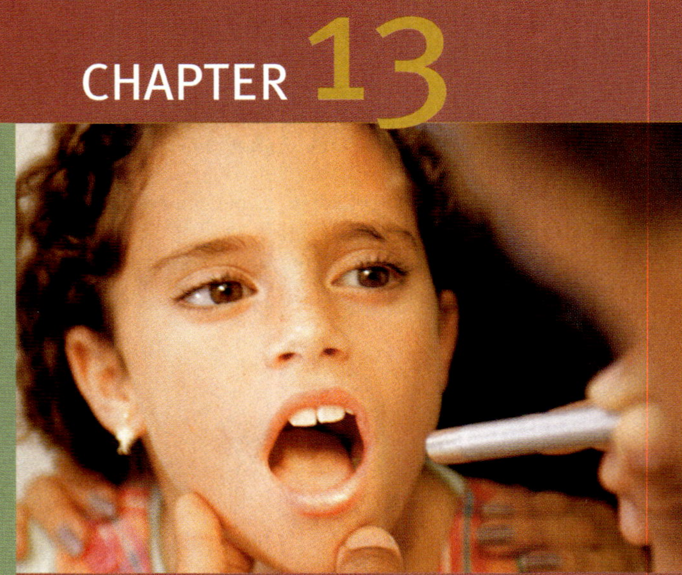

Rash

Kara N. Shah

DEFINITIONS

Dermatologists define several broad categories of skin disease based on clinical features and pathophysiology. The categories that are of primary interest from an infectious disease perspective include bacterial and mycobacterial infections, fungal infections, protozoal infections, viral infections, reactive erythemas, drug- and viral-induced hypersensitivity syndromes, and vasculitic diseases and purpura (Table 13–1).

Establishing the differential diagnosis of a rash relies both on an appropriately focused history and on correctly describing the morphology and distribution of the rash. A brief overview of common terms used in dermatology is presented in Table 13–2. Common patterns of distribution are presented in Table 13–3.

CLINICAL PRESENTATION

History

When a potential infectious etiology for a rash is considered, special attention is paid to the presence or absence of fever and other systemic symptoms. It is also important to inquire about any unusual exposures to potential infectious organisms which may occur via person-to-person transmission, through contact with arthropods or other vectors, through contact with infected animals, or as a result of an environmental exposure.

Key questions that should be part of any evaluation of a rash include the following:

Duration: When (how long ago) did the rash start? Purpura fulminans secondary to meningococcemia presents acutely.

Distribution and progression: Where (on which part of the body) did the rash begin? The cutaneous vasculitis of rocky mountain spotted fever classically starts on the ankles and wrists, and then generalizes.

Prodrome: Were there any prodromal symptoms such as fever, cough, myalgias, arthralgias, or sore throat? Stevens–Johnson syndrome may be seen in association with *Mycoplasma* infection, and fever and cough are often present.

Associated Symptoms

Are there any associated symptoms such as pain or pruritis? Bacterial cellulitis is usually painful and associated with warmth and edema of the skin, while contact dermatitis, which is a clinical mimic, is pruritic and usually lacks significant swelling and warmth.

Systemic Medications

What systemic medications has the patient been administered, including medications that were taken up to 1 month before the onset of the rash? Drug hypersensitivity reactions are often seen in the differential diagnosis of a rash. They may develop from hours to several weeks after initiation of the drug depending on the pathophysiology of the reaction and history of prior exposure to the drug. The anticonvulsants phenytoin, phenobarbitol, and carbamazepine as well as several other medications can cause a systemic hypersensitivity reaction (drug reaction with eosinophilia and systemic symptoms (DRESS)) that presents with fever, a diffuse morbilliform rash, eosinophilia, and systemic abnormalities such as renal impairment and liver dysfunction.

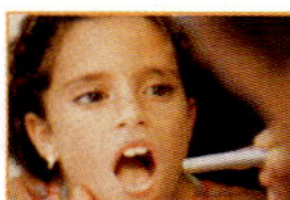

Table 13–1.

Diagnostic Categories of selected Infectious and Non-Infections Etiologies of Rashes

Diagnostic Category	Examples
Bacterial and mycobacterial infections	■ Cellulitis ■ Impetigo ■ Staphylococcal-scalded skin syndrome ■ Toxic shock syndrome ■ Ecthyma ■ Ecthyma gangrenosum ■ Meningococcemia ■ Rocky mountain spotted fever ■ Rickettsialpox ■ Cutaneous tuberculosis ■ Cutaneous anthrax ■ Nontuberculous (atypical) mycobacterial infections ■ Leprosy ■ Secondary syphilis ■ Ulceroglandular tularemia ■ Actinomycosis
Viral infections	■ Erythema infectiosum (parvovirus B19 infection) ■ Papular purpuric socks and gloves syndrome (parvovirus B19 infection) ■ Infectious mononucleosis (Epstein–Barr virus (EBV) infection) ■ Roseola infantum (human herpesvirus-6 and human herpesvirus-7 infection) ■ Rubeola (measles) ■ Hand-foot-and-mouth disease (coxsackie virus infection) ■ Herpangina (coxsackie virus infection) ■ Varicella ■ Herpes zoster ■ Cutaneous herpes and herpetic whitlow ■ Herpes labialis ■ Herpetic gingivostomatitis ■ Eczema herpeticum ■ Molluscum contagiosum ■ Warts (verruca vulgaris, verruca plana, verruca plantaris, condylomata acuminata) ■ Smallpox
Fungal infections	■ Dermatophyte infections (tinea capitis, tinea corporis, tinea pedis, onychomycosis) ■ Tinea versicolor ■ Cutaneous candidiasis ■ Subcutaneous mycoses (sporotrichosis) ■ Systemic mycoses (blastomycosis, histoplasmosis, coccidiomycosis) ■ Opportunistic mycoses (aspergillosis, mucormycosis, cryptococcosis)
Protozoal infections	■ Cutaneous leishmaniasis ■ Muocutaneous leishmaniasis
Reactive erythemas	■ Erythema multiforme ■ Urticaria ■ Serum sickness and serum sickness-like reactions ■ Erythema marginatum (acute rheumatic fever) ■ Erythema chronicum migrans (Lyme disease)
Hypersensitivity syndromes	■ Morbilliform drug eruption ■ Stevens–Johnson syndrome ■ Toxic epidermal necrolysis ■ Drug reaction with eosinophilia and systemic symptoms
Vasculitic diseases and purpura	■ Rocky mountain spotted fever ■ Erlichiosis ■ Purpura fulminans ■ Kawasaki disease ■ Hypersensitivity (leukocytoclastic) vasculitis

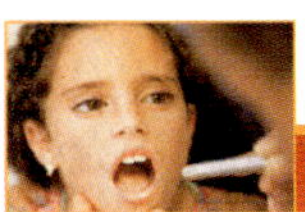

Table 13–2.

Common Morphologic Patterns of Dermatologic Disease

Morphology	Description	Examples 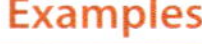
Primary lesions		
Macule 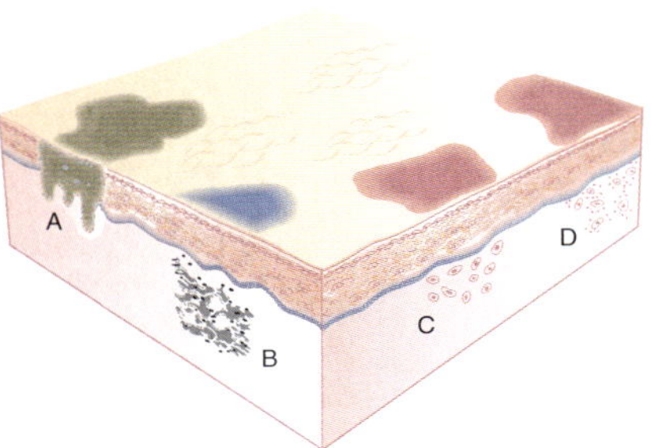	A flat lesion <1 cm in diameter	Leukocytoclastic vasculitis 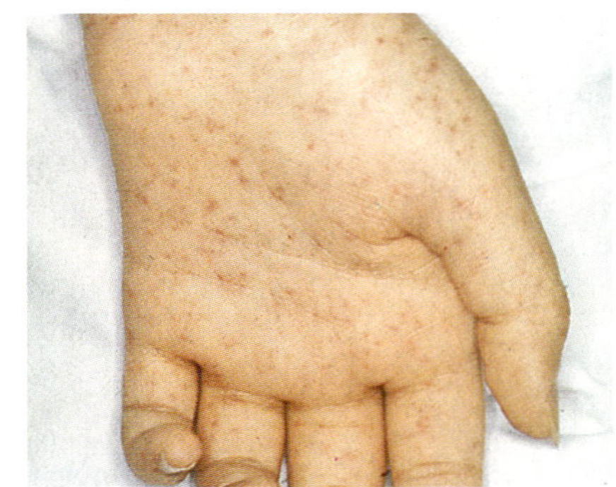
Papule 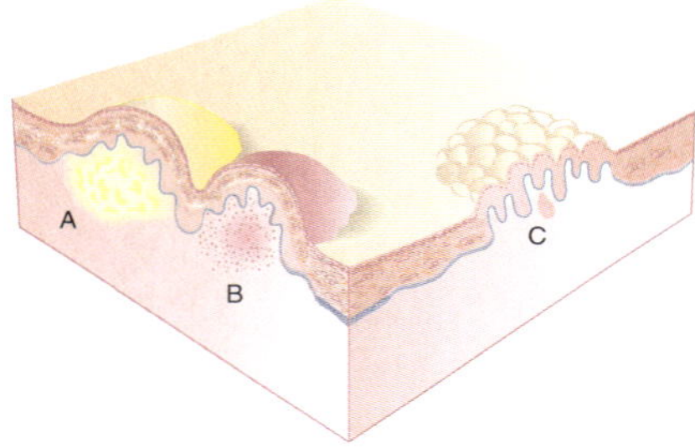	A raised lesion <1 cm in diameter	Molluscum contagiosum 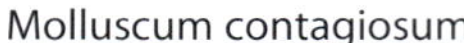 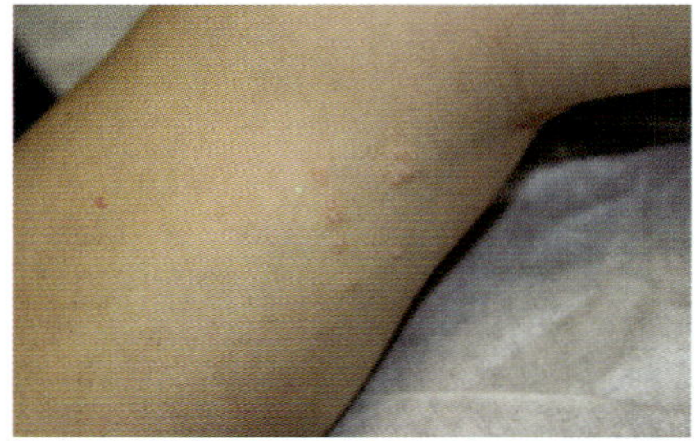
Patch 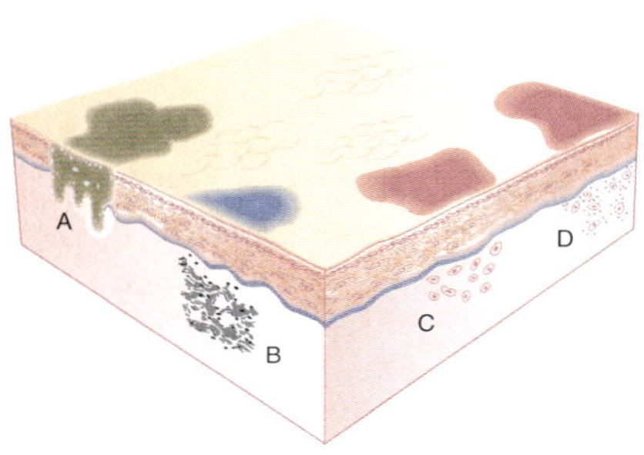	A flat lesion >1 cm in diameter	Erythema chronicum migrans (Lyme disease) 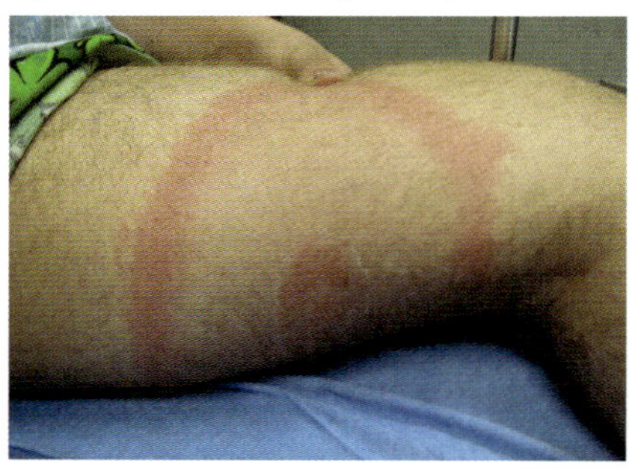
Plaque 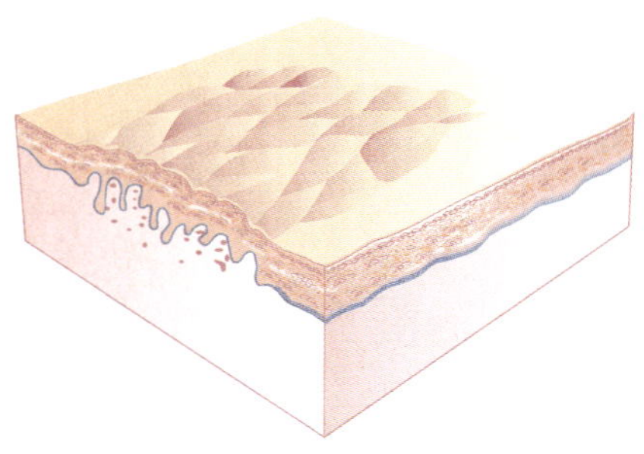	A raised lesion with a flat top >1 cm in diameter	Verucca vulgaris 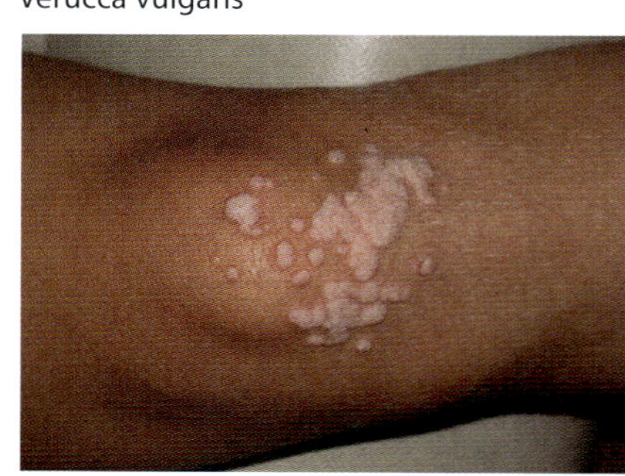

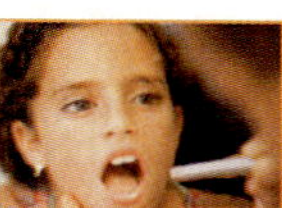

Table 13–2. (continued)

Common Morphologic Patterns of Dermatologic Disease

Morphology	Description	Examples
Nodule 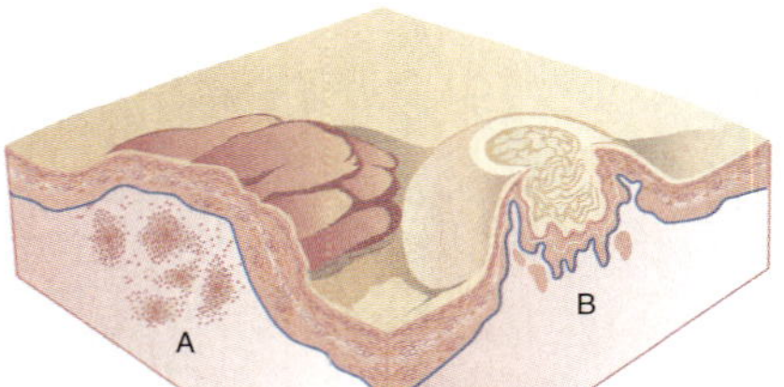	A raised lesion >1 cm in diameter	Erythema nodosum 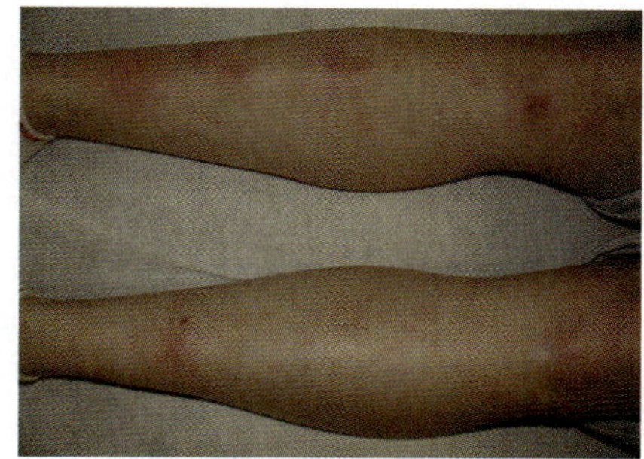
Vesicle 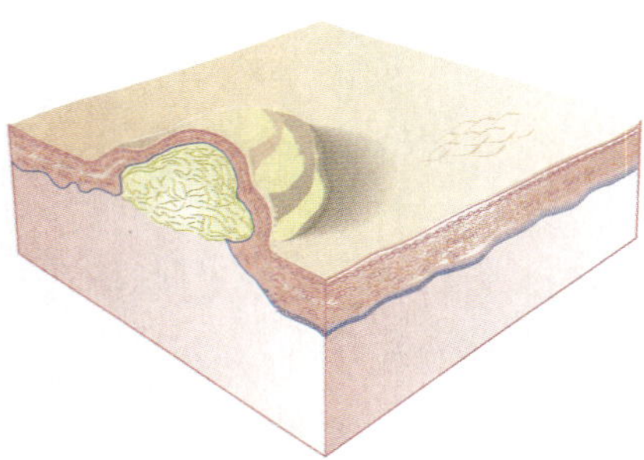	A clear fluid-filled lesion <1 cm in diameter	Herpes zoster 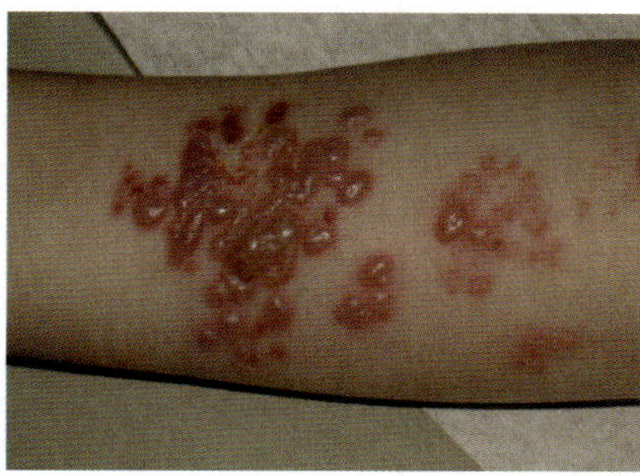
Bullae 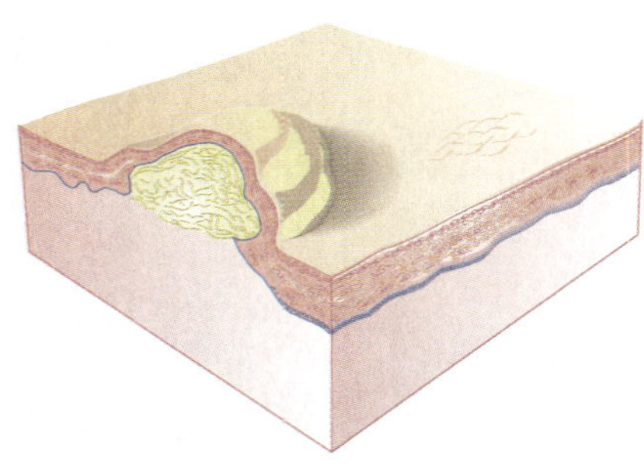	A fluid-filled lesion >1 cm in diameter	Impetigo 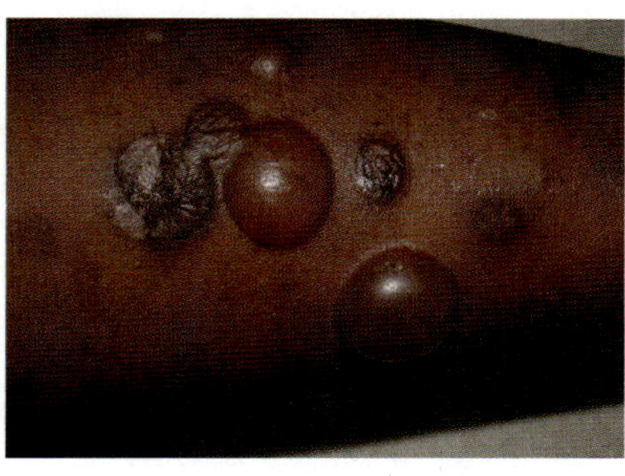
Pustule 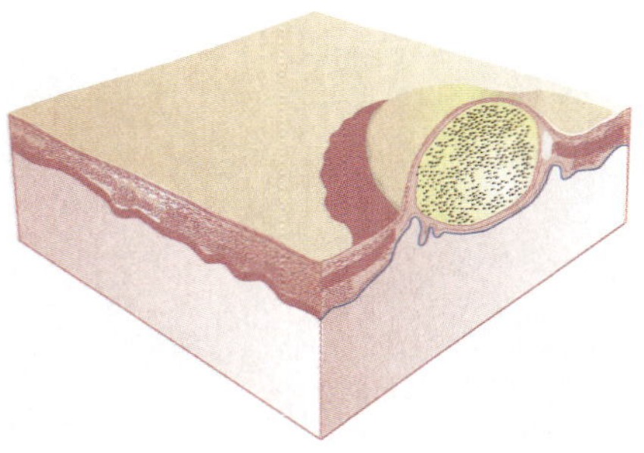	A cloudy fluid-filled lesion <1 cm in diameter	Neonatal staphylococcal pustulosis 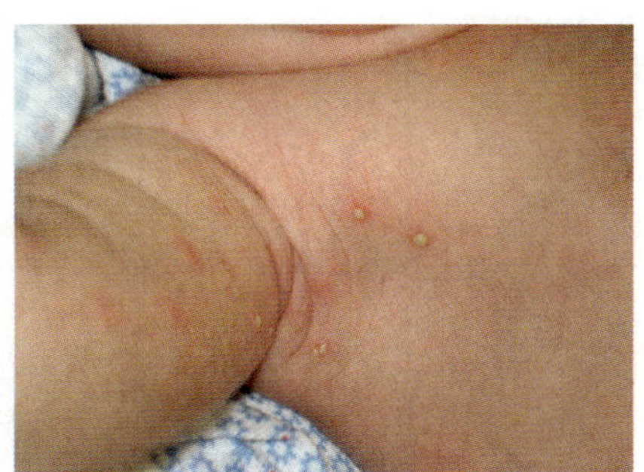

(continued)

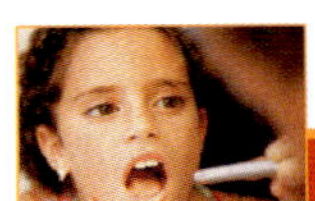

Table 13–2. (continued)

Common Morphologic Patterns of Dermatologic Disease

Morphology	Description	Examples
Erosion 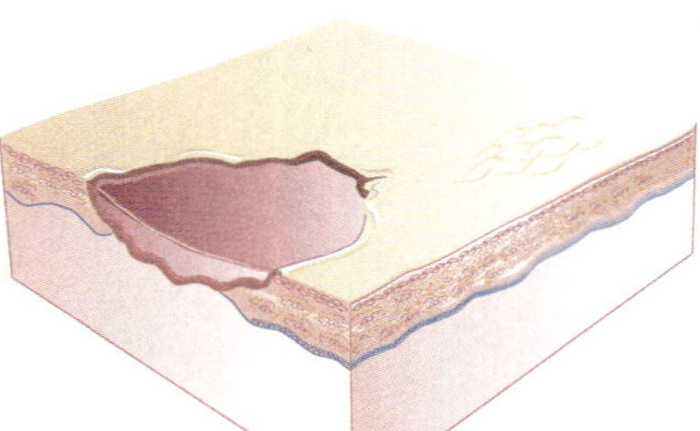	A loss of the epidermis (superficial)	Streptococcal intertrigo 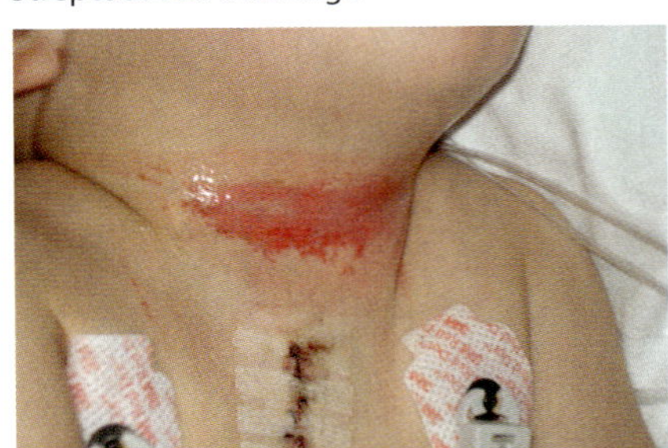
Wheal 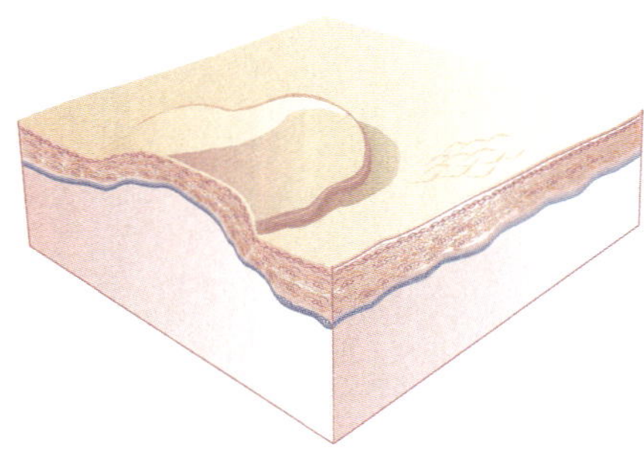	A transient edematous lesion, often with blanching or pallor centrally with surrounding erythema	Urticaria 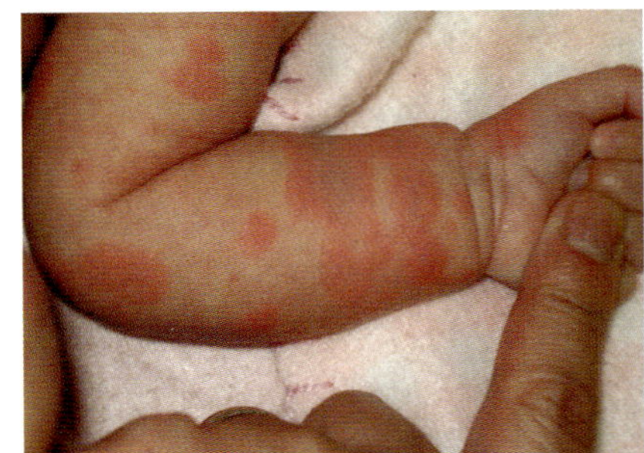
Ulcer 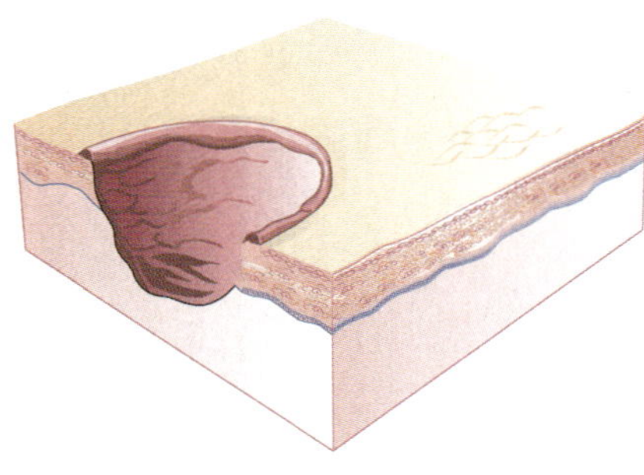	A loss of the epidermis and part of the dermis and sometimes the subcutis (deep)	Echthyma gangrenosum 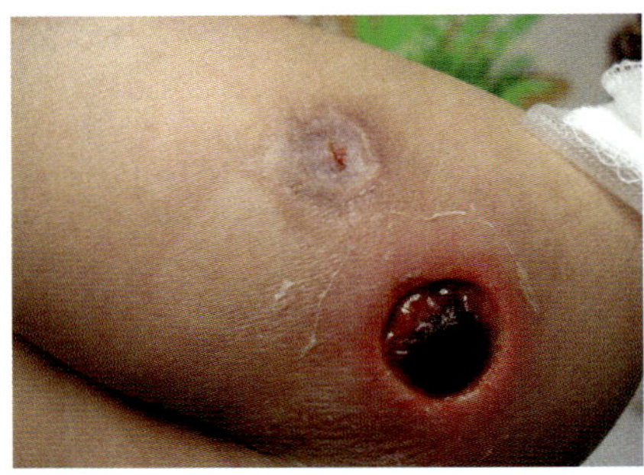
Fissure 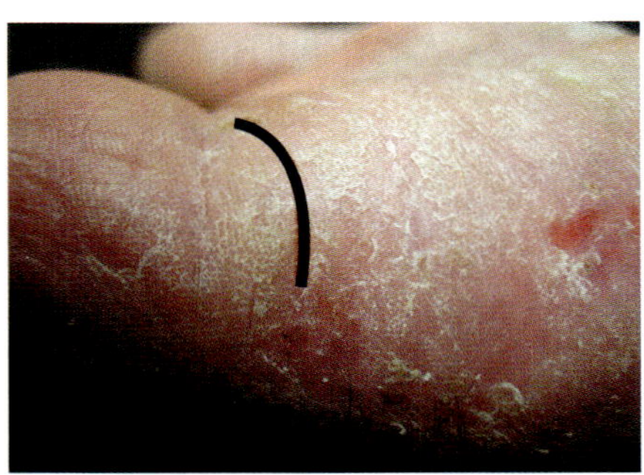	A linear cleft or ulcer	Angular chelistis (*Candida albicans*) 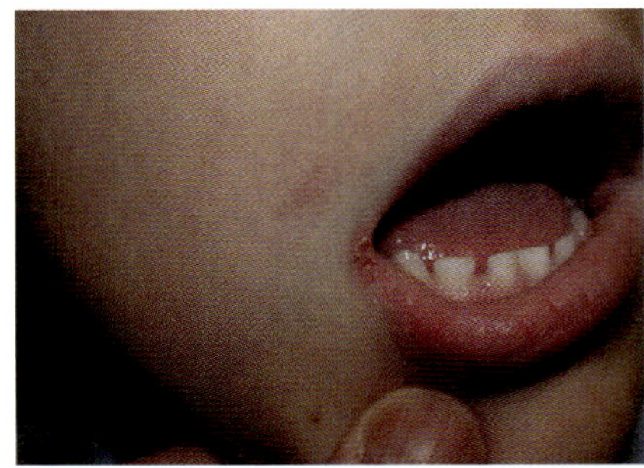

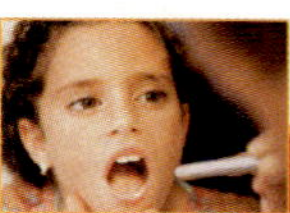

Table 13–2. (continued)

Common Morphologic Patterns of Dermatologic Disease

Morphology	Description	Examples
Erythroderma 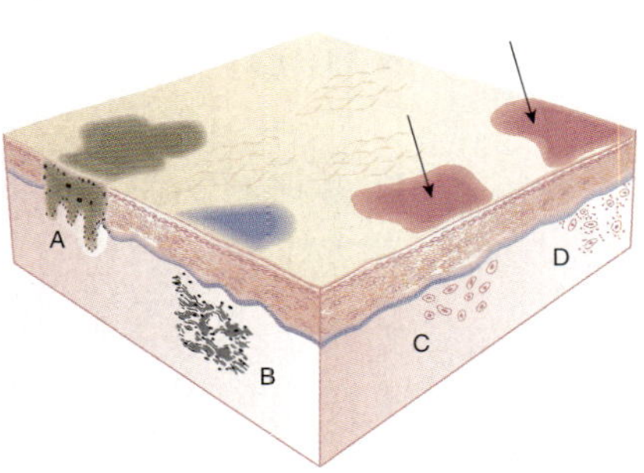	Confluent erythema resulting from vasodilation or capillary leak	Toxic epidermal necrolysis 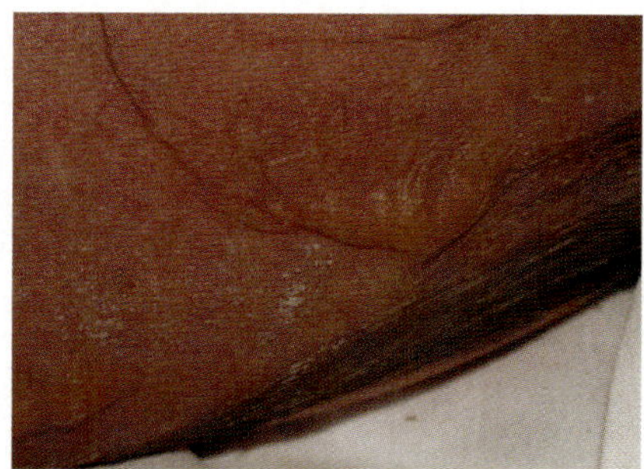
Purpura 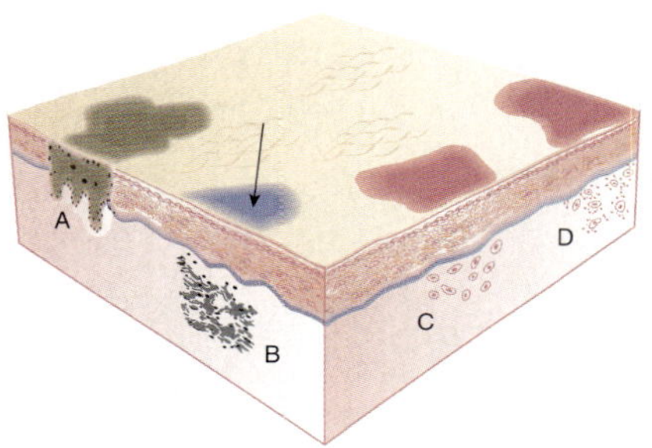	Nonblanchable erythema or violaceous areas	Cutaneous vasculitis 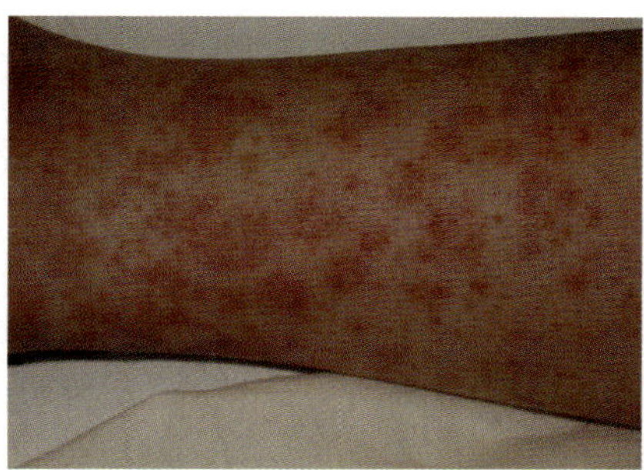
Excoriation 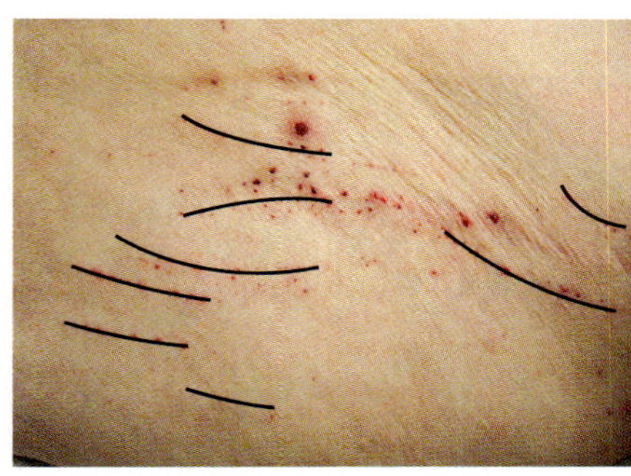	A superficial abrasion, often self-induced from scratching	Scabies 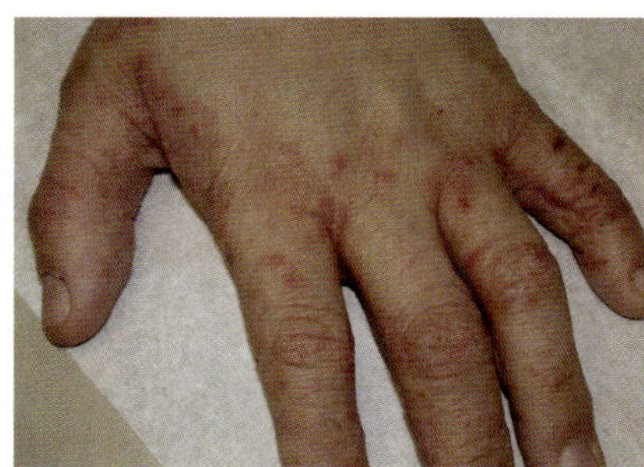
Scale 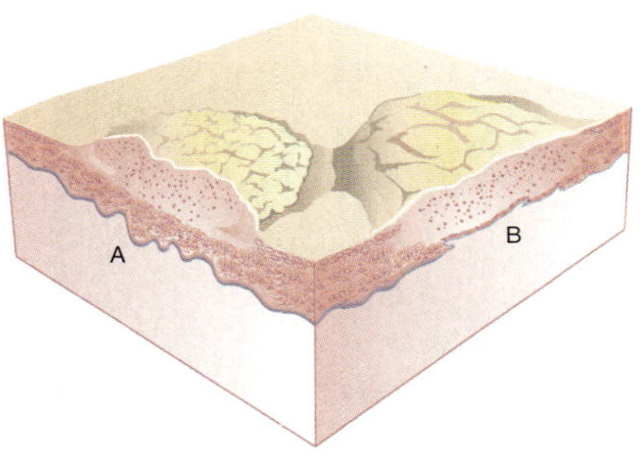	Superficial epidermal desquamation	*Tinia facei* 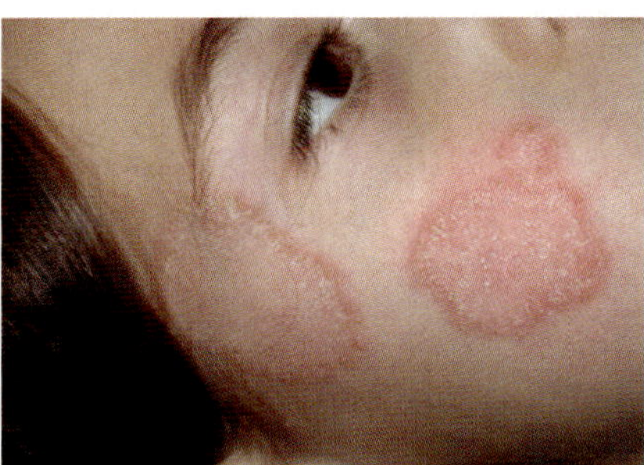

(*continued*)

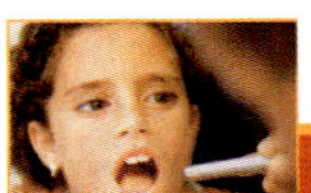

Table 13–2. (continued)

Common Morphologic Patterns of Dermatologic Disease

Morphology	Description	Examples
Crust 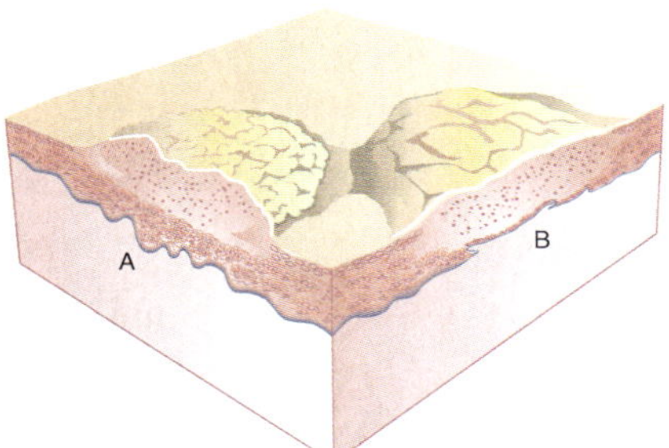	Dried exudate	Impetigo 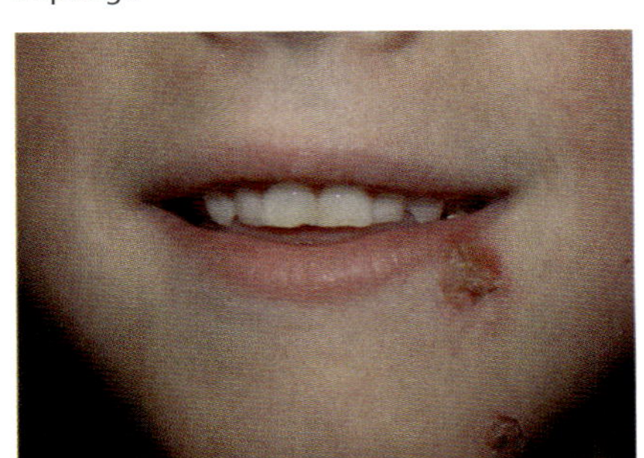
Atrophy 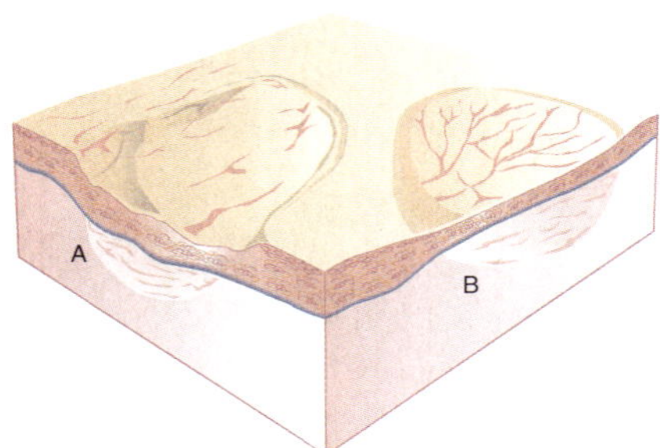	Thinning of the skin that may involve the epidermis, dermis, or subcutis; may present with hypopigmentation and a fine, wrinkled appearance to the epidermis	Lichen sclerosis et atrophicus 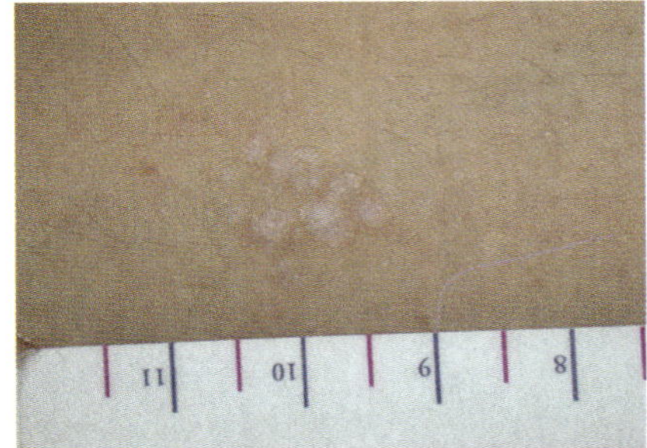
Lichenification 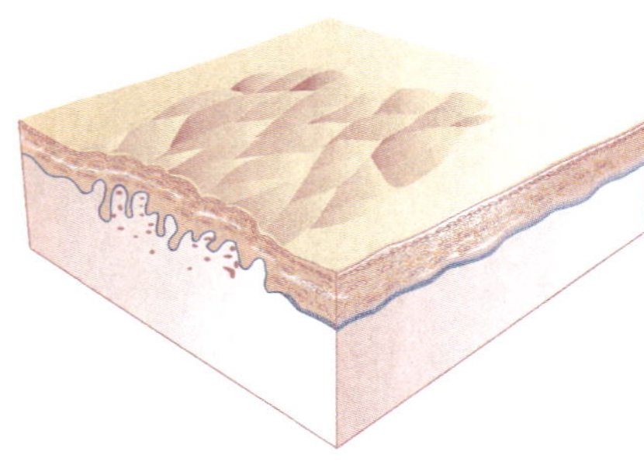	Accentuation of normal skin markings with epidermal thickening and hyperpigmentation; results from chronic rubbing or scratching	Chronic atopic dermatitis 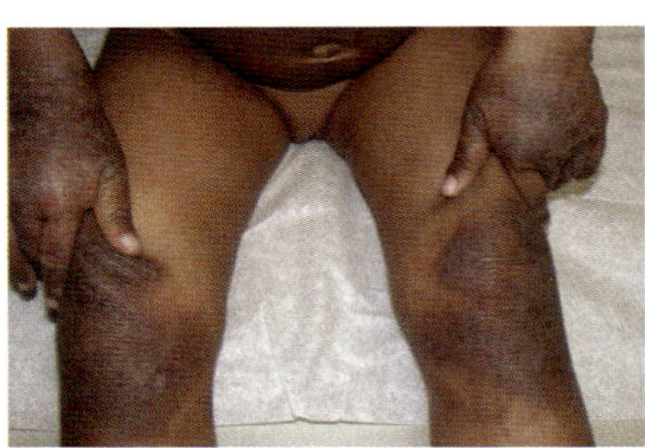
Shape and configuration		
Individual 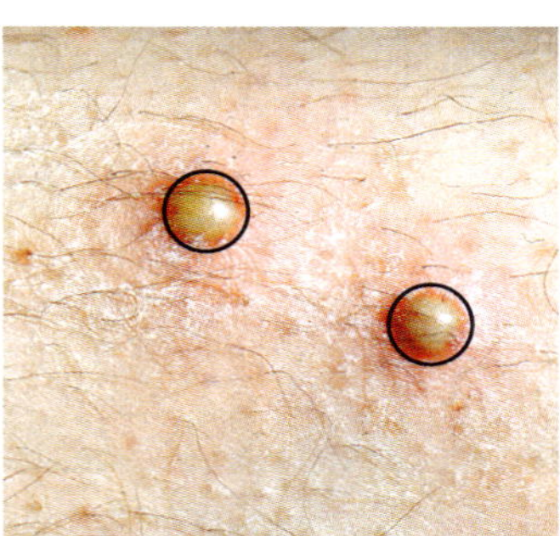	Singly dispersed lesions	Ecthyma, *S. aureus* 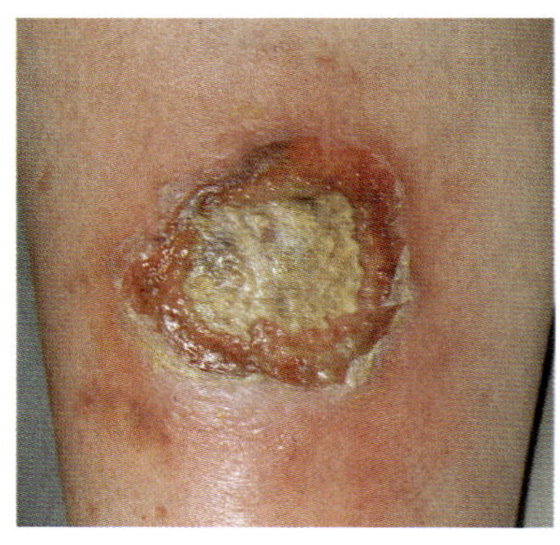

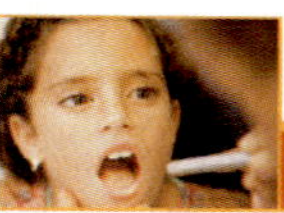

Table 13–2. (continued)

Common Morphologic Patterns of Dermatologic Disease

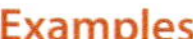

Morphology	Description	Examples
Grouped 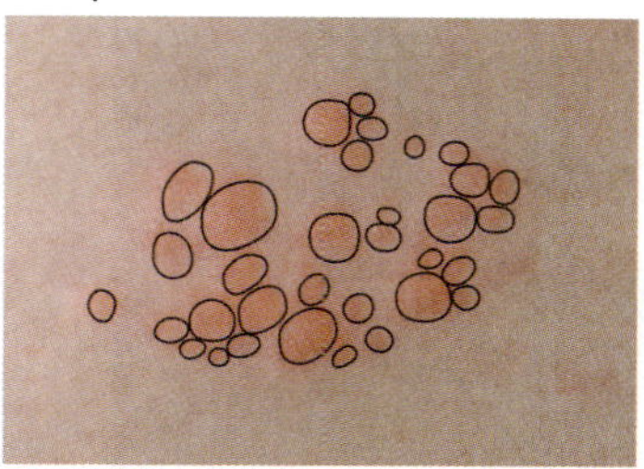	Multiple similar lesions present within a localized area	Herpes simplex virus infection 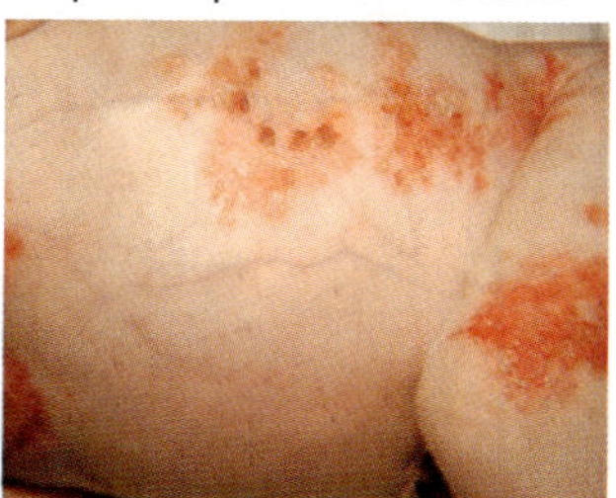
Annular 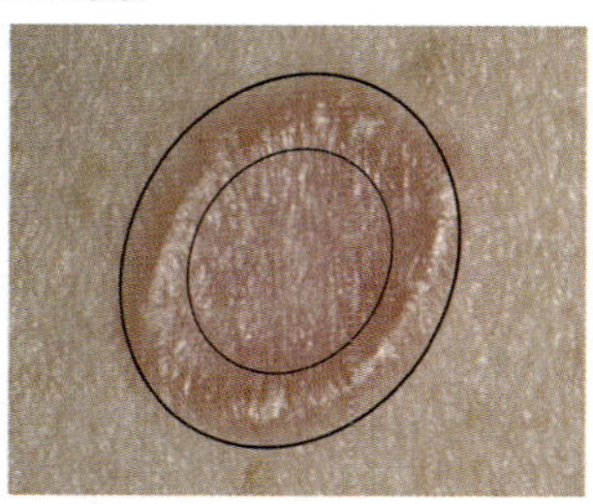	Ring-shaped	Urticaria 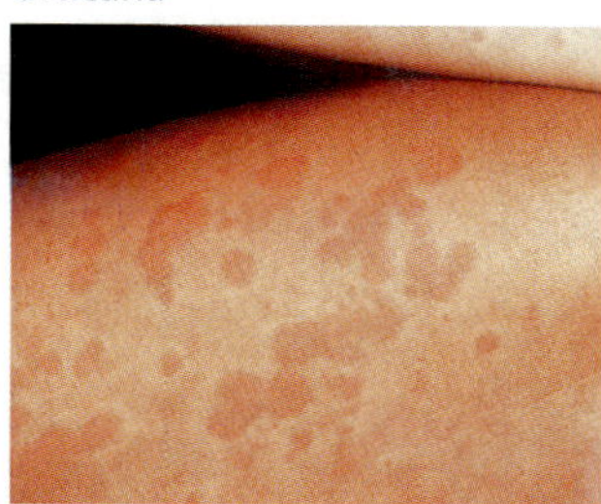
Targetoid 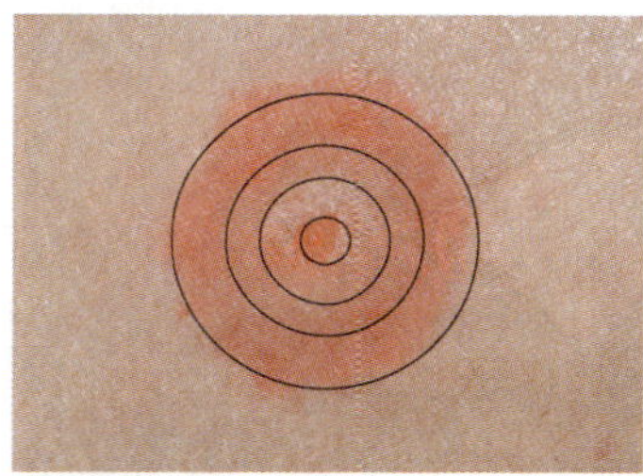	"Bulls-eye" appearance with central dusky zone surrounded by a ring of pallor (edema) and a peripheral rim of erythema	Erythema multiforme 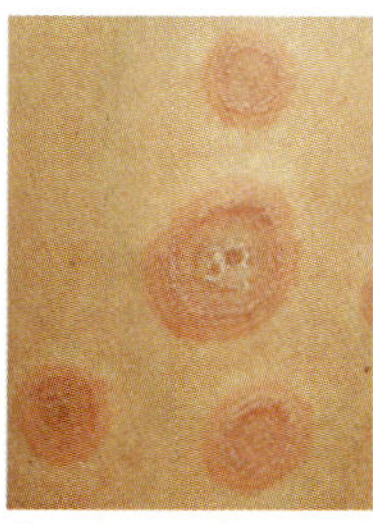
Serpiginous 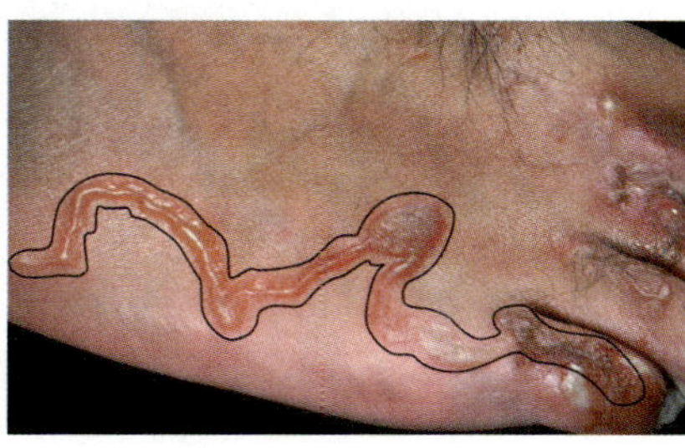	A wavy, linear grouping of lesions	Cutaneous larva migrans 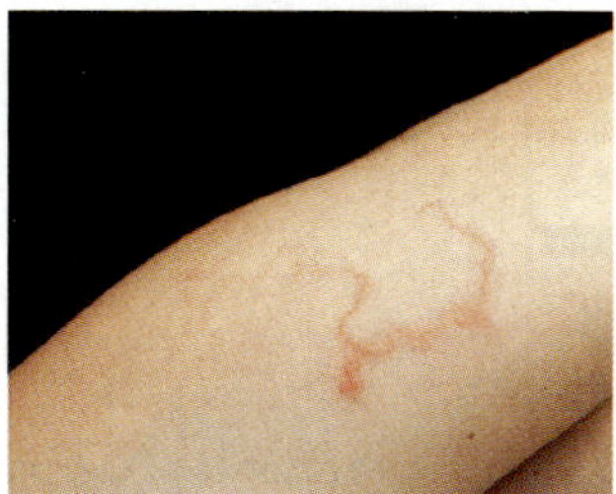
Arcuate 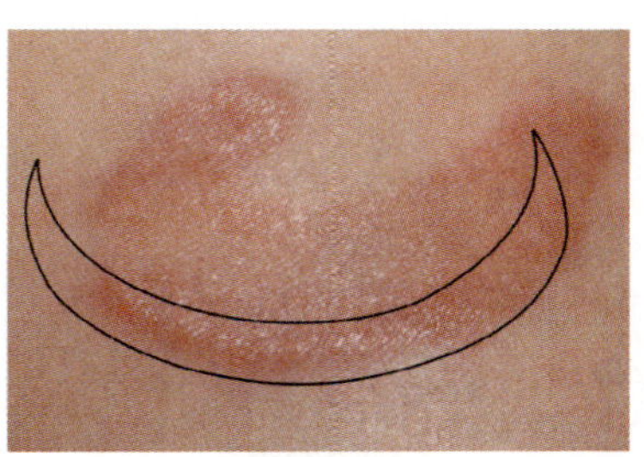	Incomplete rings and arcs	Urticaria 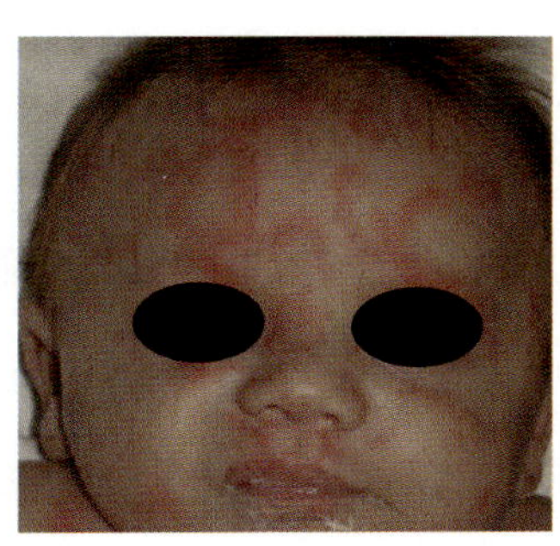

(*continued*)

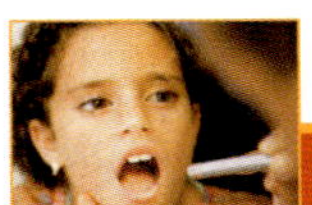

Table 13–2. (continued)

Common Morphologic Patterns of Dermatologic Disease

Morphology	Description	Examples
Polycyclic	Linked ring-shaped lesions	Urticaria 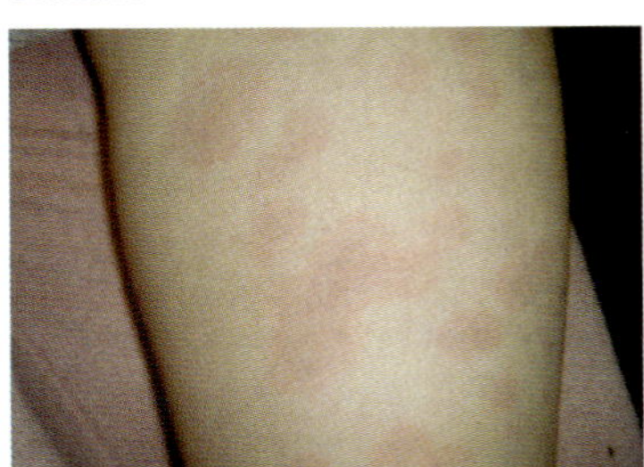
Dermatomal 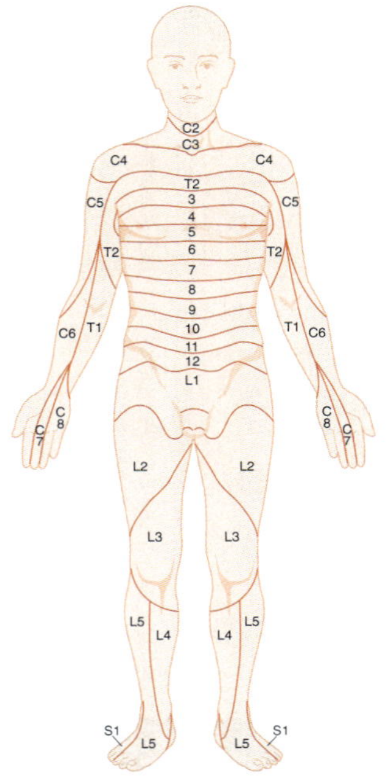	Confined to one or more areas of cutaneous sensory nerve innervation	Herpes zoster 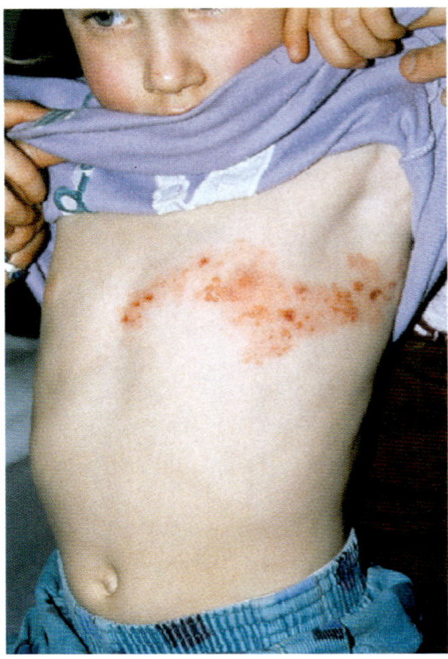

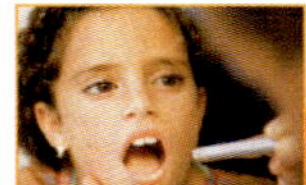

Table 13–3.

Selected Distribution Patterns of Dermatologic Disease

Distribution	Description	Examples
Exanthem	Affecting nonmucous membrane skin	Roseola (human herpes virus-6 infection) 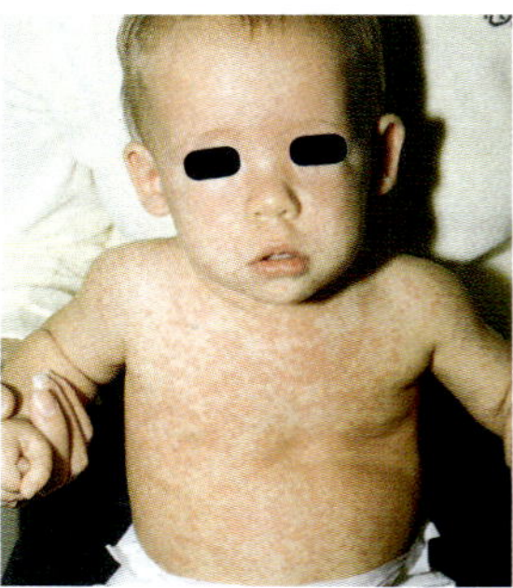

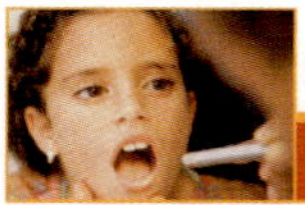

Table 13–3. (continued)

Selected Distribution Patterns of Dermatologic Disease

Distribution	Description	Examples
Enanthem	Affecting mucous membranes	Koplik spots (measles)
Acral	Affecting the distal extremities and sometimes the head	Gianotti–Crosti syndrome
Palmoplantar	Affecting the palms and soles	Erythema multiforme
Photodistributed	Affecting areas exposed to sunlight; commonly the face, upper extremities	Polymorphous light eruption
Intertriginous	Affecting skinfold areas such as the groin, axillae, and neck	Candidal intertrigo
Periorificial	Affecting the periorbital, perioral, and sometimes the perianal areas	Acrodermatitis enteropathica

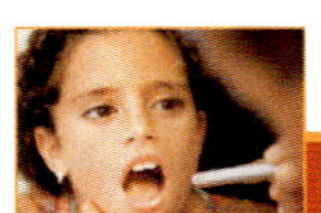

Table 13–4.

Selected Diagnostic Tests of Importance in the Evaluation of a Rash

Diagnostic Test	Procedure	Comments
Potassium hydroxide (KOH) preparation	1. Clean skin with alcohol pad 2. Use a #15 blade or a glass slide to scrape the scale from the lesion; use tangential motion 3. Place scrapings on a glass slide 4. Add 10% KOH; either warm the slide gently with a flame or allow to sit at room temperature for 5 minutes to facilitate dissolution of epithelial cells. 5. Examine under 10× power; make sure the condenser is on low	Useful in confirming a candidal or malassezia or dermatophyte infection of the skin. Candida species will appear as budding yeast. Dermatophyte species will appear as refreactile, branching hyphae. The characteristic "spaghetti and meatballs" appearance of clusters of spores in association with septate hyphae is seen with tinea versicolor infections caused by *Malassezia furfur*.
Fungal culture	1. Use a toothbrush or culture swab to rub the lesion briskly 2. Plate on mycobiotic agar (contains chlorhexidine to inhibit nondermatophyte molds)	Useful for confirmation of superficial infections with dermatophyte molds and Candidal species.
Scabies preparation	1. Use a #15 blade to briskly scrape 3–4 lesions; pick a fresh lesion 2. Place a drop of mineral oil on a glass slide 3. Spread the scrapings on the slide and examine under 4× power	Scabies mites, eggs, and scybylla (feces) can be easily seen in positive preparations. To increase diagnostic yield, scrape several lesions.
Bacterial culture	1. Swab the skin with alcohol first; allow the skin to dry 2. Puncture or unroof the pustule with a sterile needle or #11 blade 3. Obtain specimen with culture swab	Most laboratories can culture and identify common pathogenic organisms such as Staphylococcus, Streptococcus, and Pseudomonas species. Uncommon organisms may require special culture media or growth conditions. Check with your clinical laboratory if you have any questions or are trying to isolate an unusual organism.
Tzanck preparation	1. Choose an intact vesicle or pustule, if possible 2. Unroof lesion 3. Briskly scrape the base of the lesion with a #15 blade and smear onto a glass slide 4. Stain with Wright's or Giemsa stain	The presence of multinucleated giant cells suggests a herpes virus infection such as herpes simplex virus (HSV) or varizella zoster virus (VZV). Mainly of historical interest and largely supplanted by rapid diagnostic tests such as direct fluorescent antibody test (DFA) and polymerase chain reaction (PCR).
HSV/VZV direct fluorescent antibody test (DFA), PCR, and viral culture	1. Choose an intact vesicle or pustule, if possible 2. Unroof lesion with a #15 blade 3. Briskly scrape the base of the lesion with a Dacron swab 4. Place in viral culture media or smear immediately on a glass slide	Check with your clinical laboratory to verify how the specimen should be transported. PCR not available in all clinical laboratories. Viral cultures may take several days to grow. Do not delay treatment if HSV or VZV infection is suspected.
Skin biopsy	May be performed as a shave biopsy for superficial epidermal processes or as a punch biopsy for processes suspected to involve the dermis or subcutis	Consult dermatologist who can select appropriate skin lesion and perform procedure. Special immunohistochemical stains, immunofluorescence, and in situ PCR as well as bacterial, fungal, viral, and mycobacterial cultures may be performed if indicated.
Nikolsky's sign	Using your index finger, firmly stroke away from the lateral border of a bullae	Epidermal blistering processes, such as Staphylooccal-scalded skin disease and toxic epidermal necrolysis, will demonstrate additional shearing of the skin and lateral extension of the blister.
Dermatographism	Using the wooden end of a cotton-tipped applicator, briskly stroke the skin of the upper back	Often positive in children with urticaria or atopic dermatitis; essentially a form of pressure urticaria.

Topical Treatments and Products

What topical medications or other products has the patient applied to their skin, even on an intermittent basis, including any product used during the month prior to the onset of the rash? Application of topical corticosteroids may worsen a cutaneous infection or mask an inflammatory disease. A classic example is application of topical steroids to a dermatophyte infection, which leads to improvement in the associated pruritus and erythema, but allows the infection to persist and progress, often with an atypical appearance (tinea incognito).

Immunosuppression

Is the patient immunosuppressed? Patients with an underlying malignancy or any patient on chemotherapy or systemic immunosuppressive therapy are at a higher risk for both localized cutaneous infection and systemic infection, which may present in an atypical fashion. Certain organisms, such as the opportunistic molds *Aspergillus*, are seen almost exclusively in immunocompromised persons.

Exposures

Have there been any exposures to sick persons? Has there been any contact with any animals, including domestic animals, farm animals, or wildlife? Many animals harbor zoonotic infections or serve as intermediate hosts for organisms that can cause disease in humans, such as occurs with the transmission of Tularemia by exposure to wild rabbits.

Travel

Has there been any recent travel? Unusual exposures may occur in rural areas, foreign countries, or with travel to areas with endemic diseases such as Lyme disease.

Physical Examination

A key part of the physical examination is to identify a primary lesion (i.e., a new lesion) as well as any older lesions, which determine the morphologic progression of the rash. It is also important to recognize that patients may manipulate the skin in a way that alters the appearance of the rash, either through scratching or application of topical medications or other treatments. The examination should begin with an assessment of whether the patient looks well or has a toxic appearance. All areas of the skin should be examined systematically, usually beginning with the head and neck and proceeding to the trunk, buttocks and genitalia, and extremities, including the palms and soles. Examination of the mucous membranes (conjunctivae, lips and orophaynx, and urethral meatus) is important. Potentially severe drug hypersensitivity reactions such as Stevens–Johnson syndrome are differentiated from more benign drug hypersensitivity reactions on the basis of mucous membrane involvement. The examination should also include an assessment of the presence or absence of regional or systemic lymphadenopathy, which may be associated with certain infections or inflammatory conditions, and an assessment of the musculoskeletal examination, as arthralgis and arthritis are seen with several systemic inflammatory diseases and with some infections, such as parvoirus B19 infection. Finally, hair and nails should be examined, as abnormalities may indicate signs of systemic disease, such as systemic lupus erythematosus.

DIAGNOSIS

There are several useful diagnostic tests that may be helpful in diagnosing a rash (Table 13–4). Obtaining and processing the specimen correctly is important in increasing the diagnostic yield of the test. Check with your clinical laboratory if you have any questions or concerns about any special culture media or techniques that are required. In addition, in cases where a specific viral, parasitic, or bacterial infection is suspected, specific serologic tests or DNA detection tests such as polymerase chain reaction (PCR)-based assays may be available. Consult your clinical laboratory to determine which specific tests are available and whether or not they must be performed at a specialized laboratory.

CHAPTER 14

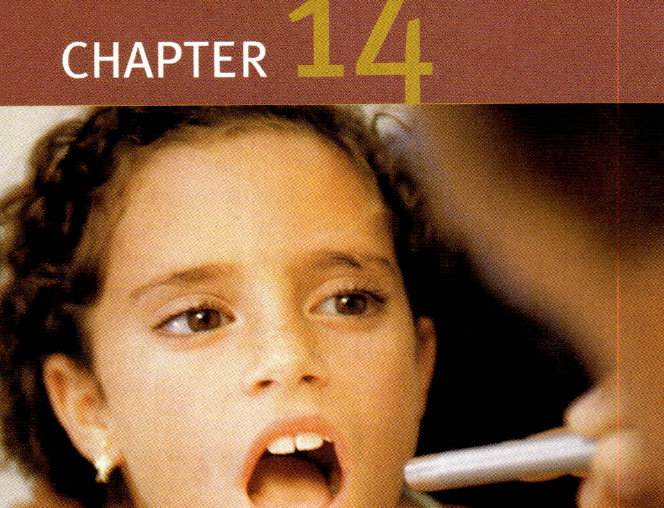

Stridor

Megan Aylor and Evan Fieldston

DEFINITION

Stridor is a harsh, high-pitched musical sound caused by oscillation of a narrowed airway while breathing, indicating partial airway obstruction. It occurs most commonly during inspiration, but may be biphasic or expiratory based on the anatomic location of the narrowing. Stridor is an important clinical finding that warrants investigation, as the etiologies range from benign, self-limited disease to severe illness leading to a rapidly progressive airway obstruction.

DIFFERENTIAL DIAGNOSIS

The differential diagnosis of stridor varies widely based on age of presentation. Stridor in neonates is nearly always caused by anatomic abnormalities, while older children and adolescents with stridor generally have underlying infectious, inflammatory, or environmental triggers.

Laryngomalacia is the most common cause of stridor in infants, accounting for approximately 60% of cases. In children with laryngomalacia, stridor begins within the first few weeks of life. It is caused by inward collapse of the supraglottic structures during inspiration; therefore, symptoms are worse with agitation, crying, and supine position. Stridor worsens over the first few months of life and begins to resolve around 6 months of age.

Subglottic stenosis is another common cause of stridor in infants. Stenosis can be congenital, or acquired from airway manipulation, such as endotracheal intubation. Stridor caused by subglottic stenosis is often biphasic and may manifest during the patient's first upper respiratory tract infection.

Vocal cord paralysis accounts for 10% of all congenital laryngeal lesions and is another common cause of stridor in infants. Vocal cord paralysis may be congenital, or acquired via birth trauma or as a complication of neonatal surgery, such as congenital heart disease or tracheoesophageal fistula repair. It is often associated with other abnormalities, such as Arnold–Chiari malformation, myelomeningocele, or hydrocephalus. Children with unilateral vocal cord paralysis may present with a weak cry or aspiration. However, with bilateral vocal cord paralysis, the cry may be normal and patients present with stridor and airway obstruction. Other causes of stridor in infants attributed to laryngeal, tracheal, vascular, or craniofacial abnormalities are listed in Table 14–1.

Stridor in older infants and children is often caused by acquired infectious or inflammatory conditions. These conditions can cause airway edema, which causes airway narrowing and an exponential increase in airway resistance. Viral croup, or laryngotracheobronchitis, is the most common cause of acute airway obstruction in older infants and children. It can be caused by a number of viral infections, the most common being parainfluenza, and occurs most commonly in patients aged 3 months to 5 years. Patients begin with upper respiratory tract symptoms, such as rhinorrhea, pharyngitis, and a low-grade fever 1–3 days prior to showing signs of airway involvement. They then develop a hoarse voice, "barking" cough, and inspiratory stridor. Symptoms resolve within 1 week. Older children are generally not as severely affected as younger children.

Though increasingly uncommon in the post-*Haemophilus influenzae* type B (Hib) vaccine era, epiglottitis is a severe, life-threatening cause of stridor and should remain on the differential for patients presenting with acute airway obstruction. The incidence of epiglottitis has fallen dramatically since the advent of

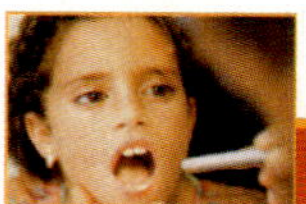

Table 14–1.

Differential Diagnosis of Stridor

Congenital Causes of Stridor	Acquired Causes of Stridor
Laryngeal abnormalities	Infectious
■ Laryngomalacia	■ Laryngotracheobronchitis (Viral croup)
■ Subglottic stenosis	■ Epiglottitis
■ Vocal cord paralysis	■ Supraglottitis
■ Laryngeal web, cyst or cleft	■ Peritonsillar abscess
■ Laryngocele	■ Retropharyngeal abscess
■ Laryngeal stenosis	■ Bacterial tracheitis
■ Subglottic hemangioma	■ Diphtheria
Tracheal abnormalities	■ Laryngeal papillomas
■ Tracheomalacia	■ Mucocutaneous candidiasis
■ Tracheoesophageal fistula	■ Endemic fungi†
■ Tracheal stenosis	■ Tuberculosis
Vascular abnormalities	Allergic/Inflammatory
■ Vascular ring*	■ Anaphylaxis
■ Pulmonary sling (i.e., aberrant left pulmonary artery)	■ Hereditary angioedema
	■ Severe asthma
Craniofacial abnormalities	■ Stevens Johnson's syndrome
■ Choanal atresia	■ Juvenile inflammatory arthritis with cricoarytenoid arthritis
■ Micrognathia	■ Dermatomyositis
■ Macroglossia	■ Allergic bronchopulmonary aspergillosis
■ Farber disease	■ Pemphigus vulgaris
■ Opitz–Frias syndrome	■ Wegener's granulomatosis
■ Apert syndrome	■ Sarcoid-laryngeal inflammation
■ Pierre–Robin sequence	■ Allergic polyps
	Miscellaneous
	■ Foreign body tracheal or esophageal
	■ Trauma/corrosive ingestion/thermal injury
	■ Lymphadenopathy
	■ Mass
	■ Laryngeal hemangioma
	■ Lingual cyst
	■ Tonsillar teratoma
	■ Nasopharyngeal angiofibroma
	■ Cystic hygroma
	■ Aberrant thyroid tissue
	■ Malignancy‡
	■ Psychogenic
	■ Spasmodic croup
	■ Laryngospasm from hypocalcemic tetany
	■ Gastroesophageal reflux
	■ Tonsillar hypertrophy

*Commonly double aortic arch, right-sided aortic arch, or aberrant (retroesophageal) subclavian artery.
†Includes Histoplasma capsulatum, Coccidioides immitis, and Blastomyces dermatitidis.
‡Such as chondrosarcoma, lymphoma, and rhabdomyosarcoma.

the Hib vaccine; however, cases of epiglottitis are still seen in unimmunized patients. Causes of epiglottitis in immunized patients include *Staphylococcus aureus*, *Streptococcus pyogenes*, and *Streptococcus pneumoniae*. The course often begins with pharyngitis, fever, and rhinorrhea, but rapidly progresses within hours to severe respiratory distress. Patients are toxic-appearing and may lean forward in a "tripod" position with their necks extended as a position of maximal comfort. Drooling can be seen because of inability to swallow. Stridor is a late finding and indicates severe airway obstruction.

Foreign body aspiration is important to consider in young children with acquired airway obstruction. Acute onset stridor occurring without other associated symptoms should raise concern for either esophageal or tracheal foreign body aspiration. Children aged 6 months to 3 years account for most cases of aspiration, though older children with developmental delay or behavior disorders are also at risk. A history of coughing, choking, or gagging should always be taken seriously even if the child does not present with stridor or respiratory distress, as some patients may have an asymptomatic interval before developing complications, such as mucosal erosion, secondary infection, or airway obstruction.[1]

HISTORY AND PHYSICAL EXAMINATION

A careful history and physical examination can help narrow the differential diagnosis of stridor. Key components of the history include the age and acuity of stridor onset, as well as the severity of symptoms. It is important to identify whether stridor is inspiratory, expiratory, or biphasic. Inspiratory stridor is caused by narrowed airway diameter during the negative pressure of inspiration and indicates a lesion above the vocal cords, while expiratory stridor suggests pathology of the intrathoracic airways. Biphasic stridor often indicates a fixed lesion that is unchanged by alterations in airway pressure.

Onset of stridor shortly after birth suggests vocal cord paralysis. In contrast, laryngomalacia is typically noted after 4 weeks of life. Previous airway manipulation, such as prolonged endotracheal intubation, predisposes to subglottic stenosis. Associated feeding difficulties, coughing during or shortly after feeds, and poor weight gain may indicate gastroesophageal reflux, poor pharyngeal tone (e.g., developmental delay, neuromuscular disorder), laryngeal cleft, tracheoesophageal fistula, or vascular ring. A hoarse cry with or without mild stridor may occur with unilateral vocal cord paralysis; bilateral vocal cord paralysis often results in severe obstruction. In older children, fever, cough, respiratory distress, drooling, and symptoms of upper respiratory tract infection, such as rhinorrhea or sore throat suggest croup, epiglottitis, or parapharyngeal abscess. Pain with neck extension also suggests parapharyngeal abscess.

The physical examination begins by observing the patient's general appearance at rest with attention to signs of respiratory distress and position of greatest comfort. Children with severe laryngeal obstruction usually hyperextend their neck as they attempt to straighten the upper airway and maximize its patency. In a neonate, certain physical examination maneuvers provide accurate assessment of the functional anatomy of the airway. Relief of stridor with placing the infant in prone position suggests supraglottic (or higher) obstruction as may occur in children with laryngomalacia, Pierre–Robin sequence (from micrognathia), or Down syndrome (from macroglossia). The latter two conditions are also relieved by pulling the infant's mandible and tongue forward. Nasal catheters should be passed to determine the patency of the nasopharyngeal airway (i.e., choanal atresia).

Any cause of neck swelling (especially diphtheria) or cervical lymphadenopathy (particularly with tuberculosis and Epstein–Barr virus infection) may cause stridor as a result of extrinsic airway compression. Cutaneous findings may be helpful, as café au lait macules raise suspicion for neurofibromatosis and associated airway neurofibromas. Cutaneous hemangiomas located in the beard distribution (any point along the preauricular, mandibular, perioral and submental areas) are also associated with a higher risk of subglottic hemangiomas that can cause stridor.

LABORATORY STUDIES

For many common causes of stridor, the diagnosis can be made clinically, without need for laboratory or radiographic studies.

Radiography

In most instances, the use of radiographic studies is not necessary in children with suspected croup. However, if the diagnosis is in question, anteroposterior and lateral neck radiographs should be obtained. In the anteroposterior view the "steeple sign," the classic finding in croup, reveals narrowing of the subglottic air column. Widening of the hypopharynx is observed in the lateral view. This finding is not present in all children with croup and can be found in some healthy children depending on the phase of inspiration. Lateral views can also reveal widening of the prevertebral soft tissues, which suggests retropharyngeal abscess (Figure 14–1) or

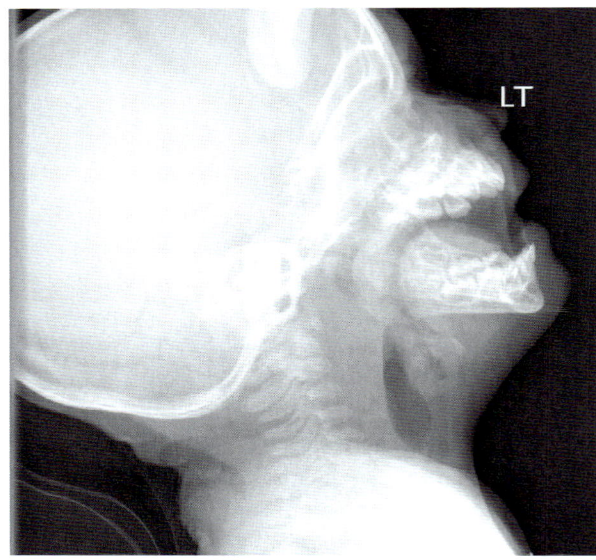

FIGURE 14–1 ■ Patient with a large retropharyngeal abscess. On a lateral neck radiograph, there is substantial widening of the prevertebral soft tissues of the retropharyngeal space with an air/fluid level. There is significant mass effect and anterior displacement of the trachea. (*Photo courtesy of Samir S. Shah, MD, MSCE.*)

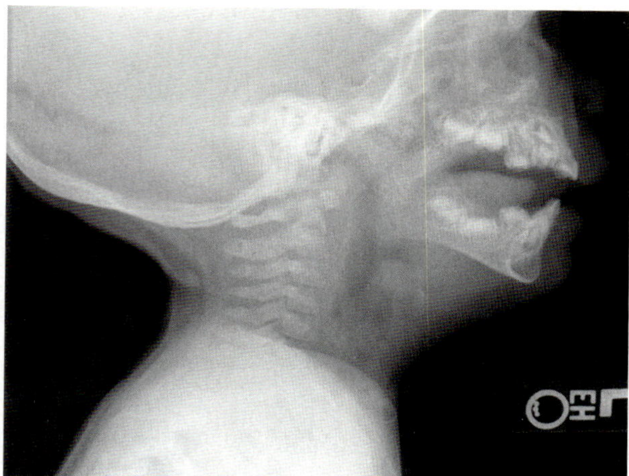

FIGURE 14–2 ■ Patient with epiglottitis caused by *Streptococcus pyogenes*. On the lateral neck radiograph, the epiglottis appears rounded and thickened (thumb print sign) with loss of the vallecular air space. (*Photo courtesy of Samir S. Shah, MD, MSCE.*)

cellulitis. Though epiglottitis can be seen on a lateral neck radiograph as a "thumb sign," this should not be used for diagnostic purposes (Figure 14–2). When epiglottitis is suspected, the child should be immediately transported to the operative suite for endotracheal intubation.

Chest radiographs can be useful in suspected foreign body aspiration. Radio-opaque objects, such as coins, can be seen both in the esophagus, and in the airway. Radiolucent objects will not be directly visualized; however, ipsilateral hyperinflation, particularly that which persists on a lateral decubitus view (with the affected side downward), suggests a foreign body in the mainstem bronchus. Additionally, chest radiographs may reveal evidence of airway bowing, as seen with either a double or a right-sided aortic arch.

Airway Fluoroscopy

Dynamic study of the airway with fluoroscopy can be helpful in localizing obstruction in patients with stridor. Fixed lesions (e.g., subglottic webs) are visualized throughout the respiratory cycle while functional lesions (e.g., laryngomalacia) change. Fluoroscopy (1) allows evaluation of hemidiaphragm movement; (2) allows assessment for air trapping; and (3) requires less patient cooperation than plain radiographs. However, when an airway foreign body is likely, airway fluoroscopy is less useful since endoscopy will be required regardless of fluoroscopy results.[2]

Flexible Fiberoptic Laryngoscopy

Flexible fiberoptic laryngoscopy provides visualization from the nasopharynx down to the vocal folds but cannot accurately evaluate the subglottis or trachea. This test is useful in diagnosing laryngomalacia as well as assessing for nasopharyngeal inflammation consistent with severe gastroesophageal reflux. For more direct assessment of the subglottic region, direct laryngoscopy and bronchoscopy with general anesthesia is required.

Barium Swallow

Barium swallow has been used for diagnosis of vascular rings in the past; however, with the advent of advanced CT angiography and MRI techniques, these newer studies are preferred when vascular rings are suspected.

Other Studies

Laboratory studies are rarely indicated in the evaluation of stridor. For patients in whom viral laryngotracheobronchitis is suspected, a viral respiratory PCR panel can be useful in identifying a viral etiology. Additionally, for patients with concern for bacterial tracheiits, culture of the exudate can be helpful in determining the bacterial pathogen.

EVALUATION

The gold standard for evaluation of stridor is direct visualization of the airway by an otorhinolaryngologist; however, not all children warrant subspecialty referral. In order to determine the children who may benefit the most from imaging or an ENT evaluation, a diagnostic approach is discussed below and an algorithm is presented in Table 14–2.[3-8]

INDICATIONS FOR CONSULTATION OR REFERRAL

While many of the common causes of stridor can be diagnosed clinically and managed as an outpatient by the primary care provider, there are several indications for subspecialty or emergency department referral.

Neonates presenting with stridor immediately after birth warrant evaluation by an otorhinolaryngologist to rule out significant laryngeal or tracheal abnormalities.[3,4] Pediatricians can monitor infants with stridor whose history and physical examination is consistent with tracheomalacia, unless they demonstrate poor weight gain, cyanosis, or respiratory distress. These findings may indicate severe malacia requiring intervention or may portend a more significant diagnosis.[5]

Children presenting with symptoms of a viral upper respiratory tract infection and stridor consistent with viral laryngotracheobronchitis can be managed as an outpatient as long as they have stridor only with

Table 14–2.

Diagnostic Algorithm for Stridor

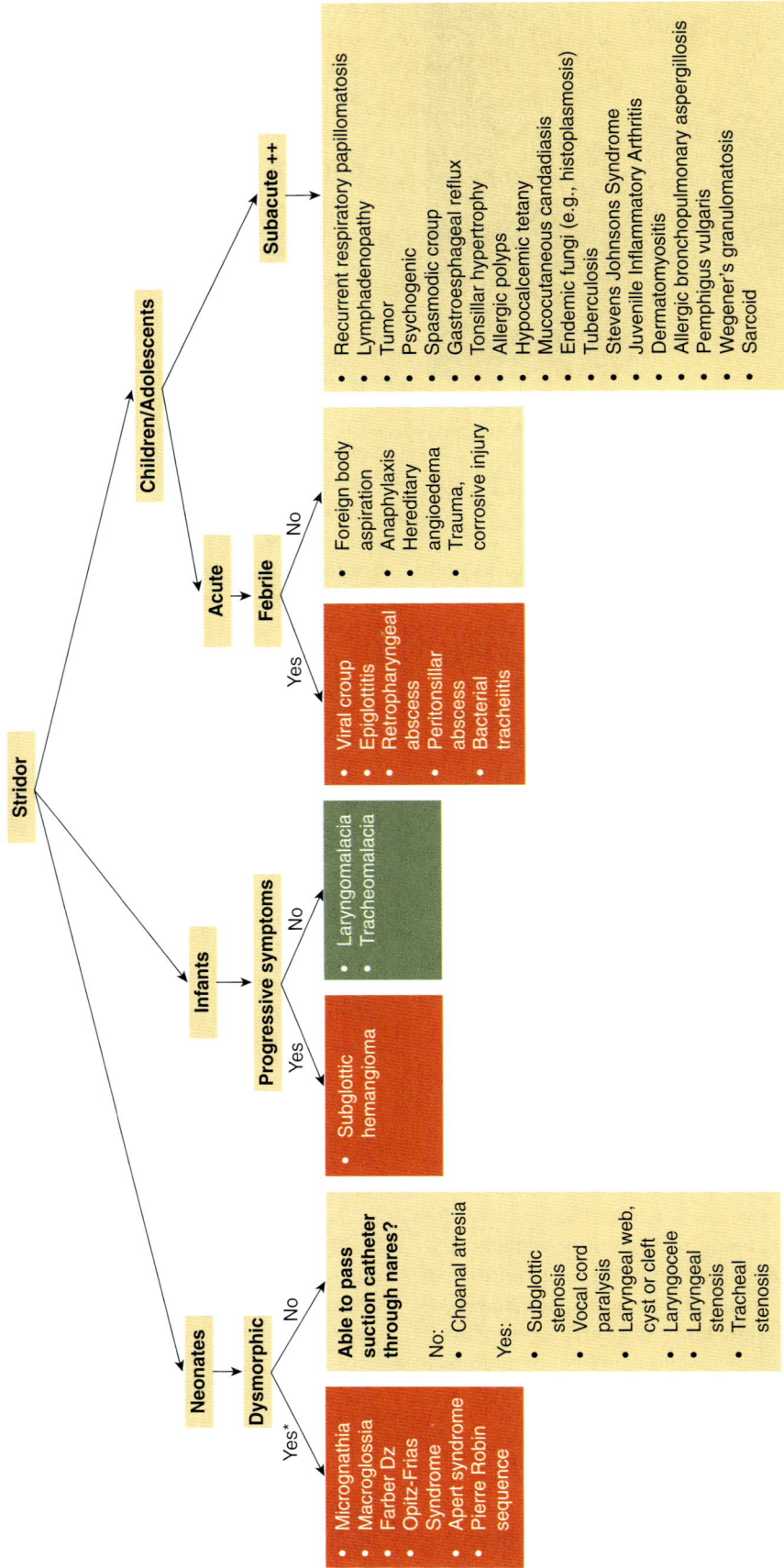

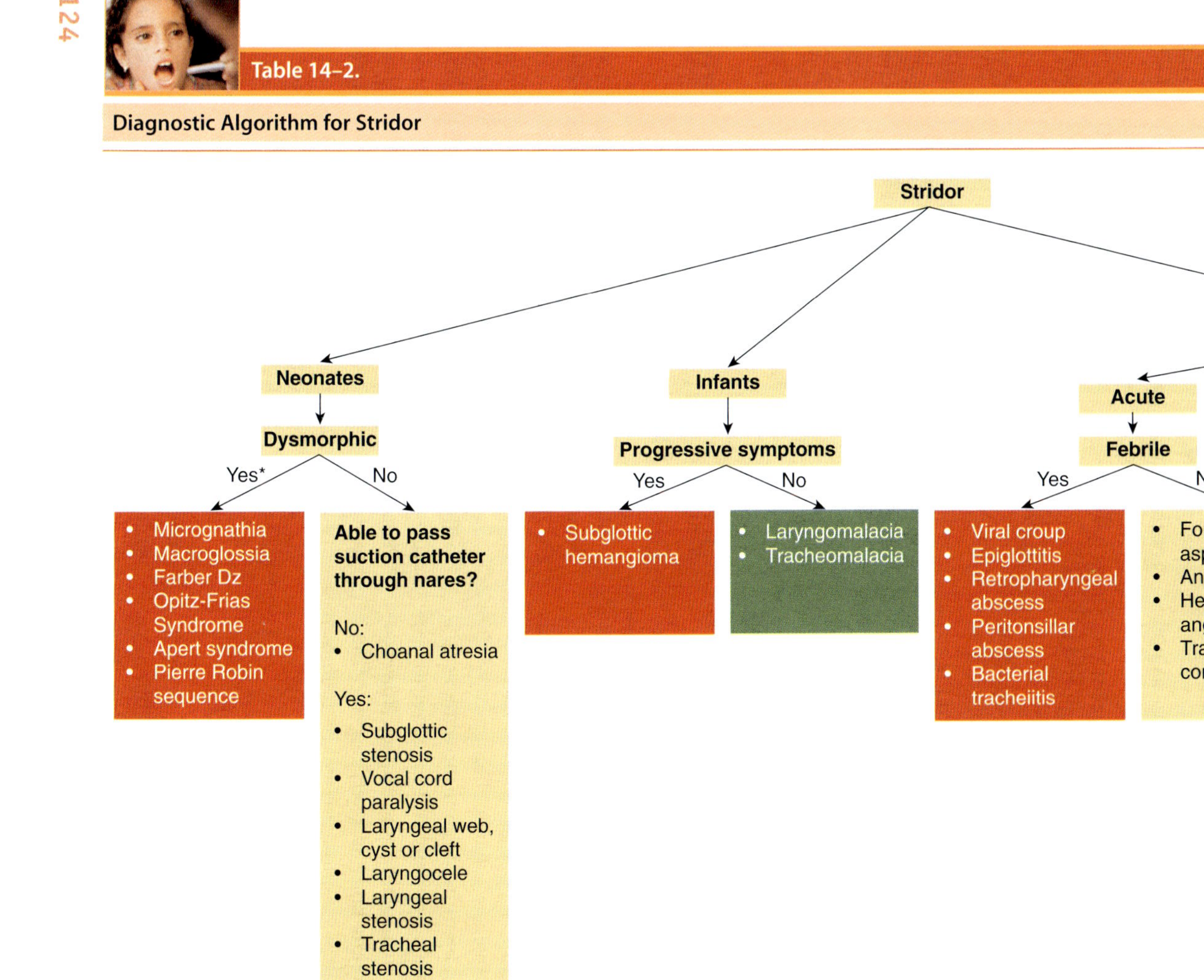

*Consider consultation with geneticist

++ Detailed history and physical to determine associated symptoms

agitation and no evidence of respiratory distress. Patients with stridor at rest, moderate subcostal retractions, decreased air entry, cyanosis, or depressed mental status require hospitalization.

Any child with suspected esophageal or tracheal foreign body aspiration, epiglottitis, or evidence of severe respiratory distress warrants immediate emergency department referral. Additionally, older children and adolescents with stridor require evaluation in the emergency department if the stridor is acute or by an otorhinolaryngologist if symptoms are insidious.

REFERENCES

1. Holinger LD. Foreign bodies of the airway. In: Behrman RE, Kliegman RM, Jenson HB, eds. *Nelson Textbook of Pediatrics.* 17th ed, Philadelphia: WB Saunders Co; 2004: 1410-1411.
2. Rudman DT. The role of airway fluoroscopy in the evaluation of stridor in children. *Arch Otolaryngol Head Neck Surg.* 2003;129(3):305-309.
3. Sie KC. Infectious and inflammatory disorders of the Larynx and Trachea. In: Wetmore RF, Muntz HR, McGill TJ, eds. *Pediatric Otolaryngology.* Thieme Medical Publishers, Inc.; 2000:811-825.
4. Hughes CA, Dunham ME. Trachea. In: Wetmore RF, Muntz HR, McGill TJ, eds. *Pediatric Otolaryngology.* Thieme Medical Publishers, Inc.; 2000:775-786.
5. Perry H. Stridor. In: Fleisher GR, Ludwig S, Henretig FM, eds. *Textbook of Pediatric Emergency Medicine.* 5th ed. Philadelphia: Lippincott Williams & Wilkins; 2006: 643-647.
6. Tunnessen WW. *Stridor in Signs and Symptoms in Pediatrics.* 3rd ed. Philadelphia: Lippincott Williams & Wilkins; 1999: 400-406.
7. Holinger LD. Congenital anomalies of the Larynx. In: Behrman RE, Kliegman RM, Jenson HB, eds. *Nelson Textbook of Pediatrics.* 17th ed. Philadelphia: WB Saunders Co; 2004:1409-1410.
8. Johnson D. Croup in Clinical Evidence Pediatrics. *BMJ Publish Group.* 2005;13:102-124.

CHAPTER 15

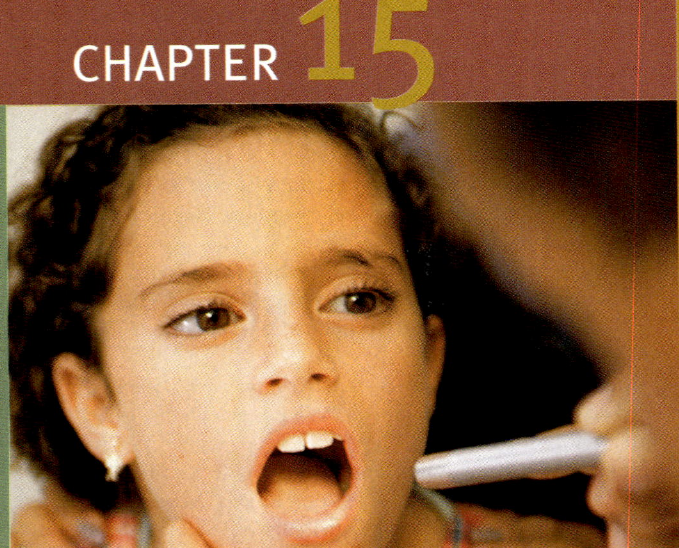

Wheezing

Evan Fieldston and Megan Aylor

DEFINITION

Wheezing is a high-pitched whistling sound heard during expiration. It occurs when air flows through narrowed or partially obstructed airways, mostly the bronchioles. It can also be heard because of narrowing of larger airways.

Wheezing is common in infants and children. An estimated 10–15% of all infants younger than 1 year have an episode of wheezing. Up to 25% of children younger than 5 years present at least once to medical attention for evaluation of wheezing.[1] Recurrent wheezing over the age of 1 year usually indicates a diagnosis of asthma.

DIFFERENTIAL DIAGNOSIS

The differential diagnosis for wheeze is broad.[2] An initial episode of wheezing typically suggests viral respiratory tract infection. Since wheezing is often associated with viral respiratory infections in infants, it is difficult to distinguish an initial episode of asthma triggered by a viral respiratory tract infection from acute viral bronchiolitis. The causes of recurrent or persistent wheezing are more diverse. Common causes of recurrent wheezing include serial viral respiratory infections, poorly controlled asthma, and gastroesopheal reflux with pulmonary aspiration. Less commonly, recurrent wheezing is caused by congenital abnormalities of the lung, diaphragm, or branches of the aorta or pulmonary vessels. Vascular rings, aberrant right subclavian artery, innominate arterial compression, aberrant left pulmonary artery (pulmonary sling), and absence of the pulmonary valve may all present with abnormal respiratory sounds and distress in infants.[3,4] Cystic fibrosis or immunologic defects may also manifest first with wheezing. In addition, wheezing may not be the reason why a caregiver brings a child to medical attention. Thus, children with wheeze can present in a variety of ways. These variable paths also provide clues to the etiology. Table 15–1 provides the most common presentations and associated signs and symptoms. Figure 15–1 provides anatomic locations of causes of wheezing.

HISTORY AND PHYSICAL EXAMINATION

A complete history and physicial examination will facilitate the accurate diagnosis of a child evaluated for wheezing. Features of the history that warrant clarification include the periodicity of the wheezing (initial, recurrent, or persistent), family history of pertinent medical conditions, relevant epidemiologic exposures, and presence of associated signs and symptoms.

For infants, a history of prematurity, mechanical ventilation (tracheal stenosis), or noisy breathing independent of symptoms of respiratory infection may suggest either bronchopulmonary dysplasia or a congenital structural airway abnormality. Investigate all perinatal screening to assess for HIV status of mother and child and pulmonary or cardiac anatomic anomaly that may have been seen on ultrasound. Delayed passage of meconium may be a clue for cystic fibrosis. Reflux, arching, or choking above the ordinary could be a sign that gastroesophageal reflux disease (GERD) or aspiration are a cause of wheezing. A history of sweating and/or difficulty with feeds suggests congenital heart disease and cardiac failure. Family history of asthma, cystic fibrosis, α1-antrypsin deficiency, immunodeficiency, or

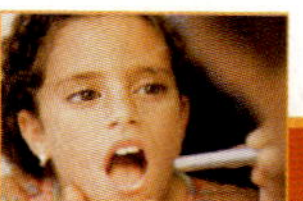

Table 15–1.

Diagnostic Tests and Expected Results in Children with Less Common Causes of Wheezing

Disease	Typical Age	Relevant Laboratory and Radiological Findings
Congenital airway anomaly, laryngomalacia, tracheomalacia	≤12 months	■ CXR and lateral neck may reveal tracheal narrowing or other airway abnormality
Foreign body aspiration	≥6 months	■ CXR (anterior-posterior, lateral, decubitus) may reveal unilateral hyperinflation, lobar or segmental atelectasis, mediastinal shift, or air-trapping (decubitus) of the dependent lung. Most foreign bodies are not radio-opaque
Anaphylaxis	Any age	■ Usually none required emergently ■ Allergy testing
Cystic fibrosis	Infancy or childhood	■ CXR may reveal hyperinflation, atelectasis, peribronchial thickening (early); diffuse interstitial disease, bronchiectasis, nodular densities of mucoid impaction (later); infiltrate ■ Sweat testing
Cardiac disease or vascular ring	Infancy	■ CXR: cardiomegaly, abnormally shaped heart, right aortic arch, tracheal deviation or compression ■ EKG ■ Echo
Aspiration syndromes: GERD, neuromuscular disease, Tracheoesophageal Fistula	Infant or child	■ CXR may reveal infiltrate, often right-sided Consider ■ Modified barium swallow ■ pH probe for reflux ■ UGI ■ Salivogram
Bronchopulmonary dysplasia	Infant or child	Consider: CXR, which may reveal increased vascular markings and increased hilar markings of chronic lung disease
Primary immunodeficiency	Variable ages of presentation	■ CXR: absence of thymus in chromosome 22q11 deletion syndromes ■ Serum immunoglobulin levels (IgA, IgE, IgG, IgM) ■ Antibody response to diphtheria, tetanus or pneumococcal vaccines ■ Lymphopenia on complete blood count

CXR, chest radiograph; EKG, electrocardiogram; Ig, immunoglobulins; UGI, upper gastrointestinal barium series

immotile cilia/Kartagener syndrome would be of interest. Relevant social history includes exposure to smoke or other exhaust, pets or animals, daycare, or travel. If tuberculosis is being considered, evaluate risk factors for exposure, including foreign travel, contact with visitors from other countries, or contact with prisoners or homeless shelters. Unusual causes of wheezing, such as histoplasmosis or other endemic fungi are more likely to occur after travel to the mid-Atlantic.

In younger children, wheezing may be hard to differentiate from stridor (harsh, high-pitched sound heard more on inspiration) or stertor (rattling and congested noise heard more on inspiration), or may accompany them. Auscultation in front of the nose and along the throat can help localize the source of the noisy breathing. Upper airway noises are also symmetrically distributed on ausculation of the chest, but wheezing can be localized or diffuse. Lack of wheezing may indicate insufficient respiratory effort by the patient or such severe narrowing of distal airways that air is not flowing to create an audible noise. Asking older children to breathe deeply or blow out, or assisting infants by compressing the chest on expiration, can make wheezing more apparent.

Physical examination should pay close attention to vital signs, with particular note of temperature, heart rate, respiratory rate, and pulse oximetry reading. Presence of fever should focus attention on infectious causes (such as pneumonia), though infants with bronchiolitis are often afebrile. Tachycardia may be a sign of signficant distress or dehydration. Preductal and postductal saturations or oxygen challenges may provide evidence

Intrinsic Airway Narrowing (1)
- Tracheobronchomalacia
- Stenosis
- Bronchopulmonary dysplasia
- Alpha-1 antitrypsin deficiency
- Bronchospasm
    - Anaphylaxis
    - Organophosphate

Inflammation (2)
- Asthma
- Bronchiolitis (respiratory syncytial virus; human metapneumovirus; parainfluenza 1,2, 3; influenza; rhinovirus; mycoplasma pneumoniae, etc.)
- Smoke exposure
- Aspiration
- Tracheoesophageal fistula
- Gastroesophageal reflux
- Swallowing disorder
- Pneumonia (bacterial, viral, atypical: mycoplasma, chlamydia)
- Hypersensitivity pneumonitis/ allergic bronchopulmonary aspergillosis
- Pulmonary edema
- Bronchiectasis
- Hemosiderosis
- Histoplasmosis, mycotic infections

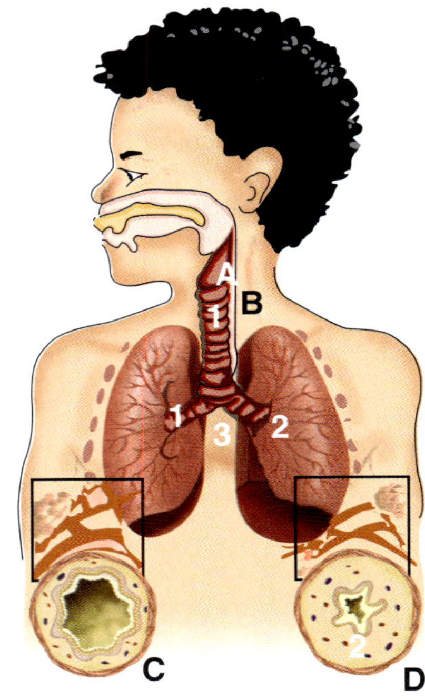

A. Throat
B. Trachea
C. Bronchiole, cross section (normal)
D. Bronchiole, cross section (inflamed)

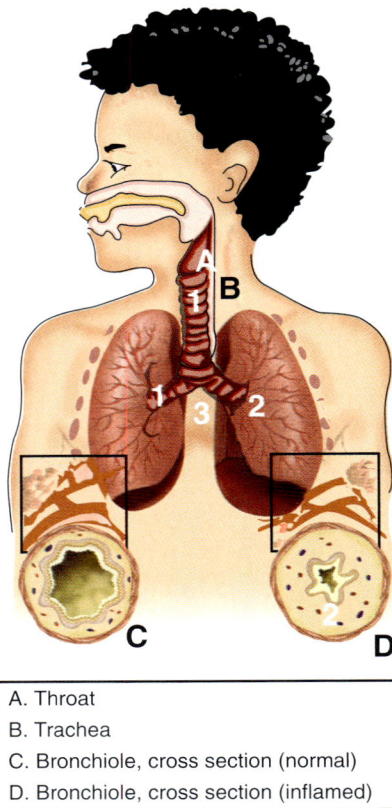

Extrinsic Airway Compression (3)
- Cystic lung malformation
- Vascular ring, aberrant right subclavian artery, innominate arterial compression, aberrant left pulmonary artery (sling), absence of pulmonary valve
- Aberrant vessels
- Cardiomegaly
- Thymus hyperplasia
- Mediastinal mass, tumors, adenopathy
- Tuberculosis
- Leukemia
- Lymphoma

Intraluminal (1)
- Foreign body

Miscellaneous
- Congestive heart failure
- Immune deficiency
- Cystic fibrosis
- Immotile cilia/Kartagener syndrome
- Factitious wheezing
- Psychogenic airway obstruction
- Pulmonary sequestration
- Pulmonary vasculitis
- Sarcoidosis
- Viscera larva migrans (toxocariasis)
- Carcinoid syndrome
- Angioneurotic edema
- Lobar emphysema
- HIV/AIDS
- Vocal cord dysfunction

FIGURE 15–1 ■ Causes of wheezing and their anatomic locations

toward heart disease. The presence of upper respiratory infection (URI) symptoms, including rhinorrhea, congestion, and sneezing may point toward a viral cause and bronchiolitis in an infant, but could also be a sign of an underlying anatomic or physiologic problem. In particular, patients with very severe illnesses that are associated with signs of URI should be evaluated in more depth.

Evidence of failure to thrive on examination should raise questions about prematurity and caloric intake, HIV status, and cystic fibrosis. Abnormal heart sounds, murmur on examination, or unequal pulses would raise the question of congenital heart disease.

Examination of a wheezing child can be done before and after bronchodilator therapy. Lack of any response to this treatment (or through history) may raise suspicion for a cause outside of the small airways. This would include congenital heart disease, aortic arch abnormalities, aberrant pulmonary veins, extrinsic compression of the trachea or bronchi, tracheobronchial anomalies, lung cysts, mediastinal masses, and thymus hyperplasia.

LABORATORY STUDIES

Chest Radiography

The need for laboratory or radiological studies depends on the presentation and level of concern. Chest radiography is often not needed in the evaluation of wheezing, especially in an infant with signs of a URI. In bronchiolitis or asthma, CXR may show hyperinflation, peribronchial thickening, and atelectasis. Plain film of the chest in anterior-posterior and lateral views may identify a right-sided or double aortic arch. The study can also delineate vascular anomaly, cardiac enlargement, or pulmonary hypertension. Plain film can also help elucidate the presence of a foreign body, but lateral decubitus films may be required (persistence of hyperinflation when lobe is down). CXR can also reveal infiltrates or masses, including mediastinal masses (Figure 15–2). Chest radiography is generally recommended in febrile patients or patients with focal findings (i.e., wheeze or rales) on pulmonary auscultation.[5] Patients with recurrent wheezing, if they have not had a

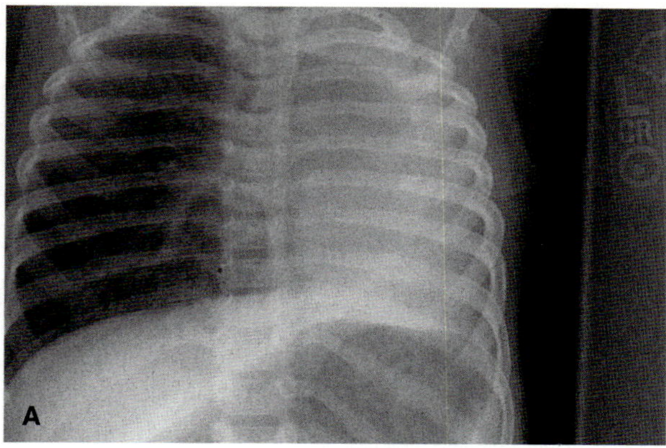

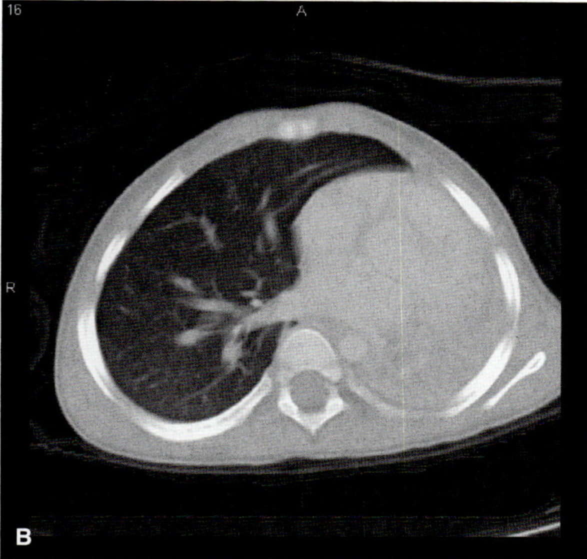

FIGURE 15–2 ■ Chest radiograph **(A)** and computed tomography of the chest **(B)** reveal collapse of left lung resulting in herniation of right lung to the contralateral side, caused by lymph node compression of left mainstem bronchus in a 3-year-old with tuberculosis. (*Courtesy of Samir S. Shah, MD, MSCE.*)

chest radiograph done, should have one to rule out an anatomic etiology for wheezing.

Other Studies

Blood-based laboratory studies are usually not needed for straightforward wheezing. A complete blood count may be indicated when evaluating for infection or anemia. Patients in severe respiratory distress, status asthmaticus, or with significant desaturations should have an arterial blood gas to evaluation for hypoxia, hypercarbia, and acidosis.

Rapid virologic testing for respiratory infections, such as influenza, RSV, and human metapneumovirus, are making their way into widespread clinical practice. The results rarely change management but can be helpful in cohorting hospitalized patients.

Other studies to consider in the wheezing patient, particularly those with chronic wheeze, would be sweat chloride test for cystic fibrosis, tuberculin skin test, allergy testing, and spirometry. Evaluation for airway and esophageal pathology (such as tracheoesophageal fistula) may be indicated in some cases. Difficult-to-control wheezing can be the result of gastroesophageal reflux disease with aspiration and studies to evaluate for those conditions may be needed.

Pulse oximetry is often used in the assessment of wheezing children, particularly those with evidence of bronchiolitis, pneumonia, and those in respiratory distress. Pulse oximetry can detect hypoxemia that is not evident on physical examination.[6]

EVALUATION

Age, severity, associated symptoms, recurrence or persistence, and knowledge of past medical history will help guide evaluation of the wheezing child. Table 15–2 provides an algorithm of features of presentation and Table 15–1 provides laboratory or radiological studies associated with various diagnoses.

INDICATIONS FOR CONSULTATION OR REFERRAL

Depending on the severity of respiratory distress, the acuity or chronicity, age of the patient, likelihood of anatomic and mechanical etiology, associated findings, and location of presentation, consultation or referral may or may not be needed.

Infants and young children without significant tachypnea, desaturation, or respiratory distress can be managed on an outpatient basis with caregiver understanding of reasons to return to medical attention and assurance of good follow-up.

Any patient in extremis, status asthmaticus, or respiratory distress should be referred to an emergency department through emergency medical services. In bronchiolitis, high-risk patients include premature infants (≤34 weeks gestational age), infants younger than 3 months, those with respiratory rate greater than 70 breaths per minute or an underlying immunodeficiency; they are at increased risk for severe disease and should be referred to a hospital for evaluation and monitoring.

Patients with chronic wheezing not associated with infections, and who are difficult to control with standard outpatient measures, may be referred to allergy or pulmonary specialists for further evaluation and management. Patients at risk for GERD or aspiration may need additional evaluation and referral to a gastroenterologist.

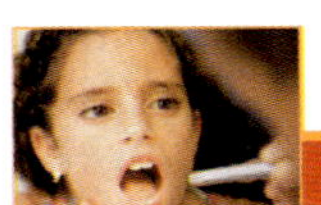

Table 15–2.

Diagnostic Algorithm for Wheezing

Nonabrupt		Abrupt	
Fever	**No Fever**	**Urticaria**	**No Urticaria**
≤1-year old ■ Bronchiolitis ■ Cystic fibrosis ■ Immune deficiency ■ Pneumonia ■ AIDS ■ Tuberculosis ■ Histoplasmosis ■ Primary immunodeficiency	■ Reactive Airways Disease ■ Anatomic heart anomaly ■ Kartagener's/immotile cilia ■ Left heart failure ■ Metabolic causes* ■ Primary immunodeficiency	■ Anaphylaxis	■ Foreign body aspiration
>1-year old **No prior wheeze** ■ Underlying anatomic variant† (worse with infection) ■ Primary immunodeficiency **Prior wheeze** ■ Asthma ■ Underlying anatomic variant† (worse with infection) ■ Viral infection ■ Tuberculosis ■ Histoplasmosis ■ Leukemia, lymphoma, lymphosarcoma ■ Kartagener syndrome ■ Hypersensitivity pneumonitis ■ Vocal cord dysfunction ■ Angioneurotic edema ■ AIDS ■ Primary immunodeficiency	**No prior wheeze** ■ RAD/Asthma ■ Primary immunodeficiency **Prior wheeze** ■ Asthma ■ Underlying anatomic variant† (worse with infection) ■ GERD ■ Smoke exposure ■ Cystic fibrosis ■ Primary immunodeficiency	■ Anaphylaxis	■ Foreign body aspiration

*Such as *Hypocalcemia, hypokalemia*
†Such as *Tracheomalacia, stenosis, compression*

REFERENCES

1. Martinati LC. Clinical diagnosis of wheezing in early childhood. *Allergy*. 1995;5(9):701-710.
2. Oski, J. Presenting signs and symptoms. In: McMillan JA, DeAngelis CD, Feigin RD, Warshaw JB, eds. *Oski's Pediatrics, 3rd ed.* Philadelphia: Lippincott Williams & Wilkins; 1999:2308.
3. Berdon WE, Baker DH. Vascular anomalies and the infant lung: rings, slings, and other things. *Semin Roentgenol.* 1972;7(1):39-63.
4. Berdon WE. Rings, slings, and other things: vascular compression of the infant trachea. Update from the Midcentury to the Millenium—the Legacy of Robert E. Gross, MD, and Edward BD. Neuhauser, MD. *Radiology*. 2000;216(3):624-632.
5. Gershel JC. The usefulness of chest radiographs in first asthma attacks. *N Engl J Med.* 1983;309(6):336-339.
6. AAP Subcommittee on Diagnosis and Management of Bronchiolitis. Diagnosis and management of bronchiolitis. *Pediatrics.* 2006;118(4):1774-1793.

SECTION 3

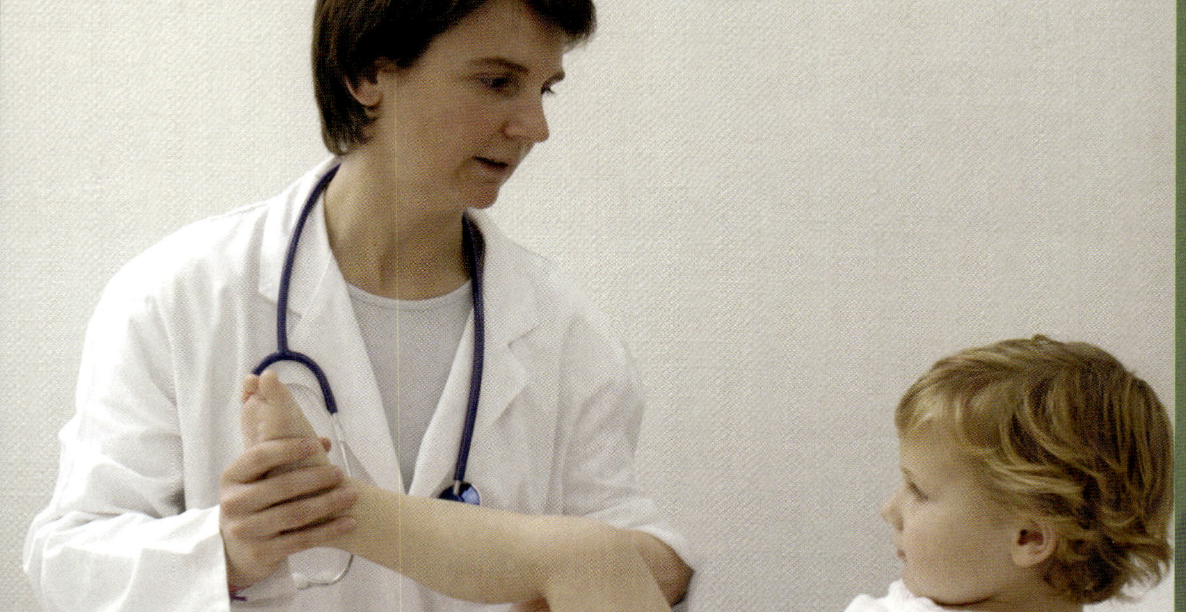

Neurologic Infections

CHAPTER 16

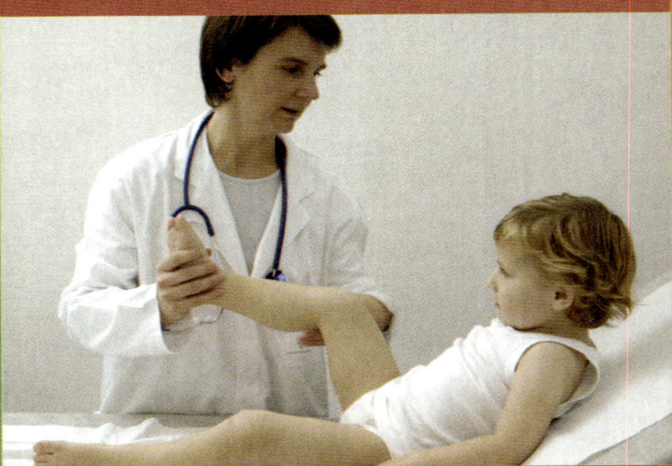

Meningitis

Marvin B. Harper

DEFINITIONS AND EPIDEMIOLOGY

Meningitis is defined as an inflammation of the leptomeninges of any cause. Bacteria, which cause meningitis by invading and replicating in the subarachnoid space, are associated with significant morbidity and mortality. Viral infections may also cause meningitis, most commonly enteroviruses, but few children with viral meningitis suffer any long-term sequelae. Therefore, the focus of this chapter will be on bacterial meningitis. Figure 16–1 displays the age and organism-specific rates of bacterial meningitis in the United States prior to the introduction of currently used conjugate vaccines (note the y-axis is a log scale). As can be seen, the greatest risk period for bacterial meningitis is in the first 6 months of life.

Overall, there has been a remarkable decline in the rate of bacterial meningitis in the developed world over the last two decades with the introduction of the *Haemophilus influenzae* type B conjugate vaccines, the *Streptococcus pneumoniae* conjugate vaccines and greater use of meningococcal vaccines. *H. influenzae* type B was once the leading cause of bacterial meningitis in children but has been virtually eliminated in countries utilizing the conjugate vaccine. In the first 2 months of life *Enterobacteriaceae* (e.g., *Escherichia coli*, *Klebsiella* spp.), group B streptococci, and occasionally *Listeria monocytogenes*, *Salmonella* spp. or enterococci will cause bacterial meningitis. Infections caused by *S. pneumoniae* occur with increasing in frequency over the second month to become the most likely cause of bacterial meningitis and continue to increase in frequency until 4 or 5 months of age when they begin to decline. *Neisseria meningitidis* is the most common cause of bacterial meningitis by 1 year of age. *S. pneumoniae*

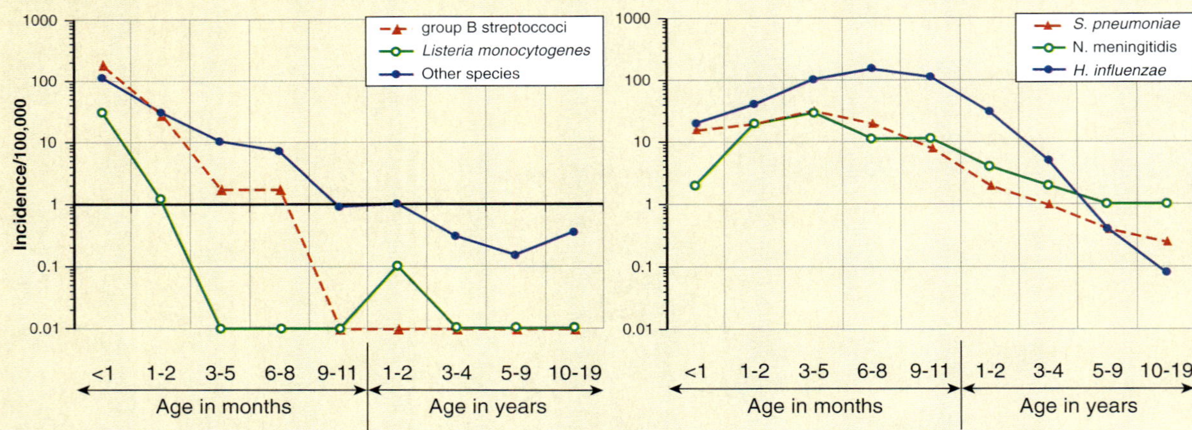

FIGURE 16–1 ■ Incidence rates of bacterial meningitis by age and pathogen prior to the introduction of the conjugate *H. influenzae* type B and heptavalent *Strep. pneumoniae* vaccines. (*From Wenger JD, Hightower AW, Facklam RR, Gaventa S, Broome CV. Bacterial meningitis in the United States, 1986: Report of a multistate surveillance study. The Bacterial Meningitis Study Group. J Infect Dis. 1990;162(6):1316–1323.*)

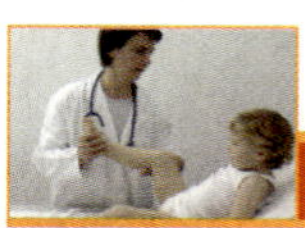

Table 16–1.

Etiology of Meningitis

Common
Enteroviruses
Neisseria meningitidis
Strep. pneumoniae
Group B streptococci
Escherichia coli
Haemophilus influenzae
Listeria monocytogenes
Less Common
Herpes simplex virus
Klebsiella spp. (and other Enterobacteriaceae)
Borrelia Burgdorferi
Candida spp..
Salmonella spp.
Mycobacterium tuberculosis
Pseudomonas aeruginosa
Staphylococcus aureus
Enterococcal spp.
Rare
Cysticercosis
Cryptococcus neoformans
Lymphocytic choriomeningitis
Mumps
Syphilis
Amoebae

remains the second most common cause after 1 year of age and all other pathogens trail behind considerably. These two pathogens occur more commonly in the winter months presumably in association with common respiratory viruses, which disrupt mucosal barriers thereby allowing these colonizing pathogens to move from the nasopharynx to the bloodstream more easily. Research is ongoing to develop vaccines that will be effective against a greater number of pneumococcal serotypes and improved meningococcal vaccines that may work for younger children and against group B strains. Table 16–1 reviews microbial causes of meningitis.

PATHOGENESIS

Bacteria most often gain access to the central nervous system via the bloodstream. Pathogens gain access to the bloodstream as a result of nasopharyngeal colonization or local infections. When these specific bacterial strains are relatively new to the host, and the child has no existing circulating antibody against that strain, the bacteria may at least temporarily evade other host defenses and cause a transient or sustained bacteremia. Some of these bacteria may traverse the blood–brain barrier and replicate in the subarachnoid space. Once bacteria begin to replicate within the central nervous system, the human host has no adequate mechanism to recover without medical intervention.

The risk for sequelae and mortality vary significantly by age of the child, pathogen, and underlying host compromise at baseline and at presentation with meningitis. Patients may have impaired neurologic function as a result of brain inflammation secondary to the bacteria and the host response to infection as well as because of cerebral hypoperfusion related to septic shock with hypotension, raised intracranial pressure, and/or disorders in local circulatory regulation including microvascular obstruction. Brain injury centers prominently on the cortex, hippocampus, and the inner ear, and the injuries are not simply the result of bacterial invasion but also occur as a result of a symphony of inflammatory mediators whose roles and control remain the focus of intense evaluation and give the promise of potential for future clinical intervention.[1]

Meningitis may also develop as the result of direct extension of pathogens from sites, such as the sinuses, mastoids, dermoid sinuses, or the skull. Recurrent episodes of bacterial meningitis should prompt immunologic evaluation as well as careful anatomic evaluation of contiguous structures (e.g., for congenital or traumatic bony, vascular, or dural defects).

CLINICAL PRESENTATION

In practice, patients present in one of two manners. The first is easier to recognize quickly but carries a worse prognosis. Approximately 25% of patients have a short clinical course of only a few hours and present with fever, mental status changes (irritability, lethargy, confusion) and the diagnosis is not elusive. The other 75% of patients with bacterial meningitis have a more insidious clinical presentation with simple fever and nonspecific symptoms that progress over 1, 2, or more days to cause signs and symptoms typical of meningitis.

SIGNS AND SYMPTOMS OF MENINGITIS

The most reliably present finding in bacterial meningitis is fever (98%) whereas complaints of headache, photophobia, or neck pain will not be heard until the child is verbal and can communicate these symptoms (around 2 years of age). Since bacterial meningitis is most common before this age, it is important to watch for other clues. Infants may initially present with irritability that is difficult for the parents to alleviate, poor feeding, sleepiness or lethargy, and possibly vomiting. Later in the illness a bulging fontanelle, nuchal rigidity, and coma may be seen.

For an older child, where neck pain can be more easily assessed, the neck pain seen with meningitis is worsened by neck flexion. The typical child can easily touch the chin to the chest without the need to open the mouth and reluctance to do so is worrisome. Patients with meningismus will often open the mouth in an attempt to reach the chest with less neck flexion. Flexion typically causes pain at the back of the neck and moving down to the upper mid-back area. It should be noted that ibuprofen and other analgesics may temporarily resolve the neck pain despite the presence of meningitis.

Seizures occur as part of the presentation in 15–30% of patients but will only rarely occur as simple (brief, nonfocal) seizures without other signs or symptoms worrisome for meningitis.[2] On the other hand, the risk of meningitis is increased significantly among febrile patients with convulsive status epilepticus (a seizure or series of seizures without recovery of consciousness between seizures lasting at least 30 minutes).[3] Therefore, if faced with a febrile patient with focal, prolonged, or recurrent seizures, or a febrile infant younger than 6 months with any type of seizure, a lumbar puncture for cerebrospinal fluid (CSF) examination should be strongly considered.

Bacterial meningitis should be considered a medical emergency and the usual attention to airway, breathing, and circulation should be applied as depressed mental status and associated septic shock may complicate management. The rapid institution of supportive measures and prompt administration of antibimicrobials is the goal.

DIFFERENTIAL DIAGNOSIS

Severe pharyngitis, parapharyngeal abscess or adenitis, musculoskeletal strain, upper lobe pneumonia, cervical spine osteomyelitis, epidural abscess, and subarachnoid hemorrhage may all produce meningismus. Depressed mental status may occur as a result of encephalitis, ingestions, mass lesions of the CNS, or simple febrile seizure.

The possibility of another primary focus for infection, which might also require specific therapy or follow-up, should be considered. This site may be distant (e.g., pyelonephritis, pleural empyema, osteomyelitis) but by causing bacteremia may have caused meningitis. In addition, a contiguous focus may also be the cause. Sinusitis, mastoiditis, osteomyelitis of the skull, or even a brain abscess may require additional intervention.

DIAGNOSIS

While the diagnosis is simple when patients come with classic symptoms of photophobia, nuchal rigidity, severe headache, or mental status changes, this is not generally the case at the initial evaluation. There is a continuum from a complete absence of clinical signs or symptoms at the time the first bacteria cross the blood–brain barrier to severe symptoms.

The point in that continuum of symptoms when the child is seen and the rate at which the disease is progressing will determine how difficult it will be for the clinician to recognize the child as having meningitis. It is for this reason that approximately half of all patients ultimately diagnosed with bacterial meningitis will visit a clinician during the course of their illness and be sent home from the encounter without meningitis being considered.[4]

The highest risk for meningitis during childhood is in the first month or two of life and at this age the clinical signs are few. Therefore, a lumbar puncture is generally warranted in the evaluation of the febrile infant younger than 2 months. After 2 months of age the diagnosis remains a challenge but more clinical cues are available to the clinician experienced in evaluating young children.

Children with prior antibiotic therapy during the illness can be more difficult to diagnose. Pretreated patients are less likely to have fever at examination, less likely to have altered mental status, and will have longer duration of symptoms at diagnosis.[5] Table 16–2

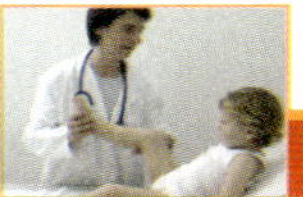

Table 16–2.

Pertinent History and Physical Examination

Important history of present illness

Fever, lethargy, irritability, headache, photophobia, neck pain or stiffness, mental status changes, focal neurologic deficits, seizures (especially focal, prolonged, recurrent)

Important past medical history

Immunocompromise, hemoglobinopathies, asplenia, chronic liver or renal disease, implanted hardware such as cochlear implants or ventriculoperitoneal shunt

Medications and allergies

Important elements of the physical examination

Assessment of airway, gag reflex, vital signs, and perfusion

Head including fontanel and head circumference

Eyes (include fundoscopic examination), ears, nose, and throat

Neck

Neurologic examination

Mental status: alertness, orientation

Skin examination for perfusion, petechiae, purpura

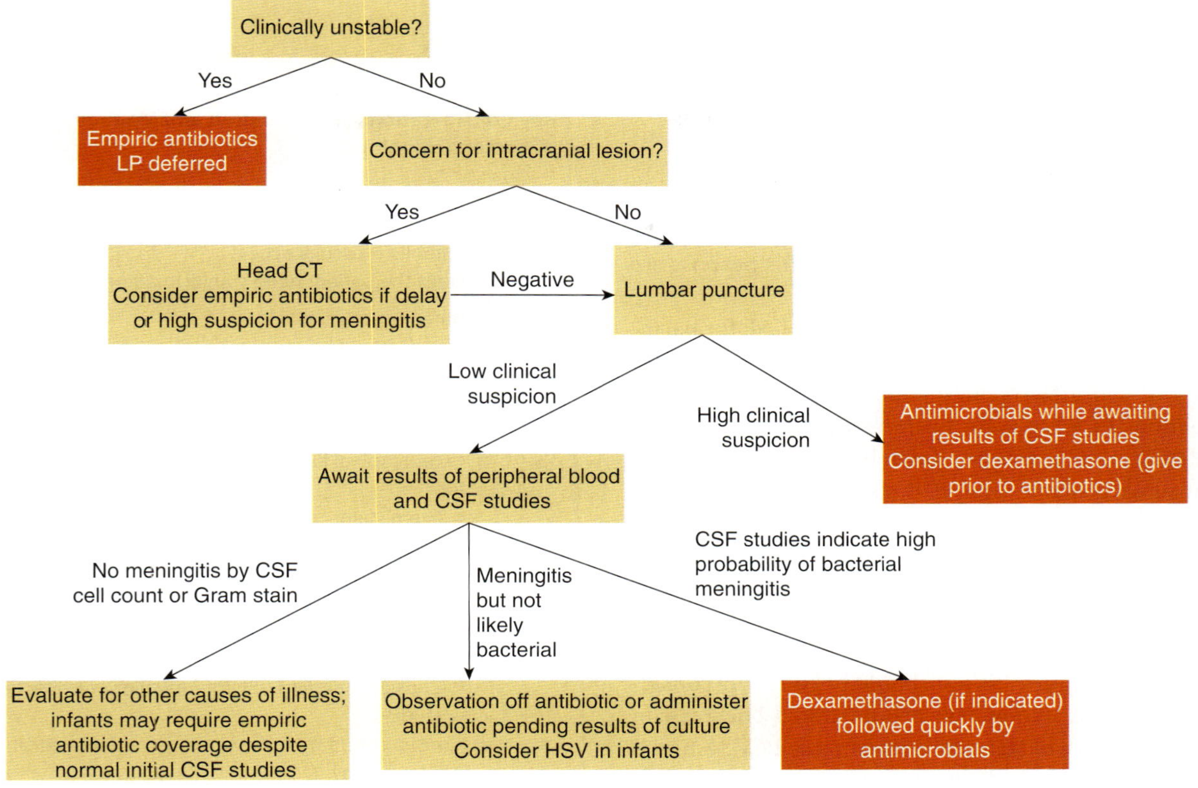

FIGURE 16–2 ■ Clinical approach to the patient with possible meningitis. (The decision to administer or delay administration of dexamethasone and empiric antimicrobials until after cranial imaging, lumbar puncture, or results of blood and CSF analysis will depend on the overall clinical appearance of the child and degree of suspicion for acute bacterial meningitis.)

summarizes the pertinent history and physical examination in the evaluation of patients suspected of having meningitis. Figure 16–2 is a flow diagram for the diagnostic approach for patients being evaluated for meningitis.

Cerebrospinal Fluid Studies

The CSF should be sent for cell count, glucose, protein, Gram stain, and bacterial culture. A CSF fungal culture should also be performed in premature infants and in children with other immunocompromising conditions. Most patients with bacterial meningitis will have an elevated CSF white blood count (WBC) count with 80% or more polymorphonuclear cells, the CSF glucose will be low in about 50% and the CSF protein concentration is generally elevated. The CSF culture is positive in about 80% of patients and the culture is positive within 24–48 hours unless antimicrobials were given prior to lumbar puncture.

For the infant under 1 month of age with CSF pleocytosis, no prediction rule can reliably exclude bacterial meningitis and these infants should be treated as possibly having bacterial meningitis until the results of CSF culture are known. Further, not even normal CSF parameters exclude bacterial meningitis as 10% of neonates with bacterial meningitis will not have a CSF pleocytosis[6–8] and a majority of very low birth weight (≤1.5 kg) neonates with bacterial meningitis have no CSF pleocytosis at diagnosis (by positive CSF culture).[6]

For older infants and children with CSF pleocytosis, a multicenter review of pediatric cases of bacterial meningitis clearly demonstrated that children older than 1 month with CSF pleocytosis (and no antibiotic pretreatment) can be considered at very low risk of bacterial meningitis if the Gram stain has no organisms, the CSF absolute neutrophil count is ≤1000 cells/mm^3, the CSF protein is ≤80 mg/dL, the peripheral blood absolute neutrophil count is ≤10,000 cells/mm^3, and there is no history of seizure before or at the time of presentation.[7] Nonetheless, even with these serially applied low-risk criteria, 2 of 121 children with bacterial meningitis had none of these risk factors for a sensitivity of 98% (95% confidence intervals: 94–100%). Both of these children were younger than 2 months of age.

Among patients beyond the first months of life, the serum procalcitonin (≥0.5 ng/mL), C-reactive protein (≥20 mg/L), CSF lactate, and the CSF glucose or CSF glucose to serum glucose ratio can all be helpful in distinguishing bacterial from nonbacterial causes of acute meningitis.[8–11] While not routinely available the CSF levels of interleukin 6 (IL-6) and tumor necrosis factor are also much higher in patients with bacterial versus aseptic meningitis.[12]

Patients with bacterial meningitis have a predominance of polymorphonuclear cells before treatment. Approximately half of patients with aseptic or demonstrated enteroviral meningitis will also have a CSF polymorphonuclear cell predominance. Symptom duration does reliably result in a change in the CSF white blood profile, so serial lumbar punctures for this purpose are not recommended.[13,14]

Latex agglutination studies of the CSF for bacterial antigens do not typically provide any benefit and are not routinely recommended.[15] Polymerase chain reaction (PCR) tests for bacteria are not readily available and have not shown much benefit beyond culture but some available viral PCR tests are faster and more sensitive than viral culture and should be considered for specific etiologies. Because enteroviruses are common causes of meningitis and enterovirus PCR tests are now readily available, it is suggested that if the turn around time for this test at your institution is usually ≤48 hours this test should be routinely considered. Previous studies have demonstrated a decrease in hospital length of stay when enterovirus PCR testing is routinely performed during enteroviral season.[16,17] Because it is slower than most routine bacterial culture or PCR tests, the routine use of viral culture is not recommended. Where herpes simplex meningoencephalitis is a possible concern a herpes simplex PCR should be sent.

A positive Gram stain or growth of a pathogen in CSF culture definitively identifies bacterial meningitis. Unfortunately the diagnosis is more difficult to establish or exclude in the patient who has received antibiotic treatment prior to obtaining CSF for examination and culture. Pretreated patients are less likely to have a positive CSF Gram stain or culture.[5]

While bacteria can be recovered in some circumstances for one or more days after initiation of antimicrobial therapy, the CSF is sterilized in 2 hours or less with meningococcal infections, in 4 to 12 hours with pneumococcal infections, and as early as 8 hours with group B streptococcal infections.[18] Table 16–3 includes suggested studies to be ordered in the evaluation of the patient with suspected meningitis.

It should be noted that it may not be possible to safely perform a lumbar puncture and the diagnosis will need to be a presumptive one in some patients. The lumbar puncture may need to be deferred if there are concerns of clinical instability, significantly elevated intracranial pressure (bradycardia, hypertension, irregular respirations, papilledema), or concern for intracranial lesion. The presence of thrombocytopenia (≤50,000 platelets/mm^3) should prompt consideration for platelet transfusion prior to lumbar puncture. The presence of skin infection in the area overlying lumbar puncture should also be considered a relative contraindication because of the concern for inoculating bacteria from the skin site to the CSF.

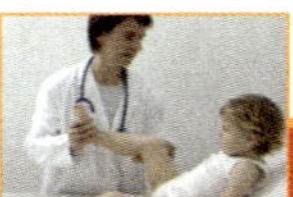

Table 16–3.

Key Considerations for Evaluation and Management of Bacterial Meningitis

Step 1: General assessment

a) Assess vital signs and perfusion
b) Establish vascular access
c) Does the patient need cranial imaging?

Step 2: Laboratory studies

a) Blood should be sent for complete cell count and culture
b) Consider blood for electrolytes, blood urea nitrogen, creatinine, and glucose
c) Cerebrospinal fluid should be obtained and sent for:
   - Gram stain
   - Bacterial culture
   - Cell count and differential
   - Glucose and protein
   - Consider sending CSF for viral studies, such as enteroviral and/or herpes simplex PCR
   - Consider sending CSF for fungal or mycobacterial studies
d) Consider sending Lyme serology based on local epidemiology

Step 3: Treat infection

a) Dexamethasone, if appropriate
b) Antimicrobials

Step 4: Subsequent management

a) Follow neurologic examination closely, especially cranial nerves
b) Daily weights and strict measurement of intake and output
c) Formal hearing evaluation
d) Consider long-term follow-up including neuropsychiatric testing

Other Studies

The decision to perform a lumbar puncture should not rest on the results of blood testing. Among infants, a very low or high peripheral WBC does increase the risk for bacterial meningitis but 41% will have peripheral WBC values in the normal range.[19] A negative peripheral blood culture does not rule out bacterial meningitis. Among patients with confirmed bacterial meningitis, no bacterial growth is seen in blood cultures in approximately one-third of cases.[13,14,18–20] Despite these limitations, blood should be routinely obtained for culture from patients evaluated for suspected meningitis. A positive blood culture will influence the choice of antimicrobial therapy in cases where the CSF does not yield growth of a pathogen. Serologic tests may be helpful and Lyme serology should be routinely ordered in the proper epidemiologic setting (e.g., areas where infection is common, opportunity for exposure).

Neuroimaging does not need to be routinely ordered but should be performed during the course of therapy when patients experience unexplained changes in mental status, focal neurologic deficits, or there is other reason for concern of intracranial abscess, empyema, hemorrhage, infarct, or thrombosis.

MANAGEMENT

Optimize supportive care to ensure adequate oxygen delivery including consideration of adequate cerebral perfusion pressure. Patients with septic shock will require appropriate resuscitation to maintain adequate oxygen and glucose delivery to the brain. In patients without the need for additional fluids to support the circulation, intravenous fluids should provide for "maintenance" needs but cautiously to avoid worsening the hyponatremia of the syndrome of inappropriate antidiuretic hormone secretion (SIADH) should it occur. Baseline and daily weight measurements and the evaluation of electrolytes may be helpful in monitoring for the development of SIADH.

When there is a high clinical suspicion for bacterial meningitis, the lumbar puncture should be performed as soon as it is clinically safe and feasible and the administration of antibiotic(s) should occur without awaiting the results of CSF studies or computed tomography (which itself is not routinely indicated unless there are focal signs or symptoms). Delays in antibiotic administration should be avoided and are associated with worsened outcome in adults.[21]

TREATMENT

Until an organism is isolated, patients should be treated with empiric antibiotic therapy that covers the range of potentially causative pathogens. Empiric antimicrobial coverage should rarely be narrowed based on the reading of the Gram stain alone as errors in interpretation are common. Conversely if the Gram stain suggests an organism not well covered by empiric therapy the coverage should be broadened awaiting the results of culture. It is important to consider *Listeria* as a potential pathogen since optimal therapy includes the use of ampicillin, which is no longer routinely included in many empiric treatment strategies.

The initial empiric antibiotic therapy for most children is listed in Table 16–4. Dosing recommendations for these antimicrobials are listed in Table 16–5. Once the specific etiologic agent causing the meningitis is known, the treatment can be focused on that organism. Recommendations by organism (and the organism antibiotic susceptibility) are listed in Table 16–6. Duration of antibiotic therapy varies depending on the causative organism, the time to CSF sterilization, the extent of CSF inflammation, and the patient's clinical response. In uncomplicated cases, parenteral antibiotic courses are typically 7 days for *N. meningitidis*, 7–10 days for *H. influenzae* type B, 10–14 days for *S. pneumoniae*, 14–21 days for group B streptococci, and 21 days for gram-negative organisms.

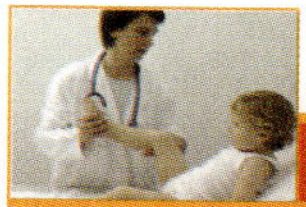

Table 16–4.

Initial Empiric Therapy of Suspected Bacterial Meningitis

Age	Common Bacterial Pathogens	Initial Empiric Therapy*
≤2 months	Group B streptococci, *E. coli* and other enterobacteriacae, *Strep. pneumoniae*, *L. monocytogenes*	Ampicillin plus cefotaxime† plus aminoglycoside
≥2 months	*N. meningitides, Strep. pneumoniae, H. influenzae* spp.	Dexamethasone‡ plus cefotaxime plus vancomycin

*Specific doses of antimicrobials vary by age and are generally higher than for other indications. Pathogens and empiric therapy will not necessarily be the same for premature infants, immunocompromised children and those post head trauma or surgery. Additional therapy will be guided by the result of CSF Gram stain and the result of blood and CSF culture.

†Meropenem may be substituted for cefotaxime in case of allergy or the need for more broad-spectrum gram-negative coverage. If gram-positive cocci are identified, the addition of vancomycin should be considered until Strep. pneumoniae and Staph. aureus have been excluded.

‡Dexamethasone should be considered if S. pneumoniae or H. influenzae type B are the suspected pathogens.

Vancomycin is a necessary component in the empiric treatment of patients with possible penicillin-resistant pneumococcus. However, one retrospective study has suggested that the use of vancomycin in the first 2 hours of treatment may be associated with an increased risk for hearing loss in pneumococcal meningitis.[22] Further corroboration is needed before changes in practice can be recommended but the priority should be to administer the dexamethasone and cefotaxime as quickly as is feasible and then administer vancomycin.

Corticosteroid Therapy

Dexamethasone when given 15 minutes prior or simultaneously with antibiotics appear to reduce mortality and sequelae among patients with *H. influenzae* type B meningitis.[23] Dexamethasone use in children with meningitis caused by *S. pneumoniae* is more controversial.[24] It is

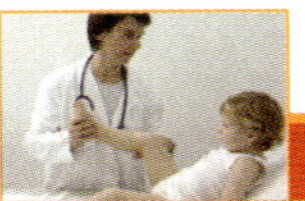

Table 16–5.

Drug Dosing by Age for Selected Medications

Medication	0–7 Days of Age*	8–28 Days of Age	Infants and Children	Adult Max. Dose
Aminoglycosides				
gentamicin	2 mg/kg/dose q12h	2 mg/kg/dose q8h	2.5 mg/kg/dose q8h	—
tobramycin	2 mg/kg/dose q12h	2 mg/kg/dose q8h	2.5 mg/kg/dose q8h	—
amikacin	10 mg/kg/dose q12h	7 mg/kg/dose q8h	7 mg/kg/dose q8h	—
Ampicillin	50 mg/kg/dose q8h	50 mg/kg/dose q6h	75 mg/kg/dose q6h	12 g/d
Cefotaxime†	50 mg/kg/dose q8h	50 mg/kg/dose q6h	50 mg/kg/dose q6h	12 g/d
Meropenem	40 mg/kg/dose q8h	40 mg/kg/dose q8h	40 mg/kg/dose q8h	6 g/d
Vancomycin	15 mg/kg/dose q12h	15 mg/kg/dose q8h	15 mg/kg/dose q6h	—

*Assumes gestational age ≥36 weeks

†Cefotaxime may be used at a dose of up to 300 mg/kg/d in pneumococcal infections

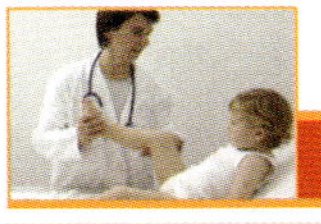

Table 16–6.

Treatment by Pathogen

Bacteria	Antibiotic(s) of Choice*
Group B streptococci	Ampicillin plus an aminoglycoside (during early therapy)
E. coli	Cefotaxime plus an aminoglycoside
L. monocytogenes	Ampicillin plus an aminoglycoside (during early therapy)
Strep. pneumoniae cefotaxime susceptible MIC ≤ 0.5 μg/mL	Cefotaxime
Strep. pneumoniae† penicillin nonsusceptible MIC ≥ 0.1 μg/mL and cefotaxime nonsusceptible MIC ≥ 1.0 μg/mL	Cefotaxime and vancomycin (also consider adding rifampin)
N. meningitidis Penicillin MIC ≤ 0.1 μg/mL	Penicillin G or ampicillin
N. meningitidis Penicillin MIC 0.1–1.0 μg/mL	Cefotaxime
H. influenzae	Cefotaxime

*Specific therapy will also be guided by clinical improvement and specific susceptibility testing performed on the bacteria recovered from the patient.

†Consultation with an infectious diseases specialist is recommended.

not known whether dexamethasone therapy has an effect on cognitive outcome. There is no demonstrated efficacy for the use of dexamethasone after antibiotics have been administered. There has been no demonstrated benefit to the use of steroids in meningococcal or neonatal meningitis.[25–27] The key steps in the evaluation and management are summarized in Table 16–3. Most authors reserve the use of dexamethasone to patients with clinical or laboratory findings highly suggestive of bacterial meningitis thought most likely to be associated with *H. influenzae* type B or *S. pneumoniae.* Dexamethasone is not routinely recommended for the child with suspected aseptic meningitis receiving antimicrobial therapy pending the results of bacterial culture. Dexamethasone has not been adequately studied or demonstrated beneficial in the treatment of neonates with bacterial meningitis.

Additional Considerations

A repeat lumbar puncture for a follow-up cerebrospinal fluid culture is not routinely recommended but should be considered when patients fail to improve within the first 24–48 hours or when the identified pathogen can be anticipated to be difficult to eliminate with conventional antibiotic therapy based on susceptibility testing or prior experience (e.g., nosocomial gram-negative infections, resistant pneumococcus).

Consultation with an infectious diseases specialist is recommended for most cases of gram-negative meningitis, fungal meningitis, meningitis in a patient with reduced immunity or indwelling intracranial hardware, and in the treatment of organisms with reduced susceptibility to antibiotics.

Meropenem is preferred to a third-generation cephalosporin for the treatment of specific gram-negative infections caused by organisms, such as *Citrobacter*-, *Enterobacter*-, or *Serratia*-related cases which may possess the ability to express extended spectrum beta-lactamases (ESBL) that may be induced by cephalosporin therapy.

COURSE AND PROGNOSIS

The mortality is associated with many factors but overall is about 5% for *H. influenzae* and meningococcal meningitis and in the vicinity of 20% for pneumococcal and *Listeria* meningitis in developed countries. The most common complications are listed in Table 16–7.

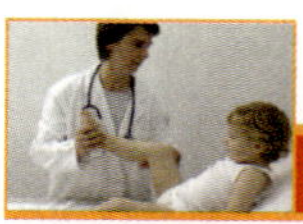

Table 16–7.

Potential Complications of Meningitis

Short-term complications
Septic shock
SIADH (syndrome of inappropriate antidiuretic hormone secretion)
Seizures
Brain infarction
Cerebral edema
Intracranial abscess
Intracranial venous thrombosis (e.g., cavernous venous thrombosis)
Intracranial hemorrhage
Cranial nerve palsies
 Most notably hearing loss

Long-term complications
Seizures
Cranial nerve palsies (including hearing loss)
Focal cerebral deficits (e.g., hemiparesis)
Cognitive impairment

The risks for mortality and sequelae are related to the severity of disease. Not surprisingly, mortality (approximately 30%) and the rate of sequelae among survivors (approximately 70%) are very high among patients requiring mechanical ventilation during therapy of acute bacterial meningitis and are highly correlated with severity of illness at admission.[28] Mortality also increases if there is a significant neurologic event during the acute phase of the illness. These may be caused by general cerebral edema, hypoperfusion, loss of microcirculatory control, and vascular thromboses, which cause secondary effects such as herniation and infarction.

The time course of presentation is also associated with severity of disease. Children who present and are diagnosed as having bacterial meningitis within the first 24 hours of illness are much more likely to have severe disease than those with a more insidious presentation that may develop over 2 days or more before diagnosis.[29]

Subdural effusions are commonly noted during the first week of therapy for bacterial meningitis of infants (approximately 30%) but do not typically require intervention.[30] Subdural empyema is a rare but important complication of meningitis which can usually be distinguished from effusion with diagnostic imaging.[31]

Monitoring of urine output, daily weights, and serum electrolytes is prudent in the early phase in order to quickly identify hyponatremia and manage patients developing the SIADH secretion. Less common complications include acute spinal cord dysfunction—myelitis.

Long-Term Sequelae

Hearing loss occurs in a large proportion (10–30% depending on the pathogen) of children and is associated with severity of infection (lower CSF glucose levels, raised intracranial pressure, nuchal rigidity, *Strep. pneumoniae* as the causative agent) with profound hearing loss in 5%.[32] Hearing loss, when it occurs, will be noted to some degree with the earliest testing.[33] While many children will experience some improvement in hearing over time, others may have further progression of hearing loss over months to years.[34] After bacterial meningitis, children are more likely to have cognitive impairments, such as poor linguistic and executive functions, and behavioral problems than their peers.[35] As a result, even after apparent complete recovery from bacterial meningitis, children benefit from formal neuropsychiatric evaluation in addition to routine tests of hearing as the findings may be subtle. Three percent to 5% of children will have seizures, mental retardation, and/or some degree of spasticity or paresis.[32]

Special Circumstances

Patients with immunocompromise, intracranial implants including cochlear implants, ventriculoperitoneal shunts, and infants in the intensive care setting are at increased risk of meningitis, including meningitis caused by bacteria or fungi not typical of other children. Therefore, they should be considered separately with regard to primary prevention and optimal initial empiric therapy.

Citrobacter meningitis in the neonate, and *Citrobacter koseri* in particular, is associated with a very high rate of mortality (30%) and sequelae (75%) and is the most common cause of neonatal abscess (Figure 16–3). Infants with *Citrobacter* meningitis should have brain imaging during the course of therapy to evaluate for this complication.

Meningitis with cranial nerve palsies, appropriate local epidemiology, or protracted symptoms, should raise suspicion for Lyme disease, and depending on the cranial nerves involved, a basilar meningitis as can be seen with tuberculous or some fungal meningitis should be considered.[36] Causes of chronic meningitis are also quite varied but pathogens such as *Brucella*, Lyme, syphilis, cryptococci, and other fungi may cause a more indolent and chronic meningitis. Noninfectious causes include malignancies, sarcoid, and autoimmune disease.

Discussion of eosinophilic meningitis ($\geq$10 eosinophils/mm^3 of CSF) is beyond the scope of this chapter but may be seen in relation to indwelling foreign body, certain parasitic diseases, malignancies, in response to medications, and with coccidioidal meningitis.

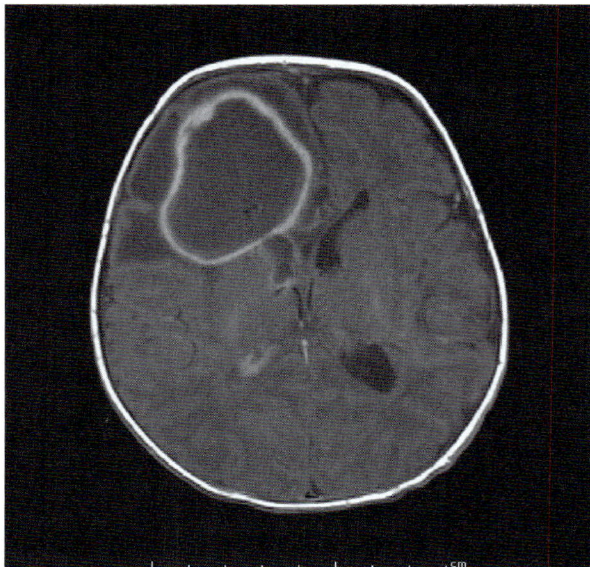

FIGURE 16–3 ■ Brain abscess complicating *Citrobacter koseri* meningitis in a 7-week-old female (T1-weighted MRI postgadolinium image).

PREVENTION

Chemoprophylaxis is recommended for close contacts of patients with disease caused by *N. meningitides* or *H. influenzae* type B. Active immunization against *H. influenzae* type B and *Strep. pneumoniae* is now part of routine childhood vaccination schedules and immunization for *N. meningitidis* is typically required prior to college entry in the United States.

Intrapartum ampicillin administered to women at high risk of transmitting group B streptococci to their infants is effective in reducing the risk of early onset but not late-onset group B streptococcal disease. Women with penicillin allergy can receive clindamycin, erythromycin, or in the absence of immediate-type hypersensitivity, a first-generation cephalosporin. Up to 20% of pregnant women require intrapartum antibiotic prophylaxis. Recurrent group B streptococcal infections occur; most of the isolates from recurrent infections are identical to the isolates from the initial infection. Recurrent infection likely occurs as a consequence of persistent mucosal group B streptococcal colonization. Attempts to eradicate mucosal colonization with oral rifampin have met with varied success. Consultation with a pediatric infectious diseases or immunology specialist should be considered in infants with recurrent group B streptococcal infections.

REFERENCES

1. Scheld WM, et al. Pathophysiology of bacterial meningitis: mechanism(s) of neuronal injury. *J Infect Dis.* 2002;186(suppl 2):S225-S233.
2. Green SM, et al. Can seizures be the sole manifestation of meningitis in febrile children? *Pediatrics.* 1993;92(4): 527-534.
3. Chin RFM, Neville BGR, Scott RC. Meningitis is a common cause of convulsive status epilepticus with fever. *Arch Dis Child.* 2005;90(1):66-69.
4. Bonsu BK, Harper MB. Fever interval before diagnosis, prior antibiotic treatment, and clinical outcome for young children with bacterial meningitis. *Clin Infect Dis.* 2001;32(4):566-572.
5. Rothrock SG, et al. Pediatric bacterial meningitis: is prior antibiotic therapy associated with an altered clinical presentation? *Ann Emerg Med.* 1992;21(2):146-152.
6. Doctor BA, et al. Clinical outcomes of neonatal meningitis in very-low birth-weight infants. *Clin Pediatr.* 2001;40(9):473-480.
7. Nigrovic LE, et al. Clinical prediction rule for identifying children with cerebrospinal fluid pleocytosis at very low risk of bacterial meningitis. *JAMA.* 2007;297(1):52-60.
8. Sormunen P, et al. C-reactive protein is useful in distinguishing Gram stain-negative bacterial meningitis from viral meningitis in children. *J Pediatr.* 1999;134(6):725-729.
9. Lembo RM, Marchant CD. Acute phase reactants and risk of bacterial meningitis among febrile infants and children. *Ann Emerg Med.* 1991;20(1):36-40.
10. Schwarz S, et al. Serum procalcitonin levels in bacterial and abacterial meningitis. *Crit Care Med.* 2000;28(6): 1828-1832.
11. Dubos F, et al. Serum procalcitonin and other biologic markers to distinguish between bacterial and aseptic meningitis. *J Pediatr.* 2006;149(1):72-76.
12. Dulkerian SJ, et al. Cytokine elevations in infants with bacterial and aseptic meningitis. *J Pediatr.* 1995;126(6): 872-876.
13. Wiswell TE, et al. No lumbar puncture in the evaluation for early neonatal sepsis: will meningitis be missed? *Pediatrics.* 1995;95(6):803-806.
14. Stoll BJ, et al. To tap or not to tap: high likelihood of meningitis without sepsis among very low birth weight infants. *Pediatrics.* 2004;113(5):1181-1186.
15. Nigrovic LE, et al. Cerebrospinal latex agglutination fails to contribute to the microbiologic diagnosis of pretreated children with meningitis. *Pediatr Infect Dis J.* 2004; 23(8):786-788.
16. Ramers C, et al. Impact of a diagnostic cerebrospinal fluid enterovirus polymerase chain reaction test on patient management. *JAMA.* 2000;283(20):2680-2685.
17. King RL, Lorch SA, Cohen DM, et al. Routine cerebrospinal fluid enterovirus polymerase chain reaction testing reduces hospitalization and antibiotic use for infants 90 days of age or younger. *Pediatrics* 2007;120(3):489-496.
18. Kanegaye JT, Soliemanzadeh P, Bradley JS. Lumbar puncture in pediatric bacterial meningitis: defining the time interval for recovery of cerebrospinal fluid pathogens after parenteral antibiotic pretreatment. *Pediatrics.* 2001; 108(5):1169-1174.
19. Bonsu BK, Harper MB. Utility of the peripheral blood white blood cell count for identifying sick young infants who need lumbar puncture. *Ann Emerg Med.* 2003;41(2): 206-214.
20. Garges HP, Moody MA, Cotten CM, et al. Neonatal meningitis: what is the correlation among cerebrospinal

fluid cultures, blood cultures, and cerebrospinal fluid parameters? *Pediatrics.* 2006; 117(4):1094-1100.

21. Aronin SI, Peduzzi P, Quagliarello VJ. Community-acquired bacterial meningitis: risk stratification for adverse clinical outcome and effect of antibiotic timing. *Ann Intern Med.* 1998;129(11):862-869.
22. Buckingham SC, et al. Early vancomycin therapy and adverse outcomes in children with pneumococcal meningitis. *Pediatrics.* 2006;117(5):1688-1694.
23. van de Beek D, et al. Corticosteroids for acute bacterial meningitis. *Cochrane Database Syst Rev.* 2007(1): CD004405.
24. Mongelluzzo J, Mohamad Z, Ten Have TR, et al. Corticosteroids and mortality in children with bacterial Meningitis. *JAMA.* 2008;299(17):2048-2055.
25. Chaudhuri A. Adjunctive dexamethasone treatment in acute bacterial meningitis. *Lancet Neurol.* 2004;3(1):54-62.
26. McIntyre PB, et al. A population based study of the impact of corticosteroid therapy and delayed diagnosis on the outcome of childhood pneumococcal meningitis. *Arch Dis Child.* 2005;90(4):391-396.
27. Grandgirard D, Leib SL. Strategies to prevent neuronal damage in paediatric bacterial meningitis. *Curr Opin Pediatr.* 2006;18(2):112-118.
28. Madagame ET, et al. Survival and functional outcome of children requiring mechanical ventilation during therapy for acute bacterial meningitis. *Crit Care Med.* 1995;23 (7):1279-1283.
29. Kilpi T, et al. Severity of childhood bacterial meningitis and duration of illness before diagnosis. *Lancet.* 1991;338(8764):406-409.
30. Snedeker JD, et al. Subdural effusion and its relationship with neurologic sequelae of bacterial meningitis in infancy: a prospective study. *Pediatrics.* 1990;86(2):163-170.
31. Chen CY, et al. Subdural empyema in 10 infants: US characteristics and clinical correlates. *Radiology.* 1998; 207(3):609-617.
32. Baraff LJ, Lee SI, Schriger DL. Outcomes of bacterial meningitis in children: a meta-analysis. *Pediatr Infect Dis J.* 1993;12(5):389-394.
33. Richardson MP, et al. Hearing loss during bacterial meningitis. *Arch Dis Child.* 1997;76(2):134-138.
34. Woolley AL, et al. Risk factors for hearing loss from meningitis in children: the Children's Hospital experience. *Arch Otolaryngol Head Neck Surg.* 1999;125(5):509-514.
35. Halket S, et al. Long term follow up after meningitis in infancy: behaviour of teenagers. *Arch Dis Child.* 2003;88(5):395-398.
36. Avery RA, et al. Prediction of Lyme meningitis in children from a Lyme disease-endemic region: a logistic-regression model using history, physical, and laboratory findings. *Pediatrics.* 2006;117(1):e1-e7.

CHAPTER 17

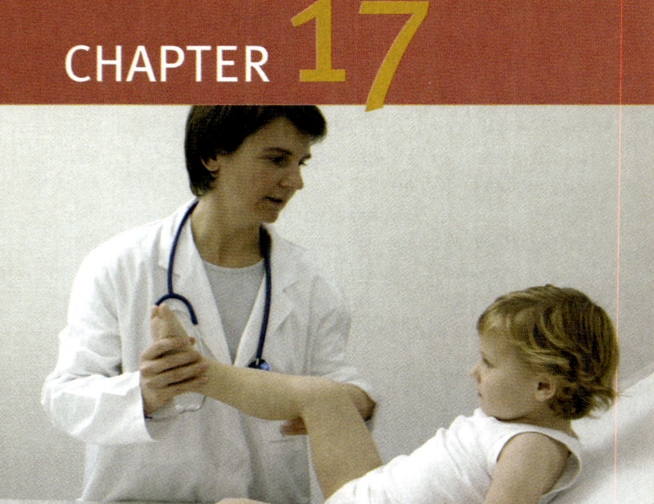

Encephalitis

Cynthia J. Campen, Sarah M. Kranick, and Daniel J. Licht

VIRAL ENCEPHALITIS

Encephalitis causes significant morbidity and mortality and raises difficult diagnostic and management challenges. The etiology is often illusive and, given the lack of literature on the subject, there is little information physicians can offer in the way of prognosis or etiology-specific treatment. This chapter defines encephalitis and describes its major causes with emphasis on the presentation, pathology, and management of viral encephalitis in pediatric populations.

DEFINITIONS AND EPIDEMIOLOGY

Encephalitis is defined as inflammation of the brain tissue, infectious or otherwise, causing alterations in cerebral function. The patient with encephalitis often presents with fever, headache, altered mental status, behavioral changes, focal neurological signs, and seizures. Meningoencephalitis describes the clinical entity in which the inflammation extends to the subarachnoid spaces and meninges. When the spinal cord is involved in the inflammatory process, the term encephalomyelitis is used. Noninfectious encephalitis is an antibody-mediated inflammation of the brain parenchyma, which may be triggered by immune response to a viral illness or tumor.

Estimating the true incidence of encephalitis is difficult, as most cases are not reported to local health departments. The most accurate estimates are those concerning the subset of arthropod-borne viral, or arboviral, encephalitides attributed to tracking efforts at the Center for Disease Control and Prevention (CDC), which estimates between 250 and 3000 cases occurring annually.[1] The California Encephalitis Project documented all hospitalized cases of encephalitis in California from 1991 to 1999 and found 35–50 cases per 100,000 people annually. Encephalitis occurred in the highest numbers in infants, followed by the elderly. A specific cause was reported in approximately 45% of 13,939 cases; HSV accounted for 14% of all cases, while arboviral disease was identified in less than 1% of the cases (West Nile Virus had not yet become established in California).[2]

PATHOPHYSIOLOGY

Because of the protection of the blood–brain barrier (BBB), the lack of a lymphatic system, and the absence of major histocompatibility complexes (antigen presenting cells), the brain was historically considered an immunologically isolated organ without the same vulnerabilities to infectious agents or immune responses as other body systems. It is increasingly apparent that the BBB is a far more dynamic entity than previously thought.

The BBB is made of capillary endothelial cells, astrocytes and pericytes with unique properties not seen in other organ systems. These anatomic differences include narrow tight junctions, lack of fenestrations, decreased transport, and a continuous basement membrane. Electrically, the surfaces of these cells are negatively charged, and therefore, repel proteins and other negatively charged molecules. Specific areas within the central nervous system (CNS) differ in their levels of BBB permeability. For example, the choroid plexus endothelium has fenestrations, allowing free entry of immune cells to the cerebrospinal fluid (CSF). The ependymal lining of the ventricles lacks tight junctions, which permits drainage of CNS antigens into the CSF.

In a study of foreign tissue graft survival in the brain parenchyma, Medawar demonstrated decreased cytotoxic T-cell response in the CNS compared with non-CNS sites.[3] Researchers have subsequently discovered that peripheral T-cell activation incites the BBB to allow lymphocyte entry to the CNS.[4–6] Immune activation releases systemic inflammatory modulators, such as nitric oxide and TNF, promoting leakiness of the BBB and leading to migration of activated macrophages and immature dendritic cells into the CNS.[7] These cells then act as antigen presenting cells for cytotoxic T cells.[8] Activated T cells infiltrate the BBB, release cytokines and chemokines, inducing the production of oxidative free radicals, excitatory neurotransmitters, and nitric oxide, culminating in an inflammatory response within the CNS. These inflammatory modulators were thought to cause neurotoxicity and, ultimately, lead to cell death.

In addition to this mechanism of defense, researchers have found an independent complement of immune cells in the CNS that act as neuroinflammatory markers, thereby defending the brain parenchyma, but also inducing injury. More recently, evidence suggests that these immune cells may offer neuroprotection as well.[9] Microglia, the resident macrophages of the CNS, are a component of this CNS immnune defense and were traditionally thought to propagate the inflammatory immune response and to phagocytize cellular debris.[10] They facilitate both the innate and adaptive immune response by upregulating the production of cytokines (IFN-γ, TNF, LPS).[10] They also act as antigen presenting cells, leading to neurotoxicity and the inflammatory response.[8,10] However, studies have shown that microglial antigen presentation can initiate immunosuppressive T cells and neuroprotective T-cell responses. T cells activated by microglia produce high levels of IL-10, which has anti-inflammatory effects.[11] IL-10 has been shown to suppress cytokines and chemokines in the setting of HSV-1 encephalitis.[12] Additional work indicates a trend toward microglial neuroprotection and modulation of the inflammatory response.[13] There is clearly a complex interplay between inflammatory markers recruiting cells to facilitate the clearance of bacterial or viral agents, and neuroprotective efforts, aimed at containing the damage these cells inflict.

DIAGNOSIS

The definitive diagnosis of encephalitis requires brain tissue, which yields a diagnosis by microscopic evaluation for inclusion bodies, isolation of the causative agent from brain tissue cultures, or detection of the infectious agent by in situ polymerase chain reaction (PCR). Detection of a serologic response or identification of the infectious agent in the CSF or other body fluids allows a presumptive diagnosis. The California Encephalitis Project reported a definitive diagnosis (brain tissue diagnosis) in 30% of cases, while a presumed diagnosis (serum, urine, or stool) was found in 12%.[14] Other sources report diagnostic rates of 50%.[15]

While isolating virus from CSF and other body fluid cultures is also helpful for definitive diagnosis, the process is cumbersome and prone to contamination. PCR testing, which detects tiny portions of the DNA in the CSF, allows diagnoses to be made more quickly and reliably. Detecting antibodies for serologic testing is limited by even small doses of immunoglobulin therapy, and because it often requires both infected samples and convalescent samples may take weeks to confirm.

Neuroimaging

All viruses affecting the CNS produce similar pathological features including inflammation and neuronal death. Thus, most viral CNS infections appear on neuroimaging as an increase in water content of the affected tissue. On CT scan, this increased water content is manifest as patchy hypodensities, and on MRI as hypointense signal on T1 and hyperintense signal on T2 and FLAIR (fluid-attenuated inversion recovery).

When imaged early in its course, viral encephalitis may first appear on MRI as restricted diffusion on diffusion-weighted imaging (DWI) (Figure 17–1). Thus, acute DWI changes may be more sensitive to abnormalities than conventional T1 or T2 imaging sequences[16–18] in early imaging. Later in the disease process, MRI often shows confluent areas of T2 hyperintensities involving white and gray matter, which may exert a variable amount of mass effect. When present, these hyperintensities enhance diffusely with gadolinium. While these findings fail to differentiate viral infections from one another, the asymmetry and the involvement of both white and gray matter structures help to differentiate viral encephalitis from primary metabolic/toxic disorders or parainfectious disorders, such as acute disseminated encephalomyelitis (ADEM) (Figure 17–2).

Though these general features apply to most viral encephalitides, certain infections show characteristic tropisms that are helpful in the differential diagnosis. Herpes simplex virus (HSV) encephalitis has been associated with hemorrhagic inflammation, frequently bilateral, of the medial temporal lobe, sylvian fissure and orbital-frontal cortex (Figure 17–3).

In neonates, the areas of inflammation are seldom as well defined as in older children or adults, and manifest as loss of distinction of the gray–white interface on T2-weighted imaging. Echo gradient imaging reveals a hemorrhagic component corresponding to

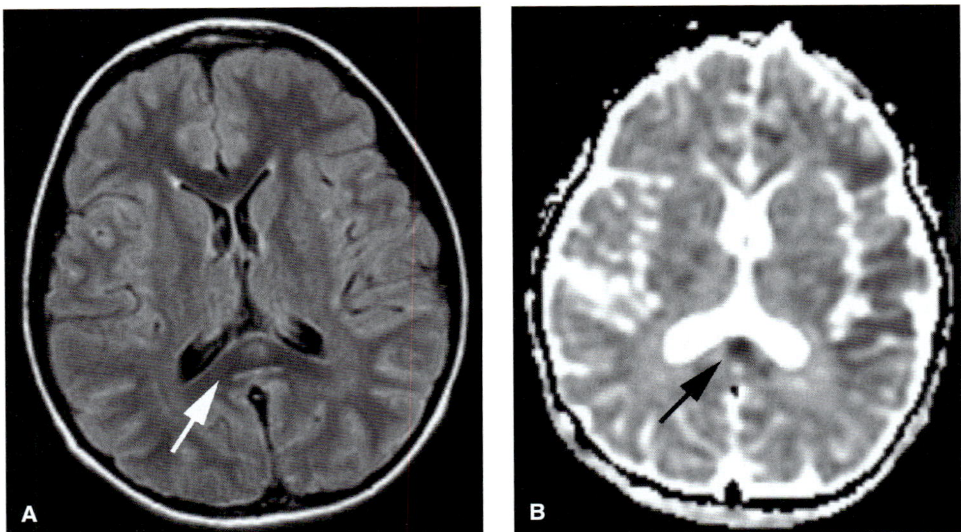

FIGURE 17–1 ■ MRI of viral encephalitis in a 7-year-old male presenting with sudden onset status epilepticus. **(A)** Hyperintensity in the splenium of the corpus callosum (white arrow) on axial FLAIR MRI. **(B)** Restriction of water diffusion demonstrated on apparent diffusion coefficient maps of the DWI examination.

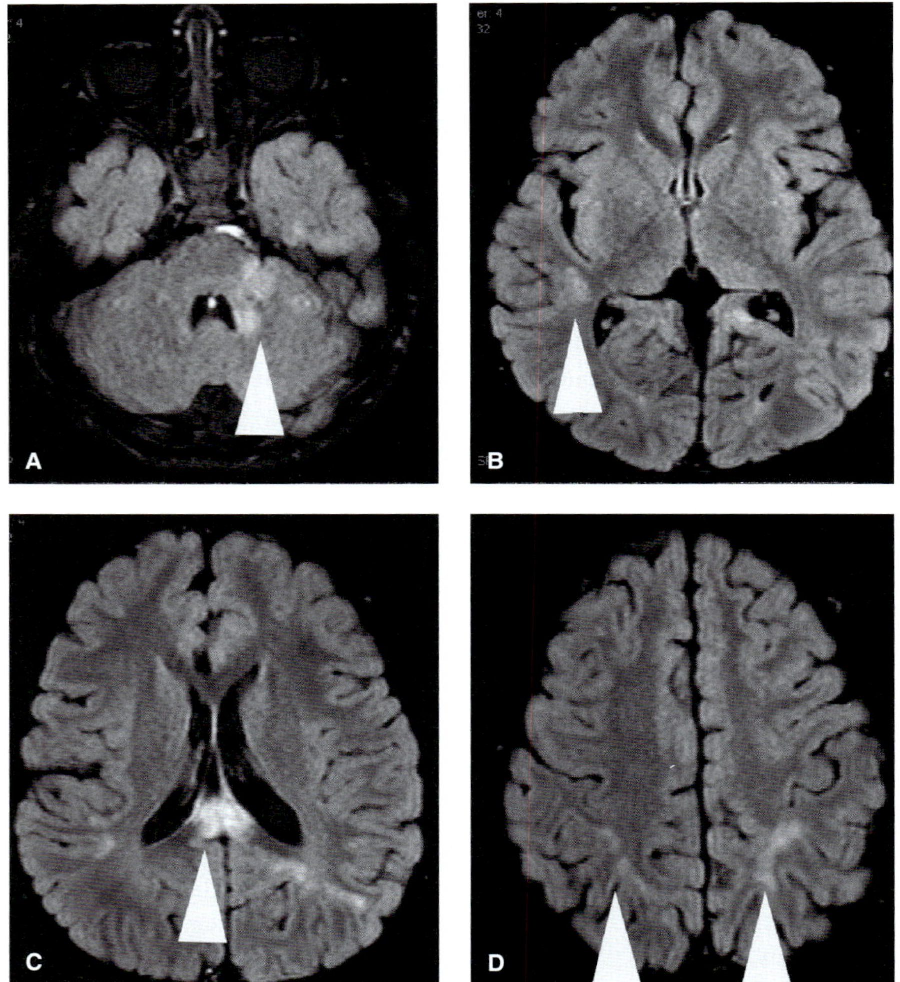

FIGURE 17–2 ■ ADEM in a 9-year-old male presenting with lethargy, irritability, and left hemiataxia. **(A)** Inflammatory lesion in the left cerebellar peduncle. **(B)** Subcortical inflammatory white matter lesion in the right temporal lobe. **(C)** Prominent lesion in the splenium of the corpus callosum. **(D)** Multiple bilateral subcortical inflammatory white matter lesions.

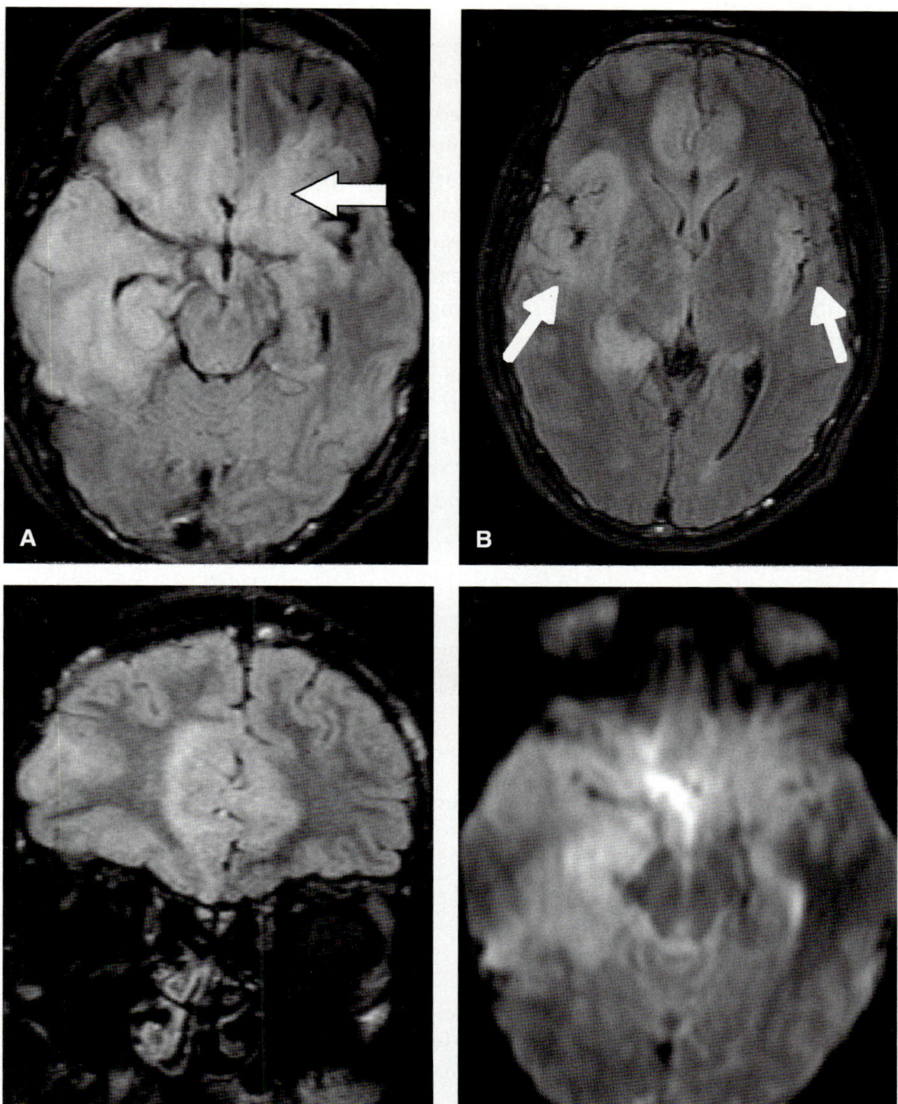

FIGURE 17–3 ■ A 14-year-old male presenting with coma and status epilepticus, diagnosed with HSV encephalitis. **(A)** Axial flair demonstrating medial temporal (hippocampus) and orbitofrontal (arrow) involvement. **(B)** Axial flair demonstrating bilateral sylvian fissure (arrows) involvement. **(C)** Coronal flair demonstrating orbitofrontal and interhemispheric involvement. **(D)** DWI (b = 1000) demonstrating infarction (cytotoxic edema) of the right temporal lobe.

infarction on DWI in the acute phase of the disease (5–7 days from insult).

Varicella-zoster virus (VZV) is an infrequent cause of encephalitis, but must be considered as a possible cause in those patients at risk either from immunocompromise or from direct inoculation via lumbar puncture. VZV is a common pathogen in other CNS infections such as transverse myelitis and cerebellitis and has been associated with transient arteriopathy of childhood and stroke.[19,20]

Other Diagnostic Testing

Electroencephalogram (EEG) must be considered early in the evaluation of patients with viral encephalitis, as subclinical seizures are a trea table cause of altered mental status. EEG may also disclose other nonspecific abnormalities including focal slowing or focal epileptiform discharges. Acute destructive lesions can produce periodic lateralized epileptiform discharges, usually in temporal leads. Periodic lateralized epileptiform discharges are considered nonspecific but are highly suggestive of HSV encephalitis.[21]

CSF profiles in encephalitis typically show mildly elevated WBC counts, with a lymphocytic predominance and, later in the course, mildly elevated protein. Elevated RBC counts and xanthochromia reflect the necrotizing nature of HSV infection, however, early in the disease CSF findings can be normal. PCR is the most common method used for CSF analysis, although PCR specificity may be as low as 94% with 98% sensitivity[22] between 72 hours and 2 weeks of symptom onset. For this reason, patients may require repeat testing.

DIFFERENTIAL DIAGNOSIS

The etiology of infectious viral encephalitis has changed significantly with the advent of widespread immunizations (Tables 17–1 and 17–2). The most common causes of viral encephalitis 30 years ago were measles, mumps, rubella and varicella, which now rarely cause neurological disease. HSV is thought to be the most common diagnosable and treatable cause of viral encephalitis in both the United States and United Kingdom, with arboviruses, varicella-zoster virus, Epstein-Barr virus (EBV), mumps, measles and enteroviruses following in prevalence. A Finnish study published in 2001 found VZV to be the most common cause of diagnosed viral encephalitis, meningitis and myelitis (29% of all confirmed agents), with HSV, enteroviruses and influenza A making up the majority of other confirmed etiological agents.[23] Even within this population, however, an etiologic agent was not identified in 60% of cases. In U.S. National Hospital Discharge Data, the pathogenic species was found in only 40% of cases.[24] According to the California Encephalitis Project, up to 70% of cases of encephalitis remain idiopathic.[2]

Postinfectious encephalitis, or ADEM is the most common white matter disease in children[25] and is usually

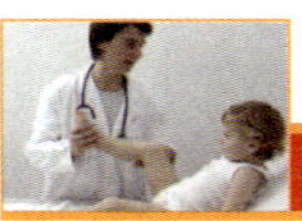

Table 17–1.

Viral Encephalitides

Double-stranded DNA viruses	Adenovirus Cytomegalovirus Epstein–Barr virus Hepatitis B Herpes simplex virus 1 and 2 Human herpesvirus 6 and 7 Varicella-zoster
Single-stranded DNA virus	Parvovirus
Arboviruses (single-stranded RNA viruses)	California (La Crosse) virus Eastern equine virus St. Louis encephalitis West Nile virus Western equine virus Powassan Colorado tick fever Venezuelan equine
Enterovirus (single-stranded RNA viruses)	Poliovirus Coxsackie Echovirus
Other RNA viruses	Hepatitis A Influenza Parainfluenza Respiratory syncytial virus Rotavirus
Paramyxovirus	Hendra Measles Mumps Nipah
Transmitted via mammals	Rabies Equine morbillivirus (Hendra) Nipah Lymphocytic choriomeningitis Encephalomyocarditis Vesicular stomatitis

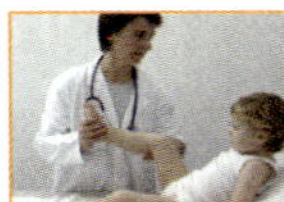

Table 17–2.

Nonviral Causes of Encephalitis

Bacterial	*Actinomyces* *Bartonella henselae* Brucellosis *Haemophilus influenzae* *Legionella* *Mycobacterium tuberculosis* *Mycoplasma pneumoniae* *Neisseria meningitidis* *Nocardia actinomyces* *Salmonella typhi* *Streptococcus pneumoniae*
Spirochetal infections:	*Treponema pallidum* *Leptospira* *Borrelia burgdorferi* *Tropheryma whippeli*
Rickettsial	Ehrlichiosis *Rickettsia rickettsii* *Rickettsia prowazeki* *Rickettsia typhi* *Coxiella burnetii* (*Q fever*)
Fungal	Aspergillosis *Candidiasis* *Coccidioides immitis* *Cryptococcus neoformans*
Parasitic	*Acanthamoeba* spp. *Balamuthia mandrillaris* Human African trypanosomiasis *Naegleria* spp. *Plasmodium* spp. Schistosomiasis *Strongyloides stercoralis* *Toxoplasma gondii* *Trypanosoma* spp. *Trichinella spiralis*
Postimmunization encephalitis	Smallpox vaccine Typhoid-paratyphoid vaccine Influenza vaccine Measles vaccine
Other	*Chlamydia psittaci* *Chlamydophila pneumoniae**

**Formerly Chlamydia pneumoniae.*

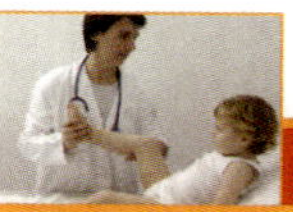

Table 17–3.

ADEM Versus Viral Encephalitis

	ADEM	Encephalitis
Age	Children ≥ Adults	Any
Recent vaccine	+++	−
Prodromal illness	+++	+
Fever	+/−	+++
Visual symptoms	+/−	−
Spinal cord/cerebellum involvement	+/−	+/−
CSF	Lymphocytic pleocytosis +/− Elevated protein Normal glucose Negative cultures + Elevated oligoclonal bands and myelin basic protein	Lymphocytic pleocytosis Elevated protein +/− Normal glucose +/− Negative cultures − Oligoclonal bands − Myelin basic protein
Serum	+/− Leucocytosis	+++ Leucocytosis
MRI	Multiple areas of white matter hyperintensity Often bilateral Often in deep brain structures (basal ganglia, brainstem, cerebellum, spinal cord) and optic nerves.	Focal areas (1 or 2) of white or gray matter Unilateral/bilateral Usually cortical

−, not present; +, present; +/−, Not consistent present; +++, consistently present.

seen days to weeks after mild viral illness or immunizations. The presumed cause of ADEM is thought to be antibodies to the offending virus cross-reacting with myelin surface proteins. The inflammation results in widespread monophasic demyelination, with a full recovery expected in the majority of pediatric cases. ADEM differs from viral encephalitis in the location of lesions on imaging: ADEM has a predilection for the cerebellum and optic nerve, which is unusual for encephalitis. Spinal cord inflammation may be noted in both, but is more frequent in ADEM than in viral encephalomyelitis. Clinical progression to coma occurs more rapidly and more commonly in ADEM than in viral encephalitis.[21]

CSF profiles in ADEM and viral encephalitis are similar and typically show elevated WBC counts with a lymphocytic predominance. To distinguish the two entities a thorough history of prodromal illnesses must be combined with MRI findings as well as negative CSF, blood, nasopharyngeal swab, urine serology and cultures (Table 17–3). ADEM is treated with immunomodulation using high-dose intravenous glucocorticoids or pooled intravenous immune globulin. The precise mechanism of action of these latter therapies is unknown.

Paraneoplastic encephalitis typically involves the limbic area with a fulminant and progressive course. The pathophysiology is thought to involve antibodies formed against a neoplasm that cross-react to brain tissue antigens. Thus paraneoplastic disorders can be diagnosed by identifying pathologic antibodies in the CSF. Paraneoplastic disorders are rare in children, but should be considered in the differential diagnosis as they can resemble HSV encephalitis. Opsoclonus-myoclonus or the "syndrome of dancing eyes and dancing feet" is perhaps the most common paraneoplastic disorder and is associated with neuroblastoma, which is invariably low grade. Opsoclonus refers to unusual and exaggerated eye movements that can be elicited on visual tracking. Myoclonus is rapid, jerky involuntary movements of the limbs or trunk.

CLINICAL PRESENTATION AND MANAGEMENT

Because the etiologic agent remains unknown in most cases of encephalitis, management is limited to symptomatic treatment. Tests to consider in the initial evaluation of the child with encephalitis are summarized in Table 17–4 while key clinical features of viral encephalitides are summarized in Table 17–5. Even for diagnosable entities, very few treatment options exist. HSV and VZV should be treated with acyclovir while cytomegalovirus (CMV) can be treated with ganciclovir (Table 17–6). In immunocompromised patients, aggressive treatment with antibiotics and antivirals is important until treatable causes of encephalitis/meningitis are ruled out.

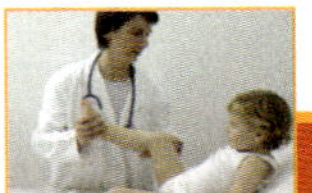

Table 17–4.

Laboratory Diagnosis of Viral Encephalitides

Virus	PCR CSF	PCR Serum	Serology: CSF	Serology: Serum	Culture Pharynx	Culture: Rectum	Culture: Blood	Culture: CSF	Other
HSV 1 & 2	CS	–	+	–	–	–	–	–	Intranuclear inclusion bodies
VZV	CS	CS	+	+	–	–	–	+	Skin vesicle (PCR)
HHV6	++	++	+/–	+/–	–	–	+	+	
EBV/CMV	++	++	CS	CS	+/–	–	+/–	+/–	
Adenovirus	++	++	+/–	+/–	CS: RAA	+	–	–	
Arbovirus*	++	++	CS	CS	–	–	CF	CF	
Enterovirus	CS	CS	–	–	+	+	–	+	Urine PCR
Measles	–	–	+	+	+	–	+	–	CS: Rapid antigen assay
Rabies	–	–	CS	CS	–	–	–	+	Negri bodies
Mycoplasma pneumoniae	++	–	+	+	CS: PCR	–	+	+	
Influenza	–	–	–	+/–	CS: DFA/PCR	–	+	+	

**Arboviruses include: St. Louis encephalitis (SLE), Western equine encephalitis (WEE), and West Nile virus (WNV)*
DFA: direct fluorescent antibody
RAA: rapid antigen assay
– Not clinically useful/not available
+/– Variable utility
+ Effective
++ Increasing clinical use
CS Clinical standard
CF Confirmatory

The development of novel antiviral agents has lagged because of the research emphasis on immunization. As the majority of cases lack an isolated causative agent, the value of developing specific antiviral drugs is questionable. The use of immunomodulatory therapy, such as steroids, to treat encephalitis is compelling; however the relative rarity of cases makes a single center study difficult, if not impossible. Acyclovir, supportive care and rehabilitative therapies remain the only treatments at this time for viral encephalitis.

HSV-1 and HSV-2

HSV-1 and HSV-2 are double-stranded DNA viruses that remain dormant in human host neurons. The clinical features distinguishing HSV-1 and HSV-2 are few; and thus, it is not clinically useful to discriminate between them.

One-third of patients with HSV encephalitis are younger than 20 years and the majority have no prior existing conditions.[26] About half of all patients with HSV encephalitis report a viral prodrome prior to the onset of neurological symptoms, with symptoms of upper respiratory and gastrointestinal illness being the most commonly reported. Neonates who acquire HSV develop CNS infection in over 50% of cases. Infection typically occurs at the time of birth (85%), but can also occur transplacentally (5%) or in the postpartum period (10%).[21] Symptoms of HSV infection in neonates range from subtle (skin vesicles) to fulminant (fever, seizures, obtundation).

HSV infects peripheral sensory neurons and then spreads to the CNS by retrograde axonal transport. The patient invariably experiences fever, headache, and altered mental status. Focal seizures at the time of presentation are common (75% of patients), while hemiparesis (45%), aphasia (75%), and cranial neuropathies are also seen. Infections can rapidly progress to involve greater areas of brain tissue.[21]

In the last 20–30 years, with the advent of acyclovir, there have been significant declines in the mortality and morbidity associated with HSV encephalitis. Prior to the use of acyclovir, approximately 70% of patients with HSV encephalitis died; this has decreased to 19% since the widespread use of acyclovir.[14] Neurological outcomes have also improved, and long-term studies demonstrate a normal outcome in 38%, moderate impairment in 9%, and severe impairment in 53%.[14,26] Outcomes were most improved in younger age groups and in patients with shorter latency to treatment.[14] The typical dose of

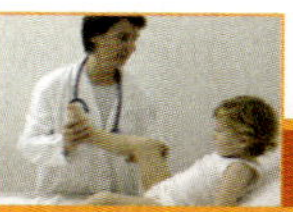

Table 17–5.

Key Features of the Viral Encephalitides

Virus	Key Clinical or Epidemiological Features
HSV	Common cause of encephalitis.
	Predilection for temporal lobes, sylvian fissure, orbital–frontal cortex.
	Associated with periodic lateralizing epileptiform disharges on EEG, vesicles on the skin, focal seizures, hemiparesis, aphasia, and cranial neuropathies.
HHV-6	Rarely causes encephalitis.
	Typically occurs in infants and small children, and has a focal onset.
VZV	Uncommon cause of encephalitis.
	Typically occurs in children. Usually associated with vesicular rash, headache, vomiting, altered mental status, and seizures. Can also cause ischemic or hemorrhagic infarcts.
EBV	Rarely causes encephalitis.
	Often associated with rash or mononucleosis.
CMV	Rarely causes encephalitis.
	More common in immunocompromised patients.
EV	Common cause of CNS infection, but rarely causes encephalitis.
	Often associated with pharyngitis, gastroenteritis, and rash.
Arboviruses	Most common causes of worldwide encephalitis.
WNV	Associated with headache, vomiting, diarrhea, abdominal pain, and rash. Presents with seizures, flaccid paralysis, and cranial neuropathies.
EEE	Rare cause of encephalitis, but children are most affected.
	Presents with sudden high fever, seizures, and altered mental status.
SLE	Rarely causes encephalitis. Presents with headache.
La Crosse	Rare cause of encephalitis, but occurs most commonly in children.
	Associated with upper respiratory illness, abdominal pain, and seizures.
Influenza	Rarely causes encephalitis in the United States.
	Presents with a prodrome of myalgias and fever, progresses to cause seizure.
Rabies	Rare in developed countries, but common throughout the world.
Encephalitic	Presents with anxiety, hydrophobia, aerophobia, hypersalivation, and seizures.
Paralytic	Presents with progressive peripheral nerve paralysis.
Measles	Rarely causes encephalitis, more commonly causes SSPE.
	SSPE occurs months to years after measles infection and presents with progressive dementia, myoclonus, seizures, and ataxia.
Mumps	Rarely causes encephalitis.
	Presents with fever, headache, and a typically mild course.
	Postinfectious encephalomyelitis: occurs 7–10 d after mumps infection and is more severe. Symptoms include seizure, hemiparesis, and altered mental status.

acyclovir is 30 mg/kg/d IV, divided every 8 hours for 14–21 days in children, and 60 mg/kg/d IV, divided every 8 hours for 21 days in neonates.

Human Herpesvirus 6

Human herpesvirus 6 (HHV-6), also known as roseola, usually infects children during infancy, with two-thirds of children seroconverting by 1 year.[27] HHV-6 encephalitis is usually focal, and thus, can be confused with HSV encephalitis. Viral invasion of the CNS is a common event during primary infection, as demonstrated by the high rate of febrile seizures. It typically causes high fever, with frank encephalitis occurring only rarely.[28] The incidence of HHV-6 encephalitis is unknown.

Varicella-Zoster Virus

Prior to widespread vaccination campaigns, 4 million cases of primary varicella-zoster virus (VZV) (chicken pox) occurred annually. Rates of serious infection-related morbidity and mortality were highest in children younger than 10 years, accounting for 60% of hospitalizations and 40% of deaths.[29] Direct infection of the CNS during a primary VZV infection is rare, but meningoencephalitis may occur by invasion of the vascular endothelium[20] leading to primary VZV encephalitis. Occurring mostly in the pediatric population, this small vessel vasculopathy presents with headache, fever, vomiting, altered mental status, seizure, and focal deficits. Encephalitis may also complicate reactivation of VZV

Table 17–6.

Antiviral Therapy

Antiviral Agent	Indication	Drug-Related Complications
Acyclovir	Herpes viruses	Nephrotoxic
Amantadine	Influenza A	Declining effectiveness, anticholinergic effects
Cidofovir	CMV retinitis Acyclovir resistant herpes	Nephrotoxic
Foscarnet	Herpes viruses: CMV (including CMV retinitis), herpes simplex viruses	Hypocalcemia Renal failure
Ganciclovir	CMV	Aplastic anemia, phlebitis, nephrotoxic, teratogenesis,
Oseltamivir*	Influenza A and B	Stevens–Johnson syndrome, hepatitis
Ribavarin	Influenza A and B, West Nile virus, Research ongoing in hepatitis B/C, polio measles, smallpox	Nephrotoxic, teratogenesis,

Currently considered first-line therapy for influenza-related complications.

(zoster or shingles), usually in elderly populations. This encephalitis, by contrast, is due to a large vessel vasculopathy, with acute focal deficits developing weeks to months after the clinical infection. MRI findings include ischemic or hemorrhagic infarcts in the cortex and subcortical gray and white matter.

The diagnosis of VZV encephalitis is made via CSF PCR for VZV or serology for VZV-specific IgM in the CSF. Treatment in children is acyclovir IV 60 mg/kg/d, divided every 8 hours for 14 days.

Epstein–Barr Virus

Epstein–Barr virus (EBV) causes severe encephalitis in less than 1% of infected patients.[30] More often, EBV causes aseptic meningitis, cerebellitis, myelitis, or ADEM with a benign course and full recovery from the infection expected. The diagnosis of EBV is made by measuring acute and convalescent serum IgM antibodies to the EBV capsid antigen. A CSF PCR test is available, but sensitivity and specificity of this test are unknown.

Cytomegalovirus

Congenitally acquired CMV causes severe and permanent brain injury, but encephalitis caused by CMV is relatively uncommon except in the immunocompromised child.[15] Serious CMV infections in the immunocompromised are treated with ganciclovir.

Enterovirus

The enterovirus (EV) family, including polioviruses, Coxsackie viruses A and B, and echoviruses, are collectively the leading viral cause of CNS disease in children in the United States, particularly affecting neonates and immunocompromised hosts.[21] Outbreaks of EV generally occur in late summer and early fall and are often associated with pharyngitis, gastrointestinal symptoms, or rash and desquamation of the hands, feet, and mouth (herpangina). Encephalitis, meningoencephalitis, cerebellitis, and a poliolike syndrome are most often seen with EV serotypes 70 and 71, but can occur with any virus in this family.[21] The viruses can be cultured directly from the CSF, but diagnosis is usually made by CSF EV PCR, which has 96–100% sensitivity and ≥99% specificity.[27] Current treatment is symptomatic and supportive, while drug trials are ongoing.

Arbovirus

Arboviruses are the most commonly identified cause of severe encephalitis worldwide.[15] Single-stranded RNA viruses are usually transmitted to humans via mosquito or tick vectors, although transmission has also been reported following blood product transfusion, organ transplantation, needle sticks, transplacentally, and via breast milk. Arboviruses have complex life cycles involving birds and other mammals, with humans being dead-end hosts. After entering the bloodstream, they reach the CNS via endothelial cell infection. The infection in the brain is diffuse, and thus the sequelae nonfocal, including altered mental status, vomiting and fever. PCR testing has not been developed for routine use, as its sensitivity in arboviruses is poor. Evaluation of virus-specific IgM from CSF or blood is the most widely used diagnostic method.

West Nile Virus

Prior to 1999 there were no reported West Nile virus (WNV) cases in the western hemisphere. In 2006, a total of 4256 infected individuals were reported with 1449 cases of confirmed West Nile meningitis/encephalitis, including 165 fatalities.[31] Roughly 80% of infected individuals experience no symptoms, while 20% have mild flu-like symptoms of fever, headache, vomiting, diarrhea, abdominal pain, myalgia, and rash.[32] Neuroinvasive disease typically includes seizures, altered mental status, meningoencephalitis, acute flaccid paralysis, cranial neuropathies, movement disorders, and optic neuritis.[21,33] In patients with neuroinvasive disease,

15% progress to coma.[33] The proportion of each presenting symptom varies with location and timing within the season. WNV meningitis and encephalitis occur more commonly in adults and are uncommon in children.

Diagnosis of neuroinvasive disease is made by CSF serology. WNV IgM is detectable in more than 90% of infected individuals 1 week after symptom onset. IgM-related immunity may persist for more than 1.5 years, complicating the diagnosis of acute disease. The presence of anti-WNV IgG peaks at 4 weeks after infection and persists throughout life. Currently, the treatment of WNV is supportive, though current clinical trials include passive immunization, interferon alpha, and ribavirin. Overall, mortality from WNV is roughly 2–14%, with encephalitis-specific mortality estimated at 12–24%.[21,33] In the United States, donor blood is screened for WNV.

Eastern Equine Encephalitis

Like WNV, Eastern equine encephalitis (EEE) can cause severe disease, with 30% mortality and 30% serious neurological sequelae in survivors.[34] It is an uncommon cause of illness in North America, with only 95 cases reported between 1995 and 2005.[35] The presentation is both sudden and fulminant, with high fever, seizures, and rapid deterioration of mental status. Young children are most severely affected and have the highest rate of neurological sequelae in recovery.

St. Louis Encephalitis Virus

St. Louis encephalitis (SLE) virus is more common than EEE and, according to the CDC, carries a risk of serious neurological morbidity in 10% of patients and 5% mortality. From 1964 to 2005, there were 4478 cases in the United States, with an annual average of 128 cases.[36] While the disease is widespread throughout North America, there is a higher risk of encephalitis and serious neurological infection in low-income areas, as well as the elderly.[37] Most individuals infected with SLE are asymptomatic, but when symptoms are present they range from simple headache to severe encephalitis.

California (La Crosse) Virus

La Crosse virus is less frequent than EEE or SLE in the United States and causes a milder form of encephalitis. Between 1964 and 2005, there were 3375 cases reported to the CDC, ranging from 41 to 167 per year.[38] Most cases are asymptomatic or result in mild illness, with rare neurological sequelae and very rare mortality ($\leq$1%).[39] It is overwhelmingly a childhood disease, with over 90% of cases occurring in children under 16 years. When symptoms occur, the presentation is a sudden onset of fever, headache, upper respiratory illness, abdominal pain, and seizures.

Influenza Virus

Influenza types A and B are common causes of illness, but rarely cause neurological complications in the United States. Influenza has been associated with Reye syndrome, encephalitis, transverse myelitis, acute necrotizing encephalopathy, Guillain–Barré syndrome, and seizures. The data regarding serious neurological sequelae differ by geography and strain. Japanese data shows that roughly 100 children die annually from influenza encephalitis.[40] Similarily, the mortality rates in influenza encephalopathy in Japan are as high as 25–37%.[41,42] A recent study suggests the prevalence of influenza encephalitis in the United States is considerably lower; this single center, retrospective chart review found only 842 laboratory-confirmed cases of influenza A and B in children from 2000 to 2004. Of those patients, 72 children experienced influenza-related neurological complications, but the authors found no cases of influenza encephalitis or influenza-related mortality.[43] The neurological complications consisted of seizures (78%), acute encephalopathy (11%), cerebral infarction after hypotension (5%), postinfectious influenza encephalopathy (3%), and aseptic meningitis (3%).[43] During 2003–2004, of the 153 deaths in children from influenza reported to state health departments, 16% were associated with altered mental status and 6% were associated with encephalopathy.[44] Treatment for influenza is primarily supportive, although rimantadine and oseltamivir have been used for CNS infections.

Rabies Virus

While relatively rare in the United States, rabies is an important cause of serious neurological illness and death. There were only 36 laboratory-confirmed cases in the United States from 1990 to 2001,[45] with half of those cases occurring in children and adolescents.[15] Worldwide, however, roughly 55,000 deaths occur because of rabies each year.[46] It is generally spread to humans by infected animal bites, although documented cases of rabies with no history or evidence of an animal bite exist. The virus spreads through retrograde axonal transport, causing progressive changes in mental status, seizures, cranial neuropathies, dysphagia, and paresis. Two forms of CNS rabies exist: one causes encephalitis, with seizures and fever, and eventually progresses to paralysis, while the other begins with paralysis of the peripheral nerves and is associated with fever, but not seizures. The paralytic form differs from Guillain–Barré syndrome by the association with fever, and the lack of sensory deficits. Once these symptoms occur, the disease almost invariably induces cardiopulmonary failure and death, in 5–7 days. Diagnosis is typically made at autopsy via serologic or PCR testing of brain tissue, and histological examination of the tissue may demonstrate Negri bodies. Viral culture may be used as a confirmatory technique. The most sensitive (100%), noninvasive, antemortem diagnostic test is PCR analysis looking for rabies RNA in the saliva of the patient, with the next most sensitive (67%) test being antigen testing of hair follicles obtained by nuchal skin biopsy.[47] Additional tests include antibody testing of CSF and serum, and antigen testing of a touch impression from the cornea.

There is no treatment available for rabies after symptom onset, but presymptomatic postexposure vaccine combined with immunoglobulin administration is highly effective if given within 24 hours after exposure,[48] and may be effective for up to 72 hours after exposure, in some cases. The only case of survival documented after symptom onset occurred in a 15-year-old girl who was placed into chemical coma with ketamine, midazolam, and barbiturates. High-dose ribavirin (33 mg/kg/load plus 64 mg/kg/d) and amantidine (200 mg/kg/d) were administered for 1 week. She had dysarthria, buccolingual choreoathetosis, intermittent dystonia, and ballismus, 5 months after hospitalization, but was able to attend high school part-time. No formal neurocognitive testing was reported at that time.[49] As of April 2007, she planned to graduate from high school, and attend college. Her persistent neurological deficits include numbness on her thumb, in the area of the bite, abnormal tone in her left arm, and a widened running gait.[49] Further attempts to utilize this treatment strategy have failed.[50]

Measles Virus

Measles is rare in the postvaccine era and progresses to encephalitis in only 0.74 per 1000 cases.[15] Its more common neurological syndrome, subacute sclerosing panencephalitis (SSPE), occurs in older children and adults months to years after a primary measles infection. This clinical syndrome presents with dementia, myoclonus, ataxia, epilepsy, and motor function decline, and progresses slowly to death. The clinical features have been divided into four stages (the Jabour stages):

- IA Behavioral, cognitive, and personality change
- IB Myoclonic spasms
- IIA Mental deterioration, myoclonic spasms (periodic, generalized, frequently causing drop spells).
- IIB Apraxias, agnosias, language difficulties, spasticity. Ambulation with assistance.
- IIIA Less speech, visual difficulties, myoclonic spasms frequent, +/− seizures
- IIIB No spontaneous speech, poor comprehension, blind, myoclonic spasms, bedridden, dysphagia, EEG with background delta, chorea, ballismus.
- IV No myoclonus, EEG low voltage with no periodic slow wave complexes, vegetative state.[51]

SSPE findings on EEG include high-voltage (300–1500 μV) and repetitive polyphasic sharp and slow wave complexes of 0.5–2-second duration recurring every 4–15 seconds. Rarely, the complexes can occur at intervals of 1–5 minutes, with the intercomplex interval shortening as the disease progresses.

Treatment for SSPE is predominantly symptomatic. Intrathecal interferon alpha initially showed promise in a case report by inducing remission for 7–8 years, but this initial success was followed by a severe neurocognitive decline.[52]

Mumps Virus

While most cases of mumps occur in areas of the world where routine childhood vaccinations do not occur, epidemics have also been seen in vaccinated populations. In the first 10 months of 2006, there were 5783 cases of mumps reported, with a median age of 22.[53] According to the CDC, 50–60% of cases of mumps show a CSF pleocytosis, despite encephalitis occurring in less than 2 per 100,000 cases.[54] Mumps occurs more often in the spring and has a low mortality rate. Patients with mumps encephalitis present with mild, nonfocal symptoms of fever and headache. Diagnosis is made by CSF and serum serology with culture of the nasopharynx, CSF, urine, and saliva.

A postinfectious encephalomyelitis because of mumps may also occur, usually 7–10 days after infection. These patients exhibit more severe symptoms, such as seizure, hemiparesis, and altered mental status. This variant carries a higher mortality rate of 10%.[21]

Emerging Viruses

Nipah and Hendra viruses are both in the family *paramyxoviridae*. The Nipah virus was identified in 1999 as the cause of a large outbreak of encephalitis among pig farmers in Malaysia and Singapore. The natural reservoir for Nipah virus is still under investigation, but preliminary data implicate bats of the genus *Pteropus* in Malaysia. In Malaysia and Singapore, humans were infected with Nipah virus through close contact with infected pigs. The Hendra virus, first isolated in 1994, is related but not identical to Nipah virus. It is predominantly known to cause fatal respiratory infections in horses and humans, but a solitary case of adult encephalitis has been reported.

PROGNOSIS

Expected outcomes vary significantly with the etiology of the encephalitis, but certain generalizations can be made. Young infants usually have more severe disease and, therefore, more significant sequelae. One study examining the prognostic indicators in 462 cases of pediatric encephalitis (including HSV, VZV, enterovirus, respiratory virus, measles, mumps, rubella, and *Mycobacterium pneumoniae* etiologies) found mortality five times greater in infants compared to older children and that patients with significantly altered mental status had four times the risk of death.[55] The majority of survivors experience seizures or cognitive and focal neurological deficits, negatively affecting their quality of life. The economic impact of encephalitis is difficult to calculate as survivors typically require intensive supportive services and, as a group, have decreased independence as adults. Overwhelmingly, the longitudinal data on outcomes in encephalitis have focused on herpes encephalitis before the advent of acyclovir. The most recent longitudinal study examined the rehabilitation of eight patients, including one child, diagnosed with encephalitis from 1990 to 1997. The study focused only on the rehabilitation scores of the patients, without mention of seizure incidence, cognitive or physical impairment, or quality of life.[56] Clearly, more investigation into the outcomes of children with viral encephalitis is required before conclusions can be drawn regarding prognosis.

REFERENCES

1. CDC. Arboviral factsheet. 2007. http://www.cdc.gov/ncidod/dvbid/arbor/arbofact.htm. Accessed May 20, 2007.
2. Trevejo RT. Acute encephalitis hospitalizations, California, 1990–1999: unrecognized arboviral encephalitis? *Emerg Infect Dis.* 2004;10(8):1442-1449.
3. Medawar P. Immunity to homologous grafted skin. III. The fate of skin homografts transplanted to the brain, to subcutaneous tissue, and to anterior chamber of the eye. *Br J Exp Pathol.* 1948;29:58-69.
4. Fujinami R, Oldstone M. Amino acid homology between the encephalitogenic site of myelin basic protein and virus: mechanism for autoimmunity. *Science.* 1985;230:1043-1045.
5. Miller S, Olson J, Croxford J. Multiple pathways to induction of virus-induced autoimmune demyelination: lessons from Theiler's virus infection. *J Autoimmun.* 2001;16:219-227.
6. Levin MC, Lee SM, Kalume F, et al. Autoimmunity due to molecular mimicry as a cause of neurological disease. *Nat Med.* 2002;8:509-513.
7. Deli M, Abraham C, Kataoka Y, Niwa M. Permeability studies on in vitro blood-brain barrier models: Physiology, pathology, and pharmacology. *Cell Mol Neurobiol.* 2005;25(1):59-127.
8. Carson M, Doose J, Melchior B, Schmid C, Ploix C. CNS immune privilege: Hiding in plain sight. *Immunol Rev.* 2006;213:48-65.
9. Stoll G, Jander S, Schroeter M. Detrimental and beneficial effects of injury-induced inflammation and cytokine expression in the nervous system. *Adv Exp Med Biol.* 2002;513:87-113.
10. Chew L, Takanohashi A, Bell M. Microglia and inflammation: impact on developmental brain injuries. *Ment Retard Dev Disabil Res Rev.* 2006;12(2):105-112.
11. Wenkel H, Streilein J, Young M. Systemic immune deviation in the brain that does not depend on the integrity of the blood-brain barrier. *J Immunol.* 2000;164(10):5125-5131.
12. Marques C, Hu S, Sheng W, Cheeran M, Cox D, Lokensgard J. Interleukin-10 attenuates production of HSV-induced inflammatory mediators by human microglia. *Glia.* 2004;47:358-366.
13. Brabb T, von Dassov P, Ordonez N, Schnabel B, Duke B, Goverman J. In situ tolerance within the central nervous system as a mechanism for preventing autoimmunity. *J Exp Med.* 2000;192(6):871-880.
14. Lewis P, Glaser C. Encephalitis. *Pediatr Rev.* 2005;26(10):353-363.
15. Feigin R, Cherry J, Demmler G, Kaplan SL. Textbook of *Pediatric Infectious Diseases.* Philadelphia: Saunders; 2004:505-517.
16. Bulakbasi N, Kocaoglu M, Tayfun C, Ucoz T. Transient splenial lesion of the corpus callosum in clinically mild influenza-associated encephalitis/encephalopathy. *AJNR Am J Neuroradiol.* 2006;27(9):1983-1986.
17. Tsuchiya K, Katase S, Yoshino A, Hachiya J. MRI of influenza encephalopathy in children: value of diffusion-weighted imaging. *J Comput Assist Tomogr.* 2000;24(2):303-307.
18. Yoshikawa H, Kitamura T. Serial changes on diffusion-weighted magnetic resonance imaging in encephalitis or encephalopathy. *Pediatr Neurol.* 2006;34(4):308-311.
19. Gilden D. Varicella zoster virus vaculopathy and disseminated encephalomyelitis. *J Neurol Sci.* 2002;195:99-101.
20. Kleinschmidt-DeMasters B, Gilden D. Varicella-Zoster virus infections of the nervous system: clinical and pathologic correlates. *Arch Pathol Lab Med.* 2001;125(6):770-780.
21. DeBiasi R, Tyler K. Viral meningitis and encephalitis. *Neurol Cont.* 2006;12(2):58-94.
22. Lakeman F, Whitley RJ. Diagnosis of herpes simplex encephalitis: application of polymerase chain reaction to cerebrospinal fluid from brain-biopsied patients and correlation with disease. National Institute of Allergy and Infectious Diseases Collaborative Antiviral Study Group. *J Infect Dis.* 1995;171(4):857-863.
23. Muttilainen M, Koskiniemi M, Linnavuori K, et al. Infections of the central nervous system of suspected viral origin: a collaborative study from Finland. *J Neurovirol.* 2001;7 (5):400-408.
24. Khetsuriani N, Holman R, Anderson L. Burden of encephalitis-associated hospitalizations in the United States, 1988–1997. *Clin Infect Dis.* 2002;35:175-182.
25. Silvia MT, Licht DJ. Pediatric central nervous system infections and inflammatory white matter disease. *Pediatr Clin North Am.* 2005;52(4):1107-1126.
26. Whitley R, Alford C, Hirsh M, et al. Vidarabine versus acyclovir therapy in herpes simplex encephalitis. *N Engl J Med.* 1986;314(3): 144-149.

27. DeBiasi RL, Tyler KL. Molecular methods for diagnosis of viral encephalitis. *Clin Microbiol Rev.* 2004;17(4):903-925.
28. Irving W, Chang J, Raymond D, Dunstan R, Grattan-Smith P, Cunningham A. Roseola infantum and other syndromes associated with acute HHV6 infection. *Arch Dis Child.* 1990;65(12):1297-1300.
29. CDC. Varicella Factsheet 2007. http://www.cdc.gov/nip/diseases/varicella/. Accessed May 20, 2007.
30. Connelly K, DeWitt L. Neurologic complications of infectious mononucleosis. *Pediatr Neurol.* 1994;10(3):181-184.
31. CDC. West Nile Virus Human Case Count 2007. http://www.cdc.gov/ncidod/dvbid/westnile/surv&controlCaseCount06_detailed.htm. Accessed May 20, 2007.
32. Mostashari F, Bunning M, Kitsutani P, et al. Epidemic West Nile encephalitis, New York, 1999: Results of a household-based seroepidemiological survey. *Lancet.* 2001;358(9278):261-264.
33. Campbell G, Marfin A, Lanciotti R, Gubler D. West Nile virus. *Lancet Infect Dis.* 2002;2(9):519-529.
34. CDC. Eastern equine encephalitis factsheet 2007. www.cdc.gov.ncidod/dvbid/arbor/eeefact.htm. Accessed May 20, 2007.
35. CDC. Eastern equine encephalitis human case count 2007. www.cdc.gov/ncidod/dvbid/arbor/arbocase.htm. Accessed May 20, 2007.
36. CDC. St. Louis encephalitis case count 2007. www.cdc.gov/ncidod/dvbid/arbor/arbocase.htm. Accessed May 20, 2007.
37. CDC. St. Louis encephalitis factsheet 2007. www.cdc.gov/ncidod/dvbid/arbor/arbofact.htm. Accessed May 20, 2007.
38. CDC. California (La Crosse) encephalitis case count 2007. www.cdc.gov/ncidod/dvbid/arbor/arbocase.htm. Accessed May 20, 2007.
39. CDC. California (La Crosse) encephalitis factsheet 2007. www.cdc.gov/ncidod/dvbid/arbor/lacfact.htm. Accessed May 20, 2007.
40. Yoshikawa H, Yamazaki S, Watanabe T, Abe T. Study of influenza-associated encephalitis/encephalopathy in children during the 1997 to 2001 influenza seasons. *J Child Neurol.* 2001;16(12): 885-890.
41. Morishima T, Togashi T, Yokota S, Okuno Y, Miyazaki C, Tashiro M. Encephalitis and encephalopathy associated with an influenza epidemic in Japan. *Clin Infect Dis.* 2002;35:512-517.
42. Togashi T, Matsuzono Y, Narita M, Morishima T. Influenza-associated acute encephalopathy in Japanese children in 1994–2002. *Virus Res.* 2004; 103:75-78.
43. Newland JG, Laurich VM, Rosenquist AW, et al. Neurologic complications in children hospitalized with influenza: characteristics, incidence, and risk factors. *J Pediatr.* 2007;150(3):306-310.
44. Bhat N, Wright J, Broder K, et al. Influenza special investigations team. Influenza-associated deaths among children in the United States, 2003-2004. *N Engl J Med.* 2005;15;353(24):2559-2567.
45. CDC. Rabies case count 2007. http://www.cdc.gov/ncidod/dvrd/rabies/Professional/publications/Surveillance/Surveillance01/Table2–01.htm. Accessed May 20, 2007.
46. CDC. Rabies factsheet 2007. www.cdc.gov/ncidod/dvrd/rabies/. Accessed May 20, 2007.
47. Plotkin S. Rabies. *Clin Infect Dis.* 2000;30:4-12.
48. American Academy of Pediatrics R. *Red Book.* In: 27th ed. Elk Grove Village: American Academy of Pediatrics; 2006:552-559.
49. Willoughby R. A cure for rabies? *Sci Am.* 2007;296(4): 88-95.
50. CDC. Human rabies–Indiana and California, 2006. *MMWR Morb Mortal Wkly Rep.* 2007;56(15):361-365.
51. Gascon G, Yamani S, Crowell J, et al. Combined oral isoprinosine-intraventricular alpha-interferon therapy for subacute sclerosing panencephalitis. *Brain Dev.* 1993;15(5):346-355.
52. Miyazaki M, Nishimura M, Toda Y, Saijo T, Mori K, Kuroda Y. Long term follow up of a patient with subacute sclerosing panencephalitis successfully treated with intrathecal interferon alpha. *Brain Dev.* 2005; 27(4):301-303.
53. CDC. Mumps factsheet 2007. www.cdc.gov/nip/diseases/mumps/default.htm. Accessed May 20, 2007.
54. CDC. Mumps factsheet complications 2007. www.cdc.gov/nip/diseases/mumps/faqs-phys-complic.htm. Accessed May 20, 2007.
55. Rautonen J, Koskiniemi M, Vaheri A. Prognostic factors in childhood acute encephalitis. *Pediatr Infect Dis J.* 1991;10:441-446.
56. Moorthi S, Schneider W, Dombovy M. Rehabilitation outcomes in encephalitis: a retrospective study 1990–1997. *Brain Inj.* 1999;13:225-229.

CHAPTER 18

Transverse Myelitis

Mark P. Gorman and
Scott L. Pomeroy

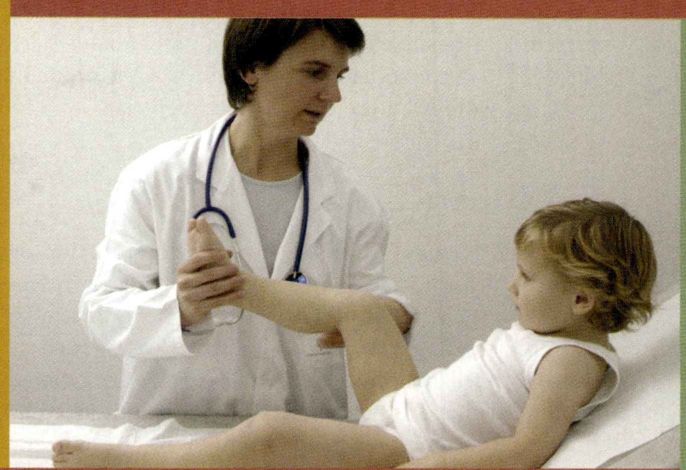

DEFINITIONS AND EPIDEMIOLOGY

Acute transverse myelopathy is a clinical syndrome consisting of progressive symptoms and signs reflecting sensory, motor, or autonomic dysfunction attributable to the spinal cord. This syndrome can be caused by a heterogeneous group of disorders, including acute transverse myelitis (ATM). Definitions of ATM have varied significantly in the literature.[1,2] To address this nonuniformity, the criteria proposed by the Transverse Myelitis Consortium Working Group[3] (Table 18–1) should be used to establish the diagnosis and guide the differential diagnosis and workup. The diagnosis of ATM can be further refined by determining whether there is partial or complete involvement of the spinal cord in the axial plane. Complete ATM is characterized by moderate to severe symmetric symptoms, while partial ATM is marked by milder, asymmetric symptoms.[4]

ATM can be associated with more diffuse central nervous system (CNS) demyelinating disorders, systemic autoimmune disorders, or specific associated infections. Idiopathic ATM is associated with a nonspecific preceding infection or no apparent cause and constitutes the most common subgroup of pediatric ATM.

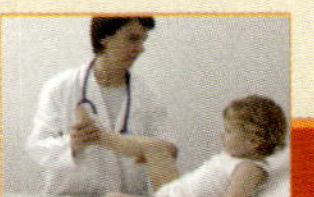

Table 18–1.

Transverse Myelitis Consortium Working Group Diagnostic Criteria

Inclusion Criteria	Exclusion Criteria
▪ Development of sensory, motor, or autonomic dysfunction attributable to the spinal cord ▪ Bilateral signs and/or symptoms (though not necessarily symmetric) ▪ Clearly defined sensory level ▪ Exclusion of extra-axial compressive etiology by neuroimaging (MRI or myelography; CT of spine not adequate) ▪ Inflammation within the spinal cord demonstrated by CSF pleocytosis or elevated IgG index or gadolinium enhancement. If none of the inflammatory criteria is met at symptom onset, repeat MRI and lumbar puncture evaluation between 2 and 7 d following symptom onset meet criteria ▪ Progression to nadir between 4 h and 21 d following the onset of symptoms (if patient awakens with symptoms, symptoms must become more pronounced from point of awakening)	▪ History of previous radiation to the spine within the last 10 y ▪ Clear arterial distribution clinical deficit consistent with thrombosis of the anterior spinal artery ▪ Abnormal flow voids on the surface of the spinal cord consistent with AVM ▪ Serologic or clinical evidence of connective tissue disease (sarcoidosis, Behçet's disease, Sjögren's syndrome, SLE, mixed connective tissue disorder, etc.)* ▪ CNS manifestations of syphilis, Lyme disease, HIV, HTLV-1, *Mycoplasma*, other viral infection (e.g., HSV-1, HSV-2, VZV, EBV, CMV, HHV-6, enteroviruses)* ▪ Brain MRI abnormalities suggestive of MS* ▪ History of clinically apparent optic neuritis*

**Do not exclude disease-associated ATM.*

AVM, arteriovenous malformation; SLE, systemic lupus erythematosus; HTLV-1, human T-cell lymphotropic virus-1; HSV, herpes simplex virus; VZV, varicella-zoster virus; EBV, Epstein–Barr virus; CMV. cytomegalovirus; HHV, human herpes virus.

Idiopathic ATM afflicts approximately 1.34 persons per million.[5] In the pediatric age group, patients present at a mean age of 8 years with an equal gender ratio.[1,2,4,6–9] Approximately 280 cases of ATM occur in pediatric patients in the United States per year.[10,11]

PATHOGENESIS

Infectious agents can cause spinal cord dysfunction by directly infecting the spinal cord parenchyma (infectious myelopathy)[12] or by triggering postinfectious, immune-mediated processes. In some cases, such as human T-cell lymphotropic virus (HTLV) associated myelitis, damage to the spinal cord may be produced by direct infection as well as the immune response to the microbe. Several agents, including cytomegalovirus (CMV) and varicella-zoster virus (VZV), are associated with direct CNS infection in certain patients (many of whom are immunocompromised) and postinfectious ATM in others.

Among all cases of ATM, the preceding infection is most commonly a nonspecific upper respiratory tract infection.[1,5,9] Approximately 50% of patients report a preceding infection with an intervening symptom-free interval of 5–11 days.[1,5,9,10] Some cases of ATM are associated with recent vaccination, although causality is difficult to prove given the paucity of cases and the frequency with which children are vaccinated.[1,6,10,13–15]

Although the precise pathophysiology of ATM is uncertain, the frequent association with preceding infections and accumulating immunological data support an inflammatory cause for the disorder.[1,5,16,17] Increased peripheral blood lymphocyte responses to myelin basic protein have been demonstrated in the research setting in patients with ATM.[18] None of the six patients who were tested in the recovery stage in this study showed significant responses to myelin basic protein, suggesting that the cellular autoimmune reaction is short-lived. In addition, the production of interleukin-6 (IL-6) by astrocytes appears to lead to nitric oxide-induced injury to spinal cord oligodendrocytes and axons in patients with idiopathic ATM. IL-6 levels are markedly elevated in the cerebrospinal fluid (CSF) of patients with ATM and correlate with long-term disability.[16]

In a specific form of ATM which also includes optic neuritis, termed neuromyelitis optica (NMO),[19] a novel biomarker (NMO-IgG) has been detected in 73% of adult patients and several pediatric patients.[20–22] This auto-antibody targets the predominant CNS water channel protein aquaporin-4, which is concentrated in astrocytic foot processes in the blood–brain barrier. The role of NMO-IgG and aquaporin-4 in the more common, idiopathic form of ATM is uncertain.

CLINICAL PRESENTATION

Seven published case series ranging in size from 9 to 50 patients disclose common symptoms in pediatric patients with ATM.[1,2,6–10] Patients universally report acute to subacute, bilateral leg weakness, which is symmetric in approximately 67% of patients.[1] Involvement of the arms occurs in about 40% of patients. Approximately 90% of patients complain of bowel and bladder dysfunction. A similar percentage of patients report sensory symptoms, including paresthesias and numbness. Back pain and fever afflict nearly 50% of patients and may prompt consideration of primary infectious etiologies, such as an epidural abscess. The symptoms of ATM develop rapidly, peaking at an average of 2 and 5 days, in two respective studies.[1,10]

The general examination, although usually unremarkable, may reveal signs suggestive of an underlying systemic infection or autoimmune disorder. Abdominal examination may reveal a distended bladder. On the neurological examination, the presence of any mental status changes suggests that the myelitis is a component of a more diffuse process, such as acute disseminated encephalomyelitis (ADEM). In the acute stages, muscle tone is flaccid in affected limbs. All sensory modalities should be carefully assessed. A spinal cord sensory level is usually located in the thoracic region (80%) and less commonly in the cervical (10%) or lumbar (10%) area.[5] In the acute phase, deep tendon reflexes are depressed in approximately 70% of patients and later become hyperactive. Similarly, Babinski responses may be negative early in the acute phase, but soon become positive, indicating upper motor neuron dysfunction.

DIFFERENTIAL DIAGNOSIS

Numerous disorders can affect the spinal cord and produce identical symptoms and signs that mimic idiopathic ATM (Table 18–2). Such conditions must be ruled out through a combination of history, physical examination, neuroimaging, and laboratory evaluation (Figure 18–1).

Isolated Spinal Cord Dysfunction

Extramedullary compressive lesions, including spinal epidural abscesses,[23] spinal epidural hematomas,[24] and tumors,[25] are neurosurgical emergencies that must be diagnosed rapidly for effective treatment. Intramedullary lesions that can mimic ATM include primary spinal cord tumors (most commonly astrocytomas and ependymomas),[26–28] radiation injury,[29] spinal cord infarction, and vascular malformations.[30] Direct infections of the spinal cord, typically viral in etiology, can also occur.

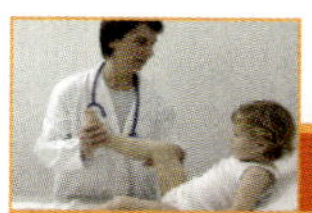

Table 18–2.

Differential Diagnosis of Idiopathic Acute Transverse Myelitis

Mimicking conditions

Common

- Traumatic spinal cord injury
- Guillain–Barré syndrome

Uncommon

- Extramedullary compressive lesions (epidural abscess, epidural hematoma, tumor)
- Intramedullary spinal cord tumors (astrocytomas, ependymomas)
- Ischemia/infarction
- Direct infectious myelopathies
- Vascular malformations
- Radiation injury

Diffuse CNS demyelinating disorders

Common

- Acute disseminated encephalomyelitis (ADEM)

Uncommon

- Multiple sclerosis (MS)
- Neuromyelitis optica (NMO)

Systemic autoimmune disorders

Uncommon

- Systemic lupus erythematosus
- Antiphospholipid antibody syndrome
- Neurosarcoidosis

The initial clinical presentation of ATM can be very similar to that of Guillain–Barré syndrome. Both can present with back pain, paraparesis, and sensory abnormalities. Although typically absent in both disorders acutely, the presence of deep tendon reflexes would point strongly toward ATM. When deep tendon reflexes are absent, the presence of a spinal cord sensory level and bowel and bladder involvement is suggestive of ATM.

Spinal Cord Dysfunction Plus Additional Neurological or Systemic Symptoms and Signs

The presence of mental status changes and cerebral white matter magnetic resonance imaging (MRI) abnormalities point toward ADEM as the correct diagnosis. Mild, asymmetric spinal cord symptoms, previous episodes of transient neurological symptoms attributable to locations other than the spinal cord, and subclinical brain MRI lesions point toward multiple sclerosis.[31] Concurrent or preceding optic neuritis suggests NMO as a possible diagnosis.[19]

ATM can also be secondary to a variety of systemic autoimmune disorders. Involvement of other organ systems, particularly the skin, lungs, kidneys, and joints, may point to a particular diagnosis, such as systemic lupus erythematosus or sarcoidosis.

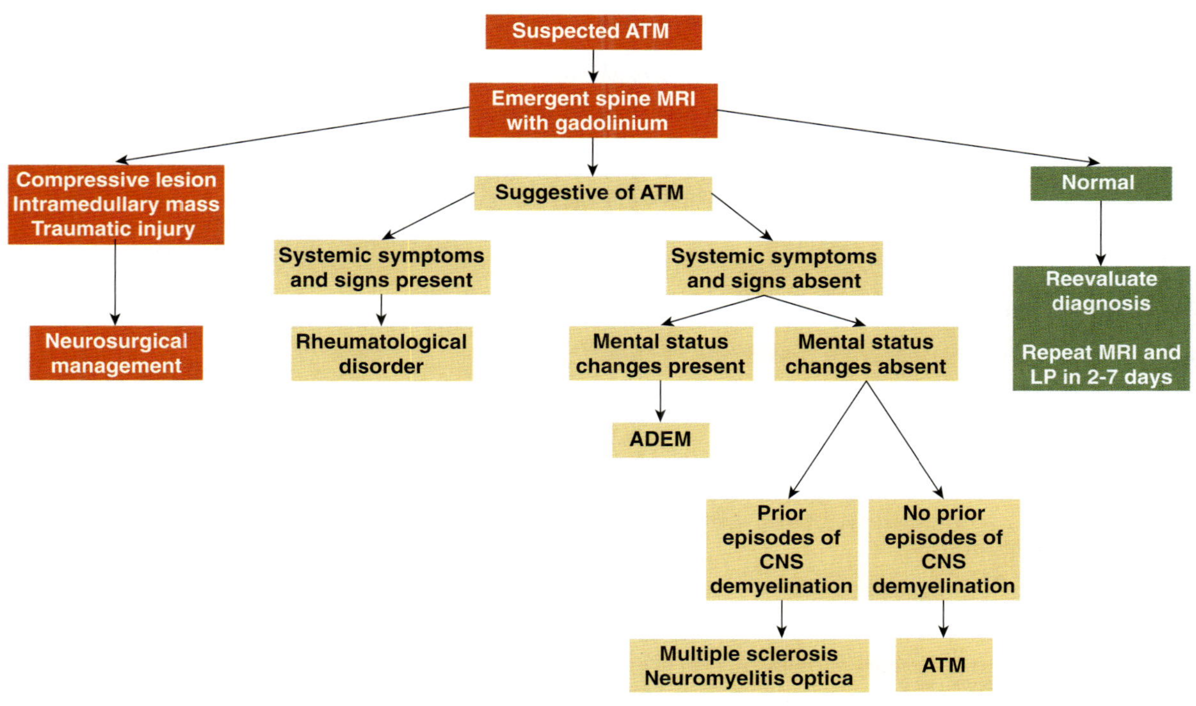

FIGURE 18–1 ■ Diagnostic algorithm for acute ATM.

DIAGNOSIS

Neuroimaging

Every patient with suspected ATM should undergo emergent gadolinium-enhanced MRI of the entire spine in order to confirm the diagnosis and rule out alternative diagnoses, particularly compressive lesions. T1- and T2-weighted sagittal imaging of the entire spine can serve as an initial screen followed by axial imaging in areas of suspected pathology.[32] All patients with ATM should also undergo gadolinium-enhanced MRI of the brain to assess for additional demyelinating lesions suggestive of ADEM or multiple sclerosis.

Spinal MRI in ATM typically reveals T1 isointense and T2 hyperintense signal over several contiguous spinal cord segments,[1] and may involve the entire spine.[32] Spinal cord swelling with effacement of the surrounding CSF spaces may be present in severe cases. Contrast enhancement is present in as many as 74% of patients.[10] In some patients with very suggestive clinical features, the initial spine MRI may be normal and should be repeated several days later.[1,2,6] In some cases, the MRI remains normal, but does not rule out the diagnosis.[10] Higher rostral levels and number of overall spinal segments predicts worse outcome.[10]

Lumbar Puncture

Unless a specific contraindication exists, all patients with ATM should undergo lumbar puncture. Approximately 50% of pediatric patients with ATM have CSF pleocytosis, typically with a lymphocytic predominance.[10] Elevated CSF protein levels, either in isolation or in conjunction with pleocytosis, are also detected in about 50% of patients.[10] Glucose is typically normal. A normal CSF profile does not rule out ATM, as this pattern is seen in approximately 25% of patients.

Additional Tests

The long list of infectious, demyelinating, and rheumatologic disorders potentially associated with ATM precludes diagnostic testing for every possible disorder (Table 18–3). The etiology of a direct infectious myelopathy is usually established by positive CSF culture or polymerase chain reaction results. In postinfectious ATM, a specific etiology can be suggested by elevated acute or rising convalescent serum titers and/or isolation of the agent from systemic sources in the setting of a suggestive clinical picture. The infectious disease workup should be focused on pathogens that are common, treatable, or suggested by particular clues in

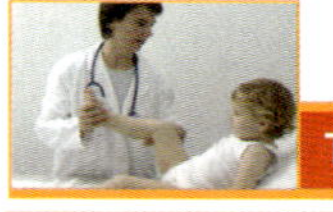

Table 18–3.

Diagnostic Workup for Suspected Acute Transverse Myelitis

All Patients	Suggestive of NMO	Also Consider
Neuroimaging	Ophthalmology consultation	**Infectious diseases**
Brain and spine MRI with gadolinium	Visual evoked potentials	Blood tests
Lumbar puncture	Formal visual field testing	Bartonella titers
Cell counts	Serum NMO-IgG	HIV antibody
Glucose, protein		HTLV-I antibody
Gram stain		Parasitic infection titers
Bacterial culture		RPR
Polymerase chain reaction testing*		CSF studies
Oligoclonal bands		Cryptococcal antigen
Cytology		HTLV antibody
Blood tests		Fungal culture
Blood cultures		VDRL
Acute and convalescent titers†		**Rheumatologic disorders**
		Blood tests
		Angiotensin converting enzyme (serum, CSF)
		Anti-dsDNA
		Anti-La
		Anti-Ro
		Anti-Smith

CMV, EBV, enterovirus, HSV, M. pneumoniae.

†Borrelia burgdorferi, CMV, EBV, M. pneumoniae, VZV.

CSF, cerebrospinal fluid; DNA, deoxyribonucleic acid; HIV, human immunodeficiency virus; HTLV, human T-cell lymphotropic virus; RPR, rapid plasma regain; VDRL, venereal disease research laboratory.

the history or examination, such as environmental exposures and immune status.

TREATMENT

There have been no randomized, controlled treatment trials in ATM. On the basis of case reports and series which have suggested a beneficial effect,[7,33,34] high-dose corticosteroids have become the standard of care in ATM. In one series of 12 children with severe ATM compared to a historical control group of 17 patients, the use of high-dose intravenous methylprednisolone significantly increased the proportion of children walking independently at 1 month (66% compared to 18%) and with full recovery at 1 year (55% compared to 12%).[7] Although a variety of agents and courses have been used, we use intravenous methylprednisolone 30 mg/kg/dose once a day for 5 days (maximum daily dose 1 g). The need for a prednisone taper is controversial and may be based on whether full or partial recovery is achieved with the intravenous steroids. For patients who do not adequately improve with intravenous methylprednisolone, intravenous immunoglobulins (IVIG)[35] or plasmapheresis can be used (Figure 18–2).

As most cases are attributed to secondary, immune-mediated mechanisms, antimicrobial treatment is not likely to have significant benefit. However, antimicrobial therapy should be considered in cases with highly suspected or proven associated infections, such as aeithromycin, doxycycline or levofloxacin for *Mycoplasma pneumoniae*,[36] ganciclovir for CMV,[37] and acyclovir for HSV and VZV.[38] When antimicrobials are used, agents with good CSF penetration are preferred as direct CNS invasion may be present in some cases.

Additional treatment includes pain management, urinary bladder catheterization, bowel regimens, peptic ulcer and deep venous thrombosis prophylaxis, physical therapy, and psychosocial support. Mechanical ventilation is required in approximately 5% of patients.

PROGNOSIS

Disability

Although the variable definitions of recovery reported in the literature preclude a definitive assessment, the prognosis for pediatric patients with ATM is generally favorable.[39] Paine and Byers' degree of recovery categories have been the most widely reported outcome scale but are limited by vague terminology.[9] Based on this scale, approximately 80% of pediatric patients who receive high-dose intravenous methylprednisolone achieve full or good recovery and 20% have a fair or poor outcome.[7,33] Among patients not treated with high-dose intravenous methylprednisolone, 60% have a full or good recovery, while 40% have a fair or poor outcome.[9]

One large, tertiary-referral, center-based study of 47 children with ATM, of whom 70% were treated with intravenous steroids, has cast doubt on the favorable prognosis of the disorder in childhood.[10] In this study, approximately 40% of patients were nonambulatory and 50% required bladder catheterization at a median follow-up of 3.2 years. These results may have been influenced by a high percentage of patients younger than 3 years and patients with cervical involvement compared to other studies. Multicenter and/or population-based studies are needed to further clarify the prognosis of ATM in childhood.

During recovery, motor function returns first, with an average time to independent ambulation of 56 days in one study[1] and 25 days in a group of patients treated with high-dose intravenous methylprednisolone.[7] Bowel/bladder control recovers more slowly with an average time to recovery of normal urinary function of 7 months in those patients with complete recovery.[1]

Recurrences

The overwhelming majority of pediatric patients with idiopathic ATM do not have any recurrences. In a series

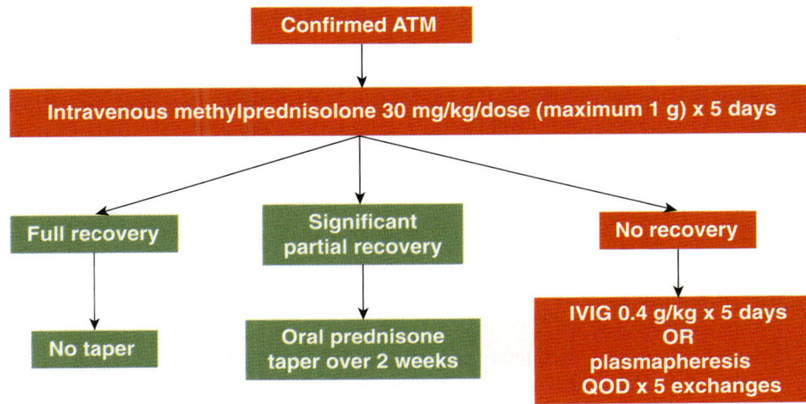

FIGURE 18–2 ■ Treatment algorithm for acute ATM.

of 24 pediatric patients with a mean follow-up of 7 years, there were no recurrences.[1] In another study of children with a variety of initial acute demyelinating events, only 2 of 29 (7%) patients with transverse myelitis had a later demyelinating event.[40,41]

REFERENCES

1. Defresne P, Hollenberg H, Husson B, et al. Acute transverse myelitis in children: clinical course and prognostic factors. *J Child Neurol.* 2003;18(6):401-406.
2. Knebusch M, Strassburg HM, Reiners K. Acute transverse myelitis in childhood: nine cases and review of the literature. *Dev Med Child Neurol.* 1998;40(9):631-639.
3. Transverse Myelitis Consortium Working Group. Proposed diagnostic criteria and nosology of acute transverse myelitis. *Neurology.* 2002;59(4):499-505.
4. Scott TF, Kassab SL, Singh S. Acute partial transverse myelitis with normal cerebral magnetic resonance imaging: transition rate to clinically definite multiple sclerosis. *Mult Scler.* 2005;11(4):373-377.
5. Berman M, Feldman S, Alter M, Zilber N, Kahana E. Acute transverse myelitis: incidence and etiologic considerations. *Neurology.* 1981;31(8):966-971.
6. Miyazawa R, Ikeuchi Y, Tomomasa T, Ushiku H, Ogawa T, Morikawa A. Determinants of prognosis of acute transverse myelitis in children. *Pediatr Int.* 2003;45(5):512-516.
7. Defresne P, Meyer L, Tardieu M, et al. Efficacy of high dose steroid therapy in children with severe acute transverse myelitis. *J Neurol Neurosurg Psychiatry.* 2001;71(2):272-274.
8. Dunne K, Hopkins IJ, Shield LK. Acute transverse myelopathy in childhood. *Dev Med Child Neurol.* 1986;28(2):198-204.
9. Paine RS, Byers RK. Transverse myelopathy in childhood. *AMA Am J Dis Child.* 1953;85(2):151-163.
10. Pidcock FS, Krishnan C, Crawford TO, Salorio CF, Trovato M, Kerr DA. Acute transverse myelitis in childhood: center-based analysis of 47 cases. *Neurology.* 2007;68(18):1474-1480.
11. Banwell BL. The long (-itudinally extensive) and the short of it: transverse myelitis in children. *Neurology.* 2007;68(18):1447-1449.
12. Berger JR, Sabet A. Infectious myelopathies. *Semin Neurol.* 2002;22(2):133-142.
13. Kelly H. Evidence for a causal association between oral polio vaccine and transverse myelitis: a case history and review of the literature. *J Paediatr Child Health.* 2006;42(4):155-159.
14. Zanoni G, Nguyen TM, Destefani E, Masala L, Nardelli E, Tridente G. Transverse myelitis after vaccination. *Eur J Neurol.* 2002;9(6):696-697.
15. Fenichel GM. Neurological complications of immunization. *Ann Neurol.* 1982;12(2):119-128.
16. Kaplin AI, Deshpande DM, Scott E, et al. IL-6 induces regionally selective spinal cord injury in patients with the neuroinflammatory disorder transverse myelitis. *J Clin Invest.* 2005;115(10):2731-2741.
17. Minami K, Tsuda Y, Maeda H, Yanagawa T, Izumi G, Yoshikawa N. Acute transverse myelitis caused by Coxsackie virus B5 infection. *J Paediatr Child Health.* 2004;40(1–2):66-68.
18. Abramsky O, Teitelbaum D. The autoimmune features of acute transverse myelopathy. *Ann Neurol.* 1977;2(1):36-40.
19. Wingerchuk DM, Lennon VA, Pittock SJ, Lucchinetti CF, Weinshenker BG. Revised diagnostic criteria for neuromyelitis optica. *Neurology.* 2006;66(10):1485-1489.
20. Lennon VA, Wingerchuk DM, Kryzer TJ, et al. A serum autoantibody marker of neuromyelitis optica: distinction from multiple sclerosis. *Lancet.* 2004;364(9451):2106-2112.
21. Lennon VA, Kryzer TJ, Pittock SJ, Verkman AS, Hinson SR. IgG marker of optic-spinal multiple sclerosis binds to the aquaporin-4 water channel. *J Exp Med.* 2005; 202(4):473-477.
22. McLinskey BA, MacAllister W, Milazzo M, Krupp L. Neuromyelitis optica in childhood. *Neuropediatrics.* 2006;26(S1):S85.
23. Auletta JJ, John CC. Spinal epidural abscesses in children: a 15-year experience and review of the literature. *Clin Infect Dis.* 2001;32(1):9-16.
24. Patel H, Boaz JC, Phillips JP, Garg BP. Spontaneous spinal epidural hematoma in children. *Pediatr Neurol.* 1998;19(4):302-307.
25. Pollono D, Tomarchia S, Drut R, Ibanez O, Ferreyra M, Cedola J. Spinal cord compression: a review of 70 pediatric patients. *Pediatr Hematol Oncol.* 2003;20(6):457-466.
26. Auguste KI, Gupta N. Pediatric intramedullary spinal cord tumors. *Neurosurg Clin N Am.* 2006;17(1):51-61.
27. Innocenzi G, Raco A, Cantore G, Raimondi AJ. Intramedullary astrocytomas and ependymomas in the pediatric age group: a retrospective study. *Childs Nerv Syst.* 1996;12(12):776-780.
28. DeSousa AL, Kalsbeck JE, Mealey J, Jr., Campbell RL, Hockey A. Intraspinal tumors in children. a review of 81 cases. *J Neurosurg.* 1979;51(4):437-445.
29. Ullrich NJ, Marcus K, Pomeroy SL, et al. Transverse myelitis after therapy for primitive neuroectodermal tumors. *Pediatr Neurol.* 2006;35(2):122-125.
30. Sure U, Wakat JP, Gatscher S, Becker R, Bien S, Bertalanffy H. Spinal type IV arteriovenous malformations (perimedullary fistulas) in children. *Childs Nerv Syst.* 2000;16(8):508-515.
31. Scott TF, Bhagavatula K, Snyder PJ, Chieffe C. Transverse myelitis. Comparison with spinal cord presentations of multiple sclerosis. *Neurology.* 1998;50(2):429-433.
32. Andronikou S, Albuquerque-Jonathan G, Wilmshurst J, Hewlett R. MRI findings in acute idiopathic transverse myelopathy in children. *Pediatr Radiol.* 2003;33(9):624-629.
33. Lahat E, Pillar G, Ravid S, Barzilai A, Etzioni A, Shahar E. Rapid recovery from transverse myelopathy in children treated with methylprednisolone. *Pediatr Neurol.* 1998;19(4):279-282.
34. Sebire G, Hollenberg H, Meyer L, Huault G, Landrieu P, Tardieu M. High dose methylprednisolone in severe acute transverse myelopathy. *Arch Dis Child.* 1997;76(2):167-168.
35. Shahar E, Andraus J, Savitzki D, Pilar G, Zelnik N. Outcome of severe encephalomyelitis in children: effect of high-dose methylprednisolone and immunoglobulins. *J Child Neurol.* 2002;17(11):810-814.

36. Tsiodras S, Kelesidis T, Kelesidis I, Voumbourakis K, Giamarellou H. Mycoplasma pneumoniae-associated myelitis: a comprehensive review. *Eur J Neurol.* 2006; 13(2):112-124.
37. Fux CA, Pfister S, Nohl F, Zimmerli S. Cytomegalovirus-associated acute transverse myelitis in immunocompetent adults. *Clin Microbiol Infect.* 2003;9(12):1187-1190.
38. Gilden DH, Beinlich BR, Rubinstien EM, et al. Varicella-zoster virus myelitis: an expanding spectrum. *Neurology.* 1994;44(10):1818-1823.
39. Pittock SJ, Lucchinetti CF. Inflammatory transverse myelitis: evolving concepts. *Curr Opin Neurol.* 2006;19(4):362-368.
40. Mikaeloff Y, Suissa S, Vallee L, et al. First episode of acute CNS inflammatory demyelination in childhood: prognostic factors for multiple sclerosis and disability. *J Pediatr.* 2004;144(2):246-252.
41. Weinshenker BG, Wingerchuk DM, Vukusic S, et al. Neuromyelitis optica IgG predicts relapse after longitudinally extensive transverse myelitis. *Ann Neurol.* 2006;59(3): 566-569.

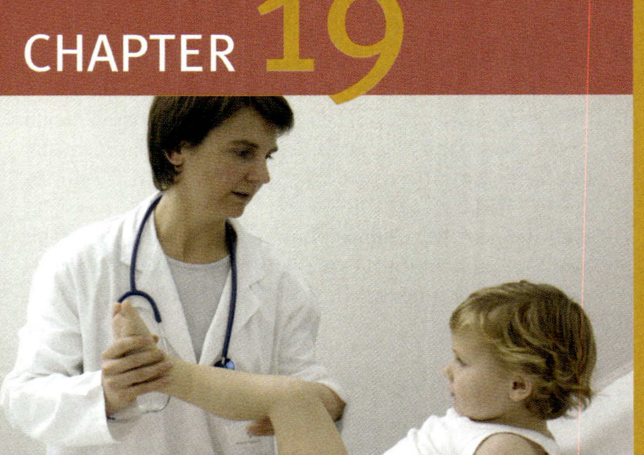

CHAPTER 19

Pediatric Movement Disorders and Infectious Disease

Samay Jain

DEFINITIONS AND EPIDEMIOLOGY

Pediatric movement disorders span a large spectrum of signs and symptoms that occur in a wide range of conditions, some of which may herald the development or sequelae of infectious disease. Accurate diagnosis of these disorders is essential for treatment, prognostication, and counseling. Interest in infectious etiologies of pediatric movement disorders has increased because of recent attention to pathophysiology involving immunologic mechanisms. This chapter will provide an overview of pediatric movement disorders, emphasizing their association with infectious diseases.

Movement disorders are traditionally defined as neurological syndromes in which there is either an excess or paucity of movements unrelated to weakness or spasticity. However, in children spasticity is included in the discussion of movement disorders because it often coexists with other movement disorders, especially in cerebral palsy.[1] There are two broad categories of movement disorders: hyperkinetic (excess of movement or tone) and hypokinetic (paucity of movement or tone) (Table 19–1). As we are classifying movement disorders by phenomenology, specific disorders will be defined in the Clinical Presentation section below. The diagnosis and treatment sections will then address each movement disorder separately in the context of infectious disease.

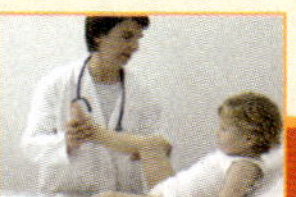

Table 19–1.

Categorization of Common Movement Disorders in Children by Phenomenology

Hypokinetic Disorders	Hyperkinetic Disorders
Bradykinesia	Dyskinesias
Apraxia	Akathesia
Cataplexy and drop attacks	Ataxia
Catatonia	Athetosis
Freezing phenomenon	Ballism
Rigidity	Chorea
Spasticity	Dystonia
	Myoclonus
	Tics
	Tremor

PATHOGENESIS

Movement disorders can be the result of dysfunction at any level of the central (brain or spinal cord) or peripheral (anterior horn cell, nerve roots, plexus, peripheral nerve, neuromuscular junction, or muscle) nervous system. Many movement disorders are associated with pathologic alterations in the basal ganglia or their connections. The basal ganglia include the caudate, putamen, pallidum, subthalamic nuclei, and substantia nigra. Table 19–2 summarizes areas of dysfunction associated with specific movement disorders.

Although the precise pathophysiology of many movement disorders is unknown, infectious and immune-mediated pathophysiology in children has garnered considerable attention. Examples include congenital infections (TORCH: *Toxoplasma gondii*, other microorganisms, rubella virus, cytomegalovirus [CMV], herpes virus, and human immunodeficiency virus [HIV]), Sydenham chorea, pediatric autoimmune neuropsychiatric disorders associated with streptococcal infection (PANDAS), and acute cerebellar dysfunction.

Congenital TORCH infections cross the placenta in utero and can cause fetal infection, resulting in

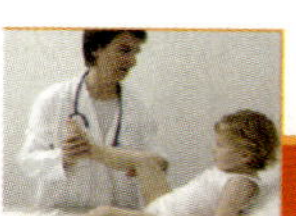

Table 19–2.

Movement Disorders and Associated Areas of the Nervous System Affected

Movement Disorders	Associated Areas
Rigidity, bradykinesia, rest tremor	Substantia nigra
Ballismus	Subthalamic nucleus
Chorea	Caudate
Dystonia	Putamen
Ataxia, asynergy, dysmetria, intention tremor	Cerebellum
Myoclonus	Central and peripheral nervous system

significant neurologic sequelae. Approximately half of infants with congenital CMV or toxoplasmosis go on to develop cerebral palsy with the associated movement disorders (Table 19–3) and two thirds of infants with congenital rubella go on to have balance and coordination problems.[2]

Sydenham chorea is considered the prototype for disorders in which an infectious process, group A β-hemolytic streptococcal infection (GABHS), triggers an autoimmune disorder that in turn causes a variety of neuropsychiatric symptoms. Sydenham chorea occurs in approximately 25% of cases of acute rheumatic fever. Antibodies to cells in the brain are found in some patients. These antibodies are absorbable with cell wall preparations from GABHS, but not group D streptococci. This led to the concept of molecular mimicry, with cross-reactivity between GABHS surface antigens and the brain. Abnormalities in cellular immunity have also been described.[3] Swedo and colleagues described a group of 50 children in whom GABHS seemed to either trigger or worsen symptoms of tic disorders and/or obsessive compulsive disorder.[3] Amidst controversy, this has since been termed PANDAS (discussed below).

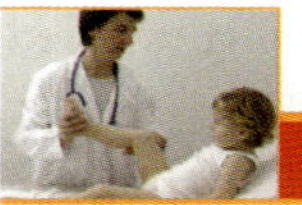

Table 19–3.

Movement Disorders Associated with Cerebral Palsy

Movement Disorder	Typical Age of Onset
Spasticity	<1 year, half resolve during early childhood
Chorea	2–5 years
Athetosis	before 5 years
Dystonia	5–10 years

Acute cerebellar dysfunction in the setting of infection is a heterogeneous set of disorders, including acute cerebellitis and acute cerebellar ataxia. In acute cerebellitis, pathological studies show T-cell infiltration within the cerebellar cortex, suggesting direct invasion of an etiologic agent.[4] On the other hand, acute cerebellar ataxia is postulated to occur as a result of a postinfectious immune mechanism, as autoantibodies may be associated with this condition. Table 19–4 summarizes infectious etiologies for movement disorders in children.

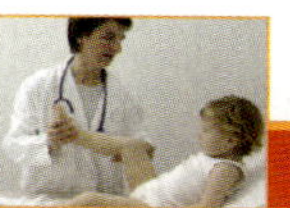

Table 19–4.

Infectious and Postinfectious Etiologies of Pediatric Movement Disorders

Spasticity
Central nervous system abscess
Encephalitis
Meningitis
Transverse myelitis
Acute disseminated encephalomyelitis (ADEM)
Dystonia
Central nervous system abscess
Encephalitis
Grisel syndrome
Chorea, ballism, and athetosis
Sydenham chorea
Encephalitis
Lyme disease
Mononucleosis
Diphtheria
Pertussis
Acquired immune deficiency syndrome
Myoclonus
Subacute sclerosing panencephalitis
Herpes simplex virus
Human immunodeficiency virus
Creutzfeldt–Jakob disease
Tics
Possibly streptococcal infection
Tremor
Encephalitis
Cerebellitis
Ataxia
Brainstem encephalitis
Acute cerebellitis
Acute cerebellar ataxia
Miller Fisher syndrome
Rigidity
Encephalitis

CLINICAL PRESENTATION

What follows are clinical descriptions of common pediatric movement disorders. This includes spasticity, dystonia, athetosis, chorea, myoclonus, tics, tremor, ataxia, and rigidity.

Spasticity

Spasticity is a velocity-dependent increased resistance to passive muscle stretch. More specifically, the Task Force on Childhood Motor Disorders defined spasticity as a hypertonia in which one or both of the following signs are present: (1) resistance to externally imposed movement increases with increasing speed of stretch and varies with the direction of joint movement or (2) resistance to externally imposed movement rises rapidly above a threshold speed or joint angle.[1] Spasticity is the result of an upper motor neuron lesion and thus often accompanied by weakness, loss of motor control, increased deep tendon reflexes, and clonus. It is much more common in cerebral disorders than spinal cord injuries. Spasticity is a dynamic condition, which changes over time based on emotional state, positions, alertness, and age. Often evident by 1 year of age, it may improve or resolve by early childhood. Although spasticity does not usually worsen during childhood, its effects usually do as the patient grows and matures. Prolonged involuntary muscle contraction may result in fixed contractures or joint dislocation.

Dystonia

Dystonia is involuntary muscle contractions that cause twisting and repetitive movements resulting in abnormal postures. The movement disorder can be sustained or intermittent. Muscle tone can fluctuate from normal or low tone to hypertonia. Dystonia can be precipitated by voluntary movement or vary with emotional state such as stress, pain, fatigue, or startle. It typically diminishes with distraction and sleep. Characteristic features of dystonia that may be present are "sensory tricks" or *geste antagoniste*, in which proprioceptive or tactile stimulation (such as touching oneself gently on the cheek) can ameliorate dystonic movement. Dystonia tends not to occur as early in life as spasticity, and typically begins in children between the age of 5 and 10 years, though it can begin as early as 2 years or later in life. The delayed onset is thought to be due to neuronal maturation or myelin formation that may be required for dystonia to manifest. Dystonia may worsen as the brain matures.[1]

Chorea, Ballism, and Athetosis

Chorea (derived from Greek khoreia, meaning dance), is involuntary, random, quick movements that flow from joint to joint. Movements are abrupt, nonrepetitive, arrhythmic, and have variable frequency and intensity. Characteristic of chorea is the inability to sustain muscular contraction, known as motor impersistence. This may manifest as the inability to keep the tongue protruded or maintain a fist resulting in a "milk-maid's" grip when patients are asked to grasp the examiner's fingers. It may affect any part of the body, with the most common causes in childhood being Sydenham chorea and cerebral palsy. *Ballism* is characterized by violent, involuntary flailing movements of the proximal muscles of the extremities. It has been considered a severe form of chorea, and is associated with damage to subcortical structures, especially the subthalamic nucleus.

Athetosis has been has been considered a slow form of chorea, and often coexists with chorea resulting in the term choreoathetosis. Athetosis is the inability to retain fingers and toes in any position because of their continual motion. This can be seen by having patients outstretch their arms with their hands held in front, demonstrating slowing moving, "piano-playing" fingers.

Myoclonus

Myoclonus presents as a sudden shock-like involuntary muscle jerk the may be focal, unilateral, or generalized. It is the fastest movement disorder, with duration of 50–200 milliseconds. It can be normal, such as hiccups or "sleep-starts" as one falls asleep. Myoclonus may be positive, meaning jerking due to active contraction of muscle groups, or negative, meaning movements due to a lapse in sustained contraction. Perhaps the most well-known form of negative myoclonus is asterixis, in which wrist extensors have a lapse in contraction, resulting in hand flapping when arms are outstretched. This is classically described with hepatic encephalopathy though can been seen with other metabolic derangements. Myoclonus may be stimulus sensitive, being brought about by tactile, postural, action, visual, or auditory stimulation, often as an "exaggerated startle." It can be due to a lesion in any level of the nervous system.

Tics

Tics are sudden, semivoluntary highly stereotyped repetitive movements. They can be simple, involving only specific muscle groups (such as excessive eye blinks or grimacing) or more complex. Tics can be anywhere in the body, but most commonly occur in the face, head, and neck. Although vocal tics associated with outbursts of profanity (copralalia) have received considerable publicity, this is rare and vocal tics may be phonations such as sorting, sniffing, sneezing, grunting, throat-clearing, or nonsensical utterances. Tics naturally wax and wane in severity, increasing with excitement, boredom, stress, and fatigue.

Tics are often described as having a premonitory urge to move, and while the movement is suppressible, the urge builds until it is unbearable and the movement must be executed, manifesting a tic. Immediately after a tic is done, there is a transient relief of the urge to move, only to be replaced by another premonitory urge, and the tic cycle repeats itself. Tics are perhaps the most common primary movement disorder in childhood, with 5–24% of school children having at least a transient tics. Often tic disorders are associated with obsessive compulsive disorder and/or attention-deficient disorder.

Tremor

Tremor is an involuntary, hyperkinetic, and rhythmic oscillatory movement of part of the body around a fixed point or place. It is important to note if tremors occur with action, rest, posture, or specific tasks, as this will influence the differential diagnosis and treatment. While the incidence of tremor in childhood is unknown, it is 1.5 in 10,000 in the general population, and in a pediatric movement disorder clinic, 19% of children had tremor as the sole or main feature of their condition.[1]

Ataxia

Ataxia is characterized by problems with muscle coordination. It can affect the trunk (truncal ataxia), walking (gait ataxia), or distal extremities (appendicular ataxia). It is often associated, but not restricted to lesions in the cerebellar pathways.

Rigidity

Rigidity is much more common in adults than children. It is hypertonia in which all of the following are true: (1) the resistance to externally imposed (passive) movement is present at low speeds and does not vary with velocity; (2) contraction of muscle groups may occur, reflected in an immediate resistance to a reversal of the direction of movement about a joint; (3) the limb does not tend to return toward a particular fixed posture or extreme joint angle; and (4) voluntary activity in distant muscle groups does not lead to involuntary movements about the rigid joints, although rigidity may worsen.[5] In children, it is most commonly associated with drug-induced side effects or juvenile Parkinsonism.

DIAGNOSIS

Any infection in the central nervous system may lead to a movement disorder, depending on which structures are involved. When approaching movement disorders, correct identification may be difficult in children where movement disorders can change in appearance given the context of growth and development. Half of all children with cerebral palsy at 1 year of age no longer have motor signs by the seventh year of life.[1] More than one movement disorder may exist within the same child especially in the presence of developmental abnormalities. Other conditions that may mimic movement disorders include epileptic seizures, gastroesophageal reflux (Sandifer's syndrome), and developmentally normal involuntary movements. These include jitteriness in neonates, rapid eye movement sleep myoclonus in young infants, ritualistic behaviors, shivering, self-stimulation, and shuddering. A videotape of the movement in question provided by the caregiver can be quite helpful. Obtaining details of birth history (especially for TORCH infections), family history, medications, as well as any exposure to toxins will help guide the workup. Referral to a pediatric neurologist and/or movement disorder specialist can be quite useful early in the course of evaluation.

During the interview and examination, it is important to be very observant, as many movements may be seen while the child is unaware that he/she is being examined. For example, playing with toys, crawling, or walking is helpful and the child must be observed both during action and at rest. All children with movement disorders should undergo a neurologic examination, and most will need neuroimaging. While computed tomography can be helpful in identifying masses, bleeds, and malformations, magnetic resonance imaging (MRI) is often the modality of choice given its greater detail. If a family history is present, genetic counseling and testing may be considered.

Testing should emphasize both common and treatable etiologies. Thus, virtually every child with no obvious cause of a movement disorder undergoes testing for Wilson disease, a disorder of copper metabolism with progressive neuropsychiatric manifestations including a wide array of movement disorders. If treated with chelating therapy, it may be reversible and further progression is prevented. In Wilson disease, serum ceruloplasmin, a protein bound to copper, is low and serum copper may be high. A 24-hour urine collection looking for copper may also be low, and ophthalmologic examination may reveal copper deposition in the cornea (Keyser–Fleisher rings, see Figure 19–1). While virtually all movement disorders may warrant the evaluation described, specific issues pertinent to each disorder will now be discussed.

Spasticity

Spasticity may be secondary to brain, spinal cord, or peripheral nerve injury from virtually any etiology. Infectious culprits include abscesses within or compressing the central nervous system, encephalitis, meningitis, and postinfectious processes such as transverse

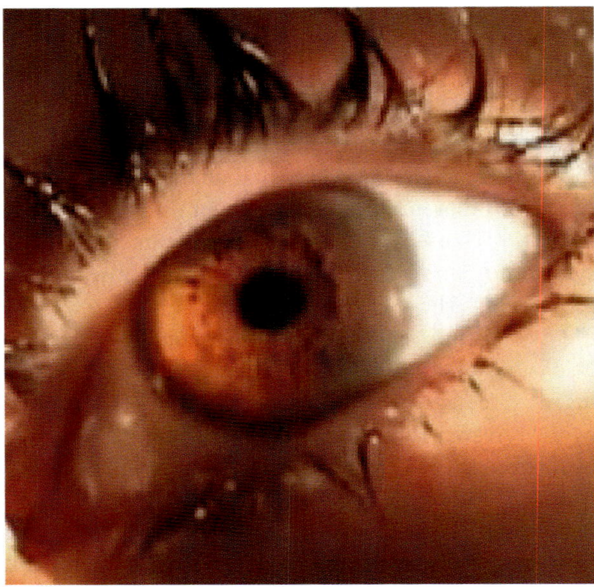

FIGURE 19–1 ■ A child with Wilson disease. The Keyser–Fleisher ring is due to copper deposition in the cornea. It appears as a cloudy gray-brown crescent along the perimeter of the iris.

myelitis and acute disseminated encephalomyelitis. Also, an infection outside of the central nervous system (e.g., otitis, urinary tact infection, pneumonia) can exacerbate preexisting spasticity. Other treatable etiologies include tethered spinal cord, spinal cord tumor, hydrocephalus and intracranial, epidural or subdural bleed. Spasticity is also present in most children with cerebral palsy, spinal cord injury, traumatic brain injury, or multiple sclerosis. For any child with spasticity, neuroimaging is indicated and joint contractures may develop. If spasticity is fluctuating or no lesion is found on imaging, infection, deep venous thrombosis, bladder distention, bowel impaction, and seizure are possibilities.

Dystonia

Dystonia may be focal or generalized and either primary, secondary, or acquired. Common focal dystonias include writer's cramp and torticollis (also known as abnormal head posture, cervical dystonia, or twisting of the neck). The term dystonia is reserved for neurologic etiologies of abnormal postures, with other causes referred to as pseudodystonia. A rare but serious and potentially infectious cause of pseudodystonia is Grisel syndrome, a nontraumatic rotatory subluxation of C1 or C2 vertebrae (atlantoaxial subluxation) without any prior history of osteopathy. This results in abnormal head and neck posture, and can appear identical to cervical dystonia (torticollis) with limited or no range of motion. It was first described as a consequence of syphilitic ulceration of the pharynx, but has since been recognized as a rare consequence of infectious, inflammatory, and/or postsurgical complications in the head and neck. It has predilection for the pediatric population, with 90% of cases below the age of 21 years. Approximately 23% of cases occur after mastoidectomy, tonsillectomy, and adenoidectomy, in that order. Upper respiration infection in the second most commonly associated syndrome.[6] Patients may present with painful torticollis or sudden onset, possibly with a history of fever. Computed tomography of the neck with contrast is necessary to confirm subluxation and look for possible infection, such as retropharyngeal abscess, odontoid osteomyelitis, or deep-space infection (Figure 19–2). Treatment usually includes cervical immobilization, airway preservation, neurosurgical consultation, antibiotics, muscle relaxants, and bed rest.

Abnormal head postures have an incidence of 1.3% in children and may benefit from a multidisciplinary approach. A recent study in 73 children ages 6 months to 8 years with this presentation found etiologies to be orthopedic in 48%, ocular in 34%, neurologic in 7%, and no cause was found in 11%.[7] Most cases presenting in the first 2 years of life were orthopedic, with congenital muscular torticollis (caused by tight neck muscles or a fibrous band) most commonly diagnosed. Ocular and neurologic causes manifested later in life. Ocular causes included abnormalities in extraocular muscles, especially superior oblique muscle palsy causing compensatory head tilting to minimize double vision.

The earlier the onset of dystonia, the more likely it will generalize and be disabling. A trial of levodopa is warranted in most cases of cryptogenic dystonia cases to evaluate the possibility of dopa-responsive dystonia (Segawa disease) or biopterin deficiency. Other etiologies of dystonia include hypoxia, trauma, encephalitis, stroke, tumor, or use of dopamine-receptor antagonists.

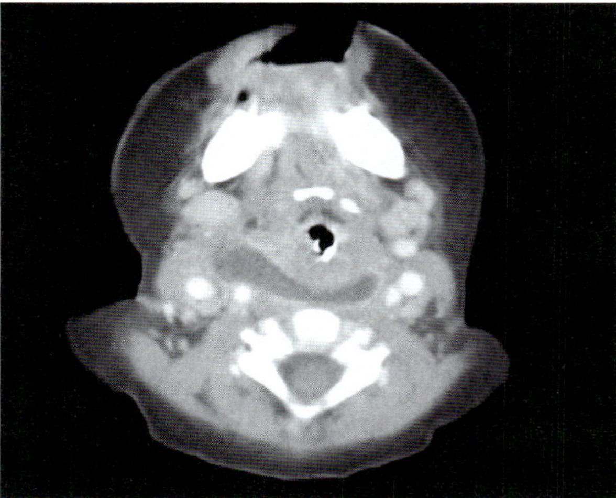

FIGURE 19–2 ■ A retropharyngeal or parapharyngeal abscess may present as pseudodystonia of the neck (Grisel syndrome). (*Image courtesy of Dr. Samir S. Shah.*)

Neuroimaging may show lesions in the basal ganglia, specifically the globus pallidus. Genetic testing may be considered if a family history is present.

Chorea, Ballism, and Athetosis

Chorea, ballism, and athetosis are often found associated with lesions in the basal ganglia. Sydenham chorea is a common cause of chorea in children and a major Jones criterion for rheumatic fever. Given its ramifications, all children presenting with chorea of unknown etiology should be asked about prior streptococcal infection and associated symptoms, such as an untreated sore throat. Sydenham chorea tends to involve the face and extremities and can begin unilaterally. If severe, ballism may be present. Children may also have behavioral abnormalities such as obsessive–compulsive symptoms that can predate chorea by weeks or months. Onset is usually between the ages of 5 and 15 years with a female predominance. The diagnosis is made strictly on clinical grounds as there is no confirmatory test. Symptoms tend to resolve in 1–6 months, though milder chorea can persist, with up to half of patients having chorea after 2 years. Chorea can recur, usually within 1–2 years after the original event.[3] If a diagnosis of Sydenham chorea is suspected, a workup for rheumatic heart disease should be done including an electrocardiogram and echocardiography. Carditis is reported in 25–80%, with higher percentages in subjects who underwent echocardiography.[3] Valvular heart disease results in antibiotic prophylaxis for medical and dental procedures. Although elevated antistreptococcal titers are found in 80% of patients, there is no consensus regarding antibiotic treatment, immunomodulatory regimens or the monitoring of antistreptococcal antibodies. However, treatments for chorea detailed below may be considered.

Chorea has many other causes, including several infectious etiologies listed in Table 19–4. It can also occur in autoimmune conditions such as sarcoidosis, systemic lupus erythematosis, and antiphospholipid syndrome. The most common causes of chorea besides Sydenham chorea include cerebral palsy and medication side effects. It is thus critical to look for secondary causes of chorea as several are treatable and reversible. If constitutional symptoms such as fever, fatigue, sweats, or lymphadenopathy or rashes are found, then an evaluation for infectious or autoimmune causes should be undertaken, including lumbar puncture. All patients with no clear etiology should also have a thyroid panel, sodium, glucose, magnesium, vitamin deficiency, and kidney function evaluated. In girls who have undergone menarche, a pregnancy test may be considered (Chorea gravidarum). A thorough medication history should also be obtained.

Ballism may be considered a severe form of chorea, and athetosis a milder variant. Thus, both have a similar differential diagnosis as chorea. Ballism is associated with lesions of the subthalamic nucleus, while athetosis is also associated with lesions in the basal ganglia due to infection, hyperbilirubinemia, ischemia, or trauma.

Myoclonus

The etiology of myoclonus is diverse, as it can originate from the cerebral cortex (cortical myoclonus), brainstem (brainstem myoclonus), or spinal cord (spinal myoclonus). Rarely, it may start in the peripheral nervous system. If an infectious or autoimmune process such as encephalitis is suspected, a lumbar puncture looking for pleocytosis and immunoglobulins in addition to neuroimaging and a complete blood count should be done. Medication and toxin exposure may also be assessed.

Cortical myoclonus may be spontaneous, occur with voluntary action or with somatosensory stimulation. Postanoxic myoclonus can be cortical in origin and stimulus sensitive with action myoclonus, which is particularly disabling as it prevents normal voluntary motion. Brainstem myoclonus, such as an exaggerated startle, is usually generalized and often triggered by auditory stimuli. Spinal myoclonus can be segmental, multisegmental, or generalized. Palatal myoclonus is a rhythmic contraction of the soft palate that occurs usually at 2–3 Hz and may persist in sleep. It may be associated with an ear-clicking sound. Some have called this palatal tremor because of its rhythmicity. There are two forms: essential and symptomatic. The essential form is self-limited and mainly occurs in children and a click may be audible. The symptomatic form results from brainstem lesions, specifically the red nucleus, inferior olive and dentate nucleus in the cerebellum, known as the Guillain–Mollaret triangle. Negative myoclonus (or asterixis) may be seen in children with diffuse encephalopathies from renal, hepatic, or pulmonary failure; malabsorption syndromes; and drug toxicity (such as phenytoin).

In virtually all cases, the possibility of epileptic activity should be evaluated. Thus an EEG should be done preferably while myoclonic movements are occurring. Video-EEG, in which a patient is videotaped during EEG recording, can be helpful in distinguishing epileptic from nonepileptic movements. Metabolic causes include kidney failure, liver failure, and hyperglycemia.

Tics

There is a wide spectrum of tic disorders, as defined by the DSM-IV criteria,[8] listed in Table 19–5. The differential is categorized by severity, duration, and the presence

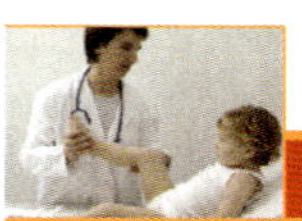

Table 19–5.

DSM-IV Criteria Tic Disorder Spectrum

Chronic motor disorder
Only motor tics, no vocal tics
Many times a day, nearly every day, for 1 year without a tic-free period of 3 months

Chronic vocal tic disorder
Only vocal tics, no motor tics
Many times a day, nearly every day, for 1 year without a tic-free period of 3 months

Transient tic disorder
If motor and/or vocal tics present more than 4 weeks and less than 1 year

Tic disorder NOS
If motor and/or vocal tics present less than 4 weeks

Tourette syndrome
Multiple motor tics and one or more vocal tics present at some time
Tics occur many times a day, nearly every day for at least 1 year without a tic-free period of 3 months before the age of 18 years

of motor and/or vocal tics. There is much debate as to whether the pathophysiology of tics is associated with streptococcal infection or autoimmunity, highlighted by the term PANDAS. Criteria for the diagnosis of PANDAS are (1) Presence of obsessive–compulsive disorder and/or a tic disorder, (2) Age of onset after 3 years but before 11 years, (3) Episodic course of symptom severity, (4) Association with GABHS infection, and (5) Association with choreaform signs is optional.[3] Much criticism of the PANDAS concept comes from the fact that Tourette syndrome and obsessive–compulsive disorder can have sudden onset or worsening without association with streptococcal infection, and isolated GABHS infection is common in children. It is thus difficult to distinguish a child with Tourette syndrome or OCD who happens to also have GABHS infection and one who may have PANDAS. Another interpretation is that PANDAS may be another form of Sydenham chorea. This controversy makes evaluation and treatment decisions difficult. If a child presents with tics or obsessive compulsive disorder in the context of recent streptococcal infection, what should be done? Certainly, if chorea is also present one should conduct an evaluation for Sydenham chorea and rheumatic fever. However, in children without chorea there is no established treatment protocol. This controversy continues to be intensely researched.

Tics usually occur in absence of any detectable pathology. Neuroimaging is normal. Unfortunately, Tourette syndrome is often misdiagnosed. However, accurate diagnosis is possible if the DSM-IV criteria are strictly followed. Tourette syndrome can only be diagnosed if both motor and vocal tics have been present for sufficient time and severity before the age of 18 years. Also, it is important to assess for and treat the common comorbidities of attention-deficit disorder and obsessive–compulsive disorder.

Tremor

Pathologic tremors can be classified by when they occur as resting, postural, action- or task-specific. Neuroimaging may reveal infection, trauma, or tumors as secondary causes and children with cerebral palsy can have any combination of tremors. Resting tremor usually has a frequency of 4–5 Hz, occurs in the absence of any voluntary movement, and is significantly reduced during volitional movement. It is relatively rare in childhood but is associated with dopa-responsive dystonia (see above), Wilson disease (dysfunction in copper metabolism), juvenile Parkinson disease, juvenile Huntington disease, basal ganglia degeneration with iron accumulation, and brain tumors.

Postural tremor has a frequency of 6–12 Hz, occurring when part of the body is maintained in a posture against gravity (i.e., arms outstretched). Two causes of postural tremor are essential tremor and enhanced physiologic tremor. Essential tremor is postural and sometimes seen during action. There may be a family history or alcohol ingestion may result in marked reduction of tremor. Essential tremor may be evident before the age of 20 years in almost one-fifth of cases, and has been reported as early as 2 years of age. Enhanced physiologic tremor may occur in children during times of stress or as a side effect of medications such as amphetamines (often used for attention-deficit disorder), bronchodilators (used in asthma and other respiratory aliments), and valproate (an antiepileptic medication). Intention, kinetic, or action tremor has a frequency of 2–4 Hz and occurs during voluntary movement and is caused by dysfunction of cerebellar pathways. Task-specific tremors occur during specific motor actions, such as writing or speaking. Psychogenic tremors occur in the context of underlying psychological disturbance, and often disappear when the patient is distracted. In almost all cases of tremor, secondary and treatable etiologies should be investigated. Thus, evaluations for Wilson disease, thyroid disease, blood glucose, electrolytes, and medications side effects should be done. In some cases, blood levels of medications can be assessed (e.g., valproate, cyclosporine, phenytoin).

Ataxia

Ataxia has several causes and like other movement disorders, in virtually all instances neuroimaging is warranted. Reversible or treatable causes include infectious or autoimmune ataxias, neoplasms, vascular etiologies, and medication-induced. In cases where an infectious, autoimmune, or neoplastic cause is suspected, a lumbar puncture for cerebrospinal fluid (CSF) analysis can be helpful. Ataxia can be classified as acute, recurrent, chronic-static, or chronic-progressive.

Infection-related etiologies include acute cerebellitis and acute cerebellar ataxia. Acute cerebellitis can present with nausea, headache, and altered mental status, including loss of consciousness in addition to acute onset of cerebellar symptoms (e.g., tremor, ataxia, dysmetria). The main symptoms of acute cerebellitis are headache, vomiting, and disturbances of consciousness varying from somnolence to coma. Fever and signs of meningeal irritation may be present. All patients show abnormal MRI findings on T2-weighted images in the cerebellar cortex. Hydrocephalus or herniation may develop owing to the obstruction of CSF flow, in which case lumbar puncture is contraindicated. CSF findings are variable, but may show increased white cell counts and/or protein. The causative agent of acute cerebellitis often remains unknown despite extensive testing, however Epstein–Barr virus (EBV) and varicella zoster virus are the most frequently identified pathogens. Associations are also reported with mumps, Lyme disease, rubella, Coxsackie B3, mycoplasma, and *Streptococcus pneumoniae*.[4] Managing acute cerebellitis requires immediate treatment with appropriate antimicrobial therapy. MRI should be done, looking for cerebellar involvement, edema, herniation, and hydrocephalus. If cerebellar swelling is seen, the patient should be treated with corticosteroids and mannitol or glycerol. If obstructive hydrocephalus is a concern, neurosurgical consultation for possible ventriculostomy or other decompressive procedures are indicated.

Acute cerebellar ataxia, unlike acute cerebellitis, is acute onset of gait ataxia *without* meningismus, seizures, alteration of mental status, or other neurologic abnormalities. Acute cerebellar ataxia is usually a self-limited benign disease showing temporary signs of gait ataxia, which may develop in children after viral infection or vaccination. It may be caused by varicella, mumps, mycoplasma, or EBV.[9] CSF in acute cerebellar ataxia may reveal oligoclonal IgG bands, and autoantibodies may be associated with this condition.[4] If acute cerebellar ataxia does not resolve or eye movements are abnormal, opsoclonus–myoclonus, which is associated with neuroblastoma, should be considered.[10]

Rigidity

Rigidity as noted above is relatively uncommon in children but can be seen in Parkinson disease, medication exposure, and infections, which affect the basal ganglia. Thus, neuroimaging is warranted as well as a thorough history of medication intake. Because childhood rigidity is often associated with juvenile Parkinson disease, other Parkinsonian signs may be seen such as bradykinesia, tremor, flexed posture, and unsteady gait. Drug-induced Parkinsonism may also be seen in the context of dopamine-receptor blocking agents such as antipsychotics and antiemetics.

Encephalitic Movement Disorders

Encephalitis has long been associated with a variety of movement disorders—both hyperkinetic and hypokinetic. This includes spasticity, Parkinsonism, dystonia, myoclonus, and ataxia. Although not always present, a distinguishing feature of encephalitic movement disorders can be oculogyric crisis, in which eyes are tonically deviated to one side. Encephalitic movement disorders may occur acutely, subacutely, or chronically. It is important to distinguish such movements from seizures, and thus an EEG is useful. Such movement disorders can be treated empirically, and may or may not be associated with MRI lesions (Figure 19–3). In the setting of HIV infection, a movement disorder may indicate an opportunistic infection or lymphoma of the central nervous system.

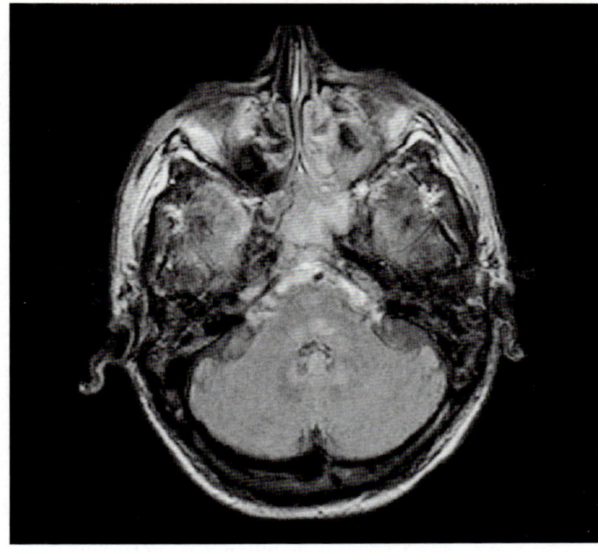

FIGURE 19–3 ■ A T2-weighted image of the brainstem demonstrating encephalitis (increased signal around the fourth ventricle). This patient developed tremor in all four limbs and myoclonus of the tongue. West Nile virus was detected in the cerebrospinal fluid.

TREATMENT

Most movement disorders are treatable. Treatment of secondary causes such as infection, autoimmunity, medication side effect, tumor, or metabolic derangement may very well lead to resolution of the movement disorder. If a primary movement disorder is diagnosed, empiric symptomatic treatment can be effective (Table 19–6). Treatment should focus on functional improvement to allow for growth and development, rather than complete resolution of movement disorder per se.

Spasticity may improve with a combination of physical therapy and muscle relaxants such as baclofen, clonidine, tizanidine, or dantroline. Focal treatment of spasticity with botulinum toxin injections can be quite effective, though careful selection of injection sites and dose are essential to avoid excessive weakness. Avoidance of contracture formation is also important. These musculoskeletal changes require surgical lengthening rather than reduction in muscle tone to improve range of motion. Intrathecal baclofen for more widespread spasticity, especially in the lower extremities may be effective.

Almost all cases of dystonia should undergo a trial of carbidopa/levodopa, in case it is a form of dopa-responsive dystonia. If this does not work, trihexyphenidyl initiated at low doses and gradually increased over the course of several weeks to months may be effective. Other muscle relaxants such as those listed above for spasticity may also be effective. Where available, dopamine-depleting medication such as tetrabenazine or reserpine may be effective, especially for tardive dyskinesia. Benzodiazepines may alleviate some dystonic symptoms, and for more focal cases, botulinum toxin injections can be very effective. Deep-brain stimulation of the globus pallidus interna has also been effective in carefully selected cases.

Often chorea, ballismus, and athetosis resolve if the underlying etiology is treated. If it persists or other nontreatable etiologies are suspected, leviteracitam, peracitam, clonazepam, valproate, tetrabenazine or reserpine can be effective. Dopamine-receptor blockers may be effective but should be avoided because of the risk of inducing tardive dyskinesia or Parkinsonism.

Myoclonus can respond to antiepileptics despite not being associated with seizure activity on EEG. Clonazepam, valproate, leviteracitam, and other antiepileptics may be tried. Potential secondary causes such as metabolic derangements and medication side effects should first be addressed.

Tic disorders naturally wax and wane, and thus it is difficult to know definitively if a particular medication is effective. Not all tics are pathologic and only tics, which confer a negative impact in a child's life socially, physically, academically, or psychologically need treatment. A multidisciplinary approach with behavioral therapy such as habit-reversal training may be helpful. Also, addressing comorbidities of attention-deficit disorder and obsessive–compulsive disorder can minimize the impact of tics. Medications that may be effective for tics include clonidine, clonazepam, and pimozide. Because of concerns of tardive dyskinesia, some consider neuroleptics such as pimozide only in severe cases refractory to other treatment. As tics spontaneously fluctuate, it is important to titrate medication based on symptomatology.

Tremor is treated by evaluation for secondary causes or based upon the type of tremor. Action, kinetic, or postural tremor that is seen in essential or familial tremor can be treated with either propranolol or primidone. Second-line treatments include topiramate, gabapentin, and benzodiazepines. Use of wrist or ankle weights may dampen the tremor. If a rest tremor is seen, then dopamine agonists or carbidopa/levodopa may be tried. In severe cases of action or rest tremor, deep-brain stimulation may be quite effective though experience in children is limited.

Ataxia may be treatable if an underlying etiology is found such as infection, autoimmunity, neoplasm, or migraine. Unfortunately, primary ataxias do not have any proven effective treatment, though physical therapy may prevent falls and allow greater independence. Rigidity, like rest tremor, may respond to dopaminergic therapy.

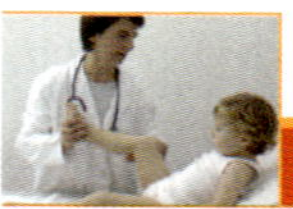

Table 19–6.

Symptomatic Treatment for Pediatric Movement Disorders

Movement Disorder	Treatment
Spasticity	Baclofen, clonidine, tizanidine, dantroline, BTX, ITB, PT
Dystonia	Carbidopa/levodopa, trihexyphenidyl, tetrabenazine, benzodiazepenes, BTX, DBS, PT
Chorea, ballismus, athetosis	Leviteracitam, peracitam, clonazepam, valproate, tetrabenazine, dopamine-receptor blockers
Myoclonus	Clonazepam, valproate, leviteracitam
Tics	Clonidine, clonazepam, pimozide, behavioral therapy
Tremor	Propranolol, primidone, topiramate, gabapentin, benzodiazepines, weights, carbidopa/levodopa, DBS
Ataxia	PT
Rigidity, bradykinesia, resting tremor	Carbidopa/levodopa, dopamine agonists, trihexyphenidyl

BTX, botulinum toxin injections; ITB, intrathecal baclofen; PT, physical therapy; DBS, deep-brain stimulation.

REFERENCES

1. Delgado MR, Albright AL. Movement disorders in children: definitions, classifications, and grading systems. *J Child Neurol.* 2003;18(suppl 1):S1-S8.
2. Chiriboga CA, De Vivo D, Percy A. Pediatric neurology: congenital infections. *Continuum.* 2000;4:52-93.
3. Pavone P, Parano E, Rizzo R, Trifiletti RR. Autoimmune neuropsychiatric disorders associated with streptococcal infection: sydenham chorea, PANDAS, and PANDAS variants. *J Child Neurol.* 2006;21(9):727-736.
4. Sawaishi Y, Takada G. Acute cerebellitis. *Cerebellum.* 2002;1(3):223-228.
5. Sanger TD, Delgado MR, Gaebler-Spira D, Hallett M, Mink JW. Classification and definition of disorders causing hypertonia in childhood. *Pediatrics.* 2003;111(1): e89-e97.
6. Battiata AP, Pazos G. Grisel's syndrome: the two-hit hypothesis–a case report and literature review. *Ear Nose Throat J.* 2004;83(8):553-555.
7. Nucci P, Kushner BJ, Serafino M, Orzalesi N. A multi-disciplinary study of the ocular, orthopedic, and neurologic causes of abnormal head postures in children. *Am J Ophthalmol.* 2005;140(1):65-68.
8. First MB, ed. *Diagnostic and Statistical Manual—Text Revision.* Washington, DC: American Psychiatric Association; 2000.
9. Shiihara T, Kato M, Konno A, Takahashi Y, Hayasaka K. Acute cerebellar ataxia and consecutive cerebellitis produced by glutamate receptor delta2 autoantibody. *Brain Dev.* 2007;29(4):254-256.
10. Tate ED, Allison TJ, Pranzatelli MR, Verhulst SJ. Neuroepidemiologic trends in 105 US cases of pediatric opsoclonus-myoclonus syndrome. *J Pediatr Oncol Nurs.* 2005;22(1):8-19.

SECTION 4

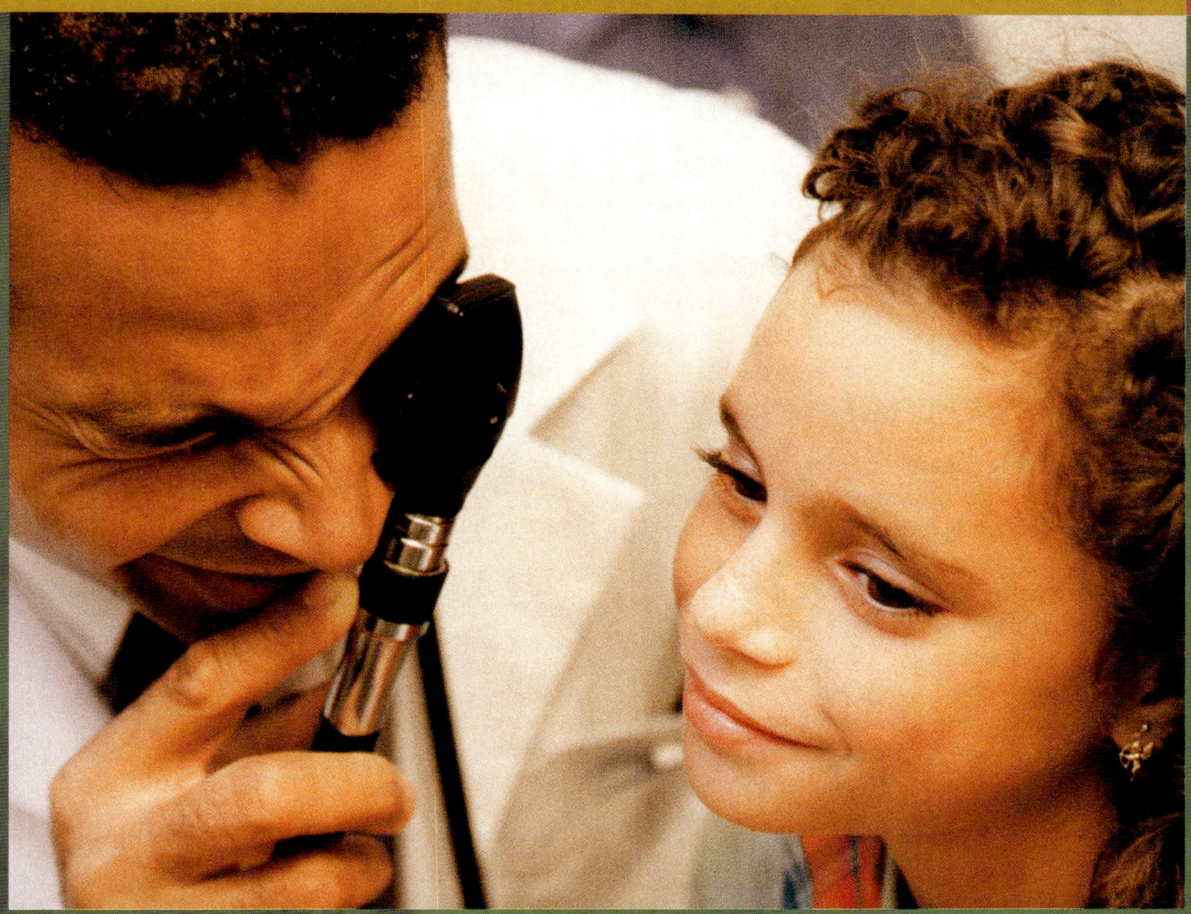

Ophthalmologic Infections

CHAPTER 20

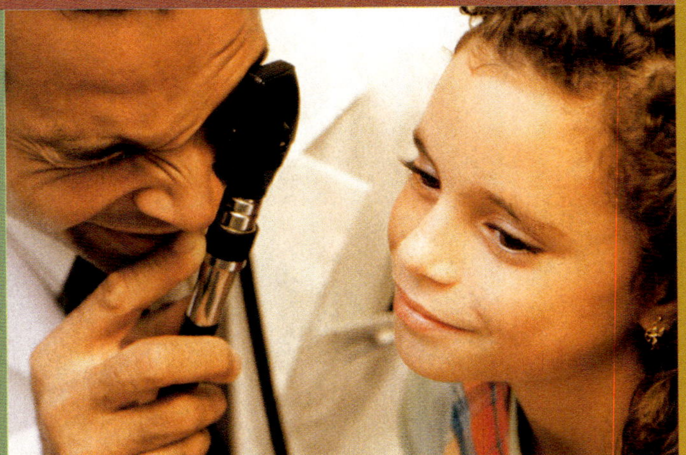

Conjunctivitis in the Neonate

Margaret R. Hammerschlag and Joseph Sleiman

DEFINITIONS AND EPIDEMIOLOGY

Neonatal conjunctivitis (ophthalmia neonatorum or neonatal blennorrhea) is a conjunctivitis that occurs in the first 4 weeks of life. It is the most common ocular disease of newborns, occurring in 1.6–12% of neonates. Neonatal conjunctivitis has been associated with a wide variety of organisms, which have varied in their relative importance over time and geographic location (Table 20–1). The introduction of neonatal ocular prophylaxis and the introduction of routine screening and treatment of pregnant women for gonorrhea and, more recently, *Chlamydia trachomatis* infection have altered the epidemiology of ophthalmia neonatorum in the United States.[3,4] In the nineteenth century, gonococcal ophthalmia was an important cause of blindness in infants; today, it is relatively uncommon in industrialized nations, although it remains a serious problem in many developing countries.[1,5–8] Before the introduction of systematic screening and treatment of *C. trachomatis* infection in pregnant women in the 1990s, *C. trachomatis* was the most frequent identifiable infectious cause of neonatal conjunctivitis in the United States.[3] Screening and treatment of pregnant women have resulted in a dramatic decrease in perinatal chlamydial infections. However, in countries where pregnant women are not routinely screened, including the Netherlands and many developing countries, *C. trachomatis* still remains the most frequent cause of neonatal conjunctivitis.[2,5]

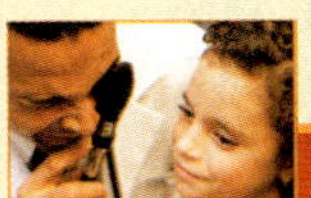

Table 20–1.

Infectious Causes of Neonatal Conjunctivitis

Organism	Prevalence (%)
Bacterial	
S. pneumoniae	0.6–7
H. influenzae	0–17
Viridans streptococci (*S. mitis* and *S. sanguis*)	5.3–17
N. gonorrhoeae	0–3.6*
C. trachomatis	0–23†
Viral	
Herpes simplex virus	<0.1

**3.6% reported from Kenya, with 42% rate of transmission from mother to infant.[1]*
†23% reported from Rotterdam.[2]

Neisseria Gonorrhoeae

The main population at risk of gonococcal conjunctivitis is neonates born to mothers with vaginal infection. The transmission rate in neonates born to infected mothers who have not received ocular prophylaxis may be as high as 42%.[1] Neonatal gonococcal ophthalmia (Figure 20–1) may cause primary disease at other mucous membrane sites or systemic disease. Gonococcal conjunctivitis in the newborn usually produces an acute purulent conjunctivitis that appears from 2 to 7 days after birth, although presentations during the second week of life are commonly described. Presentation may be earlier if there has been premature rupture of membranes, but the initial course may, occasionally, be indolent, with onset occurring later than 5 days after birth. Permanent corneal damage following gonococcal ophthalmia neonatorum was usual in the preantibiotic era.[3]

C. Trachomatis

C. trachomatis infection is acquired by the infant from his or her mother during parturition. This is based on a

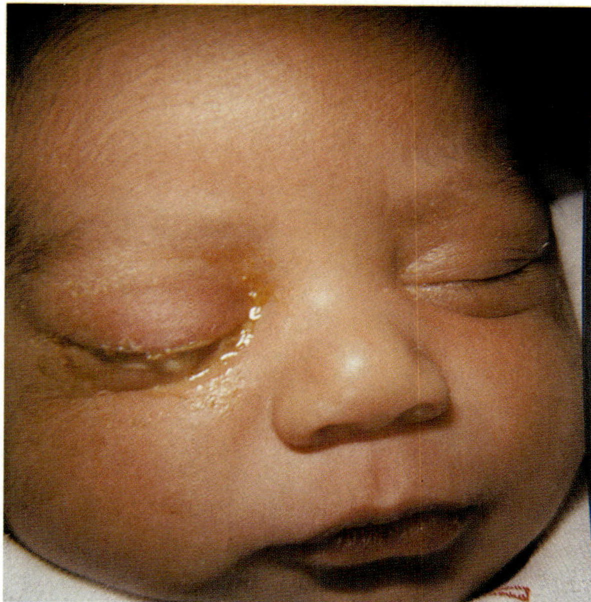

FIGURE 20–1 ■ Gonococcal ophthalmia. Profuse mulo-purulent discharge in a 5-day-old newborn. Note eryhtema and swelling of the LID. (Shah BR, Lucchesi M. *Atlas of Pediatric Emergency Medicine*, McGraw-Hill.)

number of well-controlled prospective studies of maternal–infant infection conducted in the 1970s and 1980s, where infection occurred only in those infants born to infected mothers.[3,9] Infection after cesarean delivery or through intact membranes is rare but may occur. In the former, there has usually been early rupture of the amnionic membranes. The overall risk of acquiring infection in an infant born to a mother with active chlamydial infection at any anatomical site has been approximately 50–75% in various studies.[9] Approximately one-half of infants with inclusion conjunctivitis will also be infected in the nasopharynx.[9,10] The incubation period of *C. trachomatis* conjunctivitis is 5–14 days after delivery; infection occurs earlier with premature rupture of membranes and onset as late as 60 days has been described.

Other Causes of Neonatal Conjunctivitis

Practically every known bacterial species has been implicated as a cause of ophthalmia neonatorum. Viruses, such as herpes simplex, may also cause ocular infection in neonates but is relatively uncommon. Infection is thought to occur during passage through the birth canal. A major problem in interpretation of the role of any specific bacteria is that many of these organisms are also frequently isolated from the conjunctivae of infants without conjunctivitis.

Bacteria implicated as causes of ophthalmia neonatorum include those commonly responsible for bacterial conjunctivitis in older children such as *Streptococcus pneumoniae* and *Haemophilus influenzae*. The prevalence of *S. pneumoniae* and *H. influenzae* in infants with neonatal conjunctivitis has been reported to range from 0% to 10% and 0% to 17%, respectively, compared with only 0% to <1% of infants without conjunctivitis.[3] Viridans streptococci, including *Streptococcus mitis* and *Streptococcus sanguis*, have been isolated from up to 16% of infants with conjunctivitis, but were also isolated from up to 5% of normal infants.[11]

Various gram-negative enteric rods, including *Escherichia coli*, *Klebsiella* species, and, rarely, *Pseudomonas* species have also been associated with neonatal conjunctivitis, usually in infants in intensive care. *Pseudomonas* conjunctivitis may progress to corneal ulceration and perforation and endophthalmitis. It can also disseminate systemically causing bacteremia and meningitis even in the absence of corneal perforation.[12–14]

The role of *Staphylococcus aureus* in neonatal conjunctivitis is controversial. Although the organism can be isolated from the conjunctivae of 8–46% of infants with conjunctivitis, it has also been isolated from the conjunctivae of 3–10% of age-matched infants without conjunctivitis.[3] Other organisms that are infrequent causes of neonatal conjunctivitis are *moranella catarrhalis* and *Neisseria* species including *Neisseria cinerea* and *N. meningitidis*. As these organisms are gram-negative diplococci, there is potential for confusion with *N. gonorrhoeae* if appropriate culture methods are not used.[15,16]

PATHOGENESIS

The conjunctiva is a loose connective tissue that covers the surface of the eye (bulbar conjunctiva) and forms the inner layer of the eyelids (palpebral conjunctiva). It is adherent to the underlying sclera at the limbus (corneal margin). It also contains numerous goblet cells, which secrete the mucinous layer of the tear film. Conjunctivitis is characterized by dilatation of the superficial conjunctival blood vessels, resulting in hyperemia and edema of the conjunctiva, with discharge. Fluid may accumulate beneath the loosely attached bulbar conjunctiva, causing it to swell away from the globe making eye closure difficult (chemosis), which can be seen in neonatal conjunctivitis caused by *C. trachomatis* and other bacteria.

CLINICAL PRESENTATION

The age at onset may suggest a specific etiology of conjunctivitis; however, there is substantial overlap among the various causes (Table 20–2).[14,17–20]

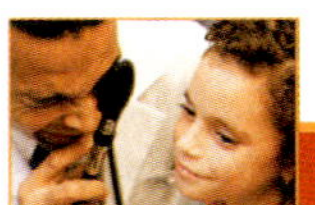

Table 20–2.

Age at Onset of Ophthalmia Neonatorum

Organism	Typical Age at Onset
Chemical conjunctivitis*	6–24 hours
H. influenzae	2–4 days
N. gonorrhoeae	2–7 days
C. trachomatis	3–14 days
Herpes simplex virus	6–14 days
P. aeruginosa†	14–20 days

*Most common with 1% silver nitrate, which is now rarely used in the United States.
†Typically affects hospitalized, premature neonates.

N. Gonorrhoeae

The infant typically develops tense edema of both lids, followed by chemosis and a progressively purulent and profuse conjunctival exudate, which literally pours or squirts out of the lids when they are separated. If treatment is delayed, the infection extends beyond the superficial epithelial layers, reaching the subconjunctival connective tissue of the palpebral conjunctivae and, more significantly, the cornea. Corneal complications include ulcerations, which may leave permanent nebulae or cause perforation and lead to anterior synechiae, panophthalmitis (rarely), and loss of the eye.

C. Trachomatis

The presentation of *C. trachomatis* conjunctivitis is variable, ranging from mild conjunctivitis with scant mucoid discharge to severe conjunctivitis with copious purulent discharge, chemosis, and pseudomembrane formation. The conjunctiva can be very friable (Figure 20–2) and may bleed when stroked with a swab.[21] Eyelid erythema and edema are frequently present. A Gram-stained conjunctival smear may initially reveal a neutrophil predominance. There can be overlap in both incubation periods and presentation. Bilateral infections are present in two-thirds of cases. A follicular reaction is not seen because infants younger than 3 months do not have the requisite lymphoid tissue present in the conjunctiva. Although uncommon, chlamydial neonatal conjunctivitis may result in long-term sequelae, including corneal neovascularization and scarring.

Conjunctivitis Caused By Gram-Negative Enteric Bacteria

Infection from these organisms presents as an acute purulent conjunctivitis in an infant in an intensive care setting. *Pseudomonas* conjunctivitis may progress to corneal ulceration and perforation and endophthalmitis. *Pseudomonas aeruginosa* can also disseminate systemically, causing bacteremia and meningitis, even in the absence of corneal perforation.[12–14]

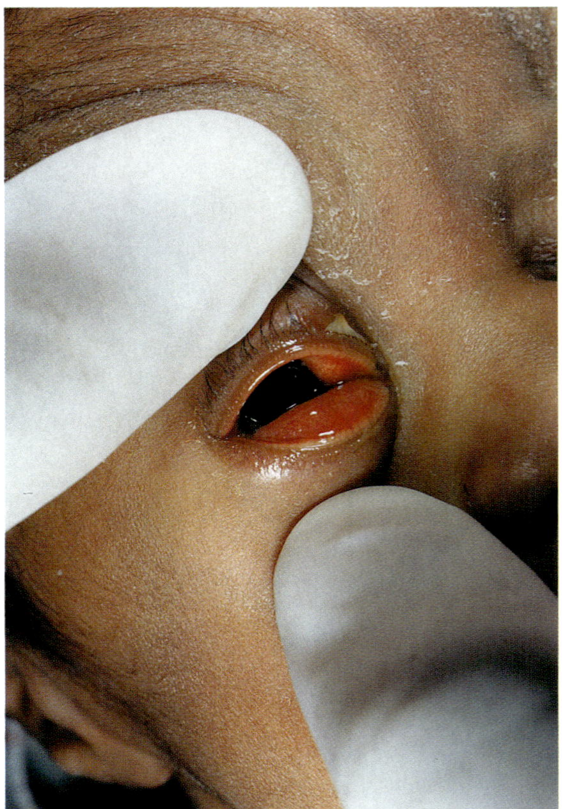

FIGURE 20–2 ■ Chlamydial conjunctivitis. Note intense hyperemia of the palpebral conjunctiva. The mucosa is very friable and may bleed when swabbed. (Shah BR, Lucchesi M. *Atlas of Pediatric Emergency Medicine*, McGraw-Hill.)

Chemical Conjunctivitis

While 1% silver nitrate is no longer manufactured or used in the United States, it is still used in many parts of the world and is associated with a mild chemical conjunctivitis, which can be easily distinguished from gonococcal conjunctivitis. Evidence of epithelial desquamation and polymorphonuclear leukocytic exudate appears usually within 6–8 hours and disappears usually within 24–48 hours.

DIFFERENTIAL DIAGNOSIS

In neonates, conjunctivitis is almost always from infection. Common infecting organisms are summarized in Table 20–1.

DIAGNOSIS

It is difficult to make an etiologic diagnosis of neonatal conjunctivitis on clinical grounds alone. There can be significant overlap in both incubation period and clinical findings. Conjunctival exudate can be directly examined by Gram stain for the presence of gram-negative intracellular bean-shaped diplococci suggestive (but not definitive) of *N. gonorrhoeae*, as other *Neisseria* spp. have also been associated with purulent ophthalmia neonatorum, as stated above. If infection with *N. gonorrhoeae* is suspected because of maternal risk factors, the diagnosis should be confirmed by culture and antibiotic susceptibility testing should be performed. Cultures for *N. gonorrhoeae* should also be obtained from the oropharynx and anal canal, since concomitant infection of these sites has been demonstrated in association with gonococcal ophthalmia neonatorum. None of the currently available nucleic acid amplification tests (NAATs) for *N. gonorrhoeae* have been evaluated or have FDA approval for use in any specimens from children including the conjunctiva.[4] Two assays, polymerase chain reaction (PCR) (Amplicor, Roche Molecular Diagnostics, Nutley, NJ) and strand displacement amplification (ProbeTec, Becton Dickson, Sparks, MD), have been reported to cross-react with other *Neisseria* species, including *N. cinerea*, *N. lactamica*, *N. sicca*, and *N. subflava*.[22] For this reason, only culture should be used for diagnosis of gonococcal conjunctivitis in infants and children.

The "gold standard" for diagnosis of *C. trachomatis* infections in infants and children remains isolation by culture of *C. trachomatis* from the conjunctiva, nasopharynx, vagina, or rectum. *C. trachomatis* culture has been defined further by the Centers for Disease Control and Prevention (CDC) as isolation of the organism in tissue culture and confirmation by microscopic identification of the characteristic inclusions, preferably by staining with a fluorescein-conjugated species-specific monoclonal antibody.[4] Several nonculture tests are approved for diagnosis of chlamydial conjunctivitis in infants, specifically enzyme immunoassays (EIAs), and direct fluorescent-antibody tests (DFAs). The only EIA and DFA assays still available in the United States are Pathfinder® Chlamydia DFA and EIA Microplate (Bio-Rad Laboratories). These tests appear to perform well with conjunctival specimens with sensitivities 90% or more and specificities 95% or more compared with culture.[3] There are currently three FDA-approved, commercially available NAATs for diagnosis of *C. trachomatis* infection: PCR (Amplicor, Roche Molecular Diagnostics, Nutley, NJ), strand displacement amplification (ProbeTec, Becton Dickson, Sparks, MD), and transcription-mediated amplification (GenProbe, San Diego, CA). These assays all have FDA approval for cervical swabs from women, urethral swabs from men, and urine from men and women.[4] Data suggest that PCR is equivalent to culture for detection of *C. trachomatis* in the conjunctiva and nasopharynx of infants with conjunctivitis; however, PCR and other NAATs do not have FDA approval for use with conjunctival specimens.[23] The identification of *C. trachomatis* and/or *N. gonorrhoeae* in a newborn infant indicates untreated infection in the parents.

INDICATIONS FOR SUBSPECIALTY REFERRAL

The patient should be referred to a subspecialist in certain cases of neonatal conjunctivitis including, but not limited to,

1. gonococcal conjunctivitis because of the potential complications;
2. suspicion or documentation of herpetic keratoconjunctivitis;
3. progression of disease despite adequate treatment;
4. lack of improvement of symptoms despite alteration of therapy;
5. development of complications during treatment, i.e., corneal perforation and endophthalmitis in infants with infections from *P. aeruginosa* or other gram-negative bacilli.

TREATMENT

The currently recommended therapy for neonatal gonococcal conjunctivitis by both the CDC and the WHO is ceftriaxone, 25–50 mg/kg IV or IM in a single dose, not to exceed 125 mg.[4] The infant should be hospitalized until the conjunctivitis has resolved, which usually occurs within 24–48 hours after treatment with ceftriaxone. Topical antimicrobial therapy is not beneficial in the presence of systemic treatment. Alternatives for the treatment of gonococcal conjunctivitis when ceftriaxone is not available are cefotaxime 25 mg/kg IM in a single dose or kanamycin 25 mg/kg (maximum 75 mg) IM in a single dose. Infants born to mothers with untreated gonorrhea at the time of delivery are at high risk of infection and should receive ceftriaxone, 25–50 mg/kg IV or IM in a single dose, not to exceed 125 mg.[4]

Oral erythromycin suspension (ethylsuccinate or stearate) (50 mg/kg/d for 14 days) is the therapy of choice for the treatment of chlamydial conjunctivitis in infants.[4] It provides better and faster resolution of the conjunctivitis as well as treats any concurrent nasopharyngeal infection. Additional topical therapy is not needed. The efficacy of this regimen has been reported to range from 80% to 90%; as many as 20% of infants may require another course of therapy.[3] Treatment with oral erythromycin has been associated with infantile hypertrophic pyloric stenosis in infants younger than 6 weeks who were given the drug for prophylaxis after nursery exposure to pertussis.[24] Data on use of other macrolides, including azithromycin or clarithromycin, for the treatment of neonatal *Chlamydia* infection are limited. There is one small study that evaluated azithromycin: It found that a short course of azithromycin suspension, 20 mg/kg/day orally, one dose daily for 3 days, was as effective as 2 weeks of erythromycin in eradication of *C. trachomatis* from the conjunctivae and nasopharynx of infants with conjunctivitis.[25] Prophylactic treatment of infants born to women with untreated chlamydial infection is not recommended, as optimum dosing and duration of treatment are not known.

Data on treatment of neonatal conjunctivitis caused by other bacteria are limited. Considering the wide range of organisms, it is difficult to treat presumptively. Once gonococcal and chlamydial infections have been ruled out, one can follow the recommendations proposed for conjunctivitis in older children. Neonatal conjunctivitis caused by *Pseudomonas* and other gram-negative bacteria should be treated with systemic antibiotics. Choices for presumptive treatment should be based on the susceptibility patterns for these organisms in your institution and should include an aminoglycoside (gentamicin, tobramycin, or amikacin) and an expanded spectrum penicillin (ticarcillin–sulbactam, piperacillin–tazobactam, imipenem, or meropenem). Final choice of antibiotics results should be based on susceptibility testing of the isolate.

COURSE AND PROGNOSIS

Neonatal conjunctivitis from bacteria such as viridans streptococci, *H. influenzae*, and *S. pneumoniae* is usually self-limited and will often resolve without specific treatment. Neonatal conjunctivitis from gram-negative bacteria including *P. aeruginosa* is potentially very serious and needs to be treated aggressively with appropriate systemic antibiotics, as described above.

Untreated neonatal gonococcal ophthalmia can lead to corneal complications including ulcerations that may leave permanent nebulae or cause perforation and lead to anterior synechiae, panophthalmitis (rarely), and loss of the eye. However, single-dose treatment with ceftriaxone is highly effective. Neonatal conjunctivitis caused by *C. trachomatis* may rarely result in long-term sequelae, including corneal neovascularization and scarring. Treatment with oral antibiotics significantly shortens the duration of symptoms and eradication of concurrent nasopharyngeal infection, which could progress to pneumonia. Herpes simplex virus (HSV) is a very rare cause of neonatal conjunctivitis. Infants with suspected HSV conjunctivitis should be hospitalized, evaluated for systemic HSV infection, and treated with parenteral acyclovir.

REFERENCES

1. Laga M, Plummer FA, Nzanze H, et al. Epidemiology of ophthalmia neonatorum in Kenya. *Lancet.* 1986;2(8516): 1145-1149.
2. Rours IG, Hammerschlag MR, Ott A, De Faber TJ, Verbrugh HA, de Groot R, Verkooyen RP. *Chlamydia trachomatis* as a Cause of Neonatal Conjunctivitis in Dutch Infants. *Pediatrics* 2008;121(2): e321-e326.
3. Hammerschlag MR. Neonatal conjunctivitis. *Pediatr Ann.* 1993;22(6):346-351.
4. Workowski KA, Berman SM. Sexually transmitted diseases treatment guidelines, 2006. *MMWR Recomm Rep.* 2006;55(RR-11):1-94.
5. Di Bartolomeo S, Mirta DH, Janer M, et al. Incidence of *Chlamydia trachomatis* and other potential pathogens in neonatal conjunctivitis. *Int J Infect Dis.* 2001;5(3): 139-143.
6. Dunn PM. Dr Carl Crede (1819–1892) and the prevention of ophthalmia neonatorum. *Arch Dis Child Fetal Neonatal Ed.* 2000;83(2):F158-F159.
7. Fransen L, Klauss V. Neonatal ophthalmia in the developing world. Epidemiology, etiology, management and control. *Int Ophthalmol.* 1988;11(3):189-196.
8. Mohile M, Deorari AK, Satpathy G, Sharma A, Singh M. Microbiological study of neonatal conjunctivitis with special reference to *Chlamydia trachomatis. Indian J Ophthalmol.* 2002;50(4):295-299.
9. Darville T. *Chlamydia trachomatis* infections in neonates and young children. *Semin Pediatr Infect Dis.* 2005;16(4): 235-244.
10. Hammerschlag MR, Chandler JW, Alexander ER, English M, Koutsky L. Longitudinal studies on chlamydial infections in the first year of life. *Pediatr Infect Dis.* 1982;1(6): 395-401.
11. Krohn MA, Hillier SL, Bell TA, Kronmal RA, Grayston JT. The bacterial etiology of conjunctivitis in early infancy. Eye Prophylaxis Study Group. *Am J Epidemiol.* 1993; 138(5):326-332.
12. Shah SS, Gloor P, Gallagher PG. Bacteremia, meningitis, and brain abscesses in a hospitalized infant: complications of *Pseudomonas aeruginosa* conjunctivitis. *J Perinatol.* 1999;19(6, pt 1):462-465.
13. Traboulsi EI, Shammas IV, Ratl HE, Jarudi NI. *Pseudomonas aeruginosa* ophthalmia neonatorum. *Am J Ophthalmol.* 1984;98(6):801-802.
14. Shah SS, Gallagher PG. Complications of conjunctivitis caused by *Pseudomonas aeruginosa* in a newborn intensive care unit. *Pediatr Infect Dis J.* 1998;17(2):97-102.
15. Denison MR, Perlman S, Andersen RD. Misidentification of *Neisseria* species in a neonate with conjunctivitis. *Pediatrics.* 1988;81(6):877-878.
16. Whittington WL, Rice RJ, Biddle JW, Knapp JS. Incorrect identification of *Neisseria gonorrhoeae* from infants and children. *Pediatr Infect Dis J.* 1988;7(1):3-10.
17. Armstrong JH, Zacarias F, Rein MF. Ophthalmia neonatorum: a chart review. *Pediatrics.* 1976;57(6):884-892.
18. Fransen L, Nsanze H, Klauss V, et al. Ophthalmia neonatorum in Nairobi, Kenya: the roles of *Neisseria gonorrhoeae* and *Chlamydia trachomatis. J Infect Dis.* 1986; 153(5):862-869.

19. Pierog S, Nigam S, Marasigan DC, Dube SK. Gonococcal ophthalmia neonatorum. Relationship of maternal factors and delivery room practices to effective control measures. *Am J Obstet Gynecol.* 1975;122(5):589-592.
20. Rusin P, Adam RD, Peterson EA, Ryan KJ, Sinclair NA, Weinstein L. *Haemophilus influenzae*: an important cause of maternal and neonatal infections. *Obstet Gynecol.* 1991;77(1):92-96.
21. Chang K, Cheng VY, Kwong NS. Neonatal haemorrhagic conjunctivitis: a specific sign of chlamydial infection. *Hong Kong Med J.* 2006;12(1):27-32.
22. Whiley DM, Tapsall JW, Sloots TP. Nucleic acid amplification testing for *Neisseria gonorrhoeae*: an ongoing challenge. *J Mol Diagn.* 2006;8(1):3-15.
23. Hammerschlag MR, Roblin PM, Gelling M, Tsumura N, Jule JE, Kutlin A. Use of polymerase chain reaction for the detection of *Chlamydia trachomatis* in ocular and nasopharyngeal specimens from infants with conjunctivitis. *Pediatr Infect Dis J.* 1997;16(3):293-297.
24. Honein MA, Paulozzi LJ, Himelright IM, et al. Infantile hypertrophic pyloric stenosis after pertussis prophylaxis with erythromycin: a case review and cohort study. *Lancet.* 1999;354(9196):2101-2105.
25. Hammerschlag MR, Gelling M, Roblin PM, Kutlin A, Jule JE. Treatment of neonatal chlamydial conjunctivitis with azithromycin. *Pediatr Infect Dis J.* 1998;17(11):1049-1050.

CHAPTER 21

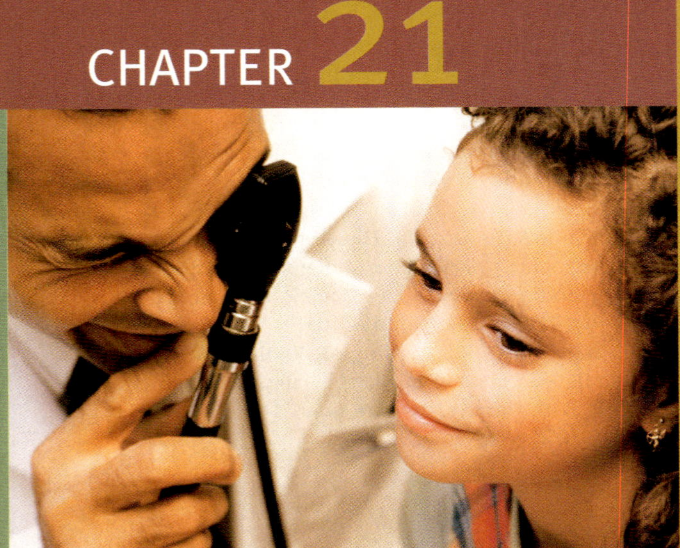

Conjunctivitis in the Older Child

Joseph Sleiman and Margaret R. Hammerschlag

DEFINITIONS AND EPIDEMIOLOGY

Conjunctivitis, commonly referred to as "red eye" or "pink eye," is a nonspecific term used to describe an inflammation of the conjunctiva, which can be caused by a wide range of conditions. The conjunctivae are the mucous membranes extending from the eyelid margin to the corneal limbus, forming the posterior layer of the eyelids and the anterior layer of the eyeball. Conjunctivitis may result from primary involvement of the conjunctival tissue or may occur as a secondary manifestation of other ocular or systemic conditions that produce conjunctival inflammation.

Conjunctivitis is prevalent worldwide. It is the most common ocular infection in childhood, usually affecting children younger than 6 years, with a peak incidence between 12 and 36 months.[1] Infectious causes of conjunctivitis may be sporadic or related to epidemic outbreaks. In most cases, conjunctivitis is benign and self-limited.

PATHOGENESIS

The conjunctiva is a loose connective tissue that covers the surface of the eye (bulbar conjunctiva) and forms the inner layer of the eyelids (palpebral conjunctiva). It is adherent to the underlying sclera at the limbus (corneal margin). It also contains numerous goblet cells, which secrete the mucinous layer of the tear film. Conjunctivitis is characterized by dilatation of the superficial conjunctival blood vessels, resulting in hyperemia and edema of the conjunctiva, with discharge. Fluid may accumulate beneath the loosely attached bulbar conjunctiva, causing it to swell away from the globe, making eye closure difficult (a phenomenon known as chemosis).

CLINICAL PRESENTATION

Patient History

The diversity of etiologies for conjunctivitis makes a detailed patient history the most important step in the differential diagnosis of conjunctivitis. The patient history should include the chief complaint such as itching, burning, tearing, discharge, pain, foreign body sensation, and photophobia. It should also include questions about the onset and course of the disease, whether it is acute or chronic and progressive or stationary. The ocular history should include questions about previous episodes, prior exposure to infected individuals, history of trauma or contact lens wear, and the use of topical legend (i.e., prescription) or over-the-counter medications or cosmetics. The general health history should include descriptions of recent upper respiratory tract infections, autoimmune disorders, atopy, skin conditions, and sexually transmitted infections. Finally, the social history such as environmental exposure and the family history of ocular diseases may contribute to the diagnosis of "red eye."

The signs and symptoms of conjunctivitis, including redness, tearing or discharge, and foreign body sensation, are similar regardless of the cause. Pain and photophobia are not symptoms of conjunctivitis; if present, they may indicate other entities, including corneal abrasion, keratitis, uveitis, or acute angle-closure glaucoma. Decreased vision is not typical in patients with conjunctivitis. Occasionally, extensive discharge may blur the visual axis intermittently, but, in general, a report of decreased acuity should prompt a search for more serious disorders.

Physical Examination

The ocular examination in a patient with conjunctivitis should include examination of the skin of the lids and the face, looking for any associated skin conditions, edema, ecchymosis, and discoloration. Certain signs and symptoms are important to consider in differentiating among the various causes of conjunctivitis. The character of the discharge may provide some diagnostic help. Serous or watery discharge usually is associated with viral or allergic etiologies. Mucopurulent discharge suggests a viral or chlamydial infection, whereas purulent discharge suggests a bacterial etiology. Close inspection of the conjunctiva may reveal follicles, suggestive of viral or chlamydial infections, or papillae, suggestive of bacterial or allergic processes. Follicles are elevations encircled by blood vessels, whereas papillae have a central vascular core.

It is also important to look for clues on physical examination, which suggest other causes of a "red eye." In general, the redness of conjunctivitis spares the limbus. If the limbus is involved, other diagnoses must be considered, including keratitis (inflammation of the cornea) and uveitis (intraocular inflammation). A comprehensive eye examination with dilation of the pupils should be performed in those patients with conjunctival hyperemia, accompanied by proptosis, optic nerve dysfunction, decreased visual acuity, diplopia, or evidence of anterior chamber inflammation.[2]

Manifestations of Common Causes of Conjunctivitis

The etiologies of conjunctivitis can be classified as infectious and noninfectious. Noninfectious causes may be primary in origin, e.g., allergic conjunctivitis, or secondary to other systemic diseases. Infectious conjunctivitis can be bacterial or viral in origin.

Bacterial conjunctivitis

Bacterial conjunctivitis (Figure 21–1) can be classified as hyperacute, acute, or chronic. It occurs when an organism is able to overcome the host's resistance, or following trauma. Most common bacterial pathogens can cause conjunctivitis. These pathogens include *Haemophilus* species (nontypable *H. influenzae*), *Streptococcus pneumoniae*, and *Moraxella* species. *S. pneumoniae* and *Haemophilus* infections occur more frequently in children.[3–5]

Symptoms of bacterial conjunctivitis typically include unilateral or bilateral conjunctival injection, purulent discharge, and matting of the eyelids. More

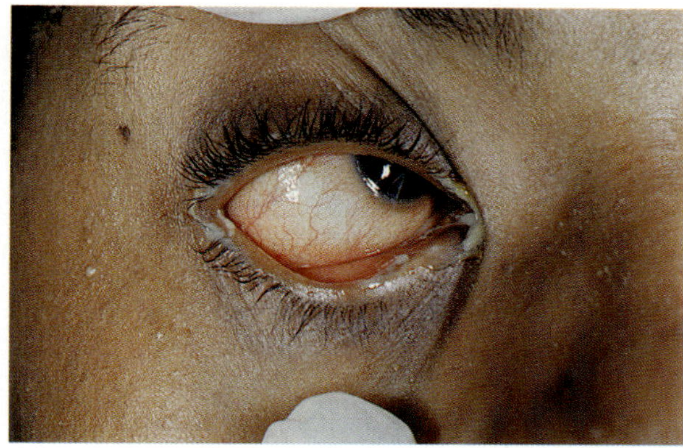

FIGURE 21–1 ■ Bacterial conjunctivitis. Note purulent discharge and conjunctival injection. (Shah BR, Lucchesi M. *Atlas of Pediatric Emergency Medicine*, McGraw-Hill.)

severe forms of bacterial conjunctivitis, as indicated by copious purulent discharge, suggest infection by more virulent organisms. These include *Neisseria gonorrhoeae*, *Neisseria meningitidis*, or *Pseudomonas aeruginosa*.

Acute or mucopurulent bacterial conjunctivitis is caused by a number of microbial agents, primarily *Staphylococcus aureus*, *S. pneumoniae*, and *Haemophilus* species. It is a common infectious condition that can affect all ages and races and both genders. This condition is usually self-limiting and generally lasts for <3 weeks. Atypical unencapsulated strains of *S. pneumoniae* are responsible for large outbreak of conjunctivitis in college campuses.[6]

Hyperacute or purulent bacterial conjunctivitis is commonly caused by *N. gonorrhoeae*, microorganisms that can penetrate an intact corneal epithelium, or, less frequently, by *N. meningitidis*. Infection by *N. gonorrhoeae* is seen most often in neonates who acquire the disease via passage through an infected birth canal; this topic is discussed in Chapter 20.[7] However, this infection can also be contracted through sexual activity and may indicate that a child has been sexually active or has been sexually abused. This organism is highly virulent and may lead to corneal ulceration and perforation. Hyperacute bacterial conjunctivitis is most commonly acquired by autoinoculation from infected genitalia and most often seen in neonates, adolescents, and young adults. It appears to be more common during warmer months of the year.[8,9] A less common cause of bacterial conjunctivitis is *P. aeruginosa*, especially in hospitalized infants, which may lead to a rapidly progressive invasive infection with corneal perforation.[10,11]

When symptoms of bacterial conjunctivitis last longer than 4 weeks, it can be considered chronic. The most common cause of chronic bacterial conjunctivitis is *S. aureus*. Chronic bacterial conjunctivitis is frequently associated with continuous inoculation of bacteria associated with blepharitis (inflammation of the eyelids, particularly at the lid margins).[12]

An unusual cause of conjunctivitis is Lyme disease, which is caused by *Borrelia burgdorferi*. Conjunctivitis usually occurs early in the disease, is mild and transient, and may be followed by other ocular manifestations of Lyme disease including keratitis, vitritis, uveitis, neuroretinitis, optic atrophy, and Bell's palsy.[13]

Parinaud oculoglandular syndrome is an entity characterized by unilateral granulomatous conjunctivitis, ipsilateral tenderness, and enlargement of the preauricular lymph nodes. It is often caused by *Bartonella henselae*[14] and less commonly by *Francisella tularensis*[12,15] but may also be associated with other infections.

The conjunctivitis–otitis media syndrome, a distinctive clinical entity, is characterized by purulent conjunctivitis associated with acute otitis media. It was initially described by Coffey[16] in 1966 and further characterized by Bodor[17] in 1982. It begins with low-grade fevers and mild upper respiratory symptoms, followed several days later by eye discharge and pain, with the development of ear pain in some cases. Sometimes otitis media may be the initial presentation with subsequent development of purulent conjunctivitis. Nontypable strains of *H. influenzae* are responsible for more than 70% of cases of conjunctivitis–otitis syndrome.[18,19] The remaining cases are usually caused by either *S. pneumoniae* or *Moraxella* species.

Viral conjunctivitis

Adenoviruses, the most common viral cause of conjunctivitis, account for 20% of all cases of conjunctivitis.[20] Other viral causes of conjunctivitis include herpes simplex virus (HSV), varicella zoster virus, and enteroviruses including coxsackievirus.

Adenoviral conjunctivitis

Adenoviral conjunctivitis is extremely contagious; transmission typically is by direct contact with infected persons or contaminated objects or instruments such as tonometers used widely in eye clinics.[21] Adenovirus conjunctivitis (Figure 21–2) is characterized by acute onset of unilateral and then bilateral, bulbar, and palpebral conjunctival hyperemia and by the formation of follicles on the palpebral conjunctiva. Petechial hemorrhages are commonly present, particularly in the bulbar conjunctiva. Follicular conjunctivitis is the most common type of adenoviral conjunctivitis. Associated findings include watery discharge, rhinitis, and preauricular lymphadenopathy usually more prominent on the side of the initially affected eye.

Depending on the stage of development, conjunctival pseudomembranes may be found on the superior or inferior tarsal conjunctiva. Lid edema may also be present.

Adenovirus infections tend to be more common in the fall and winter. Patients often have symptoms of an upper respiratory infection and may have had recent contact with another person with either a red eye or an upper respiratory tract infection.

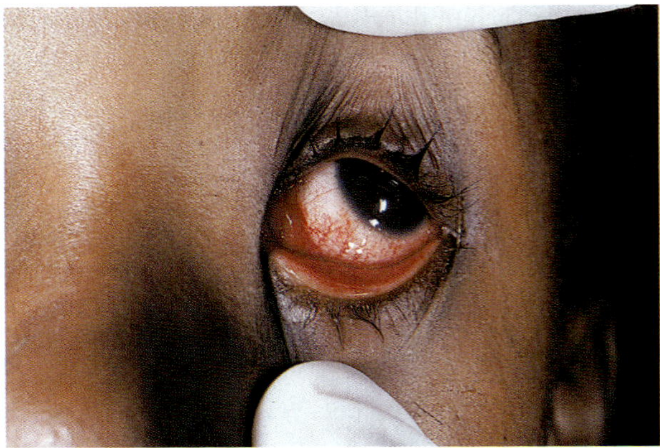

FIGURE 21–2 ■ Adenoviral conjunctivitis. Note intense bulbar and palpebral conjunctival injection and hemorrhages. (Shah BR, Lucchesi M. *Atlas of Pediatric Emergency Medicine*, McGraw-Hill.)

Other less common forms of adenoviral conjunctivitis include epidemic keratoconjunctivitis and pharyngoconjunctival fever. Epidemic keratoconjunctivitis is caused by adenoviral serotypes 8, 19, and 37.[22] Patients usually complain of severe discomfort, photophobia resulting from keratitis, and watery discharge. This form is very contagious and often occurs in epidemic outbreaks. Physical findings include injection, chemosis, follicular reaction, corneal superficial punctate defects, and eyelid edema. Corneal subepithelial infiltrates may begin to form after 2 weeks in the disease process and, if present, may last for as long as 2 years.

The third form of adenoviral conjunctivitis, the pharyngoconjunctival fever, is caused by adenoviral serotypes 3 and 7.[22] In addition to the conjunctival injection and chemosis, patients usually present with fever, pharyngitis, and preauricular lymphadenopathy. Symptoms may last for 2 weeks or more. Summertime epidemics of pharyngoconjunctival fever, linked to swimming in infected pools, have been reported.[5]

Herpetic conjunctivitis

Infection with a member of the *Herpesvirus* genus (e.g., herpes simplex, varicella zoster, or Epstein–Barr virus) can result in acute conjunctivitis. HSV conjunctivitis (Figure 21–3) may occur as either a primary or a secondary infection. Most ocular infections occur as result of HSV-1, except in neonates, in whom HSV-2 is more predominant. Transmission occurs by direct contact with another person who has an active lesion or by autoinoculation of the eye from skin lesions. Signs include a follicular conjunctival reaction, watery discharge, and preauricular lymphadenopathy. Other findings suggestive of herpes simplex infection include skin or lid vesicles, gingivostomatitis, and keratitis. Fifty

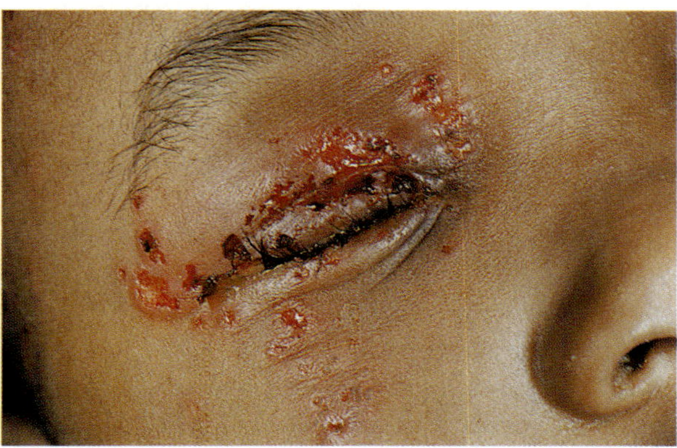

FIGURE 21–3 ■ HSV conjunctivitis. Note multiple vesicular lesions and ulcers around the eyelid margin and mucoid discharge. (Shah BR, Lucchesi M. *Atlas of Pediatric Emergency Medicine*, McGraw-Hill.)

percent of patients with herpes zoster ophthalmicus (involving the ophthalmic division of the trigeminal nerve) show involvement of the ocular structures, of which conjunctivitis is the most common manifestation.

Bulbar or palpebral conjunctivitis may occur during primary varicella zoster infection (chickenpox). The recurrence of varicella zoster infection in the distribution of the ophthalmic division of trigeminal nerve (cranial nerve V) is known as herpes zoster ophthalmicus. It involves the ocular structures, and conjunctivitis is a common manifestation of this disease. Signs and symptoms are similar to HSV infection and include conjunctival injection, follicular conjunctival reaction, vesicles, and watery discharge. Patients may also complain of pain in the cranial nerve V_1 distribution.

DIFFERENTIAL DIAGNOSIS

Causes of conjunctival inflammation in children include infectious conjunctivitis (e.g., viral, bacterial, and chlamydial), allergic conjunctivitis, blepharoconjunctivitis, trauma, foreign body, chemical reaction, and nasolacrimal duct obstruction.[2,23] The "red eye" can be the first manifestation of serious systemic disorders (Table 21–1).

Allergic conjunctivitis is mainly a hypersensitivity type I reaction mediated by IgE antibodies and involves mast cell degranulation and release of inflammatory mediators, which are responsible for the signs and symptoms present in patients with allergic conjunctivitis. This form of conjunctivitis is characterized by itching, tearing, redness, chemosis, and eyelid edema. Both eyes are usually involved, and symptoms may present seasonally. A history of other atopic diseases is frequently associated with allergic conjunctivitis.

Mechanical conjunctivitis can result from irritation of the conjunctival surface by eyelashes, sutures, and foreign bodies such as contact lenses. Conjunctivitis may also result from trauma following a direct injury that results in abrasions or lacerations. Finally, toxic conjunctivitis may occur following the administration of drugs or exposure to noxious chemicals and from overuse of eye drops, especially sulfonamide derivatives.

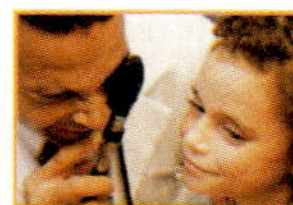

Table 21–1.

Differential Diagnosis of the Red Eye

- Conjunctivitis*
  - Bacterial (mucopurulent)
    - *H. influenzae*
    - *S. pneumoniae*
    - *S. aureus*
    - *Moraxella* species
  - Bacterial (hyperacute/purulent)
    - *N. gonorrhoeae*
    - *N. meningitidis*
    - *P. aeruginosa*
  - Other bacterial
    - *B. henselae*
    - *F. tularensis*
  - Viral
    - Adenovirus
    - Enteroviruses
    - Herpes simplex virus
    - Varicella zoster virus (herpes zoster ophthalmicus)
  - Other infectious causes
    - Loa loa
    - Onchocerca
    - Trichinella
  - Noninfectious causes
    - Giant papillary conjunctivitis (associated with contact lens wear)
    - Vernal conjunctivitis (recurrent, seasonal allergic conjunctivitis of unknown cause)
    - Systemic disease related†
- Subconjunctival hemorrhage
- Episcleritis
- Pterygium‡
- Acute angle-closure glaucoma
- Acute anterior uveitis
- Superficial keratitis
- Blepharitis
- Erythema multiforme or Stevens–Johnson syndrome
- Collagen-vascular diseases

**Only relatively common infectious causes shown.*
†Such as sarcoidosis, tuberculosis, Reiter syndrome, and Kawasaki disease.
‡A pterygium is a noninfectious, elevated, superficial, external ocular mass, which usually forms over the perilimbal conjunctiva and extends onto the corneal surface.

DIAGNOSIS

In addition to history taking, a detailed physical examination should be performed on patients with conjunctivitis. Testing of visual acuity, examination of the fundus, tonometry and biomicroscopic examination often aid in making the diagnosis and excluding other causes of conjunctivitis.

Most primary-care physicians treat conjunctivitis presumptively as bacterial in origin and do not order any diagnostic tests.[24,25] Conjunctival cultures and smears are helpful and should be considered in cases of treatment failure and for immunocompromised patients. Identification of the etiologic agent and determination of antibiotic sensitivities are essential for proper management, especially in cases of hyperacute, chronic, and recurrent conjunctivitis. If possible, cultures should be obtained prior to beginning treatment, which can help guide the selection of the initial treatment. Tympanocentesis, if indicated, may be helpful in cases of conjunctivitis–otitis syndrome because the culture of the ear exudate usually yields the causative organism.[18,19]

Conjunctival scrapings, if needed, are usually performed by a specialist. They provide a detailed examination of conjunctival epithelial cells and identification of intracellular inclusions and may also reveal the nature of the inflammatory cell response. Cell cultures can be used to diagnose viral conjunctivitis (i.e., HSV and adenovirus), but they are time consuming and not very practical in an outpatient setting. However, polymerase chain reaction using the proper primers shows an increased sensitivity over cell culture for the detection of adenoviruses in conjunctival swabs and provides results in a short time compared to cell cultures.[26]

MANAGEMENT

Clinicians nearly always treat acute conjunctivitis empirically with topical antimicrobial therapy. If the disease is mild or the patient has associated signs of upper respiratory infection, cultures are rarely obtained either because of expense or because culture results are reported days later. Social factors, including the need for children to attend day care or school and parents to go to work, the parents' desire to seek early treatment in response to their own beliefs, and advice from others that this is a contagious disease, contribute to the decision to prescribe antibiotics for children with acute infective conjunctivitis.[24,25]

TREATMENT

Bacterial Conjunctivitis

Ideally, the causative organism of bacterial conjunctivitis should be identified and effective antimicrobial treatment against the offending organism should be initiated. In the absence of a microbiological diagnosis, the etiologic agent should be considered in the context of the patient's age, environment, and related ocular findings, and the empiric treatment should be based on clinical evaluation.

Most cases of bacterial conjunctivitis are self-limited, but treatment with effective antibiotics can decrease the duration of the infection, alleviate the patient's symptoms, and reduce the chances of its recurrence compared with placebo. In randomized trials, subgroups of patients with culture-positive bacterial conjunctivitis have increased microbiological cure when treated with topical antibiotics compared with placebo.[27–29] Treatment usually consists of a broad-spectrum topical antibiotic administered four to eight times daily, depending on the type. This empirical approach is highly effective, with no major adverse consequences.[24] The available topical antibiotics have a broad spectrum of activity, including gram-positive as well as gram-negative bacteria. Topical antibiotic therapy with polymyxin–bacitracin shortens the duration of clinical disease and enhances eradication of the causative organism from the conjunctiva.[30,31] Commonly used topical antibiotics are summarized in Table 21–2.

Current Clinical Laboratory Standard Institute breakpoints for susceptibility to topical antibiotics are not available, and the appropriate formulation of combination antibiotics for in vitro testing has not been determined. Thus, evaluating antibiotic pharmacokinetics in tears may better predict efficacy for some topical antibiotics; these kinetics are usually affected by frequent tearing in children, leading to an overestimation of the concentrations in tears of younger children. Topical ointments probably deliver more sustained concentrations of antibiotic to the conjunctiva, but they are

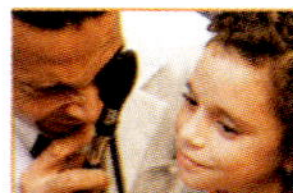

Table 21–2.

Commonly Used Topical Antibiotics

Type	Concentration
Aminoglycosides	
1. Gentamicin	0.3%
2. Amikacin	0.3%
Fluoroquinolones	
1. Ofloxacin	0.3%
2. Ciprofloxacin	0.3%
3. Levofloxacin	0.5%
Bacitracin (ointment)	500 Units/g
Erythromycin (ointment)	0.5%
Polymyxin B–neomycin	3.5 mg/mL
Polymyxin B–trimethoprim sulfate	1 mg/mL
Tetracycline	1%
Chloramphenicol*	0.5%, 1%†

**Not routinely used in the United States because of the association with aplastic anemia.*

†Solution of 0.5% and ointment of 1%.

poorly tolerated in toddlers and difficult for most parents. Alternatively, a short course of an oral beta-lactam antibiotic may possibly eradicate the conjunctival infection. In a randomized trial of oral cefixime and topical polymyxin–bacitracin, bacteriologic failure occurred in 62% for children receiving oral cefixime (orally, once daily for 3 days) and in 82% for children receiving topical polymyxin–bacitracin (topically, four times daily for 7 days); however, clinical cure rates among the 80 patients were virtually 100%, regardless of treatment group.[32] However, In cases of conjunctivitis–otitis syndrome, therapy with an appropriate oral antibiotic for the otitis media is sufficient for the cure of conjunctivitis without the addition of topical therapy.[33]

Hyperacute conjunctivitis may involve the cornea and may cause peripheral ulceration, ultimately leading to perforation if left untreated. It requires aggressive treatment and immediate referral to an ophthalmologist. Systemic treatment against gonorrhea should be instituted immediately. Current treatment recommendation is a single dose of ceftriaxone, 50 mg/kg, intramuscularly, up to a maximum of 1g.[34] Frequent saline lavage is also indicated until the purulence resolves. All children beyond the neonatal period diagnosed with gonococcal conjunctivitis should be investigated for sexual abuse.

Antimicrobial resistance is evolving rapidly especially for *H. influenzae* and *S. pneumoniae*, the two most common causative organisms of bacterial conjunctivitis in children. Nontypable strains of *H. influenzae* are also responsible for more than half of the cases of conjunctivitis–otitis syndrome. The rate of beta-lactamase producing *H. influenzae* isolated from children with acute conjunctivitis has increased from 16% in the nasopharynx during the mid-1980s, compared with rates from conjunctivitis of 44% in the late 1980s, to 69% in the late 1990s.[35,36]

On the other hand, penicillin resistance rates among *S. pneumoniae* isolates has been reported as high as 60% from conjunctival cultures.[35,36] The introduction of the heptavalent pneumococcal conjugate vaccine (PCV-7) has led to the "serotype replacement" phenomenon already described for acute otitis media and nasopharyngeal carriage promoting invasive pneumococcal disease caused by the nonvaccine serotypes. One study showed that PCV-7 would cover only 44% of *S. pneumoniae* strains isolated from conjunctival specimens and reported high penicillin resistance rates among the vaccine isolates causing conjunctivitis.[36] The penicillin resistance rate is also high among nontypable strains of *S. pneumoniae*, which are a major cause of conjunctivitis outbreaks and a common cause of sporadic acute conjunctivitis.[6,36]

Published data showed that ciprofloxacin, ofloxacin, and tetracycline are the most active drugs in vitro against both pathogens (*H. influenzae* and *S. pneumoniae*). Gentamicin, tobramycin, polymyxin B–trimethoprim, and polymyxin B–neomycin have intermediate activity.[35]

Failure of treatment should always raise the possibility of resistant organisms. In this case, conjunctival cultures should be obtained, treatment should be switched and more potent antibiotics should be used. Topical quinolones are approved by the food and drug administration for use in children to treat conjunctivitis. Their concentrations in tears remain above the minimum inhibitory concentrations described for *H. influenzae* and *S. pneumoniae*.[37] They can be used safely if first-line agents fail to cure the symptoms of conjunctivitis.

Viral Conjunctivitis

Viral conjunctivitis is usually self-limited and not routinely treated with antibiotics. Topical antiviral drugs are not indicated in adenoviral conjunctivitis.[31] The use of topical steroids in the management of this infection remains controversial. Their use is usually limited to complicated cases to reduce inflammatory reaction and prevent scarring. Corticosteroids may also prolong the disease course and may cause serious side effects such as glaucoma. Supportive therapy, including eye washing, lubricants, and cold compresses, may provide some relief, and the use of topical antibiotic is unnecessary.

The treatment of herpes simplex conjunctivitis includes topical antiviral agents such as trifluridine, which may be as effective as supportive measures.[38] Oral antiviral therapy may be used in case of complicated infections and keratitis. Topical steroids are specifically contraindicated for treating herpes simplex conjunctivitis because they may exacerbate the infection by depressing local immunity.

The treatment of herpes zoster conjunctivitis (i.e., conjunctivitis caused by reactivation of varicella zoster) includes the use of systemic antiviral therapy. This therapy should be started within 72 hours of the beginning of the symptoms to be most effective in reducing viral shedding and postherpetic neuralgia. Topical antibiotics may be used to reduce the risk of secondary bacterial infection. In contrast with herpes simplex conjunctivitis, topical steroids do not aggravate herpes zoster infections and decrease the inflammatory response.[39] They may be used in case of keratitis and uveitis.

INDICATIONS FOR SUBSPECIALTY REFERRAL

Once the primary-care physician has diagnosed conjunctivitis and initiated proper treatment, the patient requires follow-up visits, depending on the severity of the condition, the etiology considered, and the potential for ocular complications. The primary-care physician should be aware of and able to exclude other possible and serious causes of conjunctivitis that may warrant referral for a subspecialist. The patient should be referred to a subspecialist in certain cases including but not limited to

1. gonococcal conjunctivitis because of the potential complications;
2. progression of the disease despite adequate treatment;
3. lack of improvement of the symptoms despite alteration of therapy;
4. development of complications during treatment;
5. recurrent or chronic conjunctivitis;
6. monitoring of ocular pressure in case of use of topical steroids;
7. decrease in visual acuity and presence of photophobia, proptosis, or diplopia;
8. conjunctivitis diagnosed as part of other systemic disorders.

COURSE AND PROGNOSIS

Although conjunctivitis is a benign and curable disease, it may have serious complications usually related to its etiology and dependent on associated systemic and ocular disorders.

Acute forms of bacterial conjunctivitis can lead to adhesion of the eyelids to the eyeballs (symblepharon) and/or conjunctival scarring. Hyperacute forms of bacterial conjunctivitis should be monitored closely for the development of bacterial keratitis and the potential corneal perforation and visual loss. Toxic and irritative conjunctivitis, especially when the cause is unknown, has the potential to become chronic. Topical antibiotics may cause irritation of the inflamed conjunctiva and some patients may develop an allergic reaction to the instilled solution, requiring the discontinuation of the drug. If there is no improvement in the symptoms of conjunctivitis in 7–10 days, the patient should be referred to an ophthalmologist.

PREVENTION

Primary infectious conjunctivitis occurs sporadically as a result of exposure to pathogens from direct hand-to-eye contact, exposure to airborne pathogens, or sexual transmission.

Viral conjunctivitis is highly contagious. Replicating adenovirus is present in 95% of patients 10 days after the appearance of symptoms.[40] It has been recovered from nonporous surfaces for up to 49 days,[21] hence the potential transmission through sharing towels or other objects, through close contact with other persons including indirect contact (e.g., in a swimming pool), and through improperly disinfected instruments in eye clinics. Preventing the spread of infectious conjunctivitis involves, in addition to patient education, adequate infection control practices including hand washing before and after the examination, the use of protection barrier (gloves), and proper techniques for disinfection or sterilization of all equipment.

REFERENCES

1. Bodor FF. Diagnosis and management of acute conjunctivitis. *Semin Pediatr Infect Dis.* 1998;9:27-30.
2. AOA. *Care of the Patient with Conjunctivitis.* 2nd ed. St. Louis: American Optometric Association; 2002.
3. Gigliotti F, Williams WT, Hayden FG, et al. Etiology of acute conjunctivitis in children. *J Pediatr.* 1981;98(4):531-536.
4. Wald ER. Conjunctivitis in infants and children. *Pediatr Infect Dis J.* 1997;16(suppl 2):S17-S20.
5. Weiss A. Acute conjunctivitis in childhood. *Curr Probl Pediatr.* 1994;24(1):4-11.
6. Martin M, Turco JH, Zegans ME, et al. An outbreak of conjunctivitis due to atypical *Streptococcus pneumoniae. N Engl J Med.* 2003;348(12):1112-1121.
7. Westerfeld CB, Kazlas M. Pediatric conjunctivitis. *Contemp Ophthalmol.* 2007;6:1-5.
8. Brown WJ. Trends and status of gonorrhea in the united states. *J Infect Dis.* 1971;123(6):682-688.
9. Wan WL, Farkas GC, May WN, Robin JB. The clinical characteristics and course of adult gonococcal conjunctivitis. *Am J Ophthalmol.* 1986;102(5):575-583.
10. Traboulsi EI, Shammas IV, Ratl HE, Jarudi NI. *Pseudomonas aeruginosa* ophthalmia neonatorum. *Am J Ophthalmol.* 1984;98(6):801-802.
11. Shah SS, Gloor P, Gallagher PG. Bacteremia, meningitis, and brain abscesses in a hospitalized infant: Complications of *Pseudomonas aeruginosa* conjunctivitis. *J Perinatol.* 1999;19(6, pt 1):462-465.
12. Gudmundsson OG, Ormerod LD, Kenyon KR, et al. Factors influencing predilection and outcome in bacterial keratitis. *Cornea.* 1989;8(2):115-121.
13. Lesser RL. Ocular manifestations of Lyme disease. *Am J Med.* 1995;98(4A):60S-62S.
14. Escarmelle A, Delbrassine N, De Potter P. Cat's scratch disease and Parinaud's oculoglandular syndrome. *J Fr Ophthalmol.* 2004;27(2):179-183.
15. Thompson S, Omphroy L, Oetting T. Parinaud's oculoglandular syndrome attributable to an encounter with a wild rabbit. *Am J Ophthalmol.* 2001;131(2):283-284.
16. Coffey JD, Jr. Otitis media in the practice of pediatrics. Bacteriological and clinical observations. *Pediatrics.* 1966;38(1):25-32.
17. Bodor FF. Conjunctivitis–otitis syndrome. *Pediatrics.* 1982;69(6):695-698.
18. Bingen E, Cohen R, Jourenkova N, Gehanno P. Epidemiologic study of conjunctivitis–otitis syndrome. *Pediatr Infect Dis J.* 2005;24(8):731-732.

19. Bodor FF, Marchant CD, Shurin PA, Barenkamp SJ. Bacterial etiology of conjunctivitis–otitis media syndrome. *Pediatrics.* 1985;76(1):26-28.
20. Gigliotti F. Acute conjunctivitis. *Pediatr Rev.* 1995;16(6):203-207; quiz 8.
21. Nauheim RC, Romanowski EG, Araullo-Cruz T, et al. Prolonged recoverability of desiccated adenovirus type 19 from various surfaces. *Ophthalmology.* 1990;97(11):1450-1453.
22. Syed NA, Hyndiuk RA. Infectious conjunctivitis. *Infect Dis Clin North Am.* 1992;6(4):789-805.
23. Leibowitz HM. The red eye. *N Engl J Med.* 2000;343(5):345-351.
24. Manners T. Managing eye conditions in general practice. *BMJ.* 1997;315(7111):816-817.
25. McDonnell PJ. How do general practitioners manage eye disease in the community? *Br J Ophthalmol.* 1988;72(10):733-736.
26. Cooper RJ, Yeo AC, Bailey AS, Tullo AB. Adenovirus polymerase chain reaction assay for rapid diagnosis of conjunctivitis. *Invest Ophthalmol Vis Sci.* 1999;40(1):90-95.
27. Miller IM, Wittreich J, Vogel R, Cook TJ. The safety and efficacy of topical norfloxacin compared with placebo in the treatment of acute, bacterial conjunctivitis. The Norfloxacin-Placebo Ocular Study Group. *Eur J Ophthalmol.* 1992;2(2):58-66.
28. Rietveld RP, Ter Riet G, Bindels PJ, Bink D, Sloos JH, van Weert HC. The treatment of acute infectious conjunctivitis with fusidic acid: a randomised controlled trial. *Br J Gen Pract.* 2005;55(521):924-930.
29. Rose PW, Harnden A, Brueggemann AB, et al. Chloramphenicol treatment for acute infective conjunctivitis in children in primary care: a randomised double-blind placebo-controlled trial. *Lancet.* 2005;366(9479):37-43.
30. Gigliotti F, Hendley JO, Morgan J, Michaels R, Dickens M, Lohr J. Efficacy of topical antibiotic therapy in acute conjunctivitis in children. *J Pediatr.* 1984;104(4):623-626.
31. Lohr JA. Treatment of conjunctivitis in infants and children. *Pediatr Ann.* 1993;22(6):359-364.
32. Wald ER, Greenberg D, Hoberman A. Short term oral cefixime therapy for treatment of bacterial conjunctivitis. *Pediatr Infect Dis J.* 2001;20(11):1039-1042.
33. Harrison CJ, Hedrick JA, Block SL, Gilchrist MJ. Relation of the outcome of conjunctivitis and the conjunctivitis–otitis syndrome to identifiable risk factors and oral antimicrobial therapy. *Pediatr Infect Dis J.* 1987;6(6):536-540.
34. Workowski KA, Berman SM. Sexually transmitted diseases treatment guidelines, 2006. *MMWR Recomm Rep.* 2006;55(RR-11):1-94.
35. Block SL, Hedrick J, Tyler R, et al. Increasing bacterial resistance in pediatric acute conjunctivitis (1997–1998). *Antimicrob Agents Chemother.* 2000;44(6):1650-1654.
36. Buznach N, Dagan R, Greenberg D. Clinical and bacterial characteristics of acute bacterial conjunctivitis in children in the antibiotic resistance era. *Pediatr Infect Dis J.* 2005;24(9):823-828.
37. Richman J, Zolezio H, Tang-Liu D. Comparison of ofloxacin, gentamicin, and tobramycin concentrations in tears and in vitro MICs for 90% of test organisms. *Antimicrob Agents Chemother.* 1990;34(8):1602-1604.
38. Ward JB, Siojo LG, Waller SG. A prospective, masked clinical trial of trifluridine, dexamethasone, and artificial tears in the treatment of epidemic keratoconjunctivitis. *Cornea.* 1993;12(3):216-221.
39. Karbassi M, Raizman MB, Schuman JS. Herpes zoster ophthalmicus. *Surv Ophthalmol.* 1992;36(6):395-410.
40. Roba LA, Kowalski RP, Romanowski E. How long are patients with epidemic keratoconjunctivitis infectious? *Invest Ophthalmol Vis Sci.* 1993;34:848.

CHAPTER 22

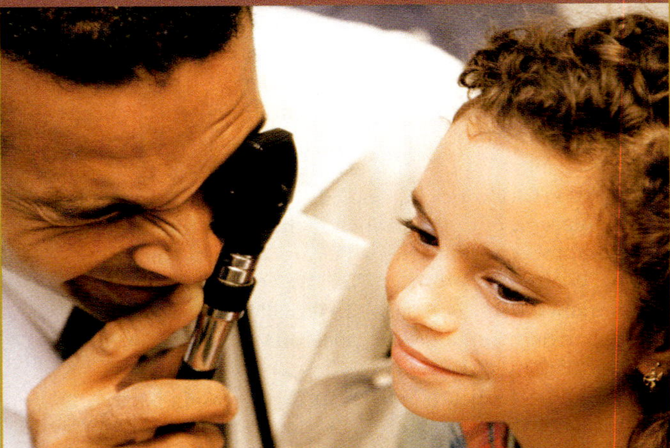

Periorbital and Orbital Infections

Latania K. Logan and Tina Q. Tan

DEFINITIONS AND EPIDEMIOLOGY

While the terms periorbital (preseptal) and orbital (postseptal) cellulitis sound similar, their pathogenesis, management, and complications are quite different. Periorbital infections refer to infections located anterior to the orbital septum, while orbital infections are infections located posteriorly.

Periorbital infections occur more frequently than orbital infections. Both infections are most commonly bacterial in origin and represent infections of the eyelid and the area surrounding the orbit. In general, these infections are caused by contiguous spread from adjacent infected structures, local trauma, or bacteremia. Noninfectious etiologies of periorbital and orbital cellulitis include inflammatory, allergic, endocrinologic, and neoplastic diseases.[1]

Prior to the advent of the *Haemophilus influenzae* type b conjugate vaccine in 1985, the majority of periorbital cellulitis in children was secondary to bacteremia from *H. influenzae* type b, which caused approximately 80% of the cases.[2] The introduction of the *H. influenzae* type b vaccine reduced pediatric cases of periorbital and orbital cellulitis by 59%.[3] Today, the most common cause of periorbital cellulitis is adjacent spread from infected neighboring structures, including skin, conjunctiva, eyelids, sinuses, respiratory tract, and teeth.[4] Other causes of periorbital cellulitis include blunt or penetrating trauma, viral infections such as adenovirus or Epstein–Barr virus, and bacteremia. In immunocompromised hosts, fungal etiologies, such as aspergillosis and phycomycosis, should be considered.[4,5]

Orbital cellulitis is an inflammation of the orbital structures, which is most commonly a complication of sinusitis, and, in more than 90% of cases, is ethmoidal in origin.[5] Other causes of orbital cellulitis include blunt or penetrating trauma, bacteremia, extension from infected adjacent structures such as dacryocystitis, or severe odontogenic infections.[1,5] Because sinusitis is more common in older than in younger children, orbital cellulitis tends to be seen more commonly in older children, and the occurrence tends to peak in the winter months when sinusitis is more prevalent (Table 22–1).[6]

PATHOGENESIS

Understanding the anatomy of the eyelid and the contiguous structures can be helpful in understanding the pathogenesis of periorbital and orbital infections. The terms preseptal and postseptal are used interchangeably with periorbital and orbital but specifically refer to infections that lie anterior or posterior to the orbital septum, respectively. The orbital septum is a fibrous extension of the periosteum of the skull located anteriorly in the orbit (periorbital). The periosteum and the orbital septum serve as barriers to prevent spread of infections from the eyelids and sinuses into the orbit (Figure 22–1).

The orbit is encompassed by the upper wall of the maxillary sinus, the lower wall of the frontal sinus, and the lateral wall of the ethmoid sinus. These bony walls of the sinuses vary in thickness; however, many are thin and porous and can be easily infiltrated, allowing for spread of infection.[1,7] One particularly thin sinus wall is the lamina papyracea of the ethmoid bone, a derivation from Latin meaning "a thin layer of paper." Thus, spread of infection from the sinuses into the orbit is often a consequence of direct extension through the wall of the ethmoid sinuses.

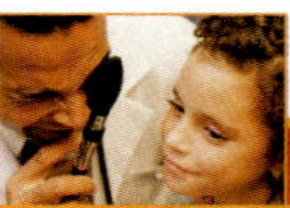

Table 22–1.

Etiologic and Demographic Characteristics of Periorbital and Orbital Cellulitis

	Periorbital Cellulitis	Orbital Cellulitis
Age	<5 y	Adolescents
Seasonal distribution	Year round	Predominately winter months
Pathogenesis	Local trauma (e.g., insect bite) Extension from adjacent infection (e.g., conjunctivitis, dental abscess, and sinusitis) Bacteremia	Sinusitis (usually ethmoidal) >90% of cases Penetrating or blunt trauma Extension from adjacent infection (e.g., dacryocystitis and severe odontogenic infection) Bacteremia
Causative organisms	Extension from skin/soft tissue infection: *S. aureus* *S. pyogenes* Extension from sinus infection: *S. pneumoniae* *H. influenzae* (nontypeable) *M. catarrhalis* *S. pyogenes* *S. aureus* Anaerobes* Extension from odontogenic infection: *Streptococcus* species Oral anaerobes Bacteremia: *S. pneumoniae*	Usually sinusitis: *S. pneumoniae* *H. influenzae* (nontypable) *M. catarrhalis* *S. pyogenes* *S. aureus* Anaerobes* Penetrating or blunt trauma: *S. aureus* *S. pyogenes* Anaerobes Gram-negative organisms Extension from skin/soft-tissue infection: *S. aureus* *S. pyogenes* Bacteremia: *S. pneumoniae*

**More likely polymicrobial in older patients with chronic sinusitis.*

In addition, the venous drainage system of the orbit is made of a valveless system, which allows the ophthalmic and ethmoidal veins to communicate directly. These veins, in turn, drain into the cavernous sinus, which can permit sinus infections to spread hematogenously into the orbit, leading to more complicated infections including thrombosis of the cavernous sinuses and meningitis.[1,2,4]

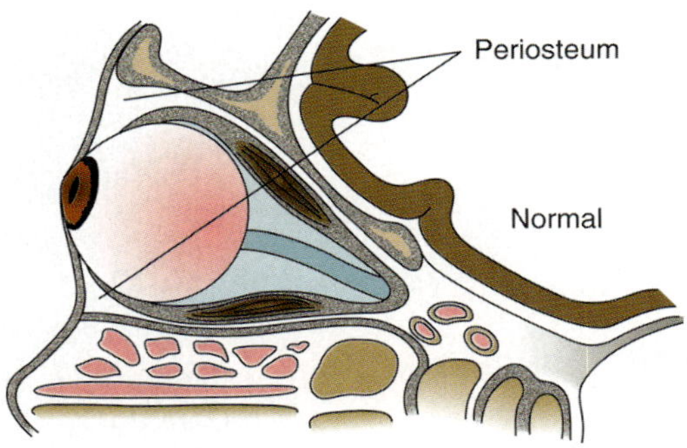

FIGURE 22–1 ■ Anatomy of eye and contiguous structures.

In nonbacteremic preseptal cellulitis, the infection remains anterior to the orbit and thus the aforementioned complications are less common. Often, the swelling seen in the soft tissues in periorbital cellulitis is not an actual "infection" of those tissues, but rather an inflammatory edema or sympathetic effusion, which is a reaction to a neighboring infection.[2] This makes it somewhat important to ascertain the location of the inciting infection, as causative organisms may be different. For example, periorbital cellulitis as a consequence of an eyelid or face trauma such as from an insect bite or from spread of infection from adjacent structures such as hordeolum, dacryocystitis, impetigo, or conjunctivitis would be more likely *Staphylococcus aureus* or *Streptococcus pyogenes*, whereas one that is caused by a sinusitis or an upper respiratory tract infection may be more commonly *Streptococcus pneumoniae*, nontypable *H. influenzae*, and other respiratory tract pathogens (Table 22–1).[5,8] Polymicrobial infections with both aerobes and anaerobes are more likely to be seen in older adolescent patients with chronic sinusitis causing orbital cellulitis and associated subperiosteal abscess.[9]

CLINICAL PRESENTATION

Differentiating between clinical signs and symptoms associated with periorbital and orbital cellulitis is critical to making a prompt diagnosis. Often, the history may not be helpful in making the diagnosis, as patients commonly might have had only vague symptoms and were not aware of any problem until the onset of overt symptoms. Patients with preseptal cellulitis may complain of symptoms associated with upper respiratory tract infection or infection of adjacent structures. The clinician should ask about recent insect bites or trauma and recent skin, soft-tissue, or eye infections such as impetigo, hordeolum, conjunctivitis, acute chalazia, acute dacryocystitis, blepharitis, or odontogenic infection.[1]

Symptoms associated with orbital cellulitis can be similar to those articulated by patients with periorbital cellulitis. Because direct extension may occur from adjacent structures, patients with orbital cellulitis may have similar inciting foci, such as a severe odontogenic infection or acute dacryocystitis. However, as the majority of patients with orbital cellulitis have sinusitis as the predominant cause, a history of a recent upper respiratory tract infection or symptoms suggestive of sinusitis may be present, such as headache, sinus tenderness, sinus pressure, and post nasal drip. Quite often, in patients presenting with sinusitis-related periorbital and orbital cellulitis, there is only a vague history of upper respiratory tract complaints. Fever may or may not be present.[5]

Periorbital and orbital cellulitis are both characterized by signs of inflammation within the periorbital tissues, including erythema, warmth, tenderness, edema, and induration (Figures 22–2 and 22–3). However, only orbital cellulitis is associated with proptosis, decreased extraocular movements or ophthalmoplegia, pain with extraocular movement, and decreased visual acuity or vision loss.[6] Photophobia is more commonly seen in orbital cellulitis, although this may be associated with conditions that cause periorbital cellulitis.

The progression of disease in orbital cellulitis can be rapid and is best described by the Chandler classification system of orbital cellulitis related to sinusitis (Table 22–2).[10] In stage 1, the patient presents with inflammatory edema and with findings similar to periorbital cellulitis, such as erythema, warmth, induration, and tenderness over the periorbital tissues. During stage 2, the patient develops true orbital cellulitis with chemosis (edema of the bulbar conjunctiva), proptosis, pain with eye movement, decreased extraocular movements, and decreased visual acuity. It is during this stage that there is extension of disease posterior to the orbital septum. In stage 3, subperiosteal abscess formation occurs, usually between the orbit and the periosteum of the sinuses. In this stage, an increase in extraocular pressure can occur, which may worsen proptosis and vision changes. Complete loss of extraocular movements or ophthalmoplegia is associated with stage 4: development of an orbital abscess, which is a true abscess of the orbital contents. Patients may complain of complete vision loss, and a marked proptosis is noted on examination. Finally in stage 5, the most serious complications occur, including cavernous sinus thrombosis,

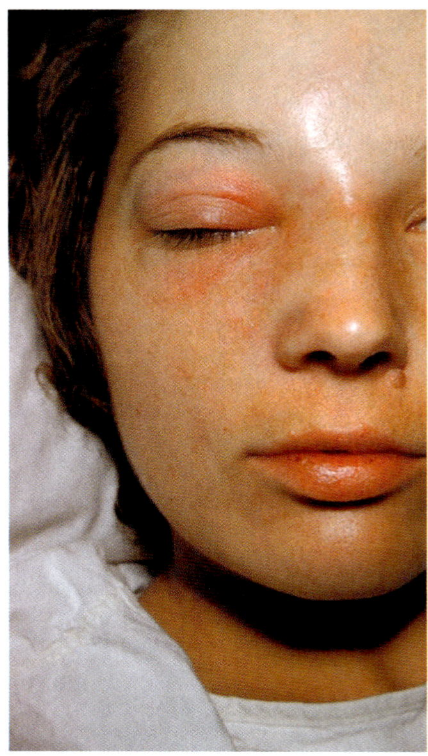

FIGURE 22–2 ■ Patient with orbital cellulitis. (From the Public Health Image Library Database [PHIL] of the U.S. Centers for Disease Control [CDC]).

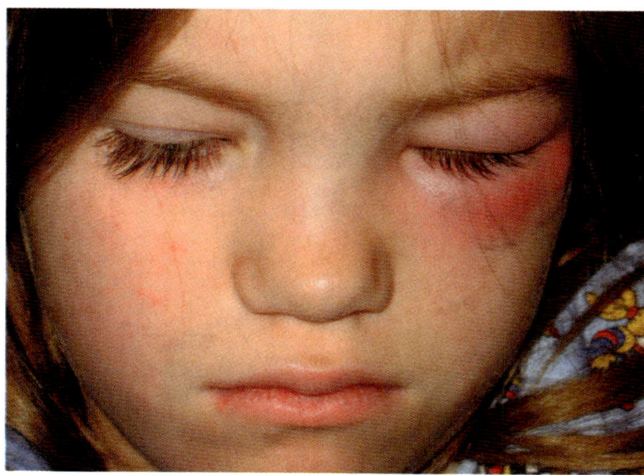

FIGURE 22–3 ■ Patient with preseptal cellulitis of the left eye. (Courtesy of Samir S. Shah, MD, MSCE.)

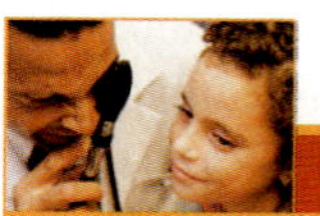

Table 22–2.

Chandler Classification of Orbital Cellulitis

Stage 1	Inflammatory edema
Stage 2	Orbital cellulitis
Stage 3	Subperiosteal abscess
Stage 4	Orbital abscess
Stage 5	Cavernous sinus thrombosis

which may present as headache, bilateral periorbital edema, cranial neuropathies, proptosis, and ophthalmoplegia with extension into the central nervous system.[1,10,11] Extension of disease into the central nervous system may also include the development of meningitis or formation of abscesses in the brain and epidural or subdural spaces.

On physical examination, it is therefore critical in any patient presenting with periorbital swelling to measure visual acuity and to assess for pain or decreased range of motion with eye movement, proptosis, chemosis, and photophobia (Table 22–3).

DIAGNOSIS

Fever and leukocytosis with a left shift are often, but not always, present in patients with periorbital and orbital cellulitis. Obtaining a complete blood count should be considered in any patient who appears ill; however, in either of these two conditions, it does not necessarily help the practitioner to differentiate between them. Blood cultures will commonly be negative in patients presenting with periorbital cellulitis and in most stages of orbital cellulitis. Cultures of wounds draining exudate may be helpful in infections caused by trauma or local infection; however, random cultures of the adjacent structures, conjunctiva, eyelids, or nasopharynx may be misleading and are generally not advised. Decisions to obtain needle aspirates of sinuses or abscesses associated with orbital cellulitis for diagnostic purposes should only be performed by consulting specialists if deemed necessary.

Radiological studies, such as computed tomography (CT) scan with intravenous contrast, should be performed in any patient with suspected orbital cellulitis to evaluate the extent of disease. Treatment modalities are often based on severity of symptoms as well as appearance on imaging.[5,11] Findings in orbital cellulitis such as opacification of the sinuses, eyelid swelling, and proptosis are easily seen on CT scan; subperiosteal abscesses generally are found on the medial orbital wall adjacent to a medially bowed periosteum, which laterally displaces a medial rectus muscle (Figure 22–4), while orbital abscesses will appear as densities within the intraconal space.[1]

DIFFERENTIAL DIAGNOSIS

Prompt differentiation and diagnosis are necessary to facilitate prompt management of periorbital and orbital cellulitis. Several noninfectious conditions can mimic these diseases, producing swelling of the eyelids and sometimes erythema. A list of these conditions is provided in Tables 22–4 and 22–5.

For periorbital cellulitis, in addition to the bacterial agents, other pathogens that should be considered include viruses (e.g., adenovirus and enteroviruses) when conjunctivitis is associated with periorbital edema, and, in immunocompromised persons, fungal organisms (e.g., aspergillus and zygomycetes) should be included in the differential diagnosis of any patient presenting with periorbital edema, erythema, and tenderness.[5]

Table 22–3.

Clinical Signs of Periorbital and Orbital Cellulitis

Periorbital inflammation	Periorbital Cellulitis	Orbital Cellulitis
Erythema	Present	Present
Warmth	Present	Present
Induration	Present	Present
Tenderness	Present	Present
Visual acuity	Normal	Decreased or visual loss
Extraocular movements	Normal	Decreased or ophthalmoplegia Pain with eye movement
Photophobia	Not usually present	Usually present
Chemosis	None	Present
Proptosis	None	Present

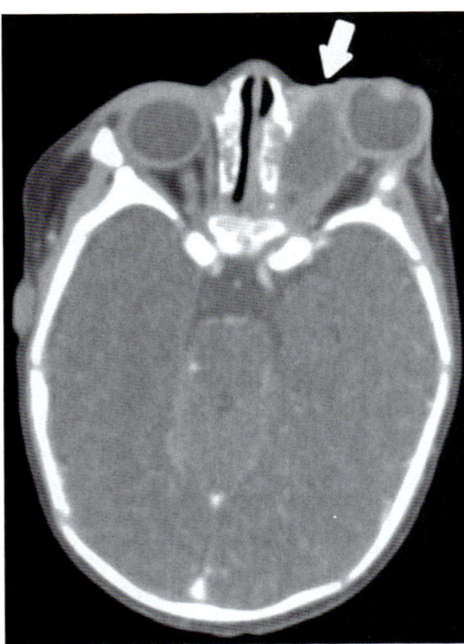

FIGURE 22–4 ■ Axial image from a computed tomography scan of the orbits performed with intravenous contrast. Note marked degree of swelling and proptosis of the left orbit with subperiosteal abscess laterally displacing medial rectus muscle. (Courtesy of Children's Memorial Hospital, Chicago, IL.)

Type I hypersensitivity reactions, such as those to animal dander and pollen, may cause acute swelling of the eyelids but typically are not erythematous or tender to palpation. Contact blepharoconjunctivitis, which is a type IV hypersensitivity reaction, is associated with ophthalmic solutions and may cause erythema, swelling, and eczematoid changes to the associated eyelid. Acute trauma, such as a basilar skull fracture, can cause unilateral or bilateral periorbital swelling, ecchymosis, and tenderness to the eyelids. The clinician must use historical data to differentiate these from infectious etiologies.[1,5]

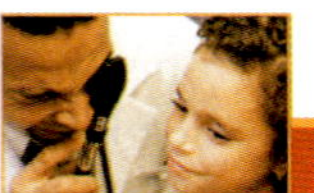

Table 22–4.

Differential Diagnosis of Periorbital Cellulitis

Condition	Distinguishing Features
Nonbacterial source such as viral or fungal organisms	Does not clear or improve on appropriate antibiotics; bilateral symptoms; patients with fungal infection usually immunocompromised
Type 1 hypersensitivity to pollen and animal hair	Does not clear or improve on appropriate antibiotics; bilateral symptoms; history consistent with allergies; not tender and not erythematous
Contact blepharoconjunctivitis	History of recent use of ophthalmic solutions
Acute trauma (e.g., basilar skull fracture)	History and physical compatible with trauma associated disease

The differential diagnosis of orbital cellulitis can be quite broad and needs to be differentiated from several conditions that cause orbital inflammation. A good general rule is in patients who are afebrile and have no evidence of sinusitis or adjacent structural disease, alternative diagnoses should be considered.

As with periorbital cellulitis, nonbacterial causes such as fungal infection should be considered in the immunocompromised patient with orbital cellulitis. Inflammatory orbital pseudotumor commonly presents with proptosis, ophthalmoplegia, and periorbital swelling. These patients are generally afebrile and without evidence of sinusitis on examination or CT. Typical CT scans reveal an intraorbital mass, not consistent with an abscess. Dacryoadenitis can mimic orbital cellulitis but is associated with nonbacterial etiologies such as viral infection or inflammatory diseases such as sarcoidosis or pseudotumor.[1,5,12] Ophthalmologic examinations revealing choroidal elevation or retinal detachment associated with exudates may be indicative of posterior scleritis.[1]

For patients presenting with cavernous sinus thrombosis, a broad workup may be necessary to find the underlying etiology. Other conditions that may present similarly to orbital cellulitis include space-occupying orbital lesions such as rapidly progressive neoplastic disorders including orbital rhabdomyosarcomas, leukemic infiltration of the orbit, or lymphoma. Other non-neoplastic lesions that may cause orbital inflammation include a ruptured dermoid cyst or a subperiosteal hematoma from trauma. These space-occupying lesions should be distinguished from orbital cellulitis based on characteristics on CT scan and/or magnetic resonance imaging; however, a biopsy may be necessary if diagnosis is uncertain.[1,13]

TREATMENT

Treatment of any periorbital or orbital cellulitis should be based on the inciting focus and should be managed in consultation with ophthalmology, otolaryngology, and infectious disease specialists. See Table 22–6 for list of treatment options. For the patient older than infancy who is nontoxic, periorbital cellulitis may be managed as an outpatient, particularly if the inciting focus is known. Patients with orbital cellulitis and ill-appearing patients should be admitted to the hospital and monitored closely with serial visual acuity examinations and for administration of intravenous antibiotics. In general, for periorbital and orbital infections thought to be caused by trauma, skin, or adjacent soft-tissue infection,

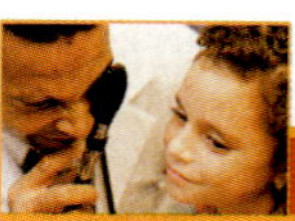

Table 22–5.

Differential Diagnosis of Orbital Cellulitis

Condition	Distinguishing Features
Nonbacterial causes such as fungal	Does not clear or improve on appropriate antibiotics; bilateral symptoms; patients usually immunocompromised
Orbital pseudotumor	Afebrile, no evidence of sinusitis
Posterior scleritis	Retinal detachment with exudates, choroidal elevation; scleral thickening on imaging
Dacryoadenitis	Other symptoms consistent with viral infection (such as parotid swelling with mumps); other symptoms or history consistent with systemic vasculitis
Cavernous sinus thrombosis (CST) not related to orbital cellulitis	A broad differential must be considered in any patient presenting with CST
Orbital tumors (e.g., rhabdomyosarcomas)	Mass lesion may be palpable; computed tomography consistent with tumor
Subperiosteal hematoma (trauma)	History and physical examination compatible with trauma associated disease
Ruptured dermoid cyst	Dermoid may be palpable at superolateral bony margin of the orbit; CT consistent with dermoid

antibiotics should be targeted at the treatment of *S. aureus* and *S. pyogenes*, recognizing that methicillin-resistant *S. aureus* is now commonly found as a causative organism of these infections. Surgical drainage of any abscesses may be necessary to achieve complete resolution of symptoms. For penetrating trauma, gram-negative and/or anaerobic coverage should also be considered. Therapy for infections thought to be occurring from an odontogenic focus should be aimed at both aerobic and anaerobic mouth flora such as *Streptococcus* species and oral anaerobes such as *Fusobacterium* and *Bacteroides* species. For sinus-related disease, therapy should be directed at aerobic respiratory flora such as *S. pneumoniae*, *H. influenzae*, *Moraxella catarrhalis*, *S. aureus*, *Streptococcus species*, as well as anaerobes.[4]

Length of therapy is dependent on inciting focus; however, typical length of therapy for periorbital cellulitis is 7–14 days, whereas 14–21 days are usually necessary for orbital cellulitis. The decision to switch from intravenous to oral antibiotics is varied between patients and is primarily based on the resolution of symptoms, cessation of fever, and ophthalmologic examination. For patients who do not improve after 24–48 hours of appropriate intravenous therapy, consider repeating radiological studies and surgical intervention.[12]

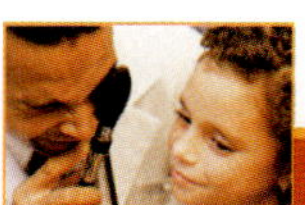

Table 22–6.

Management and Treatment of Periorbital and Orbital Cellulitis Requiring Hospitalization

General management strategies	Obtain complete blood count, blood cultures, and intravenous access Consultation with ophthalmology, otolaryngology, and infectious diseases At least twice-daily full ophthalmological examinations for the patient with orbital cellulitis Nasal drops for sinus-related disease such as ephedrine
Infections from skin and adjacent soft tissue (*S. aureus* and *S. pyogenes*)	Clindamycin 40 mg/kg/d divided every 8 h Or Alternative therapy that includes MRSA coverage
Infection extending from odontogenic focus (*Streptococcus* species and oral anaerobes)	Ampicillin/sulbactam 300 mg/kg/d divided every 6–8 h (clindamycin may be used as alternative therapy for patients with penicillin allergy)
Infection extending from sinusitis (*S. pneumoniae, H. influenzae, M. catarrhalis*, etc.)	Ampicillin/sulbactam 300 mg/kg/d divided every 6–8 h (clindamycin may be used as alternative therapy for patients with penicillin allergy)
Penetrating or blunt trauma	Broad coverage to include MRSA, *Streptococcus* species, gram-negative organisms, and anaerobes (e.g., clindamycin plus third-generation cephalosporin or aminoglycosides)
Bacteremia	Broad coverage with multiple antibiotics until organism identified

MRSA, methicillin-resistant Staphylococcus aureus.

REFERENCES

1. Lessner A, Stern GA. Preseptal and orbital cellulitis. In: Barza M, Baum J, eds. *Infectious Disease Clinics of North America.* Philadelphia: Saunders; 1992:933-952.
2. Wald ER. Periorbital and orbital infections. In: Long SS, Pickering LK, Prober CG (eds). *Principles and Practice of Pediatric Infectious Diseases.* 3rd ed. Philadelphia: Churchill Livingstone, 2008:511-516.
3. Ambati BK, Ambati JA, Azar N, et al. Periorbital and orbital cellulitis before and after the advent of *Haemophilus influenzae* type b vaccination. *Ophthalmology.* 2000;107:1450-1453.
4. Traboulsi EI. Pediatric Ophthalmology. In: McMillan JA, Feigin RD, DeAngelis CD, Jones MD Jr. *Oski's Pediatrics: Principles and Practice.* Philadelphia: Lippincott, Williams and Wilkins 2006:801-827.
5. Jain A, Rubin PA. Orbital cellulitis in children. *Int Ophthalmol Clin.* 2001;41:71-86.
6. Coats DK, Carothers TS, Brady-McCreery K, Paysse EA. Ocular Infectious Diseases. In: Feigin RD, Cherry JD, Demmler GJ, Kaplan SL (eds). *Textbook of Pediatric Infectious Diseases.* 5th ed. Philadelphia: Saunders, 2004: 787–809.
7. Givner LB. Periorbital versus orbital cellulitis. *Pediatr Infect Dis J.* 2002;21(12):1157-1158.
8. Behrman RE, Kliegman RM, Jenson HB. *Nelson Textbook of Pediatrics.* 18th ed. Philadelphia: Saunders; 2004: 2611-2612.
9. Harris GJ. Subperiosteal inflammation of the orbit: a bacteriological analysis of 17 cases. *Arch Ophthalmol.* 1988; 106:947-952.
10. Chandler JR, Langenbrunner DJ, Stevens ER. The pathogenesis of orbital complications in acute sinusitis. *Laryngoscope.* 1970;80:1414-1428.
11. Howe L, Jones NS. Guidelines for the management of periorbital cellulitis/abscess. *Clin Otolaryngol.* 2004;29: 725-728.
12. Kloek CE, Rubin PAD. Role of inflammation in orbital cellulitis. *Int Ophthalmol Clin.* 2006;46(2):57-68.
13. Ellis FD. Proptosis and orbital disease. In: Wright KW, Spiegel PH, eds. *Pediatric Ophthalmology and Strabismus.* 2nd ed. New York: Springer-Verlag; 2003.

CHAPTER 23

Infectious Keratitis in Children

Daniel J. Salchow

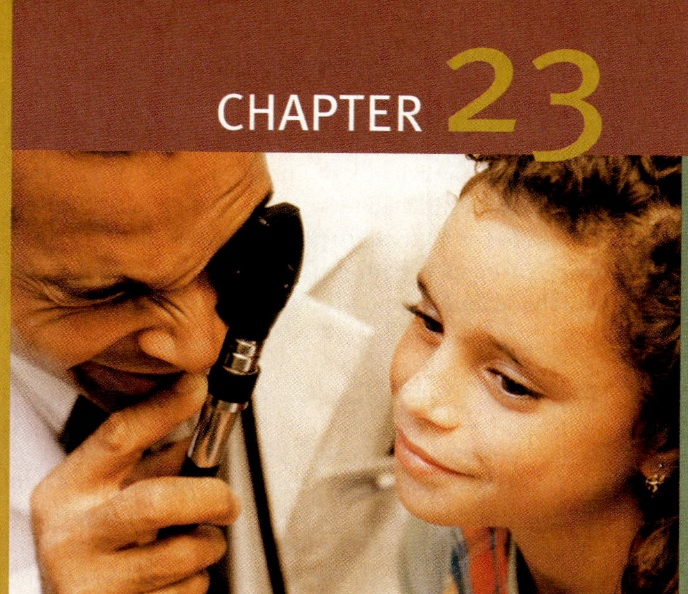

Infections of the cornea (i.e., infectious keratitis) are potentially sight threatening. They require prompt diagnosis and adequate treatment to prevent permanent compromise of vision. In the following chapter, infections causing acute corneal infections are discussed.

DEFINITIONS

Anatomy

The adult human cornea measures 10–12 mm horizontally and 10–11 mm vertically. The average corneal thickness is 555 ± 37 μm centrally,[1] and 600–690 μm peripherally.[2] The cornea has an important function in focusing light on the retina; it contributes 43.25 Diopters (approximately 75% of the total) to the total refractive power of the eye. The cornea is covered by the tear film, which functions as first-line defense against infections. The normal tear film contains components of the complement cascade, immunoglobulins, and cytokines. It lubricates and supplies the avascular cornea with essential nutrients. Proper lubrication depends on blinking, mediated by intact eyelids. Blinking helps to remove debris from the ocular surface and distributes the tear film evenly on the cornea. The corneal layers from front to back include the epithelium (4–5 layers) and its basement membrane, Bowman's layer, stroma, Descemet's membrane, and endothelium (single layer).

The transition from the cornea to the sclera (covered by the conjunctiva) is called "limbus." In the limbal area, blood vessels are present and stem cells for the corneal epithelium reside here. Behind the cornea, the anterior chamber contains a clear fluid, the aqueous humor. Anterior segment structures visible with the naked eye include the iris and crystalline lens.

Inflammation of the cornea is called keratitis. Keratitis may be infectious or noninfectious. Noninfectious keratitis is seen in ocular surface disorders such as dry eye syndrome and collagen vascular disorders such as rheumatoid arthritis. Infectious keratitis is a medical emergency, because of its potential to decrease vision permanently. Therefore, infectious keratitis requires prompt diagnosis and treatment.

Finally, whenever treating a child with ocular problems, one should recognize that amblyopia (impaired vision) can develop in an eye that receives a degraded image. Amblyopia is treated with appropriate restoration of a clear visual axis, correction of refractive errors (glasses, contact lenses), and specific treatment, such as occlusion therapy or optical/medical penalization. The risk of amblyopia development is higher in younger patients.

Superficial Versus Ulcerative Keratitis

In superficial keratitis, only the epithelial layer is involved. Mild stromal edema may be present, but the examiner can see through it and appreciate iris details. In ulcerative keratitis, an epithelial defect is present, and the underlying stroma shows whitish discoloration. This is also called a "corneal ulcer." Visualization of anterior segment structures is impeded by an ulcer. It is important to inspect the cornea with the slit lamp to assess size of the epithelial defect and depth of underlying stromal ulceration. A corneal ulcer can lead to significant thinning and even perforation of the cornea. The anterior chamber of the eye is examined for cells or layering of white blood cells (hypopyon), characteristically found in more severe cases of infectious keratitis.

EPIDEMIOLOGY

The actual prevalence of infectious keratitis is not known. It is estimated to be 11 per 100,00 in the United States,[3] but as high as 710 per 100,000 in Burma (Myanmar). In infancy, both genders are affected equally. In childhood and later in life, males predominate.[4]

PATHOGENESIS

Bacteria, fungi, viruses, and parasites can cause infectious keratitis. Most infectious agents require a breach in the corneal epithelium to infect the cornea. There are exceptions to this rule, including *Neisseria gonorrhoeae* and *Corynebacterium diphtheriae*, which are said to be able to penetrate intact corneal epithelium.

Acute Phase

Most corneal inflammations are characterized by edema. This decreases corneal transparency, makes the cornea appear hazy, and usually causes decreased vision. Because the cornea is avascular, the initial vascular reaction can be observed as perilimbal hyperemia (injection), which may involve one sector or the entire circumference. Inflammatory cells invade the cornea from limbal vessels and migrate toward the site of the inflammatory stimulus. The first wave of cellular migration consists of polymorphonuclear leukocytes (8–12 hours after injury), followed by a macrophage invasion during the next 12–16 hours. Macrophages originate from limbal vessels and through transformation of corneal stromal cells (keratocytes); they ingest microorganisms and inflammatory products.[5] In keratitis, inflammation stimulates the umyelinated endings of the sensory ciliary branches (ophthalmic division of the trigeminal nerve). Because the cornea is the most densely innervated tissue of the human body, patients with keratitis usually have pain. However, herpes simplex virus (HSV) keratitis can lead to reduced corneal sensation and, therefore, be present with mild or even no pain.

Sterilization Phase

With effective antimicrobial therapy, the inciting organism is killed and the corneal ulcer sterilized. However, the clinical findings may not improve right away, because inflammation persists and a structural lesion (stromal infiltrate) may take time to heal. Therefore, improvement can take 2–3 days to be visible. In general, stabilization of findings during this time is encouraging and the absence of progression means that the ulcer is being treated successfully.

Healing Phase

After sterilization of the ulcer, healing processes set in. Neovascularization (growth of blood vessels from the limbus into the cornea) is commonly seen in response to several inciting factors including edema, infiltration with inflammatory cells, tissue necrosis, changes in pH, oxidative processes, and enzymes from inflammatory cells. The extent of neovascularization varies with the severity and size of the corneal ulcer. Neovascularization may also occur in response to noninfectious corneal inflammation and is, therefore, not specific for infectious keratitis.[5]

The ulcer usually heals, and is covered by epithelium. Sometimes, a scar can remain and may lead to decreased vision. Up to 16% of children with microbial keratitis require surgical intervention to prevent spread of the infection or to restore a clear visual axis, which emphasizes the serious nature of infectious keratitis.[6,7]

RISK FACTORS

The risk factors for infectious keratitis vary depending on the patient's age. Trauma is an important risk factor for infectious keratitis in children and adults.[4,7,8] Trauma can cause a corneal abrasion, and microorganisms may infect the cornea through this breach in the epithelium. A corneal abrasion is painful and often presents with a red eye, but usually heals in 2–4 days. Symptoms persisting beyond this time should raise one's suspicion for an infection.

In children 12 years of age or younger, trauma is the most common predisposing factor for the development of infectious keratitis (28.9%), followed by ocular disease (22.2%) and contact lens wear (15.6%).[9] In children older than 12 years, contact lens wear is by far the most common predisposing factor (72.2%; mostly soft contact lenses—66.7%), followed by trauma (11.1%) and ocular and systemic disease (5.5% each). Gram-positive and gram-negative bacteria were isolated at similar rates for some risk factors such as trauma as well as ocular systemic diseases. Gram-negative bacteria, however, were more commonly found in contact lens wearers (55%). Fungus and *Acanthamoeba* spp. were rare causes of infectious keratitis in this study.[9]

CLINICAL PRESENTATION

Children with infectious keratitis may complain of acute onset of pain, photophobia, and impaired vision. The following historical features should be documented to identify predisposing factors:

- Contact lens wear (type of lens, wearing time, and type of disinfection system)
- Trauma (including previous eye surgery)

- Use of ocular medications
- Aqueous tear deficiencies
- Previous eye infections
- Structural abnormalities of the eyelids

Findings associated with specific pathogens are discussed below.

Adenoviral Keratoconjunctivitis

Adenovirus infections may affect mucosal surfaces throughout the body, thus, several organ systems including the upper respiratory tract, the eyes, and genitals may become involved. Some adenovirus serotypes display affinity for certain organ systems. For example, epidemic keratoconjunctivitis is most often caused by adenovirus serotypes 8, 19, and 37, but also by serotype 11 (which may also cause pharyngo-conjunctival fever, upper respiratory tract infection, and venereal disease). Epidemic keratoconjunctivitis is a common cause of ocular infection in children. A history of "pink eye" in relatives or close contacts is frequently reported. Most often, conjunctivitis is the only manifestation of adenoviral eye infection and presents with redness, photophobia, and clear mucous discharge from the involved eye. Preauricular or submandibular lymphadenopathy is usually present in the first few days of the infection and may be marked. Adenovirus infection is most often diagnosed clinically but can be confirmed using polymerase chain reaction (PCR).[10] If the eyelids are everted, one appreciates a typical pattern called "follicular conjunctivitis" (numerous small confluent nodules lacking a central vessel).

In epidemic keratoconjunctivitis, the cornea is also involved and shows fine punctate fluorescein staining within the first 3–5 days after infection. This resolves within 7–10 days. In some cases, stromal corneal opacities appear within 2 weeks and slowly resolve over the next 2–4 weeks. These stromal opacities may persist over a long time and decrease visual acuity.[11] Treatment consists of topical corticosteroids.

Herpes Simplex Virus Keratitis

The diagnosis of herpes simplex virus (HSV) keratitis is made based on clinical findings. Culture or PCR tests are available and may be helpful in some cases. In HSV keratitis, the eye is red and pain, photophobia, and tearing may be present. A history of previous HSV keratitis may be elicited. The eyelid skin sometimes shows a characteristic vesicular rash (Figure 23–1). On inspection of the cornea, one sees linear superficial corneal lesions. These may branch and are then described as "dendrites"—a finding highly characteristic of herpetic infection. In Figure 23–2, a typical corneal dendrite caused by HSV infection is shown. While the underlying stroma may be edematous, there is no purulence. Most

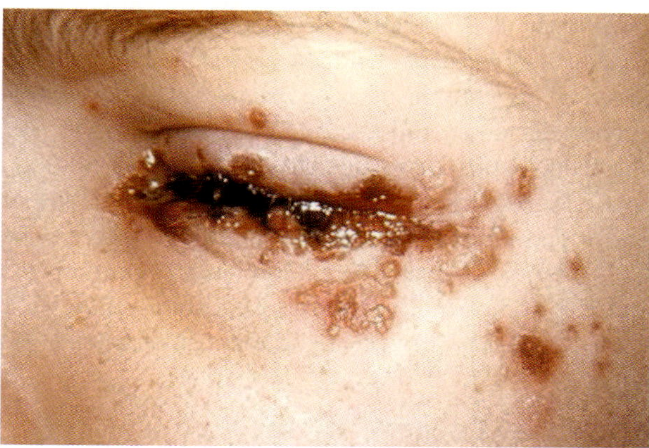

FIGURE 23–1 ■ External photograph of herpes simplex virus (HSV) dermatitis involving the margins of the upper and lower eyelid. A vesicular rash is present with crusting of the lesions. The nondermatomal distribution of the rash is characteristic for primary HSV infection in contrast to Herpes Zoster, which respects the dermatomes and therefore the midline.

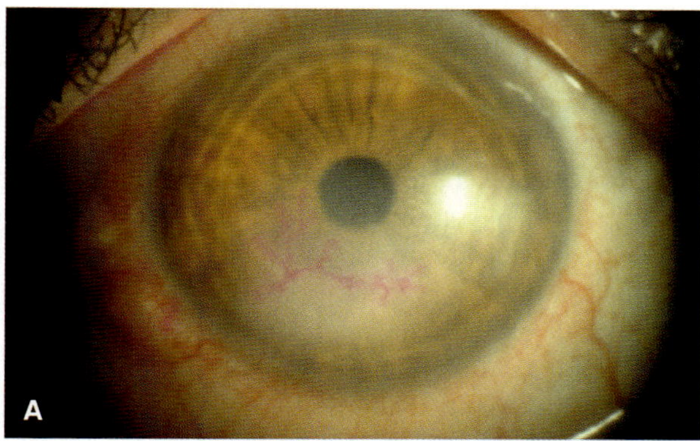

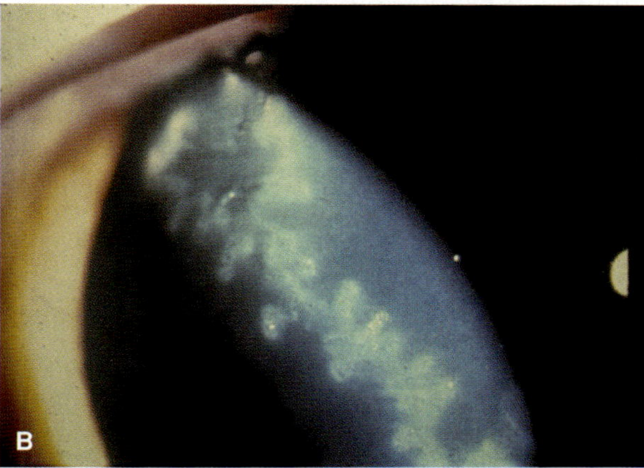

FIGURE 23–2 ■ **(A)** Photograph of herpes simplex virus corneal ulcer. Rose Bengal has been applied, the affected epithelium is stained pink. Note the branching, dendritic pattern of the staining. **(B)** Photograph of herpes simplex virus corneal ulcer. Fluorescein has been instilled, staining the epithelial defect, which appears green under blue illumination. The epithelium adjacent to the defect is slightly elevated. The underlying stroma is edematous but allows visualization of the iris. (*Courtesy of George J. Florakis, MD.*)

commonly, HSV keratitis is unilateral. If the ulcer is large, it may loose its dendritic appearance and is then called a "geographic ulcer." Corneal sensitivity is frequently decreased and needs to be tested before topical anesthetic drops are instilled. As a late complication, a corneal stromal scar can develop and decrease visual acuity permanently (disciform keratitis). In aggressive HSV keratitis, stromal inflammation may be pronounced and can lead to multiple corneal infiltrates underlying epithelial defects (necrotizing interstitial keratitis).

Bacterial Corneal Ulcer

Decreased vision, redness, photophobia, and tearing are usually present with bacterial corneal ulcers. A white or creamy appearing infiltrate underlying an epithelial defect is characteristic. The infiltrate may be deep and even extend through the full thickness of the cornea, leading to a corneal perforation. Intraocular inflammation (hypopyon) may be present. Figure 23–3 shows a typical bacterial corneal ulcer.

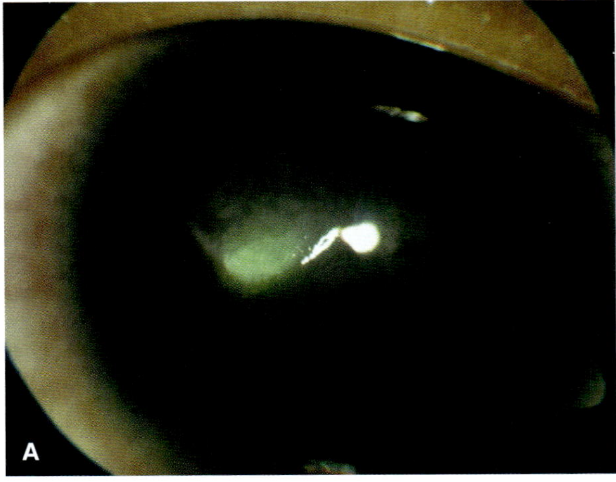

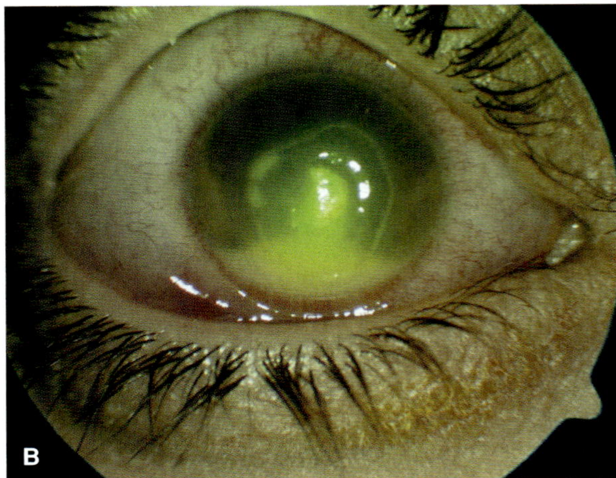

FIGURE 23–3 ■ (A) Photograph of bacterial corneal ulcer. The round central corneal opacity is visible and has a creamy appearance. **(B)** Photograph of a more severe bacterial corneal ulcer. The conjunctival vessels are hyperemic (injection), which is most pronounced inferiorly. The epithelial defect has been stained with fluorescein and appears green. Centrally, thinning of the cornea is present. This patient also has layering of white blood cells in the anterior chamber of the eye (hypopyon). (*Courtesy of Paul A. Gaudio, MD.*)

Fungal Corneal Ulcer

Pain, photophobia, redness, and tearing are common symptoms in fungal keratitis. The most important risk factor for fungal keratitis is trauma (recently, the use of some contact lens solutions has been linked with an epidemic of fungal keratitis).[12] One should ask about trauma caused by a vegetable matter such as a tree branch or thorn. The characteristic fungal corneal ulcer consists of a gray–white infiltrate with irregular, feathery borders. An epithelial defect is most often present. Satellite lesions surrounding the primary focus are frequently seen (Figure 23–4).

The etiology of fungal keratitis differs depending on the circumstances. In eyes with local risk factors such as eyelid abnormalities or dry eye syndrome, nonfilamentous fungi (typically *Candida* spp.) predominate. After trauma, filamentous fungi (*Fusarium* or *Aspergillus* spp.) are predominantly isolated.

Protozoal Infection

Acanthamoeba is a free-living protozoon commonly found in water, including bottled water, swimming pools, hot tubs, contact lens solutions, and bathroom tap water. *Acanthamoeba* spp. live in two forms, the motile trophozoite and the nonmotile cyst. They enter the cystic stage when environmental conditions are unfavorable. Corneal infection with *Acanthamoeba* should be suspected in any patient with a history of soft contact lens wear, poor contact lens hygiene, and/or swimming or hot tub use while wearing contact lenses. Corneal infection with *Acanthamoeba* is most often unilateral but may be bilateral.[13] Severe ocular pain (sometimes out of proportion to the clinical findings), redness, and photophobia develop over a period of several weeks. This contrasts the more acute time course seen in bacterial and fungal keratitis. Therefore, amoebic infection should be considered in a child when a corneal ulcer does not heal despite intensive antibacterial or antifungal therapy.

Critical signs in amoebic keratitis include corneal and anterior chamber inflammation, but less than one would expect with regard to the patient's pain. The corneal infiltrate is less dense than in fungal or bacterial keratitis. A characteristic late finding is a ring-shaped stromal infiltrate (Figure 23–5). Other, less specific signs include eyelid swelling, conjunctival injection (red eye), cells and flare in the anterior chamber.

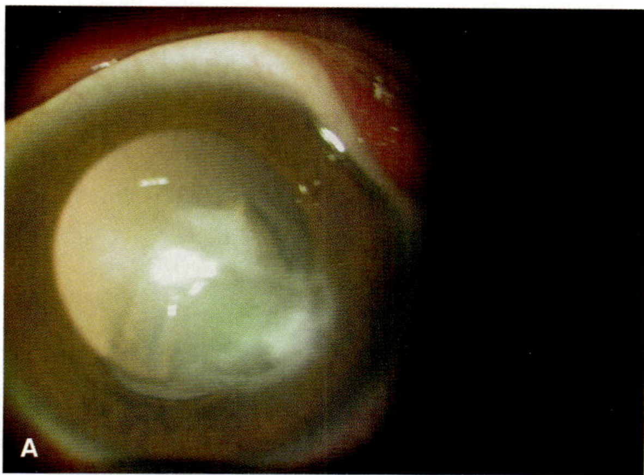

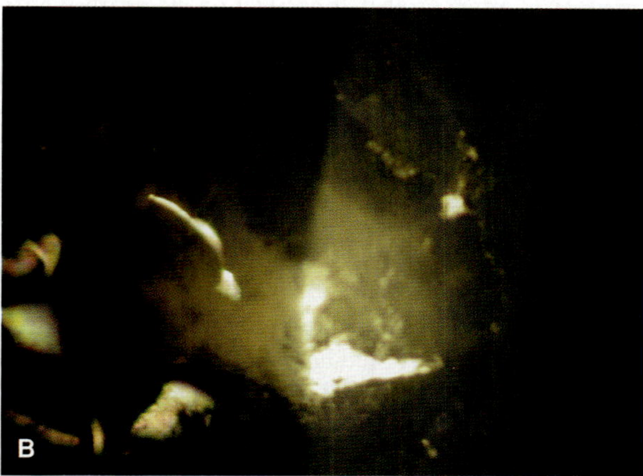

FIGURE 23–4 ■ **(A)** Photograph of fungal corneal ulcer. The whitish corneal infiltrate is not well circumscribed and has feathery borders. **(B)** Higher magnification of fungal keratitis, showing the feathery white corneal infiltrate typical for fungal keratitis. (*Courtesy of Paul A. Gaudio, MD.*)

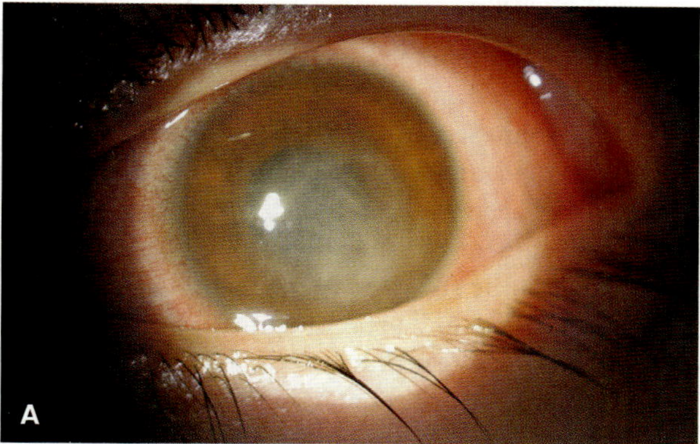

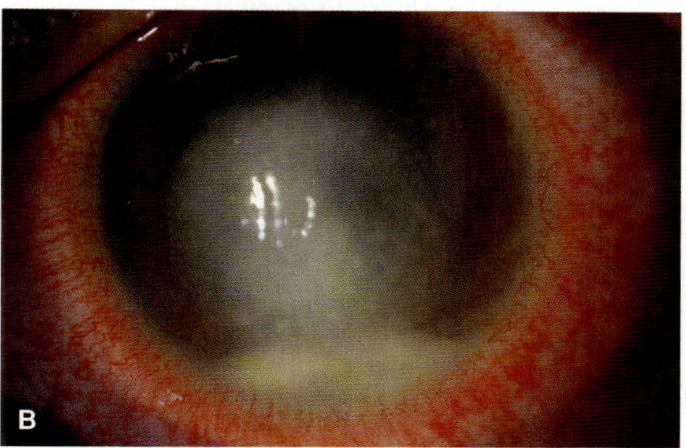

FIGURE 23–5 ■ **(A)** Photograph of corneal ulcer caused by acanthamoeba. Marked conjunctival injection is striking. The opacity in the cornea is diffuse and has a ring shape. **(B)** The same eye as in (A), 2 weeks later. Progression of the infection is seen, the conjunctival injection is very marked. A hypopyon is present. Despite its size, the ulcer is less dense than a bacterial ulcer (see Figure 23–2).

DIFFERENTIAL DIAGNOSIS

A sterile (noninfectious) corneal ulcer may be caused by systemic conditions, such as rheumatoid arthritis or other collagen vascular diseases, and local ocular disorders, such as dry eye syndrome, vernal keratoconjunctivitis, neurotrophic keratopathy, and vitamin A deficiency (rare in the developed world). Hypersensitivity to staphylococci (which populate the eyelid skin and eyelashes) can cause corneal infiltrates—these are usually peripheral, small (<1 mm in diameter), and multiple; most often, there is a clear space between these infiltrates and the limbus; blepharitis is usually present. Immune reaction to deposits on contact lenses may cause similar infiltrates, which are covered by intact epithelium (these do not stain with fluorescein). A residual rust ring after a metallic foreign body on the cornea can also result in a corneal opacity—in this case, the epithelium is also intact.

DIAGNOSIS AND MANAGEMENT

When evaluating a patient for infectious keratitis, the first step is to obtain a complete history. In infectious keratitis, signs and symptoms often appear acutely (hours to 1–2 days), whereas in noninfectious keratitis the onset is more insidious. Pain is an important symptom and is often marked in infectious keratitis. Trauma, contact lens wear or local abnormalities of the eyes and its adnexae are risk factors for infectious keratitis.

During the examination, visual acuity is measured with optimal refractive correction (glasses) at a distance of 6 m (20 ft). Alternatively, one can use a near card at 35 cm (14 inc). In children, numbers or pictures may be used according to their cognitive abilities. In preverbal or uncooperative children, fixation behavior in response to an interesting object will tell if vision is decreased (compare the two eyes). Next, the eye should be inspected in ambient light. Redness, which may be sectoral or generalized in more extensive disease, is caused by hyperemia of the perilimbal conjunctival vessels and is usually present in infectious keratitis. The cornea is inspected with a slit lamp, or if not available, with a penlight. One should look for a white or gray lesion (infiltrate), corneal edema, and hypopyon. Fluorescein eye drops (e.g., fluorescein sodium 2%) are instilled and the eye is inspected under blue illumination. Green areas represent epithelial defects. The size and shape of these areas are documented. Rose Bengal (Rose Bengal 1.3 mg sterile ophthalmic strips) may be used to stain devitalized epithelial cells and areas of epithelium that is inadequately coated by tear mucin.

The examination may be difficult to perform in young children and infants. Every effort should be made to avoid restraining the child or creating a frightening experience, because this will make subsequent examinations more difficult or even impossible. It is important to speak to child in a calming and reassuring way and to take time to explain what is done. Instillation of topical anesthetic (e.g., Proparacaine 0.5% ophthalmic drops) often alleviates the ocular discomfort, allowing the child to open the eye. When essential information cannot be obtained, restraining the child may rarely be necessary. A lid speculum and portable slit lamp can be used. On occasion, sedation or anesthesia is needed to obtain corneal scrapings for microbiological investigations (see section "Additional Investigations"), or to judge the extent of the disease process in children or uncooperative patients.

Additional Investigations

To identify the inciting organism, a corneal scraping should be performed. This is done at the slit lamp in patients that are able to cooperate. (Noncooperative patients may require sedation or even general anesthesia.) After the cornea is anesthetized with a topical anesthetic, a Tooks knife, Kimura spatula, or a Bard–Parker #15 blade is used to obtain scrapings from the ulcer. Care is taken to obtain material from the base of the ulcer, which is plated on different media or glass slides. Between different cultures, the instrument is sterilized over a flame, or a new instrument is used. The investigation for microbial agents includes:

- Glass slide for Gram stain—to stain bacteria and fungi
- Glass slide for Giemsa stain—to stain bacteria, fungi, and *Acanthamoebae*
- Blood agar—most bacteria grow on this medium
- Sabouraud dextrose agar without cycloheximide—to culture fungi
- Thioglycolate broth—for anaerobic and aerobic bacteria
- Chocolate agar (place in CO_2 jar)—for *Haemophilus* spp. and *N. gonorrhoeae*

The following culture media are optional, depending on the clinical suspicion for infections caused by the organisms listed:

- Löwenstein–Jensen medium—for mycobacteria and *Nocardia* spp.
- Nonnutrient agar with *Escherichia coli* overlay—for *Acanthamoeba* spp.
- Acid-fast stain—for mycobacteria
- Gomori methenamine silver stain or PAS stain—for fungi and *Acanthamoeba*

TREATMENT

The treatment of infectious keratitis involves the use of appropriate topical antimicrobial agents (ointment and eye drops). Systemic therapy is sometimes indicated; it is often used if the infection has spread into the eye (endophthalmitis). The concentration of the antimicrobial agent reaches higher levels in the cornea when given topically compared to systemic administration. Pathogen-specific approaches are discussed below and summarized in Figure 23–6. The specific treatment algorithm is presented in the respective sections below. Corneal ulcers are usually treated as presumed bacterial infections until culture or microbiologic investigations identify a different cause. In general, topical corticosteroid medications should be avoided in infectious keratitis, as they have the potential to worsen the infection.

If corneal thinning is present, an eye shield is taped over the eye to prevent perforation caused by minor trauma. An eye patch, however, should be avoided because it prevents oxygen from reaching the cornea and inhibits blinking. Therapy of specific infectious causes of keratitis is discussed below:

Adenoviral Keratoconjunctivitis

The best treatment of epidemic keratoconjunctivitis is prevention of spread. It is extremely contagious, so it is important that strict hygiene is observed in children with epidemic keratoconjunctivitis. This includes washing and disinfecting hands after contact with a child with epidemic keratoconjunctivitis, avoiding close contact and sharing towels or pillows. Children should be kept out of school for 2 weeks when diagnosed with adenoviral eye infection. No specific antiviral treatment is available. Supportive treatment with cold compresses, and artificial tears for foreign-body sensation is helpful. Antibiotic ophthalmic ointment to prevent bacterial superinfection is prescribed by some clinicians, although no scientific evidence exists to support this approach. Topical corticosteroids should not be given within the first 2 weeks, as they may increase viral replication. The redness and discomfort resolve within 10–14 days. If symptoms persist beyond this time, the diagnosis should be questioned. After 2 weeks, a mild corticosteroid (such as fluorometholone—Flarex®,

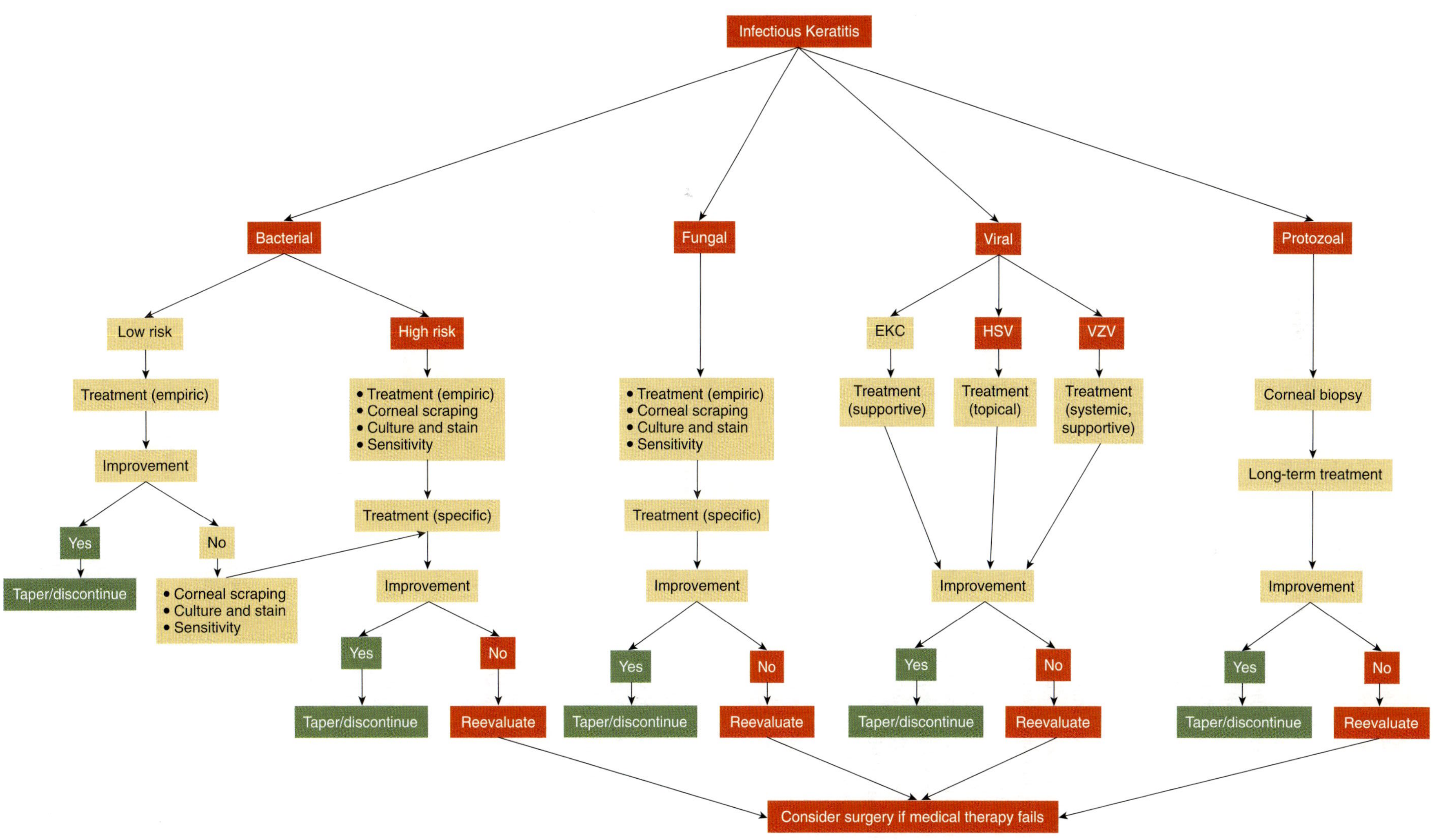

FIGURE 23–6 ■ Algorithm for evaluating and treating patients with infectious keratitis.

FML®) may be given four times a day for several days, titrated according to resolution of corneal opacities.

Herpes Simplex Virus Keratitis

The treatment of acute HSV keratitis involves antiviral medication. In many countries, acyclovir 3% (Zovirax®) ophthalmic ointment five times per day is the mainstay of therapy. In the United States, trifluorothymidine 1% (Viroptic®) drops nine times per day or vidarabine 3% (Vira-A®) ointment five times per day are prescribed for 7–14 days. In children where topical administration is not feasible, systemic acyclovir may also be used and is effective and well tolerated.[14] The recommended dosage is 20–40 mg/kg per day but may be tapered according to the clinical course. Systemic maintenance therapy should be considered if recurrences occur. If primary herpetic infection is suspected, some physicians prescribe systemic acyclovir for 7–14 days. In recurrent cases scarring of the corneal stroma may occur and lead to decreased vision. Maintenance therapy with systemic Acyclovir combined with topical steroids should be considered. Some progressive cases require corneal transplantation to reestablish a clear visual axis.

Bacterial Corneal Ulcer

If the ulcer is small (<1 mm in diameter; *low risk for visual compromise*) and superficial, empiric antibiotic topical therapy is initiated. Fourth generation fluoroquinolone eye drops (moxifloxacin 0.5%, Vigamox®, or gatifloxacin 0.3%, Zymar®) have been shown to be effective in clinical trials.[15,16] They are administered three times, 5 minutes apart upon diagnosis and then every hour for the first 24–48 hours. Depending on the clinical course, the frequency of administration is then decreased. In peripheral, intermediate size ulcers (1–1.5 mm diameter; *borderline risk for visual compromise*), fourth generation fluoroquinolone eye drops are also used.

If the corneal ulcer is larger and/or centrally located (>1.5 mm; *high risk for visual compromise*), topical treatment with fortified antibiotic eye drops is prescribed. Tobramycin or gentamicin (15 mg/mL), every hour alternating with cefazoline (50 mg/mL) or vancomycin (25–50 mg/mL) is required (this means that the patient will be placing one drop in the affected eye every 30 minutes around the clock). These solutions have to be compounded by a pharmacy. If photophobia and pain is marked, a cycloplegic agent can be added (e.g., cyclopentolate 1% [Cyclogyl®] eye drops). Depending on the results of microbiological investigations (stain, culture), the antibiotic therapy may have to be adjusted to target the specific organism.

The treatment of bacterial corneal ulcers is usually successful. Of 229 adult patients with bacterial corneal ulcer, 94% were cured, 5.2% had serious complications including perforation of the cornea or enucleation (removal of the eye).[15] In a recent study on children with microbial keratitis in Taiwan, of the eyes that had best corrected visual acuity measured, 48.5% achieved 20/25 or better.[9]

Fungal Corneal Ulcer

Antifungal treatment depends on the organism causing the infection. Since sensitivity profiles for fungi may take long to obtain, treatment with Natamycin 5% (Natacyn®) eye drops every hour while awake and every 2 hours at night is initiated as a first therapeutic approach. A sensitive and rapid PCR-based method using single-stranded conformation polymorphism was recently described for diagnosis of fungal keratitis in four patients. This may yield positive results when the conventional approach proves negative.[17] Topical steroids are strictly avoided as are eye patches. Treatment of fungal keratitis may be long and frustrating. Recently, voriconazole has shown great promise in treating fungal keratitis.[18]

If the infection involves the deep stroma or is worsening despite appropriate treatment, one or more of the following medications may be added (only natamycin is commercially available for topical ophthalmic use):

- Amphotericin B 0.15% eye drops every hour (especially effective in *Candida* infections)
- Miconazole or Clotrimazole 0.1–1% eye drops every hour
- Itraconazole 400 mg oral loading dose, then 200 mg po every day can be used in addition to topical medications.

A corneal transplant may be required when fungal keratitis progresses in a patient receiving maximal antifungal therapy or when corneal perforation is present or impending. Unfortunately, the success rate of corneal transplants is lower in children than in adults.

Protozoal Infection

The treatment of amoebic keratitis is long and sometimes ineffective. One or more of the following agents are usually combined:

- Polymyxin/neomycin/gramicidin (e.g., Neosporin®) eye drops, every 30 minutes to 2 hours
- Chlorhexidine 0.02% eye drops, every 1–2 hours
- Propamidine isethionate 0.1% (Brolene®) eye drops, every 30 minutes to 2 hours

- Polyhexamethyl biguanide 0.02% (PHMB) eye drops, every hour
- Itraconazole 400 mg orally as a loading dose, then 200 mg/d

As a first-line regimen, combination of propamidine with PHMB or chlorhexidine is recommended.[19] Additionally, clotrimazole 1% eye drops or miconazole 1% eye drops every 1–2 hours may be used. (Note: Brolene is available in the United Kingdom and may be obtained in the Unites States with approval of the Food and Drug Administration. Clotrimazole is not currently available as an ophthalmic suspension, but it can be formulated with Food and Drug Administration approval. PHMB is available in the United Kingdom and can be prepared in the Unites States from Baquacil®, a swimming pool disinfectant, on a research protocol).

Although most agents are effective against trophozoites, it is more difficult to kill the cysts, which can tolerate 2% hydrochloric acid, peroxides, and chlorine. Biguanide, diamidines, and Neosporin are recommended treatments, and oral imidazoles may also help. Polyhexamethyl biguanide can destroy most trophozoites, and chlorhexidine is more destructive to cysts.

Daily follow-up is needed to determine if the condition is improving. If this is the case, the medication may be tapered very slowly and the patient may be followed as an outpatient. The treatment is usually continued for 6–8 weeks *after* resolution of corneal inflammation, which may take up to 18 months in some cases, depending on the extent of the infection.

Other Causes of Infectious Keratitis

Other microorganisms not discussed in this chapter can cause infectious keratitis. They are rare and if found on culture or microscopy, sensitivity to antimicrobial agents should be obtained to guide treatment.

PEARLS AND SPECIAL SITUATIONS

- Contact lens wear is a major risk factor for infectious keratitis.
- Immune reactions to deposits on contact lenses may cause corneal infiltrates similar to those caused by hypersensitivity colonizing bacteria. The two reactions can be distinguished because the former usually do not stain with fluorescein.
- Patients with keratitis usually have severe eye pain. However, keratitis caused by herpes simplex virus can lead to reduced corneal sensation and, therefore, be present with mild or even no pain.
- Corneal abrasions typically heal within 2–3 days; symptoms persisting beyond this time period should raise one's suspicion for infectious keratitis.

REFERENCES

1. Muir KW, Jin J, Freedman SF. Central corneal thickness and its relationship to intraocular pressure in children. *Ophthalmology.* 2004;111:2220-2223.
2. Sanchis-Gimeno JA, Lleo-Perez A, Alonso L, Rahhal MS, Martinez-Soriano F. Anatomic study of the corneal thickness of young emmetropic subjects. *Cornea.* 2004;23: 669-673.
3. Erie JC, Nevitt MP, Hodge DO, Ballard DJ. Incidence of ulcerative keratitis in a defined population from 1950 through 1988. *Arch Ophthalmol.* 1993;111:1665-1671.
4. Keay L, Edwards K, Naduvilath T, et al. Microbial keratitis predisposing factors and morbidity. *Ophthalmology.* 2006;113:109-116.
5. Sharma S. Keratitis. *Biosci Rep.* 2001;21:419-444.
6. Cruz OA, Sabir SM, Capo H, Alfonso EC. Microbial keratitis in childhood. *Ophthalmology.* 1993;100:192-196.
7. Kunimoto DY, Sharma S, Reddy MK, et al. Microbial keratitis in children. *Ophthalmology.* 1998;105:252-257.
8. Parmar P, Salman A, Kalavathy CM, et al. Microbial keratitis at extremes of age. *Cornea.* 2006;25:153-158.
9. Hsiao CH, Yeung L, Ma DH, et al. Pediatric microbial keratitis in Taiwanese children: A review of hospital cases. *Arch Ophthalmol.* 2007;125:603-609.
10. Koidl C, Bozic M, Mossbock G, et al. Rapid diagnosis of adenoviral keratoconjunctivitis by a fully automated molecular assay. *Ophthalmology.* 2005;112:1521-1528.
11. Butt AL, Chodosh J. Adenoviral keratoconjunctivitis in a tertiary care eye clinic. *Cornea.* 2006;25:199-202.
12. Chang DC, Grant GB, O'Donnell K, et al. Multistate outbreak of Fusarium keratitis associated with use of a contact lens solution. *JAMA.* 2006;296:953-963.
13. Hassanlou M, Bhargava A, Hodge WG. Bilateral acanthamoeba keratitis and treatment strategy based on lesion depth. *Can J Ophthalmol.* 2006;41:71-73.
14. Schwartz GS, Holland EJ. Oral acyclovir for the management of herpes simplex virus keratitis in children. *Ophthalmology.* 2000;107:278-282.
15. Constantinou M, Daniell M, Snibson GR, Vu HT, Taylor HR. Clinical efficacy of moxifloxacin in the treatment of bacterial keratitis: A randomized clinical trial. *Ophthalmology.* 2007;114:1622-1629.
16. Parmar P, Salman A, Kalavathy CM, et al. Comparison of topical gatifloxacin 0.3% and ciprofloxacin 0.3% for the treatment of bacterial keratitis. *Am J Ophthalmol.* 2006;141:282-286.
17. Kumar M, Mishra NK, Shukla PK. Sensitive and rapid polymerase chain reaction based diagnosis of mycotic keratitis through single stranded conformation polymorphism. *Am J Ophthalmol.* 2005;140:851-857.
18. Sponsel W, Chen N, Dang D, et al. Topical voriconazole as a novel treatment for fungal keratitis. *Antimicrob Agents Chemother.* 2006;50:262-268.
19. Thomas PA, Geraldine P. Infectious keratitis. *Curr Opin Infect Dis.* 2007;20:129-141.

SECTION 5

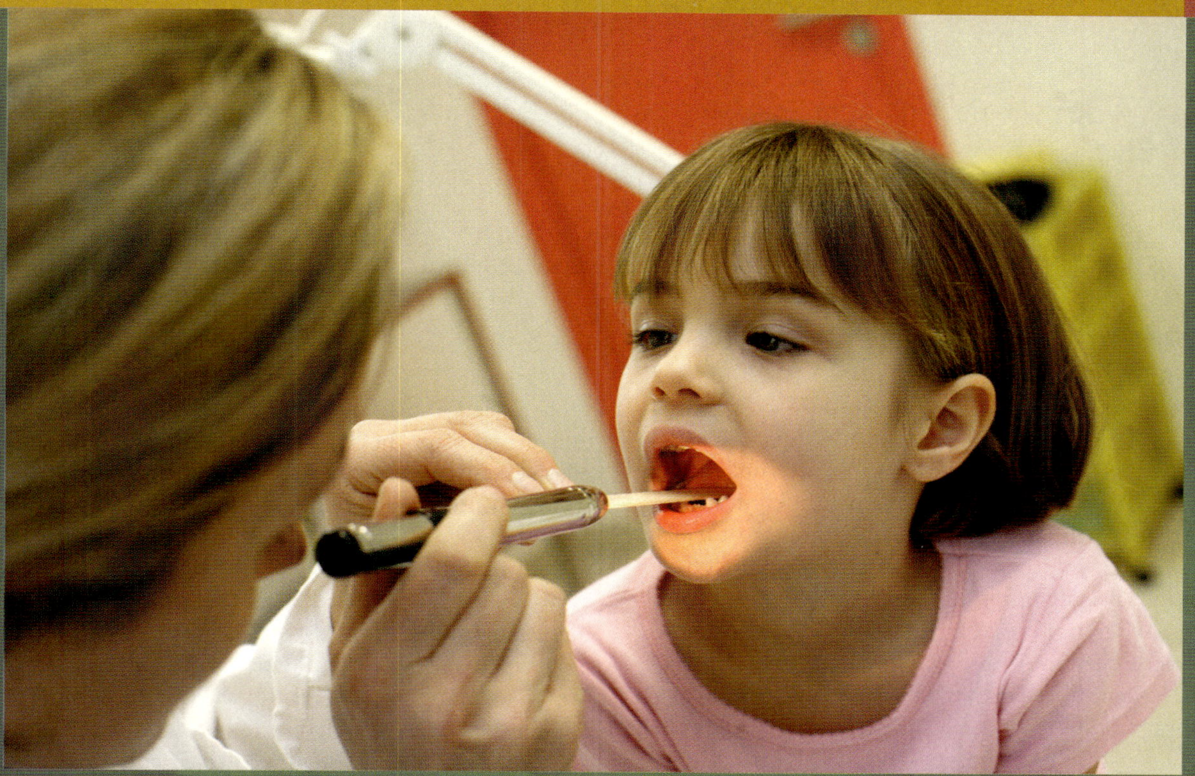

Oral Cavity and Neck Infections

CHAPTER 24

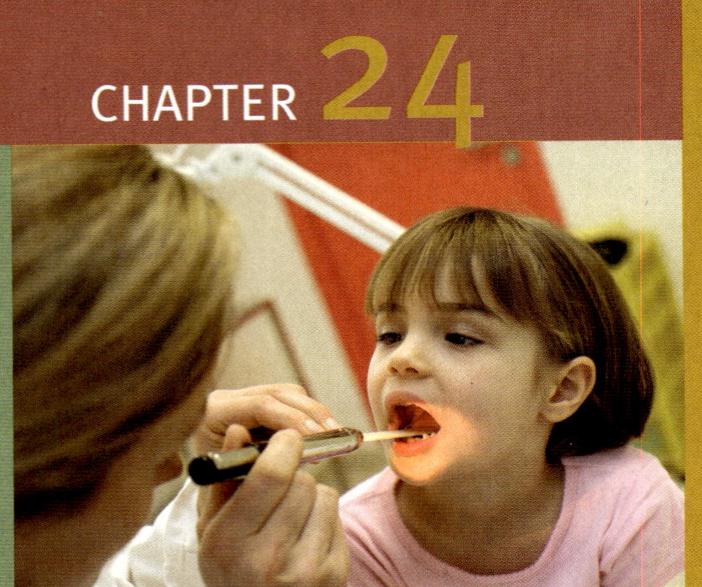

Pharyngitis and Stomatitis

Mark S. Pasternack

DEFINITIONS

Pharyngitis reflects inflammation of the mucous membranes of the pharynx and is manifested clinically as "sore throat"; inflammation of the adjoining tonsils ("tonsillopharyngitis") or isolated tonsillar infection ("tonsillitis") is commonly included in this diagnostic category. Pharyngitis may be part of a broader respiratory tract infection or one manifestation of a systemic illness. Stomatitis refers to inflammation of the mucous membranes of the oral cavity, including the buccal mucosa, palate, gingiva tongue, and lips.

EPIDEMIOLOGY

Pharyngitis is one of the most common reasons for sick visits to the pediatrician's office or other outpatient acute care settings. An estimated 6.5 million outpatient visits are made annually for evaluation of pharyngitis among children and young adults younger than age 21,[1] making this illness the third or fourth most common reason for seeking acute care in these age groups. Most episodes of pharyngitis are caused by viruses and require only supportive care. Up to 30% of acute pharyngitis episodes in children are attributable to group A beta-hemolytic streptococci (GABHS) with a peak incidence in winter and early spring.[2] GABHS frequently colonize the oropharynx of asymptomatic children (5–20%), so that recovery of GABHS by culture or rapid detection techniques does not necessarily confirm true streptococcal pharyngitis.[3]

GABHS pharyngitis is most common among young school-age children. Streptococcal pharyngitis carries a potential significance exceeding the limited morbidity of throat discomfort, since GABHS pharyngitis may trigger significant nonsuppurative complications such as acute rheumatic fever and acute glomerulonephritis. Over the last two decades, there has been a relative resurgence of acute rheumatic fever in scattered regions in the United States, particularly in the Rocky Mountains and intermountain areas, with approximately 600 cases diagnosed in Salt Lake City, UT, between 1995 and 2003.[4] This increase has brought increasing attention to the problem of streptococcal pharyngitis in the United States, although in much of the developing world, acute rheumatic fever has remained a widespread and serious clinical challenge.

GABHS are consistently detected either by rapid antigen detection testing (RADT)[5] or by the presence of beta-hemolysis and susceptibility to bacitracin following culture on blood agar plates. There is marked molecular heterogeneity among GABHS isolates. Serologic methods used to type surface proteins (e.g., M, T) have been replaced over the past decade by genotyping based on sequence analysis of the corresponding *emm* gene that has defined over 100 unique *emm* genotypes. Such strain characterization has shown that several distinct GABHS strains may circulate within a community at a particular time. The predominant circulating strains may vary both temporally and geographically within the United States.[6]

Recurrent GABHS pharyngitis may be either due to acquisition of a new *emm* type or, less commonly, due to recurrence of a previously invasive strain. Recurrent streptococcal pharyngitis is a relatively common clinical problem, especially among children entering school. The overall incidence of recurrent GABHS pharyngitis in children is approximately 1% though there is substantial variation by age. Approximately 2% of children aged 4–6 years have three or more episodes per year while 0.1% of children aged 13–15 years have recurrent GABHS infections.[7]

A number of other bacterial pathogens associated with childhood pharyngitis, including group C and G streptococci, *Mycoplasma pneumoniae*, *Chlamydophila pneumoniae* (formerly *Chlamydia pneumoniae*), *Arcanobacterium haemolyticum*, and *Corynebacterium diphtheriae*, are not detected by rapid group A streptococcal antigen detection testing nor by routine laboratory methods.[2] Thus, estimates of bacterial pharyngitis attributed to nongroup A streptococci are generally based on small clinical microbiology studies and probably do not exceed 2% of pharyngitis episodes. *M. pneumoniae* pharyngitis, which mimics GABHS infection, is considered uncommon though one study reported that *M. pneumoniae* accounted for 24% of non-GABHS episodes.[8]

Viral pharyngitis is associated with many pathogens that typically cause upper and lower respiratory tract infections (Table 24–1). The relative role of different viruses in provoking pharyngitis varies by season (e.g., respiratory viruses in winter/early spring, enteroviruses in summer) and geographic location.

Gingivostomatitis is very common and is generally caused by herpes simplex virus (HSV) type I, although a small fraction of orolabial HSV infection in children is actually due to HSV type II. HSV carriage is very common among asymptomatic adults and approaches 50% in many populations. Since culture-positive

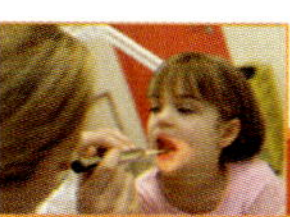

Table 24–I.

Differential Diagnosis

Stomatitis	*Candida albicans*
	Coxsackie virus
Noninfectious	Aphthous ulcers
	Erythema multiforme/Stevens Johnson syndrome (may be seen with/without HSV, *M. pneumoniae*) chemotherapy-associated mucositis
	Marshall's syndrome (PFAPA syndrome: periodic fever with aphthous ulcers, pharyngitis and cervical lymphadenopathy)
Gingivostomatitis	Herpes simplex virus type I
	Herpes simplex virus type II
Noninfectious	Aphthous ulcers
	Erythema multiforme/Stevens Johnson syndrome (may be seen with/without HSV, *M. pneumoniae*)
Rare	*Treponema pallidum*
	Crohn's disease
	Bullous disorders: pemphigus vulgaris, pemphigoid
	Behcet's syndrome
Pharyngitis	
Bacterial	Group A streptococci (may have associated scarlet fever)
	Group C streptococci (may have scarlatiniform rash)
	Arcanobacterium haemolyticum (teenagers/young adults, often with fine rash on extensor surfaces of extremities)
	Mycoplasma pneumoniae (with/without typical lower respiratory tract findings)
	Chlamydia pneumoniae (with/without typical lower respiratory tract findings)
	Chlamydia psittaci (generally with lower respiratory tract findings)
	Vincent's angina (mixed anerobic infection of gingivae/pharynx)
Rare	*Corynebacterium diphtheriae* (thick membranous disease, airway compromise)
	Neisseria gonorrheae (exudative pharyngitis; in sexually active teenagers/child abuse)
	Tularemia (oropharyngeal form due to ingestion of contaminated water/meat)
	Plague
Viral	Rhinoviruses
	Parainfluenza viruses 1–4 (may see bronchiolitis, croup)
	Adenovirus (often prominent conjunctivitis; may see pneumonitis, hepatitis)
	Enterovirus (esp. coxsackie A) (herpangina, hand-foot-mouth disease)
	Influenza A
	Influenza B
	Respiratory syncytial virus (often with bronchiolitis)
	Human metapneumovirus
	Coronaviruses
	Epstein–Barr virus (infectious mononucleosis, typically teenagers/young adults)
	Cytomegalovirus (heterophile-negative mononucleosis)
	Human immunodeficiency virus (as part of primary HIV infection)

(*continued*)

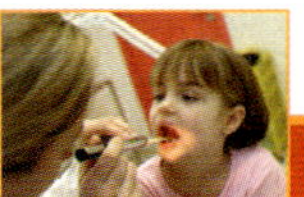

Table 24–I. (Continued)

Differential Diagnosis	
Additional oropharyngeal infections mimicking as pharyngitis	Epiglottis: <5 years, drooling, hot potato voice, 'sniffing' neck extension, now rare due to universal infant conjugate *H. influenzae* vaccination Peritonsillar abscess: Quinsy; may complicate GABHS pharyngitis and/or infectious mononucleosis Retropharyngeal abscess (Younger children, often without prior pharyngitis) Parapharyngeal abscess Lemierre's syndrome (suppurative thrombophlebitis of internal jugular vein, with *Fusobacterium necrophorum* bacteremia, and metastatic infection, especially to lungs)
Noninfectious	Kawasaki disease (may have prominent oropharyngeal and cervical lymphadenopathy findings) Marshall's syndrome (PFAPA syndrome: periodic fever with aphthous ulcers, pharyngitis and cervical lymphadenopathy)

asymptomatic viral shedding may occur in approximately 1% of these adults (and up to 30% of patients' saliva is HSV-positive by polymerase chain reaction (PCR)) at any time without a clear seasonal pattern, infection of susceptible children by direct contact occurs commonly.[9]

PATHOGENESIS

In general, bacteria and viruses causing pharyngitis are disseminated by direct contact with respiratory secretions and through contaminated airborne droplets produced with coughing or sneezing. Many viral pathogens, including influenza, parainfluenza viruses, and respiratory syncytial virus, are also transmitted by contact with contaminated surfaces. Virions bind to specific receptor moieties on respiratory epithelium, leading to their internalization, uncoating, and escape into the intracellular milieu of infected cells where viral replication occurs. Viral respiratory infections generate local and systemic immune responses though clinically significant reinfections can be seen with certain agents (e.g., Respiratory Syncytial Virus (RSV)). In contrast, orolabial herpes simplex, which spreads beyond the epithelium to infect sensory neurons, leads to latent infection within dorsal root ganglion cells, thus providing a viral reservoir for reactivation within neurons and recurrent mucocutaneous disease.

Bacterial pathogens similarly interact with respiratory epithelial cells in a highly specific manner. GABHS express pili and several distinct adhesion proteins on the bacterial surface that facilitate binding to respiratory epithelium[10] and secrete biofilms to enhance their growth.[11] In addition to their surface growth, adherent GABHS bind fibronectin via the M protein and in turn are internalized via the epithelial fibronectin receptor, integrin $\alpha_5\beta_1$.[12] Such intracellular sequestration of viable GABHS may contribute to persistent pharyngeal colonization despite antibiotic therapy, as most antibiotics used to treat streptococcal pharyngitis do not achieve significant intracellular concentrations. *C. diphtheriae* also express pili, which adhere to respiratory epithelium, leading to dense pseudomembrane formation, which can progress to life-threatening airway obstruction. The secretion and systemic dissemination of bacterial toxins (streptococcal pyrogenic exotoxin and diphtheria toxin) are responsible for the systemic features of these diseases (e.g., scarlet fever, diphtheria). Acute rheumatic fever, the major nonsuppurative complication of GABHS pharyngitis, is thought to result from the development of antistreptococcal cellular and humoral immune responses that cross-react with proteins expressed in target organs such as the heart and basal ganglia.[13] The risk of acute rheumatic fever depends on the infecting strain of GABHS and likely also depends on host immunological features.

CLINICAL FEATURES

Pharyngitis

Viral Pharyngitis

Viral pharyngitis is generally associated with broad and progressive involvement of upper and often lower respiratory tract disease. Thus, a variety of additional respiratory tract symptoms such as rhinorrhea, nasal congestion, conjunctivitis, laryngitis, cough, and wheezing, or gastrointestinal symptoms (diarrhea) or cutaneous manifestations (exanthem) may accompany a complaint of sore throat. These symptoms evolve over the course of 2–3 days and children come to attention primarily because of worsening throat pain or persistent fever. The pharyngeal findings are often quite nonspecific, with tonsillopharyngeal erythema, and variable tonsillomegaly; shotty cervical lymphadenopathy may be noted as well. The presence of small palatal or pharyngeal vesicles or ulcers strongly suggests enteroviral infection but is infrequently seen. The development of

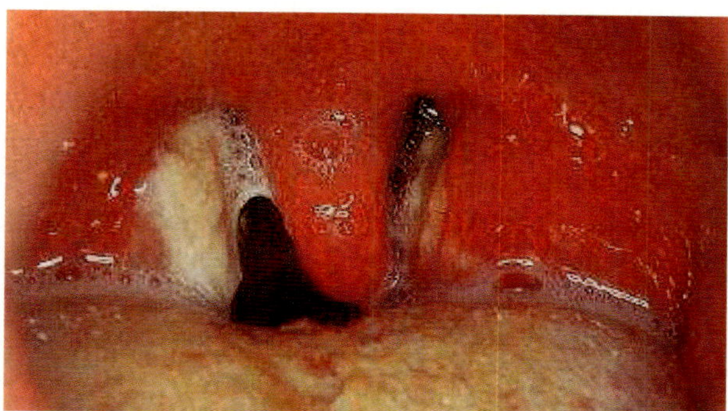

FIGURE 24–1 ■ Acute infectious mononucleosis. The exudative tonsillopharyngitis closely resembles severe streptococcal pharyngitis (*Courtesy of Hugh Hazenfield, MD.*)

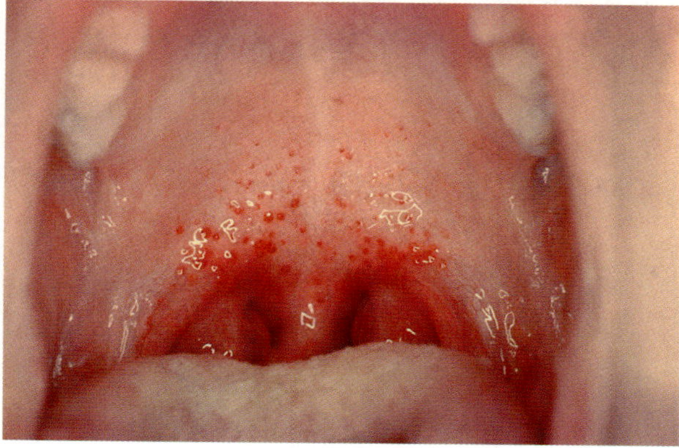

FIGURE 24–2 ■ Group A streptococcal pharyngitis. Note the prominent tonsillar edema, erythema, and palatal petechiae. Exudative pharyngitis is often prominent. (*Courtesy of Heinz Eichenwald, MD, CDC Public Health Image Library.*)

bronchospasm strongly supports a viral process. Generalized rash may be seen in either viral or bacterial pharyngitis, but discrete maculopapular or vesicular lesions on the palms and soles accompany pharyngitis or oropharyngeal ulcerations (herpangina) in "hand-foot-mouth" syndrome caused by Coxsackie A16 or enterovirus 71. Exudative pharyngitis is less common with viral disease but occurs commonly in younger children with adenoviral infection.[14]

Epstein–Barr virus (EBV) pharyngitis (Figure 24–1), as part of the infectious mononucleosis syndrome, resembles the exudative pharyngitis of GABHS infection; coinfections with both pathogens are well known.[15] Older children and teenagers typically present with severe exudative tonsillopharyngitis, with persistent fever and significant tender cervical lymphadenopathy. In contrast to patients with streptococcal infection, illness may persist for 7–21 days, with the common development of palpable splenomegaly, less common hepatomegaly, and regularly observed anicteric hepatitis. Primary cytomegalovirus infection and HIV infection may mimic severe cases of EBV-induced infectious mononucleosis, although in the case of HIV, rash and headache are more prominent than with EBV or other forms of acute pharyngitis. Among younger children, the pharyngeal manifestations of EBV infection may be less prominent: Preschoolers may present with prolonged undifferentiated fever, sometimes with adenopathy, splenomegaly, myelosuppression or periorbital edema.

Bacterial Pharyngitis

In contrast to viral processes and the nonexudative pharyngitis associated with respiratory tract infection by *M. pneumoniae* and *C. pneumoniae*, group A streptococcal disease classically presents as a "pure" exudative pharyngitis (Figure 24–2). The onset of symptoms is quite abrupt, with progression of pain and dysphagia over hours with or without fever. Clinical scoring systems accurately predict high-probability classic GABHS infection and low-probability typical viral disease but yield indeterminate scores for many patients.[16] Younger patients often have prominent gastrointestinal symptoms of abdominal pain or vomiting.

In toddlers, upper respiratory symptoms of coryza and copious serous rhinorrhea predominate while findings of exudative pharyngitis are uncommon; younger children rarely develop nonsuppurative complications of streptococcal pharyngitis such as acute rheumatic fever. In older children, physical findings of streptococcal pharyngitis include marked pharyngeal erythema, enlarged tonsils, uvular swelling, and a patchy white tonsillopharyngeal exudate. Petechiae may be present on the soft palate. Tender cervical lymphadenopathy is common. Exudative pharyngitis accompanied by "strawberry tongue," scarlatinaform rash (diffuse "sandpaper" erythroderma), and petechiae in flexor creases (Pastia's lines) suggests scarlet fever due to GABHS expressing pyrogenic exotoxin.

Nongroup A beta-hemolytic streptococci cause exudative tonsillopharyngitis in severe cases. However, nongroup A streptococci are not associated with rheumatic fever or poststreptococcal glomerulonephritis. *A. haemolyticum* typically causes infection in adolescents and young adults. Pharygeal erythema and tonsillar exudate are common. Bilateral anterior cervical or submandibular lymphadenopathy occurs in up to half of infected patients. Classifically, the rash associated with *A. haemolyticum* manifests on the extensor surfaces of the extremities and occasionally the neck and trunk; the palms and soles are spared.

Diphtheria is now vanishingly rare in the United States, but must remain a consideration when evaluating recent immigrants, particularly from the former Soviet Union where population migration and decreased childhood immunization rates have contributed to a widespread epidemic. Sore throat is a common initial manifestation but fever is characteristically absent or low grade. Nasopharyngeal and laryngotracheal inflammation

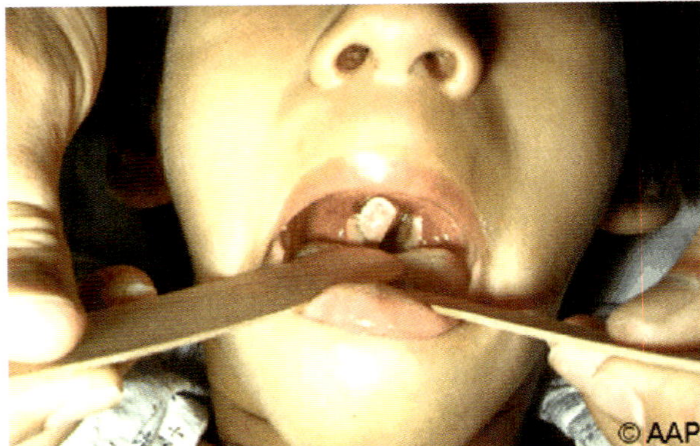

FIGURE 24–3 ■ Diphtheritic pharyngitis in a 15-year-old girl. Note the dense membranous pharyngitis involving the tonsil and uvula. (*Source*: *AAP 2006 Red Book, with permission of the American Academy of Pediatrics*.)

are followed by the development of a thick exudative tonsillar membrane that may extend to the uvula, soft palate, and posterior pharynx (Figure 24–3). Marked neck swelling develops as a consequence of soft tissue edema and massive cervical adenopathy ("bull neck" appearance). Airway obstruction due to neck edema and pseudomembrane formation occurs in severe cases.[17]

Stomatitis

Orolabial herpes simplex infections begin with the development of crops of small vesicles with adjoining erythema involving part or occasionally most of the vermilion border of the lips (Figure 24–4). These superficial thin-roofed vesicles are readily unroofed following minimal local trauma (e.g., eating), so children may present with localized crusting lesions that obscure the primary viral process and resemble impetigo. Additional herpetic vesicles may be present on adjoining facial skin, the anterior buccal mucosa, and the anterior gingivae, but posterior pharyngeal herpetic lesions are rare; the presence of discrete soft palatal and posterior pharyngeal vesicles or ulcerations suggests enteroviral infection. Intraoral disease may interfere with normal oral intake, and children may come to attention primarily for dehydration. There is a broad range of systemic reaction, with no or little fever in some cases and significant fever and acute illness in other cases particularly in toddlers with severe primary infection. Following primary infection, HSV gingivostomatitis may recur at the sites of primary infection. Although children younger than 5 years may have very frequent, even monthly recurrences, most children experience mild focal recurrent HSV infections only sporadically, typically after incidental respiratory tract infection ("cold sores" and "fever blisters") or after local trauma such as sunburn or scalding. In contrast, aphthous ulcers are even more painful, generally larger in size than herpetic vesicles (from 3 to 4 mm superficial lesions to ⩾1 cm more deeply ulcerated lesions), often somewhat irregular in shape, and occur as solitary lesions or as part of a group of a few lesions scattered on the buccal mucosa, palate, or gingival mucosa.[18] Systemic manifestations such as fever are uncommon. Superficial lesions heal over days, but large deeper lesions may require a month or more to heal. Aphthous ulcers may recur quite frequently for reasons that are not entirely clear (Figure 24–5). Stress, exposure to irritant substances such as toothpaste cleansers (sodium lauryl sulfate), and a variety of other substances have been proposed as triggering agents.

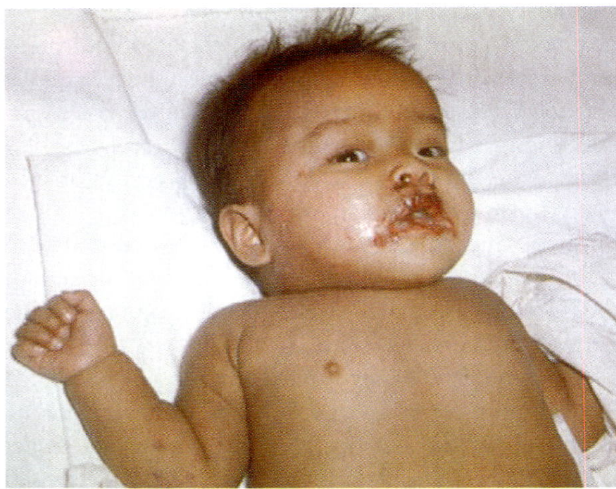

FIGURE 24–4 ■ Herpes simplex gingivostomatitis in a 10-month-old child. Note the nearly confluent involvement of the lips and scattered facial and upper extremity vesicles. (*Source: CDC, J.D. Millar, Public Health Image Library #2903*).

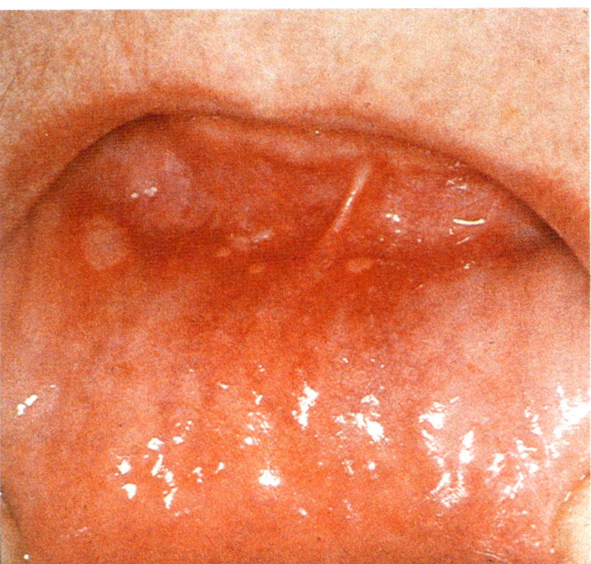

FIGURE 24–5 ■ Aphthous stomatitis. Note the irregularly shaped, shallow ulcerations distributed at the base of the gingival sulcus. (*Source: Generously provided by Dr. Michael Cunningham, Massachusetts Eye and Ear Infirmary*).

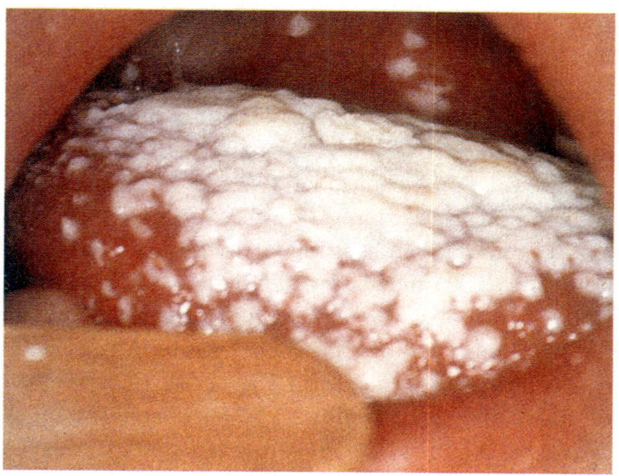

FIGURE 24–6 ■ Oral candidiasis. There are widespread plaques of adherent white material involving the tongue and palate. The lesions are densely adherent and are not removed by gentle debridement. *(Courtesy of Michael Cunningham, MD.)*

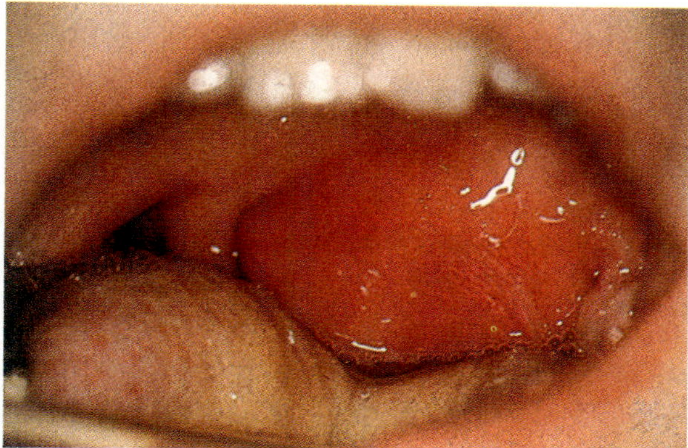

FIGURE 24–7 ■ Peritonsillar abscess. The left tonsil is displaced forward and the uvula is displaced to the right. *(Courtesy of Michael Cunningham, MD.)*

Candidal infection can also produce focal or rather diffuse infection of the lips, tongue, buccal mucoasa, and/or palate. In contrast to the ulcerative and crusted lesions of HSV, candidiasis displays an adherent white exudate on involved mucosa (Figure 24–6), and is not associated with fever or other signs of systemic toxicity. It may occur in otherwise healthy infants, but certainly occurs commonly after antibiotic therapy. Candidiasis as a harbinger of cell-mediated immunodeficiency is uncommon given its frequent incidence in healthy infants.

DIFFERENTIAL DIAGNOSIS

Invasive focal bacterial infections of the oral cavity include epiglottitis; peritonsillar, parapharyngeal, and retropharyngeal abscesses; Lemierre's syndrome; and Vincent's and Ludwig's angina. These focal infections are associated with high fever, increased clinical toxicity, as well as localizing or lateralizing pain, tenderness, drooling, stridor, and occasionally alterations in voice. These syndromes represent otolaryngologic emergencies due to possible airway obstruction. Epiglottitis (now very rare) and retropharyngeal abscess occur primarily in preschool-age children. Epiglottitis typically presents with drooling, dysphagia, and respiratory distress. Retropharyngeal abscesses may present with torticollis or pain with neck extension; stridor is a rare manifestation of retropharyngeal abscess. Peritonsillar (Figure 24–7) and parapharyngeal abscesses typically develop in older children as suppurative complications of pharyngitis. Lemierre's syndrome is a rare but life-threatening infection typically caused by *Fusobacterium necrophorum*. Lemierre's syndrome consists of internal jugular septic thrombophlebitis accompanied by septic emboli to the lung and other sites and occurs almost exclusively in adolescents and young adults.[19] Lemierre's syndrome should be suspected in a child with persistent or progressive pharyngitis associated with neck stiffness, torticollis, or systemic toxicity.

The differential diagnosis of pharyngitis is summarized in Table 24–1. Although several clinical features point toward streptococcal pharyngitis (palatal petechiae, exudative tonsillitis, tender cervical lymphadenopathy, and fever) or viral disease (conjunctivitis, coryza, cough, laryngitis, wheezing, and viral exanthem), the diagnostic accuracy of clinical examinations, even by experienced clinicians, is limited (50–60%).

DIAGNOSIS

Pharyngitis

Diagnostic approaches are summarized in Table 24–2 and in Figure 24–8. The diagnostic challenge of pharyngitis lies in distinguishing bacterial from viral infections. While most (>70%) episodes of pharyngitis are self-limited viral infections, children with untreated GABHS infection are at increased risk of suppurative as well as nonsuppurative sequelae. Clinical judgment is inadequately sensitive and specific for the diagnosis of GABHS pharyngitis, so laboratory confirmation is required to support antibiotic therapy. RADTs offer relatively quick turnaround, especially in office practice, and have high specificity (i.e., false-positives are uncommon). However, most RADT methodologies have a sensitivity of approximately 85%, so children with a strong clinical likelihood of streptococcal pharyngitis with negative RADT require throat culture to confirm the diagnosis.[5,20] Throat cultures streaked on blood agar plates containing bacitracin disks should be inspected after overnight incubation at 37°C, as well as

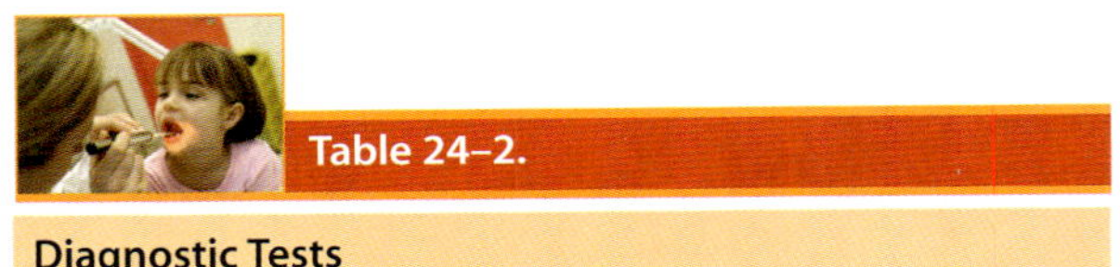

Table 24–2.

Diagnostic Tests

Gingivostomatitis:
Clinical diagnosis usually satisfactory
In atypical cases, can consider
(1) direct immunofluorescence or
(2) viral culture or
(3) HSV PCR
depending on study availability
Oropharyngeal candidiasis:
Clinical diagnosis usually satisfactory
In immunocompromised children failing to respond to standard therapy, can consider fungal culture and sensitivity testing of candidal isolates
Group A streptococcal pharyngitis:
Laboratory confirmation necessary for definitive therapy
Consider rapid antigen detection testing (several commercial products) if available
If negative, proceed to throat culture for group A *Streptococcus* (streptococcal serology, test of cure cultures, and monitoring of asymptomatic patients are not helpful except in special circumstances)

after another 24 hours at room temperature. Even throat cultures to identify GABHS have limited sensitivity and specificity due to the limitations of bacitracin susceptibility testing. A small percentage of presumptive GABHS throat culture isolates may be false-positives, and a small percentage of true group A streptococcal isolates may be missed.[2] Serologic testing for the presence of antistreptococcal antibody responses (antistreptolysin-O, DNase B, or antihyaluronidase) may be helpful in assessing past invasive streptococcal infection, but does not assist in the diagnosis of acute pharyngitis and is not routinely useful in managing acute episodes of pharyngitis.

Although comprehensive microbiologic testing to identify and treat other bacterial pathogens responsible for pharyngitis would be desirable, the time and effort required and the limited clinical benefit of the therapy makes comprehensive testing in the outpatient setting impractical. Some clinical laboratories report the presence of abundant group C or group G hemolytic streptococci, but this identification often requires 48 hours or more, by which time many children have improved clinically in the absence of antibiotic therapy.[21] In the proper clinical setting, specialized testing for *Neisseria gonorrheae* (throat culture on Thayer Martin medium), *C. diphtheriae* (throat culture), *M. pneumoniae* (PCR of throat swab and of nasopharyngeal aspirate), and the other listed bacterial pathogens can be performed; in these situations, the laboratory should be notified as specialized media for growth of these bacteria are not routinely used. Similarly, respiratory viral antigen testing, viral PCR testing, or viral cultures can be performed, but the cost, limited availability, delayed turnaround, and absence of impact on management make such studies impractical. Heterophile testing for infectious mononucleosis is readily available and quite helpful in clinical management, but may not turn positive until the convalescent phase of illness, or even remain negative despite EBV infection, particularly in preteenage children and a small fraction of teenagers and young adults.

Stomatitis

The diagnosis of herpes gingivostomatitis is generally established by clinical criteria alone in view of the unique physical findings. Rapid diagnostic testing for HSV (PCR, direct immunofluorescence or, less commonly, Tzanck testing) is often difficult to perform on intraoral or labial ulcers; it is preferable to unroof an undisturbed

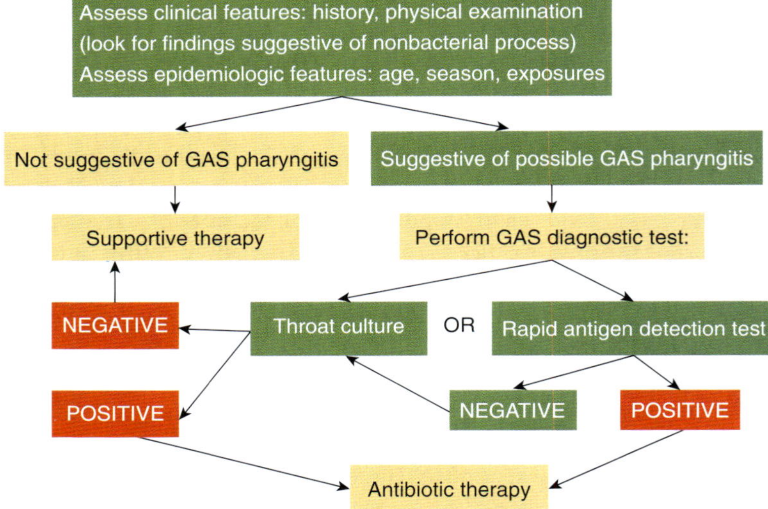

FIGURE 24–8 ■ Algorithm for the management of acute pharyngitis.

cutaneous vesicle to harvest vesicular fluid and to scrape the vesicle base for cellular material for these studies and for viral culture, if desired. In rare problematic cases of refractory or severe recurrent disease, local biopsy is helpful to assess possible herpes simplex infection from the variety of noninfectious, inflammatory processes, which can produce ulcerative stomatitis.

TREATMENT

The goals of therapy of streptococcal pharyngitis include (1) ameliorate symptoms, (2) prevent suppurative and nonsuppurative complications, (3) decrease spread of group A streptococci to family members and other contacts, (4) reduce long-term carriage of group A streptococci, and (5) minimize antibiotic utilization and selection pressure for resistant bacteria.[2,22] Symptomatic streptococcal pharyngitis is usually a self-limited process with resolution of symptoms within 4 days or so even in the absence of therapy. Prompt antibiotic therapy may hasten recovery by 1–2 days. The development of acute rheumatic fever can be prevented by initiating proper antibiotic therapy any time within 9 days of the start of symptomatic illness. Thus, treatment for mild to moderate episodes of streptococcal pharyngitis is focused on the prevention of acute rheumatic fever and may be safely delayed until throat culture results are available. In cases of severe symptomatic disease consistent with streptococcal pharyngitis, antibiotic therapy may be initiated at the time of evaluation even if RADT is negative, and then stopped after 48 hours if the throat culture is negative.

Oral penicillin therapy remains the mainstay of treatment for nonallergic children, based on its long record of efficacy, safety, and low cost (Table 24–3). Amoxicillin is commonly prescribed for younger children because of the enhanced palatability and absorption of amoxicillin suspension. Erythromycin is still generally recommended as second line therapy for patients with immediate hypersensitivity to beta lactams. Although high rates of erythromycin resistance have been reported during clonal outbreaks over small geographic regions (e.g., a private school in Pittsburgh, PA),[23] the general rate of erythromycin resistance among group A streptococcal pharyngeal isolates in the United States is still below 5%.[24] Patients with nonurticarial rash allergy to penicillin may receive oral first generation cephalosporin therapy. A variety of additional cephalosporins have been approved for the therapy of streptococcal pharyngitis, with potential treatment regimens lasting only 5 days or requiring only one or two medication doses/day.[25] Although more convenient, these alternate regimens are more costly and have had limited experience when compared with penicillin therapy. Routine follow-up cultures to assess microbiological cure are not indicated, since persistent positive cultures obtained after a full 10-day course of therapy are ascribed to streptococcal carriage rather than persistent infection. The rarity of posttherapy nonsuppurative sequelae despite streptococcal carriage strongly supports this perspective.

Recurrent symptomatic pharyngitis following a 10-day antibiotic course may occur soon after completion of therapy, suggesting true antibiotic failure and relapse,[26] or may occur after extended intervals of weeks to months. Early antibiotic failure is commonly attributed to poor compliance with multidose 10-day antibiotic regimens, since children are often entirely well halfway into their course of therapy. However, the possibility that penicillin or amoxicillin may fail to eradicate streptococcal pharyngitis despite excellent compliance has been raised by Brook[27] and others. They suggest that resident oral cavity microorganisms are "copathogens" that frequently secrete beta-lactamase, which in turn inactivates penicillin or amoxicillin, requiring therapy with beta-lactamase-resistant agents such as cephalosporins. The management of children with short-term recurrent streptococcal pharyngitis has been addressed by expert panels.[2,28] Treatment for apparent relapsing infection may include repeat oral courses of penicillin or amoxicillin, parenteral benzathine penicillin to overcome possible compliance issues, as well as consideration of macrolide or first-generation cephalosporin therapy.

For the patient with multiple episodes of streptococcal pharyngitis per year, distinguishing between episodes of viral pharyngitis with positive streptococcal testing due to asymptomatic long-term carriage and true recurrent streptococcal pharyngitis can be challenging. The presence of elevated antibody responses to group A streptococcal antigens and the absence of positive cultures between episodes of pharyngitis suggest true recurrent bacterial pharyngitis, while low-level antibody titers and persistently positive surveillance cultures suggest streptococcal carriage. Although *emm* genotyping can clarify questions of streptococcal carriage versus recurrent infection, this methodology is available in research settings only. In situations where frequent relapsing infection is raised, treatment of pharyngitis with penicillin (oral or pareneral) combined with rifampin, or oral therapy with clindamycin or azithromycin have been suggested.[2] Penicillin prophylaxis is recommended only for children who have had previous episodes of acute rheumatic fever or have siblings with previous acute rheumatic fever.

Tonsillectomy has been studied as adjunctive therapy for children with very frequent recurrent episodes of GABHS pharyngitis.[29] Among children with three or more episodes per year for 3 years, five or more episodes per year for 2 years, or seven or more episodes in a single

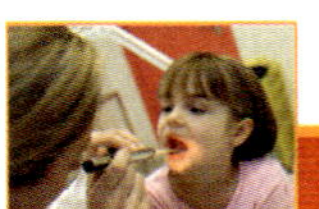

Table 24–3.

Treatment Regimens

Treatment Regimens
GABHS pharyngitis treatment
Preferred regimens:
Oral:
< 60 lb: Penicillin VK 250 mg twice or three times daily × 10 days
Amoxicillin 250 mg twice or three times daily × 10 days
>60 lb: Penicillin VK 500 mg twice or three times daily × 10 days
Amoxicillin 250–500 mg twice or three times daily × 10 days
Parenteral:
Benzathine penicillin G
600,000 U IM for children < 60 lb as single dose
1,200,000 U IM for children > 60 lb as single dose
In penicillin-allergic children (immediate hypersensitivity):
Erythromycin (20–40 mg/kg/d in 2 to 4 divided doses, depends on formulation) × 10 days
Additional options:
In penicillin-allergic children (nonimmediate hypersensitivity):
Erythromycin (dose depends on formulation) × 10 days or
Cephalexin 25–50 mg/kg/d in 2–3 divided doses × 10 days
[Clindamycin (20 mg/kg/d in 2–3 divided doses × 10 days]
Additional options (more expensive, less experience in preventing nonsuppurative sequelae of GABHS pharyngitis):
Clarithromycin 15 mg/kg/d in 2 divided doses × 10 days (max. 250 mg twice daily)
Azithromcyin 12 mg/kg/d × 5 days (max. 500 mg/day)
Cefuroxime 20 mg/kg/d in 2 divided doses × 10 days (max. dose 250 mg twice daily)
Cefadroxil 30 mg/kg/d in 1 dose or 2 divided doses × 10 days (max. 1 g twice daily)
Cefdinivir 14 mg/kg/d in 2 divided doses × 5–10 days or once daily × 10 days
Herpes simplex gingivostomatitis
Acyclovir 20 mg/kg orally 4 times daily (80 mg/kg/d)
If oral route is compromised by pain and dysphagia, administrer acyclovir 10mg/kg every 8 hours (30 mg/kg/d)
Oral candidiasis
Nystatin suspension (100,000 U/mL) swish and swallow (efficacy enhanced in cooperative older children) 5 mL at least 4 times daily continue for 2–3 days following resolution of thrush
Nystatin suspension apply directly 2 mL 4–6 times daily in infants
Clotrimazole troches (10 mg) dissolve one orally up to 5 times daily × 14 days (usually limited to children >3 years of age)
Fluconazole suspension 6 mg/kg loading dose then 3 mg/kg/d × 7–14 days continue therapy for several days beyond resolution of visible candidiasis
Aphthous stomatitis
Symptomatic supportive therapy
Mixture of diphenhydramine and kaolin–pectin suspensions applied directly several times daily

year, tonsillectomy reduces the frequency of GABHS pharyngitis substantially over the 2 postoperative years. The incidence of GABHS pharyngitits tends to wane significantly at 2 years with or without surgery, which thus limits indications for tonsillectomy to children with both frequent and severe disease. Tonsillectomy for children with less frequent GABHS pharyngitis offers only marginal benefit with increased cost and risk and is not generally recommended.[30]

HSV gingivostomatitis responds rapidly to acyclovir therapy, and new vesicles or ulcers generally stop appearing within 36–48 hours of starting treatment. Acyclovir can be administered as an oral suspension, but if children require hospitalization for dehydration, therapy is usually administered intravenously until comfortable oral intake is reestablished; topical acyclovir therapy is not effective. Newer nucleoside agents such as famciclovir and valacyclovir, requiring only two to three doses daily, are not formulated for intravenous or oral suspension use, and are used only in older children who can swallow pills. Children with sporadic recurrences can repeat short courses of acyclovir with each recurrence, but on occasion, children with very frequent recurrences are offered suppressive treatment with twice daily acyclovir for 12 months or more. Although this has no direct effect on the rate of recurrence, the recurrence rate often subsides following a prolonged period of suppression as part of the natural history of this process.

Oral candidiasis can be treated with topical nystatin or azole antifungal agents. Infants and toddlers are unable to "swish and swallow," of course, and compliance with multiple directly applied doses of topical therapy may be problematic. The availability of systemic therapy with oral fluconazole, available as a suspension for younger children, has facilitated treatment of refractory, severe, and frequently recurring episodes. True failure due to fluconazole resistance has been rare in the absence of underlying immunodeficiency and recurrent severe disease. Formal susceptibility testing can be performed for these patients; in many of these cases, newer azole agents (itraconazole, posaconazole, and voriconazole) may be effective.

REFERENCES

1. Cherry DK, Woodwell DA, Rechtsteiner EA. National Ambulatory Medical Care Survey: 2005 summary. Advance Data from Vital and Health Statistics No. 387. Hyattsville, MD: National Center for Health Statistics, 2007:1-39.
2. Bisno AL, Gerber MA, Gwaltney JM, Jr, Kaplan EL, Schwartz RH. Infectious Diseases Society of America. Practice guidelines for the diagnosis and management of group A streptococcal pharyngitis. Infectious Diseases Society of America. Clin Infect Dis 2002;35:113-25.
3. Martin JM, Green M, Barbadora KA, Wald ER. Group A streptococci among school-aged children: Clinical characteristics and the carrier state. Pediatrics 2004;114:1212-9.
4. Hillman ND, Tani LY, Veasy LG, et al. Current status of surgery for rheumatic carditis in children. Ann Thorac Surg 2004;78:1403-8.
5. Gerber MA, Shulman ST. Rapid diagnosis of pharyngitis caused by group A streptococci. Clin Microbiol Rev 2004;17:571,80.
6. Shulman ST, Tanz RR, Kabat W, et al. Group A streptococcal pharyngitis serotype surveillance in North America, 2000–2002. Clin Infect Dis 2004;39:325-32.
7. St Sauver JL, Weaver AL, Orvidas LJ, Jacobson RM, Jacobsen SJ. Population-based prevalence of repeated group A beta-hemolytic streptococcal pharyngitis episodes. Mayo Clin Proc 2006;81:1172-6.
8. Esposito S, Cavagna R, Bosis S, Droghetti R, Faelli N, Principi N. Emerging role of *Mycoplasma pneumoniae* in children with acute pharyngitis. Eur J Clin Microbiol Infect Dis 2002;21:607-10.
9. Miller CS, Danaher RJ. Asymptomatic shedding of herpes simplex virus (HSV) in the oral cavity. Oral Surg Oral Med Oral Pathol Oral Radiol Endod 2008;105:43-50.
10. Cunningham MW. Pathogenesis of group A streptococcal infections. Clin Microbiol Rev 2000;13:470-511.
11. Baldassarri L, Creti R, Recchia S, et al. Therapeutic failures of antibiotics used to treat macrolide-susceptible *Streptococcus pyogenes* infections may be due to biofilm formation. J Clin Microbiol 2006;44:2721-7.
12. Bisno AL, Brito MO, Collins CM. Molecular basis of group A streptococcal virulence. Lancet Infect Dis 2003;3:191-200.
13. Guilherme L, Kalil J. Rheumatic fever: From innate to acquired immune response. Ann NY Acad Sci 2007;1107:426-33.
14. Dominguez O, Rojo P, de Las Heras S, Folgueira D, Contreras JR. Clinical presentation and characteristics of pharyngeal adenovirus infections. Pediatr Infect Dis J 2005;24: 733-4.
15. Rush MC, Simon MW. Occurrence of Epstein–Barr virus illness in children diagnosed with group A streptococcal pharyngitis. Clin Pediatr (Phila) 2003;42:417-20.
16. Wald ER, Green MD, Schwartz B, Barbadora K. A streptococcal score card revisited. Pediatr Emerg Care 1998;14:109-11.
17. American Academy of Pediatrics. Diphtheria. In: Pickering LK, Baker CJ, Long SS, McMillan JA (eds.) Red Book: 2006 Report of the committee on infectious diseases, 27th edition. Elk Grove Village, IL: American Academy of Pediatrics, 2006:277-281.
18. Scully C. Clinical practice. Aphthous ulceration. N Engl J Med 2006;355:165-72.
19. Venglarcik J. Lemierre's syndrome. Pediatr Infect Dis J 2003;22:921-3.
20. Mirza A, Wludyka P, Chiu TT, Rathore MH. Throat culture is necessary after negative rapid antigen detection tests. Clin Pediatr (Phila) 2007;46:241-6.
21. Lindbaek M, Hoiby EA, Lermark G, Steinsholt IM, Hjortdahl P. Clinical symptoms and signs in sore throat patients with large colony variant beta-haemolytic streptococci groups C or G versus group A. Br J Gen Pract 2005;55:615-9.
22. Brunton S, Pichichero M. Considerations in the use of antibiotics for streptococcal pharyngitis. J Fam Pract 2006;Suppl:S9-S16.
23. Martin JM, Green M, Barbadora KA, Wald ER. Erythromycin-resistant group A streptococci in schoolchildren in Pittsburgh. N Engl J Med 2002;346:1200-6.
24. Tanz RR, Shulman ST, Shortridge VD, et al. Community-based surveillance in the United States of macrolide-resistant pediatric pharyngeal group A streptococci during 3 respiratory disease seasons. Clin Infect Dis 2004;39:1794-801.
25. Adam D, Scholz H, Helmerking M. Short-course antibiotic treatment of 4782 culture-proven cases of group A streptococcal tonsillopharyngitis and incidence of post-streptococcal sequelae. J Infect Dis 2000;182:509-16.
26. Casey JR, Pichichero ME. Symptomatic relapse of group A beta-hemolytic streptococcal tonsillopharyngitis in children. Clin Pediatr (Phila) 2007;46:307-10.
27. Brook I. Overcoming penicillin failures in the treatment of Group A streptococcal pharyngo-tonsillitis. Int J Pediatr Otorhinolaryngol 2007;71:1501-8.
28. Group A Streptococcal Infections. In: Pickering LK, Baker CJ, Long SS, McMillan JA, eds. Red Book: 2006 Report of the Committee on Infectious Diseases, 27th ed. Elk Grove Village, IL: American Academy of Pediatrics; 2006:550-60.
29. Paradise JL, Bluestone CD, Bachman RZ, et al. Efficacy of tonsillectomy for recurrent throat infection in severely affected children. Results of parallel randomized and nonrandomized clinical trials. N Engl J Med 1984;310:674-83.
30. Paradise JL, Bluestone CD, Colborn DK, Bernard BS, Rockette HE, Kurs-Lasky M. Tonsillectomy and adenotonsillectomy for recurrent throat infection in moderately affected children. Pediatrics 2002;110:7-15.

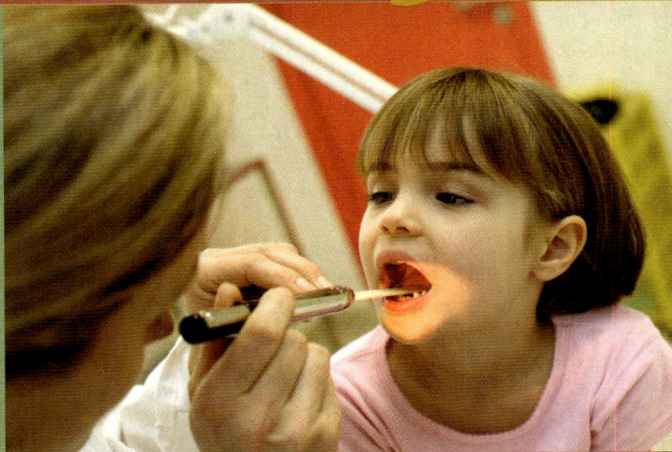

CHAPTER 25

Peritonsillar and Retropharyngeal Abscess

Udayan K. Shah

INTRODUCTION

Peritonsillar and retropharyngeal abscesses (PTA and RPA, respectively) are commonly seen in children. The intent of this chapter is to help the clinician establish an accurate diagnosis early and to achieve cure by the judicious and adjunctive use of antibiotics, radiography, and surgery.

DEFINITIONS AND EPIDEMIOLOGY

Peritonsillar Abscess

The pharyngeal tonsils are paired organs, which serve as the lateral lymphoid guardians at the posterior aspect of the oropharynx. PTA is an infected collection in the potential space surrounding the palatine tonsils. PTA usually presents with a pointing collection at the superior tonsillar pole.[1,2] The loose areolar tissue surrounding the tonsils provides a potential space into which infections may spread.

In 1995, Herzon and Hassis estimated that children accounted for approximately one-third of the 45,000 episodes of PTA that occur annually.[3] Most children with PTA present in the early teen years.[4] While group A beta-hemolytic *Streptococcus* (GABHS) is the most commonly cultured organism, isolated in approximately one-third of cases,[5] it is not the only bacterial pathogen identified. Most PTAs are polymicrobial, with GABHS, *Staphylococcus aureus* and *Haemophilus influenzae* accounting for most of the aerobic organisms and *Prevotella* spp., *Porphyromonas* spp., *Fusobacterium* spp., and *Peptostreptococcus* spp. comprising the common anaerobes.[2,4]

Retropharyngeal Abscess

The retropharyngeal space is a potential space located between the visceral layer of deep cervical fascia anteriorly and the alar division of deep cervical fascia posteriorly.[6]

Suppuration of lymphoid tissue imbricated between these layers is responsible for retropharyngeal infections. The lateral retropharyngeal nodes traditionally associated with RPA are eponymously referred to as the nodes of Rouviere.[7] Infections may spread readily from the oropharynx to mediastinum via this "highway" of the neck. The retropharyngeal nodes regress around the age of 3–5 years.[6,8]

Consistent with nodal regression by the age of 5 years, most children present before age of 6 years with RPA, with the median age of around 3 years.[4,6,9] The prevalence is in general thought to be increasing and was 4.94 cases/10,000 population in the Wayne State experience.[8] RPA accounted for approximately 5% of deep neck space infections in Papua, New Guinea.[10]

Acute upper respiratory infection is the usual antecedent cause of RPA in children, as opposed to adults in whom foreign bodies, trauma, and dental infections are considered etiologic. Microbiology of RPA demonstrates a mixture of aerobic and anaerobic organisms. Common aerobic organisms include alpha- and beta-hemolytic streptococcal species, *S. aureus*, *Neisseria* spp., *Eikenella* spp., and nontypable *H. influenzae*. Common anaerobes include *Bacteroides* spp., peptostreptococci, *Fusobacterium* spp., and *Prevotella* spp. An increase over the past decade in the prevalence of GABHS has been noted.[8] Less common organisms responsible for RPA include Epstein–Barr virus and *Mycobacterium tuberculosis*.[6,11]

PATHOGENESIS

PTAs typically occur when infectious tonsillopharyngitis progresses from cellulitis to abscess. RPAs may also develop as a consequence of antecedent pharyngitis. The lymphatics drain the nasopharynx, posterior sinuses, and adenoids. Purulent infections in these regions spread to the retropharynx by lymphatic drainage. Retropharyngeal lymph node inflammation may be complicated by necrosis and abscess formation. Rarely, RPAs are caused by penetrating neck injury or by extension of cervical osteomyelitis. The retropharyngeal lymph nodes atrophy by 4–5 years of age, making RPAs less common in older children.

CLINICAL PRESENTATION

General Considerations

Relevant history includes review of prodromal symptoms, recent travel and ill contacts, immunization status, airway and swallowing concerns, ability to maintain hydration, and response to supportive and pharmacologic therapy.

Physical examination may show serous otitis media as part of a usually antecedent upper respiratory infection. Oral examination should note the degree of trismus, which may be measured roughly in finger breadths or centimeters; the color and hydrations status of mucosa; and tonsillar size, symmetry, color, and exudate. The neck should be assessed for fullness, tenderness, adenopathy, and range of motion. Skin examination should focus on stigmata of complicated GABHS infections such as the scarlet fever rash.

Examination of the oropharynx is best achieved by first asking the child to open his or her mouth without protruding the tongue. This permits for a measurement of trismus (difficult with opening the mouth, measured in fingerbreadths or in centimeters) and can allow for a view of the posterior pharynx. Gentle depression of the mid portion of the tongue with a tongue depressor allows for a better view of the tonsils and posterior pharynx while avoiding gagging and allows examination even in the setting of trismus (Figures 25–1 and 25–2).

Flexible nasopharyngolaryngoscopy is useful when oral opening is limited or when there is a concern over pharyngeal edema or airway stability. Should supraglottitis be a concern, physical examination must be handled very carefully, as supraglottic contact by a tongue depressor or nasopharyngolaryngoscopy against inflamed and protuberant tissues may trigger immediate and life-threatening laryngospasm. Agitating a marginally stable child should be avoided.

Adequate lighting is critical to good oropharyngeal examination. Most often, the most expedient lighting is provided by an otoscope, penlight, or small flashlight, held by the examiner. A separate person to hold the light is useful. Stronger illumination without a second set of hands may be provided by a headlamp such as that worn by hikers, a set of lenses that magnify and illuminate (LumiView™, Welch Allyn, Skaneateles Falls, NY), or a headlight or head mirror.

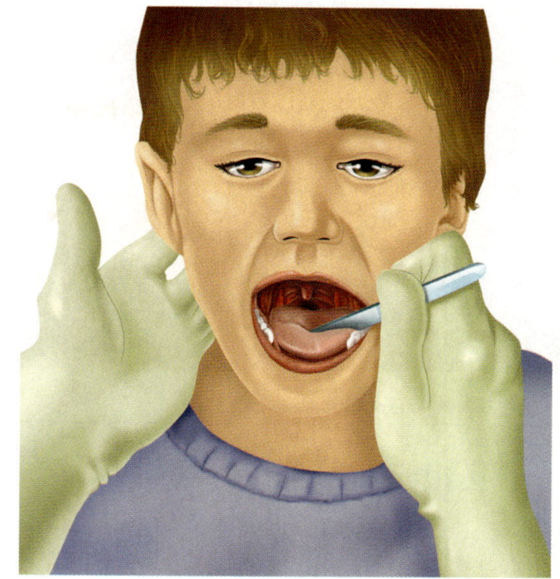

FIGURE 25–1 ■ Examination of the tonsils and posterior oropharynx.

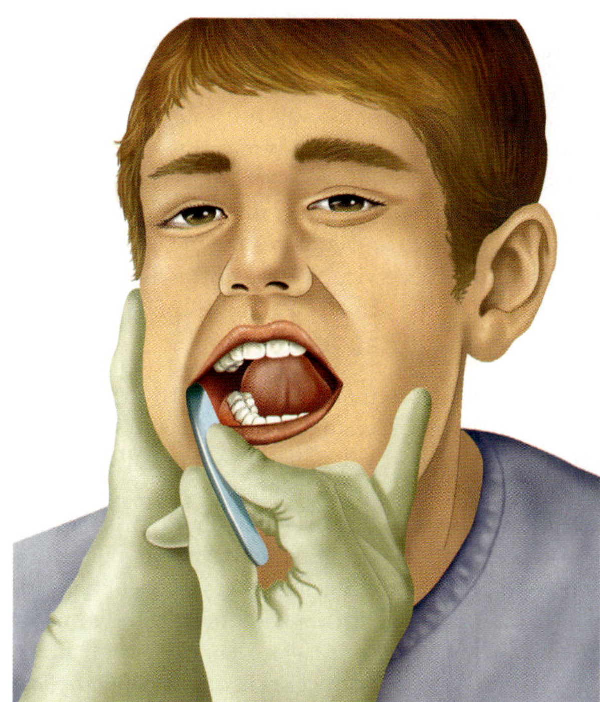

FIGURE 25–2 ■ Examination of the oral mucosa and anterior mouth.

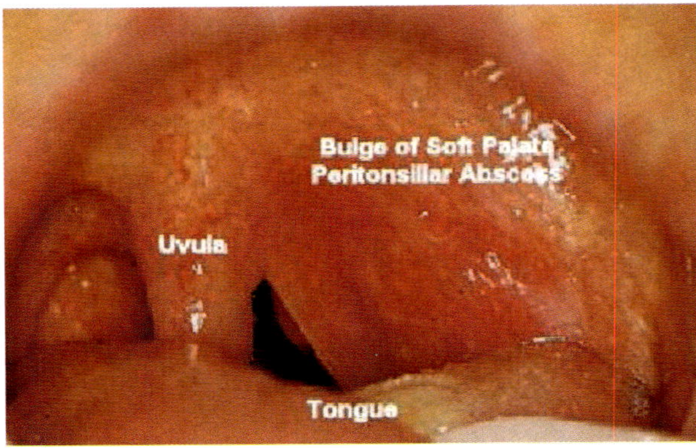

FIGURE 25–3 ■ Peritonsillar abscess.

Peritonsillar Abscess

Children usually present with several days of fever, dysphagia, or odynophagia. Ipsilateral otalgia and neck pain may be present.[2] A characteristic voice change, described as muffled or "hot potato voice," is frequently noted. Trismus, reported in two-thirds of patients with PTA in one series, results from irritation and reflex spasm of the internal pterygoid muscle.[12] Physical examination shows an erythematous bulging of the soft palate above the tonsil, possibly with medial displacement of the tonsil, and/or uvular deviation away from its usual midline position (Figure 25–3). Trismus may limit examination, and so the previously described technique for oral examination is recommended, rather than attempting to force the mandible down and compressing the entire anterior tongue. Ipsilateral cervical adenopathy is also common.

Retropharyngeal Abscess

Retropharyngeal infections present similarly to peritonsillar infections with fever, drooling, dysphagia, odynophagia, and tender neck adenopathy. Many children have pharyngitis or tonsillitis,[12] although pain with neck extension is a key finding that should raise suspicion for RPA rather than streptococcal or viral pharyngitis; as a consequence, the head is generally maintained in a neutral position, although in some children torticollis may be evident. Meningismus or stridor occurs in fewer than 5% of children. Airway obstruction is a possible complication.[9] Diagnosis is suspected by a bulging of the posterior pharyngeal wall and confirmed by radiography.

LABORATORY AND RADIOLOGIC STUDIES

Laboratory Studies

Children in whom intravenous therapy or hospitalization is considered should have a baseline urinalysis, and blood should be checked for a serum metabolic panel and a complete blood count with differential and may also be tested for serum markers of inflammation such as C-reactive protein and/or an erythrocyte sedimentation rate. Laboratory evaluation shows a leukocytosis with a propensity to immature cells. Monospot, as well as a throat culture or rapid strep test, should also be performed.

Radiologic Studies

Peritonsillar abscess

Plain radiography has a limited role in the initial assessment of cases of peritonsillar cellulitis or abscess and may be reserved for cases in which fiberoptic nasopharyngolaryngoscopy is not available or possible. Contrast-enhanced computed tomography (CT) or gadolinium-enhanced magnetic resonance imaging (MRI) is useful in assessing young children with suspected PTA who are not cooperative with examination. It is also helpful for persistent symptoms (after 24–48 hours of therapy), especially if needle aspiration or surgical drainage had been performed initially. Imaging may reveal an unusual manifestation such as an inferior pole PTA.[1] CT has a high sensitivity (approximately 90%) but modest specificity (60%) in detecting abscesses (as opposed to cellulitis) compared with operative findings.[12]

Retropharyngeal abscess

In contrast to peritonsillar infections, radiologic studies are usually required for precise anatomic diagnosis of RPA. Lateral neck radiography provides only limited information and may show bulging of the retropharyngeal soft tissues, with resultant airway narrowing, loss of cervical lordosis, and a wide retropharyngeal space. The width of an abnormal retropharynx was defined by Wholey et al. in a 1958 paper as >7 mm in children 15 years of age or younger at the anteroinferior aspect of C2 and a wide retrotracheal space measured forward from the anteroinferior aspect of C6 of >14 mm (Figure 25–4).[8]

Contrast-enhanced CT and MRI are most useful, as these permit differentiation of abscess from phlegmon and anatomically localize the process to facilitate aspiration and surgical treatment. An abscess is identified by a rim-enhancing fluid collection, while a hypolucent area without ring enhancement is defined as phlegmon (Figures 25–5 and 25–6). Radiography may also localize a collection and indicate other sites of abscess formation as well as provide a means for objectively measuring abscess size and for following the progress of infection when clinical complaints are difficult to elicit, such as for a child with developmental delays.

Repeat imaging is generally not necessary for children who demonstrate unequivocal clinical improvement. Sequential radiography may be useful in monitoring the efficacy of therapy, particularly when surgery is not used initially or the patient is difficult to assess

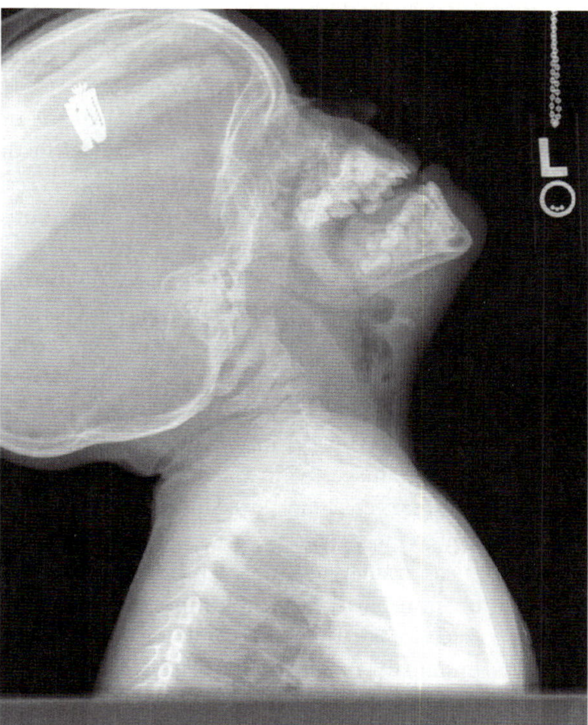

FIGURE 25–4 ■ Retropharyngeal abscess, lateral neck radiograph.

clinically because of age or cognitive development. Interventional radiologic techniques may have a role in some cases, for either therapeutic drainage or to provide diagnostic material for microbial culture. Consideration of the long-term effects of low-dose diagnostic irradiation should be weighed when selecting which type of study (e.g., CT that requires diagnostic irradiation vs. MRI that does not administer irradiation).[13]

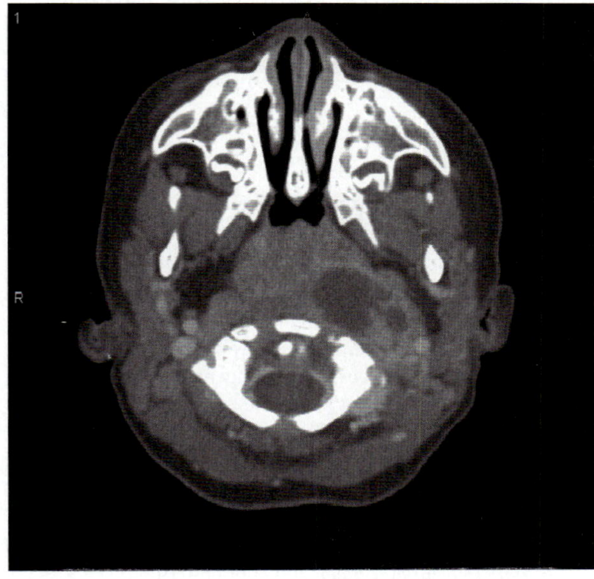

FIGURE 25–5 ■ CT Scan, Retropharyngeal abscess.

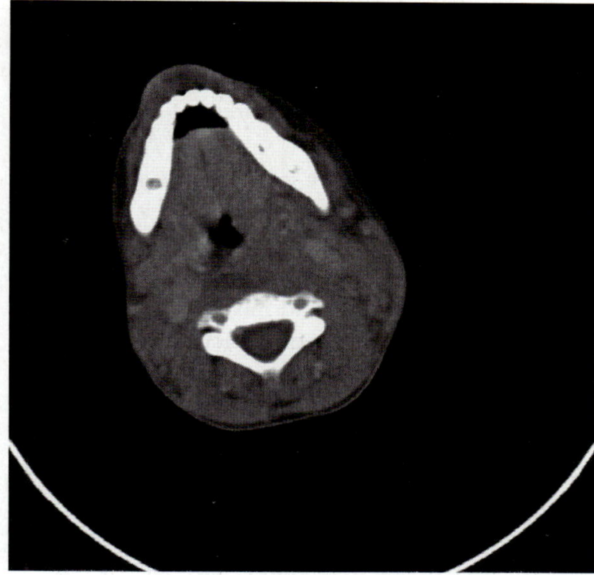

FIGURE 25–6 ■ CT Scan, Retropharyngeal phlegmon.

MANAGEMENT

Peritonsillar Abscess

Treatment aims to resolve discomfort, maintain the airway, and prevent abscess rupture. A ruptured PTA may result in the aspiration of purulence and lead to bronchopneumonia.[2] The sixth century Byzantine physician Aetius of Amida treated spontaneously draining abscesses with gargles of honey, milk, and herbs, or with rose extract.[14] Today, oral antibiotics are recommended to begin with, such as penicillin, amoxicillin/clavulanic acid, cephalosporins, and clindamycin. Antibiotic selection should be culture directed when possible. Hospitalization may be necessary for rehydration, analgesia, intravenous antibiotics, and/or airway observation.

Intravenous corticosteroid therapy may be considered to reduce inflammation in children with airway compromise, administered at the dose of 0.5 mg/kg of dexamethasone intravenously up to a maximum single dose of 10 mg, every 8 hours, for up to three total doses.

Many PTAs require either needle aspiration or incision and drainage (I&D). Needle aspiration may be performed diagnostically to confirm abscess formation, to identify the best point at which to perform I&D, or as a therapeutic measure to relieve symptoms and provide material for microbial culture. Needle aspiration is a rapid means of relieving the painful bulging of the abscess and may speed the course of recovery. Bacterial culture results are not clinically useful in most cases, but the cultures are valuable when there is a concern over antibiotic resistance, such as for immunodeficient children or those who have been recently treated with broad-spectrum antibiotics.[15] CT guidance of needle aspiration is indicated after an unsuccessful surgical attempt and for an abscess that is located in an atypical location or that may be difficult to reach with standard surgical approaches.

I&D permits a more complete evacuation than that allowed by needle aspiration. I&D is performed trans-orally and is indicated for the older, more cooperative patients who may more easily permit a longer procedure. I&D may be performed awake, with the aid of local and topical anesthetic, with conscious sedation protocols or under general anesthesia in the operating room, the latter usually caused by a child's inability to cooperate. Acute tonsillectomy ("quinsy" tonsillectomy) may be necessary for relief of obstructive symptoms, a history of recurrent streptococcal pharyngotonsillitis, or an exposure of the abscess. Quinsy tonsillectomy is necessary in approximately one out of three cases of PTA in children.[2,16]

For both PTA and RPA, a proactive and coordinated airway management plan is critical when considering sedation, imaging, and surgery. A plan should be communicated between all providers, including physicians, anesthesiologists, and nursing and support staff. Appropriate preparation should be made for a variety of intubating laryngoscopes as well as flexible fiberoptic bronchoscopes. A discussion should be considered with the family of potential airway risks as well as the option for tracheotomy in the most dire circumstances.

When treating PTA, attention should be paid to the tissue characteristics of tonsillar and peritonsillar tissues. Fleshy, granular, or pale tissue may indicate a neoplasm presenting as a PTA.[17] In such cases, tissue should be sent for immunohistopathologic evaluation. Follow-up should confirm resolution of fullness in the peritonsillar region along with normalization of swallowing and airway status.

Retropharyngeal Abscess

Management of small collections—whether abscess or phlegmon—may be initiated with oral or intravenous antibiotics. Usually, children who present with RPA are dehydrated and receive intravenous fluid. Initial inpatient antimicrobial therapy via the intravenous route is therefore easily achieved and is advised until clinical improvement is clearly demonstrated by at least 24 hours without fever and the child is able to swallow secretions, liquids, and medications. Inpatient stay allows for rehydration and antimicrobial care while permitting for airway observation with expedient airway intervention, imaging, or surgical drainage if necessary. Length of stay is generally less than 2 weeks and is often shorter than 5 days.[9]

RPA may often be treated by antibiotics alone, particularly when the abscess is small and there is no airway compromise. Antibiotic therapy may empirically begin with clindamycin with or without cefuroxime or ceftriaxone, or ampicillin/sulbactam.[8,9] Duration of therapy should be for 10–21 days and, in some cases, may require placement of an indwelling intravenous catheter for outpatient administration of antibiotics. As with PTA, antibiotic choice should be guided by microbiologic cultures when possible. Intravenous corticosteroid therapy may be considered for children with airway compromise, with the dosing detailed above for children with PTA.

RPAs that are extensive or refractory to antibiotics require surgical drainage, by the trans-oral route for RPA medial to the great vessels and/or transcervically for collections lateral to the great vessels. Airway considerations during surgical drainage include difficult laryngoscopy during intubation caused by neck stiffness and a limited view as a result of forward bulging of retropharyngeal tissues. Spontaneous or iatrogenic abscess rupture may permit foul secretions to pour into the tracheobronchial tree and lead to aspiration pneumonia.

COURSE AND PROGNOSIS

PTA recurs in 10–15% of patients undergoing drainage by needle aspiration. Recurrence is more common in patients with a history of recurrent tonsillitis prior to developing PTA; among 290 patients, PTA recurrence occurred in 40% of those with a history of recurrent tonsillitis compared with 9.6% of those with no such history.[18]

Suppurative complications of RPA include rupture of the abscess with aspiration of purulent secretions into the tracheobronchial tree, extension of inflammation into the mediastinum, jugular vein thrombophlebitis, erosion of carotid or vertebral arteries, and sepsis.[8,9]

REFERENCES

1. Licameli GR, Grillone GA. Inferior pole peritonsillar abscess. *Otolaryngol Head Neck Surg.* 1998;118(1):95-99.
2. Schraff S, McGinn JD, Derkay CS. Peritonsillar abscess in children: a 10-year review of diagnosis and management. *Int J Pediatr Otorhinolaryngol.* 2001;57(3):213-218.
3. Herzon FS, Harris P. Mosher award thesis. Peritonsillar abscess: incidence, current management practices, and a proposal for treatment guidelines. *Laryngoscope.* 1995;105 (8, pt 3 suppl 74):1-17.
4. Schweinfurth JM. Demographics of pediatric head and neck infections in a tertiary care hospital. *Laryngoscope.* 2006;116(6):887-889.
5. Brook I. The role of anaerobic bacteria in tonsillitis. *Int J Pediatr Otorhinolaryngol.* 2005;69(1):9-19.

6. Takoudes TG, Haddad J, Jr. Retropharyngeal abscess and Epstein–Barr virus infection in children. *Ann Otol Rhinol Laryngol.* 1998;107(12):1072-1075.
7. Rouviere H. Lymphatic system of the head and neck. In: Tobias MJ, ed. *Anatomy of the Human Lymphatic System.* Ann Arbor, MI: Edward Brothers; 1938:3-28.
8. Abdel-Haq NM, Harahsheh A, Asmar BL. Retropharyngeal abscess in children: the emerging role of group A beta hemolytic *Streptococcus. South Med J.* 2006;99(9): 927-931.
9. Craig FW, Schunk JE. Retropharyngeal abscess in children: clinical presentation, utility of imaging, and current management. *Pediatrics.* 2003;111(6, pt 1):1394-1398.
10. Larawin V, Naipao J, Dubey SP. Head and neck space infections. *Otolaryngol Head Neck Surg.* 2006;135(6): 889-893.
11. Nalini B, Vinayak S. Tuberculosis in ear, nose, and throat practice: Its presentation and diagnosis. *Am J Otolaryngol.* 2006;27(1):39-45.
12. Ungkanont K, Yellon RF, Weissman JL, Casselbrant ML, Gonzalez-Valdepena H, Bluestone CD. Head and neck space infections in infants and children. *Otolaryngol Head Neck Surg.* 1995;112(3):375-382.
13. Berrington de Gonzalez A, Darby S. Risk of cancer from diagnostic X-rays: estimates for the UK and 14 other countries. *Lancet.* 2004;363(9406):345-351.
14. Shah UK. Tonsillitis and peritonsillar abscess. In: AJ G, Talavera F, Allen GC, Slack CL, Meyers AD, eds. *Otolaryngology and Facial Plastic Surgery.* WebMD; 2001:http://www.emedicine.com/ent/topic314.htm. Accessed June 25, 2007.
15. Cherukuri S, Benninger MS. Use of bacteriologic studies in the outpatient management of peritonsillar abscess. *Laryngoscope.* 2002;112(1):18-20.
16. Bauer PW, Lieu JE, Suskind DL, Lusk RP. The safety of conscious sedation in peritonsillar abscess drainage. *Arch Otolaryngol Head Neck Surg.* 2001;127(12):1477-1480.
17. Windfuhr J. Malignant neoplasia at different ages presenting as peritonsillar abscess. *Otolaryngol Head Neck Surg.* 2002;126(2):197-198.
18. Kronenberg J, Wolf M, Leventon G. Peritonsillar abscess: recurrence rate and the indication for tonsillectomy. *Am J Otolaryngol.* 1987;8(2):82-84.

CHAPTER 26

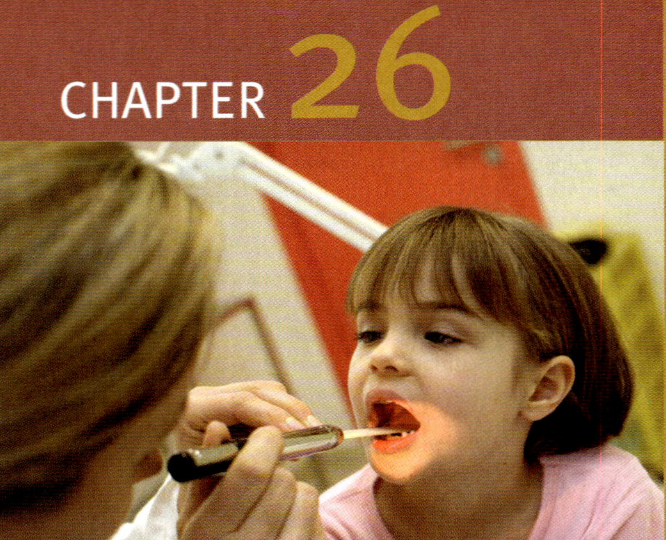

Cervical Lymphadenitis

Yodit Belew and Rebecca E. Levorson

DEFINITIONS AND EPIDEMIOLOGY

Lymphadenopathy, or enlarged lymph nodes, may be the result of acute inflammation, chronic inflammation, or infiltration via malignant cells. Lymphadenitis is the term used to describe inflammation of lymph nodes.

Most cases of acute cervical lymphadenitis are caused by either staphylococcal or streptococcal infections, and the changing epidemiology of acute unilateral cervical adenitis has been well documented in the literature. In 1944, Powers and Boisvert reported that 79% of cervical abscesses were caused by group A beta-hemolytic *Streptococcus* (GABHS; *Streptococcus pyogenes*) and only 17% were caused by *Staphylococcus aureus* (formerly *S. pyogenes*). In 1969, Scobie reported that *Staphylococcus* species caused most (67%) cases of cervical adenitis, and only 7% were caused by streptococci.[1]

Nontuberculosis mycobacterium (NTM) infections in the head and neck are common among children.[2] NTM includes mycobacterial species *Mycobacterium avium-intracellulare* complex, *Mycobacterium scrofulaceum*, *Mycobacterium fortuitum*, and *Mycobacterium chelonei.* NTM are ubiquitous in the environment and can be found in soil, contaminated water, dairy products, eggs, and dust. NTM are endemic in certain regions of the United States such as the mid-west and southwest. Ingestion of contaminated materials is likely to be the main route for introduction of NTM. This explains why cervicofacial lymph nodes are the sites primarily affected by NTM infections.[2] Until approximately 50 years ago, adenitis caused by *Mycobacterium tuberculosis* (TB) and *Mycobacterium bovis* were more common than NTM adenitis. However, as TB and *M. bovis* disease decreased in the United States and other developed countries, NTM became a major cause of chronic lymphadenitis in children. Cessation of Bacille Calmette–Guerin vaccination in the United States has decreased collateral immunity against NTM. Chlorination of water has also been attributed to decrease in number of infections caused by *M. scrofulaceum.*[3]

Peripheral tuberculous lymphadenitis involves mainly the cervical lymph nodes. It is the most common form of extrapulmonary tuberculosis in children from tuberculosis-endemic areas. Lymphadenitis is thought to occur secondary to a lymphatic spread of organisms from a primary pulmonary focus. However, it can occasionally occur from primary focus in the mouth, tonsils, oropharynx, or tissues of the head and neck.[4]

Cat-scratch disease (CSD) was first reported by Debre in 1950 as a syndrome of regional lymphadenopathy after a cat scratch. CSD is caused by infection with *Bartonella henselae*, a zoonotic disease.[5,6] Cat fleas *Ctenocephalides felis* transmit *B. henselae* between cats who remain asymptomatic. Humans become infected after exposure to infected cats, usually after scratches or bites from kittens. Dogs have also been known to be the vector for transmitting the disease. The true incidence of CSD is unknown. Most cases occur in people younger than 20 years. More than 90% of patients with CSD have a history of recent contact with cats, often kittens.[7] Infection is reported to occur more often during the autumn and winter. The incubation period from the time of the scratch to appearance of the primary cutaneous lesion is 7–12 days; the period from the appearance of the primary lesion to the appearance of lymphadenopathy is 5–50 days (median, 12 days).[8]

Toxoplasma gondii, a parasite, is distributed throughout the world. Cats are definitive hosts and acquire the infection by feeding on infected animals such as mice or uncooked meats.[7,8] After the parasite sexually replicates in the intestine, it is excreted as a oocyst in stools. After excretion and maturation, the oocytes are capable of infecting if ingested by the oral route. Intermediate hosts such as sheep, pigs, and cattle can have tissues infected with the cysts, which are viable for the lifetime of the host. Humans become infected by consumption of raw or undercooked meat that contains cysts or by accidental ingestion of sporulated oocysts from soil or in contaminated food. Primary infection with *T. gondii* is usually benign. The most common presentation is nontender and nonsuppurative lymphadenopathy. Infection usually causes regional enlargement of lymph nodes (most commonly suboccipital and cervical) rather than generalized lymphadenopathy.[7,8] The incubation period of acquired infection is estimated to be 7 days (range: 4–21 days).

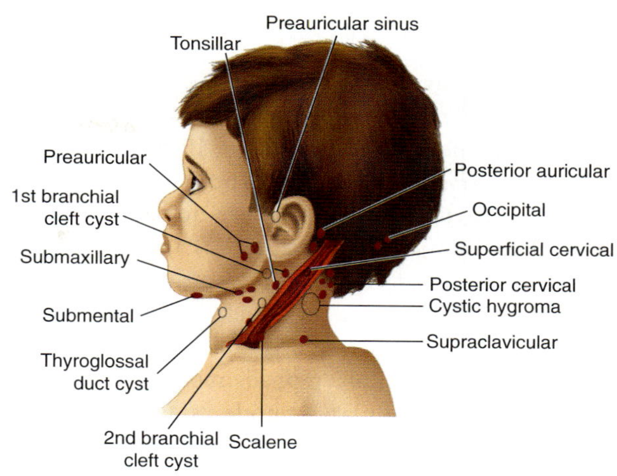

FIGURE 26–1 ■ Diagram of cervical lymph node anatomy.

PATHOGENESIS

Based on the location of infection, lymphatic vessels drain infectious agents and inflammatory mediators to regional lymph nodes. An initial inflammatory response involves hyperplasia of the lymphoid tissue and recruitment of phagocytic cells, cytokine release, and vascular edema. This leads to enlargement of the regional nodes. In acute adenitis, this rapid expansion increases pressure on the lymph node capsule, resulting in pain at the site of the swollen lymph node. Involvement of adjacent lymph nodes and surrounding soft tissue can lead to cellulitis, suppuration, necrosis, or fixation to nearby structures. In chronic adenitis, pain at the site of lymph node enlargement is less common because lymphoid hyperplasia is more gradual, inflammatory responses are less robust, and the body attempts to wall off the infection with fibrosis and granuloma formation.

Lymph Node Drainage in the Head

Figure 26–1 illustrates the regional lymph nodes affected in children with cervical adenitis. Five important lymph node groups found in the head include the postauricular (mastoid), occipital, preauricular, parotid, and facial nodes. The postauricular nodes drain temporal and parietal scalp and the posterior ear canal. Occipital nodes are responsible for the posterior scalp and neck. Scalp dermatitis or infection may cause regional occipital lymphadenitis. However, in generalized lymphadenopathy, occipital nodes are often enlarged. Preauricular nodes drain the anterior and temporal scalp, ear canal and pinna, and lateral conjunctivae. The parotid and facial nodes drain the midface, parotid gland, external auditory canal, middle ear, posterior palate, conjunctivae, eyelids, and nasopharynx.

Lymph Node Drainage in the Neck

Lymph tissue of the neck is divided into five regions of local drainage, which include the submental, submandibular (submaxillary), superficial cervical, and the superior and inferior deep cervical groups. Submental nodes lie on the inferior aspect of the chin and are responsible for draining the intraoral region. The submandibular lymph nodes lie next to the submandibular salivary gland and receive a large proportion of lymphatic drainage from the head, including from the lateral aspect of the lower lip, vestibule of the nose, cheeks, medial parts of the eyelids, and the forehead. The superficial cervical nodes are three vertical chains that lie along the posterior border of the sternomastoid muscle, external jugular vein, and midline from the chin to the suprasternal notch. These are responsible for draining the superficial anterior neck tissues, including the skin, lower larynx, thyroid, lower ear canal, and parotid regions. Deep cervical nodes of the neck lie deep to the sternomastoid muscle and are divided into the superior and inferior regions. The superficial deep nodes drain the palatine tonsils and submental nodes. The lower deep cervical nodes drain the larynx, trachea, thyroid, and esophagus. The supraclavicular nodes, also part of the inferior deep cervical chain, are responsible for draining the lungs and abdomen. Enlargement of supraclavicular nodes most often indicates thoracic or abdominal pathology, including Hodgkin and non-Hodgkin lymphomas. Prompt evaluation and biopsy are necessary with supraclavicular nodal enlargement.

The majority of the lymphatics of the head and neck drain to the deep cervical and submandibular nodes. Therefore, these are the nodes most often (80%) involved in cervical lymphadenitis in children.

CLINICAL PRESENTATIONS

Most normal infants and children have palpable cervical, inguinal, and axillary lymph nodes. In general, a lymph node measuring greater than 10 mm in longest diameter is considered enlarged. There are three exceptions to this rule: (1) epitrochlear nodes measuring more than 5 mm are abnormal; (2) inguinal nodes measuring more than 15 mm are abnormal; and (3) palpable supraclavicular, iliac, or popliteal nodes are always considered abnormal.[9]

Regarding cervical lymphadenopathy, it is important to classify the enlarged node as either acute or chronic and unilateral or generalized. These criteria can help guide the decision-making process in a differential diagnosis.

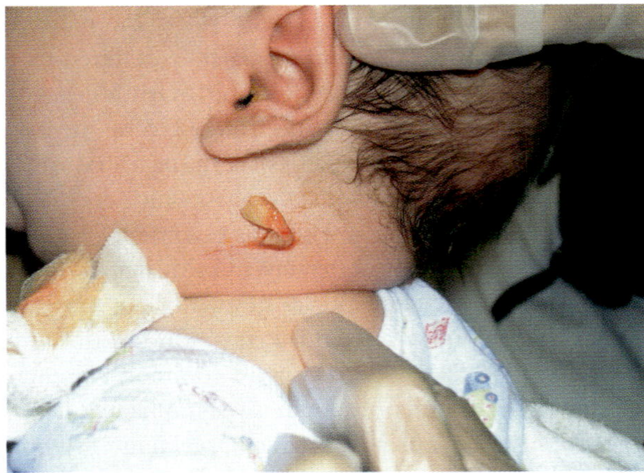

FIGURE 26–2 ■ Patient with acute unilateral cervical adenitis. (Photo courtesy of N Singh, MD, MPH, and S Nicholas, MD.)

History

Important details of the history include location, onset, duration, and rate of enlargement of lymph node. Epidemiologic clues as to the etiology include exposure to animal bites or scratches, especially cats or kittens, risk factors for HIV infection, contact with tuberculosis infection, and travel outside of the geographical region of residence. Weight loss, protracted fever, rash, hepatosplenomegaly, and generalized lymphadenopathy signify systemic disease.

Asking if the patient received antibiotics and the clinical response with the prescribed antibiotics are important. Past history of tuberculin testing skin with results and date of test is an essential part of the history.

Physical Examination

A comprehensive physical examination is necessary to determine whether the lymphadenopathy is isolated or generalized. The skin and soft tissue near the enlarged lymph node should be evaluated for evidence of inflammation such as erythema, induration, tenderness, or fluctuance. Areas distal to the adenopathy may yield important information regarding scars, nodules, or papules.

Characteristics of the lymph node are important in helping to identity the etiology of the lymphadenopathy. Viral hyperplastic lymph nodes are typically small, discrete, mobile, nontender, and bilateral. No superficial cellulitis or periadenitis should be present. Pyogenic lymphadenitis is typically unilateral, warm, large, and tender with surrounding erythema and edema (Figure 26–2). Lymph node characteristics associated with specific infectious causes are discussed further in the "Differential Diagnosis" section of this chapter. Chronic lymphadenitis is characterized by discrete margins and adherence to underlying tissue with minimal signs of inflammation. Characteristic malignant lymphadenopathy is firm, discrete, and nontender, with a classic description of "rubbery texture" without inflammation. After a period of time, the surrounding tissue becomes matted together and fixed in place to the skin and underlying structures. Malignancy should not suppurate.

The rest of the physical examination should focus on a detailed head and neck examination including sources for infection—scalp, dental, oropharyngeal, otitic, and conjunctival sources. Range of motion of the neck should be evaluated. All lymph chains should be palpated for lymphadenopathy. Liver and spleen should be palpated. Inspection for rash and peripheral extremity changes could signal Kawasaki syndrome, malignancy, or viral etiology. See Table 26–1 for important aspects of the history and physical examination.

DIFFERENTIAL DIAGNOSIS

Infectious and noninfectious etiologies of cervical lymphadenopathy are summarized in Tables 26–2 and 26–3.

Infectious Causes of Lymphadenitis by Lymph Node Location

Acute bilateral cervical lymphadenitis

Acute bilateral lymphadenitis is commonly associated with other constitutional symptoms including fever, cough, rhinorrhea, conjunctivitis, or pharyngitis of upper respiratory or oropharyngeal infections. Viral etiologies include adenovirus, rhinovirus, parainfluenza, influenza, respiratory syncytial virus, and coronavirus. In adenoviral infections, anterior and posterior cervical nodal enlargements are more common than preauricular lymphadenopathy.[9]

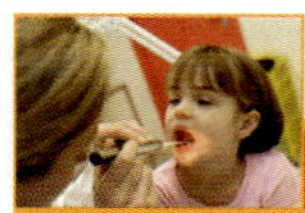

Table 26–1.

Pertinent History and Physical Examination Features

History

Constitutional: weight loss, anorexia, fevers, night sweats, and rash
Lymph node: onset, location, duration, and rate of enlargement
Exposure to animals (cats, kittens, dogs, rabbits, cows, and fleas)
Exposure to HIV or tuberculosis
Travel history: endemic areas for TB, leishmaniasis, scrub typhus, trypanosomiasis
Dietary history: unpasteurized milk and other dairy products
Previous TB skin test results
Previous use of antibiotics, compliance to regimen, and response of symptoms

Physical examination

Complete lymph node examination: isolated or generalized lymphadenopathy
Character of the lymph node
Viral: small, discrete, mobile, nontender, bilateral, and absence of cellulitis
Acute bacterial: unilateral, warm, large, tender, surrounding erythema, and edema
Chronic bacterial or parasitic: discrete margins, adherence to underlying tissue, and minimal inflammation
Tubercular: violet, thin skin above node
Malignant: firm, discrete, nontender, rubbery to matted and fixed, no inflammation, and no suppuration
Skin and soft tissue near enlarged node: evidence of inflammation, scars, nodules, papules, and rash
Detailed head and neck examination: scalp, dental, oropharyngeal, otic, and conjunctival
Liver and spleen

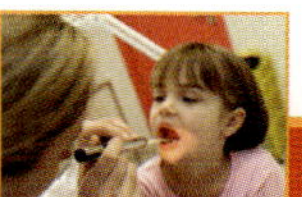

Table 26–2.

Infectious Etiologies of Cervical Lymphadenopathy

Bacterial

Staph. aureus
Group A *Streptococcus*
Group B *Streptococcus*
M. tuberculosis
Atypical mycobacteria (e.g., *Mycobacterium kansasii* and *Mycobacterium avium-intracellulare*)
B. henselae (cat-scratch disease)
Anaerobic bacteria
Gram-negative enterics
Y. pestis
Actinomyces israelii
F. tularensis
Treponema pallidum (syphilis)
C. diphtheriae (diphtheria)
Brucella spp.
Salmonella spp.

Viral

Epstein–Barr virus
Cytomegalovirus
Herpes simplex virus
Varicella zoster virus
Adenovirus
Human immunodeficiency virus
Human herpes virus 6
Measles
Mumps
Rubella
Coxsackie virus

Fungal

Aspergillus spp.
Candida spp.
Cryptococcus neoformans
Endemic fungi (e.g., *Histoplasma capsulatum, Coccidioides immitis,* and *Blastomyces dermatitidis*)
Sporothrix schenckii (sporotrichosis)

Parasitic

T. gondii

Both Epstein–Barr Virus (EBV) and cytomegalovirus (CMV) can cause acute bilateral cervical adenitis associated with infectious mononucleosis. EBV is more commonly the cause of cervical adenitis than is CMV.[9] In both EBV and CMV infections, posterior cervical nodes are more commonly enlarged than are anterior cervical nodes. Cervical lymphadenitis may present prior to generalized lymphadenopathy in many cases of EBV or CMV infectious mononucleosis.[9]

Other infectious etiologies responsible for bilateral cervical lymphadenitis include HIV, rubella, varicella, HSV, measles, coxsackie, and roseola (HHV-6) viruses. Associated symptoms are important factors in arriving at the correct diagnosis. Gingovistomatitis caused by HSV or herpangia from coxsackie virus infection is commonly associated with bilateral enlargement of the anterior cervical, submental, and submandibular nodes.[9] In addition, many of these viral agents, which cause generalized infections, will also produce generalized lymphadenopathy.

Acute unilateral cervical lymphadenitis

Acute, unilateral, suppurative bacterial cervical lymphadenitis is the classic form of cervical lymphadenitis brought to medical attention. *S. aureus* and GABHS are responsible for the majority of these infections. Reports of 40–80% of isolated organisms were *S. aureus* or GABHS in studies where fine needle aspiration or excision was performed.[10–13] These infected lymph nodes may result from upper respiratory, throat, dental, or

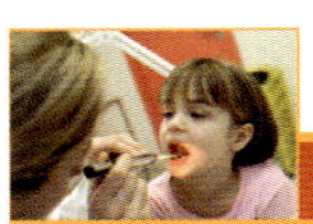

Table 26–3.

Noninfectious Etiologies of Cervical Lymphadenopathy

Malignancy
Hodgkin disease
Non-Hodgkin lymphoma
Leukemia
Thyroid tumors
Neuroblastoma
Metastatic malignancy (e.g., metastatic papillary thyroid carcinoma)
Rhabdomyosarcoma
Parotid tumors
Nasopharyngeal carcinoma

Other
Collagen vascular disease
Kawasaki syndrome
Sarcoidosis
Primary immunodeficiency diseases (e.g., chronic granulomatous disease and hyper-IgE syndrome)
Langerhans cell histiocytosis
Storage disorders (e.g., Gaucher disease)
Serum sickness
Sinus histocytosis with massive lymphadenopathy (Rosai–Dorfman disease)
Kikuchi–Fugimoto syndrome
Pediatric fever, aphthous stomatitis, pharyngitis, and adenitis syndrome (PFAPA)
Castleman disease
Isoniazid
Dilantin
Post vaccination

Congenital masses mistaken for lymphadenopathy or lymphadenitis
Branchial cleft cyst
Cystic hygroma
Thyroglossal duct cyst
Epidermoid cyst
Sternocleidomastoid tumor

scalp infections. In children aged 1–4 years, *S. aureus* and GABHS are common etiological agents. In older children, GABHS and anaerobic infections are most frequently seen.[9] Streptococcal infections in this age group appear to represent the natural incidence of streptococcal pharyngitis in this group. Anaerobic organisms associated with dental abscesses, gingival infections, and mucositis have been cultured from biopsied lymph nodes. *Bacteroides, Peptostreptococcus, Proteus, Escherichia coli, Pseudomonas,* mixed infections of both *Staphylococcus* and *Streptococcus,* coagulase-negative staphylococcal species, *Actinomyces israelii, Streptococcus milleri* group, *Haemophilus influenzae, Francisella tularensis, Aspergillus* spp., *Nocardia* spp., and NTM have all been isolated from pediatric patients with acute cervical adenitis or abscess.[1,9,13–16]

The primary sites of acute cervical lymphadenitis are submandibular (50–75%), cervical (13–39%), submental (5–8%), and occipital (2–3%).[1,15] Suppuration occurs most commonly with *Staph. aureus* infection, with a rate of 25% of all acute bacterial cervical adenitis.[15,16]

Subacute or chronic unilateral cervical lymphadenitis

The most common causes of subacute or chronic lymphadenitis are mycobacterial infection, CSD, and toxoplasmosis.[17]

Cervical lymphadenitis is the most common mycobacterial infection found in children. These infections are typically caused by NTM rather than *M. tuberculosis*; *M. avium-intracellulare* complex is isolated most often. Adenitis caused by mycobacteria generally affects healthy children between the ages of 1 and 5 years. The involved cervical lymph nodes are frequently located in the submandibular and preauricular nodal groups. The size of the node can vary between 1 and 7 cm in diameter. Symptoms may have been ongoing for several weeks to months before seeking medical attention.[2] In the early phase of the infection, the lymph nodes are firm with minimal tenderness, erythema, or warmth. Later, a necrotic center develops. Without treatment, the infection leads to progressive lymph node necrosis, overlying violaceous skin discoloration with a papyraceous or cigarette paper-like appearance, and, subsequently, draining skin sinus.[2,18]

CSD is usually a localized, self-limited disease but may be complicated by encephalitis, neuroretinitis, or Parinaud oculoglandular syndrome, a syndrome of unilateral conjunctivitis associated with regional lymphadenopathy and a characteristic neuroretinitis that occurs after conjunctival inoculation.[6–8,19] The primary clinical feature is lymphadenitis, which is single or regional and restricted to the drainage area of the site of the inoculation. The involved nodes tend to be as large as several centimeters in diameter. These may be elastic, mobile, and tender. Spontaneous regression of the nodes usually occurs in 2 weeks to 2 months. A primary lesion or papule may be located at the site of a scratch. This lesion typically precedes the development of lymphadenitis. CSD is generally associated with systemic symptoms such as fever and malaise. There is usually a history of contact with a kitten or a cat.[6–8]

Lymphadenopathy without fever is the most frequent clinical manifestation of acute acquired infection with *T. gondii* in the immunocompetent individual. The majority of acquired *T. gondii* infections are asymptomatic. The adenopathy may be present for months and tends to be nonsuppurative and only occasionally tender. Toxoplasmic lymphadenitis most frequently involves a solitary lymph node in the head and neck regions, without systemic symptoms.[8]

Cervical lymphadenitis caused by TB is uncommon in the United States. However, in endemic areas, TB remains a significant cause of cervical lymphadenitis.[4]

Subacute or chronic bilateral cervical lymphadenitis

Viral etiologies such as EBV, CMV, and HIV infections can cause bilateral subacute chronic cervical lymphadenitis. Syphilis can also cause lymphadenitis. However, the above infections account for only a small proportion of the clinically diagnosed cervical lymphadenopathies.

Infectious Causes of Lymphadenitis by Demographic Characteristics and Epidemiologic Exposures

Age

The most common cause of acute cervical lymphadenitis in infants is *S. aureus*. However, group B *Streptococcus* can cause a late-onset cellulitis-adenitis syndrome in neonates. Presenting features of cellulitis-adenitis syndrome include poor feeding, irritability, fever, and unilateral facial, preauricular, or submandibular swelling with overlying erythema. Adenitis presents within 2–3 days after onset of soft-tissue infection. Reported cases have a male predominance (72%). Blood culture and culture of the soft tissue or lymph node are almost always positive. This syndrome had previously been thought not to be associated with meningitis, but, in 1998, two cases of meningitis were reported in association with group B *Streptococcus* cellulitis-adenitis syndrome in afebrile, well-appearing neonates.[20,21]

Staph. aureus and GABHS are the most common etiologies (80%) of acute cervical adenitis in children aged 1–4 years. The majority of cases of acute cervical lymphadenitis occur in this age group. Children aged 5 years and older are more likely to have lymphadenitis caused by NTM, *T. gondii*, *B. henselae*, EBV, CMV, and tularemia.[9]

Immunization status

Lack of immunizations can predispose patients to preventable causes of cervical adenitis including measles, rubella, varicella, *H. influenzae* type b, and *Corynebacterium diphtheriae*. In rare cases, cervical lymphadenopathy has been reported following immunization with some vaccines (diphtheria–pertussis–tetanus, poliomyelitis, typhoid fever, and Bacille Calmette–Guerin).[1,7,17]

Contact with animals

Zoonoses are a common cause of cervical lymphadenitis in children. History of exposure to animals is very important in the diagnosis of CSD, toxoplasma, tularemia, anthrax, brucellosis, and plague.

Pasturella multocida can cause acute adenitis following bites or scratches from animals.[16] Tularemia results from infection with *F. tularensis* via insect vectors, direct contact with infected animals or carcasses, or ingestion of contaminated food or water. Approximately 250 animal species can be infected with tularemia including the rabbit. Occurrence is seasonal (June through September and November through February), which corresponds to vector and rabbit-hunting activities. Tularemia is highly infectious, with as few as 10 organisms being needed to cause infection. The ulceroglandular form is most common (75% cases) and causes ulcer at site of inoculation with regional lymphadenopathy. Exposure to *F. tularensis* through the conjunctiva can result in Parinaud oculoglandular syndrome, which is indistinguishable from that caused by *B. henselae*.[22]

Cutaneous anthrax begins as a focal pustule at the site of skin wound, and within 2–3 days, the lesion rapidly progresses with ulceration and eschar formation. Regional lymphadenitis may develop.[22] Brucellosis is contracted via direct contact with animals or ingestion of unpasteurized dairy products. In rare cases, brucellosis causes chronic lymphadenopathy with chronic fatigue-like syndrome. *Yersinia pestis* is endemic in rodents and several notable outbreaks in the southwest United States have occurred in the recent years. Bubonic plague, the most common form of the disease, is transmitted to humans via flea bites, leading to regional lymphadenitis characteristic of the classic bubo.[22]

Contact with sick individuals

GABHS and the respiratory viral pathogens are all highly communicable via respiratory droplet transmission. History of a close contact with symptoms suggestive of TB, travel to endemic parts of the world, or history of incarceration should prompt evaluation for *M. tuberculosis* infection. Both congenital HIV and acute retroviral syndrome are characterized by lymphadenopathy.

Underlying illness or predisposing condition

Patients with underlying undiagnosed immunodeficiency disease may present with lymphadenopathy or lymphadenitis. For example, suppurative lymphadenitis is one of the common initial presentations for patients with either chronic granulomatous disease or Job syndrome (hyperimmunoglobulin E syndrome). HIV infection may also present with generalized lymphadenopathy.

Noninfectious Causes of Lymphadenitis

PFAPA (periodic fever, aphthous stomatitis, pharyngitis, and cervical adenitis) is characterized by the onset of fever, malaise, chills, headaches, aphthous ulcers, pharyngitis, and tender cervical adenopathy. This cluster of symptoms cyclically recurs at 4–6-week intervals, and the episodes resolve spontaneously approximately 4–5 days.[7] PFAPA is discussed further in the "Periodic Fever Syndromes" chapter (Chapter 61).

Kawasaki Syndrome (discussed in Chapter 62) manifests with nonsuppurative cervical lymphadenopathy (usually a single, large node). The other associated symptoms of fever, conjunctival injection, rash, and subsequent desquamation suggest the diagnosis. However, diagnosis may be difficult if unilateral lymphadenitis precedes mucocutaneous manifestations.[23]

Kikuchi disease (histocytic necrotizing lymphadenitis) is a self-limited condition characterized by cervical lymphadenopathy and fever. It usually occurs in women of Asian decent.[7] Other inflammatory diseases such as juvenile rheumatoid arthritis may present with lymphadenopathy.

Infected congenital cysts such as bronchial cleft cysts, cystic hygromas, or thyroglossal duct cysts can mimic lymphadenitis. Congenital cysts should be considered, especially in cases when there appears to be recurrent cervical lymphadenitis.

Malignancy should be considered in the cases of indolent adenopathy, especially with a history of anorexia, weight loss, and other systemic symptoms.

DIAGNOSIS

The need for diagnostic evaluation depends on the history and clinical presentation. Most childhood cases of cervical lymphadenitis are benign and self-limited.

If the patient appears ill with systemic infection and has suggestive history, complete blood count, blood culture, liver enzymes, inflammatory markers such as erythrocyte sedimentation rate or c-reactive protein, and serologies for EBV, CMV, HIV, *T. gondii*, and *Brucella* spp. may be helpful.

Radiologic Studies

Ill-appearing patients with acute unilateral lymphadenitis should be evaluated for abscess via either ultrasound or CT. Ultrasound has a 90–95% sensitivity for identifying presence of liquefaction and abscess formation, and CT adds information about osseous involvement, in addition to the nature of the nodal tissue.[13] Chest radiograph should be obtained to assess for pulmonary tuberculosis and hilar lymphadenopathy.

Tuberculin Skin Testing

A tuberculin skin test should be placed if NTM or TB is considered. Induration >5 mm in a low-risk population suggests NTM. TB should be considered if induration is >14 mm. However, usefulness of purified protein derivative (PPD) is limited even in the United States as subpopulations, such as those who live in major metropolitan areas, have a high risk of TB exposure.[3]

Serologic Studies

Serologic testing is available for *B. henselae*, *T. gondii*, HIV, EBV, CMV, tularemia, brucella, and plague. Details of testing for HIV (Chapter 52), EBV (Chapter 63), and CMV (Chapter 63) are discussed elsewhere in this text.

Specific serologic diagnostic tests can support the diagnosis of CSD. One of these, the indirect fluorescent antibody test, was shown to be 98% sensitive and 98% specific in a population of patients who met the classic case definition of CSD. Enzyme immunoassay testing for immunoglobulin (Ig) M and IgG antibodies to *B. henselae* is also commercially available. A high antibody titer (>1:64) suggests recent infection. An elevation in titer between acute and convalescent sera may be confirmatory. Paired sera are particularly useful in cat owners who may have a background rate of *Bartonella* antibody seropositivity greater than the general population (2–6%). The most sensitive technique currently available to diagnose *B. henselae* infection is polymerase chain reaction. This species-specific test detects *B. henselae* DNA in blood or tissue specimens (e.g., lymph nodes and bone). The Centers for Disease Control and Prevention and some commercial laboratories perform *B. henselae* polymerase chain reaction testing. This test should be considered when an atypical manifestation is suspected. It is also useful to diagnose CSD in immunocompromised patients who may not be able to mount a significant antibody response.

The presence of *T. gondii*-specific IgM antibodies suggests recent infection. IgM antibodies can be detected 2 weeks after infection. The concentration peaks in 1 month and is generally undetectable within 6–9 months. The lack of *T. gondii*-specific IgM antibodies indicates infection more than 6 months ago. Enzyme immunoassay tests are the more sensitive assays compared to indirect fluorescent antibody tests. False-positive IgM tests do occur, particularly with the use of commercial laboratory kits. This has been documented, particularly, in pregnant women. It is recommended that retesting be done by reference laboratory if there is a positive IgM test.[24,25] IgG-specific antibodies achieve a peak concentration 1–2 months after infection and remain positive indefinitely.[8]

Throat Cultures

Viral cultures are expensive and not typically helpful. Throat culture for GABHS is warranted in cases of acute lymphadenitis. Patients have been reported to have negative throat cultures but positive nodal cultures with GABHS; therefore, a negative throat culture does not rule out GABHS, nor does a positive throat culture confirm the diagnosis.[15] However, since approximately 15% of children have asymptomatic throat carriage of GABHS, detection of these bacteria from the throat does not necessarily mean that it is the cause of lymphadenitis.

Biopsy, Histology, and Culture

Up to 10% of patients with acute unilateral infection without abscess who are treated with oral antibiotics may still need incision and drainage as a result of progression to suppurative infection.[26] Aspiration of the node is safe and reliable in both solid and cystic lesions (Table 26–4). Nodal aspirate should be sent for Gram stain, acid-fast bacilli (AFB) stain, and aerobic, anaerobic, and mycobacterial cultures. Complete blood count and throat and blood cultures should also be sent. However, yield of blood cultures in children with cervical abscesses is low, with rates of 3.8–10.5%.[10,27]

Definitive diagnosis of NTM adenitis depends on isolating the organisms.[28] Excisional biopsy can help make the definitive diagnosis. Fine needle aspiration has been shown as an alternative mode for obtaining sample for diagnostic culture. Incision and drainage are contraindicated if NTM is suspected, as it may lead to chronically draining sinus tract. NTM is found in the environment and can commonly be a contaminant of specimens. However, its recovery from sterile site such as lymph node is considered diagnostic.

When the diagnostic suspicion is TB, mycobacterial culture remains the standard for definitive diagnosis of tuberculosis. A positive TB polymerase chain reaction, stain with AFB, and granulomas on histopathology may aid in the diagnosis but are not definitive.

In CSD, lymph node histology may also be helpful in suggesting the diagnosis. Histologically, lymphocytic infiltration is present in the early phase followed by polymorphonuclear leukocyte infiltration with necrotic granulomas.[6,8,19] Warthin–Starry silver stain may show bacilli although not specific for *B. henselae.*

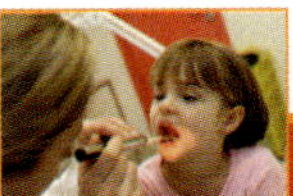

Table 26–4.

How to Perform Needle Aspiration of a Lymph Node

Identify the largest node with most direct access
Enter the node through an area of healthy skin
Aspirate material with sterile technique
Examine aspirated material by Gram stain and acid-fast stain
Culture for aerobic, anaerobic, and mycobacteria
If no purulent material aspirated, inject a small amount (1 cc) of nonbacteriostatic saline into the node and aspirate fluid
Etiologic agent can be recovered in 60–88% cases via this procedure[16]

MANAGEMENT

Strategies for the management of acute and subacute cervical lymphadenitis are summarized in Figures 26–3 and 26–4.

TREATMENT

Treatment is based on presumed or known etiology. It is neither important nor possible to identify all etiologies for acute lymphadenitis. Empiric therapy is based on history and clinical presentation, assessment of risk factors, and review of the current antibiotic susceptibility patterns in the population.

Therapy for acute bacterial lymphadenitis should begin with oral or parenteral antistaphylococcal and streptococcal antibiotics based on patient's clinical appearance. Prevalence of community-acquired methicillin-resistant *S. aureus* (CA-MRSA) is important in deciding empiric antibiotic coverage. Many institutions in areas with a high MRSA prevalence use clindamycin or a combination of trimethoprim–sulfamethoxazole (to cover MRSA) and penicillin (to cover GABHS). The usual course of antibiotics is 7–14 days. Clinical response should be noted within 72 hours of starting the therapy. If no improvement is noted after 72 hours or symptoms worsen, this should prompt evaluation for abscess or reconsideration of the diagnosis. If abscess is identified, incision and drainage may be required. If a dental infection is present, empiric therapy should include coverage for Gram-positive cocci, anaerobes, and Gram-negative organisms. Once a specific etiology is identified, treatment should be based on review of current literature or a consultation with an infectious disease specialist (Table 26–5). If a patient completes a full antibiotic course and has no regression in nodal size, excisional biopsy should be considered.

Fine needle aspiration has been suggested as an initial step of the evaluation of chronic cervical lymphadenitis in patients who are stable. If the culture result yields NTM, surgery remains the best-established treatment, as it provides cure for localized NTM disease. If excision of the node is incomplete or the disease recurs, medical management with antimicrobials is recommended: clarithromycin or azithromycin plus ethambutol with rifampin or rifabutin.[8] The utility of macrolide-based antimicrobial therapy as an alternative to surgery (or as an additive) has not been fully established. More recent studies suggest surgical excision to be more effective than antibiotic treatment.[29] The study results

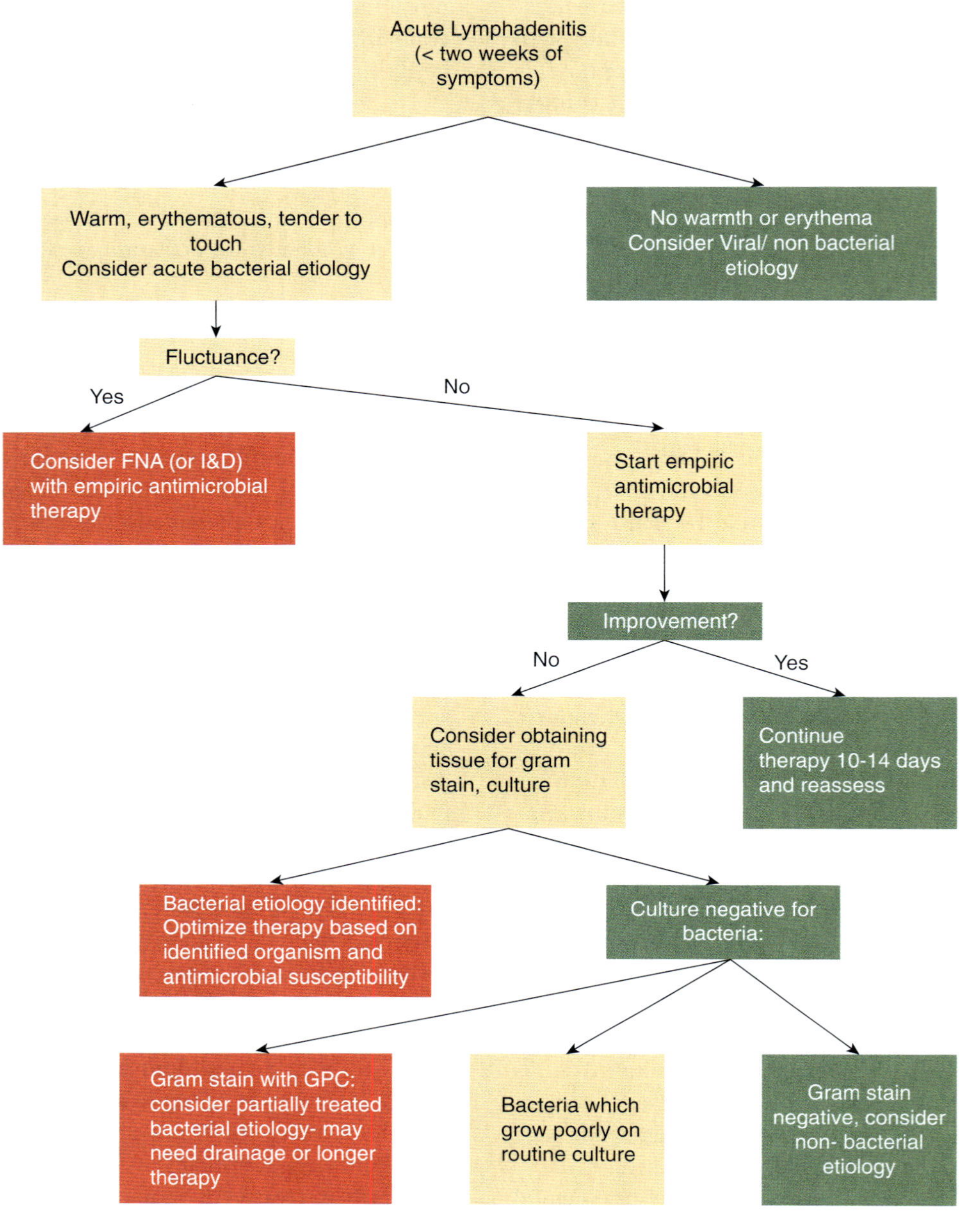

FIGURE 26–3 ■ Algorithm for the management of acute cervical lymphadenitis.

showed that surgical excision was more effective than antibiotic therapy, with cure rates of 96% and 66%, respectively (95% confidence interval for the difference, 16–44%). Treatment failures in the antibiotic group could not be explained by noncompliance or development of resistance (to clarithromycin or rifabutin). Adverse events were also lower in the surgical group (28%) compared to the antimicrobial group (78%).

If TB is suspected, empiric antituberculosis therapy should be promptly started after the needle aspiration. Three-drug combination therapy is recommended for the first 2 months. Isoniazid, rifampin, and pyrazinamide (plus ethambutol or an aminoglycoside if resistance is suspected) are the initial choices of therapy. The fourth drug may be discontinued once susceptibility is known. Additional treatment for at least 4 months with isoniazid and rifampin is indicated for susceptible *M. tuberculosis*.[8] The local Department of Health should be informed of cases of tuberculous lymphadenitis.

Treatment is supportive for lymphadenitis caused by *B. henselae*, as it is primarily a self-limited disease.[6,8] Symptoms usually resolve in 2–4 months. A prospective, randomized, double-blind, placebo-controlled study to evaluate benefit of treatment (with azithromycin) showed that there is treatment benefit within the first month of treatment (defined by lymph

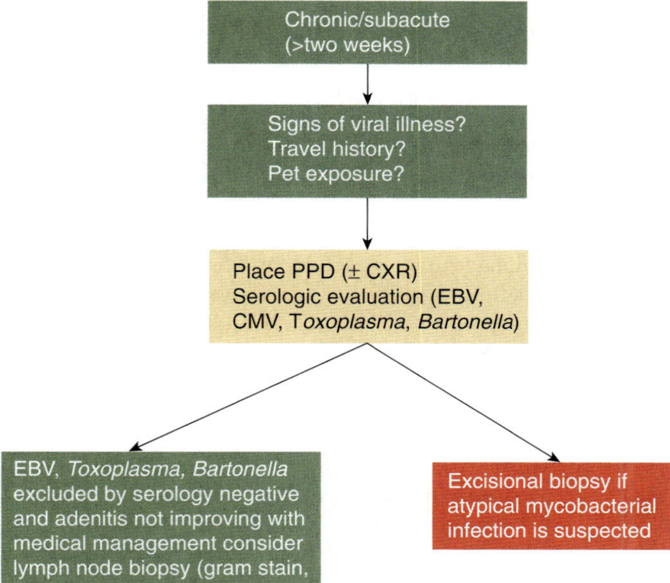

FIGURE 26–4 ■ Algorithm for the management of subacute cervical lymphadenitis.

node volume); after the 30 days, there was no significant difference between the two groups.[30] Fine needle aspiration may be indicated to relieve pressure from painful suppurative lymph nodes. Antimicrobial therapy may be necessary for patients with severe or systemic disease or for those who are immunocompromised. Optimal choice of antimicrobial therapy or its length has not been established. Choices of antimicrobial therapies include erythromycin, azithromycin, gentamicin, trimethroprim–sulfamethoxazole, rifampin, and ciprofloxacin.[7,8]

Lymphadenitis caused by acquired *T. gondii* infection in a nonpregnant, immunocompetent host does not require antimicrobial therapy.[8]

Table 26–5.

Table of Current Antibiotic Treatments with Doses

	Empiric Oral Therapy	Empiric IV Therapy
*S. aureus**	Cephalexin or cloxacillin	Oxacillin 150 mg/kg/d divided Q6h Or Cefazolin 100 mg/kg/d divided Q8h
MRSA†	Clindamycin, TMP-SMX, or linezolid	Clindamycin 30 mg/kg/d divided Q8h Or Vancomycin 40 mg/kg/d divided Q8h
S. pyogenes	Amoxicillin or penicillin VK Total course po + IV of 7–14 d	Penicillin G IV or IM
Non-TB mycobacterium	Excision is curative	
TB adenitis	INH 10–15 mg/kg/d po/IV × 6 months and rifampin 10–20 mg/kg/d po/IV × 6 months and pyrazinamide 20–40 mg/kg/day po × first 2 months If multidrug resistance is suspected, add ethambutol 20 mg/kg/d po Qday	

**Based on community antibiotic sensitivities.*
†*If high prevalence of community Staph. aureus is methicillin resistant, treat empirically for MRSA.*
MRSA, methicillin-resistant *Staph. aureus;* INH, isoniazid.

COURSE AND PROGNOSIS

Most cases of acute unilateral lymphadenitis resolve with appropriate antibiotic therapy. Up to 10% of patients may need incision and drainage despite appropriate management.[26] Described risk factors that predict need for surgical intervention include patient aged <1 year and symptoms present approximately 48 hours prior to presentation.[13,31] Abscess formation is a common complication of cervical lymphadenitis. Rapid progression or failure to treat adenitis can result in cellulitis, septicemia, or toxin-mediated sequelae. Poststreptococcal glomerulonephritis occurs occasionally. Rare complications include cervical fasciitis, carotid artery aneurysm with rupture, jugular vein thrombosis, septic embolization, mediastinal abscess, and purulent pericarditis.[31] These complications stress the need for appropriate treatment with the first signs of lymphadenitis.

REFERENCES

1. Scobie WG. Acute suppurative adenitis in children: a review of 964 cases. *Scott Med J.* 1969;14(10):352-354.
2. Albright JT, Pransky SM. Nontuberculous mycobacterial infections of the head and neck. *Pediatr Clin North Am.* 2003;50(2):503-514.
3. Hill AR. The tuberculin skin test: a useful screen for nontuberculous mycobacterial lymphadenitis in regions with a low prevalence of tuberculosis? *Clin Infect Dis.* 2006;43(12):1552-1554.
4. Marais BJ, Wright CA, Schaaf HS, et al. Tuberculous lymphadenitis as a cause of persistent cervical lymphadenopathy in children from a tuberculosis-endemic area. *Pediatr Infect Dis J.* 2006;25(2):142-146.
5. Reynolds MG, et al. Epidemiology of cat-scratch disease hospitalizations among children in the United States. *Pediatr Infect Dis J.* 2005;24(8):700-704.
6. Conrad DA. Treatment of cat-scratch disease. *Curr Opin Pediatr.* 2001;13(1):56-59.
7. Thorell EA, Chesney PJ. Cervical lymphadenitis and neck infections. In: Long SS, Pickering LK, Prober CG, eds. *Principles and Practice of Pediatric Infectious Diseases.* 3rd ed. Philadelphia: Churchill Livingstone, 2008;143-155.
8. Florin TA, Zaoutis TE, Zaoutis LB. Beyond cat-scratch disease: widening the spectrum of Bartonella henselae infection. *Pediatrics.* 2008; 121:e413-e425.
9. Kelly CS, Kelly RE, Jr. Lymphadenopathy in children. *Pediatr Clin North Am.* 1998;45(4):875-888.
10. Cengiz AB, et al. Acute neck infections in children. *Turk J Pediatr.* 2004;46(2):153-158.
11. Tanir G, et al. Soft tissue infections in children: a retrospective analysis of 242 hospitalized patients. *Jpn J Infect Dis.* 2006;59(4):258-260.
12. Serour F, Gorenstein A, Somekh E. Needle aspiration for suppurative cervical lymphadenitis. *Clin Pediatr (Phila).* 2002;41(7):471-474.
13. Simo R, et al. Microbiology and antibiotic treatment of head and neck abscesses in children. *Clin Otolaryngol Allied Sci.* 1998;23(2):164-168.
14. Lane RJ, Keane WM, Potsic WP. Pediatric infectious cervical lymphadenitis. *Otolaryngol Head Neck Surg.* 1980;88(4):332-335.
15. Barton LL, Feigin RD. Childhood cervical lymphadenitis: a reappraisal. *J Pediatr.* 1974;84(6):846-852.
16. Gosche JR, Vick L. Acute, subacute, and chronic cervical lymphadenitis in children. *Semin Pediatr Surg.* 2006;15(2):99-106.
17. Leung AK, Robson WL. Childhood cervical lymphadenopathy. *J Pediatr Health Care.* 2004;18(1):3-7.
18. Panesar J, et al. Nontuberculous mycobacterial cervical adenitis: a ten-year retrospective review. *Laryngoscope.* 2003;113(1):149-154.
19. Margileth AM. Cat scratch disease: nonbacterial regional lymphadenitis. The study of 145 patients and a review of the literature. *Pediatrics.* 1968;42(5):803-818.
20. Albanyan EA, Baker CJ. Is lumbar puncture necessary to exclude meningitis in neonates and young infants: lessons from the group B streptococcus cellulitis-adenitis syndrome. *Pediatrics.* 1998;102(4, pt 1):985-986.
21. Edwards MS, Nizet V, Baker, CJ. Group B Streptococcal Infections. In: Remington JS, Klein JO, Wilson CB, Baker CJ, eds. *Infectious Diseases of the Fetus and Newborn Infant.* 6th ed. Philadelphia: Elsevier Saunders, 2006:403-464.
22. Mattix ME, et al. Clinicopathologic aspects of animal and zoonotic diseases of bioterrorism. *Clin Lab Med.* 2006;26(2):445-489, x.
23. Stamos JK, et al. Lymphadenitis as the dominant manifestation of Kawasaki disease. *Pediatrics.* 1994;93(3):525-528.
24. Garry DJ, et al. Commercial laboratory IgM testing for *Toxoplasma gondii* in pregnancy: a 20-year experience. *Infect Dis Obstet Gynecol.* 2005;13(3):151-153.
25. Public Health Service, Department of Health and Human Services (US), Food and Drug Administration. FDA Public Health Advisory: limitations of Toxoplasmosis IgM Commercial Test Kits [Letter]. Washington, USA: Department of Health and Human Services; 1997. (http://www.fda.gov/cdrh/toxopha.html)
26. Peters TR, Edwards KM. Cervical lymphadenopathy and adenitis. *Pediatr Rev.* 2000;21(12):399-405.
27. Brook I. Microbiology of abscesses of the head and neck in children. *Ann Otol Rhinol Laryngol.* 1987;96(4):429-433.
28. Lindeboom JA, et al. Tuberculin skin testing is useful in the screening for nontuberculous mycobacterial cervicofacial lymphadenitis in children. *Clin Infect Dis.* 2006;43(12):1547-1551.
29. Lindeboom JA, et al. Surgical excision versus antibiotic treatment for nontuberculous mycobacterial cervicofacial lymphadenitis in children: a multicenter, randomized, controlled trial. *Clin Infect Dis.* 2007;44(8):1057-1064.
30. Bass JW, et al. Prospective randomized double blind placebo-controlled evaluation of azithromycin for treatment of cat-scratch disease. *Pediatr Infect Dis J.* 1998;17(6):447-452.
31. Luu TM, et al. Acute adenitis in children: clinical course and factors predictive of surgical drainage. *J Paediatr Child Health.* 2005;41(5-6):273-277.

CHAPTER 27

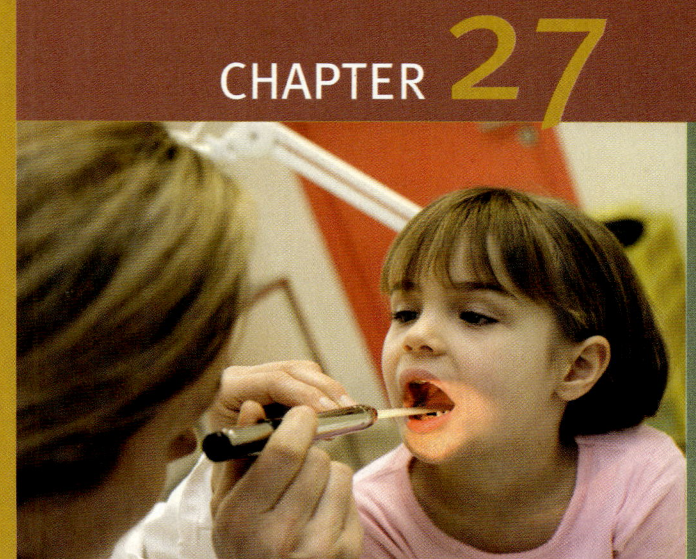

Gingival and Periodontal Infections

Nadeem Karimbux and David Kim

INTRODUCTION

Gingivitis and periodontitis are inflammatory conditions of the tooth-supporting structures (periodontium). The transition from primary to permanent dentition, and the hormonal changes associated with puberty present unique periodontal conditions in children.[1] In adults, these diseases are of a chronic nature, whereas in children they can be aggressive in nature. Thus, early diagnosis and treatment are critical. The nondestructive nature of gingival inflammation of childhood can progress to the more significant periodontal disease seen in the adult population if left untreated.[1]

DEFINITION

Gingivitis and periodontitis are the two major forms of inflammatory diseases affecting the periodontium.[2] Broadly speaking, gingivitis refers to reversible inflammation of the gingiva that does not result in clinical attachment loss. In contrast, periodontitis implies inflammation of both the gingiva and the adjacent attachment apparatus, and is characterized by loss of connective tissue attachment and alveolar bone. Each of these diseases may be further classified based upon etiology, clinical presentation, rate of progression, or associated complication factors as follows[3,4]:

- Dental plaque-induced gingival diseases
- Chronic periodontitis
- Aggressive periodontitis
- Periodontitis as a manifestation of systemic diseases
- Necrotizing periodontal diseases

CLINICAL PRESENTATIONS AND DIAGNOSIS

Dental Plaque-Induced Gingival Disease

Dental plaque-induced gingival disease can be characterized by redness and edema of the gingival tissue, bleeding upon provocation, changes in contour and consistency, presence of calculus and/or plaque, without radiographic evidence of crestal bone loss (Figure 27–1).[5]

Chronic Periodontitis

Chronic periodontitis is more prevalent in adults, but can occur in children and adolescents. Chronic periodontitis is characterized by edema, erythema, gingival bleeding upon tissue manipulation, and suppuration with variable degrees of clinical attachment loss. In addition, radiographic evidence of bone loss and increased tooth mobility might be present.[6] Chronic periodontitis can be classified based on disease severity

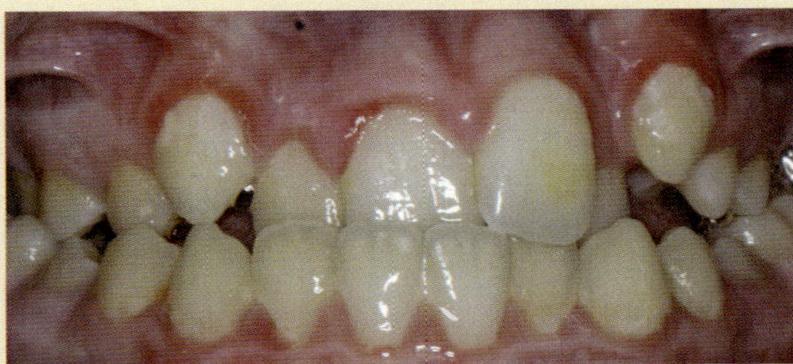

FIGURE 27–1 ■ Dental plaque-induced gingival disease in the mixed dentition.

and extent of involvement. Disease severity can be categorized into mild (1–2 mm clinical attachment loss), moderate (3–4 mm clinical attachment loss), or severe (≥5 mm clinical attachment loss).[3] The disease can be localized (less than 30% of the dentition affected) or generalized (greater than 30% of the dentition affected), and is characterized by a slow to moderate rate of progression that may include periods of rapid destruction.[4]

Aggressive Periodontitis

Aggressive periodontitis encompasses the distinct type of periodontitis that affect children, who, in most cases, appear healthy. Aggressive periodontitis can be presented in localized (LAgP) or generalized (GAgP) pattern. The localized version has a circumpubertal onset with familial aggregation, and there is a rapid rate of disease progression around first molars and incisors (Figure 27–2).[7] However, atypical pattern of affected teeth are possible.[7] Characteristically, the amounts of microbial deposits are inconsistent with the severity of periodontal tissue destruction.[7] Thus, the primary features of localized aggressive periodontitis include a rapid clinical attachment and bone loss with familial aggregation.[4] Secondary features include phagocyte abnormalities and a hyperresponsive macrophage phenotype.[4] Generalized aggressive periodontitis is classically a disease of adolescent and young adults, but it can begin at any age. There is generalized interproximal attachment loss affecting at least three permanent teeth other than the first molars and incisors.[7] Smoking may be a risk factor for this disease.

Systemic Causes of Periodontitis

Periodontitis as a manifestation of systemic disease in children is a rare disease that often begins between the time of eruption of the primary teeth (at about 6 months of age) up to the age of 5 years.[8,9] Systemic etiologic components may be suspected in children who exhibit periodontal inflammation or destruction, which appears disproportionate to the local irritants.[10] Conditions that make children more susceptible to periodontal disease include hematologic and genetic disorders (Table 27–1). This category of periodontitis can occur in localized and generalized forms. In the localized form, affected sites exhibit rapid bone loss and minimal gingival inflammation.[8,9] In the generalized form, there is rapid bone loss around nearly all teeth and marked gingival inflammation.[8,9] In some forms of this disease, the primary and permanent dentitions can be affected. In addition, gingival enlargement or gingival overgrowth can be associated with drugs such as anticonvulsants (e.g., phenytoin), calcium channel blockers (e.g., nifedipine), and immunosuppressants (e.g., cyclosporin).

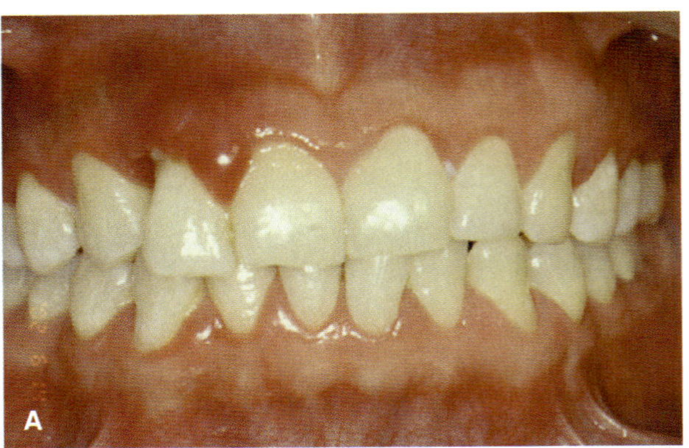

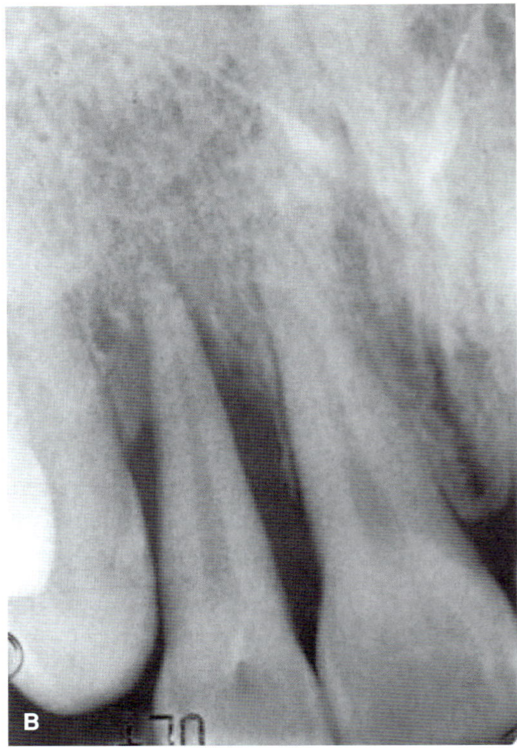

FIGURE 27–2 ■ (A) Clinical picture of localized aggressive periodontitis (around lateral incisor). (B) Radiographic evidence of bone loss around lateral incisor.

Necrotizing Periodontal Diseases

Necrotizing periodontal diseases are caused by abnormal overgrowth of normal oral bacteria as a consequence of poor oral hygiene.[11] Necrotizing periodontal diseases manifest in two different forms: necrotizing ulcerative gingivitis and necrotizing ulcerative periodontitis.[12] Necrotizing ulcerative gingivitis (also known as Trench mouth or Vincent's infection) is an acute infection of the gingiva, and when necrotizing ulcerative gingivitis has progressed to include attachment loss, it is known as necrotizing ulcerative periodontitis. The two most significant findings used in the diagnosis of necrotizing

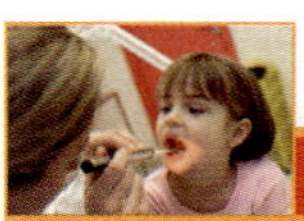

Table 27–1.

Periodontitis as a Manifestation of Systemic Disease[13]

Diabetes mellitus
Human immunodeficiency virus infection
Tobacco use and drug abuse
Stress
Leukemias
Neutropenia and agranulocytosis
Langerhans cell histiocytosis
Acrodynia
Genetic abnormalities
- Trisomy 21 (Down syndrome)
- Hypophosphatasia
- Leukocyte adhesion deficiency
- Papillon–Lefèvre syndrome
- Chédiak–Higashi syndrome
- Ehlers–Danlos syndrome

periodontal diseases are the presence of interproximal gingival tissue necrosis and ulceration, and the rapid onset of halitosis and gingival pain.[4] Other findings often include lymphadenopathy, fever, and malaise.[12]

Specific Considerations and Presentations

Periodontal abscess is an acute suppurative infection of the deeper periodontal tissues that may lead to the destruction of periodontal ligament and alveolar bone.[12] Patients may complain of localized pain and swelling with progression over hours or days, heat sensitivity, fever, and gingival bleeding. Clinical features may include a smooth, shiny swelling of the gingiva; pain with the area of swelling tender to touch; a purulent exudate; and/or increase in pocket depth.[12] In addition, the tooth may be sensitive to percussion and may be mobile.[12] More severe infections lead to trismus, dysphagia, respiratory difficulty, face or neck swelling, and regional lymph node involvement. Treatments include irrigation and mechanical debridement of the pocket, drainage and debridement of the lesion, and administration of antibiotics.[13]

Linear gingival erythema is a manifestation of human immunodeficiency virus (HIV) infection. This condition is distinguished by 2–3 mm marginal band of intense erythema in the free gingiva, which may extend into the attached gingiva as a focal or diffuse erythema and extend beyond the mucogingival line into the alveolar mucosa.[14] Treatments include improving oral hygiene, scaling and root planing, chlorhexidine rinses, and frequent dental cleaning.[13]

PATHOGENESIS

Inadequate brushing and flossing are by far the most common causes of gingivitis and periodontitis. Without proper brushing, plaque (a film-like substance made up primarily of bacteria) remains along the gum line of the teeth. Plaque also accumulates in faulty fillings and around the teeth next to poorly cleaned partial dentures, bridges, and orthodontic appliances. When plaque stays on the teeth for more than 72 hours, it hardens into tartar (calculus), which cannot be completely removed by brushing and flossing. Long-term accumulation of plaque and tartar leads to the creation of pockets between the teeth and gums. These pockets extend downward between the root of the tooth and the underlying bone, leading to destruction of the supporting bone and loosening of the tooth.

Dental plaque-induced gingival disease is compounded by bacterial accumulation that induces pathological changes in the tissues by direct (i.e., bacterial-derived byproducts) and indirect paths (i.e., host-derived inflammatory mediators). Although the microbiology of dental plaque has not been completely characterized, increased subgingival concentrations of *Actinomyces* spp., *Capnocytophaga* spp., *Leptotrichia* spp., and *Selenomonas* spp. have been found in experimental gingivitis in children when compared with gingivitis in adults.[15,16] Histopathological observations have led to the subdivision into three stages that consist of vasodilation, increased gingival crevicular fluid, emigration of neutrophils, and activation of monocytes, lymphocytes, and fibroblasts.[11] In addition, normal and abnormal fluctuation in hormone levels can modify the gingival inflammatory response to dental plaque, leading to a diagnosis of puberty or menopausal gingivitis.[17,18]

The pathology of *chronic periodontitis* lesions are characteristic of, and consistent with a subversion of host defenses against bacterial plaque pathogens and subsequent activation of bacterially induced host mediated processes that destroy periodontal tissues.[11] The predominance of a gram-negative bacterial flora (*Actinobacillus actinomycetemcomitans, Tannerella forsythensis, Porphyromonas gingivalis, Prevotella intermedia*, and *Fusobacterium nucleatum*) in combination with the cellular and cytokine profiles of the lesions, indicate the likelihood that bacterial lipopolysaccharide activation of monocytes and subsequent production of tissue destructive cytokines is likely a major pathway for connective tissue attachment loss and bone loss.[11]

Highly virulent strains of *A. actinomycetemcomitans* in combination with *Bacteriodes*-like species are involved in localized aggressive periodontitis.[19–21] In addition, a variety of functional defects have been reported in neutrophils from patients with LAgP.[22,23] These include anomalies of chemotaxis, phogocytosis, bactericidal activity, superoxide production, FcγRIIIB (CD 16) expression, leukotriene B_4 generation and Ca2+ channel, and second messenger activation.[4] Even though the influence of these functional defects on the susceptibility of individuals to LAgP is unknown, it is possible that they play a role in the clinical course of disease in some patients.[4] Generalized aggressive periodontitis is also frequently associated with periodontal pathogens *A. actinomycetemcomitans* and *P. gingivalis*, and neutrophils function abnormalities.[4,7] For example, a poor serum antibody response to infecting agents is frequently detected.[7] Smoking can increase the progression of periodontitis, and is sometimes an attribute to generalized aggressive periodontitis.

Neutrophils from some children with *periodontitis as a manifestation of systemic disease* have abnormalities in a cell surface glycoprotein (LFA-1 and Mac-1).[4] Thus, the neutrophils in these patients having leukocyte adhesion deficiency are likely to have a decreased ability to move from the circulation to sites of inflammation and infection.[24] In addition, affected sites harbor elevated percentages of putative periodontal pathogens, such as *A. actinomycetemcomitans*, *P. intermedia*, *Eikenella corrodens*, and *Capnocytophage sputigena*.[25,26] Since there are several systemic diseases that cause periodontitis in young patients, health care providers need to be cognizant of all of possible hematologic and genetic disorders. In addition, health care providers need to determine appropriate clinical and laboratory tests that need to be performed in order to determine specific etiology of disease. Unfortunately, sometimes both the primary and permanent dentition can be lost due to underlying systemic conditions, such as Down syndrome and Papillon–Lefèvre syndrome, a rare autosomal recessive disorder characterized by palmoplantar keratoderma with periodontitis followed by premature shedding of both deciduous and permanent teeth (Table 27–1).

Necrotizing ulcerative periodontal disease sites harbor high levels of spirochetes and *P. intermedia*.[27,28] The role of an impaired host response in necrotizing ulcerative gingivitis has long been recognized. For example, factors that predispose children to *necrotizing periodontal disease* include an altered immune system (response), viral infections, malnutrition, emotional stress, lack of sleep, and a variety of systemic diseases.[29–31]

TREATMENT

In general, the therapeutic goals of periodontal treatment are to alter or eliminate the microbial etiology and contributing risk factors for periodontal disease, thereby arresting the progression of disease and preserving the dentition.[6] In addition, appropriate supportive periodontal maintenance that includes personal and professional care is important in preventing reinitiation of inflammation.[2] Since contributing systemic risk factors may affect treatment and therapeutic outcomes, elimination, alteration, or control of these risk factors should be attempted, and consultation with the patient's physician will likely be indicated to coordinate medical care in conjunction with periodontal therapy (Figure 27–3).[6] For example, early nontraumatic tooth loss in children 3–18 years of age warrants evaluation for systemic causes of periodontitis.

Periodontal therapy will likely include patient education and hygiene.[5] For gingivitis, rinsing several times a day with a hydrogen peroxide solution (3% hydrogen

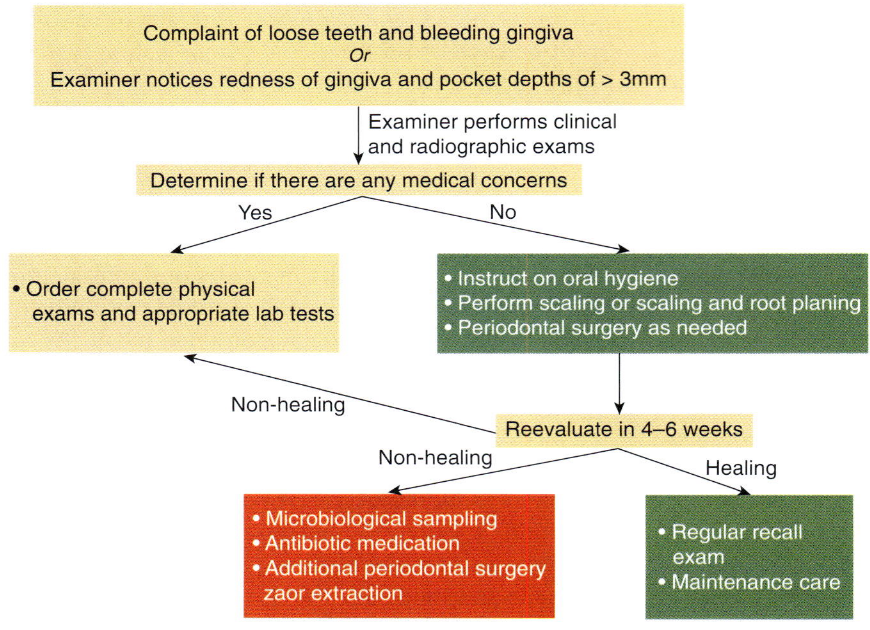

FIGURE 27–3 ■ Screening and treatment strategy for children and adolescents.

peroxide mixed with equal parts water) or chlorhexidine will reduce bacterial burden and hasten disease resolution. For periodontitis, debridement of tooth surfaces to remove supragingival and subgingival plaque and calculus is necessary. Unlike gingivitis, which usually resolves with improved oral hygiene, periodontitis requires professional care. A person using good oral hygiene can clean only 2–3 mm below the gum line. A dentist can clean pockets up to 4–6 mm deep using scaling and root planing which thoroughly remove tartar and the diseased root surface. In some cases (e.g., localized aggressive periodontitis), antibiotics, such as tetracycline in combination with scaling and root planing, are beneficial. Correction of ill-fitting restorations, caries, and tooth malposition will reduce the likelihood of plaque retention. Gingival deformities may require surgical correction using one of the following approaches[6]:

- Gingival augmentation therapy
- Regenerative therapy (i.e., bone replacement grafts, guided tissue regeneration, combined regenerative techniques)
- Resective therapy (i.e., flaps with or without osseous surgery, gingevectomy)

COURSE AND PROGNOSIS

Long-term outcomes in children with periodontal diseases depend on patient compliance with treatment regimens and the delivery of professional periodontal maintenance at appropriate intervals.[7] A satisfactory response to therapy should result in a significant reduction in clinical signs of gingival inflammation, stability of clinical attachment levels, and reduction of clinically detectable plaque to a level compatible with gingival health. An appropriate initial interval for follow-up care and dental prophylaxis should be determined by the clinician; typically, a return visit occurs within 4–6 weeks.

If the patient is not better, there may be continuing clinical signs of disease progression with the possible development of periodontal defects. Factors that may contribute to the periodontal condition not resolving include lack of effectiveness and/or patient's noncompliance in controlling plaque, untreated underlying systemic disease, presence of calculus buildups, and patient's noncompliance with dental prophylaxis interval.

In the management of patients where the periodontal condition does not resolve, treatment may include additional sessions of oral hygiene instruction and education, additional or alternative methods or devices for plaque removal, medical/dental consultation, additional tooth debridement, increasing the frequency of dental prophylaxis, microbial assessment, and continuous monitoring and evaluation to determine further periodontal treatment needs.

REFERENCES

1. Duperon D, Takei HH. Gingival diseases in childhood. In: Newman MG, Takei HH, Klokkevold PR, Carranza FA, eds. *Carranza's Clinical Periodontology.* 10th ed. St. Louis, MO: Saunders Elsevier; 2006:404-410.
2. The American Academy of Periodontology. Treatment of plaque-induced gingivitis, chronic periodontitis, and other clinical conditions (academy report). *J Periodontol.* 2001;72:1790-1800.
3. Armitage GC. Development of a classification system for periodontal diseases and conditions. *Ann Periodontol.* 1999;4:1-6.
4. The American Academy of Periodontology. Periodontal diseases of children and adolescents (position paper). *J Periodontol.* 2003;74:1696-1704.
5. The American Academy of Periodontology. Parameter on plaque-induced gingivitis (parameters of care). *J Periodontol.* 2000;71:851-852.
6. The American Academy of Periodontology. Parameter on chronic periodontitis with slight to moderate loss of periodontal support (parameters of care). *J Periodontol.* 2000;71:853-855.
7. The American Academy of Periodontology. Parameter on aggressive periodontitis (parameters of care). *J Periodontol.* 2000;71:867-869.
8. Page RC, Bowen T, Altman L, et al. Prepubertal periodontitis. I. Definition of a clinical entity. *J Periodontol.* 1983;54:257-271.
9. Watanabe K. Prepubertal periodontitis: a review of diagnostic criteria, pathogenesis, and differential diagnosis. *J Periodont Res.* 1990;25:31-48.
10. The American Academy of Periodontology. Parameter on periodontitis associated with systemic conditions (parameters of care). *J Periodontol.* 2000;71:876-879.
11. The American Academy of Periodontology. The pathogenesis of periodontal diseases (academy report). *J Periodontol.* 1999;70:457-470.
12. The American Academy of Periodontology. Parameter on acute periodontal diseases (parameters of care). *J Periodontol.* 2000;71:863-866
13. Mariotti AJ. In: Bimstein E, Needleman HL, Karimbux N, Van Dyke TE, eds. *Periodontal and Gingival Health and Diseases.* London, UK: Martin Dunitz Ltd; 2001:31-48.
14. Winkler JR, Grassi M, Murray PA. Clinical description and etiology of HIV-associated periodontal diseases. In: Robertson PB, Greenspan Js, eds. Perspectives of Oral Manifestations of AIDS. Proceedings of the First International Symposium on Oral manifestations of AIDS. Littleton, MA: PSG Publishing; 1988:49-70.
15. Moore W, Holdeman L, Smibert R, et al. Bacteriology of experimental gingivitis in children. *Infect Immun.* 1984;46:1-6.
16. Slots J, Möenbo D, Langebaek J, Frandsen A. Microbiota of gingivitis in man. *Scand J Dent.* 1978;86:174-181.
17. Nakagawa S, Fujii H, Machida Y, Okuda K. A longitudinal study from prepuberty to puberty of gingivitis. Correlation between the occurrence of *Prevotella intermedia* and sex hormones. *J Clin Periodontol.* 1994;21:658-665.
18. De Pommereau V, Dargent-Paré C, Robert JJ, Brion M. Periodontal status in insulin-dependent diabetic adolescents. *J Clin Periodontol.* 1992;19:628-632.

19. Haraszthy V, Hariharan G, Tinoco E, et al. Evidence for the role of highly leukotoxic *Actinobacillus actinomycetemcomitans* in the pathogenesis of localized and other forms of early-onset periodontitis. *J Periodontol.* 2000;71:912-922.
20. Kornman KS, Robertson PB. Clinical and microbiological evaluation of therapy for juvenile periodontitis. *J Periodontol.* 1985;56:443-446.
21. Genco RJ, Zambon JJ, Christersoon LA. The origin of periodontal infections. *Adv Dent Res.* 1988;2:245-259.
22. Daniel MA, Van Dyke TE. Alteration in phagocyte function and periodontal infection. *J Periodontol.* 1996;67:1070-1075.
23. Dennison DK, Van Dyke TE. The acute inflammatory response and the role of phagocytic cells in periodontal health and disease. *Periodontol 2000.* 1997;14:54-78.
24. Page RC, Beatty P, Waldrop TC. Molecular basis for the functional abnormality in neutrophils from patients with generalized prepubertal periodontitis. *J Periodont Res.* 1987;22:182-183.
25. Sweeney EA, Alcoforado GAP, Nyman S, Slots J. Prevalence and microbiology of localized prepubertal periodontitis. *Oral Microbiol Immunol.* 1987;2:65-70.
26. Delaney DE, Kornman KS. Microbiology of subgingival plaque from children with localized prepubertal periodontitis. *Oral Microbiol Immunol.* 1987;2:71-76.
27. Loesche WJ, Syed SA, Laughon BE, Stoll J. The bacteriology of acute necrotizing ulcerative gingivitis. *J Periodontol.* 1982;53:223-230.
28. Listgarten M. Electron microscopic observations on the bacterial flora of acute necrotizing ulcerative gingivitis. *J Periodontol.* 1965;36:328-339.
29. Taiwo JO. Severity of necrotizing ulcerative gingivitis in Nigerian children. *Periodontal Clin Investig.* 1995;17:24-27.
30. Contreras A, Falkler WA, Jr., Enwonwu CO, et al. Human Herpesviridae in acute necrotizing ulcerative gingivitis in children in Nigeria. *Oral Microbiol Immunol.* 1997;12:259-265.
31. Horning G, Cohen M. Necrotizing ulcerative gingivitis, periodontitis, stomatitis: clinical staging and predisposing factors. *J Periodontol.* 1995;66:990-998.

SECTION 6

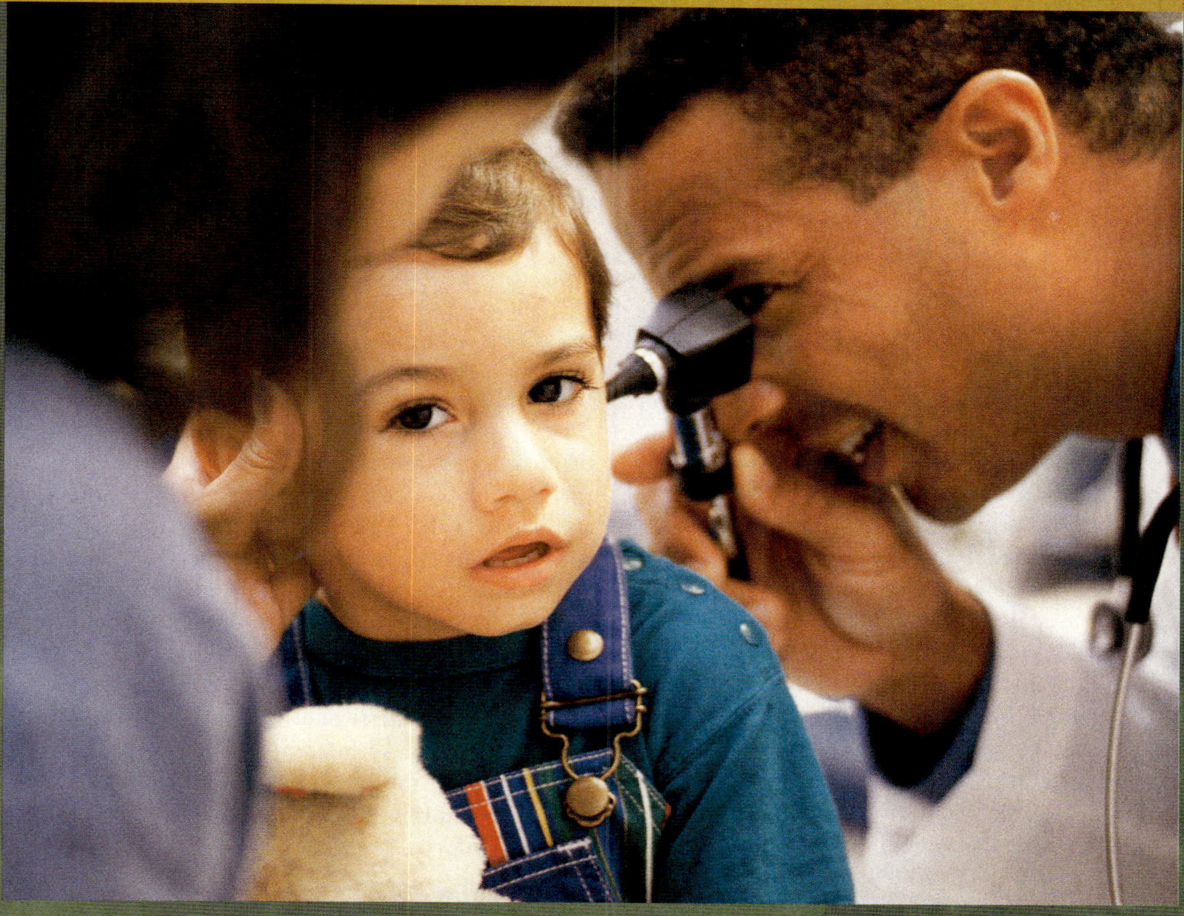

Upper Respiratory Infections

CHAPTER 28

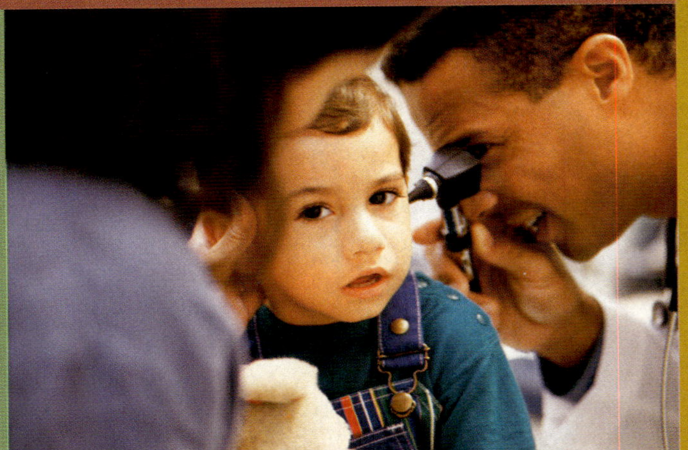

Otitis Media

Donald H. Arnold and David M. Spiro

INTRODUCTION

The term otitis media (OM) has been used to describe multiple disorders of the middle ear, including acute otitis media (AOM), otitis media with effusion (OME), chronic OME, and the umbrella designation including all of these terms. This chapter uses the term otitis media in its historic usage as an umbrella term including AOM and OME, and uses the terms AOM and OME as specific disease processes as defined below. The purpose of the chapter is to describe the contemporary approach to diagnosis and management of AOM and to discuss OME as it relates to AOM.

As few as 50% of pediatricians in the United States are aware of recent guidelines for diagnosis and management of AOM. Only 28% of those aware of these guidelines changed their practice as a result.[1] University-affiliated pediatricians' diagnoses of AOM complied with Centers for Disease Control and Prevention diagnostic criteria only 38% of the time during the winter of 1999–2000.[2] Additionally, tympanometry as an adjunct to otoscopy did not improve diagnostic accuracy or decrease antibiotic usage.[3] In Finland, implementation of a national guideline for OM resulted in health benefits and lower direct costs.[4] One conclusion from the Finnish data is that adherence to such guidelines may improve care and reduce use of antibiotics.

DEFINITIONS

OME is usually the result of AOM. Therefore, AOM and OME are pathologic processes along the same disease continuum. This relationship has resulted in diagnostic uncertainty and variations in the definition of AOM over time. However, establishing a uniform and appropriate definition is of utmost importance if AOM is to be diagnosed and managed appropriately. The most important distinction is that OME is not treated with antibiotics, whereas AOM may be treated with antibiotics. This difference exemplifies the need for uniform and appropriate definitions, diagnostic criteria, and management schema for AOM and OME.[5,6]

With the above caveat in mind, the American Academy of Pediatrics Subcommittee on Management of AOM and the Agency for Healthcare Research and Quality has established a definition of AOM.[7–9] This definition requires the presence of three equally important elements[8]:

1. Acute onset (<48 hours) of signs and symptoms, and
2. Middle-ear effusion (MEE), and
3. Signs and symptoms of middle-ear inflammation.

Methods and criteria for the diagnosis of AOM pertaining to each of these diagnostic elements are included in the following sections and in Table 28–1.

In similar fashion the Agency for Healthcare Research and Quality has convened an expert panel to define and develop clinical practice guidelines for OME. OME is defined as the presence of middle ear fluid without signs or symptoms of AOM.[5,10] Implicit in this definition is the absence of evidence of middle-ear inflammation. OME occurs without an inflammatory component as a result of Eustachian tube dysfunction or, alternatively, during the period following AOM in which inflammation has resolved but effusion persists.

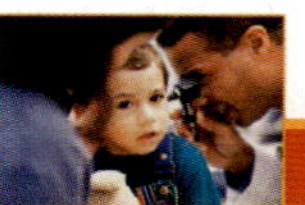

Table 28–1.

Diagnostic Elements, Method, and Criteria for Diagnosing AOM[7]

Diagnostic Element	Method	Criteria
Acute onset	History of illness	<48 h
MEE	Pneumatic otoscopy *or*	Bulging of the TM
	Otorrhea *or*	Limited TM mobility
	Tympanometry	Air fluid level behind TM
Middle ear inflammation	History/physical examination	At least one: fever, otalgia, irritability in infant, red TM *not because of crying or fever*[42]

TM, tympanic membrane.

EPIDEMIOLOGY

AOM, OME, and other processes comprising the designation OM are second only to upper respiratory infections (URIs) as a reason for ambulatory care visits in patients younger than 15 years, and account for 13% of all emergency department visits.[11] These data reflect a statistically significant decrease in the age-adjusted visit rate, reported by the National Ambulatory Medical Care surveys between the years 1993–1995 and 2001–2002.[11,12] However, accurate data on the epidemiology of AOM are lacking because these surveys do not make the critical distinction among AOM, OME, or eustachian tube dysfunction.[8] OM has previously been reported as the most frequent reason for antibiotic prescribing in childhood and accounted for $4.1 billion in the US expenditures in 1992.[13,14]

There is overlap of presenting signs and symptoms of AOM with those of other upper respiratory illnesses, and over recent decades there has been considerable variability in diagnostic criteria published for AOM. As a result, AOM is one of the most frequent diagnoses in infants and children.[9] Age-specific rates of AOM since introduction of the 7-valent pneumococcal conjugate vaccine (PCV7) (Prevnar®), in 2000, are lacking. Although previous studies have noted that as many as 60% of children have an episode before 1 year and 80% by 3 years of age, these rates may no longer be accurate.[14,15] Paradise et al.[16] followed a large cohort of infants from age 2 months until 2 years with frequent expert examinations, using pneumatic otoscopy and tympanometry. Middle ear effusion (MEE) was noted in 48%, 79%, and 91% by 6, 12, and 24 months, respectively. Although the investigators did not use strict criteria for defining AOM, these rates provide an indication of the frequency of MEE in the first 2 years of life.

PATHOGENESIS

The middle ear is a laterally compressed space within the temporal bone, bounded by the tympanic membrane (TM) and the eustachian tube.[17] It is normally aerated and contains the ossicular chain, essential for transmission of sound energy to the inner ear. The eustachian tube is shorter and more horizontally oriented in children, thus allowing easier egress of nasopharyngeal secretions into the middle ear cavity.

The common pathway in AOM pathogenesis is dysfunction or edema of the eustachian tube, for instance from a viral URI or environmental smoke, that in turn results in development of negative middle ear pressure and MEE. The fluid may then become secondarily infected with viruses or bacteria, provoking an inflammatory response and resulting in AOM.[18] Alternatively, the fluid may remain sterile and persist as OME.[5]

The relatively high incidence and spontaneous resolution of OME and AOM indicate these may be natural occurrences as the child's anatomy and immune system develop.[18] However, environmental insults such as tobacco smoke lead to episodes that would otherwise not occur. Prevention of much of the disease burden of AOM in children is possible.

Although viral URIs appear to frequently initiate eustachian tube dysfunction and AOM, they have been reported as primary pathogens in only 0–13% of cases.[19,20] At a minimum, viral–bacterial interaction appears to occur frequently in the cascade of events leading to AOM.[20] Viral–bacterial coinfection of the middle ear is common, occurring in up to 30–60% of cases.[19,20] The most frequently isolated viral agents are rhinoviruses; respiratory syncytial virus (RSV); influenza A and B; parainfluenza types 1,2, and 3; and adenovirus.[19] Studies utilizing culture and antigen detection have noted RSV (41%) as the most common

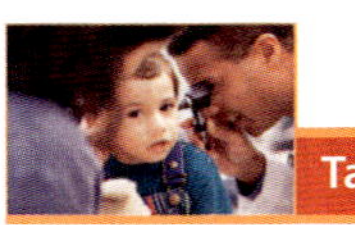

Table 28–2.

Bacterial Pathogens From Middle Ear Fluid Pre- and Post-PCV7 Vaccine

Organism	Pre-PCV7[20] (%)	Post-PCV7[25] (%)	β-Lactamase Producing[26] (%)
S. pneumoniae	20–40	31	—
H. influenzae	10–30	56	64
M. catarrhalis	5–15	11	100

PCV7, 7-valent pneumococcal conjugate vaccine.

virus isolated from middle ear fluid, whereas those utilizing polymerase chain reaction have noted human rhinovirus (24%) as most prevalent with RSV (18%) less frequently isolated.[21,22]

When meticulous isolation technique (tympanocentesis) and bacteriologic isolation methods have been employed, bacteria were isolated from the middle ear in up to 95% of cases of AOM in the pre-PCV7 era.[23,24] The major bacterial pathogens have been constant over time, and include *Streptococcus pneumoniae*, nontypable *Haemophilus influenzae*, and *Moraxella catarrhalis*. However, the relative frequencies of these pathogens subsequent to introduction of PCV7 appear to be changing (Table 28–2).

In a prospective cohort of children 7–24 months of age with severe or refractory AOM, Block et al.[25] compared isolates from the pre-PCV7 era with those of vaccinated children in the post-PCV7 era in a rural setting. Statistically significant decreases in *S. pneumoniae* (48–31%) and increases in nontypable *H. influenzae* (41–56%) were noted, such that nontypable *H. influenza* had supplanted *S. pneumoniae* as the predominant bacterial pathogen. Casey and Pichichero[26] conducted a prospective study of infants and children with persistent or treatment-failure AOM in a suburban practice. Similar post-PCV7 era decreases occurred in *S. pneumoniae* (44–31%) and increases in nontypable *H. influenzae* (43–57%) isolates.

The relative frequencies of major bacterial pathogens may change yet again as the prevalence of non-vaccine serotypes causing AOM increase.[27] Of particular relevance in considering antibiotic treatment, a statistically significant increase of β-lactamase producing organisms (32–47%) occurred, and both investigations noted nonsignificant trends toward penicillin-susceptible *S. pneumoniae* in the post-PCV7 era.

The natural history of AOM has been intensely scrutinized in prospective studies and as part of randomized trials of antibiotic treatment.[28] MEE is a natural consequence of AOM, and resolves in approximately two-thirds of children within 1 month and in 90% within 3 months. In the pre-PCV7 era, the mean cumulative proportion of days with MEE was 20% and 17% in the first and second years of life, respectively.[16]

RISK FACTORS

Hereditary and Demographic Risk Factors

Genetic predisposition and premature birth are variables that contribute to anatomic and immunologic aspects of risk for AOM. The unique and developing anatomy of the middle ear system, as well as immunologic immaturity in infants and young children, are primary determinants of young age as a risk factor. Children of age 7–36 months are at greatest risk.[14] Male gender appears to confer additional risk of AOM, although studies have not consistently demonstrated this risk.[7,16]

Although these associations are biologically plausible, investigations of race and ethnicity have inconsistently controlled for other statistically significant variables, including socioeconomic status, environmental tobacco smoke (ETS), and numbers of exposures to siblings and other infants and young children.[16] There has also been variable diligence in observation for and diagnostic accuracy of middle ear disease in studies examining these variables.[28] Native American, Inuit, and Native Alaskan children appear to have higher rates of middle ear disease than Caucasian children.[7]

Environmental Risk Factors

Exposure to older siblings or attendance at day care increases exposure to upper respiratory viruses, thereby influencing risk in infants and young children. Risk conferred by some exposures, in particular tobacco smoke, have been more difficult to assess because some studies have not controlled for other statistically significant variables, most importantly socioeconomic status. Importantly, the influence of certain of these risk factors may be changed through primary prevention.[29]

Aspects of breast feeding suggest that it might be protective against AOM. These include the upright positioning during feeding, resulting in less reflux of milk through the eustachian tube, and possible immune modulating and antimicrobial constituents of breast milk. This appears to be the case for exclusive breast feeding during the first 3–6 months. This protection continues until 1 year of age when the effect of breast feeding was adjusted for other variables.[16]

ETS is both biologically plausible and consistently demonstrated in numerous investigations to be associated with increased risk for both AOM and persistent

MEE.[16,30] Household members may underestimate the amount of ETS or deny smoking. Investigations using cotinine as a biomarker for ETS consistently demonstrate an association between cotinine levels and the risk of middle ear disease.[31–33] Although the effect of ETS is confounded by socioeconomic status, a meta-analysis of prospective cohort studies adjusting for this and other potential confounders found a pooled RR (relative risk) of 1.19 (95% CI, 1.05–1.35, $p < 0.01$) for ETS and middle ear disease, and estimated that 13% of middle ear disease may be accounted for by ETS.[30] Of the modifiable risk factors for AOM, ETS appears to be the most significant, and efforts are warranted to prevent exposure of infants and children to ETS.

Group day care and the number of older siblings both confer risk of AOM, although studies of the association between numbers of older siblings and middle ear disease have not consistently demonstrated such an association. What appears significant is not the location of exposure to other children (and upper respiratory viral illnesses), but rather the number and intensity of exposures.[16]

Immunoprophylaxis with the live trivalent intranasal influenza vaccine may prevent as much as 30% of AOM during the upper respiratory viral season and was 90–97% effective in preventing episodes of AOM associated with influenza.[34,35] However, trivalent killed influenza vaccine did not decrease the incidence of AOM either during influenza season or during the subsequent 1-year period.[36] PCV7 has been demonstrated to reduce the number of episodes of AOM from all causes by 6–8%, those episodes as a result of vaccine serotypes by 51–67%, and placement of tympanostomy tubes by 24%.[37–39] In addition, a large study examining Medicaid and insurance databases found a decrease in AOM rates of 6% in Tennessee and 20% in upstate New York as a result of PCV7 use.[40]

CLINICAL PRESENTATION

Features of the medical history, signs, and symptoms of AOM are familiar to clinicians. Although some of these are relatively specific for middle ear disease (e.g., otalgia), many are nonspecific and are associated with other disease processes. If clinicians are to make an accurate diagnosis of AOM and, in turn, manage AOM and other upper respiratory illnesses appropriately, the various elements of the history and physical examination must be employed correctly. Of importance to clinicians are features of the history and physical examination found to be predictive of AOM using validated criterion measures such as tympanometry.[41]

A necessary first step in establishing the presence of relevant physical findings is a properly conducted otoscopic examination. This includes comfortable immobilization of the patient and the use of an otoscope with a bright light source and properly fitting speculum.[9] An atraumatic examination is helpful because crying or irritation of the external auditory canal will cause redness of the TM.[42]

Cerumen in the external ear canal can be a significant diagnostic barrier for the clinician. Minimal-to-moderate cerumen in the external canal may not prevent the clinician from visualizing part of the TM, but impacted cerumen may need to be removed. Techniques for removal of cerumen include a soft speculum or gentle irrigation of the canal with warm sterile water or saline. Both procedures induce some risk of discomfort, pain, abrasion of the skin of the external canal (which may lead to bleeding) or traumatic perforation of the TM. An additional adjunct is the use of cerumenolytic agents such as docusate (Colace®) or triethanolamine polypeptide. The technique involves instillation of 1 mL of the agent into the ear canal for 15 minutes, followed by irrigation with saline if necessary. Trials of this technique have been of variable quality and have provided inconsistent evidence of efficacy.[43–46] The examiner is more likely to be successful if the child's head is immobile while removing the cerumen. While no technique is always successful or risk free, it is nonetheless imperative that the clinician properly visualize the TM and assess mobility in order to confirm the presence or absence of an effusion in the middle ear space.

In addition to the position of the TM, the examiner should assess color, landmarks and mobility. For the latter, pneumatic otoscopy is invaluable, and may be supplanted with tympanometry or acoustic reflectometry. In this way, the examiner may achieve an examination approaching the validity of the criterion standard, tympanocentesis, although these individual elements of the otoscopic examination do not provide the diagnostic certainty of tympanocentesis and culture of middle ear fluid.

The normal TM has a pearl to pink color. Red coloration alone does not alone indicate inflammation, as crying will result in hyperemia with red coloration.[42] The normal TM is neither retracted nor bulging. The TM is relatively translucent, allowing for visualization of some middle ear structures, including the handle and lateral process of the malleus, umbo, pars flaccida, long limb of the incus, chorda tympani nerve, as well as the light reflex (Figure 28–1). AOM is indicated by a red, bulging (with exudate), and immobile TM (Figure 28–2). A bluish or yellow coloration may indicate MEE, a finding supported by a TM that is bulging, retracted, or that has decreased mobility on pneumatic otoscopy (Figures 28–3 and 28–4). The TM may become perforated as a result of AOM, trauma, or prior PET insertion, and such perforations allow an avenue of egress for middle ear fluid (Figures 28–5 and 28–6).

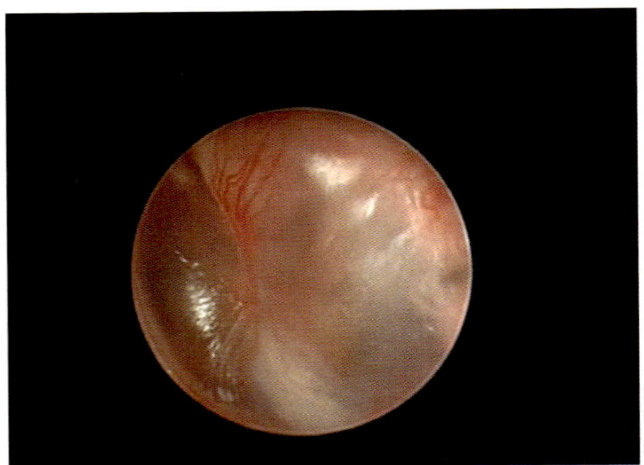

FIGURE 28–1 ■ Normal right TM in 6-year-old child (*All TM images courtesy of Dr. Shelagh Cofer, Department of Otolaryngology, Vanderbilt Children's Hospital.*)

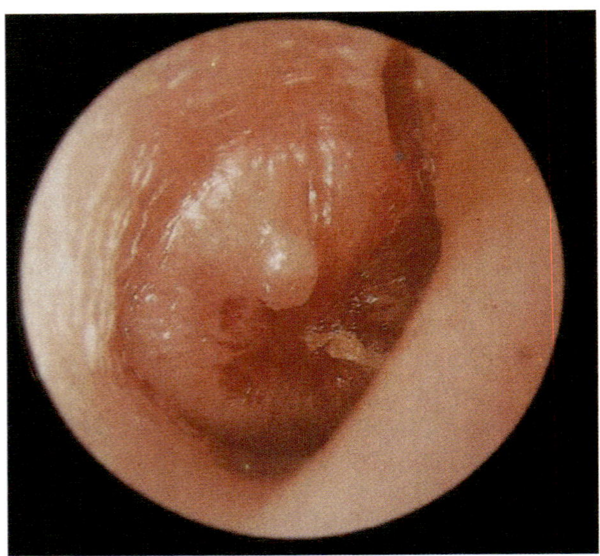

FIGURE 28–2 ■ Acute OM in a 3-year-old child.

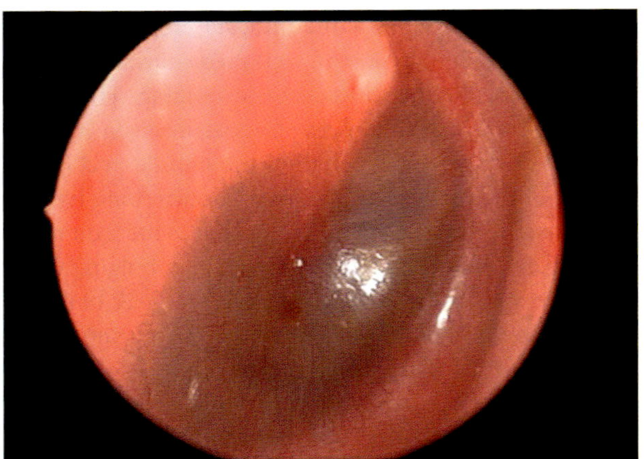

FIGURE 28–3 ■ An 18-month-old toddler with MEE. Note bluish discoloration and slight bulging of TM.

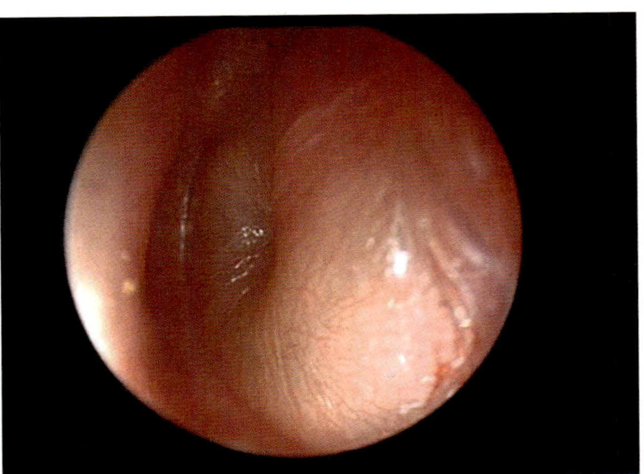

FIGURE 28–4 ■ An 18-month-old toddler with MEE. Note marked bulging of TM and white coloration of effusion. Purulent effusion does not always indicate AOM.

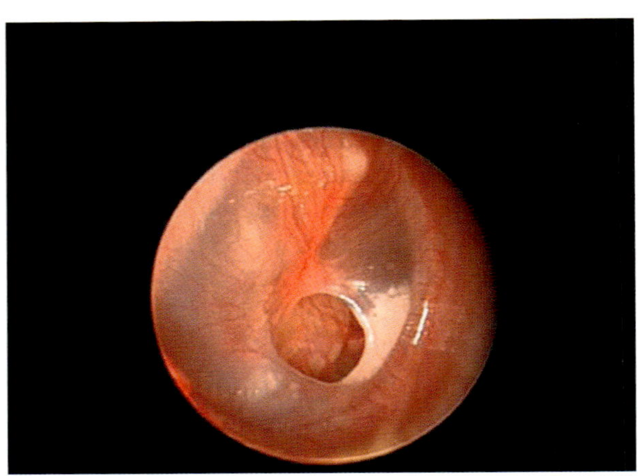

FIGURE 28–5 ■ A 6-year-old with TM perforation. Note tympanosclerosis along anterior border of perforation.

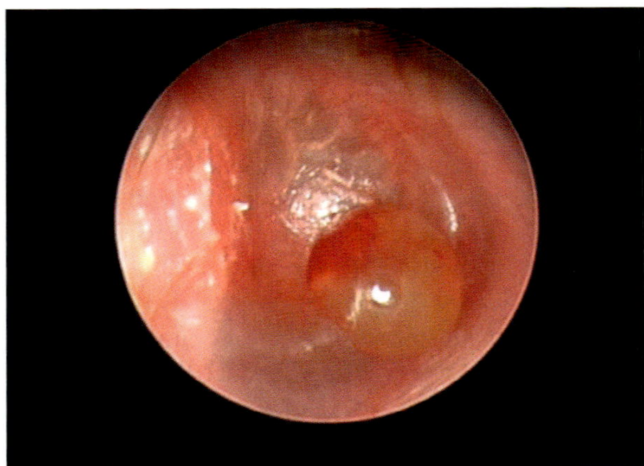

FIGURE 28–6 ■ A 19-month-old toddler with serous discharge through TM perforation.

Rothman et al.[9] have performed a systematic review of the literature pertaining to the precision and accuracy of the history and physical examination for diagnosis of AOM. Of 17 studies that specifically investigated signs and symptoms in the diagnosis of AOM, 5 met inclusion criteria. The presence of URI symptoms was sensitive (96%) for AOM but had low specificity (8–43%), and other signs and symptoms, including fever, cough, and excess crying had poor sensitivity and specificity.[9] The presence of otalgia was 54–100% sensitive and 82–92% specific for AOM. However, although otalgia appeared to be the only symptom useful in establishing the diagnosis of AOM, 15% of children with otalgia did not have AOM in a well-performed prospective study.[41] In addition, although it may appear that parental suspicion is highly predictive of the presence of AOM, 20% of parents suspected AOM in the presence of URI alone.[41] The findings of this systematic review emphasize the need to fulfill all three diagnostic criteria in making a diagnosis of AOM (see section on "Definitions").

DIFFERENTIAL DIAGNOSIS FOR AOM

The differential diagnosis for AOM is large and includes both common and uncommon entities encountered by the clinician (Table 28–3). Common diagnoses include foreign body in the external ear canal and otitis externa. Foreign body in the external ear canal may present with otalgia in the preverbal or developmentally delayed child. This diagnosis is usually confirmed with otoscopy. However, blood in the ear canal can obscure a foreign body. Otitis externa is more likely with a history of aural exposure to water. In this case, pain is usually produced with gentle movement of the pinna or with pressure on the tragus. An edematous external canal or a foul smelling exudate found within the canal seen via otoscopy helps confirm the diagnosis. Uncommon diagnoses include: brain abscess, accidental and nonaccidental trauma including perforation of the TM, Lemiere disease, Herpes zoster oticus (Ramsey Hunt Syndrome), peri-tonsillar abscess, sinusitis, mastoiditis (although usually associated with AOM) Wegener's granulomatosis, referred pain from oral cavity diseases, rhabdomyosarcoma of the ear and temporal bone, and cholesteatoma.

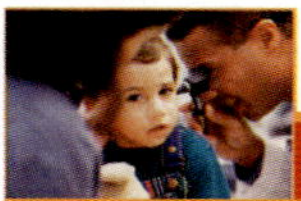

Table 28–3.

Differential Diagnoses of Acute Otalgia

Common

Foreign body in the external ear canal
Otitis externa

Less Common

Accidental trauma (e.g., perforation of TM)
Nonaccidental trauma
Oral cavity diseases (referred pain)
Cholesteatoma
Peri-tonsillar abscess
Sinusitis

Rare

Mastoiditis*
Brain abscess
Lemiere disease
Herpes zoster oticus (Ramsey Hunt syndrome)
Wegener's granulomatosis
Rhabdomyosarcoma of the ear or temporal bone

**Although rare, the most common suppurative complication of AOM.*

MANAGEMENT

Otalgia is present in the majority of children that present with AOM, yet clinicians frequently prescribe antibiotics for AOM without addressing the pain often associated with this condition.[47] A recent consensus practice guideline published by the American Academy of Pediatrics strongly recommends the assessment and treatment of otalgia in children diagnosed with AOM.[7] However, there are few controlled studies that specifically evaluate the use of pain modalities for AOM. Table 28–4 describes the various medications used to treat pain associated with AOM.

Various home remedies, such as oils placed into the external canal, have been used for centuries. No controlled studies have demonstrated effectiveness of home remedies compared to placebo. Topical therapy applied directly to the TM using a combination of antipyrene as an analgesic agent and benzocaine as an anesthetic agent (Auralgan®) has been demonstrated in a small, randomized controlled trial to provide short-term relief of pain compared to the placebo olive oil.[48] Auralgan® also contains glycerin, which may reduce middle ear pressure via fluid osmosis through the TM. This medication does not discolor the TM and will not alter otoscopic landmarks after application. Auralgan® may also facilitate the removal of cerumen but is contraindicated in children who have perforation of the TM.

Systemic medications such as acetaminophen and ibuprofen are the primary medications used to treat otalgia and also offer antipyretic relief, which is usually associated with AOM. Only ibuprofen has been shown to be superior to placebo in one randomized study.[49] Combining ibuprofen and Auralgan® drops may be a beneficial combination to address otalgia in the outpatient setting.[50] The effects of topical therapy are likely to be immediate whereas systemic therapy may take 30–60 minutes to

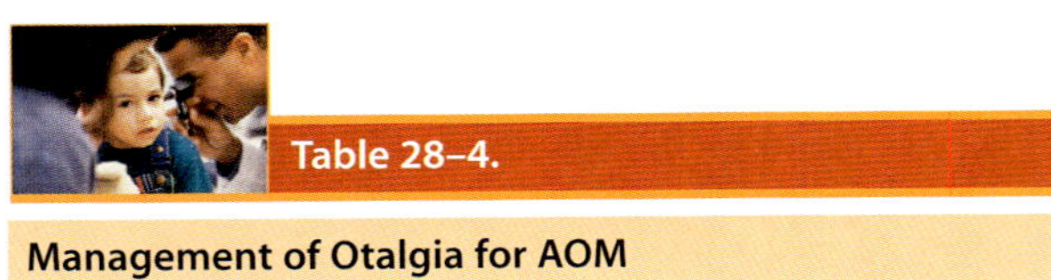

Table 28–4.

Management of Otalgia for AOM

Medication	Dose	Comments
Systemic		
Acetaminophen	15 mg/kg/ dose po/pr q4h prn	May reduce fever, generally well tolerated
Ibuprofen	10 mg/kg/ dose po q6h prn	May reduce fever, may cause GI upset, take with food
Codeine	1.0 mg/kg/ dose po/sq/im q6h prn	Indicated for moderate-severe otalgia
Hydrocodone	0.2 mg/kg/ dose po q8h	Lortab® contains acetominophen
Topical		
Antipyrene/ Benzocaine	2–4 gtts q2h prn pain	Moisten cotton pledget with solution and insert into external canal after drops applied

relieve pain. Codeine and its analogs may be used for moderate-to-severe otalgia especially at night to help reduce pain when sleeping, although side effects of this pharmacologic class may limit its usefulness as a scheduled medication. Both ibuprofen and codeine may have adverse effects on the gastrointestinal system including nausea and emesis. Taking these medications with food may reduce these adverse effects.

TREATMENT

AOM is the most common condition for which antimicrobials are prescribed for children. Clinicians write an estimated 15 million antibiotic prescriptions annually in the United States for AOM alone.[51] Most cases of AOM will resolve spontaneously. Therefore, the benefit of antimicrobials must be weighed against adverse reactions.[52] Approximately 15 children need to be treated with antibiotics to reduce or eliminate otalgia in one child within a week of treatment. This statistic should temper enthusiasm for immediate treatment with antibiotics. Antimicrobial resistance is a major public health concern, which is strongly associated with the use of antibiotics.[53]

The clinician may choose to give a wait-and-see prescription (WASP) for the antimicrobial treatment of AOM. This alternative form of therapy empowers the parent to make a decision about filling or not filling the prescription based on whether the child has worsened or not improved 48 hours after the initial visit. This model has been evaluated both in the outpatient clinic and emergency department settings.[50,54,55] Children older than 6 months who are well appearing, do not have another suspected bacterial illness, are nonimmunocompromised, have access to medical care and no recent treatment with antibiotics may be suitable for a WASP (see Figure 28–7). Approximately two-thirds of children given a WASP will not fill their antibiotic prescriptions. Outcomes are similar compared to immediate treatment with antibiotics.[50] Widespread use of an optional prescription for antibiotics in the United States may lead to a reduction in antimicrobial resistance.

When the child is younger than 6 months, or optional therapy is not warranted, immediate treatment of AOM with an antibacterial agent may be prescribed (see Table 28–5). High dose amoxicillin (80–90 mg/kg/day) is recommended as the initial antibacterial medication for uncomplicated AOM.[7] This recommendation is based on middle ear concentrations of high dose amoxicillin that exceed the minimum inhibitory concentration for most resistant forms of *S. pneumoniae*.[56] Children who have completed a recent course of antibiotics are at a higher risk of resistance to amoxicillin.[57] High-dose amoxicillin-clavulanate may be considered for children with high fever or as a second tier medication if high-dose amoxicillin fails, a reasonable option given the relatively high prevalence of β-lactamase producing organisms discussed in the "Pathogenesis" section.[7] However, the addition of clavulanic acid to amoxicillin increases the likelihood of gastrointestinal side effects including diarrhea, and these adverse effects should be explained to the family prior to prescribing this medication. For patients unable to tolerate oral medications, ceftriaxone (50 mg/kg/ day) intramuscularly or intravenously for 3 days may be considered.[58] In patients with a history of type 1 allergy to penicillin, azithromycin, or erythromycin-sulfasoxizole should be considered; it should be noted that both medications have a high incidence of nausea and vomiting. The latter medication has a high incidence of drug eruptions associated with its use. In patients who fail both oral and intramuscular medications, either clindamycin or tympanocentesis (with culture) should be considered.

The clinician may consider various options for duration of antimicrobial therapy for AOM. A shortened course of antibiotics (5–7 days) compared to a standard course (10 days) may reduce the likelihood of resistance

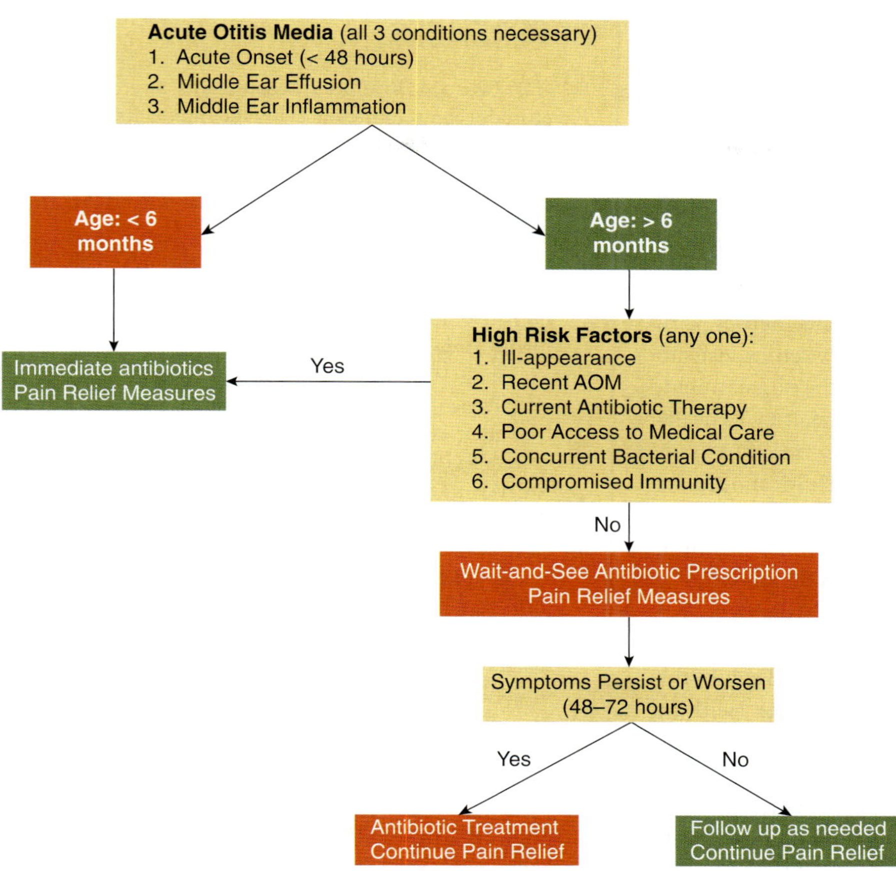

FIGURE 28–7 ■ Initial treatment algorithm for AOM.[7,50]

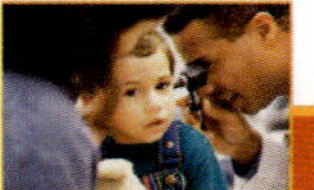

Table 28–5.

Frequent Antimicrobials Used for AOM

Medication	Dose	Comments
Amoxicillin (high dose)	80–90 mg/kg po per d	First-line agent; well tolerated, narrow spectrum, inexpensive
Amoxicillin-clavulanate	80–90 mg/kg po per d amoxicillin component ÷ q12h	High rates of diarrhea, first-line agent with ill appearing child or amoxicillin failure
Azithromycin	10 mg/kg po d 1 then 5 mg/kg po d 2–5	Can be used for type I allergy to penicillin, nausea, and diarrhea are common side effects
Cefdinir	14 mg/kg po daily for 5 d	Second-or third-line agent; expensive
Ceftriaxone	50 mg/kg IM/IV/ d	3 Daily doses; option if unable to tolerate po medication; expensive
Cefuroxime	30 mg/kg po per d ÷ q12h	Second-or third-line agent; expensive
Clarithromycin	15 mg/kg po per d ÷ q12h	Can be used for type I allergy to penicillin; nausea and diarrhea are common side effects
Clindamycin	10–30 mg/kg/d ÷ q8h	Third-line agent; diarrhea a common side effect

to antibiotics by reducing the total dose exposure. This may also reduce unwarranted side effects that are known to be associated with their use. Approximately 44 children would need to be treated with a long course of antibiotics to avoid one short-course treatment failure for uncomplicated AOM.[59] Standard course antimicrobial therapy should be prescribed in children younger than the age of 2 years or those who present with severe AOM. Discharge instructions to the family should describe the expected clinical response to therapy with antibiotics in order to avoid unnecessary return visits to the office. During the first 24–48 hours of treatment, fever and or otalgia may persist or worsen. If by 72 hours the child's condition does not improve, treatment failure should be considered and the child should be promptly re-evaluated in the office.

Effusions of the middle ear are part of the natural resolution of AOM and are visualized in the majority of children, weeks after AOM is diagnosed (Figures 28–3 and 28–4).[60] There is no need for a scheduled follow up examination if symptoms of AOM have resolved. In the children diagnosed with uncomplicated OME (with or without a recent diagnosis of AOM), there are no indications for the use of antibiotics.[61] If OME is present for greater than 3 months referral for placement of tympanostomy tubes may be warranted, although recent evidence suggests that this practice may not alter long-term developmental outcomes.[62]

COMPLICATIONS

Mastoiditis is the most frequent suppurative complication of AOM with an estimated frequency in the United States of approxiamately 1–2 cases per 100,000 person-years.[63] Rates of mastoiditis are similar in countries whose physicians regularly prescribe antibiotics for AOM, such as the United States, compared to countries where physicians do not routinely prescribe antibiotics immediately for AOM, such as the Netherlands.[63] Clinical signs include erythema, warmth and edema over the mastoid space with protrusion of the auricle. Less common findings include cranial nerve palsies (VI and VII) with extension of the infection into the intracranial space. The bacterial pathogens isolated in children with acute mastoiditis include those commonly found in AOM. Other common bacterial organisms isolated with mastoiditis include *Pseudomonas aeruginosa* and *Streptococcus pyogenes*.[64] The treatment of mastoiditis includes antimicrobial therapy directed against the most common bacterial pathogens and may also include myringotomy. Mastoidectomy is recommended with antimicrobial treatment failure, the presence of a cholesteatoma in the middle ear space or with intracranial extension.[65]

REFERENCES

1. Christakis DA, Rivara FP. Pediatricians' awareness of and attitudes about four clinical practice guidelines. *Pediatrics.* 1998;101(5):825-830.
2. Garbutt J, Jeffe DB, Shackelford P. Diagnosis and treatment of acute otitis media: an assessment. *Pediatrics.* 2003;112(1, pt 1):143-149.
3. Spiro DM, King WD, Arnold DH, Johnston C, Baldwin S. A randomized clinical trial to assess the effects of tympanometry on the diagnosis and treatment of acute otitis media. *Pediatrics.* 2004;114(1):177-181.
4. Koskinen H, Rautakorpi UM, Sintonen H, et al. Cost-effectiveness of implementing national guidelines in the treatment of acute otitis media in children. *Int J Technol Assess Health Care.* 2006;22(4):454-459.
5. American Academy of Pediatrics. Otitis media with effusion. *Pediatrics.* 2004;113(5):1412-1429.
6. Get Smart: know When Antibiotics Work. http://www.cdc.gov/drugresistance/community/files/ads/otitis_media.htm. Accessed January 6, 2007.
7. Subcommittee on Management of Acute Otitis Media. Diagnosis and management of acute otitis media. *Pediatrics.* 2004;113(5):1451-1465.
8. Marcy M, Takata G, Chan LS, et al. Management of acute otitis media. *Evid Rep Technol Assess (Summ).* 2000;15:1-4.
9. Rothman R, Owens T, Simel DL. Does this child have acute otitis media? *JAMA.* 2003;290(12):1633-1640.
10. Shekelle P, Takata G, Chan LS, et al. Diagnosis, natural history, and late effects of otitis media with effusion. *Evid Rep Technol Assess (Summ).* 2002;2(55):1-5.
11. Schappert SM, Burt CW. Ambulatory care visits to physician offices, hospital outpatient departments, and emergency departments: United States, 2001-2002. *Vital Health Stat 13.* 2006(159):1-66.
12. Freid VM, Makuc DM, Rooks RN. Ambulatory health care visits by children: principal diagnosis and place of visit. *Vital Health Stat13.* 1998(137):1-23.
13. Finkelstein JA, Stille C, Nordin J, et al. Reduction in antibiotic use among US children, 1996–2000. *Pediatrics.* 2003;112(3, pt 1):620-627.
14. Bondy J, Berman S, Glazner J, Lezotte D. Direct expenditures related to otitis media diagnoses: extrapolations from a pediatric medicaid cohort. *Pediatrics.* 2000;105(6):e72.
15. Teele DW, Klein JO, Rosner B. Epidemiology of otitis media during the first seven years of life in children in greater Boston: a prospective, cohort study. Comment. *J Infect Dis.* 1989;160(1):83-94.
16. Paradise JL, Rockette HE, Colborn DK, et al. Otitis media in 2253 Pittsburgh-area infants: Prevalence and risk factors during the first two years of life. *Pediatrics.* 1997;99(3):318-333.
17. *Anatomy of the Human Body.* Philadelphia, PA: Lea & Febiger; 2000. Also available at www.bartleby. com/107/. Accessed January 7, 2007.
18. Rovers MM, Schilder AG, Zielhuis GA, Rosenfeld RM. Otitis media. *Lancet.* 2004;363(9407):465-473.
19. Heikkinen T, Chonmaitree T. Importance of respiratory viruses in acute otitis media. *Clin Microbiol Rev.* 2003;16(2):230-241.

20. Ruuskanen O, Heikkinen T. Otitis media: etiology and diagnosis. *Pediatr Infect Dis J.* 1994;13(1 Suppl 1):S23-S26; discussion S50-S54.
21. Heikkinen T, Thint M, Chonmaitree T. Prevalence of various respiratory viruses in the middle ear during acute otitis media. *N Engl J Med.* 1999;340(4):260-264.
22. Pitkaranta A, Virolainen A, Jero J, Arruda E, Hayden FG. Detection of rhinovirus, respiratory syncytial virus, and coronavirus infections in acute otitis media by reverse transcriptase polymerase chain reaction. *Pediatrics.* 1998;102(2, pt 1):291-295.
23. Rodriguez WJ, Schwartz RH, Thorne MM. Increasing incidence of penicillin- and ampicillin-resistant middle ear pathogens. *Pediatr Infect Dis J.* 1995;14(12):1075-1078.
24. Del Beccaro MA, Mendelman PM, Inglis AF, et al. Bacteriology of acute otitis media: a new perspective. *J Pediatr.* 1992;120(1):81-84.
25. Block SL, Hedrick J, Harrison CJ, et al. Community-wide vaccination with the heptavalent pneumococcal conjugate significantly alters the microbiology of acute otitis media. *Pediatr Infect Dis J.* 2004;23(9):829-833.
26. Casey JR, Pichichero ME. Changes in frequency and pathogens causing acute otitis media in 1995-2003. *Pediatr Infect Dis J.* 2004;23(9):824-828.
27. Jenson HB, Baltimore RS. Impact of pneumococcal and influenza vaccines on otitis media. *Curr Opin Pediatr.* 2004;16(1):58-60.
28. Daly KA, Giebink GS. Clinical epidemiology of otitis media. *Pediatr Infect Dis J.* 2000;19(suppl 5):S31-S36.
29. Gordis L. Epidemiology. Philadelphia, PA: WB Saunders; 2000.
30. DiFranza JR, Lew RA. Morbidity and mortality in children associated with the use of tobacco products by other people. *Pediatrics.* 1996;97(4):560-568.
31. Etzel RA, Pattishall EN, Haley NJ, Fletcher RH, Henderson FW. Passive smoking and middle ear effusion among children in day care. *Pediatrics.* 1992;90(2, pt 1):228-232.
32. Strachan DP, Jarvis MJ, Feyerabend C. Passive smoking, salivary cotinine concentrations, and middle ear effusion in 7 year old children. *BMJ.* 1989;298(6687): 1549-1552.
33. Ilicali OC, Keles N, De er K, Sa un OF, Guldiken Y. Evaluation of the effect of passive smoking on otitis media in children by an objective method: urinary cotinine analysis. *Laryngoscope.* 2001;111(1):163-167.
34. Belshe RB, Mendelman PM, Treanor J, et al. The efficacy of live attenuated, cold-adapted, trivalent, intranasal influenzavirus vaccine in children. *N Engl J Med.* 1998;338(20):1405-1412.
35. Vesikari T, Fleming DM, Aristegui JF, et al. Safety, efficacy, and effectiveness of cold-adapted influenza vaccine-trivalent against community-acquired, culture-confirmed influenza in young children attending day care. *Pediatrics.* 2006;118(6):2298-2312.
36. Hoberman A, Greenberg DP, Paradise JL, et al. Effectiveness of inactivated influenza vaccine in preventing acute otitis media in young children: a randomized controlled trial. *JAMA.* 2003;290(12):1608-1616.
37. Eskola J, Kilpi T, Palmu A, et al. Efficacy of a pneumococcal conjugate vaccine against acute otitis media. *N Engl J Med.* 2001;344(6):403-409.
38. Black S, Shinefield H, Fireman B, et al. Efficacy, safety and immunogenicity of heptavalent pneumococcal conjugate vaccine in children. Northern California Kaiser Permanente Vaccine Study Center Group. *Pediatr Infect Dis J.* 2000;19(3):187-195.
39. Fireman B, Black SB, Shinefield HR, Lee J, Lewis E, Ray P. Impact of the pneumococcal conjugate vaccine on otitis media. *Pediatr Infect Dis J.* 2003;22(1):10-16.
40. Poehling KA, Lafleur BJ, Szilagyi PG, et al. Population-based impact of pneumococcal conjugate vaccine in young children. *Pediatrics.* 2004;114(3):755-761.
41. Kontiokari T, Koivunen P, Niemela M, Pokka T, Uhari M. Symptoms of acute otitis media. *Pediatr Infect Dis J.* 1998;17(8):676-679.
42. Pichichero ME. Acute otitis media: part I. Improving diagnostic accuracy. *Am Fam Physician.* 2000;61(7):2051-2056.
43. Singer AJ, Sauris E, Viccellio AW. Ceruminolytic effects of docusate sodium: a randomized, controlled trial. *Ann Emerg Med.* 2000;36(3):228-232.
44. Lemon HM, Mazyck-Brown J, Cancellaro TA, Darden PM, Basco WT, Jr. Review of a randomized trial comparing 2 cerumenolytic agents. *Arch Pediatr Adolesc Med.* 2003;157(12):1181-1183.
45. Burton MJ, Doree CJ. Ear drops for the removal of ear wax. *Cochrane Database Syst Rev.* 2003;(3):CD004400.
46. Whatley VN, Dodds CL, Paul RI. Randomized clinical trial of docusate, triethanolamine polypeptide, and irrigation in cerumen removal in children. *Arch Pediatr Adolesc Med.* 2003;157(12):1177-1180.
47. Hayden GF, Schwartz RH. Characteristics of earache among children with acute otitis media. *Am J Dis Child.* 1985;139(7):721-723.
48. Hoberman A, Paradise JL, Reynolds EA, Urkin J. Efficacy of Auralgan for treating ear pain in children with acute otitis media. *Arch Pediatr Adolesc Med.* 1997;151(7):675-678.
49. Bertin L, Pons G, d'Athis P, et al. A randomized, double-blind, multicentre controlled trial of ibuprofen versus acetaminophen and placebo for symptoms of acute otitis media in children. *Fundam Clin Pharmacol.* 1996;10(4):387-392.
50. Spiro DM, Tay K-Y, Arnold DH, Dziura JD, Baker MD, Shapiro ED. Wait-and-see prescription for the treatment of acute otitis media: a randomized controlled trial. Comment. *JAMA.* 2006;296(10):1235-1241.
51. McCaig LF, Besser RE, Hughes JM. Trends in antimicrobial prescribing rates for children and adolescents. *JAMA.* 2002;287(23):3096-3102.
52. Glasziou PP, Del Mar CB, Hayem M, Sanders SL. Antibiotics for acute otitis media in children. *Cochrane Database Syst Rev.* 2004;(1):CD000219.
53. Whitney CG, Farley MM, Hadler J, et al. Increasing prevalence of multidrug-resistant *Streptococcus pneumoniae* in the United States. Comment. *N Engl J Med.* 2000;343(26): 1917-1924.
54. Little P, Gould C, Williamson I, Moore M, Warner G, Dunleavey J. Pragmatic randomised controlled trial of two prescribing strategies for childhood acute otitis media. *BMJ.* 2001;322(7282):336-342.
55. McCormick DP, Chonmaitree T, Pittman C, et al. Nonsevere acute otitis media: a clinical trial comparing outcomes of watchful waiting versus immediate antibiotic treatment. *Pediatrics.* 2005;115(6):1455-1465.

56. Dagan R, Hoberman A, Johnson C, et al. Bacteriologic and clinical efficacy of high dose amoxicillin/clavulanate in children with acute otitis media. *Pediatr Infect Dis J.* 2001;20(9):829-837.
57. Wald ER, Mason EO, Jr., Bradley JS, Barson WJ, Kaplan SL, Group USPMPS. Acute otitis media caused by *Streptococcus pneumoniae* in children's hospitals between 1994 and 1997. *Pediatr Infect Dis J.* 2001;20(1):34-39.
58. Leibovitz E, Piglansky L, Raiz S, Press J, Leiberman A, Dagan R. Bacteriologic and clinical efficacy of one day vs. three day intramuscular ceftriaxone for treatment of nonresponsive acute otitis media in children. *Pediatr Infect Dis J.* 2000;19(11):1040-1045.
59. Kozyrskyj AL, Hildes-Ripstein GE, Longstaffe SEA, et al. Treatment of acute otitis media with a shortened course of antibiotics: a meta-analysis. *JAMA.* 1998;279(21):1736-1742.
60. Rosenfeld RM. Natural history of untreated otitis media. *Laryngoscope.* 2003;113(10):1645-1657.
61. Dowell SF, Marcy SM, Phillips WR, Gerber MA, Schwartz B. Otitis media—principles of judicious use of antimicrobial agents. *Pediatrics.* 1998;101(1):165-171.
62. Paradise JL, Feldman HM, Campbell TF, et al. Tympanostomy tubes and developmental outcomes at 9–11 years of age. Comment. *N Engl J Med.* 2007;356(3):248-261.
63. Van Zuijlen DA, Schilder AG, Van Balen FA, Hoes AW. National differences in incidence of acute mastoiditis: relationship to prescribing patterns of antibiotics for acute otitis media? Comment. *Pediatr Infect Dis J.* 2001;20(2):140-144.
64. Butbul-Aviel Y, Miron D, Halevy R, Koren A, Sakran W. Acute mastoiditis in children: *Pseudomonas aeruginosa* as a leading pathogen. *Int J Pediatr Otorhinolaryngol.* 2003;67(3):277-281.
65. Taylor MF, Berkowitz RG. Indications for mastoidectomy in acute mastoiditis in children. *Ann Otol Rhinol Laryngol.* 2004;113(1):69-72.

CHAPTER 29

Otitis Externa

Rahul K. Shah and Udayan K. Shah

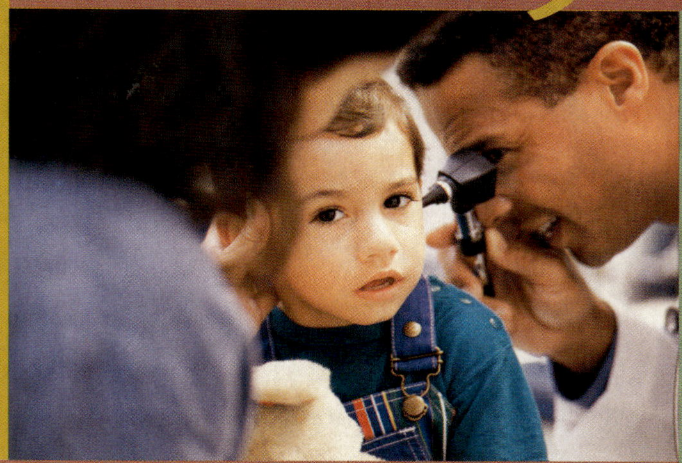

Otitis externa (OE) or "swimmer's ear" is commonly defined as an inflammation of the external auditory canal (EAC).* Up to 10% of all persons may experience an episode of OE during their lifetime.[1,2] OE most often besets children during the summer months, and can be painful and difficult to manage because of the confines of the ear canal. Early diagnosis and a stepwise treatment approach, including debridement and ototopical therapy, and on occasion systemic antimicrobials, are critical to expedient management. This chapter will review the epidemiology, pathogenesis, management, and complications of OE to facilitate an expeditious and cost-effective treatment for this common disease.

PATHOGENESIS

The EAC is comprised of a thin lining of sebum containing epithelium over a bony and cartilaginous canal. This warm dark tunnel is a perfect culture medium for bacterial and fungal growth if the protective acidic cerumen or epithelial barrier is violated by aggressive cleaning, soapy water, skin conditions such as eczema or a heavy bacterial load.[1,3]

Almost all acute otitis externa (AOE) in North America is bacterial (98%). The most common offending organisms in AOE include *Staphylococcus aureus*, *Pseudomonas aeruginosa* and other gram-negative organisms; many infections are polymicrobial organisms.[1,4,5] *Candida* spp. rarely cause primary AOE, however, they are much more prevalent in chronic OE and in partially treated AOE.[1]

CLINICAL PRESENTATION

History

Conditions predisposing to AOE include recent water exposure (e.g., swimming), travel, immunocompromised states (e.g., diabetes mellitus), otologic trauma (from cotton swab use), and dermatologic conditions such as eczema. Affected patients often complain of pain limited to the ear canal which ranges from mild to severe intensity; the pain is exacerbated with auricular traction or tragal pressure. Occasionally, pain occurs with mouth opening because of the motion of the temporomandibular joint, which abuts the anterior EAC. Aural discharge may be present, and may be clear or murky colored, rarely bloody, and can be sweet or foul smelling. Fever is uncommon.

Physical Examination

Because of the exquisite tenderness children may exhibit with OE, physical examination may be best approached initially without instrumenting the ear canal. A magnifying, illuminating loupe or headlight, with the child lying on its contralateral side may allow for external assessment prior to instrumentation of the ear canal. The otologic examination should focus on the external ear for erythema, edema, and tenderness to palpation. Unlike children with mastoiditis in which the pinna may be protruberant, children with OE rarely have a displaced auricle. Skin surrounding the EAC and auricle may reveal cellulitis. The concha may have crusted drainage, which has collected or dried as it drips from the EAC. Many families will not clean this external part

*While strictly speaking the auricle is part of the external ear, infections of this area are less common and are dealt with below.

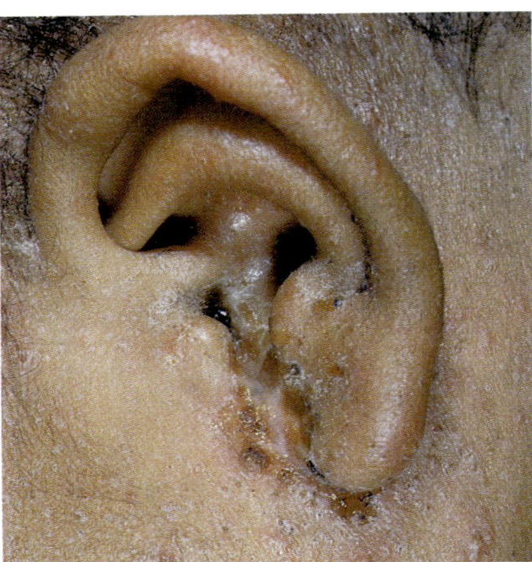

FIGURE 29–1 ■ Yellow–white discharge often seen in EAC in OE.

prior to a visit to a health care provider, as they want the provider to see the quality of discharge.

EAC examination should be performed with a smaller diameter speculum, taking care to avoid contacting the tender skin lining the EAC, and tragal pressure should be avoided. The external ear canal may be occluded, partially or completely, by a pink to red boggy edema of the EAC skin, and usually will exhibit a flaky or cheesy yellow–white exudate which may be cultured (Figure 29–1).[5] EAC edema and tragal pain may limit the view of the tympanic membrane (TM) as well as debridement of the exudate.

If the TM is visible, it may be coated with a thin layer of debris and/or appear thickened. Evaluation for middle ear effusion may therefore be difficult.

Cranial neuropathies should heighten concern for the diagnosis of necrotizing or "malignant" otitis externa (NOE).[6] NOE is characterized by granulation tissue in the EAC. NOE must be differentiated from a tuberculous or neoplastic process, or an inflammatory condition such as Langerhans cell histiocytosis, by biopsy with histopathologic analyis and culture (for bacteria, fungi, and mycobacteria).[6]

LABORATORY EVALUATION

Microscopic evaluation of drainage may reveal the causative organism. Gram staining typically detects both bacteria and yeast. Yeast can also be detected by potassium hydroxide preparation or Gomori methenamine silver staining. Such assessments, along with bacterial and fungal culture, are useful when first- or second-line ototopical therapy and debridement as outlined below have been unsuccessful.

Hearing assessment shows a conductive hearing loss in the affected ear, either by tuning fork testing or by formal audiometry. Audiometric evaluation is not required to establish the diagnosis of OE. Audiologic assessment may be difficult to perform because of the tenderness of the external ear, and may show conductive hearing loss caused by the debris and swelling in the EAC. Testing of the auditory nerve for sensorineural hearing levels (the "bone conduction" hearing test) may be uncomfortable because of the tenderness in this region, but should indicate normal auditory nerve function.

There is not a role for routine imaging by computed tomography (CT) or MRI scan for most cases of OE, unless there is concern for spread beyond the ear canal such as intracranial complications. For NOE, gallium scan for diagnosis and thallium scan to follow the disease course may be considered.[6]

DIFFERENTIAL DIAGNOSIS

Causes of chronic otorrhea are summarized in Table 29–1. The differential diagnosis of an AOE includes a localized skin infection of the hair bearing lateral portion of the EAC, caused by a furuncle or an infected sebaceous cyst. These infections are usually restricted to an area of the EAC rather than involving the entire length of the EAC as in the case of OE, and are usually staphylococcal rather than *pseudomonal* in origin.

More extensive infections of the external ear may involve the pinna or auricle. These infections are usually caused by posttraumatic subperichondrial collections of

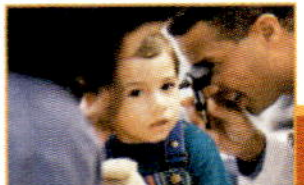

Table 29–1.

Differential Diagnosis for Chronic or Recurrent Otorrhea

Infection
- Bacterial*
- Fungal
- Mycobacterial (especially Mycobacterium tuberculosis)
- Viral†

Cerebrospinal fluid leak

Foreign body

Tumor
- Benign neoplasm (e.g., cholesteatoma)
- Malignant neoplasm

Other causes
- Infected branchial remnant
- Langerhan's cell histiocytosis
- Sebaceous cyst (usually infected)‡
- Seborrheic dermatitis
- Wegener's granulomatosis

**Especially S. aureus or P. aeruginosa.*

†Especially herpes simplex virus or herpes zoster (caused by varicella).

‡Characteristically restricted to one segment of the EAC rather than involving the entire length.

blood which become infected. Infected collections around the cartilage of the auricle may result, if untreated, in the deformity termed "wrestler's" or "cauliflower" ear. Management involves prompt and aggressive incision and drainage, with placement of bolsters to reappose the skin and cartilage, and an anti-pseudomonal antibiotic.

Embryologic persistence of the first or second branchial arch may result in preauricular cyst or fistulas. An infected branchial remnant would require antibiotic therapy followed by incision and drainage, and/or eventual complete surgical removal of the lesion to prevent recurrence. A pit or fistula in the region of the EAC, or a preauricular cyst, would indicate the possibility of an infected branchial remnant. Imaging with an MRI or CT scan may be required in such cases for diagnosis when infections are not responsive to culture-directed therapy and aural debridment, to assess for the extent and depth of a tract or canal duplication.

Infection from trauma may occur from violation of the dermal barrier by cotton swabs or other paraphernalia, such as "wax spoons" which may be used to instrument the ear. In addition, EAC skin can become inflamed or irritated from iatrogenic causes, such as ototopical solutions which alter the pH and commensal organisms of the EAC. Sensitivity to metals in ear piercings (most commonly nickel) can have a similar effect on the skin. In cases of suspected atopic dermatitis, removal of the offending allergen and topical antibiotic and steroid therapy may be considered.

Chronic myringitis presents with TM granulation (Figure 29–2) and aural discharge. Treatment is difficult and includes ototopical medications and debridement of the granulation tissue.[7] Biopsy for tumor and mycobacterial processes may also be considered particularly for a child with a chronic or recurrent process.

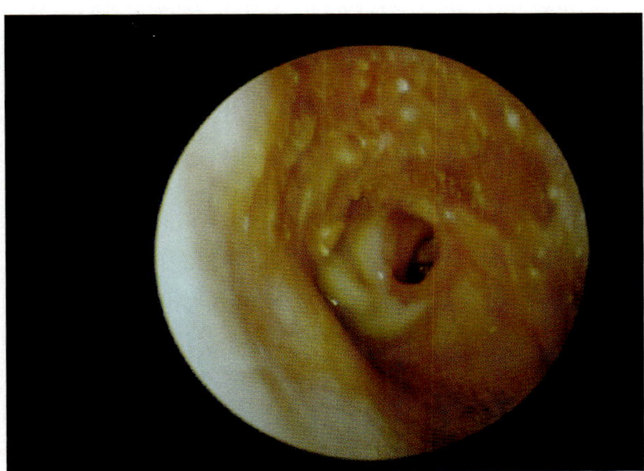

FIGURE 29–2 ■ Granulation against the tympanic membrane.

MANAGEMENT AND TREATMENT

Effective initial management of OE involves the "four *D*'s": Prompt *D*iagnosis, *D*ebridement, *D*irected drop and drug therapy, and promoting a *D*ry environment (water precautions and drying agents) (Table 29–2 and Figure 29–3).

Debridement

Aural debridement is accomplished by curette or suction in the ambulatory setting. Treatment may require several weeks to a month's time. Cleaning may be accomplished through the otoscope, using the illuminated magnifying loupes, or a microscope. Hospitalization may be necessary for disease refractory to outpatient care, for complications, or when pain cannot be managed by oral medications. Pain can be severe, requiring narcotics, particularly in adolescent patients.

Directed Drop and Antimicrobial Therapy

Topical otic drops are useful to change the pH of the EAC and as antimicrobials. Initial cure may begin using dilute white vinegar (3 parts of vinegar to 1 part water) or a 1:1 mixture of vinegar and rubbing alcohol, particularly if a family is not able to readily fill a prescription because of distance (e.g., while on vacation and a "telephone diagnosis" is made). This "camper's cure" is available as a prescription form (Vosol), which permits acidification of the EAC with topical solution of 2% acetic acid. In addition to acetic acid, other ototopicals for which there has been demonstrated clinical efficacy include boric acid, aluminum acetate, silver nitrate, topical steroids without antimicrobials, anitfungals, and *N*-cholortaurine.[1]

Antimicrobial therapy focuses on targeting the most common offending organism—*P. aeruginosa.* This is usually achieved by using topical ofloxacin as a first line, or less commonly by initial use of ciprofloxacin drops.[8] Oral ciprofloxacin is indicated for auricular chondritis or cellultitis complicating OE.

Oral antibiotics are not the first line of therapy for uncompliated AOE. Rather, these may be used for

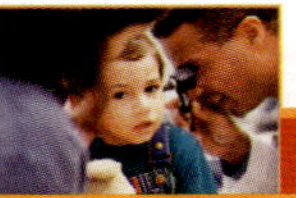

Table 29–2.

The Four D's of OE Management
*D*iagnosis
*D*ebridement
*D*irected therapy with drops and antimicrobials
*D*ryness

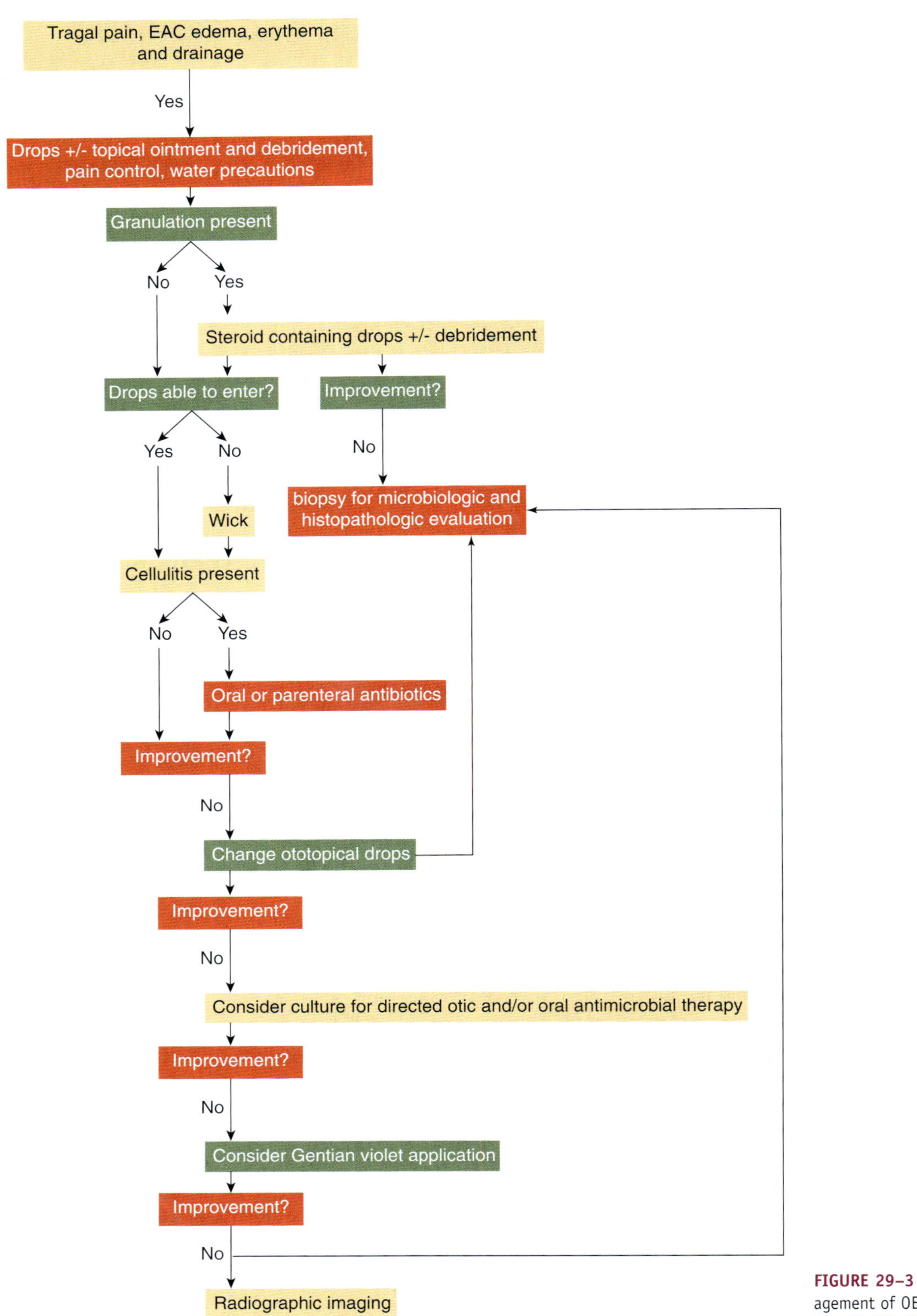

FIGURE 29–3 ■ Algorithm for management of OE.

cellulitis involving the adjacent cutaneous structures of the pinna, erythema extending beyond the confines of the EAC, in an immunocompromised patient or for children with osteitis, abcess formation, middle ear disease, or recurrent infections.[1]

Steroid therapy via topical drops reduces canal edema and is advised for children with bloody otorrhea, canal edema which limits the view of the TM, and for OE in which pain and otorrhea are not diminished by a week of nonsteroid drop therapy. Steroid drops are particularly useful when granulation is present. Management of granulation is best accomplished by initial reduction of the bulk of granular tissue by debridement, or complete removal if possible in the office, followed by topical therapy. Topical steroids may be delivered as part of a combination antibacterial–steroid preparation (such as Ciprodex) or as a separate ototopical (e.g., Dexacidin).[9] Ototopical therapy is considered to achieve clinical resolution in 65% to 90% of patients within 7–10 days.[1]

For OE refractory to debridement and drops after approximately 2 weeks, culture and Gram stain for aerobic and fungal organisms may be considered. Fungal OE is strongly suspected when black spores are seen, or when a white fuzzy layer coats the EAC. Suspicion of fungal OE may be aroused as well by the familiar sweet "athlete's foot" odor of fungal dermatitis. Fungal OE is usually managed effectively by debridement and by topical antifungal drops (e.g., Lotrimin), or by a combination antifungal/steroid-containing cream (e.g., Mycolog cream, containing Nystatin and triamcinolone), which may be applied by a small cotton applicator (fashioned in the office or commercially available).

Bacterial and fungal OE that are not responding promptly to debridement and culture-directed drop therapy, may be treated by painting the EAC with a cotton applicator, dipped in Gentian violet. This purple stain is effective against a wide variety of microorganisms. Caution is advised regarding the relative permanence of this stain on office furniture and clothing.

This stepwise approach to treating OE with a logical progression of ototopical agents is advised to limit antimicrobial resistance. Furthermore, topical antimicrobial therapy for OE is less likely than oral treatment to contribute to the emergence of resistant organisms colonizing at distant sites caused by limited systemic absorption of ototopical antimicrobial agents.[1]

Frequency of drop therapy depends upon tolerance to therapy, and the severity of the OE, and may vary from five drops, twice a day to four times daily. Effective therapy is achieved—regardless of the actual "drop count"—by seeing the drops welling up in the EAC, and by compressing the tragus to medialize the drops. Analgesic premedication is advised because of the extreme tenderness which can characterize OE.

Caution should be exercised in ototopical selection in cases where there is a concern that the TM is not intact (e.g., in a child with a history consistent with a preceding rupture of the TM from AOM caused by fever, and pain relief upon discharge evidencing ruptured TM, or in a child with a recently seen patent tympanostomy tube). Specific agents to avoid in such cases include those preparations which contain alcohol or which are acidifying.

Edema of the EAC may limit examination, cleaning, and entry of ear drops. Occlusive EAC edema may require placement of a wick so that drops can reach the medial EAC. The wick may be composed of tightly rolled cotton or a commercially available cellulose wick (Pope Merocel Wick, Medtronic, Jacksonville, FL, USA). In general, the commercially available wick is easier to place and less likely to shred than cotton upon removal, which may leave a nidus for infection. Merocel Wick placement may be accomplished simply by pushing a dry 1.5 cm length of wick medially using one's thumb. The Wick does not need to contact the TM, in fact, such medial positioning of the wick may be both painful and harmful to the TM.

Drops may be applied after wick placement. The dry wick will expand from its approximately 2 mm diameter to approximately 4 mm diameter, and remain soft. As the EAC edema regresses, the wick may lateralize and be removed by the child, the family, or a provider, or simply fall out. Replacement is not required so long as drops are felt to be reaching the medial EAC.

Dryness

Dry ear precautions prevent further moisture from exacerbating the maceration of the EAC skin and allow for effective topical drop therapy. Lambswool, or more often a cotton ball impregnated by petrolatum jelly, may be placed against the concha to occlude the meatus of the EAC to limit water exposure during bathing or hair washing. Swimming is generally contraindicated since wax and silicone plugs are painful to place and difficult to retain, even with the use of a retentive headband (such as the Ear Band-It®, Jaco Enterprises, Phoenix, AZ, USA). The vicious cycle of moisture begetting inflammation and exudate must be stressed to children and their parents as OE is most frequently seen during the swim season. An expedient return to swimming will be achieved only by curing the OE; water exposure only prolongs the painful condition and need for continued office visits with potentially uncomfortable debridements. The use of a hair dryer to remove moisture from the external canal after swimming and showering will also help in preventing and managing OE although care must be taken as thermal injuries may occur. Avoiding otologic trauma by limiting Q-tip use, and by avoiding the insertion of a hearing aid, may also help by protecting the epithelium of the EAC and allowing for aeration of the EAC.[3]

Special Consideration: NOE

In diabetic or immunocompromised patients, malignant OE can develop; *P. aeruginosa* is the usual offending organism in such cases. Severe otalgia, cranial neuropathies, and OE point to a diagnosis of NOE. Otologic findings include friable granulation tissue in the EAC. In the setting of concerning symptoms and signs, an underlying malignancy should be considered, and therefore a biopsy for histopathologic assessment is indicated. Diagnosis of NOE requires CT scan which demonstrates bony erosion. Serial gallium scanning may help to monitor disease resolution, which can take many months.[6] The treatment of NOE includes long-term intravenous antibiotic treatment with an antipseudomonal such as ceftazidime or ciprofloxacin (may be administered orally). Debridement of the granulation tissue and bony sequestra must be performed, and adjuvant hyperbaric oxygen therapy may be considered.

CONCLUSION

OE is a commonly seen disorder in children that can most often be effectively managed by early diagnosis, debridement, a logical progression of ototopical therapy, and maintenance of dry ear precautions.

REFERENCES

1. Rosenfeld RM, Brown L, Cannon CR, Dolor R, et al. Clinical practice guideline: acute otitis externa. *Otolaryngol Head Neck Surg.* 2006;134:S4-S23.
2. Beers SL, Abramo TJ. Otitis externa review. *Ped Emerg Care.* 2004;20(4):250-253.
3. Sander R. Otitis externa: a practical guide to treatment and prevention. *Am Fam Physician.* 2001;63(5):927–936, 941-942.
4. McCoy SI, Zell ER, Besser RE. Antimicrobial prescribing for otitis externa in children. *Pediatr Infect Dis J.* 2004;23(2):181-183.
5. Manolidis S, Friedman R, Hannley M, Roland PS, et al. Comparative efficacy of aminoglycoside versus fluoroquinolone topical antibiotic drops. *Otolaryngol Head Neck Surg.* 2004;130:S83-S88.
6. Shah RK, Blevins NK. Otalgia. *Otolaryngol Clin North Am.* 2003;36(6):1137-1151.
7. Blevins NH, Karmody CS. Chronic myringitis: prevalence, presentation, and natural history. *Otol Neurotol.* 2001;22(1):3-10.
8. Schwartz RH. Once-daily ofloxacin otic solution versus neomycin sulfate/polymyxin B sulfate/hydrocortisone otic suspension four times a day: a multicenter, randomized, evaluator-blinded trial to compare the efficacy, safety, and pain relief in pediatric patients with otitis externa. *Curr Med Res Opin.* 2006;22(9)1725-1736.
9. Osguthorpe JD, Nielsen DR. Otitis externa: review and clinical update. *Am Fam Physician.* 2006;74(9):1510-1516.

CHAPTER 30

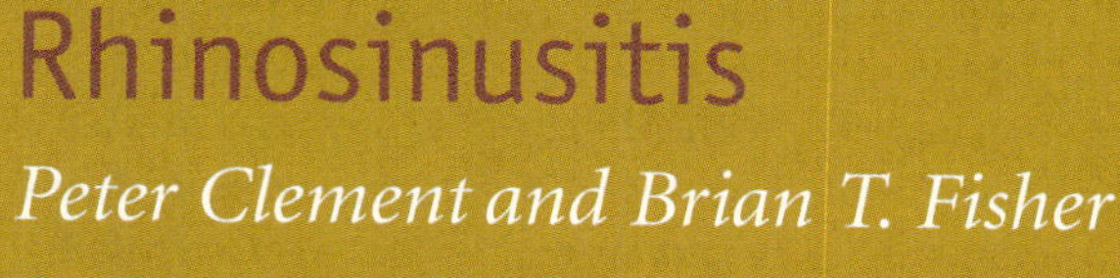

Rhinosinusitis

Peter Clement and Brian T. Fisher

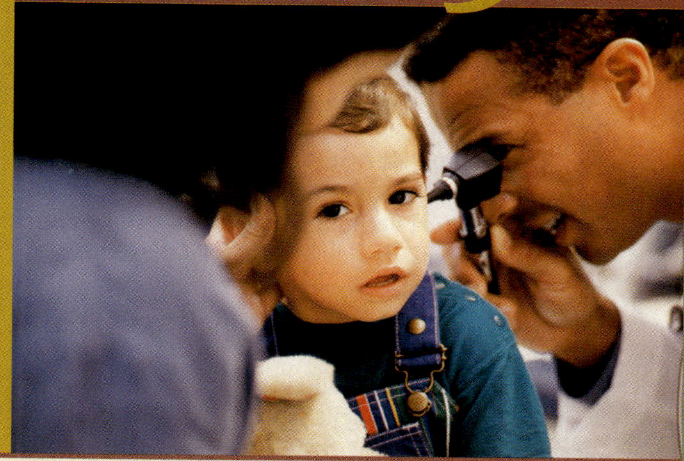

DEFINITIONS AND EPIDEMIOLOGY

Rhinitis and sinusitis are frequently referred to as two separate and distinct disease processes. However, since the mucosa of the nasal cavity and sinuses are contiguous, rhinitis and sinusitis often coexist, making a distinction on clinical presentation difficult. Therefore, rhinosinusitis may serve as a more appropriate term[1] to define a "group of disorders characterized by inflammation of the mucosa of the nose and paranasal sinuses."[2]

The inflammation resulting in rhinosinusitis can be multifactorial including viral infections, bacterial infections, and allergic processes. This varied etiology of rhinosinusitis in children makes the management of the condition challenging for pediatricians. Defining the etiology of rhinosinusitis is paramount to guiding therapeutic interventions. Definitions based on the patient's history and clinical presentation have been created to categorize rhinosinusitis as acute, subacute, recurrent, chronic, and acute superimposed on chronic (Table 30–1).[2,3] Practitioners are encouraged to utilize these definitions to guide their therapeutic decisions.

Estimates of the incidence and prevalence of rhinosinusitis are varied. This is likely attributable to the inclusion of different subcategories of rhinosinuisitis in various estimates of disease burden. In adults suffering

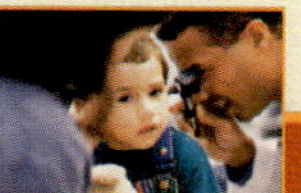

Table 30–1.

Classification of Rhinosinusitis

Classification	Duration	Symptoms and Signs
Acute rhinosinusitis		
Viral	<10–14 days	Upper respiratory symptoms that peak in severity and start to improve by 10 days
Bacterial	>10 days to less than 30 days	Persistent nasal or postnasal discharge or fever with purulent discharge for 3–4 days in an ill-appearing child
Subacute rhinosinusitis		
Bacterial process	4–12 weeks	Similar symptoms to acute bacterial rhinosinusitis just persisting for longer
Recurrent acute rhinosinusitis		
Bacterial process	4 or more episodes per year; each <30 days	Similar symptoms to acute bacterial rhinosinusitis; each episode separated by 7–10 days of symptom free interval
Chronic rhinosinusitis		
Isolated episode	>12 weeks	Persistent symptoms that include cough, rhinorrhea, or nasal obstruction; etiology may be nonbacterial
Acute on chronic episode	>12 weeks	Acute exacerbation of symptoms beyond the baseline persistent symptoms noted above

an acute viral upper respiratory infection there is often concominant evidence of paranasal sinus inflammation, a finding that supports the diagnosis of viral rhinosinusitis.[4,5] Based on this, there are over 1 billion episodes of all-cause rhinosinusitis each year in the United States.[4] More important to the practitioner is the rate at which a viral process progresses to acute bacterial rhinosinusitis. Approximately 0.5–2% of patients with viral upper respiratory infections progress to bacterial rhinosinusitis. This translates into 5–20 million cases of acute bacterial rhinosinusitis each year.[4]

Attempts to quantify the burden of acute bacterial rhinosinusitis in children have also been performed. Progression from viral upper respiratory infection to bacterial disease is thought to be more frequent in pediatric cases at a rate of 5–10%.[6] The rate of progression to a bacterial infection may be as high as 13% in children attending daycare.[7] In one prospective study, 135 (6.7%) of 2013 children aged 2–15 years presenting with upper respiratory symptoms had radiographic evidence of maxillary sinusitis and met the definition for acute or subacute bacterial rhinosinusitis.[8] In 35 (26%) of 135 patients, acute bacterial rhinosinusitis was thought to be preceded by allergic symptoms while all others were thought to be preceded by a viral illness.[8] These data support earlier evidence suggesting that acute bacterial rhinosinusitis usually occurs as a superinfection following inflammation secondary to a viral illness or less commonly from allergic symptoms.[9] The peak incidence of acute bacterial sinusitis in this pediatric population was in patients 3–6 years of age.[8]

Few data exist regarding the prevalence of chronic sinusitis in children. One published account suggested that 24% of children presenting for evaluation at an Ear Nose and Throat clinic was related to the complaint of a "chronic runny nose."[10] This dearth of information likely reflects the difficulty in identifying patients with chronic rhinosinusitis versus patients with recurrent acute episodes of viral or bacterial rhinosinusitis. Additionally, the primary etiologies for chronic rhinosinusitis are often noninfectious, making it even more challenging.[3]

Regardless of the etiology, it is clear that the health expenditures related to rhinosinusitis are substantial. The costs attributed to the treatment of rhinosinusitis in 1996 were estimated at $5.8 billion of which $1.8 billion was for children younger than 12 years.[11]

As discussed above, viral infections are a predominant cause of upper respiratory infections that also involve the sinuses. It is reasonable to assume that the pathogens causing viral rhinosinusitis are the same as those seen in the common cold. In one adult study, rhinovirus was isolated in over half of the patients with viral rhinosinusitis.[12] Other common viral pathogens include coronavirus, respiratory syncytial virus, influenza, parainfluenza, and adenovirus.[13]

The bacterial organisms implicated in acute and subacute bacterial rhinosinusitis are similar to the pathogens seen in acute otitis media. Results from maxillary aspirates in 79 children diagnosed with acute bacterial rhinosinusitis revealed 28% with *Streptococcus pneumoniae*, 19% with *Moraxella catarrhalis*, and 19% with nontypeable *Haemophilus influenzae*. Group A and C *Streptococcus*, *Eikenella corrodens*, and *Peptostreptococcus* were each isolated from fewer than 2% of cultures; approximately 30% of children had negative cultures.[14] Similar bacteriology was noted in 40 children undergoing sinus aspirate for subacute rhinosinusitis.[15]

A number of studies attempting to define the pathogens associated with chronic rhinosinusitis have been performed.[16–21] However, the results of these studies were not consistent. This is likely a result of the varied inclusion criteria adopted by the authors and methods for culture attainment and processing. The initial study evaluating bacterial pathogens in children with chronic rhinosinusitis showed anaerobes in all children cultured.[16] Subsequent studies also showed anaerobes but at a much lower rate.[17] Similar to acute and subacute rhinosinusitis, *S. pneumoniae*, *M. catarrhalis*, and nontypeable *H. influenzae* are frequently isolated in patients with more chronic symptoms.[19,21] *Staphylococcus aureus* has also been isolated in a small percentage of children with chronic rhinosinusitis.[17,18,21]

PATHOGENESIS

Sinus Anatomy and Development

Knowledge of the development of the paranasal sinuses is helpful to the clinician to understand the pathogenesis of rhinosinusitis. There are four paired sinuses: maxillary, ethmoid, sphenoid, and frontal. It is often taught that infants and small children do not yet have paranasal sinuses and therefore cannot have sinusitis. In reality, the ethmoid, maxillary, and sphenoid sinuses although small are present at birth (Figure 30–1). The overall growth of the sinuses is slow in the first 6 years of life. The ethmoid sinuses are the first to become pneumatized, which takes place at birth. The maxillary sinuses are pneumatized at age 4 and by the time a child reaches the age of 7–8 years, the inferior portion of the maxillary sinuses has extended to the level of the nasal cavity floor. Further growth into the maxilla is a continued process and dependent on the loss and descent of teeth. The sphenoid sinuses are pneumatized at the age of 5. The frontal sinuses are the last sinuses to develop. The point of origin of the frontal sinuses is the primary frontal sinus ostium. When the upper edge of the infundibulum frontalis (cupola) reaches the same level as the roof of the orbit, one can start to distinguish a real frontal sinus. This is often evident on radiograph

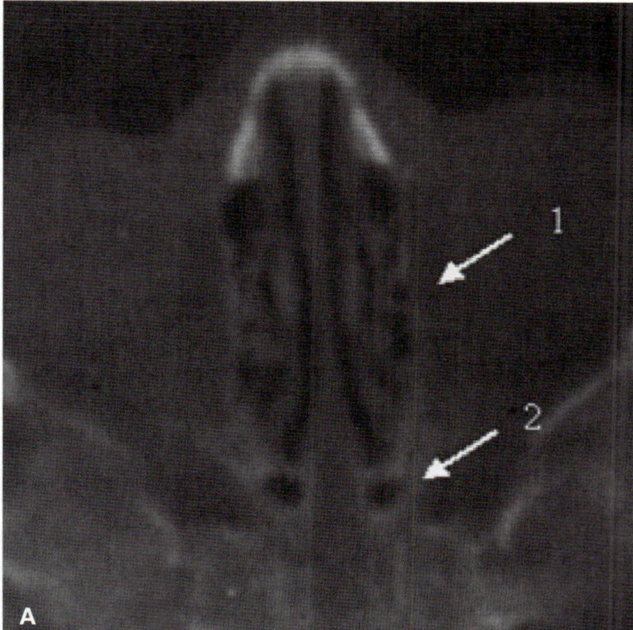

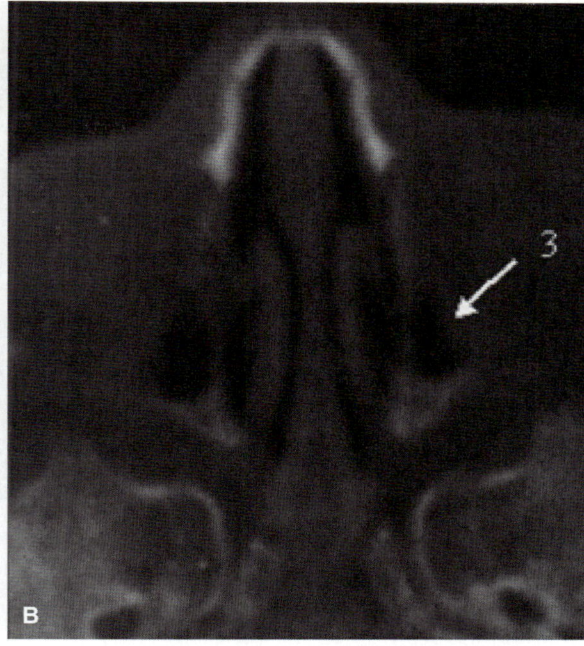

FIGURE 30–1 ■ Axial CT-scan (bone window settings) of 16-month-old child. **(A)** 1. Ethmoidal cells; 2. Sphenoidal cells. **(B)** 3. Maxillary sinus.

between 7 and 8 years of age. Maturation of the frontal sinuses is not until late adolescence.[22]

Sinus Physiology

Three components are thought to be necessary for the normal functioning of the paranasal sinuses[23]: (1) patency of the sinus ostia, (2) function of the mucociliary apparatus, and (3) quality of the secretions. Obstruction of the ostia or impaired mucociliary function can result in impaired sinus drainage, leading to the development of rhinosinusitis.

There are two sinus meati. The first is the middle meatus, which drains the maxillary, anterior ethmoid, and frontal sinuses. The second is the superior meatus, which drains posterior ethmoid and sphenoid sinuses.[24] The narrow caliber of the ostia and the narrow passageways in the ethmoids predispose children younger than 8 years of age to obstruction resulting in more diffuse sinus involvement.[25,26] Factors influencing ostial obstruction can be divided into those that cause mucosal edema and those due to mechanical obstruction (Table 30–2).[23,27] The most frequent etiology in children for ostial obstruction is a viral upper respiratory infection. As discussed above, inflammation second to allergies is less common but still a frequent cause of mucosal edema in children.[9] There is a three- to fourfold increased risk for recurrent coryza and sinus problems in children with smoking mothers compared to children from nonsmoking families.[28] Some specific mechanical factors include a deviated septum and hyperinflation of local structures shown in Figure 30–2.

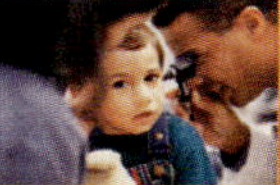

Table 30–2.

Predisposing Factors to Sinus Ostial Obstruction in Children

Mucosal Swelling	Mechanical Obstruction
Infection	Congenital/craniofacial anomalies:
Viral upper respiratory infection	Choanal atresia
Odotogenic infection	Cleft palate
Allergy	Foreign bodies
Immune disorders (e.g., common variable immune deficiency)	Anatomical abnormalities:
Genetic/congenital disorders:	Deviated septum
Cystic fibrosis	Tumors or polyps
Trisomy 21	Concha bullosa
Cyanotic congenital heart disease	Hyperinflated structures
Primary ciliary dyskinesia	Trauma related
Environmental exposures:	
Swimming	
Passive smoke exposure	
Hypothyroidism	
Gastroesophageal reflux	
Drug induced (general and topical medications)	

Under normal circumstances the sinuses are thought to be sterile with intermittent and transient

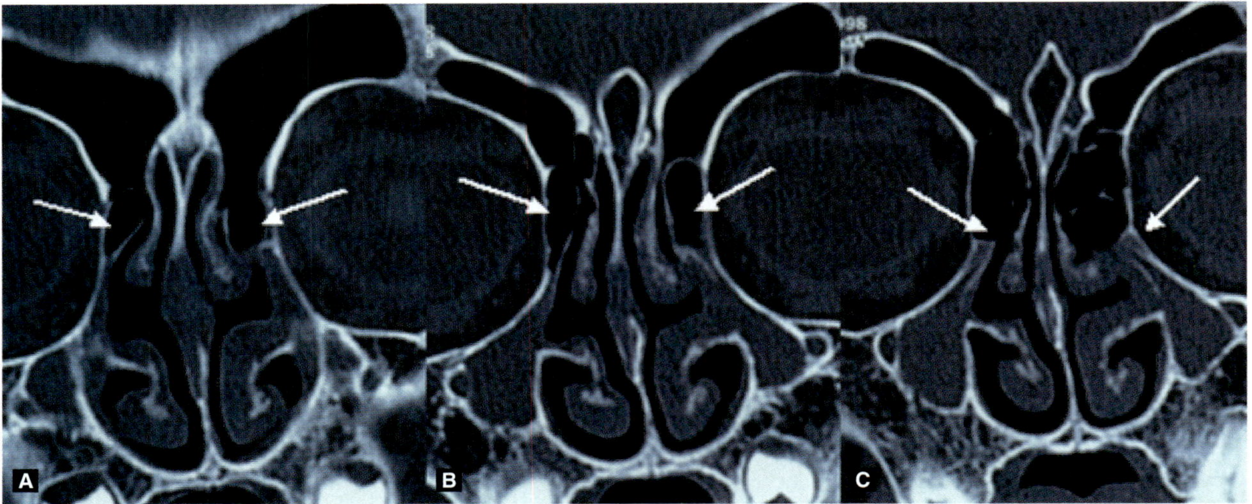

FIGURE 30–2 ■ Coronal CT-scan (bone window settings). Note hyperinflated structures. (**A** and **B**): Uncinate process = white arrows and **(C)** ballooning of lamina orbitalis, hyperinflated bulla ethmoidalis bilaterally, sealing of the infundibulum ethmoidalis and the drainage of the maxillary sinuses.

colonization by nasopharyngeal bacteria. The mucociliary apparatus functions to clear the sinuses of this transient contamination of bacteria. When the nasal ostia are obstructed and/or mucociliary activity is impaired, bacterial growth can ensue, leading to acute bacterial rhinosinusitis.[29]

CLINICAL PRESENTATION

History and Physical

Current definitions of rhinosinusitis are primarily based on the duration of symptoms in patients and clinical presentation, making the practitioner's history and physical examination integral to the diagnosis. The history should focus on the duration and trend of current symptoms, presence of predisposing conditions, environmental exposures, and history of sick contacts (Table 30–3). The history associated with rhinosinusitis is often dependent on age. Younger children are frequently unable to completely communicate with their parents or the physician. Therefore, the clinician should be alert to less specific symptoms, such as irritability, anorexia, frequent throat clearing, and severe halitosis. Older children and adolescents have complaints similar to adults, such as headache, facial pain, and pressure, maxillary dental pain, anosmia, and pharyngitis.[30]

Although there is not one physical finding that allows for definitive diagnosis of rhinosinusitis, a number of pertinent positives can aid in the diagnosis. The focused physical examination should include evaluation of the patient's facial appearance. Specifically, the clinician should look for the presence of periorbital edema or evidence of allergic shiners. Percussion of the maxillary and frontal sinuses may reveal facial tenderness. Upon examination of the oropharynx halitosis, tonsillar and adenoid hyperplasia, pharyngitis or lymphoid hyperplasia of the posterior pharynx would support the presence of rhinosinusitis. The cervical lymph nodes may be

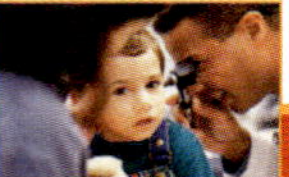

Table 30–3.

Historical Information for Diagnosing Rhinosinusitis

Identify the presence or absence and duration of the following symptoms:
- Rhinorrhea/nasal congestion
- Cough
- Headache/facial pain
- Fever
- Periorbital edema
- Halitosis

Inquire about presence of potential predisposing conditions (see Table 30–3)

Identify potential underlying allergies:
- Itching of the nose, ears and eyes
- Paroxysm of sneezing
- History of infantile eczema, food allergies during infancy, previous good response to antiallergic treatment (antihistamines and corticosteroids)
- Family history of atopy in a first degree relative
- Pets in the house

Identify environmental exposures:
- Smokers in the household
- Other sick contacts
- Daycare attendance

If there is a history of rhinosinusitis inquire about the following:
- Number of prior episodes and means of diagnosis
- Management methods including types of antibiotics prescribed for prior episodes

moderately enlarged or slightly tender. Transillumination is most helpful when there is asymmetry, however, the sensitivity of this finding is relatively poor (i.e., many children with bacterial sinusitis will not have asymmetric findings on transillumination).

Anterior rhinoscopy, although sometimes technically difficult in a young child, should be routinely performed. Direct visualization can be obtained in a simple way by tilting the nose tip upwards. Toddlers have wide noses with round nostrils, allowing for examination of the head of the inferior turbinates and assessment for the presence and character of secretions. For a more thorough examination, an otoscope should be used. When examining the nares, the clinician should note the appearance of the mucosa and presence of any draining fluid. The nasal and pharyngeal mucosa often appears erythematous while any drainage is typically yellow to greenish and of varying viscosity.

In some cases, endoscopy may be necessary and provides more useful information compared to anterior rhinoscopy. This is especially true if the history suggests the presence mechanical obstruction such as with polyps, foreign bodies, tumors, or septal deviations. Moreover, it allows a direct sampling of the middle meatus in cases where a bacterial culture is desired. Fiberoscopy has been shown possible under local anaesthesia for a majority of children. Those of toddler age may be more prone to resist such an examination.[31] Nasal endoscopy can be performed with a flexible fiberscope or rigid nasal scope. Fiberoscopy is a good tool in viewing the nasal cavity and the nasopharynx (including the size and condition of the adenoids), but it is not very adequate for visualising the middle meatus in a child. Rigid nasal endoscopy allows better visualization of the middle meatal structures. This procedure in children can only be performed under general anesthesia (Figure 30–3). In general, endoscopy should be reserved for more complicated rhinosinusitis cases and be performed by an experienced ear, nose, and throat (ENT) physician.

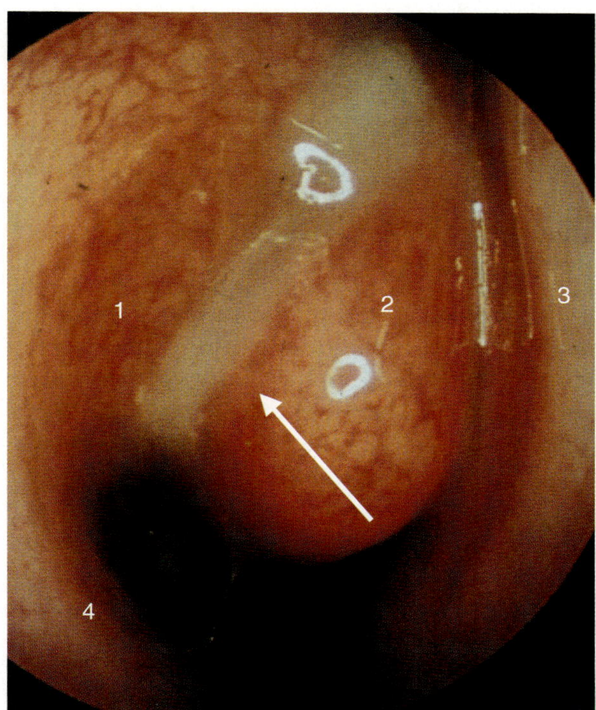

FIGURE 30–3 ■ Endoscopic view of sinusitis (right nasal cavity). 1 = Uncinate process; 2 = middle turbinate; 3 = septum; 4 = attachment of inferior turbinate.

Signs and Symptoms of Rhinosinusitis

Rhinorrhea and cough are the most frequent presenting symptoms in all forms of sinusitis occurring in 54–80% and 50–83% of cases, respectively. Cough is present during the day and night, although it is often noted to be worse at nighttime. Persistence of daytime cough is frequently the symptom that brings a child to medical attention. Fever and pain are less common but still frequent complaints appearing in 50–63% and 29–32% of cases, respectively.[32] Certain symptoms may help the clinician categorize acute sinusitis as severe or nonsevere (Table 30–4). In severe sinusitis, the fever is often high (more than 39°C), the nasal discharge is purulent and copious, and there may be associated periorbital swelling and facial pain.

Chronic rhinosinusitis should be suspected in children with very protracted symptoms including nasal discharge or cough that lasts for more than 12 weeks. Although the nasal discharge is purulent, it may be thin and clear, and occasionally it is minimal or absent. Cough and throat clearing is more prominent, present during the daytime and reported to be more common at night. Furthermore, nasal obstruction or mouth breathing are frequent (70–100%) and often accompanied by otitis media or otitis media with effusion. Morning

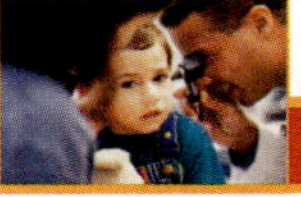

Table 30–4.

Acute Rhinosinusitis

Nonsevere	Severe
Rhinorrhea (of any quality)	Purulent rhinorrhea (thick, colored, opaque)
Nasal congestion	Nasal congestion
Headache, facial pain	Nasal pain and headache
Irritability (variable degree)	Periorbital edema (variable)
Cough	High fever (≥39°C)
Low grade or no fever	

periorbital swelling may be noted by the parents because of secondary compression of the superior ophthalmic veins in the context of ethmoid sinus inflammation.

DIFFERENTIAL DIAGNOSIS AND UNDERLYING CONDITIONS

The differential diagnosis for rhinosinusitis should focus on illnesses that result in rhinorrhea such as a viral upper respiratory infection or allergies. A foreign body should be considered in a child with persistent foul-smelling unilateral drainage. Patients with unilateral periorbital swelling may be suffering from preseptal or orbital cellulitis. The presence of headache or vomiting in addition to fever should prompt consideration of an intracranial complication of sinusitis (Table 30–5).

Equally important as the differential diagnosis is the number of underlying conditions that can predispose a patient to recurrent bacterial rhinosinusitis or result in rhinosinusitis that is recalcitrant to appropriate therapy (Table 30–2).[33] Allergies can be contributing factors in the severity and persistence of rhinosinusitis. If a careful history suggests the possibility of allergic rhinosinusitis, then it is reasonable to refer the patient for allergic testing.

Recurrent and chronic rhinosinusitis can be a common clinical presentation of various immune deficiencies. Common variable immune deficiencies have been found in children with recurrent infections including rhinosinusitis. Children with recurrent infections were shown to have significantly lower IgG2 and IgG4 levels, reduced specific pneumococcal antibodies in the IgG2 class, or reduced opsonization for staphylococci and *H. influenzae*.[33] Additionally, some patients who lack IgA antibodies and patients with acquired immune deficiencies (e.g. treatment for malignancies, organ transplants, acquired immunodeficiency syndrome (AIDS), drug-induced immune suppression) have an increased number of more severe respiratory infections. Patients suspected of having an underlying immune deficiency because of recurrent or persistent rhinosinusitis may require some of the following laboratory analyses: complete blood count with differential, quantitative immunoglobulins with IgG subclasses, and vaccine specific IgG levels for tetanus, diphtheria, pneumococcus, and *H. influenzae* type b, and HIV testing. In addition, sinus aspirate for culture may be useful to guide subsequent antibiotic therapy.

Sinusitis is a common problem in children with cystic fibrosis (CF). CF patients commonly have nasal polyps in the middle meatus[34] with partial or complete opacification of the anterior complex (anterior ethmoid, maxillary and frontal sinuses) and sometimes opacification of the posterior complex (posterior ethmoid and/or sphenoid sinuses) (Figures 30–4 and 30–5). When suspected, a pilocarpine sweat test should be ordered.

Primary ciliary dyskinesia (PCD) is an inherited condition in which there are functional or structural abnormalities of the patient's cilia (Figure 30–6). PCD is often associated with rhinosinusitis and bronchiectasias, which typically develop later in life. This diagnosis should be considered in any neonate with recurrent bronchial or nasal symptoms beyond what would be typically expected. At least half of children diagnosed with PCD had respiratory or ENT symptoms soon after birth.[35] In the older child, PCD may present as atypical asthma, severe gastroesophageal reflux, chronic rhinosinusitis (rarely with polyps), or chronic and severe otitis media with effusion. Diagnosis is confirmed by inspection of ciliary beat frequency from a biopsy of the nasal mucosa.

Gastroesophageal reflux disease (GERD) may be a cause of chronic nasal discharge and obstruction. Patients suffering from GERD may present with chronic cough, hoarseness and stridulous respiration, recurrent croup, and pharyngotracheitis.[36] Upper endoscopy may reveal cobblestone appearance of the mucosa of the laryngohypopharynx, inflammation of the upper airway, posterior glottic erythema, or edema. The diagnosis can also be confirmed by 24-hour esophageal pH monitoring.

Craniofacial disorders can contribute to chronic sinus disease. The most common craniofacial anomalies causing chronic rhinosinusitis are cleft palate and choanal atresia. Other factors might be regurgitation of food and saliva into the nasal cavity, inducing chronic irritation of the mucosa. Septal deviations and anomalies of the middle meatus (concha bullosa, oversized bulla etc.) are more frequently seen in older children (Figure 30–2). These anomalies do not directly result in

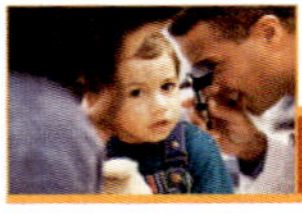

Table 30–5.

Differential Diagnosis for Acute Bacterial Rhinosinusitis Presenting with Fever and Headache

Disease Process	Presenting Symptoms
Epidural abscess	Dull headache, fever and normal CSF studies
Subdural abscess or empyema	Fever, usually toxic patient, intensive headache, meningeal signs, nuchal rigidity, altered consciousness
Brain abscess	Fever, lack of neurological signs in the frontal lobe, lethargy, headache, cranial nerve palsies
Meningitis	Headache, fever, nuchal rigidity, abnormal CSF studies

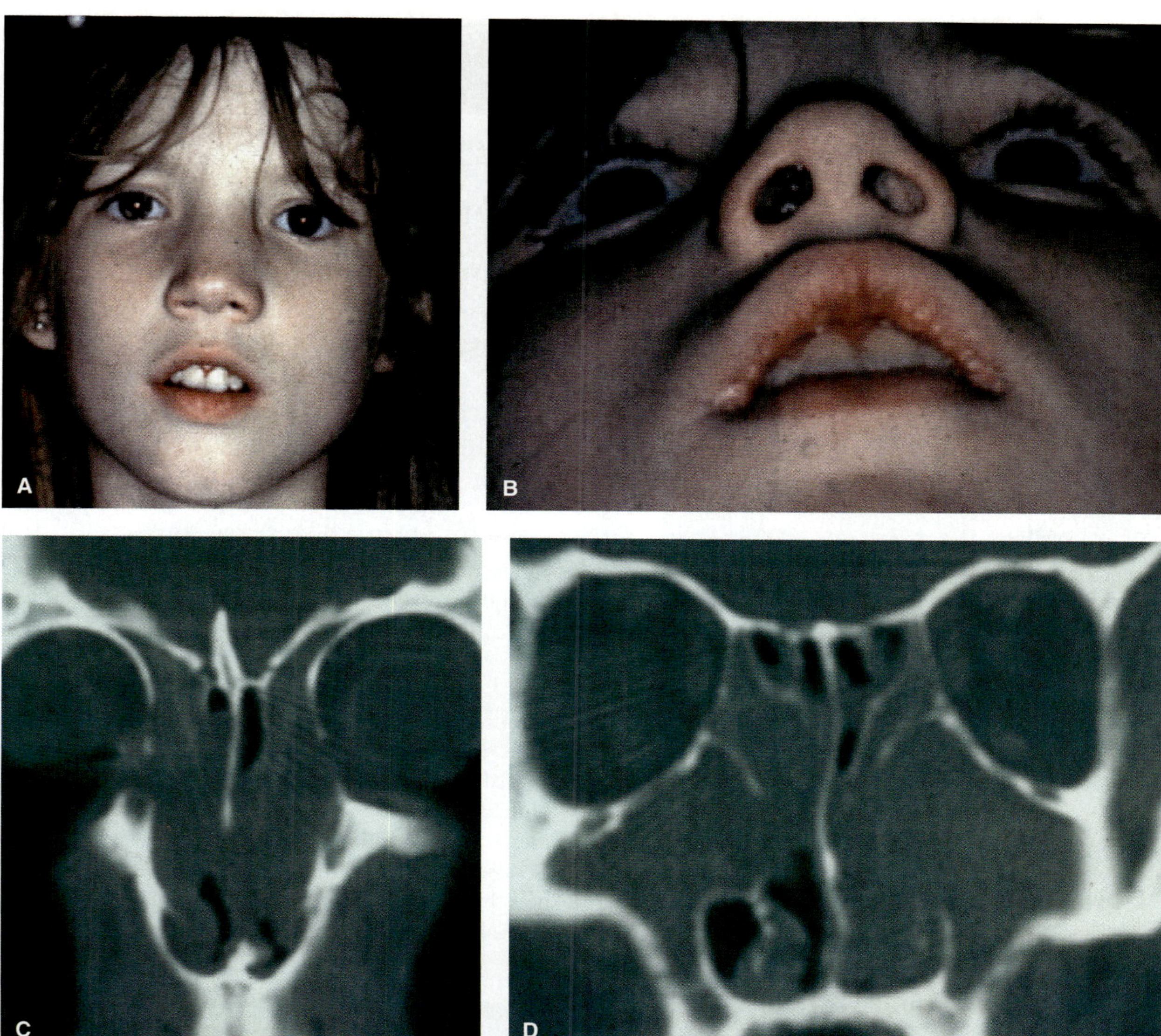

FIGURE 30–4 ■ (**A** and **B**): An 8-year-old girl with cystic fibrosis and massive nasal polyposis. Note in A the mouth breathing and hypertrophy of the gum. In B, the polyps can be visualized by tilting the head of the patient. **(C)** + **(D)**: Coronal CT-scan (bone windows setting) of same patient. Note the complete disappearance of all bony structures of the lateral nasal wall (complete "white out") due to demineralization of the thin bony structures of the ethmoid because of the chronic inflammation.

rhinosinusitis. However, on occasion, the anomaly can lead to obstruction of the middle meatus, allowing for development of rhinosinusitis.

Acquired mechanisms of mechanical obstruction can include trauma, adenoid hyperplasia, prolonged nasogastric tube placement, polyps, and tumor. Similar to the obstruction from the congenital disorders listed above, these acquired conditions can result in the development of rhinosinusitis. An acquired mechanical obstruction can be suspected by careful history and physical examination and confirmed by endoscopy or computed tomography imaging. When polyps are identified in a child, an evaluation for CF should be done.

There is growing evidence that rhinosinusitis may be linked to refractory asthma. In some patients with longstanding asthma, airway remodelling can result in a component of irreversible airflow obstruction. Most of the asthmatic children with chronic and recurrent rhinosinusitis show changes in the respiratory tract and on computed tomography examination. These changes include sinus-mucosal thickening and concha hypertrophy.[37] The improvement of asthma after treatment of rhinosinusitis suggests that rhinosinusitis may actually be a trigger for asthma.[38]

DIAGNOSIS

Most experts agree that the diagnosis of rhinosinusitis should be based primarily on a careful history and physical examination. In patients where symptoms persist

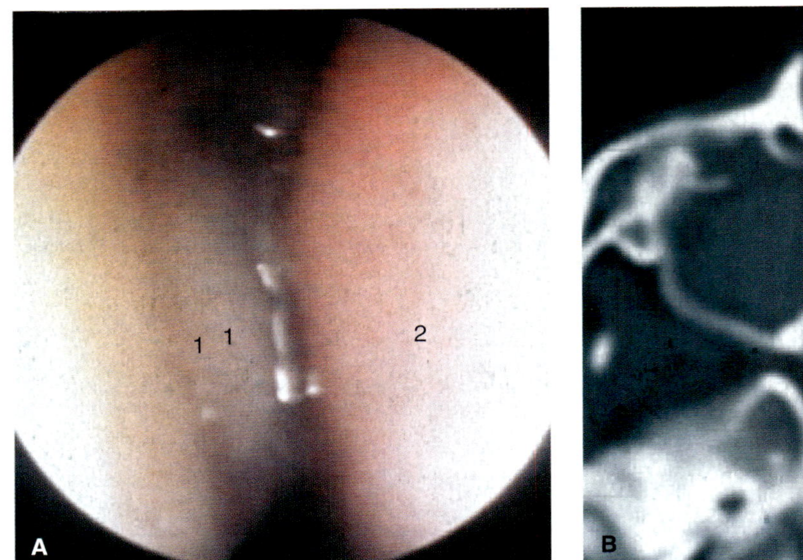

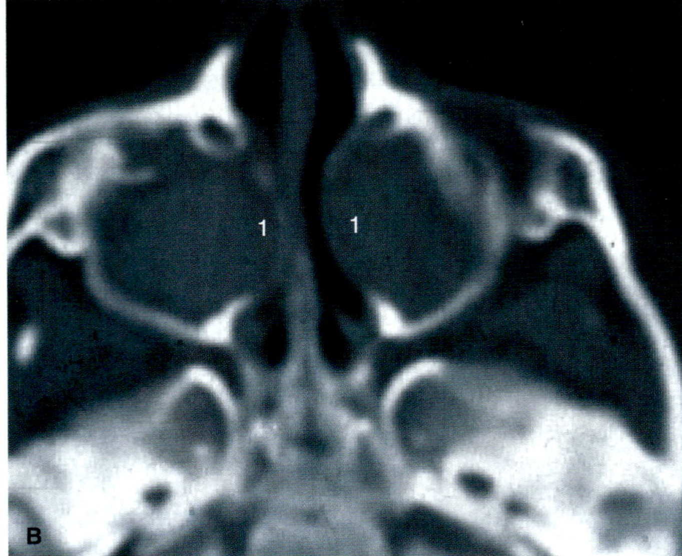

FIGURE 30–5 ■ **(A)** Endoscopic view of the right nasal cavity in a 6-year-old girl with cystic fibrosis. 1=fontanel region (none osseus part of the medial maxillary sinus wall), deviating medially touching the septum (=2). **(B)** Coronal CT-scan of same child. Bilateral maxillary mucopy-osinusitis with extreme deviation of fontanel region towards the nasal septum.

despite appropriate interventions, further studies including sinus samples for culture and radiographic imaging may be warranted.[1–3]

Microbiology

Although culture is the gold standard for diagnosis of bacterial rhinosinusitis, it is often not performed because of the necessity of a somewhat invasive procedure.[4,39] When sinus cultures are desired, endoscopically guided middle meatal sampling is preferable to antral puncture sampling as it does not require general anesthesia. The indication for microbiological sampling are (1) a severe illness or a toxic condition, (2) an acute illness that does not improve with medical therapy within 48–72 hours, (3) an immunocompromised host, and (4)

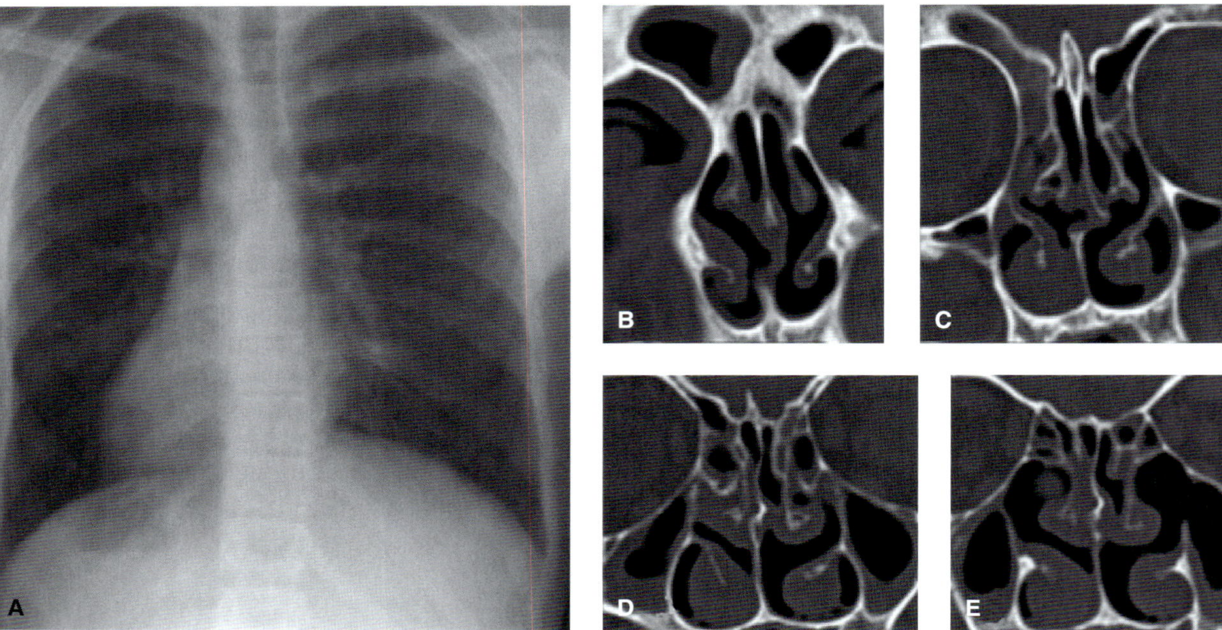

FIGURE 30–6 ■ **(A)**: Thorax standard X-ray of a 13-year-old child with Kartegener syndrome (PCD), note dextrocardy. **(B–E)**: Coronal CT-scans (bone window settings program): Note signs of chronic sinusitis (soft tissue swelling in all sinuses).

presence of suppurative intraorbital or intracranial complications.[1] Only the recovery of a high density of bacteria (>10^4 colony-forming units per mL) ensures that the culture results reflect actual sinus infection. Isolation of an organism at a density below 10^4 colony-forming units suggests the presence of sinus colonization or culture contamination from nasopharyngeal organisms.[4,39]

Radiographic Imaging

The use of radiographic imaging for diagnosis of rhinosinusitis remains controversial. Most experts agree that in the initial evaluation of rhinosinusitis, imaging is unnecessary. Certainly the diagnosis of rhinosinusitis should never be based on radiograph results alone. When ordered, radiographs should only support a diagnosis that is based on the history and physical examination. Various imaging modalities such as plain radiographs, computed tomography scans, and magnetic resonance imaging have been used to evaluate the sinuses. A negative result on plain radiograph supports the absence of bacterial sinusitis and may direct the clinician to an alternative diagnosis.[40] However, in children, a clinical examination consistent with rhinosinusitis was found to highly correlate with abnormalities on sinus radiographs.[41] Given the high correlation between the physical examination and radiograph results as well as the fact that radiographs can only evaluate the maxillary and frontal sinuses, they are likely not necessary to make a diagnosis.[3,42]

Computed tomography imaging can provide the clinician with a more detailed evaluation of the all paranasal sinuses as well as the local anatomy. The indications for ordering a computed tomography scan in a child are the same as the indications listed above for microbiological sampling.[1] Additionally, computed tomography scans are often necessary whenever surgical intervention may be considered.[3] Magnetic resonance imaging should never be used in routine sinus evaluation because diffuse sinus mucosal thickening is often an incidental finding. Magnetic resonance imaging is most useful when intracranial complications of rhinosinusitis are suspected or in an immunocompromised patient when invasive fungal rhinosinusitis is a concern. Additionally, magnetic resonance imaging may also be helpful when differentiating a tumor from surrounding edema.[43]

MANAGEMENT/TREATMENT

Depending on the recent history of the patient and the clinical presentation, a number of therapeutic options exist for the clinician managing rhinosinusitis. The potential role of antibiotics, adjuvant therapies, and surgical management are each discussed below. Initial categorization of the patient with rhinosinusitis as viral or bacterial in origin as well as acute, subacute, or chronic is necessary before proceeding with therapeutic decisions.

Antibiotics

Patients with symptoms lasting for less than 10 days likely have a viral illness or suffer from allergic rhinosinusitis and thus will not benefit from antibiotics. These patients may or may not improve with symptomatic therapies such as oral or topical decongestants, oral analgesics, and topical antiinflammatory drugs. Those patients with persistent or worsening symptoms beyond 10 days are more likely to have a bacterial rhinosinusitis.

Clearly patients presenting with a severe illness or toxic condition or patients with a suspected or proven suppurative complication of rhinosinusitis should receive parenteral antibiotics. However, significant controversy exists as to the necessity of antibiotics for the child with bacterial rhinosinusitis in the outpatient setting. The initial randomized controlled trial comparing antibiotics with placebo in pediatric outpatients with clinical and radiographic diagnosis of acute bacterial rhinosinusitis showed more rapid and complete recovery in those receiving antibiotics. Interestingly, 60% of the children receiving placebo did ultimately recover without antibiotics.[41] More recently, pediatric[44] and adult[45] randomized controlled trials reported no difference in the antibiotic treatment group versus the placebo group with regard to timing and completeness of recovery. Unfortunately, the pediatric study was limited because of the use of low-dose antibiotic therapy while the adult study included a number of patients who did not have at least 10 days of symptoms at presentation.

In an attempt to limit outpatient antibiotic prescribing practices, the 2001 American Academy of Pediatric guidelines recommend the initiation of antibiotics only when a child is diagnosed with acute bacterial rhinosinusitis based on clinical examination and duration of symptoms.[3] Similarly other expert panels suggest reserving outpatient antibiotic use for patients with severe acute rhinosinusitis and in some patients when nonsevere acute rhinosinusitis accompanies other comorbid illnesses (i.e. asthma, acute otitis media).[1]

Definitive data guiding the duration of therapy once antibiotics are initiated are lacking. Current recommendations include 10 days,[3] 10–14 days or longer if symptoms persist[1], or 7 days beyond symptom resolution.[46] Some evidence does exist in adults to suggest the effectiveness of shorter durations such as 3–5 days.[47] Randomized controlled trials are needed to further define the most appropriate duration. At this time, 10 days of therapy is likely adequate. Most important to the clinician is that the patient show clinical improvement after 48–72 hours of therapy. If improvement does not take place, the patient should be reevaluated.

Choice of Antibiotics

As previously stated, the bacterial pathogens most frequently isolated in acute and subacute bacterial rhinosinusitis are *S. pneumoniae*, nontypeable *H. influenzae*, and *M. catarrhalis*. The reader should be aware that a vast majority of nontypeable *H. influenzae* and all *M. catarrhalis* isolates are beta-lactamase producers making amoxicillin ineffective. Despite this, the American Academy of Paediatrics still recommends amoxicillin at a dose of 45 mg/kg/d as a first-line agent because of its general effectiveness, safety and tolerability, low costs and narrow spectrum.[3] Furthermore, based on acute otitis media data, infections secondary to nontypeable *H. influenzae* and *M. catarrhalis* are more likely to resolve spontaneously.[48]

Increasing rates of *S. pneumoniae* resistance to penicillin may warrant the initial use of high-dose amoxicillin (80–90 mg/kg/d). Patients who attend daycare, those younger than 2 years of age, or those who have received antibiotics in the past 90 days are more likely to have a pneumococcal infection that is resistant to amoxicillin. [49,50] The reader should consult their local resistance patterns for pneumococcus as they can vary from region to region. Patients with more severe symptoms at presentation (Table 30–4) or those who do not respond to initial amoxicillin therapy should be given high-dose amoxicillin therapy in conjunction with clavulanate at 6.4 mg/kg/d. The clinician should be aware that only certain preparations of combination amoxicillin/clavulanate allow for increasing the dose of amoxicillin to 80–90 mg/kg/d while maintaining the appropriate dose of clavulanate. This is important because administration of clavulanate above 6.4 mg/kg/d may result in gastrointestinal side effects.

Patients with a nontype 1 allergic history to amoxicillin can be prescribed a third-generation oral cephalosporin such as cefdinir (14 mg/kg/d). In cases of serious allergic reactions, clindamycin (25 mg/kg/d) or clarithromycin (15 mg/kg/d) can be used. Clindaymcin will only have activity against *S. pneumoniae* and will not be effective against nontypeable *H. influenzae* or *M. catarrhalis*. Recent analysis of pneumococcal isolates from across the United States suggests a high rate of resistance to trimethoprim/sulfamethoxazole, cefuroxime, and azithromycin.[51,52] These agents should be avoided when possible for empirical therapy of bacterial rhinosinusitis. Ceftriaxone at 50 mg/kg/d either intravenously or intramuscularly can be used in children with vomiting. Once vomiting subsides, oral therapy can be initiated to complete the antibiotic course.[3]

Although fluoroquinolones, especially levofloxacin, have good activity against the bacterial pathogens of rhinosinusitis, they are not routinely recommended for use in children. In cases where resistant organisms require the use of a fluoroquinolone, the physician should consider consultation with an infectious disease specialist.

Antibiotic Prophylaxis

Antibiotic prophylaxis is often not recommended given the concerns for promoting antimicrobial resistance. Certain high-risk children (immunodeficiency, CF, PCD, and craniofacial anomalies) may require prophylaxis in the setting of recurrent disease. The decision to initiate prophylaxis in these patients should be weighed against the risk of limiting antibiotic options over time secondary to resistance.

Antibiotics and Chronic Rhinosinusitis

Children suffering from chronic rhinosinusitis are likely to have an underlying condition that predisposes them to persistent obstruction of the sinus ostia, resulting in chronic symptoms.[53] The use of antibiotics in this setting is controversial. Antibiotics have been shown to stop the purulent rhinorrhea for a short period of time, but on long-term follow-up, they do not have a significant curative effect.[19] In children with chronic rhinosinusitis complicated by frequent acute exacerbations, an initial course of antibiotics may be prudent. In this setting, antibiotic therapy should be directed at the organisms commonly associated with acute or subacute rhinosinusitis. The choice of antibiotic should also cover *Streptococcus pyogenes, S. aureus,* and anaerobes, which are sometimes isolated in patients with chronic symptoms. Amoxicillin/clavulanate is a reasonable first-line choice in this setting.

If symptoms do not improve after 1 week of therapy, it is unlikely that bacterial infection is the cause for the chronic symptoms. The physician should instead evaluate for other predisposing conditions (Table 30–2).[53] Patients with suspected or confirmed methicillin-resistant *S. aureus* should be referred to an infectious disease specialist for further management.

Adjuvant Therapy

A number of adjuvant therapies for rhinosinusitis exist including antihistamines, decongestants, topical intranasal steroids, and saline nasal irrigation. Unfortunately, there is little scientific evidence for the effectiveness of any of them. Recently, the Food and Drug Administration (FDA) has recommended against the use of systemic cough and cold remedies in children younger than 2 years of age and questioned their safety in children older than 2.[54] Given this recommendation and the lack of efficacy data, the use of systemic antihistamines and decongestants in children should be avoided.

Theoretically the use of intranasal corticosteroids should improve acute rhinosinusitis by reducing tissue inflammation and relieving ostial obstruction.[30] However, based on the few studies to date, there are little data to support their use in acute bacterial rhinosinusitis. Two adult studies showed that the use of flunisolide or mometasone in combination with antibiotics provided only a modest benefit in reduction of symptoms.[55,56] A single pediatric study evaluating budesonide nasal spray also showed just modest improvements during the second week of therapy.[57] In studies of chronic rhinosinusitis, minimal to no benefit was appreciated when compared to placebo.[58] These agents should be reserved for the treatment of nasal inflammation secondary to allergies.

Nasal saline sprays and nasal saline drops have not been rigorously evaluated. Using saline washes at body temperature twice a day may help decrease the viscosity of nasal cavity secretions and enhance sinus drainage and ventilation.[59] Given the limited side effects and minimal cost, it is reasonable to suggest them to patients for potential symptomatic relief.

Physicians can aid their patients in discussing proper techniques for nose blowing as nose blowing has been identified as a potential risk factor for the development of acute bacterial sinusitis. This is based on the observation in adults where after nose blowing contrast was seen in one or more of the sinuses of all volunteers.[60] If one blows the nose with both nostrils closed, intranasal pressures can be very high and potentially result in hyperinflated ethmoid air cells.[61] Therefore, patients should be advised not to blow the nose with both nostrils closed. On the contrary, keeping one nostril open during nose blowing can help to clear the nasal cavity from secretions without generating excessively high pressures.

Surgical Management

Surgical interventions are often emergently necessary for various complications (see the section on Complications) of rhinosinusitis and sometimes are performed electively in patients with symptoms that persist after attempts at medical management fail (Table 30–6). Elective surgery should be considered as a last resort therapy for pediatric patients with isolated rhinosinusitis and only after consultation with a pediatric ENT physician. Various surgical approaches have been implemented for the relief of rhinosinusitis. Adenoidectomy is one of the oldest, fastest, and simplest of all ENT operations, and carries minimal risk and morbidity. It is most often performed if the amount of adenoid tissue in the nasal pharynx seems large enough to cause obstruction, to serve as a reservoir for bacterial pathogens, or when almost the entire surface area of the adenoid is covered with biofilm.[62] Overall, an adenoidectomy can be expected to improve the symptoms in approximately 50% of patients with chronic rhinosinusitis.[63–65]

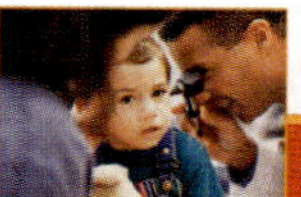

Table 30–6.

Indications for Surgery in Children with Rhinosinusitis

Absolute indications
Intracranial complications
Antrachoanal polyp
Mucocoeles and mucopyocoeles
Fungal sinusitis
Total nasal obstructions due to massive nasal polyposis or medialization of the lateral nasal wall in cystic fibrosis
Anatomical anomalies impeding proper nasosinus ventilation and drainage
Possible indication
Orbital abscess
Chronic rhinosinusitis with frequent exacerbations resistant to optimal medical therapy

When maximal medical therapy and adenoidectomy have failed, functional endoscopic sinus surgery (FESS) may be performed. "Functional" implies that the surgery's goal is for the restoration of ventilation and drainage of all sinuses (Figure 30–7B). With this technique, the ethmoid is cleared from disease endonasally with the help of rigid endoscopes. A nasoantral window is created in the middle meatus, allowing for removal of diseased mucosa. FESS should be individually tailored to each case by the pediatric ENT specialist.

COMPLICATIONS

Complications of rhinosinusitis occur more frequently in children, young adolescents, and patients with depressed immune function. The most concerning complications of rhinosinusitis in children are infections of the orbital content and intracranial abscesses. A high index of suspicion for these complications is mandatory as they can be life-threatening when not diagnosed early and adequately treated. Other less severe complications are bony osteitis, osteomyelitis, and local complications such as mucoceles and antrachoanal polyps.

Orbital Complications

Unilateral orbital symptoms in the presence of purulent rhinorrhea are highly suggestive of orbital complications of rhinosinusitis. In rare cases, bilateral orbital

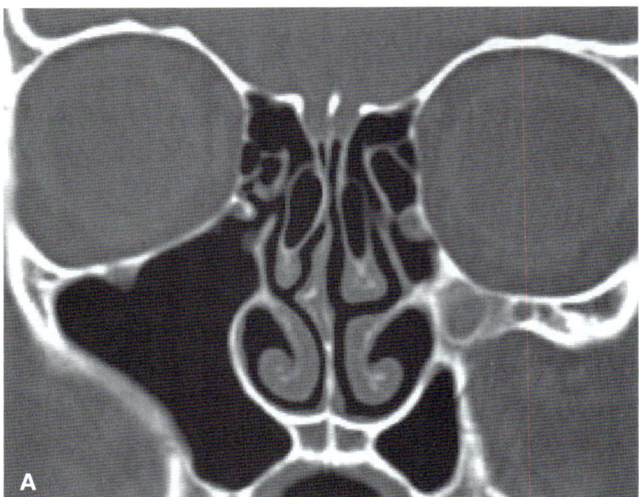

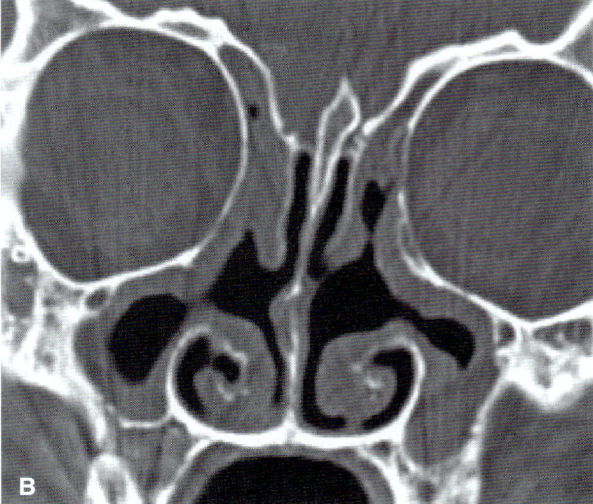

FIGURE 30–7 ■ **(A)** Coronal CT-scan (bone window settings) of an adult operated as a child for left acute maxillary sinusitis, using a Caldwell-Luc approach. Note the severe distortion of the bony framework of the maxillary sinus on that side. **(B)** Coronal CT-scan of an adult patient with cystic fibrosis and operated upon as a child for massive nasal polyposis using a FESS technique (complete sphenoethmoidectomy). Note the preservation of the bony framework of the sinuses. The persisting swollen mucosa is of course due to the systemic disease.

edema may exist from the start.[66] The routes of expansion of an infection in the ethmoid toward the orbit can be direct via a bony dehiscence at the level of the lamina orbitalis (papyracea) or os lacrimale or indirect via arterial, venous, or lymphatic seeding. The most common germs for orbital complications in children are *H. influenzae*, streptococci species, and staphylococci species. When orbital cellulitis progresses rapidly or fails to respond to intravenous antibiotics, a subperiostal abscess should be suspected. Asymmetric proptosis and limitations of ocular mobility are symptoms that suggest the presence of a subperiostal abscess (Figure 30–8).

Less frequently, compression of the optic nerve can result in color impairment and vision loss requiring emergent surgical intervention. When the initial unilateral signs progressively become bilateral, a posterior extension beyond the limits of the orbit with associated cavernous sinus thrombosis must be suspected. In this setting, there may be bilateral axial proptosis in combination with cranial nerve III, IV, and VI palsies. Diagnosis can usually be made on clinical examination, but should be confirmed with magnetic resonance imaging. Presence of a subperiostal abscess that does not respond to intravenous antibiotics should be drained via an endonasal endoscopic approach (Figure 30–9).

Intracranial Complications

Intracranial complications are present in 3% of the patients admitted into the hospital for treatment of severe

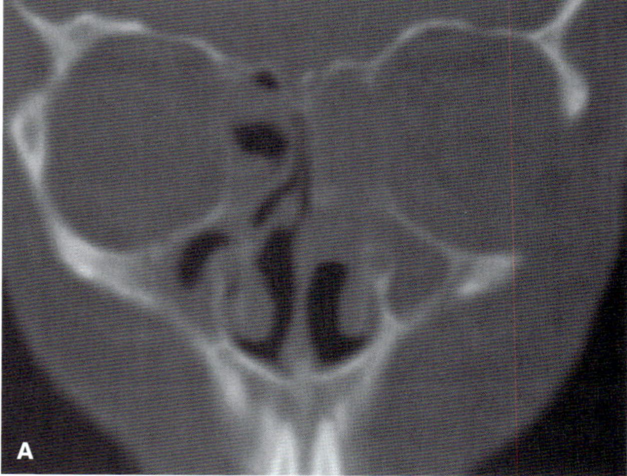

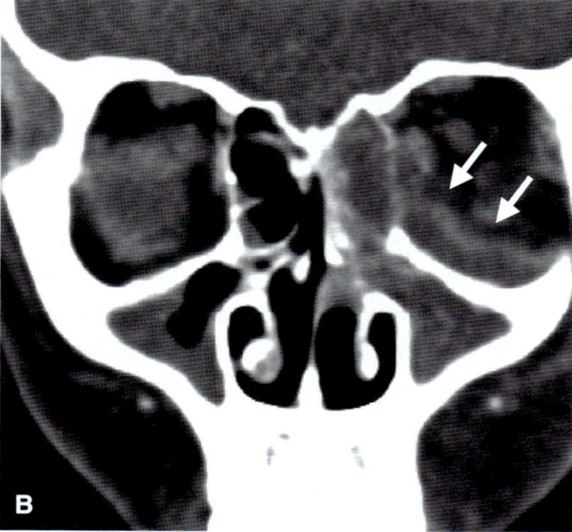

FIGURE 30–8 ■ A 6-year-old girl with a subperiostal abscess of the orbita. **(A)** Coronal CT-scan (bone window settings) acute pansinusitis left side with subperiostal abscess of the left orbit. The latter is not well visualized with this bone window settings. **(B)** Coronal CT-scan (soft tissue window settings) of the same child. Now the subperiostal abscess in the left orbit is visualized very clearly.

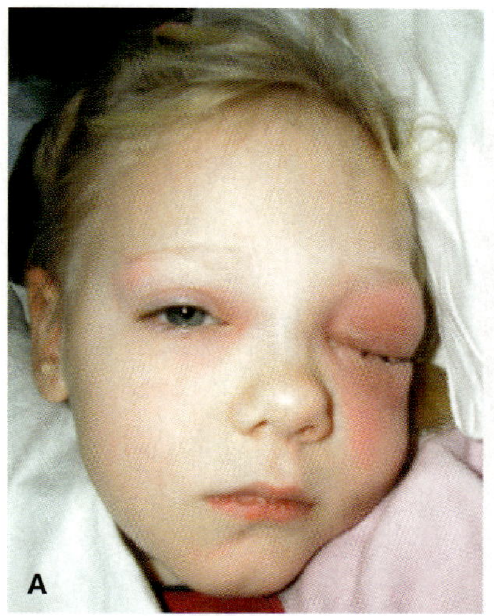

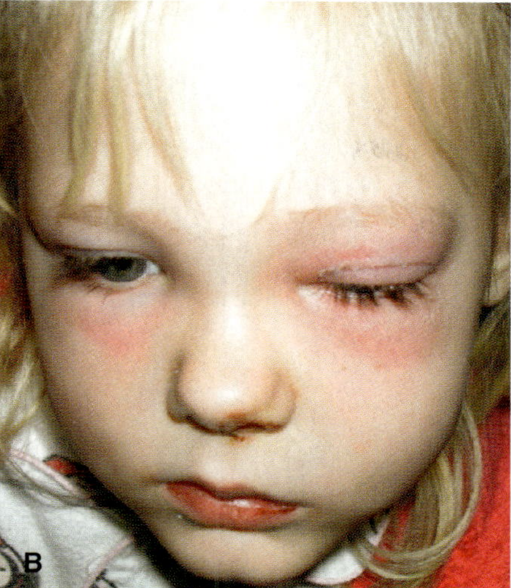

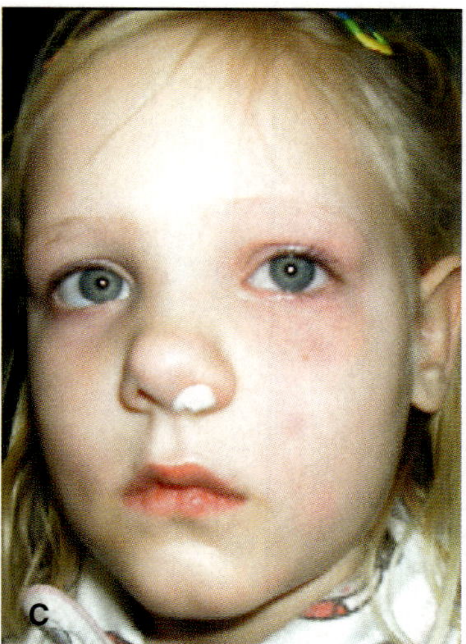

FIGURE 30–9 ■ Same child as in Figure 30–8. **(A)** With an acute pansinusitis and left subperiostal abscess. Before surgery. **(B)** Same child 1 day after surgery. **(C)** Same child, 5 days after surgery.

rhinosinusitis[67] (Figures 30–10 and 30–11). The most common presenting signs and symptoms apart from nasal and orbital symptoms are headache (75%), fever (44%), mental status changes (30%), motor deficit (38%), seizures (19%), nausea and vomiting (19%), and respiratory distress or arrest (6%).[68] The clinician should also be aware of signs of increased intracranial pressure such as bradycardia, pappilloedema, hypertension, nausea, vomiting, decreased consciousness, and dilated pupil(s) (ominous sign suggesting transtentorial herniation).

These patients almost always have involvement of the frontal sinuses and frequently suffer from pansinusitis. In rare cases, isolated sphenoiditis (cerebellar abscess via the sinus petrosus inferior) or maxillary sinusitis (cerebellar abscess via the plexus venosus pterigoideus) can cause intracranial complications (Figure 30–11). Osteomyelitis of the anterior wall of the frontal bone (tabula externa) will cause a subperiostal abscess of the forehead via venous vessels. This is often referred to as "Pott's puffy tumor" (Figure 30–12). Osteomyelitis of the posterior wall (tabula interna) will induce a thrombophlebitis of the valveless diploic veins of "Breshet,"which serve as a conduit for the spread of the infection to the intracranial space.[68,69]

When intracranial complications are suspected, the clinician should seek consultation with an infectious disease specialist, an ENT surgeon, and potentially a neurosurgeon. Empiric antibiotics should include vancomycin (active against Gram-positive organisms), a third-generation cephalosporin (active against Gram-negative microbes), and metrodinazole (active against anaerobes). Surgical intervention is often necessary in

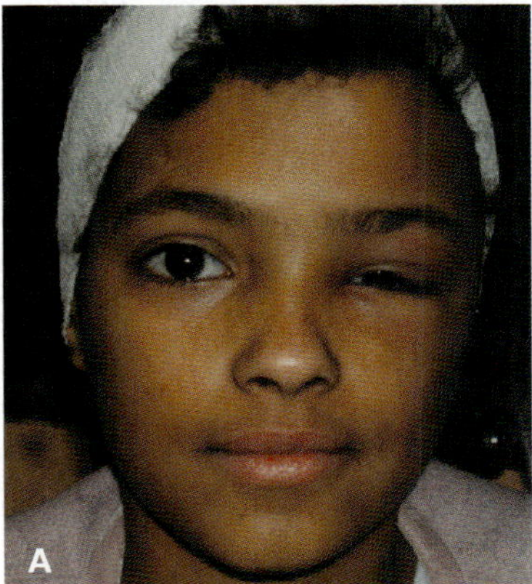

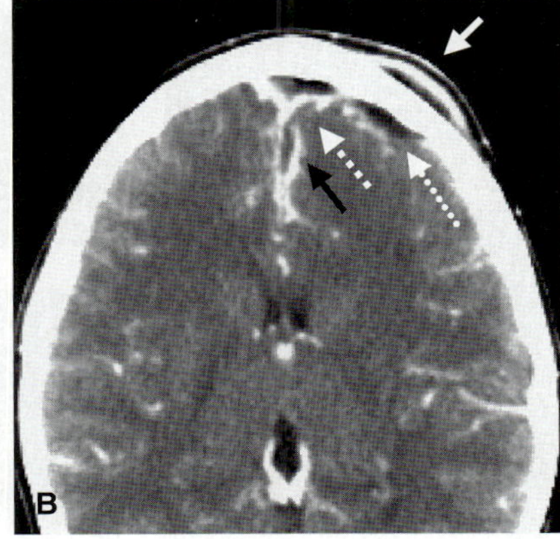

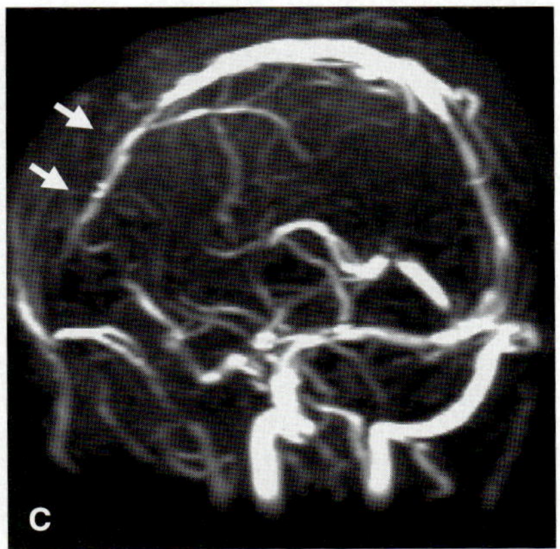

FIGURE 30–10 ■ Thirteen-year-old girl with dual complication of sinusitis. **(A)** Orbital cellulitis. **(B)** Axial CT-scan + contrast. 1=Presence of one Pott's puffy tumor (solid white arrow); 2=epi- and subdural abscess (dotted whitearrow); 3=sagital abscess (black arrow). **(C)** MRI venogram: No thrombosis of superior sagital sinus (with arrows).

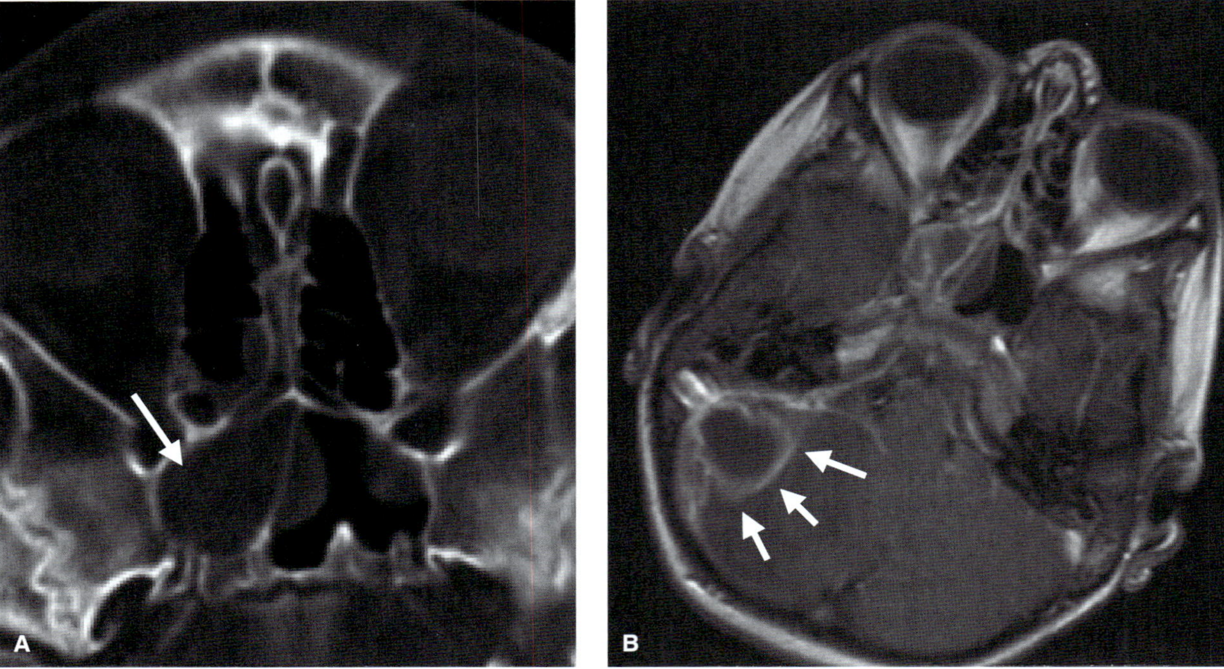

FIGURE 30–11 ■ **(A)** Axial CT-scan (bony program) of a 6-year-old child with isolated sphenoiditis left side. **(B)** MRI T_1-weighted image. Note presence of cerebellar abscess (left side). Route of spread probably via the sinus petrosus inferior.

addition to antibiotics. All involved sinuses need to be drained especially the frontal sinus, which needs adequate postoperative ventilation and drainage. Additionally, intracranial fluid collection (especially subdural and cerebral abscesses) need to be drained neurosurgically[69] (Figure 30–13).

Rare Complications

An extremely rare intracranial complication of rhinosinusitis is an extradural hematoma, which presents as a combination of extradural hematoma and rhinosinusitis in the absence of trauma (Figure 30–14). Hematologic

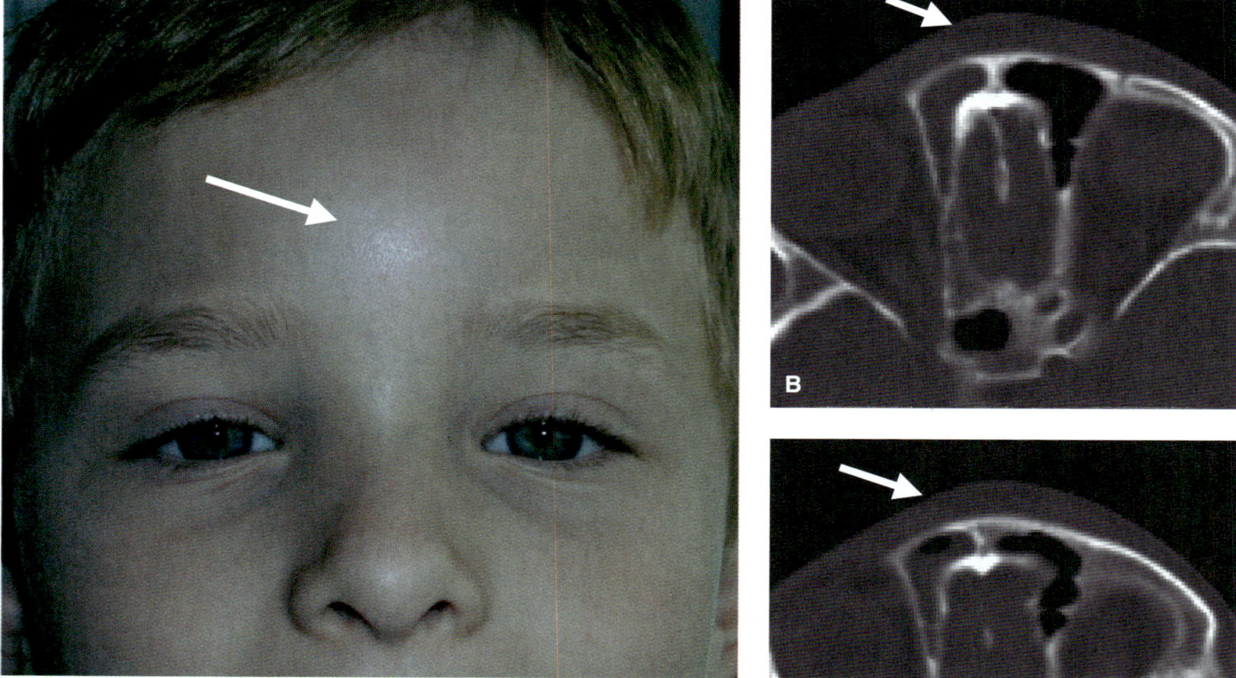

FIGURE 30–12 ■ **(A)** A 7-year-old boy with Pott's puffy tumor of the forehead (white arrow). (**B** and **C**) Axial CT-scan (bone window settings) showing left frontal sinusitis and swelling of the skin (abscess) over the frontal sinus.

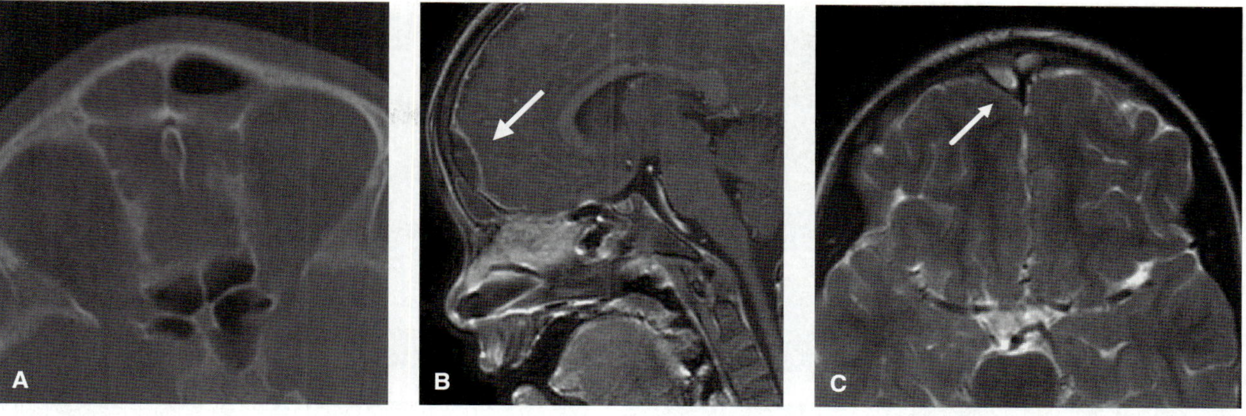

FIGURE 30–13 ■ A 9-year-old boy with epidural abscess. **(A)** Axial CT-scan (bony program) showing complete opaque frontal sinus on the left side and fluid level on the right side. (**B** and **C**) Sagittal, coronal: MRI T_1-weighted image of same case.

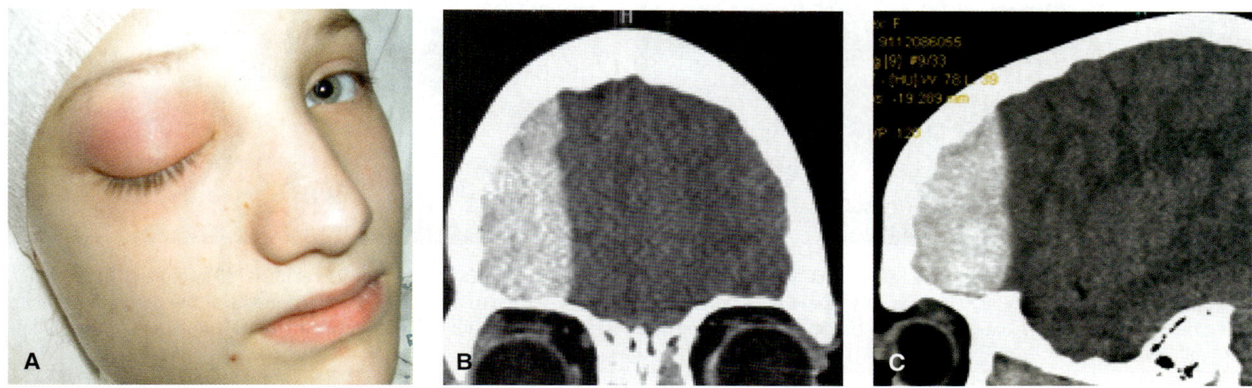

FIGURE 30–14 ■ Dual complication of sinusitis in a 15-year-old girl. **(A)** Presence of orbital cellulitis. **(B)** + **(C)** CT-scan + contrast: Note the presence of a huge extradural hematoma (extremely rare complication).

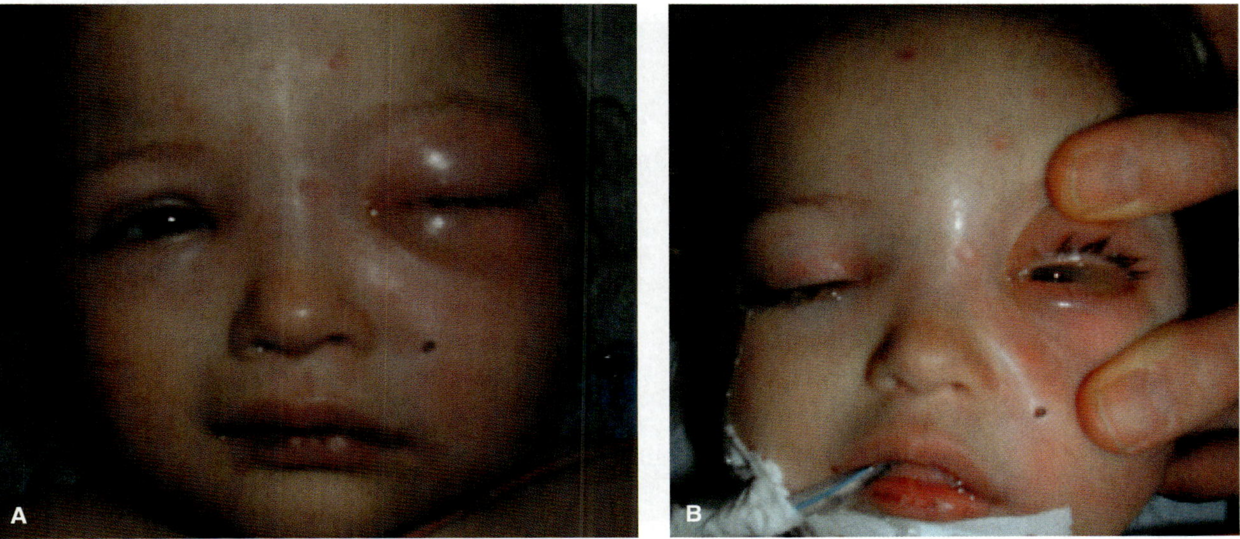

FIGURE 30–15 ■ **(A)** A 2-year-old girl with osteomyelitis of the maxilla from dental origin (coronitis of dorsal molar). Note the edema at the level of the cheek and the left eye. **(B)** Forceful opening of the eyes shows chemosis of the conjunctiva.

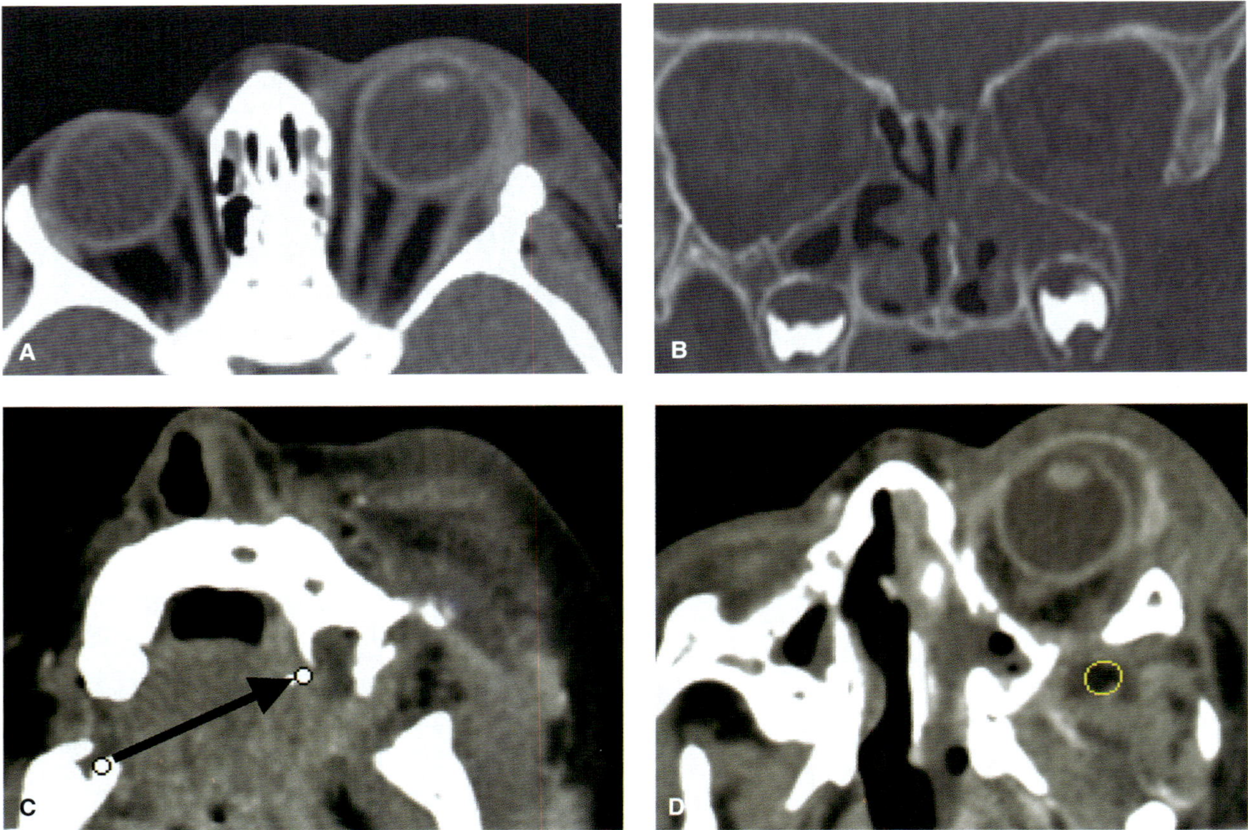

FIGURE 30–16 ■ Same child as Figure 30–15. **(A)** Axial CT-scan (soft window settings). Extraconal orbital cellulitis. **(B)** Coronal CT-scan (bone window settings). Note maxillary sinusitis. **(C)** Axial CT-scan (soft tissue window settings), arrow shows extraction site of the dorsal molar, note premaxillary oedema. **(D)** Axial CT-scan (soft tissue window settings). Involvement of the orbit via retromaxillary space and fissura orbitalis inferior (yellow circle).

studies and lumbar puncture are required after a computed tomography scan or magnetic resonance image have excluded the possibility of herniation.

Osteomyelitis of the maxilla in infancy is primarily a staphylococcal infection of an unerupted tooth (coronitis) and the surrounding bone. The swelling of the soft tissue over the maxilla is considerably more extensive than in acute sinusitis and involves the soft tissues of the maxillary region and eyelids. Appropriate antibiotics are indicated (Figures 30–15 and 30–16).

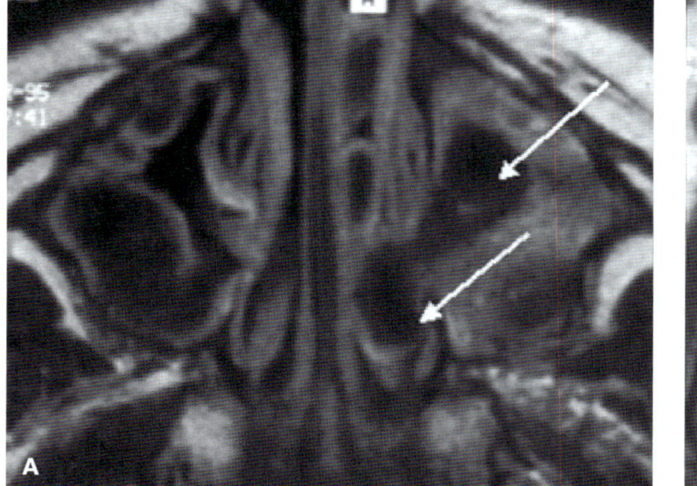

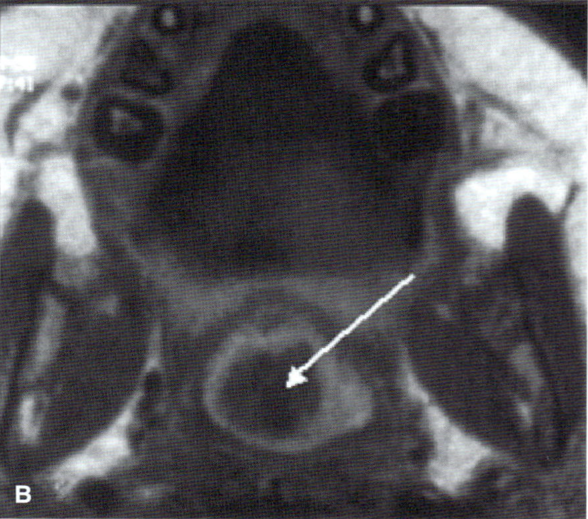

FIGURE 30–17 ■ MRI T_1-weighted image. Antrachoanal polyp in a 5-year-old child. **(A)** Arrows point to the cystic character of the antrachoanal polyp (right side). Right nasal cavity obstructed, left nasal cavity is free. **(B)** Choanal part of the polyp obstructing the nasopharynx.

Mucoceles are epithelial-lined mucus-containing sacs that fill the whole sinus or a compartment of the sinus. They can originate from the sinus mucosa after chronic infection, or iatrogenic or external trauma of the sinuses. Pressure on the bone from the mucocele can flatten or deform the bony contour of the sinuses. The diagnosis is confirmed by computed tomography scan (to visualize the bony structures) and magnetic resonance imaging (to confirm compartmentalization). It is important to know before the surgery the existence of compartmentalization to get an adequate surgical drainage of the mucocele during surgery.

Antrachoanal polyps are mucous polyps protruding from the choana. They are mostly unilateral and originate in the majority of cases from the maxillary sinus and can obstruct the nasopharynx (Figure 30–17). They mostly occur in children older than 10 years but the youngest patient seen by the author was only 3 years of age.[70] The cause of the disease is unclear but some theorize that the disease is a result of reflux. The symptoms are mainly unilateral purulent nasal secretions with a history of mouth breathing and snoring. The diagnosis is done by rigid endoscopy or fiberoscopy. Computed tomography scans will show the origin of the antrachoanal polyp, which is necessary for adequate surgical removal.

REFERENCES

1. Clement PA, Bluestone CD, Gordts F, et al. Management of rhinosinusitis in children: consensus meeting, Brussels, Belgium, September 13, 1996. *Arch Otolaryngol Head Neck Surg* .1998;124(1):31-34.
2. Meltzer EO, Hamilos DL, Hadley JA, et al. Rhinosinusitis: establishing definitions for clinical research and patient care. *Otolaryngol Head Neck Surg.* 2004;131(suppl 6):S1-62.
3. Clinical practice guideline: management of sinusitis. *Pediatrics.* 2001;108(3):798-808.
4. Gwaltney JM, Jr. Acute community-acquired sinusitis. *Clin Infect Dis.* 1996;23(6):1209-1223; quiz 24-5.
5. Gwaltney JM, Jr, Phillips CD, Miller RD, Riker DK. Computed tomographic study of the common cold. *N Engl J Med.* 1994;330(1):25-30.
6. Wald ER. Sinusitis in children. *Israel J Med Sci.* 1994;30 (5-6):403-407.
7. Wald ER, Guerra N, Byers C. Upper respiratory tract infections in young children: duration of and frequency of complications. *Pediatrics.* 1991;87(2):129-133.
8. Ueda D, Yoto Y. The ten-day mark as a practical diagnostic approach for acute paranasal sinusitis in children. *Pediatr Infect Dis J.* 1996;15(7):576-579.
9. Fireman P. Diagnosis of sinusitis in children: emphasis on the history and physical examination. *J Allergy Clin Immunol.* 1992;90(3, pt 2):433-436.
10. Clement PA, Gordts F. Epidemiology and prevalence of aspecific chronic sinusitis. *Int J Pediatr Otorhinolaryngol.* 1999;49(suppl 1):S101-S103.
11. Ray NF, Baraniuk JN, Thamer M, et al. Healthcare expenditures for sinusitis in 1996: contributions of asthma, rhinitis, and other airway disorders. *J Allergy Clin Immunol.* 1999;103(3, pt 1):408-414.
12. Puhakka T, Makela MJ, Alanen A, et al. Sinusitis in the common cold. *J Allergy Clin Immunol.* 1998;102(3):403-408.
13. Makela MJ, Puhakka T, Ruuskanen O, et al. Viruses and bacteria in the etiology of the common cold. *J Clin Microbiol.* 1998;36(2):539-542.
14. Wald ER, Milmoe GJ, Bowen A, Ledesma-Medina J, Salamon N, Bluestone CD. Acute maxillary sinusitis in children. *N Engl J Med.* 198126;304(13):749-754.
15. Wald ER, Byers C, Guerra N, Casselbrant M, Beste D. Subacute sinusitis in children. *J Pediatr.* 1989;115(1):28-32.
16. Brook I. Bacteriologic features of chronic sinusitis in children. *Jama.* 1981;246(9):967-969.
17. Muntz HR, Lusk RP. Bacteriology of the ethmoid bullae in children with chronic sinusitis. *Arch Otolaryngol Head Neck Surg.* 1991;117(2):179-181.
18. Orobello PW, Jr, Park RI, Belcher LJ, et al. Microbiology of chronic sinusitis in children. *Arch Otolaryngol Head Neck Surg.* 1991;117(9):980-983.
19. Otten FW, Grote JJ. Treatment of chronic maxillary sinusitis in children. *Int J Pediatr Otorhinolaryngol.* 1988;15(3):269-278.
20. Otten HW, Antvelink JB, Ruyter de Wildt H, Rietema SJ, Siemelink RJ, Hordijk GJ. Is antibiotic treatment of chronic sinusitis effective in children? *Clin Otolaryngol Allied Sci.* 1994;19(3):215-217.
21. Tinkelman DG, Silk HJ. Clinical and bacteriologic features of chronic sinusitis in children. *Am J Dis Child (1960).* 1989;143(8):938-941.
22. Anon JB, Rontal M, Zinreich SJ. *Anatomy of the Paranasal Sinuses.* New York: Thieme; 1996.
23. Wald ER. Rhinitis and acute and chronic sinusitis. In: Bluestone CD, Stool SE, Alper CM, et al., eds. *Pediatric Otolaryngology.* 4th ed. Philadelphia: Elsevier Science; 2003:995-1012.
24. Wald ER. Sinusitis. In: Long SS, ed. *Principles and Practice of Pediatric Infectious Disease.* 2nd ed. Philadelphia: Churchill Livingstone; 2003.
25. van der Veken PJ, Clement PAR, Buisseret TH. Age-related CT-scan study of the incidence of sinusitis in children. *Am J Rhinol.* 1992;6:45-48.
26. Gordts F, Clement PA, Destryker A, Desprechins B, Kaufman L. Prevalence of sinusitis signs on MRI in a non-ENT paediatric population. *Rhinology.* 1997;35(4):154-157.
27. Rachelefsky GS, Katz RM, Siegel SC. Chronic sinusitis in the allergic child. *Pediatr Clin North Am.* 1988;35(5): 1091-1101.
28. Barr MB, Weiss ST, Segal MR, Tager IB, Speizer FE. The relationship of nasal disorders to lower respiratory tract symptoms and illness in a random sample of children. *Pediatr Pulmonol.* 1992;14(2):91-94.
29. Esposito S, Bosis S, Bellasio M, Principi N. From clinical practice to guidelines: how to recognize rhinosinusitis in children. *Pediatr Allergy Immunol.* 2007;18 (suppl 18):53-55.
30. Zacharisen M, Casper R. Pediatric sinusitis. *Immunol Allergy Clin North Am.* 2005;25(2):313-332, vii.
31. Wang D, Clement P, Kaufman L, Derde MP. Fiberoptic examination of the nasal cavity and nasopharynx in children. *Int J Pediatr Otorhinolaryngol.* 1992;24(1):35-44.
32. Clement PAR. Management of sinusitis in infants and young children. In: Schaefer SD, ed. *Rhinology and Sinus Disease: A Problem-Oriented Approach.* St. Louis, MO: Mosby; 1998:105-134.

33. Lund VJ, Neijens HJ, Clement PA, Lusk R, Stammberger H. The treatment of chronic sinusitis: a controversial issue. *Int J Pediatr Otorhinolaryngol.* 1995;32 (suppl):S21-S35.
34. Brihaye P, Clement PA, Dab I, Desprechin B. Pathological changes of the lateral nasal wall in patients with cystic fibrosis (mucoviscidosis). *Int J Pediatr Otorhinolaryngol.* 1994;28(2-3):141-147.
35. Bush A. Primary ciliary dyskinesia. *Acta Otorhinolaryngol Belg.* 2000;54(3):317-324.
36. Gilger MA. Pediatric otolaryngologic manifestations of gastroesophageal reflux disease. *Curr Gastroenterol Rep.* 2003;5(3):247-252.
37. Nuhoglu Y, Nuhoglu C, Sirlioglu E, Ozcay S. Does recurrent sinusitis lead to a sinusitis remodeling of the upper airways in asthmatic children with chronic rhinitis? *J Investig Allergol Clin Immunol.* 2003;13(2):99-102.
38. Smart BA, Slavin RG. Rhinosinusitis and pediatric asthma. *Immunol Allergy Clin North Am.* 2005;25(1):67-82.
39. Wald ER. Microbiology of acute and chronic sinusitis in children. *J Allergy Clin Immunol.* 1992;90(3, pt 2):452-456.
40. Kovatch AL, Wald ER, Ledesma-Medina J, Chiponis DM, Bedingfield B. Maxillary sinus radiographs in children with nonrespiratory complaints. *Pediatrics.* 1984;73(3):306-308.
41. Wald ER, Chiponis D, Ledesma-Medina J. Comparative effectiveness of amoxicillin and amoxicillin–clavulanate potassium in acute paranasal sinus infections in children: a double-blind, placebo-controlled trial. *Pediatrics.* 1986;77(6):795-800.
42. Antimicrobial treatment guidelines for acute bacterial rhinosinusitis. Sinus and Allergy Health Partnership. *Otolaryngol Head Neck Surg.* 2000;123(1, pt 2):5-31.
43. Mafee MF, Tran BH, Chapa AR. Imaging of rhinosinusitis and its complications: plain film, CT, and MRI. *Clin Rev Allergy Immunol.* 2006;30(3):165-186.
44. Garbutt JM, Goldstein M, Gellman E, Shannon W, Littenberg B. A randomized, placebo-controlled trial of antimicrobial treatment for children with clinically diagnosed acute sinusitis. *Pediatrics.* 2001;107(4):619-625.
45. Williamson IG, Rumsby K, Benge S, et al. Antibiotics and topical nasal steroid for treatment of acute maxillary sinusitis: a randomized controlled trial. *Jama.* 2007;298(21): 2487-2496.
46. Wald ER. Sinusitis. *Pediatr Ann.* 1998;27(12):811-818.
47. Pichichero ME. Short course antibiotic therapy for respiratory infections: a review of the evidence. *Pediatr Infect Dis J.* 2000;19(9):929-937.
48. Diagnosis and management of acute otitis media. *Pediatrics.* 2004;113(5):1451-1465.
49. Block SL, Harrison CJ, Hedrick JA, et al. Penicillin-resistant *Streptococcus pneumoniae* in acute otitis media: risk factors, susceptibility patterns and antimicrobial management. *Pediatr Infect Dis J.* 1995;14(9):751-759.
50. Levine OS, Farley M, Harrison LH, Lefkowitz L, McGeer A, Schwartz B. Risk factors for invasive pneumococcal disease in children: a population-based case–control study in North America. *Pediatrics.* 1999;103(3):E28.
51. Critchley IA, Brown SD, Traczewski MM, Tillotson GS, Janjic N. National and regional assessment of antimicrobial resistance among community-acquired respiratory tract pathogens identified in a 2005-2006 U.S. Faropenem surveillance study. *Antimicrob Agents Chemother.* 2007; 51(12):4382-4389.
52. Sahm DF, Benninger MS, Evangelista AT, Yee YC, Thornsberry C, Brown NP. Antimicrobial resistance trends among sinus isolates of *Streptococcus pneumoniae* in the United States (2001–2005). *Otolaryngol Head Neck Surg.* 2007;136(3):385-389.
53. Wald ER. Chronic sinusitis in children. *J Pediatr.* 1995;127(3):339-347.
54. Kuehn BM. FDA warns of adverse events linked to smoking cessation drug and antiepileptics. *Jama.* 2008;299(10): 1121-1122.
55. Meltzer EO, Charous BL, Busse WW, Zinreich SJ, Lorber RR, Danzig MR. Added relief in the treatment of acute recurrent sinusitis with adjunctive mometasone furoate nasal spray. The Nasonex Sinusitis Group. *J Allergy Clin Immunol.* 2000;106(4):630-637.
56. Meltzer EO, Orgel HA, Backhaus JW, et al. Intranasal flunisolide spray as an adjunct to oral antibiotic therapy for sinusitis. *J Allergy Clin Immunol.* 1993;92(6):812-823.
57. Barlan IB, Erkan E, Bakir M, Berrak S, Basaran MM. Intranasal budesonide spray as an adjunct to oral antibiotic therapy for acute sinusitis in children. *Ann Allergy Asthma Immunol.* 1997;78(6):598-601.
58. Scadding GK. Recent advances in the treatment of rhinitis and rhinosinusitis. *Int J Pediatr Otorhinolaryngol.* 2003;67(suppl 1):S201-S204.
59. Steele RW. Chronic sinusitis in children. *Clin Pediatr (Phila).* 2005;44(6):465-471.
60. Gwaltney JM, Jr, Hendley JO, Phillips CD, Bass CR, Mygind N, Winther B. Nose blowing propels nasal fluid into the paranasal sinuses. *Clin Infect Dis.* 2000;30(2):387-391.
61. Clement P, Chovanova H. Pressures generated during nose blowing in patients with nasal complaints and normal test subjects. *Rhinology.* 2003;41(3):152-158.
62. Coticchia J, Zuliani G, Coleman C, et al. Biofilm surface area in the pediatric nasopharynx: chronic rhinosinusitis vs obstructive sleep apnea. *Arch Otolaryngol Head Neck Surg.* 2007;133(2):110-114.
63. Ramadan HH. Adenoidectomy vs endoscopic sinus surgery for the treatment of pediatric sinusitis. *Arch Otolaryngol Head Neck Surg.* 1999;125(11):1208-1211.
64. Ungkanont K, Damrongsak S. Effect of adenoidectomy in children with complex problems of rhinosinusitis and associated diseases. *Int J Pediatr Otorhinolaryngol.* 2004;68(4):447-451.
65. Adappa ND, Coticchia JM. Management of refractory chronic rhinosinusitis in children. *Am J Otolaryngol.* 2006;27(6):384-389.
66. Mitchell R, Kelly J, Wagner J. Bilateral orbital complications of pediatric rhinosinusitis. *Arch Otolaryngol Head Neck Surg.* 2002;128(8):971-974.
67. Hermann BW, Chung JC, Eisenbeis JF, Forsen JWJ. Intracranial complications of pediatric frontal sinusitis. *Am J Rhinol.* 2006;20:320-324.
68. Herrmann BW, Forsen JW, Jr. Simultaneous intracranial and orbital complications of acute rhinosinusitis in children. *Int J Pediatr Otorhinolaryngol.* 2004;68(5):619-625.
69. Lerner DN, Choi SS, Zalzal GH, Johnson DL. Intracranial complications of sinusitis in childhood. *Ann Otol Rhinol Laryngol.* 1995;104(4, pt 1):288-293.
70. Gordts F, Clement PA. Unusual choanal polyps. *Acta Otorhinolaryngol Belg.* 1997;51(3):177-180.

CHAPTER 31

Croup

Robert Bruce Wright and Terry Klassen

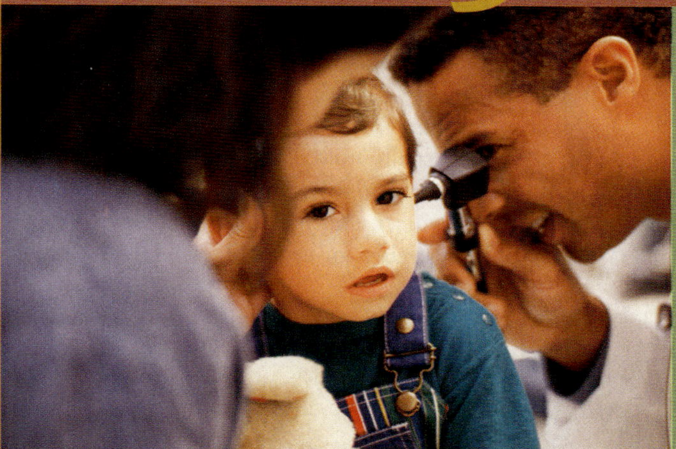

DEFINITION AND EPIDEMIOLOGY

Croup (acute laryngotracheobronchitis) is a respiratory illness of childhood and one of the most common causes of upper airway obstruction in children. Physicians should be comfortable with the disease as it will be one of the most frequent presentations of acute stridor in children to the office or emergency setting. In the United States, it is estimated to affect around 3% of the population and is most common in children aged 6 months to 6 years with the largest number of cases seen in those between 1 and 2 years of age.[1] Reinfection and recurrence of croup is common. The ratio of males to females with croup is 1.43:1.[1] There are two seasonal peaks of croup in North America, the first in autumn and the second in late winter.[1] Because of biennial increases in viral epidemics, the number of croup cases is 50% higher in odd-numbered years when compared to even-numbered years.[2]

Clinical symptoms of croup include a hoarse voice, a seal-like barky cough and stridor. As croup symptoms worsen, respiratory distress and occasionally cyanosis can appear. Symptoms typically worsen when the child is agitated and at nighttime. Fortunately croup symptoms are short-lived with the majority (60%) having resolution within 48 hours,[3] and only a small portion having symptoms lasting up to 1 week.[3] The majority of children with croup can be managed as outpatients with less than 5% requiring admission.[4–6] For those children requiring hospitalization, the need for endotracheal intubation is rare (1–5%)[7] and mortality is extremely rare.[7,8]

PATHOGENESIS

Localized inflammation of the upper airway caused by an upper respiratory tract infection leads to varying degrees of airway obstruction and the range of symptoms seen in croup. Specifically, the infection causes the mucosa of the vocal folds and subglottis become erythematous and swollen.[9] The subglottic area is the narrowest part of the airway and any edema affects the lumen negatively. This narrowing disrupts airflow resulting in the barky seal-like cough, stridor and increased work of breathing (indrawing).

The most common viral etiologic agents for croup are parainfluenza viruses types 1 and 3. One study showed they were responsible for greater than 65% of the cases of croup.[1] Most recently, human metapneumovirus has been identified as another etiologic agent for croup.[10]

Table 31–1 lists the most common infectious and noninfectious causes of croup.

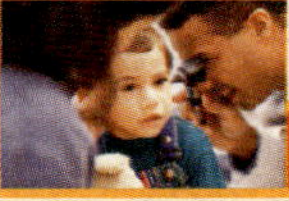

Table 31–1.

Etiologic Agents of Croup

Infectious
Parainfluenza types 1 and 3
Respiratory syncytial virus (RSV)
Parainfluenza type 2
Influenza type A and B
Mycoplasma pneumoniae
Human metapneumovirus
Noninfectious
Gastroesophageal reflux disease (GERD)
Postintubation
Foreign body aspiration

Adapted from Denny FW, Murphy TF, Clyde WA, Jr., Collier AM, Henderson FW. Croup: An 11-year study in a pediatric practice. Pediatrics. 1983;71(6):871–876; and Crowe JE, Jr. Human metapneumovirus as a major cause of human respiratory tract disease. Pediatr Infect Dis J. 2004;23(11 Suppl):S215–S221.

CLINICAL PRESENTATION

The clinical history for children that present with croup is fairly typical. Parents will tell the health care providers that their child was well during the day apart from upper respiratory tract infection symptoms. If fever is present, it is usually mild. They may or may not have symptoms of a hoarse voice. Within 24 hours the symptoms acutely worsen and the child often develops stridor. This rapid change prompts the family to seek medical attention.

Croup symptoms are usually classified into mild, moderate, and severe and are based upon the Westley croup score (Table 31–2).[11] Symptoms of croup (barky seal-like cough and stridor) almost always begin in the night time. If the child develops severe respiratory distress, they may appear agitated but do not drool or appear toxic. Respiratory failure is often preceded by a change in mental status such as fatigue, pallor or cyanosis, and decreasing stridor, breath sounds, and chest wall retractions.[11–14]

DIFFERENTIAL DIAGNOSIS

The diagnosis of croup is a clinical one. Most children presenting with an acute onset of upper airway obstruction with hoarse voice, barky 'seal like' cough and stridor will have croup.[3,6] Table 31–3 lists the most common differential diagnoses for croup. Of those listed, particular note should be made of both bacterial tracheitis and epiglottitis. These two diseases may be confused with croup but often the symptoms are more severe and the child appears much more toxic. Bacterial tracheitis, a true infection of the trachea and a complication of croup,[15] occurs as a secondary bacterial superinfection in patients with a viral respiratory disease.[16–18] The most common bacterial agents that have been implicated in bacterial tracheitis are: *Staphylococcus aureus,* group A *Streptococcus,* and *Moraxella catarrhalis. Streptococcus pneumoniae* and *Haemophilus influenzae* have also been cultured but are less common because of current immunization practices.[15,18–22] Children who have a high fever, appear toxic, and have a poor response to initial treatment of croup should be considered to have bacterial tracheitis.[15,18] Administration of broad-spectrum antibiotics is the mainstay of treatment in bacterial tracheitis along with close monitoring of the patients airway status in the intensive care unit. Intubation rates vary from 57% to 80% and mortality figures are zero to 21%.[16,17,23,24]

Epiglottitis, although rare since wide spread use of the *H. influenzae* B vaccine,[25,26] is another important

Table 31–2.

Westley Croup Score

Symptom	Score	
Stridor	None	0
	When agitated	1
	At rest	2
Retractions	None	0
	Mild	1
	Moderate	2
	Severe	3
Air entry	Normal	0
	Decreased	1
	Markedly decreased	2
Cyanosis in room air	None	0
	With agitation	4
	At rest	5
Level of consciousness	Normal	0
	Disorientated	5
Total score		0–17

Note: *Mild croup, 1–2; Moderate croup, 3–8; Severe croup, >8*

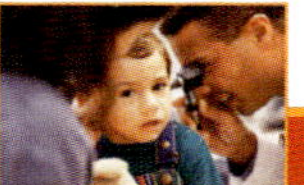

Table 31–3.

Differential Diagnoses of Croup and Associated Symptoms

Common	
Bacterial Tracheitis	Prolonged symptoms of croup Toxic appearing Poor response to standard treatment or requires repeated doses of racemic epinephrine
Epiglottitis	Short history Very sore throat, drooling, and dysphagia Toxic appearing Cough absent
Peritonsilar abscess	Sore throat Muffled voice with drooling and dysphagia
Retropharyngeal abscess	Fever Sore neck with lateral movement or extension
Foreign Body Aspiration	Coughing spell prior to symptoms Stridor is often biphasic
Rare	
Hereditary angioedema	Sudden onset Nontoxic appearing
Uvulitis	Sore throat
Hemangioma	Seen on endoscopy
Neoplasm	May have other systemic signs (weakness, pallor)

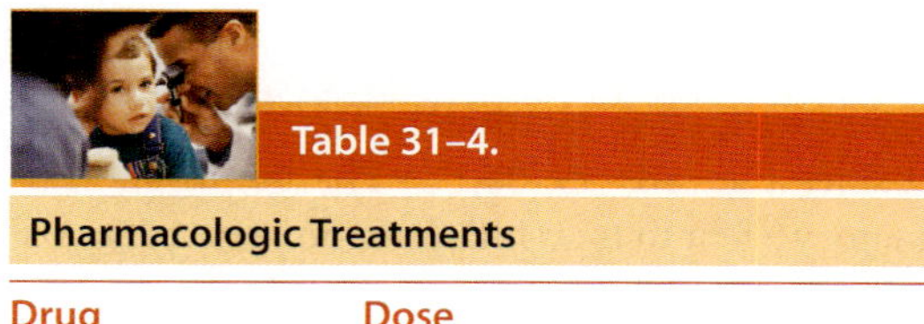

Table 31–4.

Pharmacologic Treatments

Drug	Dose
Epinephrine	0.5 mL in 2.5 mL of a 2.25% racemic solution via nebulizer 5 mL of L-epinephrine (1:1000) solution via nebulizer
Dexamethasone	0.6 mg/kg orally or intramuscular once (May be repeated if symptoms still persistent >24 h for an additional dose)
Budesonide	2 mg (2 mL) solution via nebulizer

potential diagnosis. Children present with a high fever and toxic appearance that is typically abrupt in onset. They will also have symptoms of stridor, drooling, and dysphagia and may be quite anxious. Children often sit in the forward "sniffing" position which aids in maintaining airway patency. If epiglottitis is suspected, leave the child in a position of comfort (usually with the parent), decrease stimuli, and have someone who is skilled in advanced airway management prepare to secure the child's airway.

DIAGNOSIS

As mentioned earlier, the diagnosis of croup is a clinical one. Radiological studies are useful to help exclude other diagnoses but are rarely helpful in diagnosing croup.[27] Therefore, for those patients who present with the classic history and clinical symptoms of croup, treatment should not be delayed for radiographs.[28] If radiographs are preformed after initial management, the lateral and anteroposterior neck X-rays will show the classic "steeple sign" which is caused by subglottic narrowing (Figure 31–1). A membrane in the trachea as well as a ragged tracheal contour suggests bacterial tracheitis[15,20,29,30] (Figure 31–2). Findings of thickened aryepiglottic folds and epiglottis suggest epiglottitis.[31] A widened soft tissue space of the posterior pharynx is suspicious for retropharyngeal abscess[31] (Figure 31–3).

Two Canadian studies recommended against the use of routine bronchoscopy in croup and stated that bronchoscopy should only be used when the diagnosis is severely in question, when the case is prolonged, or nonresolving in spite of optimal medical management.[32,33] Both studies also stated that if endoscopy is used, caution should be taken to avoid further damage to the vocal chords and subglottic area.[32,33]

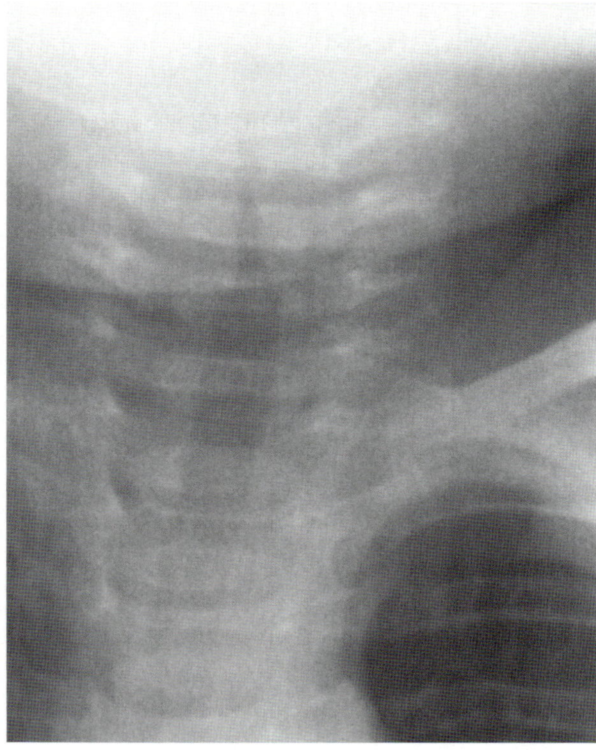

FIGURE 31–1 ■ AP radiograph showing the classic "steeple sign" caused by subglottic narrowing in croup.

MANAGEMENT

Table 31–4 and Figure 31–4 outline recommended medications and management used in the treatment of croup in the emergency department (ED) setting.

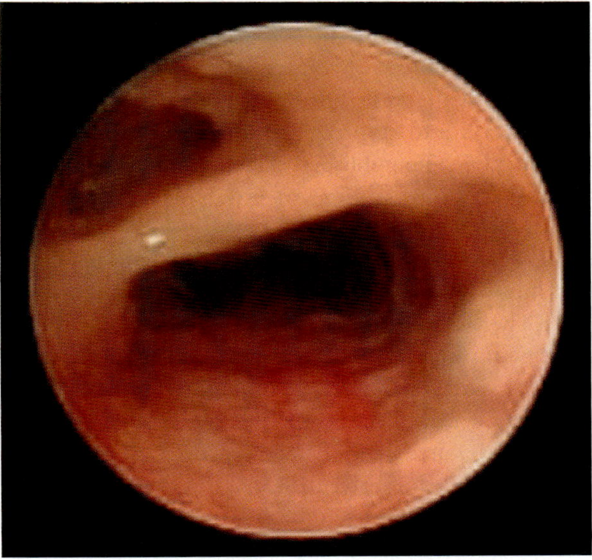

FIGURE 31–2 ■ Photograph of tracheal endoscopy showing pseudomembrane in bacterial tracheitis.

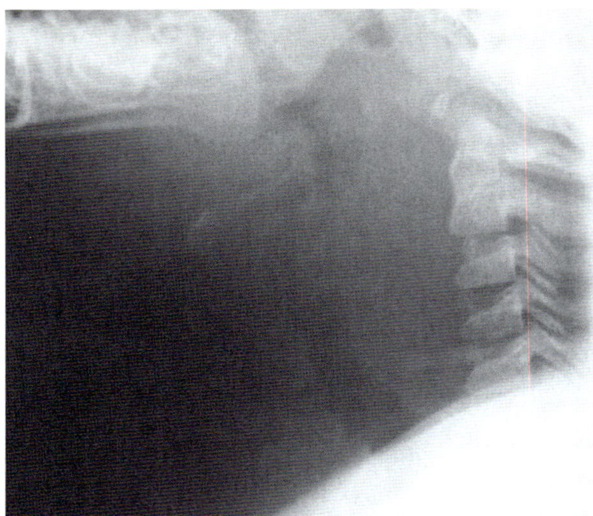

FIGURE 31–3 ■ Soft tissue neck radiograph showing a widened soft tissue space suggestive of a retropharyngeal abscess.

TREATMENT

Cold Air

Of those children who present to the ED with croup, the parents will often state that their child's symptoms have improved en route to the hospital. Although not clinically or scientifically proven, parents will anecdotally attribute the resolve of symptoms to cold air exposure. It is hypothesized that the cold air soothes the airway and helps to decrease the swelling of the subglottic area.

Mist Therapy

Often parents will also state that they have tried some form of mist therapy prior to arrival in the ED. It is thought that the act of comforting the child in the parent's arms while mist is being administered may soothe the airways and improve symptoms. Unfortunately, there has been no published evidence to support the use of mist in the treatment of croup.[14,34–37] In 2007, a Cochrane review by Moore and Little concluded that the croup score of children that are managed in the ED will not improve greatly with the inhalation of humidified air.[35] There are also potential risks to using mist in the treatment of croup. Several studies have demonstrated that there may be bacterial contamination in the mist that may cause infection or hypersensitivity reactions that could worsen the disease process.[38–41] Mist tents, often used to administer mist therapy, are also discouraged because they worsen the child's anxiety by separating him from the parents, preclude rapid and accurate evaluation of the child, and may precipitate bronchospasm in susceptible children, potentially compounding the croup-related respiratory distress.

Corticosteroids

Corticosteroids for the treatment of croup have been debated since the early 1970s.[42–44] The use of an anti-inflammatory agent to treat inflammation and edema of the subglottic area makes intuitive sense.[45] Several forms of corticosteroids have been used in the treatment of croup; the most common being dexamethasone followed by budesonide.[46] However methylprednisolone, betamethasone, and fluticasone have also been used[46,47] (Table 31–4). The onset of action of corticosteroids to decrease symptoms in croup was initially thought to be approximately 6–8 hours, but recent studies have demonstrated that the beneficial effects of corticosteroids occur as early as 2 hours after corticosteroid administration.[48–50] One dose of dexamethasone is usually all that is needed because of its long half-life and bioavailability (up to 82 h).[51] Most children will have resolution of symptoms approximately 72 hours after medical assessment and administration of corticosteroids.[52]

Several well-designed, randomized, placebo-controlled clinical trials and systematic reviews have all demonstrated the effectiveness of corticosteroids in reducing symptoms in all forms of croup (mild, moderate, and severe) in both the inpatient and outpatient setting.[4,46,52–55] For mild croup (Westley score < 3), there have been three studies that have demonstrated a clear benefit in the administration of corticosteroids.[52,56,57] In one study patients received a single dose of 0.15 mg/kg of dexamethasone compared to placebo. The treatment group had a significant reduction in repeat visits to medical care with ongoing croup symptoms compared with the placebo group.[56] Another study looked at those patients with mild croup and allocated them to receive either 0.6 mg/kg of oral dexamethasone, 160 μg of inhaled budesonide, or placebo. Both steroid groups had a faster resolution of croup symptoms compared with the placebo group and were less likely to seek medical attention in the week-after treatment.[57] The most recent study by Bjornson et al. demonstrated that those children who received a single dose of 0.6 mg/kg of dexamethasone when compared to placebo had a significantly less chance of returning to medical care and faster resolution of symptoms.[52] Other added benefits in the 48 hours after treatment was a decrease in parental anxiety and less lost sleep.[52] The authors also concluded that there was a small but significant economic benefit to both the health care system and families in the dexamethasone group.[52] An average savings of $21 was seen per child.[52]

In treatment of patients with moderate croup (Westley score 3–8), a systematic review found that there was a significant reduction in the Westley score at both 6 and 12 hours posttreatment. Fewer readmissions and/or return visits to medical care as well as decreased length of stay in the ED or hospital were also noted. Of note

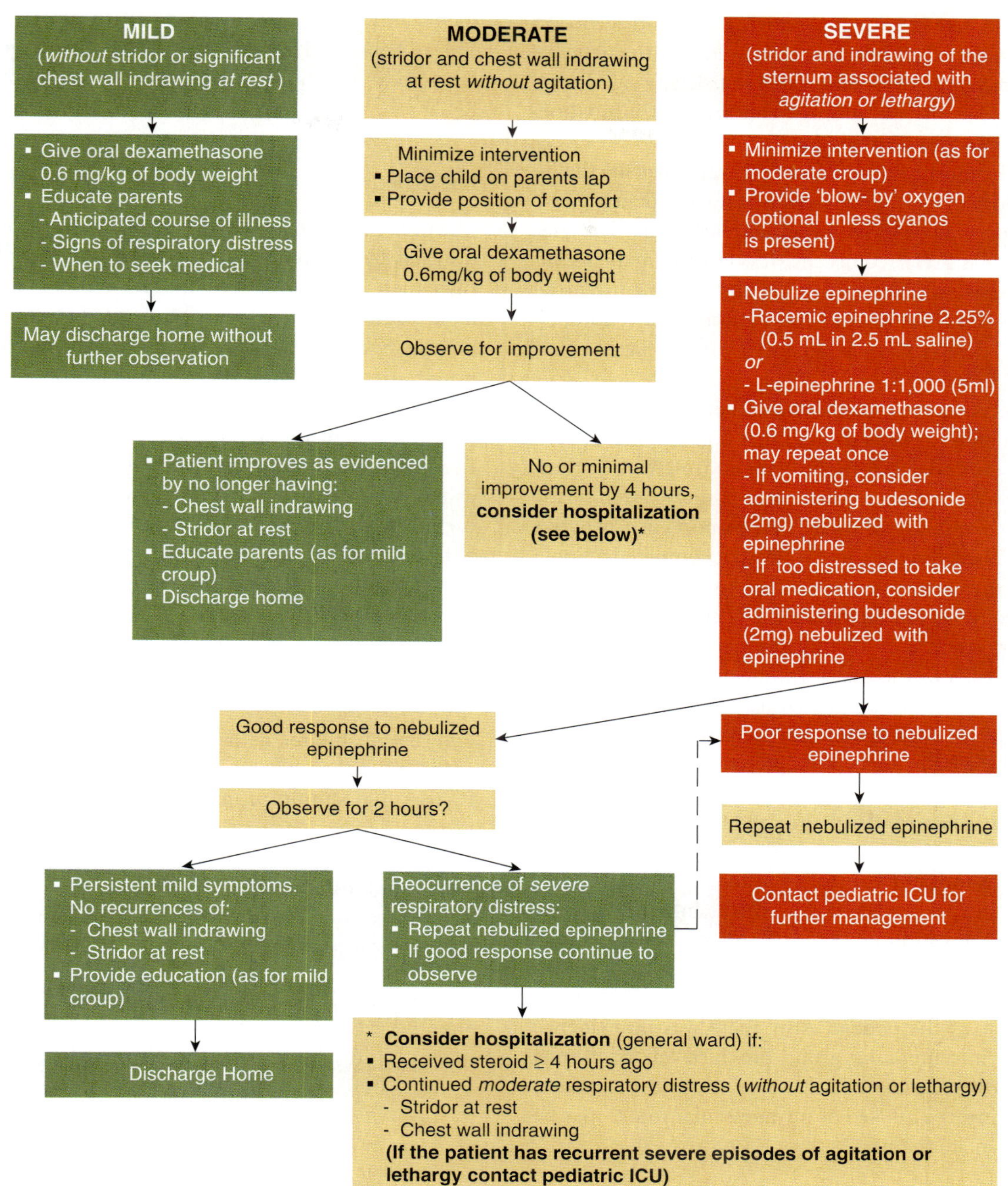

MILD
(without stridor or significant chest wall indrawing at rest)
▪ Give oral dexamethasone 0.6 mg/kg of body weight
▪ Educate parents
- Anticipated course of illness
- Signs of respiratory distress
- When to seek medical
May discharge home without further observation
MODERATE
(stridor and chest wall indrawing at rest without agitation)
Minimize intervention
▪ Place child on parents lap
▪ Provide position of comfort
Give oral dexamethasone 0.6mg/kg of body weight
Observe for improvement
▪ Patient improves as evidenced by no longer having:
- Chest wall indrawing
- Stridor at rest
▪ Educate parents (as for mild croup)
▪ Discharge home
No or minimal improvement by 4 hours, consider hospitalization (see below)*
SEVERE
(stridor and indrawing of the sternum associated with agitation or lethargy)
▪ Minimize intervention (as for moderate croup)
▪ Provide 'blow- by' oxygen (optional unless cyanos is present)
▪ Nebulize epinephrine
-Racemic epinephrine 2.25% (0.5 mL in 2.5 mL saline)
or
- L-epinephrine 1:1,000 (5ml)
▪ Give oral dexamethasone (0.6 mg/kg of body weight); may repeat once
- If vomiting, consider administering budesonide (2mg) nebulized with epinephrine
- If too distressed to take oral medication, consider administering budesonide (2mg) nebulized with epinephrine
Good response to nebulized epinephrine
Observe for 2 hours?
▪ Persistent mild symptoms. No recurrences of:
- Chest wall indrawing
- Stridor at rest
▪ Provide education (as for mild croup)
Discharge Home
Reocurrence of severe respiratory distress:
▪ Repeat nebulized epinephrine
▪ If good response continue to observe
Poor response to nebulized epinephrine
Repeat nebulized epinephrine
Contact pediatric ICU for further management
* Consider hospitalization (general ward) if:
▪ Received steroid ≥ 4 hours ago
▪ Continued moderate respiratory distress (without agitation or lethargy)
- Stridor at rest
- Chest wall indrawing
(If the patient has recurrent severe episodes of agitation or lethargy contact pediatric ICU)

FIGURE 31–4 ■ Proposed management plan for croup in the emergency department setting. (*From Johnson DW, Klassen TP, Kellner JD, et al. "Croup" Working Committee. Guideline for the diagnosis and management of croup. Alberta Med Associat Clin Pract Guide. 2008.*)

there was also a decrease in the usage of racemic epinephrine treatment when compared with placebo.[46]

For inpatients that had severe croup (Westley score >8), several well-designed studies promote the use of steroids for treatment. First, a 1989-meta-analysis found that in those patients who received corticosteroid treatment when compared to placebo, there was a significant reduction in symptoms and clinical improvement at both 12 and 24 hours posttreatment.[55] There were also significantly fewer intubations of patients with croup for the same time period.[55] This was additionally supported by a second study from Western Australia.[48] This study reviewed admitted croup patients over a 16-year period that received corticosteroids. The authors found them to have a decrease in number of ICU days, intubations, and overall length of stay in the hospital[48]; therefore, leading to their recommendation that all patients should receive corticosteroids in the treatment of croup.[48] Finally, two randomized controlled trials by Rivera[58] and Tibballs[59] comparing intubated croup patients receiving either placebo or prednisolone until extubation showed that the patients who received prednisolone had a statistically significant reduction in the duration of endotracheal intubation and the need for reintubation.[58,59]

The most common dose of dexamethasone that is used today is 0.6 mg/kg. This is most frequently given orally but may be given intramuscularly if needed. The oral route is preferred because it is less traumatic to the patient, has excellent absorption and serum concentrations peak as fast as with intramuscular injection.[51,60] The oral dose is also tolerated well with vomiting being a rare occurrence.[52]

As far as the dose that is most effective in croup, a meta-analysis in 1989 showed that higher doses of corticosteroids (0.3–0.6 mg/kg) are more effective than lower doses.[55] This resulted in a clinically significant improvement of patients at 12 hours post corticosteroid dose.[55] There has been one study that compared a single dose of 0.15 mg/kg versus 0.3 mg/kg versus 0.6 mg/kg in the effectiveness in the treatment of croup. The authors found no difference in improvement of croup symptoms in each of the treatment groups.[61] Unfortunately the study was not designed to test equivalence and the study size in each group may have been too small to detect a clinically important difference between all three dosing groups.[46,61]

The route of administration of corticosteroids has been debated also. As a result, there have been a total of seven randomized controlled studies comparing parenteral, intramuscular or oral, versus inhaled corticosteroid administration.[26,49,57,62–66] All studies concluded that the oral route was superior to the intramuscular route with regards to ease of administration and was less traumatic to the patient. Also, there was no evidence that the intramuscular group provided any additional benefit when compared to the oral route. If the patient is vomiting, the inhaled or intramuscular routes may be used as an alternative.

Racemic Epinephrine

The first description of using racemic epinephrine in the treatment of croup was back in 1971 by Adair and colleagues.[67] A dose of 0.5 mL of a solution of 2.25% of racemic epinephrine is given via nebulizer over 5–10 minutes. If racemic epinephrine is not available, a dose of 5 mL of L-epinephrine (1:1000) may be given to achieve the same effect.[68,69] Since then, there have been several studies demonstrating the effectiveness of racemic epinephrine when compared to placebo in improving croup scores within the first 30 minutes after receiving treatment.[11,12,26,34,70] The clinical effect of racemic epinephrine is present for at least 1 hour and essentially nonexistent after 2 hours.[11,12,34] With the addition of oral dexamethasone or inhaled budesonide, the child, who has been treated with racemic epinephrine and observed for a period of 2–4 hours if symptom free, may be safely discharged home from the ED.[50,62,71–73]

Heliox

The use of helium for therapy in upper airway obstruction has been reported since 1934 by Barach.[74] Since then there have been several small studies that have looked at its use in the form of heliox (a helium–oxygen mixture at a ratio of 80:20 or 70:30) administered by a non–rebreather mask for the alleviation of croup symptoms. Heliox is thought to provide increased laminar airflow through the narrowed airway, thereby decreasing the mechanical work of breathing. Heliox cannot be used to treat children who require supplemental oxygen >30%. Most authors concluded that although heliox may alleviate symptoms of croup, it is not superior to other conventional treatments (i.e., racemic epinephrine).[75–78]

COURSE AND PROGNOSIS

Only 2% of children with croup require hospitalization; of these, less than 1.5% require endotracheal intubation. Factors that should prompt hospitalization include a history of severe obstructive symptoms prior to presentation, a congenital or acquired airway anomaly (e.g., subglottic stenosis), age younger than 6 months, stridor at rest, inadequate oral intake, extreme parental anxiety, or worsening symptoms.

REFERENCES

1. Denny FW, Murphy TF, Clyde WA, Jr., Collier AM, Henderson FW. Croup: an 11-year study in a pediatric practice. *Pediatrics.* 1983;71(6):871-876.
2. Marx A, Torok TJ, Holman RC, Clarke MJ, Anderson LJ. Pediatric hospitalizations for croup (Laryngotracheobronchitis): biennial increases associated with human parainfluenza virus 1 epidemics. *J Infect Dis.* 1997;176(6):1423-1427.
3. Johnson DW. Croup: duration of symptoms and impact on family functioning. *Pediatr Res.* 2001;49:83A.
4. Segal AO, Crighton EJ, Moineddin R, Mamdani M, Upshur RE. Croup hospitalizations in ontario: A 14-year time-series analysis. *Pediatrics.* 2005;116(1):51-55.
5. To T, Dick P, Young W, et al. Hospitalization rates of children with croup in ontario. *Paediatr child health.* 1996;1:103-108.
6. Johnson DW. Health care utilization by children with croup in alberta. *Pediatr Res.* 2003;53:185.
7. Baugh R, Gilmore BB, Jr. Infectious croup: a critical review. *Otolaryngol Head Neck Surg.* 1986;95(1):40-46.
8. Mceniery J, Gillis J, Kilham H, Benjamin B. Review of intubation in severe laryngotracheobronchitis. *Pediatrics.* 1991;87(6):847-853.

9. Jd C. *Croup (Laryngitis, Laryngotracheitis, Spasmodic Croup, Laryngotracheobronchitis, Bacterial Tracheitis and Laryngotracheobronchopneumonitis)*. 4th ed. Philadelphia: WB Saunders; 1998.
10. Crowe JE, Jr. Human metapneumovirus as a major cause of human respiratory tract disease. *Pediatr Infect Dis J.* 2004;23(11 suppl):S215-S221.
11. Westley CR, Cotton EK, Brooks JG. Nebulized racemic epinephrine by IPPB for the treatment of croup: a double-blind study. *Am J Dis Child.* 1978;132(5): 484-487.
12. Taussig LM, Castro O, Beaudry PH, Fox WW, Bureau M. Treatment of laryngotracheobronchitis (croup). Use of intermittent positive-pressure breathing and racemic epinephrine. *Am J Dis Child.* 1975;129(7): 790-793.
13. Leipzig B, Oski FA, Cummings CW, Stockman JA, Swender P. A prospective randomized study to determine the efficacy of steroids in treatment of croup. *J Pediatr.* 1979;94(2):194-196.
14. Bourchier D, Dawson KP, Fergusson DM. Humidification in viral croup: a controlled trial. *Aust Paediatr J.* 1984;20(4):289-291.
15. Jones R, Santos JI, Overall JC, Jr. Bacterial tracheitis. *JAMA.* 1979;242(8):721-726.
16. Liston SL, Gehrz RC, Jarvis CW. Bacterial tracheitis. *Arch Otolaryngol.* 1981;107(9):561-564.
17. Liston SL, Gehrz RC, Siegel LG, Tilelli J. Bacterial tracheitis. *Am J Dis Child.* 1983;137(8):764-767.
18. Donnelly BW, Mcmillan JA, Weiner LB. Bacterial tracheitis: report of eight new cases and review. *Rev Infect Dis.* 1990;12(5):729-735.
19. Edwards KM, Dundon MC, Altemeier WA. Bacterial tracheitis as a complication of viral croup. *Pediatr Infect Dis.* 1983;2(5):390-391.
20. Bernstein T, Brilli R, Jacobs B. Is bacterial tracheitis changing? A 14-month experience in a pediatric intensive care unit. *Clin Infect Dis.* 1998;27(3):458-462.
21. Hopkins A, Lahiri T, Salerno R, Heath B. Changing epidemiology of life-threatening upper airway infections: the reemergence of bacterial tracheitis. *Pediatrics.* 2006;118(4):1418-1421.
22. Kasian GF, Shafran SD, Shyleyko EM. Branhamella catarrhalis bronchopulmonary isolates in picu patients. *Pediatr Pulmonol.* 1989;7(3):128-132.
23. Gallagher PG, Myer CM, IIIrd. An approach to the diagnosis and treatment of membranous laryngotracheobronchitis in infants and children. *Pediatr Emerg Care.* 1991;7(6):337-342.
24. Kasian GF, Bingham WT, Steinberg J, et al. Bacterial tracheitis in children. *CMAJ.* 1989;140(1):46-50.
25. Shah RK, Roberson DW, Jones DT. Epiglottitis in the Hemophilus influenzae type B vaccine era: changing trends. *Laryngoscope.* 2004;114(3):557-560.
26. Progress towards eliminating Haemophilus influenzae type B disease among infants and children-United States, 1987-1997. *MMWR Morb Mortal Wkly Rep* 1998;47(46): 993-998.
27. Kaditis AG, Wald ER. Viral croup: current diagnosis and treatment. *Pediatr Infect Dis J.* 1998;17(9):827-834.
28. Johnson DW, Klassen TP, Kellner JD, et al. "Croup" Working Committee. Guideline for the diagnosis and management of croup. *Alberta Med Associat Clin Pract Guide.* 2008. Available: http://www.topalbertadoctors.org/top/cpg/croup
29. Friedman EM, Jorgensen K, Healy GB, Mcgill TJ. Bacterial tracheitis-two-year experience. *Laryngoscope.* 1985;95(1): 9-11.
30. Han BK, Dunbar JS, Striker TW. Membranous laryngotracheobronchitis (Membranous Croup). *AJR.* 1979; 133(1):53-58.
31. Le S. *Emergency Imaging of the Acutely Ill or Injured Child.* Philadelphia, PA: Lippincott, Williams, & Wilkins; 2000:624.
32. Sendi K, Crysdale WS, Yoo J. Tracheitis: outcome of 1700 cases presenting to the emergency department during 2 years. *J Otolaryngol.* 1992;21(1):20-24.
33. Tan AK, Manoukian JJ. Hospitalized croup (Bacterial and viral): the role of rigid endoscopy. *J Otolaryngol.* 1992;21(1):48-53.
34. Kristjansson S, Berg-Kelly K, Winso E. Inhalation of racemic adrenaline in the treatment of mild and moderately severe croup. Clinical symptom score and oxygen saturation measurements for evaluation of treatment effects. *Acta Paediatr.* 1994;83(11):1156-1160.
35. Moore M, Little P. Humidified air inhalation for treating croup. *Cochrane Database Syst Rev.* 2006;3:CD002870.
36. Neto GM, Kentab O, Klassen TP, Osmond MH. A randomized controlled trial of mist in the acute treatment of moderate croup. *Acad Emerg Med.* 2002;9(9):873-879.
37. Scolnik D, Coates AL, Stephens D, Da Silva Z, Lavine E, Schuh S. Controlled delivery of high vs low humidity vs mist therapy for croup in emergency departments: a randomized controlled trial. *JAMA.* 2006;295(11):1274-1280.
38. Chung JC, Choi JM, Lee HW, Hong SI, Kim CS. Hypersensitivity pneumonitis by a cool-mist vaporizer: a detailed microbiologic and immunologic study. *Korean J Intern Med.* 1989;4(2):174-177.
39. Hodges GR, Fink JN, Schlueter DP. Hypersensitivity pneumonitis caused by a contaminated cool-mist vaporizer. *Ann Intern Med.* 1974;80(4):501-504.
40. Van Assendelft A, Forsén KO, Keskinen H, Alanko K. Humidifier-associated extrinsic allergic alveolitis. *Scand J Work Environ Health.* 1979;5(1):35-41.
41. Dale BA, Williams J. Pseudomonas paucimobilis contamination of cool mist tents on a paediatric ward. *J Hosp Infect.* 1986;7(2):189-192.
42. Coffin LA, III. Corticosteroids in croup: is there a reply from the ivory tower? *Pediatrics.* 1971;48(3):493.
43. Menachof L. Corticosteroids in croup: reply from ground level. *Pediatrics.* 1972;49(1):154.
44. Tenenbein M. The steroid odyssey in croup. *Pediatrics.* 2005;116(1):230-231.
45. Wright RB, Rowe BH, Arent RJ, Klassen TP. Current pharmacological options in the treatment of croup. *Expert Opin Pharmacother.* 2005;6(2):255-261.
46. Russell K, Wiebe N, Saenz A, et al. Glucocorticoids for croup. *Cochrane Database Syst Rev.* 2004(1):CD001955.
47. Amir L, Hubermann H, Halevi A, Mor M, Mimouni M, Waisman Y. Oral betamethasone versus iIntramuscular dexamethasone for the treatment of mild to moderate viral croup: a prospective, randomized trial. *Pediatr Emerg Care.* 2006;22(8):541-544.
48. Geelhoed GC. Sixteen years of croup in a western Australian teaching hospital: effects of routine steroid treatment. *Ann Emerg Med.* 1996;28(6):621-626.

49. Johnson DW, Jacobson S, Edney PC, Hadfield P, Mundy Me, Schuh S. A comparison of nebulized budesonide, intramuscular dexamethasone, and placebo for moderately severe croup. *N Engl J Med.* 1998;339(8):498-503.
50. Kuusela AL, Vesikari T. A randomized double-blind, placebo-controlled trial of dexamethasone and racemic epinephrine in the treatment of croup. *Acta Paediatr Scand.* 1988;77(1):99-104.
51. Duggan DE, Yeh KC, Matalia N, Ditzler CA, Mcmahon FG. Bioavailability of oral dexamethasone. *Clin Pharmacol Ther.* 1975;18(2):205-209.
52. Bjornson CL, Klassen TP, Williamson J, et al. A randomized trial of a single dose of oral dexamethasone for mild croup. *N Engl J Med.* 2004;351(13):1306-1313.
53. Ausejo M, Saenz A, Pham B, et al. The effectiveness of glucocorticoids in treating croup: meta-analysis. *BMJ.* 1999;319(7210):595-600.
54. Griffin S, Ellis S, Fitzgerald-Barron A, Rose J, Egger M. Nebulised steroid in the treatment of croup: a systematic review of randomised controlled trials. *Br J Gen Pract.* 2000;50(451):135-141.
55. Kairys SW, Olmstead EM, O'connor GT. Steroid treatment of laryngotracheitis: a meta-analysis of the evidence from randomized trials. *Pediatrics.* 1989;83(5):683-693.
56. Geelhoed GC, Turner J, Macdonald WB. Efficacy of a small single dose of oral dexamethasone for outpatient croup: a double blind placebo controlled clinical trial. *BMJ.* 1996;313(7050):140-142.
57. Luria JW, Gonzalez-Del-Rey JA, Digiulio GA, Mcaneney CM, Olson JJ, Ruddy RM. Effectiveness of oral or nebulized dexamethasone for children with mild croup. *Arch Pediatr Adolesc Med.* 2001;155(12):1340-1345.
58. Rivera R, Tibballs J. Complications of endotracheal intubation and mechanical ventilation in infants and children. *Crit Care Med.* 1992;20(2):193-199.
59. Tibballs J, Shann FA, Landau LI. Placebo-controlled trial of prednisolone in children intubated for croup. *Lancet.* 1992;340(8822):745-748.
60. Richter O, Ern B, Reinhardt D, Becker B. Pharmacokinetics of dexamethasone in children. *Pediatr Pharmacol (New York).* 1983;3(3-4):329-337.
61. Geelhoed GC, Macdonald WB. Oral dexamethasone in the treatment of croup: 0.15 Mg/Kg versus 0.3 Mg/Kg versus 0.6 Mg/Kg. *Pediatr Pulmonol.* 1995;20(6):362-368.
62. Cetinkaya F, Tufekci BS, Kutluk G. A comparison of nebulized budesonide, and intramuscular, and oral dexamethasone for treatment of croup. *Int J Pediatr Otorhinolaryngol.* 2004;68(4):453-456.
63. Geelhoed GC. Budesonide offers no advantage when added to oral dexamethasone in the treatment of croup. *Pediatr Emerg Care.* 2005;21(6):359-362.
64. Geelhoed GC, Macdonald WB. Oral and inhaled steroids in croup: a randomized, placebo-controlled trial. *Pediatr Pulmonol.* 1995;20(6):355-361.
65. Klassen TP, Craig WR, Moher D, et al. Nebulized budesonide and oral dexamethasone for treatment of croup: a randomized controlled trial. *JAMA.* 1998;279(20): 1629-1632.
66. Pedersen LV, Dahl M, Falk-Petersen HE, Larsen SE. Inhaled budesonide versus intramuscular dexamethasone in the treatment of pseudo-croup. *Ugeskr Laeger.* 1998;160(15):2253-2256.
67. Adair JC, Ring WH, Jordan WS, Elwyn RA. Letter: racemic epinephrine in croup (Continued). *Pediatrics.* 1974;53(3):448.
68. Fraser B. Nebulized levo-epinephrine as an alternative to racemic epinephrine in pediatrics. *Can J Hosp Pharm.* 1995;48(5):303.
69. Waisman Y, Klein BL, Boenning DA, et al. Prospective randomized double-blind study comparing L-epinephrine and racemic epinephrine aerosols in the treatment of laryngotracheitis (croup). *Pediatrics.* 1992;89(2): 302-306.
70. Gardner HG, Powell KR, Roden VJ, Cherry JD. The evaluation of racemic epinephrine in the treatment of infectious croup. *Pediatrics.* 1973;52(1):52-55.
71. Kelley PB, Simon JE. Racemic epinephrine use in croup and disposition. *Am J Emerg Med.* 1992;10(3):181-183.
72. Ledwith CA, Shea LM, Mauro RD. Safety and efficacy of nebulized racemic epinephrine in conjunction with oral dexamethasone and mist in the outpatient treatment of croup. *Ann Emerg Med.* 1995;25(3):331-337.
73. Rizos JD, Digravio BE, Sehl MJ, Tallon JM. The disposition of children with croup treated with racemic epinephrine and dexamethasone in the emergency department. *J Emerg Med.* 1998;16(4):535-539.
74. Barach AL, Eckman M. The effects of inhalation of helium mixed with oxygen on the mechanics of respiration. *J Clin Invest.* 1936;15(1):47-61.
75. Beckmann KR, Brueggemann WM, Jr. Heliox treatment of severe croup. *Am J Emerg Med.* 2000;18(6):735-736.
76. Duncan PG. Efficacy of helium-oxygen mixtures in the management of severe viral and post-intubation croup. *Can Anaesth Soc J.* 1979;26(3):206-212.
77. Terregino CA, Nairn SJ, Chansky ME, Kass JE. The effect of heliox on croup: a pilot study. *Acad Emerg Med.* 1998;5(11):1130-1133.
78. Weber JE, Chudnofsky CR, Younger JG, et al. A randomized comparison of helium-oxygen mixture (Heliox) and racemic epinephrine for the treatment of moderate to severe croup. *Pediatrics.* 2001;107(6):E96.

SECTION 7

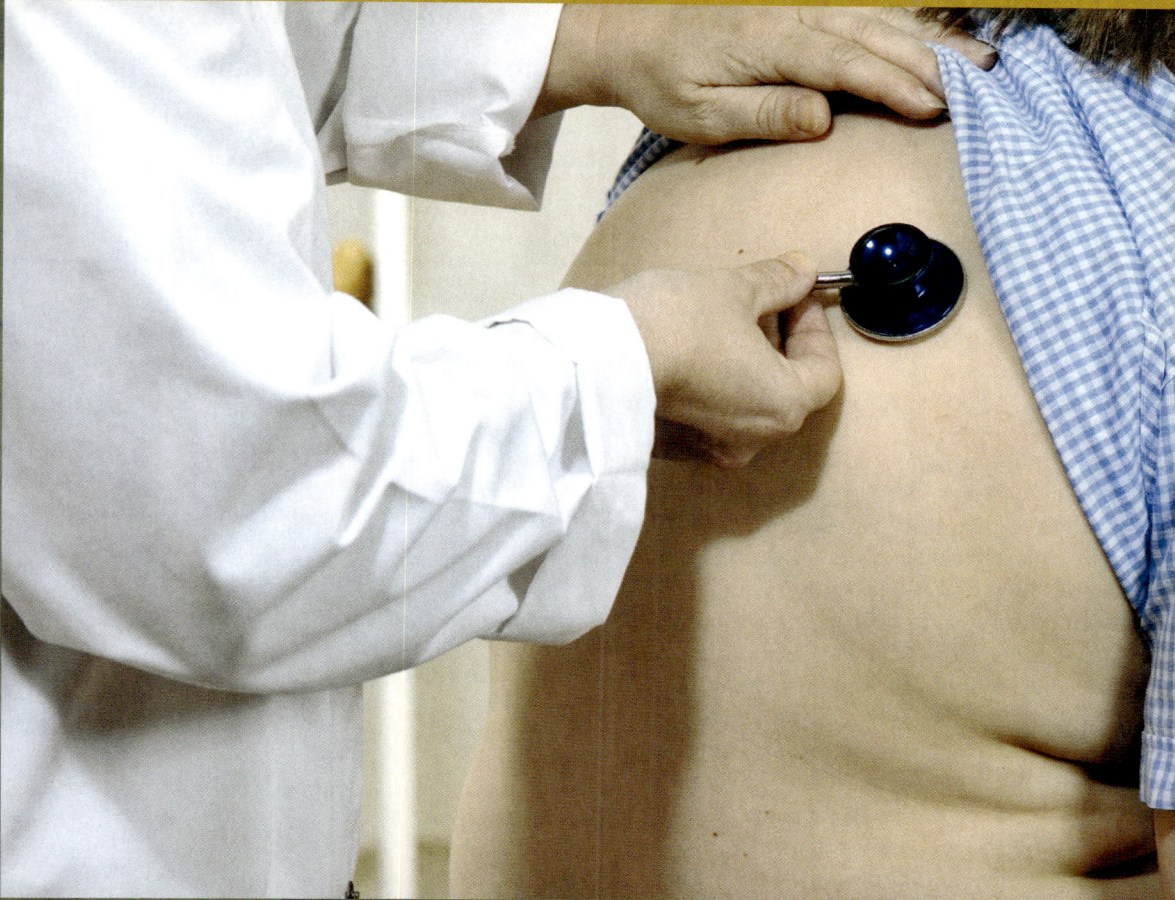

Lower Respiratory Infections

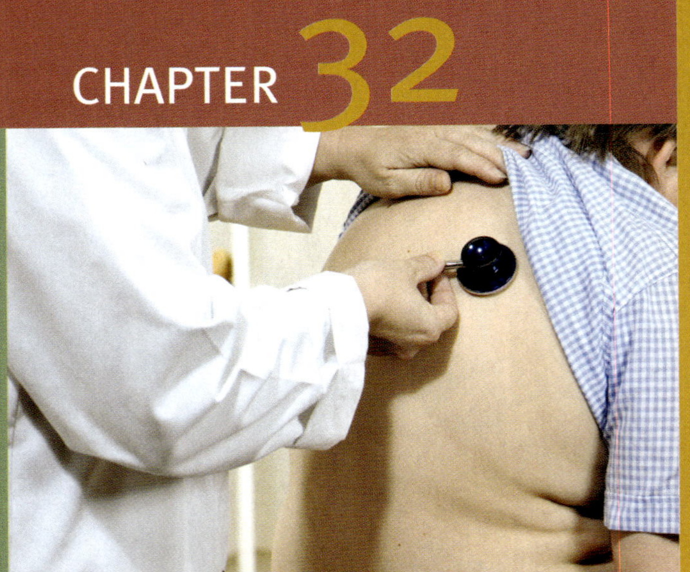

CHAPTER 32

Bronchiolitis

Brian K. Alverson

DEFINITIONS AND EPIDEMIOLOGY

Bronchiolitis, a common communicable respiratory illness manifesting with signs of small airways inflammation, primarily affects children younger than 2 years. Over one in five children will have bronchiolitis-associated wheezing in the first year of life.[1] Bronchiolitis is the most common cause of hospitalization of children in the United States. Between 1% and 3% of all children are hospitalized as a result of bronchiolitis; one in four infants hospitalized for bronchiolitis are younger than 6 weeks of age, and over half are younger than 6 months of age. The mean length of hospital stay for children is 3 days (interquartile range 2–5 days), and the cost for care is estimated at over a half billion dollars annually.[2–4] Despite the high prevalence of the disease and high rates of hospitalization, bronchiolitis is responsible for only about 100 pediatric deaths each year in the United States.[5]

Respiratory syncytial virus (RSV) causes 50–70% of bronchiolitis-related illness (Table 32–1).[6] Recently identified causes of bronchiolitis include human metapneumovirus (hMPV) and human bocavirus (HBoV), a human parvovirus. These viruses have been detected in 20–25% for hMPV[7,8] and 5% for HBoV[9] of children with bronchiolitis and negative direct fluorescent antibody testing of nasal aspirates for RSV, parainfluenza types 1 to 3, influenza A and B, and adenovirus.

Bronchiolitis is more predominant in the winter months though the timing of disease onset within a particular season and the duration of the respiratory virus season vary by geographic location. For example, RSV season in the southern United States begins earlier and lasts longer than the RSV season in the rest of the nation. Between 1990 and 2000, the median onset of RSV season (defined as the first 2 consecutive weeks where more than 10% of nasal wash specimens tested at a regional reference laboratory were positive for RSV) was late November for the South and late December for the rest of the country.[10] The median duration of RSV seasons during this 10-year time period was 16 weeks for states located in the South compared with 13 weeks for states in the Midwest.[10] There is also significant season-to-season variation in RSV with the period of peak prevalence varying by as much as 7 weeks (ranging from early January to late February) between seasons.[10] While the majority of bronchiolitis seasonality is caused by dramatic annual spikes in RSV prevalence, other viruses exhibit different seasonal outbreak patterns (Figure 32–1).[11]

Several factors place children at increased risk of severe bronchiolitis. Shortly after recognition of hMPV as a causative agent in bronchiolitis, a group in England noted that 70% of RSV-positive children who required

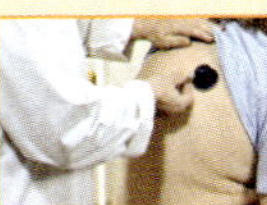

Table 32–1.

Pathogens Commonly Identified in Patients with Bronchiolitis

Viruses
Respiratory syncytial virus
Influenza A and B
Parainfluenza types 1, 2, and 3
Adenovirus
Coronaviruses
Rhinovirus
Human metapneumovirus
Human bocavirus
Bacteria*
Chlamydia trachomatis
Mycoplasma pneumoniae

**Bacteria are less common causes of bronchiolitis.*

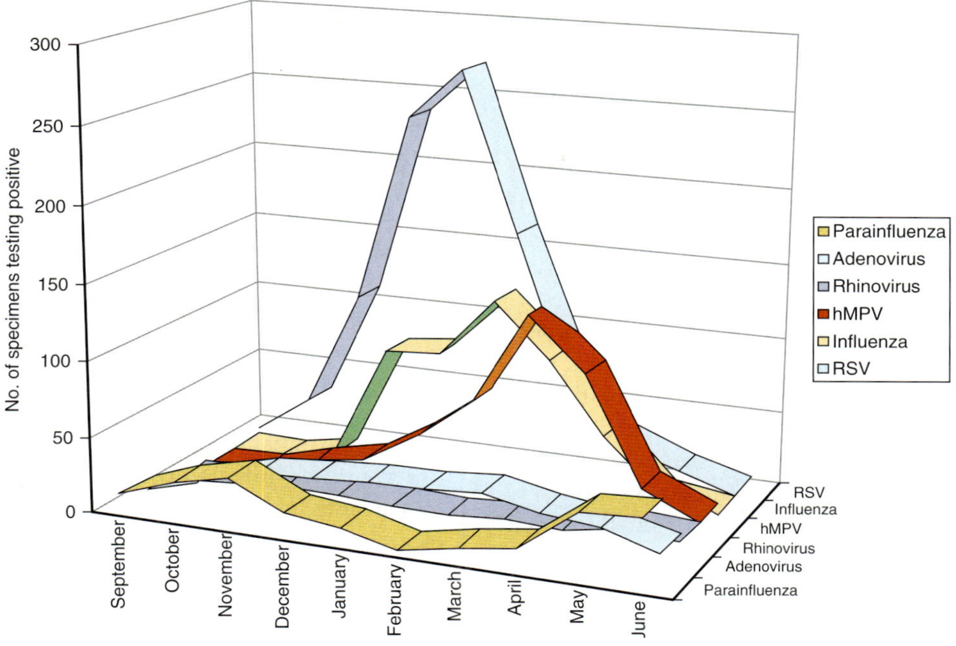

FIGURE 32–1 ■ Seasonal variation of selected viruses that cause bronchiolitis.

admission to the intensive care unit were coinfected with hMPV, suggesting that coinfection with these two viruses was a risk factor for a more severe disease course.[12] In another study, hMPV was detected in 50 (8.5%) of 589 children with respiratory tract infections; 15 (30%) of hMPV-infected children were coinfected with RSV. Coinfected patients had a 3-day longer length of hospitalization than patients infected by either hMPV or RSV alone.[13] While hMPV and RSV coinfection may lead to more severe illness, most studies have found very low rates of hMPV coinfection among RSV-infected children.[14,15]

Infants of Hispanic or Native American descent are at increased risk for severe bronchiolitis.[16] Additionally, boys are slightly more likely to develop severe bronchiolitis than girls, a finding that may be associated with sex-related differences in lung volume at the end of tidal expiration.[17] Infants who are formula-fed are three times as likely to be hospitalized for bronchiolitis as those who are breastfed, even when adjusting for other risk factors for bronchiolitis such as smoking and socioeconomic status.[18] Infants exposed to secondhand smoke are between two and four times as likely to suffer an early wheezing episode.[19] Among children with RSV bronchiolitis, disease course is more severe in infants exposed to maternal cigarette use.[20]

Residence at high altitudes also increases the risk of severe bronchiolitis. The normal physiologic effects of altitude on the respiratory tract are multiple. Baseline oxygen saturation values decrease with increasing altitude, an expected response to the decreased fraction of inspired oxygen. In addition, nasal obstruction and impaired ciliary activity exhibited at high altitude,[21] in conjunction with low humidity, can impair the ability to clear respiratory secretions associated with viral lower respiratory tract infections. In Colorado, RSV-specific hospitalization rates increased 25% among infants younger than 1 year and 53% among children 1–4 years of age for every 1000-m increase in altitude; the risk of RSV-associated hospitalization was highest at elevations above 2500 m.[22] The stronger effect of altitude on child compared with infant hospitalization is likely because infants decompensate more readily with illness than older children. Thus, clinicians may have a lower threshold for hospital admission at baseline for younger infants, mitigating the additional effect of altitude on the hospitalization decision in younger infants.

Other Factors Predisposing to Severe Bronchiolitis-Related Illness

Underlying conditions such as prematurity, complex congenital heart disease, cystic fibrosis, bone marrow and solid organ transplantation, and human immunodeficiency virus infection contribute to a worsened disease course. Premature infants are at high risk for severe illness as a result of bronchiolitis[23,24] because of immune compromise related to immunologic immaturity compounded by incomplete placental transfer of maternal IgG before birth.[25] Furthermore, incomplete formation of the alveoli of the lung leads to pulmonary fibrosis and decreased lung compliance. As a consequence, premature infants with bronchiolitis are more likely to require hospitalization and endotracheal intubation than infants born at term gestation. These infants will also have prolonged hospitalization and incur a much higher cost of care.[23,25] Children with chronic lung disease, especially those requiring home oxygen therapy, are at highest risk for severe illness, intensive care unit hospitalization, and prolonged length of stay.[23,26,27]

Children with congenital heart disease have a lower tolerance for increased pulmonary vascular resistance, which accompanies lower respiratory tract infection. They also may not tolerate the higher cardiac output precipitated by the active disease state. One-third of children with congenital heart disease hospitalized with RSV require admission to an intensive care unit and 3.4% die from bronchiolitis-related complications.[28,29] Children with cystic fibrosis suffer from thickened mucous secretions and decreased pulmonary ciliary function, placing them at increased risk for a severe illness in the context of any lower respiratory tract infection; RSV is responsible for one-third of hospitalizations in the first year of life in this population.[30,31] The median duration of hospitalization for infants with cystic fibrosis and viral respiratory illness is 14 days. Infection with RSV may also precipitate a permanent deterioration in lung function.[32] Mortality rates of RSV pneumonia range from 60% to 78% in recipients of both bone marrow and solid organ transplants. Patients with impaired T-cell function, including those with congenital immunodeficiency, those on steroids, and patients undergoing chemotherapy, also have a more severe disease course.[32]

PATHOGENESIS

Multiple etiologic agents have been implicated as causes of bronchiolitis (Table 32–1).[6] Following direct inoculation of the eye or nose, or through inhalation of viral particles, the virus directly invades the respiratory epithelium. Progressive infection of the respiratory mucosa leads to lymphocytic infiltration of peribronchial epithelial cells and enhanced goblet cell mucous production. Necrosis and subsequent desquamation of the ciliated respiratory epithelial cells lead to small airway obstruction as intraluminal cellular debris accumulates and mucosal edema worsens. This degraded material, a composite of fibrin and inflammatory debris, may cause plugging of the small airways, further worsening airflow obstruction.[33] According to Poiseuille's law, the flow of air through a lumen is proportional to the fourth power of the airway's radius. Thus, even a small deposition of material in the airway will dramatically limit airflow and cause significant obstruction.

CLINICAL PRESENTATION

The average incubation period for bronchiolitis is 5–7 days, although there is variability of incubation periods between the causal viral pathogens; incubation periods are shorter for parainfluenza and influenza viruses.[33] Bronchiolitis in infants usually begins with symptoms of upper respiratory tract infection including rhinorrhea, cough, nasal congestion, and fever. Younger children often exhibit posttussive emesis. Children who are more ill may have anorexia and irritability. Diarrhea is present in a minority of cases. As the disease progresses, however, and as inflammatory material accumulates in the lower airways, infants develop signs of lower airway obstruction. Infants may appear barrel-chested because of air trapping. Tachypnea, flaring of the alae nasi, grunting, and respiratory accessory muscle use are evident on physical examination. On auscultation, most infants have a prolonged expiratory phase, wheezing and rales or rhonchi.[8,34,35] The respiratory sounds may be loud enough to obscure auscultation of the heart sounds. Patients with severe disease may develop hypoxia associated with cyanosis.

Approximately one in 30 infants younger than 6 months of age have apnea as their initial manifestation of bronchiolitis. Apnea is more common in younger and premature infants.[36] Rarely, bronchiolitis is associated with pneumothorax, subcutaneous emphysema, and subglottic inflammation.[37,38] Severe RSV infections may be associated with extrapulmonary complications such as cardiovascular failure, arrhythmias, seizures, focal neurological deficits, hyponatremia, hepatitis, and intussusception.[39,40]

Approximately half the patients with bronchiolitis also have acute otitis media (AOM).[41–43] Among 42 RSV-infected patients followed prospectively, 21 (50%) patients had AOM at study enrollment, an additional five (12%) patients developed AOM within the next 10 days.[42] In this study, 10 (24%) additional patients had otitis media with effusion. Bacteria were isolated from the middle ear fluid of all 25 patients with AOM who underwent tympanocentesis; RSV was isolated concurrently from the middle ear fluid in 8 (32%) of these patients.[42] Presence of an AOM does not have any impact on the outcome of bronchiolitis.[43] Treatment of AOM is discussed in Chapter 28 (Otitis Media).

DIAGNOSIS

The diagnosis of bronchiolitis can be made on the basis of history and physical examination. Routine laboratory or radiologic testing in not necessary for the diagnosis or management of bronchiolitis.[44]

Laboratory Testing

A variety of tests are available for identification of the causative virus in children with bronchiolitis. The most widely used tests are rapid antigen tests (such as direct florescence antibody testing). Additionally, some centers perform polymerase chain reaction (PCR)-based testing to detect viral genome from nasal aspirates or swabs; influenza, parainfluenza, adenovirus, RSV, hMPV, HBoV, and rhinovirus can all be detected by PCR. Multiple studies have demonstrated a high sensitivity and specificity of rapid testing, and a high concordance with viral culture techniques.[45] Knowledge of viral pathogen, however, is unlikely to affect clinical management.

Pulse Oximetry

Pulse oximetry is an important tool in the management of infants with bronchiolitis. Infants with hypoxia will have a more serious disease course,[11,26,46] and pulse oximetry reliably detects hypoxemia that is not suspected on physical examination. However, appropriate lower limits for oxygen saturation in children with bronchiolitis are not known and transient desaturation occurs in healthy, full-term infants.[47] Among outpatients, mild reductions in percutaneous oxygen saturation at initial evaluation are associated with higher return visits for additional care. Among inpatients, the perceived need for supplemental oxygen, based on continuous pulse oximetry measurements, is associated with prolonged hospitalization. Restricting pulse oximetry to intermittent rather than continuous measurements shortens length of stay without adverse consequences.[48] Furthermore, clinicians should be wary about using pulse oximetry as the sole surveillance tool for the detection of respiratory failure. Percutaneous oxygen saturation measurements do not accurately predict which infants will become apneic.[36] Pulse oximetry measurements do not detect hypoventilation, which, despite the presence of significant hypercapnia, results in only modest decreases in percutaneous oxygenation saturation. Furthermore, small amounts of supplemental oxygen will restore partial pressure of oxygen (PO_2), thereby normalizing oxygen saturation; this allows unrecognized inadequate ventilation to progress without further derangements in pulse oximeter readings until the development of significant respiratory acidosis and worsening hypercapnia. Physical examination at this point would reveal somnolence and tachypnea with shallow respirations and apnea or bradypnea.

Arterial Blood Gas Measurements

Arterial blood gases are sometimes used to evaluate severity of respiratory distress in bronchiolitis. A low PaO_2 (partial pressure of oxygen, arterial) indicates the need for supplemental oxygen; however, in the setting of bronchiolitis, this can usually be inferred from pulse oximetry in the absence of severe anemia. Partial pressure of carbon dioxide (PCO_2) measurements are more valuable in informing mechanical ventilation decisions. Expected derangements in the arterial blood gas values range from hypocapnia associated with tachypnea and hyperventilation to the normal-range PCO_2 to hypercapnia and respiratory acidosis. A "normal" PCO_2 in the setting of hyperventilation is inappropriate and is an early indication of respiratory insufficiency.

Radiologic Studies

Chest radiography is not routinely required in the diagnosis or management of infants with bronchiolitis. However, radiographs are indicated in the setting of a severe illness, when a patient is not improving as expected or if another diagnosis is suspected.[44] Peribronchial cuffing or thickening may be present. Other typical radiographic findings in children with bronchiolitis include hyperinflation with flattening of the diaphragm (Figure 32–2) and scattered areas of consolidation. The consolidation, present in 40% of patients with bronchiolitis undergoing radiography, may represent either atalectasis or true alveolar infiltrates. While most of these alveolar infiltrates are likely related to viral pneumonitis, distinguishing viral from bacterial etiology in an individual patient can be difficult. In a subset of RSV-infected patients with radiographic infiltrates who required intensive care unit admission, 42% had lower airway secretions positive for bacteria.[49] The implications of this finding are unclear but it is possible that critically ill patients with RSV are more likely to have bacterial superinfection than other RSV-infected patients. Subcutaneous emphysema and pneumomediastinum are rare complications of bronchiolitis (Figure 32–3). Studies assessing the utility of radiography in predicting disease course have been mixed, with some showing marked increased risk for a severe course among those with infiltrates,[11,41] and another showing no predictive value.[50]

Complete Blood Count

Higher white blood cell counts and absolute neutrophil counts are associated with an increased risk of bacterial disease but the results rarely affect the diagnosis or management of bronchiolitis.[45] An ANC above $10{,}000/mm^3$

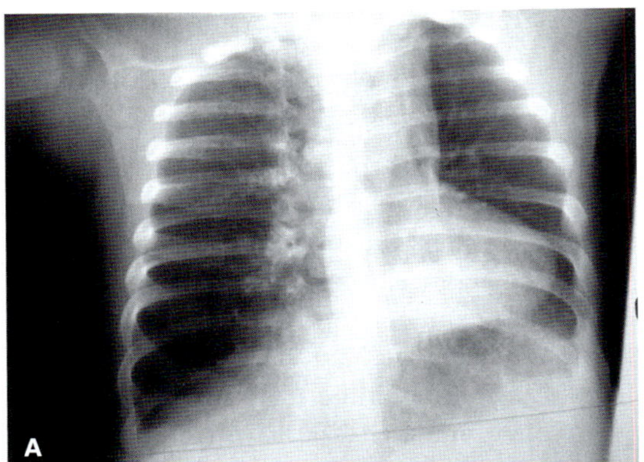

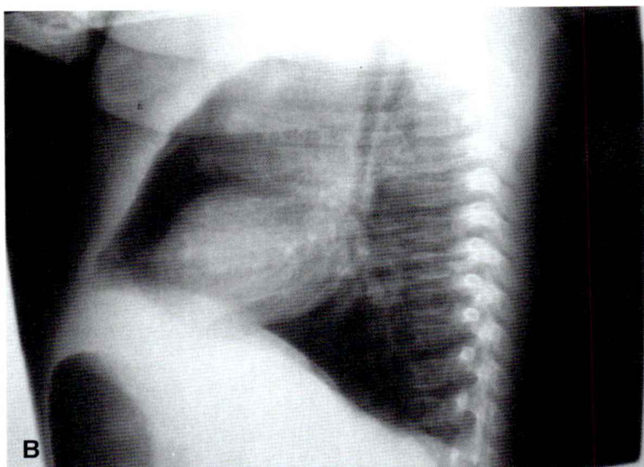

FIGURE 32–2 ■ Chest radiograph with **(A)** anterior-posterior and **(B)** lateral views showing hyperinflation in a patient with bronchiolitis. Note the inversion of the curve of the diaphragms on the lateral view, resulting from pronounced hyperinflation. Peribronchial thickening or "cuffing" and diffuse perihilar infiltrates suggest small airway edema.

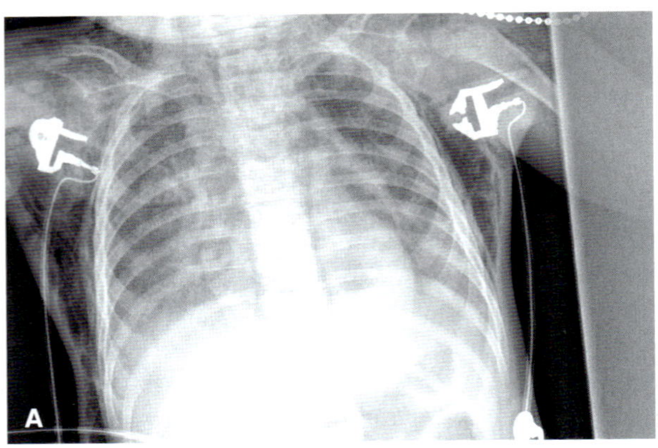

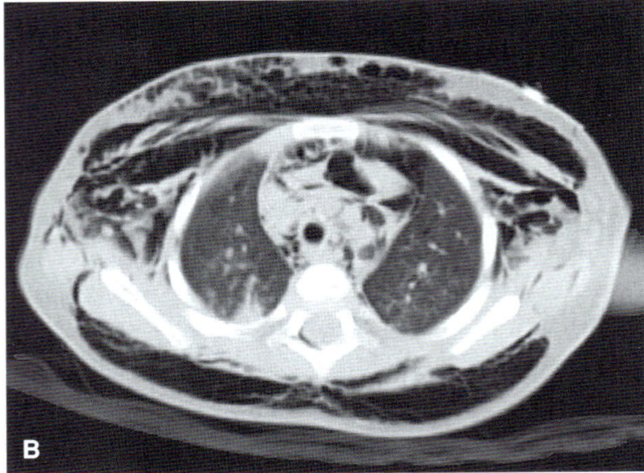

FIGURE 32–3 ■ Both chest radiograph **(A)** and computed tomography of the chest **(B)** demonstrate extensive bilateral subcutaneous emphysema of the neck and chest wall with pneumomediastinum extending both anteriorly and posteriorly in a child with bronchiolitis caused by human metapneumovirus. (*Both figures courtesy of Dr. Samir S. Shah.*)

increases the likelihood of bacterial infection (8% vs. 0.8% for those with an ANC $<10{,}000/\text{mm}^3$)[51] though the positive predictive value of an elevated ANC is low, particularly in infants who received the heptavalent pneumococcal conjugate vaccine. Routine complete blood counts are not recommended.

Lumbar Puncture

Meningitis is rare in well-appearing infants and children with fever, particularly in the context of bronchiolitis. In older children, the risk of meningitis is quite low and a lumbar puncture is not warranted unless the child has signs or symptoms that suggest meningitis. The decision to perform lumbar puncture routinely in young infants is more controversial. Febrile infants younger than 2 months with bronchiolitis appear to be at lower risk for meningitis than those without bronchiolitis. However, the risk is not zero and clinicians must balance the risk of missing a case of bacterial meningitis against the risk of the procedure in an infant with a respiratory illness. In a prospective, multicenter study of febrile infants younger than 2 months, the prevalence of bacterial meningitis was 0% [95% confidence interval (CI): 0–1.2%] in RSV-positive infants and 0.9% (95% CI: 0.4–1.7%) in RSV-negative infants.[52] Other studies addressing the issue were conducted retrospectively and contain important methodologic flaws that limit their generalizability.[53–56] It is prudent to consider meningitis in ill-appearing young infants with fever, however care should be taken not to impede respiratory effort during the procedure, and lumbar puncture (but not empiric antibiotic therapy) should be deferred in children with significant respiratory distress and suspected meningitis.

Blood Culture

Blood cultures are performed in one-third of all infants with bronchiolitis.[57] However, rates of bacteremia in infants have dramatically decreased since the introduction of the heptavalent pneumococcal vaccine.[58] The prevalence of bacteremia in infants with fever is low, particularly in the presence of overt signs of bronchiolitis. In older infants, a blood culture is more likely to reveal a contaminant than a pathogenic organism.[58] However, the prevalence is higher among young children with high fever, immunization delay, or ill appearance. In the previously mentioned multicenter study of infants younger than 2 months, the prevalence of bactermia was 1.1% in RSV-positive infants and 2.3% in RSV-negative infants.[52] Therefore, infants in these higher risk categories may warrant blood culture as part of their initial evaluation.

Urinalysis and Urine Culture

Rates of urinary tract incontinence (UTI) in infants with bronchiolitis have been reported between 1.9% and 12% with higher rates in the youngest infants.[52, 55, 59–61] Among febrile infants younger than 2 months, rates of UTI were 5.4% in RSV-positive infants and 10.1% in RSV-negative infants.[52] Empiric testing of the urine in young febrile children may be indicated, even in the presence of bronchiolitis.[62] UTIs are discussed further in Chapter 42.

MANAGEMENT

Guidelines and Pathways

There is a wide variation in the way practitioners and hospitalists manage bronchiolitis.[63,64] The American Academy of Pediatrics has published evidence-based guidelines for management of this common disease.[44] Institution of evidence-based guidelines or pathways for therapy has reduced unnecessary care, reduced bed occupancy, shortened length of stay, and decreased costs of care at several institutions.[65–67] An example of a pathway for the management of infants with bronchiolitis is shown in Figure 32–4. Sustainability of these benefits has been demonstrated.[68] Inpatient management strategies are summarized in Table 32–2.

Supplemental Oxygen

Hospitalized children with bronchiolitis often receive supplemental oxygen therapy. While the normal mean percutaneous oxygen saturation exceeds 95%, infants may exhibit transient decreases as a result of periodic breathing, physiologic apnea, and gastroesophageal reflux.[47] In the context of bronchiolitis, airway edema and necrosis of respiratory epithelial cells causes ventilation–perfusion mismatch and subsequent hypoxia. Because of longitudinal variation, continuous pulse oximetry measurements may demonstrate a variability that makes distinction between normal physiology and disease pathology difficult. The increased rates of hospitalization for bronchiolitis over the past two decades have been attributed to the improved ability to noninvasively determine oxygen saturation levels rather than to an increased disease burden.[69] Continuous pulse oximetry has been shown to prolong length of stay in the hospital unnecessarily, and has been estimated to incur a cost of $1500 per patient as a result.[48]

From a management standpoint, data support the position that otherwise healthy infants with bronchiolitis with a percutaneous oxygen saturation at or above 90% at sea level while breathing room air gain little benefit from increasing PaO_2 with supplemental oxygen.[44] As infants recover, improvement of low percutaneous oxygen saturation may lag behind other indicators like accessory muscle use. Though home oxygen therapy requires further assessment of safety, one study found low complication rates and high parental satisfaction with a strategy of 8-hour emergency department observation followed by home oxygen therapy for infants with bronchiolitis.[70] This study excluded patients with prior wheezing, corticosteroid receipt, apnea, significant underlying medical conditions, and focal radiographic infiltrates and residence more than 30 minutes from the health care facility.

Hydration

Symptoms of bronchiolitis can be a double-edged sword against an infant's ability to maintain adequate hydration. Patients suffer increased insensible losses via fever and tachypnea. Increased respiratory effort and upper airway mucous obstruction may render feeding difficult. Viral illness may also decrease appetite. Furthermore, in normal infants with increased respiratory effort secondary to bronchiolitis, aspiration of food products is possible, worsening respiratory distress.[71] To render the picture more complicated, however, patients with bronchiolitis have increased plasma levels of antidiuretic hormone, placing them at risk for fluid overload. There may be an increased propensity specifically for RSV to generate an inappropriately elevated level of antidiuretic hormone[72] Thus, while rapid correction of clinical dehydration is appropriate, clinicians should monitor the infants' intake and urinary output to ensure that the infant is not retaining fluid, which can lead to hyponatremia. In patients with ongoing poor feeding, intravenous maintenance fluids are indicated, however patients with adequate oral intake do not require parenteral hydration.[44] While in many cases of dehydration, the nasogastric route is preferred over the intravenous route, nasogastric tube placement may impede respiratory effort in infants with bronchiolitis.

Rhode Island Hospital
A Lifespan Partner

Bronchiolitis Scoring Sheet
Hasbro Children's Hospital

Date				
Oxygen Saturation (%)				
O2 Flow Rate / Delivery Device				
Heart Rate				

SUCTIONING OR TREATMENT IS RECOMMENDED ONLY FOR A SCORE OF 3 OR HIGHER

SUCTIONING									
Suction Device (circle one) *Initial use of bulb followed by NP suction only if needed!*		Bulb NP	Bulb NP	Bulb NP	Bulb NP	Bulb NP	Bulb NP	Bulb NP	Bulb NP
		Pre Suction Score	**Post Suction Score**	**Pre Suctio n Score**	**Post Suction Score**	**Pre Suction Score**	**Post Suction Score**	**Pre Suction Score**	**Post Suctio Scor**
Time (military)									
Respiratory Rate	0) Normal 1) Tachypneic (>50 bpm)								
Accessory Muscles	0) Normal 1) Retractions (subst/subcst/intercst) 2) Neck or Abdominal Muscles								
Air Exchange	0) Normal 1) Localized Decreased 2) Multi Areas Decreased								
Wheezes	0) None/End Expiratory 1) Entire Expiratory 2) Entire Expiratory and Inhalation								
I:E Ratio	0) Less or Equal to 1:2 1) Greater than 1:2								
Total									
Further Treatment Recommended? (Y/N)									
Initials:									

TREATMENT									
Treatment (circle one)		Albuterol Racemic Epi		Albuterol Racemic Epi		Albuterol Racemic Epi		Albuterol Racemic Epi	
		Pre Rx Score	**15-30 Min Post Rx**	**Pre Rx Score**	**15-30 Min Post Rx**	**Pre Rx Score**	**15-30 Min Post Rx**	**Pre Rx Score**	**15-30 Min Post R**
Time (military)									
Respiratory Rate	0) Normal 1) Tachypneic (>50 bpm)								
Accessory Muscles	0) Normal 1) Retractions (subst/subcst/intercst) 2) Neck or Abdominal Muscles								
Air Exchange	0) Normal 1) Localized Decreased 2) Multi Areas Decreased								
Wheezes	0) None/End Expiratory 1) Entire Expiratory 2) Entire Expiratory and Inhalation								
I:E Ratio	0) Less or Equal to 1:2 1) Greater than 1:2								
Total									
Further Treatment Recommended? (Y/N)									
Initials:									

Initial:_____ **Print:**________________ **Signature:**______________ **Initial:**_____ **Print:**________________ **Signature:**______________
Initial:_____ **Print:**________________ **Signature:**______________ **Initial:**_____ **Print:**________________ **Signature:**______________
Initial:_____ **Print:**________________ **Signature:**______________ **Initial:**_____ **Print:**________________ **Signature:**______________

FIGURE 32–4 ■ Sample pathway for the management of infants with bronchiolitis.

TREATMENT

Beta-Agonists

It is often difficult to clinically distinguish, in advance, children with bronchiolitis who are normal infants with an infectious process causing wheezing, and children who have an underlying predisposition to wheezing, which has been triggered by an infectious process. There is no role for oral albuterol in the management of bronchiolitis.[73,74] Many clinicians have argued for use of nebulized or inhaled beta-agonists such as albuterol in the management of bronchiolitis. In the ambulatory setting, Flores and Horwitz[75] found

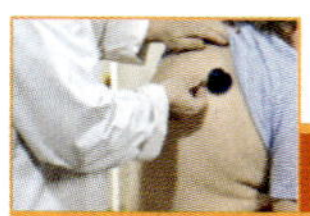

Table 32–2.

Summary of Inpatient Management Strategies for Bronchiolitis

- Do not routinely utilize chest radiography or laboratory data in diagnosis or management of patients
- Use an objective respiratory score to track changes in patient status
- Employ intermittent pulse oximetry (performed with routine vital signs), rather than continuous pulse oximetry
    - Establish hospitalwide consensus of acceptable level and duration of desaturation
    - Initiate or increase supplemental oxygen therapy only in cases of increasing respiratory distress or when other maneuvers such as stimulation, suctioning, or repositioning fail to improve oxygenation level
- Trial of neublized racemic epinephrine or albuterol may be indicated, but only continue use if an objective improvement in clinical score is noted
- Do not treat patients with steroids, decongestants, or antihistamines
- Be very conservative in the management of patients with underlying immune deficiency, pulmonary disease, or cardiac disease
- Employ bulb suctioning with saline. Reserve nasopharyngeal suctioning for cases of severe respiratory distress
- Criteria for patient discharge:
    - Comfortable breathing without hypoxia
    - Able to maintain adequate hydration
    - Resolution of apnea
    - Caregiver expresses understanding of disease process and follow-up

no difference in respiratory rate and a statistically significant but clinically unimportant improvement in percutaneous oxygen saturation (by 1.2%) following nebulized albuterol therapy. Kellner et al.[76] found a modest short-term reduction in severity of illness among infants with bronchiolitis, however, the benefit was not sustained and respiratory effort returned to pretreatment levels within an hour. Albuterol use in the ambulatory setting does not affect hospitalization rates.[75,76]

In the hospital setting, albuterol use does not decrease the length of hospital stay or the frequency of bronchiolitis-associated adverse outcomes.[77] Although beta-agonists are usually well tolerated, adverse reactions such as tachycardia, flushing, and tremor occur commonly. Albuterol may also cause a ventilation–perfusion mismatch immediately after therapy, leading to transient oxygen desaturation.[78] Despite its unproven efficacy, beta-agonist use for RSV bronchiolitis has been estimated to cost over $37 million annually.[79]

In summary, beta-agonist therapy is not routinely indicated for the treatment of bronchiolitis. While practitioners may use this as a trial therapy, it should only be continued if a significant objective clinical benefit to the patient has been demonstrated.[44] While ipratropium bromide has been found to be a useful adjuvant in the treatment of asthma, there is no role for anticholinergic therapy in the management of bronchiolitis, either alone or in combination with beta-agonists.[44]

Racemic Epinephrine

Inhaled racemic epinephrine caries a theoretical advantage over inhaled beta-agonists in bronchiolitis because the drug not only carries the beta-agonist benefits of bronchodilation, but also the alpha-agonist effect of reducing edema and mucous production through vasoconstriction.[34] One randomized trial found a decreased admission rate for children who were administered racemic epinephrine (33%) compared with those administered albuterol (81%) during emergency department evaluation.[80] However, most other studies in the ambulatory setting have failed to find any differences.[81] Among hospitalized patients, while racemic epinephrine use resulted in minor improvements in respiratory assessment score or respiratory rate compared with either placebo or albuterol, there was no difference in length of hospital stay.[81] Racemic epinephrine is not used outside the hospital setting. In hospitalized patients, the American Association of Pediatrics (AAP) currently recommends a carefully monitored trial of racemic epinephrine with continuation of the drug only in those who demonstrate clear and objective improvement.[44]

Corticosteriods

Despite the high prevalence of corticosteroid usage, there is very little evidence that steroids improve the clinical course of patients with bronchiolitis.[82] Most trials and a Cochrane database review have failed to demonstrate an improvement in length of stay in the hospital, clinical breathing scores, oxygenation, readmission rates, or duration of illness regardless of route of corticosteroid administration.[82–86] In a meta-analysis that included six studies, infants receiving corticosteroids had a mean length of stay that was 0.43 days less than those who received the placebo treatment (95% confidence interval: –0.81 to –0.05 days); however, this difference was not statistically significant when only studies that excluded children with prior wheezing were included.[87]

Ribavirin

Ribavirin, a guanosine analog, disrupts the replication of RSV viral RNA, thereby inhibiting replication of the virus. While its efficacy has been demonstrated in vitro, its therapeutic utilization remains controversial. One small study demonstrated decreased length of stay and decreased time of mechanical ventilation in patients, however the authors used nebulized sterile water, a known precipitant of bronchospam, as a control for comparison.[88] Another study demonstrated a reduction in rates of future wheezing in patients treated with ribavirin during acute illness but two others failed to replicate this result.[44] Because ribavirin is a potential teratogen, administration to patients requires either positive pressure ventilation or a specialized vacuum exhaust hood system.[89] The cost of this medicine is estimated at $1100 per day and use of the drug is not cost-effective.[90, 91] In practice, ribavirin use is limited to small subsets of immunocompromised or critically ill patients.

Helium–Oxygen Mixtures

In diseases where an obstruction of air flow causes increased respiratory effort, helium, an inert gas with no bronchodilatory or anti-inflammatory properties, has been proposed as a possible solution. Mixing oxygen with low-density helium at a helium:oxygen ratio of 80:20 or 70:30 (heliox) results in easier, more laminar flow past obstructions in the airway compared with ambient air, which is comprised of higher density nitrogen.[92] While use in asthma is still controversial, it is effective in diseases of upper airway obstruction, such as croup. In bronchiolitis, several small trials have studied its efficacy at relieving respiratory distress. By improving laminar flow in the lungs, it becomes easier for infants to move a larger quantity of air, which in turn reduces respiratory effort. Most of these studies have shown that heliox reduces respiratory effort[93–95] and decreases intensive care unit length of stay,[94] and one argued that heliox may reduce the likelihood of endotracheal intubation.[93]

Other Drugs

In animal models, RSV infection has altered the production of endogenous surfactant. In mechanically ventilated infants with bronchiolitis, treatment with surfactant decreased the duration of ventilatory support.[96] However, surfactant is still considered an experimental treatment for critically ill children with bronchiolitis. Other therapies including decongestants, antihistamines, and dextromethorphan offer no benefit to children with bronchiolitis.[97–99]

Other Therapeutic Considerations

The accrual of mucous in the upper airway can contribute to the respiratory distress of infants with bronchiolitis. Nasal bulb suctioning preceded by saline administration is a mainstay of clearing the upper airway for infants; this technique may be taught to parents as a method of managing their children's illness at home. Optimally, patients should be suctioned in this manner prior to feedings and prior to any inhalational therapy that has been demonstrated to be efficacious.[62] In the hospital setting, respiratory therapists may be inclined to use vacuum-assisted nasopharyngeal suctioning by catheter. This technique is more traumatic and painful than bulb suction, and may cause bleeding and may worsen gastroesophageal reflux,[100] and has been reported as a cause of pneumothorax, apnea, worsened bronchospasm, and even intraventricular hemorrhage of the newborn.[101] It may be prudent to limit invasive suctioning to patients with significant respiratory distress, as the efficacy of this modality on moderately ill patients has never been demonstrated.

While patients with bronchiolitis may demonstrate areas of atalectasis on chest radiography and secretions may obstruct airflow, chest physiotherapy is contraindicated. Infantile chest physiotherapy has been associated with adverse events such as rib fractures and does not improve respiratory effort or reduce hospital length-of-stay.[102]

COURSE AND PROGNOSIS

Ninety percent of infants will acquire RSV in their first two years of life, and almost half of these will develop bronchiolitis.[44] Much effort has been spent in trying to prospectively determine which patients with bronchiolitis will have a more severe course of illness. Roughly 0.5% of infants who acquire bronchiolitis will be hospitalized.[2] Of these, 14% will require mechanical ventilation for apnea or respiratory failure.[41] It is difficult, but important, to be able to predict which patients are likely to deteriorate, and thus warrant observation in the hospital setting. Infants younger than 1 month, who were premature or who have witnessed apnea, require careful observation for apnea or a repeated episode of apnea.[36] Children with high fever are more likely to have a more severe and prolonged hospital course.[103] Patients who have underlying pulmonary or cardiac conditions, especially cystic fibrosis, pulmonary hypertension, and chronic lung disease of prematurity are also at risk for severe bronchiolitis-related illness. These patients warrant a lower threshold for admission and close monitoring.[44]

The typical acute bronchiolitis illness lasts 3–7 days. Infants hospitalized early in the course of illness may worsen clinically for several days before improving. Potential complications include cardiac arrhythmia (2%) and electrolyte imbalance (20%).[41] Apnea associated with bronchiolitis usually resolves within 48–72 hours, although some infants may require longer periods of hospitalization and monitoring. In general, improvement is gradual. For infants younger than 24 months, the median length of illness is 12 days, but up to 9% of patients will still have persistence of symptoms at 28 days of illness.[104]

Bronchiolitis in infancy has long-term implications. In mice, infection with either RSV and hMPV in the perinatal period results in asthma in adult mice.[105,106] While causality is difficult to determine in humans, RSV exposure in infancy is strongly associated with development of asthma. In one study, 47 children hospitalized for bronchiolitis and 93 age-matched controls were followed prospectively. At 13 years of age, 48% of the children hospitalized with RSV in infancy had suffered wheezing in the past 12 months, compared with 8% of their age-matched controls.[107] Additionally, among children who develop persistent wheezing, encountering a first-time wheezing episode early in life is correlated with having more severe disease.[108]

PREVENTION

Infection Control and Patient Safety

During the peak of the bronchiolitis season, there is a high risk of nosocomial transmission of infection. Approximately 5% of RSV-infected children acquire their RSV in a health care setting.[109] Transmission rates approach at least 45% of contacts within the hospital in the absence of infection control measures.[110] Nosocomially acquired RSV leads to a median 8-day increase in the length-of-hospital stay.[111] A program consisting of early recognition of patients with respiratory symptoms, cohorting nursing staff to care for isolated patients, and widespread use of gown and glove barrier precautions has proven cost-effective in reducing nosocomial RSV transmission.[111] Isolating patients in private rooms more effectively reduces nosocomial transmission than cohorting patients by type of virus isolated because infants with bronchiolitis (1) do not generate a robust immunoglobulin response to RSV; (2) may be infected by different strains of RSV simultaneously or within the span of the same viral season;[112] and (3) shed multiple unrelated respiratory viruses in 20% of cases.[113]

Alcohol-based hand sanitizers are an easy, effective technique for cleansing after caring for patients with bronchiolitis.[114] Family members with viral symptoms should remained confined to their child's room, wear face masks when venturing outside their child's room,[115] and refrain from any contact with other patients. Other visitors with viral symptoms should be restricted from visiting hospitalized patients. Clinicians should also educate families about the importance of hand hygiene to prevent spread of disease.[44] In the home setting, secondary transmission rates were 0.63 respiratory illnesses per susceptible person-month.[116] Alcohol-based hand sanitizers and hand hygiene education can reduce transmission of illness within the home setting.[116, 117] Chapters 5 (Hospital Infection Control) and 4 (Office Infection Control) provide additional guidance on infection control issues.

In addition to risks for nosocomial infection, children hospitalized for bronchiolitis have a high rate of preventable adverse events during hospitalization. One study found that 10% of admitted patients with bronchiolitis suffered a near miss or adverse event. The rate was higher among critically ill patients. These included a range of severity from unwarranted phlebotomy to infection of central catheters and the acquisition of serious nosocomial infection.[118]

Palivizumab

Palivizumab (Synagis™) is a humanized mouse antibody directed against a glycoprotein specific for the

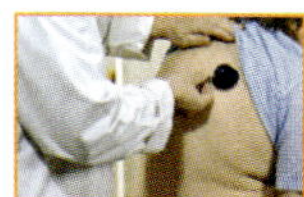

Table 32–3.

Indications for Prophylaxis Against Respiratory Syncytial Virus with Palivizumab

1. Under 24 months with chronic lung disease who have required medical therapy in the 6 months prior to start of RSV season
2. Infants born on or before the 32nd week of gestation, even if no chronic lung disease
   a. If 28 weeks or earlier, give during RSV season for first 12 months of life
   b. If 29–32 weeks, give during RSV season if in the first 6 months of life
3. Infants born between 32 and 35 weeks gestation who satisfy 2 of the following criteria
   a. Child care attendance
   b. School age sibling
   c. Exposure to environmental air pollutants
   d. Congenital abnormalities of the airways
   e. Severe neuromuscular disease
4. Children with hemodynamically significant cyanotic or acyanotic heart disease
   a. Once a child satisfies criteria during one particular season, they should continue until the end of that season
   b. If a child receiving palivizumab during the season gets RSV anyway, he/she should continue to receive the drug through the end of the season
   c. Palivizumab is administered in 5 monthly doses, generally November through March, depending on timing of local seasonality

Summarized from American Academy of Pediatrics. Respiratory syncytial virus. In: Pickering LK, Baker CJ, Long SS, McMillan JA, eds. Red Book: 2006 Report of the Committee of Infectious Diseases. 27th ed. Elk Grove Village, IL: American Academy of Pediatrics; 2006: 560–6.

RSV virus. The use of this drug has replaced RSV-IG, which is no longer available. Palivizumab is administered as an intramuscular injection on a monthly basis during the course of the RSV season, usually a 5-month course. Administration is highly effective at preventing RSV infection and also at curtailing severity of disease. Compared with placebo, palivizumab decreases by half an infant's risk for hospitalization (from 10.6% to 4.8%), and reduces length of stay and oxygen utilization in those who are hospitalized.[29, 119] Among 1287 infants with hemodynamically significant heart disease, hospitalization rates were lower among palivizumab recipients (5.3%) compared with placebo recipients (9.7%; $P = 0.003$). For a 5-kg child, a 5-month course of therapy costs over $3000. It is estimated that for every 7.4 patients treated, one hospitalization is averted.[120] When given to selected patients, palivizumab costs $12,000 per averted hospitalization, however the money saved by administration does not likely cover the cost of the drug across a given population.[121] Thus, administration of palivizumab is recommended only in certain patients at increased risk for significant disease (Table 32–3). Among children with hemodynamically significiant heart disease, the estimated cost per year-of-life saved is over $100,000.[29, 122] Palivizumab is well tolerated and rates of complaints after administration are similar to placebo.[119] There is no therapeutic role for Palivizumab in children acutely infected with RSV.[123]

REFERENCES

1. Glezen WP, Taber LH, Frank AL, Kasel JA. Risk of primary infection and reinfection with respiratory syncytial virus. *Am J Dis Child.* 1986;140(6):543-56.
2. Shay DK, Holman RC, Newman RD, Liu LL, Stout JW, Anderson LJ. Bronchiolitis-associated hospitalizations among US children, 1980-1996. *Jama.* 1999;282(15): 1440-1446.
3. Stang P, Brandenburg N, Carter B. The economic burden of respiratory syncytial virus-associated bronchiolitis hospitalizations. *Arch Pediatr Adolesc Med.* 2001;155(1): 95-96.
4. Pelletier AJ, Mansbach JM, Camargo CA. Direct medical costs of bronchiolitis hospitalizations in the United States. *Pediatrics.* 2006;118:2418-2423.
5. Shay DK, Holman RC, Roosevelt GE, Clarke MJ, Anderson LJ. Bronchiolitis-associated mortality and estimates of respiratory syncytial virus-associated deaths among US children, 1979-1997. *J Infect Dis.* 2001;183(1):16-22.
6. Legg JP, Warner JA, Johnston SL, Warner JO. Frequency of detection of picornaviruses and seven other respiratory pathogens in infants. *Pediatr Infect Dis J.* 2005; 24(7):611-616.
7. Esper F, Boucher D, Weibel C, Martinello RA, Kahn JS. Human metapneumovirus infection in the United States: clinical manifestations associated with a newly emerging respiratory infection in children. *Pediatrics.* 2003;111(6, pt 1):1407-1410.
8. Williams JV, Harris PA, Tollefson SJ, et al. Human metapneumovirus and lower respiratory tract disease in otherwise healthy infants and children. *N Engl J Med.* 2004;350(5):443-450.
9. Kesebir D, Vazquez M, Weibel C, et al. Human bocavirus infection in young children in the United States: molecular epidemiological profile and clinical characteristics of a newly emerging respiratory virus. *J Infect Dis.* 2006;194(9):1276-1282.
10. Mullins JA, Lamonte AC, Bresee JS, Anderson LJ. Substantial variability in community respiratory syncytial virus season timing. *Pediatr Infect Dis J.* 2003;22(10): 857-862.
11. Shaw KN, Bell LM, Sherman NH. Outpatient assessment of infants with bronchiolitis. *Am J Dis Child.* 1991; 145(2):151-155.
12. Greensill J, McNamara PS, Dove W, Flanagan B, Smyth RL, Hart CA. Human metapneumovirus in severe respiratory syncytial virus bronchiolitis. *Emerg Infect Dis.* 2003;9(3):372-375.
13. Foulongne V, Guyon G, Rodiere M, Segondy M. Human metapneumovirus infection in young children hospitalized with respiratory tract disease. *Pediatr Infect Dis J.* 2006;25(4):354-359.
14. Lazar I, Weibel C, Dziura J, Ferguson D, Landry ML, Kahn JS. Human metapneumovirus and severity of respiratory syncytial virus disease. *Emerg Infect Dis.* 2004; 10(7):1318-1320.
15. van Woensel JB, Bos AP, Lutter R, Rossen JW, Schuurman R. Absence of human metapneumovirus co-infection in cases of severe respiratory syncytial virus infection. *Pediatr Pulmonol.* 2006;41(9):872-874.
16. Boyce TG, Mellen BG, Mitchel EF, Jr, Wright PF, Griffin MR. Rates of hospitalization for respiratory syncytial virus infection among children in medicaid. *J Pediatr.* 2000;137(6):865-870.
17. Martinez FD, Morgan WJ, Wright AL, Holberg CJ, Taussig LM. Diminished lung function as a predisposing factor for wheezing respiratory illness in infants. *N Engl J Med.* 1988;319(17):1112-1117.
18. Bachrach VR, Schwarz E, Bachrach LR. Breastfeeding and the risk of hospitalization for respiratory disease in infancy: a meta-analysis. *Arch Pediatr Adolesc Med.* 2003;157(3):237-243.
19. Stocks J, Dezateux C. The effect of parental smoking on lung function and development during infancy. *Respirology.* 2003;8(3):266-285.
20. Bradley JP, Bacharier LB, Bonfiglio J, et al. Severity of respiratory syncytial virus bronchiolitis is affected by cigarette smoke exposure and atopy. *Pediatrics.* 2005;115 (1):e7-e14.
21. Barry PW, Mason NP, O'Callaghan C. Nasal mucociliary transport is impaired at altitude. *Eur Respir J.* 1997;10(1):35-37.
22. Choudhuri JA, Ogden LG, Ruttenber AJ, Thomas DS, Todd JK, Simoes EA. Effect of altitude on hospitalizations for respiratory syncytial virus infection. *Pediatrics.* 2006;117(2):349-356.
23. Horn SD, Smout RJ. Effect of prematurity on respiratory syncytial virus hospital resource use and outcomes. *J Pediatr.* 2003;143(5 suppl):S133-S141.

24. Sampalis JS. Morbidity and mortality after RSV-associated hospitalizations among premature Canadian infants. *J Pediatr.* 2003;143(5 suppl):S150-S156.
25. Weisman LE. Populations at risk for developing respiratory syncytial virus and risk factors for respiratory syncytial virus severity: infants with predisposing conditions. *Pediatr Infect Dis J.* 2003;22(2 suppl):S33-S37; discussion S7-S9.
26. Wang EE, Law BJ, Stephens D. Pediatric Investigators Collaborative Network on Infections in Canada (PICNIC) prospective study of risk factors and outcomes in patients hospitalized with respiratory syncytial viral lower respiratory tract infection. *J Pediatr.* 1995;126(2): 212-219.
27. Groothuis JR, Gutierrez KM, Lauer BA. Respiratory syncytial virus infection in children with bronchopulmonary dysplasia. *Pediatrics.* 1988;82(2):199-203.
28. Navas L, Wang E, de Carvalho V, Robinson J. Improved outcome of respiratory syncytial virus infection in a high-risk hospitalized population of Canadian children. Pediatric Investigators Collaborative Network on Infections in Canada. *J Pediatr.* 1992;121(3):348-354.
29. Feltes TF, Cabalka AK, Meissner HC, et al. Palivizumab prophylaxis reduces hospitalization due to respiratory syncytial virus in young children with hemodynamically significant congenital heart disease. *J Pediatr.* 2003;143 (4):532-540.
30. Abman SH, Ogle JW, Butler-Simon N, Rumack CM, Accurso FJ. Role of respiratory syncytial virus in early hospitalizations for respiratory distress of young infants with cystic fibrosis. *J Pediatr.* 1988;113(5):826-830.
31. Wang EE, Prober CG, Manson B, Corey M, Levison H. Association of respiratory viral infections with pulmonary deterioration in patients with cystic fibrosis. *N Engl J Med.* 1984;311(26):1653-1658.
32. Meissner HC. Selected populations at increased risk from respiratory syncytial virus infection. *Pediatr Infect Dis J.* 2003;22(2 suppl):S40-S44; discussion S4-S5.
33. Domachowske JB, Rosenberg HF. Respiratory syncytial virus infection: immune response, immunopathogenesis, and treatment. *Clin Microbiol Rev.* 1999;12(2): 298-309.
34. Wohl ME, Chernick V. State of the art: bronchiolitis. *Am Rev Respir Dis.* 1978;118(4):759-781.
35. Welliver RC. Review of epidemiology and clinical risk factors for severe respiratory syncytial virus (RSV) infection. *J Pediatr.* 2003;143(5 suppl):S112-S117.
36. Willwerth BM, Harper MB, Greenes DS. Identifying hospitalized infants who have bronchiolitis and are at high risk for apnea. *Ann Emerg Med.* 2006;48(64):441-447.
37. Piastra M, Caresta E, Tempera A, et al. Sharing features of uncommon respiratory syncytial virus complications in infants. *Pediatr Emerg Care.* 2006;22(8):574-578.
38. Lipinski JK, Goodman A. Pneumothorax complicating bronchiolitis in an infant. *Pediatr Radiol.* 1980;9(4): 244-246.
39. Moore FO, Berne JD, Slamon NB, Penfil SH, Dunn SP. Intussusception in a child with respiratory syncytial virus: a new association. *Del Med J.* 2006;78(5):185-187.
40. Eisenhut M. Extrapulmonary manifestations of severe RSV bronchiolitis. *Lancet.* 2006;368(9540):988.
41. Willson DF, Landrigan CP, Horn SD, Smout RJ. Complications in infants hospitalized for bronchiolitis or respiratory syncytial virus pneumonia. *J Pediatr.* 2003;143(5 suppl):S142-S149.
42. Andrade MA, Hoberman A, Glustein J, Paradise JL, Wald ER. Acute otitis media in children with bronchiolitis. *Pediatrics.* 1998;101(4, pt 1):617-619.
43. Shazberg G, Revel-Vilk S, Shoseyov D, Ben-Ami A, Klar A, Hurvitz H. The clinical course of bronchiolitis associated with acute otitis media. *Arch Dis Child.* 2000; 83(4):317-319.
44. Diagnosis and management of bronchiolitis. *Pediatrics.* 2006;118(4):1774-1793.
45. Bordley WC, Viswanathan M, King VJ, et al. Diagnosis and testing in bronchiolitis: a systematic review. *Arch Pediatr Adolesc Med.* 2004;158(2):119-126.
46. Mulholland EK, Olinsky A, Shann FA. Clinical findings and severity of acute bronchiolitis. *Lancet.* 1990;335 (8700):1259-1261.
47. Hunt CE, Corwin MJ, Lister G, et al. Longitudinal assessment of hemoglobin oxygen saturation in healthy infants during the first 6 months of age. Collaborative Home Infant Monitoring Evaluation (CHIME) Study Group. *J Pediatr.* 1999;135(5):580-586.
48. Schroeder AR, Marmor AK, Pantell RH, Newman TB. Impact of pulse oximetry and oxygen therapy on length of stay in bronchiolitis hospitalizations. *Arch Pediatr Adolesc Med.* 2004;158(6):527-530.
49. Thorburn K, Harigopal S, Reddy V, Taylor N, van Saene HK. High incidence of pulmonary bacterial co-infection in children with severe respiratory syncytial virus (RSV) bronchiolitis. *Thorax.* 2006;61(7):611-615.
50. Dawson KP, Long A, Kennedy J, Mogridge N. The chest radiograph in acute bronchiolitis. *J Paediatr Child Health.* 1990;26(4):209-211.
51. Kuppermann N, Fleisher GR, Jaffe DM. Predictors of occult pneumococcal bacteremia in young febrile children. *Ann Emerg Med.* 1998;31(6):679-687.
52. Levine DA, Platt SL, Dayan PS, et al. Risk of serious bacterial infection in young febrile infants with respiratory syncytial virus infections. *Pediatrics.* 2004;113(6):1728-1734.
53. Liebelt EL, Qi K, Harvey K. Diagnostic testing for serious bacterial infections in infants aged 90 days or younger with bronchiolitis. *Arch Pediatr Adolesc Med.* 1999;153 (5):525-530.
54. Purcell K, Fergie J. Concurrent serious bacterial infections in 2396 infants and children hospitalized with respiratory syncytial virus lower respiratory tract infections. *Arch Pediatr Adolesc Med.* 2002;156(4):322-324.
55. Purcell K, Fergie J. Concurrent serious bacterial infections in 912 infants and children hospitalized for treatment of respiratory syncytial virus lower respiratory tract infection. *Pediatr Infect Dis J.* 2004;23(3): 267-269.
56. Antonow JA, Hansen K, McKinstry CA, Byington CL. Sepsis evaluations in hospitalized infants with bronchiolitis. *Pediatr Infect Dis J.* 1998;17(3):231-236.
57. Christakis DA, Cowan CA, Garrison MM, Molteni R, Marcuse E, Zerr DM. Variation in inpatient diagnostic testing and management of bronchiolitis. *Pediatrics.* 2005;115(4):878-884.

58. Herz AM, Greenhow TL, Alcantara J, et al. Changing epidemiology of outpatient bacteremia in 3- to 36-month-old children after the introduction of the heptavalent-conjugated pneumococcal vaccine. *Pediatr Infect Dis J.* 2006;25(4):293-300.
59. Melendez E, Harper MB. Utility of sepsis evaluation in infants 90 days of age or younger with fever and clinical bronchiolitis. *Pediatr Infect Dis J.* 2003;22(12):1053-1056.
60. Titus MO, Wright SW. Prevalence of serious bacterial infections in febrile infants with respiratory syncytial virus infection. *Pediatrics.* 2003;112(2):282-284.
61. Kuppermann N, Bank DE, Walton EA, Senac MO, Jr., McCaslin I. Risks for bacteremia and urinary tract infections in young febrile children with bronchiolitis. *Arch Pediatr Adolesc Med.* 1997;151(12):1207-1214.
62. Bronchiolitis Guideline Team CCsHMC. Evidence based clinical practice guideline for medical management of bronchiolitis in infants 1 year of age or less presenting with a first time episode. 2005(Guideline 1):1-13.
63. Wang EE, Law BJ, Boucher FD, et al. Pediatric Investigators Collaborative Network on Infections in Canada (PICNIC) study of admission and management variation in patients hospitalized with respiratory syncytial viral lower respiratory tract infection. *J Pediatr.* 1996;129(3):390-395.
64. Behrendt CE, Decker MD, Burch DJ, Watson PH. International variation in the management of infants hospitalized with respiratory syncytial virus. International RSV Study Group. *Eur J Pediatr.* 1998;157(3):215-220.
65. Kotagal UR, Robbins JM, Kini NM, Schoettker PJ, Atherton HD, Kirschbaum MS. Impact of a bronchiolitis guideline: a multisite demonstration project. *Chest.* 2002;121(6):1789-1797.
66. Perlstein PH, Kotagal UR, Bolling C, et al. Evaluation of an evidence-based guideline for bronchiolitis. *Pediatrics.* 1999;104(6):1334-1341.
67. Muething S, Schoettker PJ, Gerhardt WE, Atherton HD, Britto MT, Kotagal UR. Decreasing overuse of therapies in the treatment of bronchiolitis by incorporating evidence at the point of care. *J Pediatr.* 2004;144(6):703-710.
68. Perlstein PH, Kotagal UR, Schoettker PJ, et al. Sustaining the implementation of an evidence-based guideline for bronchiolitis. *Arch Pediatr Adolesc Med.* 2000;154(10):1001-1007.
69. Mallory MD, Shay DK, Garrett J, Bordley WC. Bronchiolitis management preferences and the influence of pulse oximetry and respiratory rate on the decision to admit. *Pediatrics.* 2003;111(1):e45-e51.
70. Bajaj L, Turner CG, Bothner J. A randomized trial of home oxygen therapy from the emergency department for acute bronchiolitis. *Pediatrics.* 2006;117(3):633-640.
71. Khoshoo V, Edell D. Previously healthy infants may have increased risk of aspiration during respiratory syncytial viral bronchiolitis. *Pediatrics.* 1999;104(6):1389-1390.
72. van Steensel-Moll HA, Hazelzet JA, van der Voort E, Neijens HJ, Hackeng WH. Excessive secretion of antidiuretic hormone in infections with respiratory syncytial virus. *Arch Dis Child.* 1990;65(11):1237-1239.
73. Gadomski AM, Aref GH, el Din OB, el Sawy IH, Khallaf N, Black RE. Oral versus nebulized albuterol in the management of bronchiolitis in Egypt. *J Pediatr.* 1994;124(1):131-138.
74. Gadomski AM, Lichenstein R, Horton L, King J, Keane V, Permutt T. Efficacy of albuterol in the management of bronchiolitis. *Pediatrics.* 1994;93(6, pt 1):907-912.
75. Flores G, Horwitz RI. Efficacy of beta2-agonists in bronchiolitis: a reappraisal and meta-analysis. *Pediatrics.* 1997;100(2, pt 1):233-239.
76. Kellner JD, Ohlsson A, Gadomski AM, Wang EE. Efficacy of bronchodilator therapy in bronchiolitis. A meta-analysis. *Arch Pediatr Adolesc Med.* 1996;150(11):1166-1172.
77. Dobson JV, Stephens-Groff SM, McMahon SR, Stemmler MM, Brallier SL, Bay C. The use of albuterol in hospitalized infants with bronchiolitis. *Pediatrics.* 1998;101(3, pt 1):361-368.
78. Ho L, Collis G, Landau LI, Le Souef PN. Effect of salbutamol on oxygen saturation in bronchiolitis. *Arch Dis Child.* 1991;66(9):1061-1064.
79. Gadomski AM, Bhasale AL. Bronchodilators for bronchiolitis. *Cochrane Database Syst Rev.* 2006;3:CD001266.
80. Menon K, Sutcliffe T, Klassen TP. A randomized trial comparing the efficacy of epinephrine with salbutamol in the treatment of acute bronchiolitis. *J Pediatr.* 1995;126(6):1004-1007.
81. Hartling L, Wiebe N, Russell K, Patel H, Klassen TP. Epinephrine for bronchiolitis. *Cochrane Database Syst Rev.* 2004;(1):CD003123.
82. Patel H, Platt R, Lozano JM, Wang EE. Glucocorticoids for acute viral bronchiolitis in infants and young children. *Cochrane Database Syst Rev.* 2004;(3):CD004878.
83. Roosevelt G, Sheehan K, Grupp-Phelan J, Tanz RR, Listernick R. Dexamethasone in bronchiolitis: a randomised controlled trial. *Lancet.* 1996;348(9023):292-295.
84. De Boeck K, Van der Aa N, Van Lierde S, Corbeel L, Eeckels R. Respiratory syncytial virus bronchiolitis: a double-blind dexamethasone efficacy study. *J Pediatr.* 1997;131(6):919-921.
85. Bulow SM, Nir M, Levin E, et al. Prednisolone treatment of respiratory syncytial virus infection: a randomized controlled trial of 147 infants. *Pediatrics.* 1999;104(6):e77.
86. Berger I, Argaman Z, Schwartz SB, et al. Efficacy of corticosteroids in acute bronchiolitis: short-term and long-term follow-up. *Pediatr Pulmonol.* 1998;26(3):162-166.
87. Garrison MM, Christakis DA, Harvey E, Cummings P, Davis RL. Systemic corticosteroids in infant bronchiolitis: A meta-analysis. *Pediatrics.* 2000;105(4):E44.
88. Smith DW, Frankel LR, Mathers LH, Tang AT, Ariagno RL, Prober CG. A controlled trial of aerosolized ribavirin in infants receiving mechanical ventilation for severe respiratory syncytial virus infection. *N Engl J Med.* 1991;325(1):24-29.
89. Bradley JS, Connor JD, Compogiannis LS, Eiger LL. Exposure of health care workers to ribavirin during therapy for respiratory syncytial virus infections. *Antimicrob Agents Chemother.* 1990;34(4):668-670.
90. Feldstein TJ, Swegarden JL, Atwood GF, Peterson CD. Ribavirin therapy: Implementation of hospital guidelines and effect on usage and cost of therapy. *Pediatrics.* 1995;96(1, pt 1):14-17.
91. Ventre K, Randolph A. Ribavirin for respiratory syncytial virus infection of the lower respiratory tract in infants and young children. *Cochrane Database Syst Rev.* 2004;(4):CD000181.

92. Gupta VK, Cheifetz IM. Heliox administration in the pediatric intensive care unit: an evidence-based review. *Pediatr Crit Care Med.* 2005;6(2):204-211.
93. Hollman G, Shen G, Zeng L, et al. Helium-oxygen improves clinical asthma scores in children with acute bronchiolitis. *Crit Care Med.* 1998;26(10):1731-1736.
94. Martinon-Torres F, Rodriguez-Nunez A, Martinon-Sanchez JM. Heliox therapy in infants with acute bronchiolitis. *Pediatrics.* 2002;109(1):68-73.
95. Cambonie G, Milesi C, Fournier-Favre S, et al. Clinical effects of heliox administration for acute bronchiolitis in young infants. *Chest.* 2006;129(3):676-682.
96. Ventre K, Haroon M, Davison C. Surfactant therapy for bronchiolitis in critically ill infants. *Cochrane Database Syst Rev.* 2006;3:CD005150.
97. Hutton N, Wilson MH, Mellits ED, et al. Effectiveness of an antihistamine-decongestant combination for young children with the common cold: a randomized, controlled clinical trial. *J Pediatr.* 1991;118(1):125-130.
98. Clemens CJ, Taylor JA, Almquist JR, Quinn HC, Mehta A, Naylor GS. Is an antihistamine–decongestant combination effective in temporarily relieving symptoms of the common cold in preschool children? *J Pediatr.* 1997;130(3):463-466.
99. Paul IM, Yoder KE, Crowell KR, et al. Effect of dextromethorphan, diphenhydramine, and placebo on nocturnal cough and sleep quality for coughing children and their parents. *Pediatrics.* 2004;114(1):e85-e90.
100. Demont B, Escourrou P, Vincon C, Cambas CH, Grisan A, Odievre M. [Effects of respiratory physical therapy and nasopharyngeal suction on gastroesophageal reflux in infants less than a year of age, with or without abnormal reflux]. *Arch Fr Pediatr.* 1991;48(9):621-625.
101. Macmillan C. Nasopharyngeal suction study reveals knowledge deficit. *Nurs Times.* 1995;91(50):28-30.
102. Perrotta C, Ortiz Z, Roque M. Chest physiotherapy for acute bronchiolitis in paediatric patients between 0 and 24 months old. *Cochrane Database Syst Rev.* 2007;(1):CD004873.
103. El-Radhi AS, Barry W, Patel S. Association of fever and severe clinical course in bronchiolitis. *Arch Dis Child.* 1999;81(3):231-234.
104. Swingler GH, Hussey GD, Zwarenstein M. Duration of illness in ambulatory children diagnosed with bronchiolitis. *Arch Pediatr Adolesc Med.* 2000;154(10):997-1000.
105. Hamelin ME, Prince GA, Gomez AM, Kinkead R, Boivin G. Human metapneumovirus infection induces long-term pulmonary inflammation associated with airway obstruction and hyperresponsiveness in mice. *J Infect Dis.* 2006;193(12):1634-1642.
106. You D, Becnel D, Wang K, Ripple M, Daly M, Cormier SA. Exposure of neonates to respiratory syncytial virus is critical in determining subsequent airway response in adults. *Respir Res.* 2006;7:107.
107. Sigurs N, Gustafsson PM, Bjarnason R, et al. Severe respiratory syncytial virus bronchiolitis in infancy and asthma and allergy at age 13. *Am J Respir Crit Care Med.* 2005;171(2):137-141.
108. Martinez FD. Respiratory syncytial virus bronchiolitis and the pathogenesis of childhood asthma. *Pediatr Infect Dis J.* 2003;22(2 suppl):S76-S82.
109. Langley JM, LeBlanc JC, Wang EE, et al. Nosocomial respiratory syncytial virus infection in Canadian pediatric hospitals: a Pediatric Investigators Collaborative Network on Infections in Canada Study. *Pediatrics.* 1997;100(6):943-946.
110. Hall CB, Douglas RG, Jr, Geiman JM, Messner MK. Nosocomial respiratory syncytial virus infections. *N Engl J Med.* 1975;293(26):1343-1346.
111. Macartney KK, Gorelick MH, Manning ML, Hodinka RL, Bell LM. Nosocomial respiratory syncytial virus infections: The cost-effectiveness and cost-benefit of infection control. *Pediatrics.* 2000;106(3):520-526.
112. Scott PD, Ochola R, Ngama M, et al. Molecular analysis of respiratory syncytial virus reinfections in infants from coastal Kenya. *J Infect Dis.* 2006;193(1):59-67.
113. Andreoletti L, Lesay M, Deschildre A, Lambert V, Dewilde A, Wattre P. Differential detection of rhinoviruses and enteroviruses RNA sequences associated with classical immunofluorescence assay detection of respiratory virus antigens in nasopharyngeal swabs from infants with bronchiolitis. *J Med Virol.* 2000;61(3):341-346.
114. Boyce JM, Pittet D. Guideline for hand hygiene in health-care settings. Recommendations of the Healthcare Infection Control Practices Advisory Committee and the HICPAC/SHEA/APIC/IDSA Hand Hygiene Task Force. Society for Healthcare Epidemiology of America/Association for Professionals in Infection Control/Infectious Diseases Society of America. *MMWR Recomm Rep.* 2002;51(RR-16):1-45, quiz CE1-4.
115. Hall CB. Nosocomial respiratory syncytial virus infections: the "Cold War" has not ended. *Clin Infect Dis.* 2000;31(2):590-596.
116. Lee GM, Salomon JA, Friedman JF, et al. Illness transmission in the home: A possible role for alcohol-based hand gels. *Pediatrics.* 2005;115(4):852-860.
117. Sandora TJ, Taveras EM, Shih MC, et al. A randomized, controlled trial of a multifaceted intervention including alcohol-based hand sanitizer and hand-hygiene education to reduce illness transmission in the home. *Pediatrics.* 2005;116(3):587-594.
118. McBride SC, Chiang VW, Goldmann DA, Landrigan CP. Preventable adverse events in infants hospitalized with bronchiolitis. *Pediatrics.* 2005;116(3):603-608.
119. Palivizumab, a humanized respiratory syncytial virus monoclonal antibody, reduces hospitalization from respiratory syncytial virus infection in high-risk infants. The IMpact-RSV Study Group. *Pediatrics.* 1998;102(3, pt 1):531-537.
120. Joffe S, Ray GT, Escobar GJ, Black SB, Lieu TA. Cost-effectiveness of respiratory syncytial virus prophylaxis among preterm infants. *Pediatrics.* 1999;104(3, pt 1):419-427.
121. Stevens TP, Sinkin RA, Hall CB, Maniscalco WM, McConnochie KM. Respiratory syncytial virus and premature infants born at 32 weeks' gestation or earlier: hospitalization and economic implications of prophylaxis. *Arch Pediatr Adolesc Med.* 2000;154(1):55-61.
122. Yount LE, Mahle WT. Economic analysis of palivizumab in infants with congenital heart disease. *Pediatrics.* 2004;114(6):1606-1611.
123. Fuller H, Del Mar C. Immunoglobulin treatment for respiratory syncytial virus infection. *Cochrane Database Syst Rev.* 2006;(4):CD004883.

CHAPTER 33

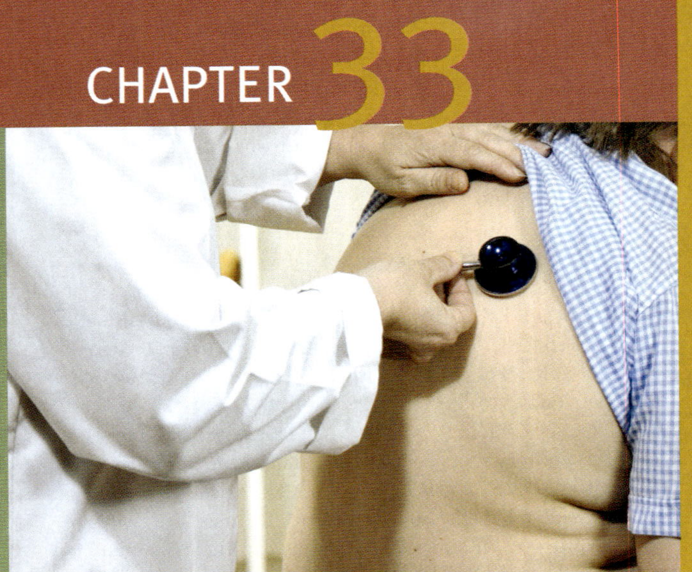

Uncomplicated Pneumonia

Gary Frank and Samir S. Shah

DEFINITIONS AND EPIDEMIOLOGY

The World Health Organization defines pneumonia as the presence of cough and fast or difficult breathing (above 50 breaths per minute for children 2 to 12 months of age; above 40 breaths per minutes for children 12 months to 5 years of age).[1] This broad definition may encompass other causes of lower respiratory tract infection including bronchiolitis as well as noninfectious causes of respiratory distress such as asthma. A more specific definition for pneumonia is "the presence of fever, acute respiratory symptoms, or both, plus evidence of parenchymal infiltrates on chest radiography."[2] This definition allows for the possibility of bacterial as well as viral causes of pneumonia.

Over 4 million children are diagnosed with pneumonia each year in the United States.[3] The annual incidence of pneumonia of 34–56 per 1000 in children <5 years of age is higher than at any other time of life except perhaps in adults >75 years of age.[3–6] This incidence decreases to approximately 16 cases per 1000 children 5 years of age or older.[7] In 1996, the incidence of death from community-acquired pneumonia (CAP) in US children was <5 per 100,000; this figure represents a mortality rate of <1% per episode of pneumonia that requires hospitalization. Though mortality rates attributable to CAP have decreased by 97% over the past 50 years,[8] more than 600,000 children annually require hospitalization for the management of CAP and its complications.[3,9]

A predisposition for respiratory tract infections seems to be a risk factor for developing pneumonia as evidenced by a study of 201 children with CAP between 3 months and 15 years of age.[10] Compared to a cohort of healthy controls, children with CAP were more likely to have a history of recurrent respiratory infections during the past year, wheezing episodes, otitis media, and tympanocentesis before the age of 2 years.

Relatively common causes of childhood pneumonia are summarized in Table 33–1. Viruses are an important cause of childhood pneumonia.[11–14] Respiratory viruses may be the primary cause of pneumonia or viral infection may predispose to bacterial superinfection by causing extensive tracheobronchial inflammation. *Streptococcus pneumoniae* remains the most common bacterial cause of lobar pneumonia outside of the perinatal period though its frequency may be decreasing as a result of the seven valent pneumococcal protein–polysaccharide conjugate vaccine (PCV7) licensed in 2000.[15] Three randomized, double-blind controlled trials, one in the United States and two in developing countries, have demonstrated that vaccination with a pneumococcal conjugate vaccine decreased the incidence of CAP.[16–18] The Kaiser Permanente trial in Northern California enrolled 37,868 children; 11% of control patients developed CAP during the study period.[16] The decrease in pneumonia among PCV7 vaccinated patients was 20.5% when pneumonia was defined by the presence of clinical symptoms plus an abnormal chest radiograph.[16] A subsequent observational study revealed that pneumonia-associated hospitalizations decreased by 39% in the United States from 2001 to 2004.[19]

Once considered to occur primarily among adolescents and young adults,[20–22] *Mycoplasma pneumoniae* is increasingly being recognized as a cause of lower respiratory tract disease in young children[7,11,13,14,23–26]. In a study of CAP in Finland, *M. pneumoniae* was the causative pathogen in 9% of children 0–4 years of age and in 40% of children 5–9 years of age.[13] Although the frequency of pneumonia due to any respiratory pathogen decreases

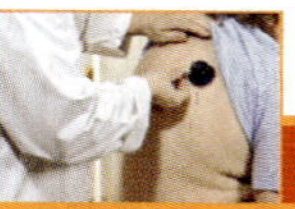

Table 33–1.

Bacteria Commonly Implicated in Childhood Pneumonia

Neonates	1–3 Months	3 Months to 5 Years	>5 Years
Group B *Streptococcus*	Lower respiratory viruses*	Lower respiratory viruses*	*Mycoplasma pneumoniae*
Enteric Gram-negative bacilli	*Streptococcus pneumoniae*	*Streptococcus pneumoniae*	*Chlamydophila pneumoniae*
Cytomegalovirus	*Chlamydia trachomatis*	*Mycoplasma pneumoniae*	*Streptococcus pneumoniae*
Herpes simplex virus†	*Bordetella pertussis*	*Chlamydophila pneumoniae*	Influenza A and B
Listeria monocytogenes	*Staphylococcus aureus*	*Haemophilus influenzae*	
Streptococcus pneumoniae	*Ureaplasma urealyticum*		
Ureaplasma urealyticum			
Treponema pallidum†			

**Includes respiratory syncytial virus, adenovirus, parainfluenza (types 1, 2, and 3), influenza (A and B), human metapneumovirus, human bocavirus, and less commonly rhinovirus.*

†As part of perinatal (e.g., disseminated herpes simplex virus) or congenital (e.g., syphilis) infection.

in children older than 5 years of age, the relative importance of *M. pneumoniae* as a cause of pneumonia increases with patient age. *M. pneumoniae* accounts for approximately 20–40% of cases of acute pneumonia in junior high and high school students and for up to 50% of cases among college students.[27–31]

PATHOGENESIS

Bacterial Pneumonia

S. pneumoniae is the leading bacterial cause of CAP in children. Pneumococci gain access to the lung by aspiration or inhalation. They lodge in bronchioles, proliferate, and initiate an inflammatory process that begins in alveolar spaces with an outpouring of protein-rich fluid. The fluid acts as culture medium for the bacteria and helps spread them to neighboring alveoli, typically resulting in lobar pneumonia.[32] In some cases, bacteremia leads to hematogenous seeding of the lung with subsequent development of pneumonia. This latter mechanism is thought to be more common for *Staphylococcus aureus.*

CAP-related complications may occur by several overlapping mechanisms. First, progressive disease may lead to subpleural bacterial replication, endothelial injury, fibrin deposition, impaired lung perfusion (causing necrosis), and extension of infection to contiguous sites (e.g., empyema, bronchopleural fistula).[33] Second, as leukocytes control bacterial multiplication, dying bacteria release cell wall and other components, which lead to overwhelming lung inflammation and, in some cases, respiratory failure.[34] Third, bacteremia may lead to metastatic infection (e.g., endocarditis, meningitis) and organ dysfunction. Mortality, though rare, usually results from sequelae of bacteremia.[35] Local complications of pneumonia are discussed in Chapter 34.

Atypical Pneumonia

Organisms such as *M. pneumoniae* and *Chlamydophila pneumoniae* gain access to the respiratory tract through aerosolized droplets spread among close contacts. Specific attachment to the respiratory epithelial tissue occurs primarily through interaction between a host epithelial cell receptor and the organisms attachment proteins.[36–38] Following attachment, hydrogen peroxide and superoxide radicals synthesized by the atypical pathogens act in concert with endogenous toxic oxygen molecules generated by host cells to induce oxidative stress in the respiratory epithelium.[39] In the lower respiratory tract, the organism may be opsonized by complement or antibodies. Activated macrophages begin phagocytosis and undergo chemotactic migration to the site of infection. $CD4^+$ T lymphocytes, B lymphocytes, and plasma cells infiltrate the lung. Further amplification of the immune response occurs in association with lymphocyte proliferation, production of immunoglobulins, and release of tumor necrosis factor alpha, gamma interferon, and various interleukins.[40] Lymphocyte activation and cytokine production may either minimize disease by enhancing host defense mechanisms or exacerbate disease by stimulating immune-mediated lung injury.[41] Extrapulmonary complications of *M. pneumoniae* infection may occur as a consequence of either immune-mediated injury or direct invasion. Effects of cross-reactive antibody remain the proposed mechanism for hemolysis and cutaneous manifestations.[42]

Neonatal Pneumonia

Neonatal pneumonia can be acquired in three main ways: Congenital, during birth, or after birth. Congenital causes of pneumonia include *Toxoplasma gondii*, rubella, herpes simplex virus, mumps, adenoviruses, *Listeria monocytogenes*, and *Mycobacterium tuberculsosis*. Group B streptococci are responsible for most cases of bacterial pneumonia acquired at delivery. *Chlamydia trachomatis* is acquired during passage through an infected birth canal though cases occasionally occur in infants born by cesarean section after prolonged membrane rupture. Pneumonia develops in 5–20% of infants born to mothers with *C. trachomatis* infection.

CLINICAL PRESENTATION

The classic presentation of pneumonia is the sudden onset of fever, cough, and tachypnea. However, the clinical presentation of pneumonia in children can be diverse, and differentiating upper respiratory tract from lower respiratory tract infection can be especially challenging. Additionally, childhood pneumonia may be preceded by symptoms of viral upper respiratory tract infection.

Clinical examination findings of bacterial pneumonia include tachypnea, rales, and retractions. Tachypnea is the most sensitive sign of pneumonia with a sensitivity ranging from 64% to 81%[43–48] (i.e., most patients with pneumonia have tachypnea at initial evaluation); however, its specificity is poor (i.e., most patients with tachypnea do not have pneumonia). The sensitivity of rales is lower (43–57%) but the specificity is higher (60–70%).[43] Thus, pneumonia should be considered in any child with unexplained tachypnea, even if the lungs are clear to auscultation.

Abdominal pain is a well-recognized presenting symptom in children with basilar pneumonias.[49] This occurs because the T9 dermatome is shared by the lung and the abdomen.[50] The abdominal symptoms can be quite impressive and pneumonia has been inadvertently detected on abdominal computed tomography in children evaluated for suspicion of appendicitis.

Wheezing is more typical of viral respiratory infections and reactive airways disease, but may occur in childhood pneumonia, especially those cases caused by atypical bacteria such as *M. pneumoniae* and *C. pneumoniae.*[11,51] Children infected with these atypical bacteria may present with the gradual onset of headache, malaise, fever, and pharyngitis with the subsequent development of cough and dyspnea, indicating the development of bronchopneumonia. However, more acute presentations occur in up to 25–40% of patients.[52] A typical course for infections caused by atypical pathogens includes a dry, nonproductive cough, which develops approximately 3–5 days after the initial symptoms; it can become productive of mucopurulent or blood-streaked sputum. The cough usually brings the patient to medical attention 5–7 days after onset of symptoms. Coughing from either tracheobronchitis or pneumonia can persist for 2 or more weeks after resolution of fever and other constitutional signs and symptoms, resulting in a month-long illness that may resemble pertussis.[53] Physical findings associated with lower respiratory tract disease such as wheezing may be absent during the first week of the illness, the time when cough and constitutional symptoms are most troublesome. As sputum production begins in the second week of illness, fever, myalgias, and other constitutional symptoms have resolved, but auscultation of the chest frequently reveals crackles or wheezes or both, thus the designation "walking pneumonia."

An association between atypical bacteria and asthma has been proposed in a study which identified *M. pneumoniae* in 50% of children hospitalized with their first asthma attack and in 20% with a prior episode of wheezing.[51] In that study,[51] children with *M. pneumoniae* or *C. pneumoniae* infection during their first asthma attack were far more likely to have asthma recurrences.

Pneumonia caused by *C. trachomatis* typically manifests between 4 and 12 weeks of life. Infants are usually afebrile with tachypnea and diffuse rales; wheezing is not usually present. Approximately half of infants with pneumonia also have conjunctivitis.

DIFFERENTIAL DIAGNOSIS

Pneumonia due to an infectious etiology is by far the most likely diagnosis in a patient presenting with fever, cough, and focal consolidation. However, a number of noninfectious conditions may mimic pneumonia (Table 33–2) including foreign body aspiration, heart failure, malignancy (e.g., lymphoma), atelectasis, pulmonary embolus, pulmonary hemorrhage (e.g., idiopathic pulmonary hemosiderosis, Wegner's granulomatosis), and sarcoidosis. Collagen vascular diseases including systemic lupus erythematosus, scleroderma, and rheumatoid arthritis may cause interstitial lung disease with pulmonary fibrosis. Other causes of interstitial lung disease include environmental irritants such as noxious gases, radiation, and certain drugs. Hydrocarbons (e.g., gasoline, kerosene, charcoal lighter fluid) may be accidentally ingested by young children, leading to a secondary pneumonitis. Congenital lung anomalies, which can lead to pneumonia, include pulmonary sequestration, congenital lobar emphysema, and congenital cystic adenomatoid malformations.

Aspiration pneumonia should be considered in children with underlying neuromuscular disorders, swallowing difficulties, or gastroesophageal reflux. Infection is typically caused by oral flora and may include anaerobes such as *Peptostreptococcus* spp., *Fusobacterium* spp., and *Bacteroides* spp. Gram-negative rods that cause aspiration pneumonia include *Escherichia coli, Pseudomonas aeruginosa*, and *Klebsiella pneumoniae.*

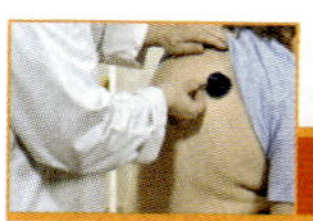

Table 33–2.

Mimics of Pneumonia

Atelectasis
Collagen vascular diseases
  Systemic lupus erythematosus
  Scleroderma
  Rheumatoid arthritis
Congenital lung anomalies
  Pulmonary sequestration
  Congenital lobar emphysema
  Congenital cystic adenomatoid malformations.
Environmental irritants
  Noxious gases
  Radiation
  Drugs
  Hydrocarbons (e.g., gasoline, kerosene, charcoal lighter fluid)
Foreign body aspiration
Heart failure
Malignancy (e.g., lymphoma)
Pulmonary embolus
Pulmonary hemorrhage
  Idiopathic pulmonary hemosideroiss
  Wegner's granulomatosis
Sarcoidosis

Specific animal exposure may suggest a less common infectious etiology of pneumonia (Table 33–3). Exposures to consider include pigeons (*Chlamydia psittaci*, *Cryptococcus neoformans*), animal urine (leptospirosis), and rabbits (*Francisella tularensis*). *Bacillus anthracis* is associated with wool sorting and may be seen in animal handlers and veterinarians as well as in the context of bioterrorism.

Plague is an infection of rodents caused by *Yersinia pestis* and transmitted to humans by infected fleas. Symptoms of pneumonic plague include high fever, chills, myalgias, malaise, headache followed within 24 hours by cough and hemoptysis. Human-to-human transmission occurs by inhaling infected droplets from patients with pulmonary infection.

Hantavirus pulmonary syndrome is a disease that begins with a viral prodrome and can rapidly progress to respiratory failure and circulatory collapse. Hantavirus is carried by rodents such as deer mice and is spread through the inhalation of aerosolized urine or dried excreta.

DIAGNOSIS

Radiologic Imaging

The clinical manifestations of CAP are diverse and are shared by other infectious and noninfectious respiratory conditions, therefore chest radiography (CXR) should be used to confirm the presence and determine the location of a pulmonary infiltrate in all children with suspected CAP evaluated in the emergency department as well as those requiring hospitalization. Both posterior–anterior (PA) and lateral views should be obtained since nonlobar infiltrates may be missed using only frontal view CXRs.[54] We recognize that routine performance of CXRs in children with suspected CAP in the ambulatory setting is neither practical nor possible. Furthermore, in children with relatively mild symptoms, it is unlikely that the CXR results will alter management or outcome. In the office setting, CXRs should be performed in moderately ill patients, including those with hypoxia, and in those whose symptoms persist despite antibiotic therapy.

The radiographic pattern of the infiltrate does not reliably differentiate among various causes. For example, an alveolar infiltrate (disease affecting the terminal air space characterized by a lobar or segmental distribution

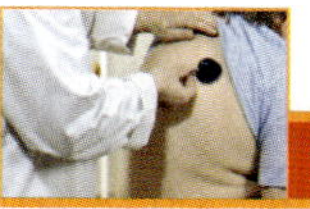

Table 33–3.

Animal Exposures Causing Pneumonia

Infectious Agent	Source	Syndrome
Yersinia pestis	Reservoir is rodents; transmission by infected fleas	Pneumonic plague
Leptospira interrogans	Urine of infected wild and domestic animals	Leptospirosis—pneumonia is an uncommon presentation
Chlamydia psittaci	Birds (e.g., pigeons, parrots)	Psittacosis
Hantavirus	Rodents (e.g., deer mice)	Hantavirus pulmonary syndrome.
Francisella tularensis	Rabbits	Tularemia
Bacillus anthracis	Primarily herbivores such as cattle, sheep, goats, horses; associated with wool sorting	Anthrax
Cryptococcus neoformans	Soil contaminated with pigeon droppings	Cryptococcosis

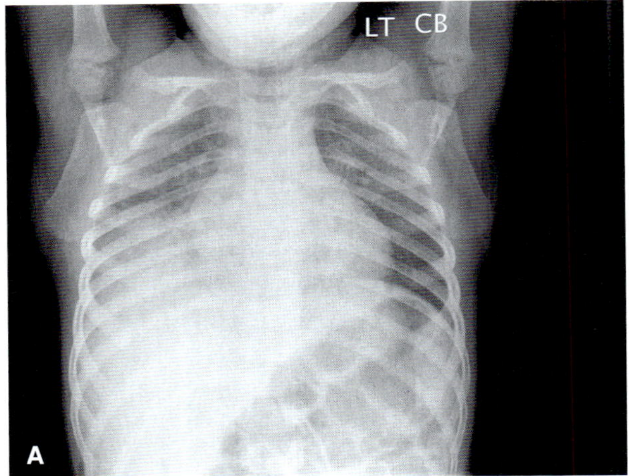

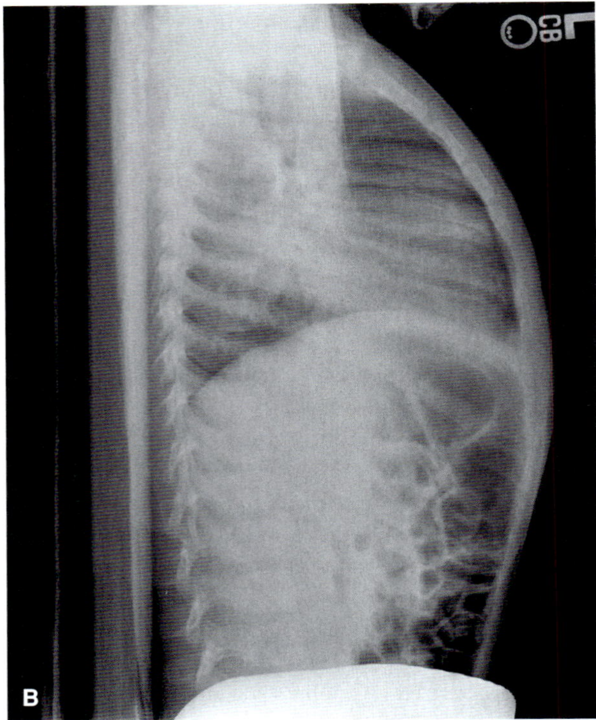

FIGURE 33–1 ■ Chest radiograph of a 2-year-old boy with pneumonia. An area of consolidation is evident in the right lower lobe on both the **(A)** posterior–anterior and **(B)** lateral chest radiograph views. On the posterior–anterior view, the right hemidiaphragm is completely obscured.

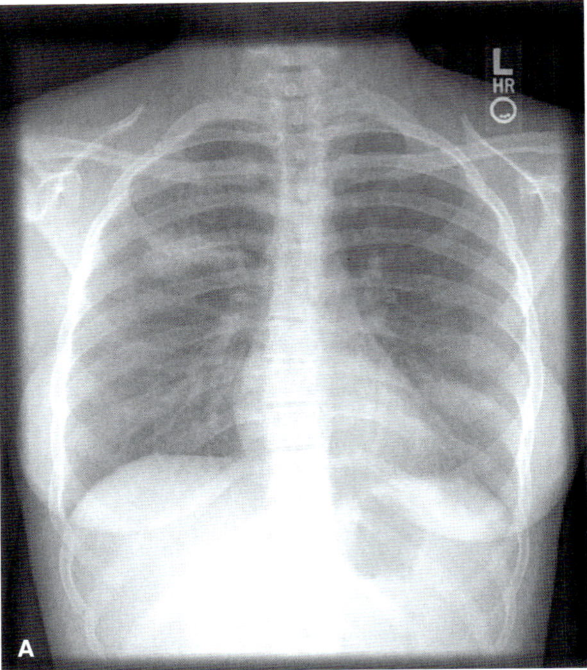

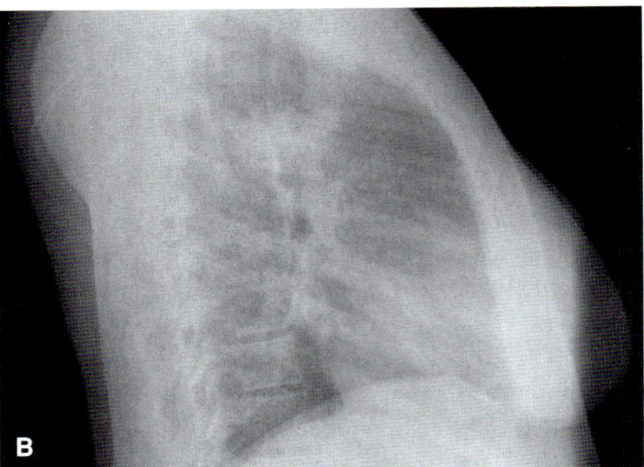

FIGURE 33–2 ■ Chest radiograph of a 15-year-old girl with pneumococcal pneumonia. A focal opacity consistent with a round pneumonia is visualized on the **(A)** posterior–anterior and **(B)** lateral chest radiographs. *Streptococcus pneumoniae* was isolated from this patient's blood culture.

with a tendency to coalesce) (Figures 33–1 and 33–2) may represent viral pneumonitis rather than bacterial pneumonia. While interstitial infiltrates are more typical of *M. pneumoniae* (Figure 33–3), patchy, unilateral, segmental, or subsegmental consolidation also occur (Figure 33–4). The presence of specific findings may serve to raise the suspicion of specific pathogens (Table 33–4). Pneumatoceles (air-filled cavities resulting from alveolar rupture) are detected in approximately two-thirds of patients with pneumonia caused by *S. aureus* (Figure 33–5).[55] The presence of hilar adenopathy, especially bilateral, out of proportion to the extent of parenchymal consolidation should raise suspicion for infection caused by *M. tuberculosis*, endemic fungi (e.g., *Histoplasma capsulatum*), and *M. pneumoniae*. Nodular infiltrates, though more common with infections caused by *Pneumocystis jiroveci* (formerly *P. carnii*) and endemic fungi, may also be caused by viruses and atypical bacteria.

An important caveat is that variation exists among radiologists on the presence or absence of radiographic features used for diagnosis of CAP. When radiographs for 34 children with a diagnosis of CAP and 34 children without CAP were reviewed without knowledge of the prior interpretation or clinical history, there was variation in the radiographic confirmation of pneumonia in 24%

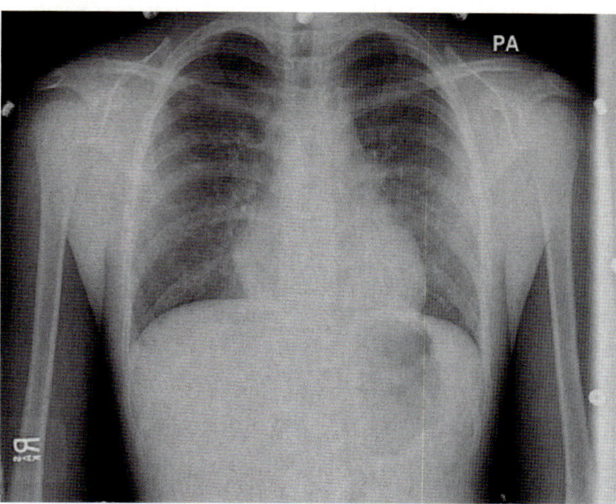

FIGURE 33–3 ■ Chest radiograph showing a diffuse interstitial infiltrate in an 11-year-old boy with pneumonia caused by *Mycoplasma pneumoniae*.

of cases and variation regarding the location of the lesion in 50% of cases.[56] In a study of adults with suspected CAP, there was fair to good interobserver reliability in detecting the presence of an infiltrate or pleural effusion; however, the interobserver reliability of other radiographic characteristics such as the pattern of the infiltrate (alveolar vs. interstitial) and the presence of air bronchograms and hilar lymphadenopathy was poor.[57] Computed tomography (CT) of the chest should be performed to more clearly define specific abnormalities such as nodular infiltrates, lung abscesses, necrotizing pneumonia, and pleural effusions.

Blood Cultures

Blood cultures are positive for pathogenic bacteria in <2% of patients with pneumonia who are well enough to be managed in the outpatient setting.[16,58,59] Blood cultures are more commonly positive in patients requiring hospitalization for pneumonia (7–10%) and in patients with pneumonia complicated by pleural effusion (up to 25%).[55,60,61] Despite the low overall yield of blood cultures in patients who require hospitalization, information on the causative organism may provide information that allows for directed narrowing or broadening of the spectrum of antibiotic therapy. Therefore, we believe that blood cultures are not required for patients with CAP who are well enough to be treated in the outpatient setting but should routinely be obtained from children with CAP requiring hospitalization.

Other Microbiologic Investigations

Gram stain and culture of expectorated sputum is infrequently performed in children with CAP because

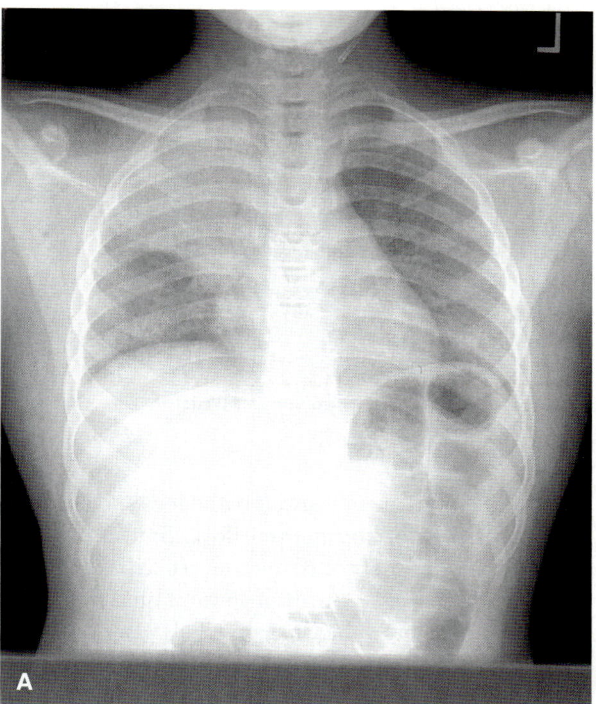

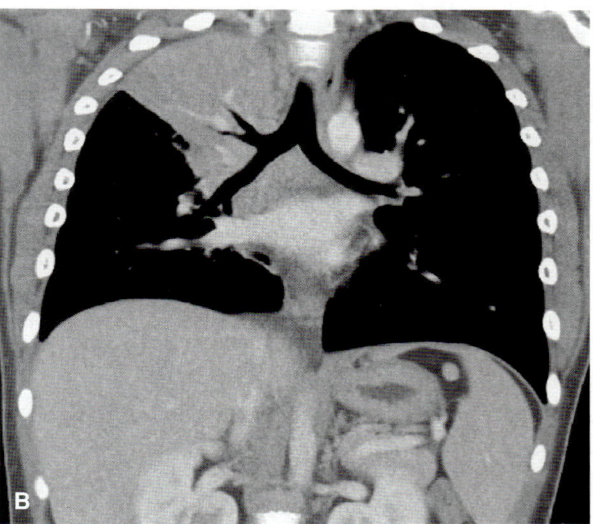

FIGURE 33–4 ■ Chest radiograph and computed tomography of a 12-year-old girl with pneumonia caused by *Mycoplasma pneumoniae*. **(A)** Posterior–anterior chest radiograph reveals a right upper lobe opacity with air bronchograms. **(B)** Contrast-enhanced computed tomography of the chest (coronal view) shows that the right upper lobe is almost completely opacified. There is also mild blunting of the right costophrenic angle indicating the presence of a pleural effusion.

children cannot always provide adequate specimens for testing. Gram stain and culture of expectorated sputum should be considered in patients with cavitary lesions, failure of outpatient therapy, and intensive care unit hospitalization if a good quality specimen can be provided. Expectorated sputum should be visibly purulent and transported to the laboratory as soon as possible (within 2 hours) since delayed transport times decrease

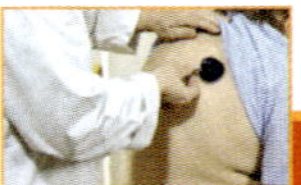

Table 33–4.

Radiographic Findings of Pneumonia

Cause	Lobar	Alveolar	Interstitial	Nodular	Hilar Adenopathy
Bacterial	++	++	−	−	+
Atypical	+	+	++	+	+
Viral	−	+	++	+	+
Tuberculosis	+	−	−	−	++
P. jiroveci	−	+	−	++	−
Endemic fungi	−	−	+	++	++

−, Uncommon manifestation; +, occasional manifestation; ++, typical manifestation.

the viability of many important pathogens and allow for the overgrowth of commensal flora. Sputum culture results must be interpreted in concert with the Gram stain. Laboratory assessment of sputum quality is based on the number of squamous epithelial cells (<10/high power field) and white blood cells (WBCs) (>25 per high power field) on Gram stain. In our experience, cooperative children 8 years of age or older with a productive cough can usually provide an adequate sputum sample. Sputum production can be induced with administration of nebulized hypertonic (5%) saline.

In young infants, *C. trachomatis* can be detected by direct fluorescent antibody testing or by culture of a nasopharyngeal (NP) or conjunctival swab. Polymerase chain reaction (PCR) testing of a NP aspirate is very sensitive for *B. pertussis* whereas culture is time-consuming and direct fluorescent antibody testing has poor sensitivity. In a patient with diffuse wheezing, *M. pneumoniae* and *C. pneumoniae* can be detected by PCR testing of a NP aspirate; if PCR is not available, acute and convalescent serum antibody titers are appropriate. Viruses can be detected in NP aspirates by PCR or immunofluorescence, but identification of a virus does not exclude the possibility of bacterial superinfection. Nasopharyngeal bacterial cultures are of no value in the etiologic diagnosis of childhood pneumonia since *S. pneumoniae* and other lower respiratory tract pathogens commonly colonize the nasopharynx in healthy children.

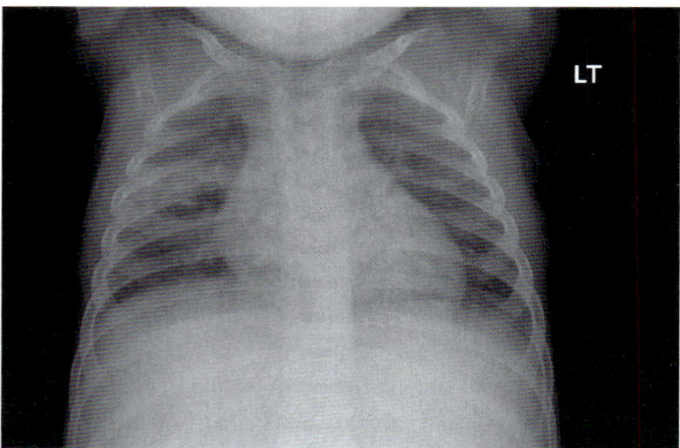

FIGURE 33–5 ■ Posterior–anterior chest radiograph shows several round lucencies consistent with pneumatocele formation in the right upper lobe at the site of a resolving pneumonia.

Urinary antigen tests for the detection of *S. pneumoniae* are routinely used to diagnose pneumococcal pneumonia in adults.[62] *S. pneumoniae* can be isolated from sputum culture in up to 80% of adults with a productive cough and a positive pneumococcal urinary antigen test.[63,64] These tests have good sensitivity in identifying children with pneumococcal bacteremia (sensitivity, 77–100%).[65] They were also positive in 47 of 62 (76%) patients with lobar pneumonia; however, since the etiology of pneumonia could not be confirmed in these patients, the relevance of this finding is not clear.[65] Additionally, false positives, attributable to pneumococcal nasopharyngeal colonization, occur in 15% of children. Pneumococcal urinary antigen tests are not routinely recommended since the results are difficult to interpret in the absence of a true gold standard.

Acute Phase Reactants

Acute phase reactants, including peripheral WBC count with differential, C-reactive protein (CRP), and erythrocyte sedimentation rate (ESR), do not reliably distinguish bacterial from viral infections. Korppi et al. found that the WBC count, CRP, and ESR were significantly higher in children with pneumococcal pneumonia compared with viral or atypical pneumonia.[66] However, the number of patients with pneumococcal disease was relatively small ($n = 29$), there was considerable overlap in values between the two groups, and the sensitivity and positive predictive value for their cutoffs were low. The sensitivity for a CRP >6.0 mg/dL or an ESR >35 mm/h was 26% and 25%, respectively. The positive predictive value for CRP >6.0 mg/dL or an ESR >35 mm/h was 43% and 38%, respectively.[66] Nohynek et al. found wide variation in WBC count, CRP, and ESR values between children with CAP attributable to bacteria and viruses; the values did not differ significantly between the two groups.[67] Therefore, we feel that acute phase reactants can be measured at baseline for patients requiring hospitalization and may then be useful in conjunction with clinical findings in assessing response to antibiotic therapy; however, they are not useful in differentiating bacterial versus viral etiologies.

Other Laboratory Tests

Other laboratory tests include serum electrolytes and arterial or venous blood gas measurements. Serum electrolytes should be measured in ill, appearing patients and in those with clinical evidence of dehydration. Inappropriate secretion of antidiuretic hormone, leading to hyponatremia, is relatively common in children with severe pneumonia.[68,69] The likely mechanism is latent vasopressin-dependent impairment of renal water excretion.[70] Resolution of hyponatremia correlates with clinical recovery. Other electrolyte abnormalities, including hypernatremia and hyper- or hypokalemia, are much less common. Blood gas measurements allow detection of hypoxemia and metabolic acidosis. Most instruments also provide crude (but rapid) measurements of the patient's hemoglobin and serum sodium; abnormalities in these parameters detected by bedside instruments should always be confirmed in the clinical laboratory.

TREATMENT

Treatment of CAP is usually empiric since definitive information about the causative pathogen is seldom available (Table 33–5).

Outpatient Therapy

For outpatients, amoxicillin remains appropriate first-line therapy. Alternate antibiotics for patients with penicillin allergy include clindamycin, levofloxacin, third-generation cephalosporins or macrolide derivatives such as clarithromycin or azithromycin. Amoxicillin-clavulanate, while providing coverage against beta-lactamase producing *Haemophilus influenzae* and *Moraxella catarrhalis*, does not provide expanded coverage against *S. pneumoniae*, the most likely bacterial pathogen. Pneumococcal resistance to beta-lactam antibiotics is mediated by alterations in penicillin-binding proteins; increasing the dose of amoxicillin or penicillin can overcome this mechanism of resistance but adding a beta-lactamase inhibitor such as clavulanic acid does not. If a patient with CAP initially managed in the outpatient setting fails to improve, a CXR should be performed to

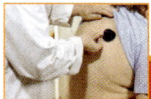

Table 33–5.

Empiric Treatment for Community Acquired Pneumonia

	Inpatient	Outpatient
Neonate	First line: Ampicillin + aminoglycoside Alternate: Ampicillin + cefotaxime; piperacillin-tazobactam ± vancomycin*	Outpatient therapy not recommended
1-3 months	First line: Ampicillin or cefotaxime Alternate: Add erythromycin or azithromycin if *Chlamydia trachomatis* or *Bordetella pertussis* suspected	Outpatient therapy not recommended
>3 months to 5 years	First line: Ampicillin Alternate: cefotaxime or ceftriaxone or clindamycin; add azithromycin or clarithromycin for diffuse wheezing to cover for atypical bacteria	First line: Amoxicillin Alternate: clindamycin or oral third-generation cephalosporins†; consider azithromycin or clarithromycin for diffuse wheezing to cover for atypical bacteria
>5 years	First line: Ampicillin or clindamycin Alternate: Levofloxacin or cefotaxime; for extremely ill patients, use azithromycin plus cefotaxime; consider adding vancomycin for patients with hypotension	First line: Amoxicillin or clindamycin Alternate: Oral third-generation cephalosporins† or levofloxacin‡; switch to levofloxacin or add azithromycin or clarithromycin for diffuse wheezing to cover for atypical bacteria

**If hospital-acquired rather than perinatally or community-acquired.*

†Efficacy against resistant pneumococci is not known.

‡Not currently approved by the food and drug administration for children <18 years though there is published evidence to support its use in younger children.

assess for the presence of local complications such as pleural effusions that require hospitalization for further management. The typical duration of treatment is 10 days (5 days can be used for azithromycin).

Inpatient Therapy

For hospitalized patients, ampicillin remains appropriate first-line therapy for uncomplicated pneumonia. For moderately or severely ill patients, cefotaxime, ceftriaxone, and levofloxacin provided broader coverage against penicillin-resistant pneumococci. Azithromycin, clarithromycin, or levofloxacin should be added to cover atypical pathogens for patients who do not respond to beta-lactam therapy; these may be administered orally. Vancomycin should be considered in patients with hypotension or necrotizing pneumonia where methicillin-resistant *S. aureus* (MRSA) is possible. Other options for coverage against MRSA include clindamycin or linezolid. The typical duration of therapy for uncomplicated pneumonia is 10–14 days. Patients may be switched to oral therapy at the time of discharge.

Changing Drug Resistance Patterns and Selection of Empiric Therapy

A key question is whether the changing patterns of pneumococcal drug resistance should change our empiric antibiotic choices for uncomplicated CAP. The alarming increase in the prevalence of penicillin resistance among *S. pneumoniae* has been well publicized. Prior to PCV7 licensure, approximately one-third of pneumococcal isolates obtained from children were resistant to penicillin.[71] This changing antibiotic resistance pattern has prompted clinicians to administer other antibiotics to patients with CAP, including more frequent use of cephalosporin and macrolide class antibiotics.[72] However, virtually all penicillin-resistant isolates were also resistant to second-generation cephalosporin antibiotics and 60% were resistant to erythromycin, a macrolide antibiotic.[71] A reduction in drug-resistance among pneumococci has been noted in studies conducted shortly after PCV7 licensure.[73–75] Kyaw et al.,[76] using data from Active Bacterial Core surveillance from 1996 to 2004, identified a significant decrease in the incidence of penicillin-nonsusceptible pneumococcal infections (by 57%) and in the incidence of strains nonsusceptible to multiple antibiotics (by 59%) beginning in 1999.[76] However, the incidence of invasive pneumococcal disease caused by penicillin-nonsusceptible vaccine-related and nonvaccine serotypes increased by 54% and 195%, respectively.[76]

The precise contributions of antibiotic-resistant *S. pneumoniae* and specific antimicrobial agents to clinical outcomes are not known. Some studies have failed to find a difference in clinical outcomes for children with pneumonia caused by penicillin-susceptible versus penicillin-nonsusceptible *S. pneumoniae*.[77,78] However, these studies have generally included patients with low levels of drug resistance; it is possible that higher levels of drug resistance are more likely to lead to treatment failure than lower levels of drug resistance. Additionally, pediatric studies have included few patients receiving discordant therapy (i.e., receipt of antibiotics that are inactive in vitro against the isolated organism), a limitation that precludes specific assessment of the effect of drug resistance on outcomes. In contrast, Yu et al. reported that clinical outcome following discordant therapy depended on the class of antibiotic administered.[79] Among 844 adult patients with pneumococcal bacteremia, cefuroxime (a second-generation cephalosporin) therapy was associated with higher mortality in the setting of cefuroxime resistance. However, therapy with penicillin or third-generation cephalosporins, such as cefotaxime and ceftriaxone, was not associated with increased mortality in the setting of penicillin or third-generation cephalosporin resistance, respectively. Other studies have documented treatment failure with macrolide-class antibiotics in the treatment of adults with pneumococcal pneumonia.[80,81] In summary, the degree to which empiric antibiotic selection affects the clinical outcome of children with pneumonia is not known. In adults, use of second-generation cephalosporin or macrolide antibiotics is associated with higher rates of treatment failure and mortality compared with use of other antibiotic classes.

Some experts advocate using higher doses of cefuroxime to overcome cefuroxime resistance. While this strategy may be effective, there is no data to suggest that such a strategy would be any more effective than using penicillin, amoxicillin, or ampicillin. When broader pneumococcal coverage is desired, third-generation cephalosporins may be more appropriate than second-generation cephalosporins.

COURSE AND PROGNOSIS

Hospitalization Decisions

Selection of the initial site of care, whether outpatient or inhospital, is one of the most important management decisions as it directly affects the intensity of subsequent testing and therapy. CAP-related admission rates vary significantly among nearby regions; within Pennsylvania, admission rates for children with CAP differ by as much as fivefold between adjacent counties.[82] These data suggest that physicians do not use consistent criteria to make site of care decisions. Unnecessary hospitalization has disadvantages, including increased likelihood of exposure to ionizing radiation and increased health care costs. However, outpatient management of high-risk patients may increase CAP-associated morbidity.

Generally agreed upon indications for hospitalization include percutaneous oxygen saturation ≤92%, marked tachypnea (>70/min in infants or >50/min in older children), difficulty in breathing, grunting, dehydration, or poor oral intake, and when the family is unable or unwilling to provide close observation and recognize clinical worsening.[4]

Follow-up Radiographs

Routine follow-up CXRs are not warranted in children who recover uneventfully from an episode of CAP. CXRs performed 3–7 weeks after an episode of radiographically confirmed CAP revealed residual or new changes in 59 (30%) of 196 children; persistence of interstitial infiltrates and the interval development of atelectasis were the most commonly noted findings.[83] Follow-up 8–10 years later did not reveal any illnesses attributable to the initial episode of CAP.[83] Among 41 children with CAP, repeat CXRs 4–6 weeks later were normal in 37 children and revealed resolving infiltrates in the remaining four children.[84] In a prospective study of adults hospitalized with severe CAP, CXRs were repeated 7 and 28 days after admission.[85] At day 7, 75% of patients still had abnormal findings on CXR. At day 28, 47% of patients still had abnormal findings on CXR. Delayed resolution of radiographic abnormalities was associated with multilobar disease, dullness to percussion on examination, higher CRP levels, and documented pneumococcal infection. However, delayed resolution of radiographic abnormalities did not portend failure of therapy or a worse clinical outcome. In summary, routine follow-up CXRs do not seem to provide additional clinical value. A subset of patients, such as those with lobar collapse or recurrent pneumonia involving the same lobe, may benefit from repeat CXRs.

PEARLS

- Tachypnea is the most sensitive sign of pneumonia.
- Abdominal pain is a well-recognized presenting symptom in children with basilar pneumonia.
- Blood cultures are not required for patients with CAP who are well enough to be treated in the outpatient setting, but should routinely be obtained from children with CAP requiring hospitalization.
- *M. pneumoniae* may cause lobar or segmental infiltrates on CXR.

REFERENCES

1. UNICEF. *Pneumonia: The Forgotten Killer of Children.* New York: UNICEF/WHO; 2006.
2. McIntosh K. Community-acquired pneumonia in children. *N Engl J Med.* 2002;346:429-437.
3. Peck AJ, Holman RC, Curns AT, et al. Lower respiratory tract infections among American Indian and Alaska Native children and the general population of U.S. children. *Pediatr Infect Dis J.* 2005;24:342-351.
4. British Thoracic Society Guidelines for the Management of Community Acquired Pneumonia in Childhood. *Thorax.* 2002;57(suppl)1:i1-24.
5. Jokinen C, Heiskanen L, Juvonen H, et al. Incidence of community-acquired pneumonia in the population of four municipalities in eastern Finland. *Am J Epidemiol.* 1993;137:977-988.
6. Murphy TF, Henderson FW, Clyde WA, Jr., Collier AM, Denny FW. Pneumonia: an eleven-year study in a pediatric practice. *Am J Epidemiol.* 1981;113:12-21.
7. Heiskanen-Kosma T, Korppi M, Jokinen C, et al. Etiology of childhood pneumonia: serologic results of a prospective, population-based study. *Pediatr Infect Dis J.* 1998;17:986-991.
8. Dowell SF, Kupronis BA, Zell ER, Shay DK. Mortality from pneumonia in children in the United States, 1939 through 1996. *N Engl J Med.* 2000;342:1399-1407.
9. DeFrances CJ, Hall MJ. 2002 National Hospital Discharge Survey. *Adv Data.* 2004:1-29.
10. Heiskanen-Kosma T, Korppi M, Jokinen C, Heinonen K. Risk factors for community-acquired pneumonia in children: a population-based case-control study. *Scand J Infect Dis.* 1997;29:281-285.
11. Michelow IC, Olsen K, Lozano J, et al. Epidemiology and clinical characteristics of community-acquired pneumonia in hospitalized children. *Pediatrics.* 2004;113:701-707.
12. Korppi M, Heiskanen-Kosma T, Jalonen E, et al. Aetiology of community-acquired pneumonia in children treated in hospital. *Eur J Pediatr.* 1993;152:24-30.
13. Korppi M, Heiskanen-Kosma T, Kleemola M. Incidence of community-acquired pneumonia in children caused by Mycoplasma pneumoniae: serological results of a prospective, population-based study in primary health care. *Respirology.* 2004;9:109-114.
14. Wubbel L, Muniz L, Ahmed A, et al. Etiology and treatment of community-acquired pneumonia in ambulatory children. *Pediatr Infect Dis J.* 1999;18:98-104.
15. Preventing pneumococcal disease among infants and young children. Recommendations of the Advisory Committee on Immunization Practices (ACIP). *MMWR Recomm Rep.* 2000;49:1-35.
16. Black SB, Shinefield HR, Ling S, et al. Effectiveness of heptavalent pneumococcal conjugate vaccine in children younger than five years of age for prevention of pneumonia. *Pediatr Infect Dis J.* 2002;21:810-815.
17. Cutts FT, Zaman SM, Enwere G, et al. Efficacy of nine-valent pneumococcal conjugate vaccine against pneumonia and invasive pneumococcal disease in The Gambia: randomised, double-blind, placebo-controlled trial. *Lancet.* 2005;365:1139-46.
18. Klugman KP, Madhi SA, Huebner RE, Kohberger R, Mbelle N, Pierce N. A trial of a 9-valent pneumococcal

conjugate vaccine in children with and those without HIV infection. *N Engl J Med.* 2003;349:1341-1348.
19. Grijalva CG, Nuorti JP, Arbogast PG, Martin SW, Edwards KM, Griffin MR. Decline in pneumonia admissions after routine childhood immunisation with pneumococcal conjugate vaccine in the USA: a time-series analysis. Lancet. 2007;369:1179-1186.
20. Foy HM, Grayston JT, Kenny GE, Alexander ER, McMahan R. Epidemiology of *Mycoplasma pneumoniae* infection in families. *Jama.* 1966;197:859-866.
21. Fernald GW, Collier AM, Clyde WA, Jr. Respiratory infections due to *Mycoplasma pneumoniae* in infants and children. *Pediatrics.* 1975;55:327-335.
22. Alexander ER, Foy HM, Kenny GE, et al. Pneumonia due to *Mycoplasma pneumoniae.* Its incidence in the membership of a co-operative medical group. *N Engl J Med.* 1966;275:131-136.
23. Block S, Hedrick J, Hammerschlag MR, Cassell GH, Craft JC. *Mycoplasma pneumoniae* and *Chlamydia pneumoniae* in pediatric community-acquired pneumonia: Comparative efficacy and safety of clarithromycin vs. erythromycin ethylsuccinate. *Pediatr Infect Dis J.* 1995;14:471-477.
24. Gendrel D. Antibiotic treatment of *Mycoplasma pneumoniae* infections. *Pediatr Pulmonol Suppl.* 1997;16:46-47.
25. Harris JA, Kolokathis A, Campbell M, Cassell GH, Hammerschlag MR. Safety and efficacy of azithromycin in the treatment of community-acquired pneumonia in children. *Pediatr Infect Dis J.* 1998;17:865-871.
26. Glezen WP, Loda FA, Clyde WA, Jr., et al. Epidemiologic patterns of acute lower respiratory disease of children in a pediatric group practice. *J Pediatr.* 1971;78:397-406.
27. Mogabgab WJ. *Mycoplasma pneumoniae* and adenovirus respiratory illnesses in military and university personnel, 1959-1966. *Am Rev Respir Dis.* 1968;97:345-358.
28. Evans AS, Allen V, Sueltmann S. *Mycoplasma pneumoniae* infections in University of Wisconsin students. *Am Rev Respir Dis.* 1967;96:237-244.
29. Foy HM. Infections caused by *Mycoplasma pneumoniae* and possible carrier state in different populations of patients. *Clin Infect Dis.* 1993;17(suppl 1):S37-S46.
30. Foy HM, Kenny GE, Cooney MK, Allan ID. Long-term epidemiology of infections with *Mycoplasma pneumoniae.* *J Infect Dis.* 1979;139:681-687.
31. Feikin DR, Moroney JF, Talkington DF, et al. An outbreak of acute respiratory disease caused by *Mycoplasma pneumoniae* and adenovirus at a federal service training academy: new implications from an old scenario. *Clin Infect Dis.* 1999;29:1545-1550.
32. Harford C, Hara M. Pulmonary edema in influenzal pneumonia of the mouse and the relation of fluid ni the lung to the inception of pneumococal pneumonia. *J Exp Med.* 1950;91:245-259.
33. Tuomanen EI, Austrian R, Masure HR. Pathogenesis of pneumococcal infection. *N Engl J Med.* 1995;332: 1280-1284.
34. Tuomanen E, Rich R, Zak O. Induction of pulmonary inflammation by components of the pneumococcal cell surface. *Am Rev Respir Dis.* 1987;135:869-874.
35. Tilghman R, Finland M. Clinical significance of bacteremia in pneumococcic pneumonia. *Arch Inter Med.* 1937;59:602-19.
36. Collier AM, Hu PC, Clyde WA, Jr. Location of attachment moiety on *Mycoplasma pneumoniae. Yale J Biol Med.* 1983;56:671-677.
37. Kahane I. In vitro studies on the mechanism of adherence and pathogenicity of mycoplasmas. *Isr J Med Sci.* 1984;20:874-877.
38. Krause DC, Baseman JB. Inhibition of *Mycoplasma pneumoniae* hemadsorption and adherence to respiratory epithelium by antibodies to a membrane protein. *Infect Immun.* 1983;39:1180-1186.
39. Almagor M, Yatziv S, Kahane I. Inhibition of host cell catalase by *Mycoplasma pneumoniae*: a possible mechanism for cell injury. *Infect Immun.* 1983;41:251-256.
40. Waites KB, Talkington DF. *Mycoplasma pneumoniae* and its role as a human pathogen. *Clin Microbiol Rev.* 2004;17: 697-728, table of contents.
41. Shah SS. *Mycoplasma pneumoniae.* In: Long SS, Pickering LK, Prober CG, eds. *Principles and Practice of Pediatric Infectious Diseases.* 3rd ed. Philadelphia: Churchill Livingstone; 2008:979-985.
42. Lind K. Manifestations and complications of *Mycoplasma pneumoniae* disease: *a review. Yale J Biol Med.* 1983;56: 461-468.
43. Palafox M, Guiscafre H, Reyes H, Munoz O, Martinez H. Diagnostic value of tachypnoea in pneumonia defined radiologically. *Arch Dis Child.* 2000;82:41-45.
44. Berman S, Simoes EA, Lanata C. Respiratory rate and pneumonia in infancy. *Arch Dis Child.* 1991;66:81-84.
45. Leventhal JM. Clinical predictors of pneumonia as a guide to ordering chest roentgenograms. *Clin Pediatr (Phila).* 1982;21:730-734.
46. Zukin DD, Hoffman JR, Cleveland RH, Kushner DC, Herman TE. Correlation of pulmonary signs and symptoms with chest radiographs in the pediatric age group. *Ann Emerg Med.* 1986;15:792-796.
47. Grossman LK, Caplan SE. Clinical, laboratory, and radiological information in the diagnosis of pneumonia in children. *Ann Emerg Med.* 1988;17:43-6.
48. Taylor JA, Del Beccaro M, Done S, Winters W. Establishing clinically relevant standards for tachypnea in febrile children younger than 2 years. *Arch Pediatr Adolesc Med.* 1995;149:283-287.
49. Ravichandran D, Burge DM. Pneumonia presenting with acute abdominal pain in children. *Br J Surg.* 1996;83: 1707-1708.
50. Leung AK, Sigalet DL. Acute abdominal pain in children. *Am Fam Physician.* 2003;67:2321-2326.
51. Biscardi S, Lorrot M, Marc E, et al. *Mycoplasma pneumoniae* and asthma in children. *Clin Infect Dis.* 2004;38:1341-1346.
52. Esposito S, Blasi F, Bellini F, Allegra L, Principi N. *Mycoplasma pneumoniae* and *Chlamydia pneumoniae* infections in children with pneumonia. Mowgli Study Group. *Eur Respir J.* 2001;17:241-245.
53. Davis SF, Sutter RW, Strebel PM, et al. Concurrent outbreaks of pertussis and *Mycoplasma pneumoniae* infection: clinical and epidemiological characteristics of illnesses manifested by cough. *Clin Infect Dis.* 1995;20: 621-628.
54. Rigsby CK, Strife JL, Johnson ND, Atherton HD, Pommersheim W, Kotagal UR. Is the frontal radiograph alone sufficient to evaluate for pneumonia in children? *Pediatr Radiol.* 2004;34:379-383.

55. Freij BJ, Kusmiesz H, Nelson JD, McCracken GH, Jr. Parapneumonic effusions and empyema in hospitalized children: a retrospective review of 227 cases. *Pediatr Infect Dis.* 1984;3:578-591.
56. Stickler GB, Hoffman AD, Taylor WF. Problems in the clinical and roentgenographic diagnosis of pneumonia in young children. *Clin Pediatr (Phila).* 1984;23:398-399.
57. Albaum MN, Hill LC, Murphy M, et al. Interobserver reliability of the chest radiograph in community-acquired pneumonia. PORT Investigators. *Chest.* 1996;110:343-350.
58. Shah SS, Alpern ER, Zwerling L, McGowan KL, Bell LM. Risk of bacteremia in young children with pneumonia treated as outpatients. *Arch Pediatr Adolesc Med.* 2003; 157:389-392.
59. Hickey RW, Bowman MJ, Smith GA. Utility of blood cultures in pediatric patients found to have pneumonia in the emergency department. *Ann Emerg Med.* 1996;27:721-725.
60. Hoff SJ, Neblett WW, Edwards KM, et al. Parapneumonic empyema in children: decortication hastens recovery in patients with severe pleural infections. *Pediatr Infect Dis J.* 1991;10:194-199.
61. Byington CL, Spencer LY, Johnson TA, et al. An epidemiological investigation of a sustained high rate of pediatric parapneumonic empyema: risk factors and microbiological associations. *Clin Infect Dis.* 2002;34:434-440.
62. Mandell LA, Wunderink RG, Anzueto A, et al. Infectious Diseases Society of America/American Thoracic Society consensus guidelines on the management of community-acquired pneumonia in adults. *Clin Infect Dis.* 2007;44 (suppl 2):S27-S72.
63. Roson B, Fernandez-Sabe N, Carratala J, et al. Contribution of a urinary antigen assay (Binax NOW) to the early diagnosis of pneumococcal pneumonia. *Clin Infect Dis.* 2004;38:222-226.
64. Ishida T, Hashimoto T, Arita M, Tojo Y, Tachibana H, Jinnai M. A 3-year prospective study of a urinary antigen-detection test for *Streptococcus pneumoniae* in community-acquired pneumonia: utility and clinical impact on the reported etiology. *J Infect Chemother.* 2004;10:359-363.
65. Neuman MI, Harper MB. Evaluation of a rapid urine antigen assay for the detection of invasive pneumococcal disease in children. *Pediatrics.* 2003;112:1279-1282.
66. Korppi M, Heiskanen-Kosma T, Leinonen M. White blood cells, C-reactive protein and erythrocyte sedimentation rate in pneumococcal pneumonia in children. *Eur Respir J.* 1997;10:1125-1129.
67. Nohynek H, Valkeila E, Leinonen M, Eskola J. Erythrocyte sedimentation rate, white blood cell count and serum C-reactive protein in assessing etiologic diagnosis of acute lower respiratory infections in children. *Pediatr Infect Dis J.* 1995;14:484-490.
68. Dhawan A, Narang A, Singhi S. Hyponatraemia and the inappropriate ADH syndrome in pneumonia. *Ann Trop Paediatr.* 1992;12:455-462.
69. Singhi S, Dhawan A. Frequency and significance of electrolyte abnormalities in pneumonia. *Indian Pediatr.* 1992; 29:735-740.
70. Dreyfuss D, Leviel F, Paillard M, Rahmani J, Coste F. Acute infectious pneumonia is accompanied by a latent vasopressin-dependent impairment of renal water excretion. *Am Rev Respir Dis.* 1988;138:583-589.
71. Whitney CG, Farley MM, Hadler J, et al. Increasing prevalence of multidrug-resistant *Streptococcus pneumoniae* in the United States. *N Engl J Med.* 2000;343:1917-1924.
72. Metlay JP, Shea JA, Asch DA. Antibiotic prescribing decisions of generalists and infectious disease specialists: thresholds for adopting new drug therapies. *Med Decis Making.* 2002;22:498-505.
73. Kaplan SL, Mason EO, Jr., Wald ER, et al. Decrease of invasive pneumococcal infections in children among 8 children's hospitals in the United States after the introduction of the 7-valent pneumococcal conjugate vaccine. *Pediatrics.* 2004;113:443-449.
74. Pelton SI, Loughlin AM, Marchant CD. Seven valent pneumococcal conjugate vaccine immunization in two Boston communities: changes in serotypes and antimicrobial susceptibility among *Streptococcus pneumoniae* isolates. *Pediatr Infect Dis J.* 2004;23:1015-1022.
75. Talbot TR, Poehling KA, Hartert TV, et al. Reduction in high rates of antibiotic-nonsusceptible invasive pneumococcal disease in Tennessee after introduction of the pneumococcal conjugate vaccine. *Clin Infect Dis.* 2004;39: 641-648.
76. Kyaw MH, Lynfield R, Schaffner W, et al. Effect of introduction of the pneumococcal conjugate vaccine on drug-resistant *Streptococcus pneumoniae. N Engl J Med.* 2006; 354:1455-1463.
77. Kaplan SL, Mason EO, Jr., Barson WJ, et al. Outcome of invasive infections outside the central nervous system caused by *Streptococcus pneumoniae* isolates nonsusceptible to ceftriazone in children treated with beta-lactam antibiotics. *Pediatr Infect Dis J.* 2001;20:392-396.
78. Tan TQ, Mason EO, Jr., Barson WJ, et al. Clinical characteristics and outcome of children with pneumonia attributable to penicillin-susceptible and penicillin-nonsusceptible *Streptococcus pneumoniae. Pediatrics.* 1998;102: 1369-1375.
79. Yu VL, Chiou CC, Feldman C, et al. An international prospective study of pneumococcal bacteremia: correlation with in vitro resistance, antibiotics administered, and clinical outcome. *Clin Infect Dis.* 2003;37:230-237.
80. Peterson LR. Penicillins for treatment of pneumococcal pneumonia: does in vitro resistance really matter? *Clin Infect Dis.* 2006;42:224-233.
81. Lonks JR, Garau J, Gomez L, et al. Failure of macrolide antibiotic treatment in patients with bacteremia due to erythromycin-resistant *Streptococcus pneumoniae. Clin Infect Dis.* 2002;35:556-564.
82. Gorton CP, Jones JL. Wide geographic variation between Pennsylvania counties in the population rates of hospital admissions for pneumonia among children with and without comorbid chronic conditions. *Pediatrics.* 2006; 117:176-180.
83. Virkki R, Juven T, Mertsola J, Ruuskanen O. Radiographic follow-up of pneumonia in children. *Pediatr Pulmonol.* 2005;40:223-227.
84. Heaton P, Arthur K. The utility of chest radiography in the follow-up of pneumonia. *N Z Med J.* 1998;111:315-317.
85. Bruns AH, Oosterheert JJ, Prokop M, Lammers JW, Hak E, Hoepelman AI. Patterns of resolution of chest radiograph abnormalities in adults hospitalized with severe community-acquired pneumonia. *Clin Infect Dis.* 2007; 45:983-991.

CHAPTER 34

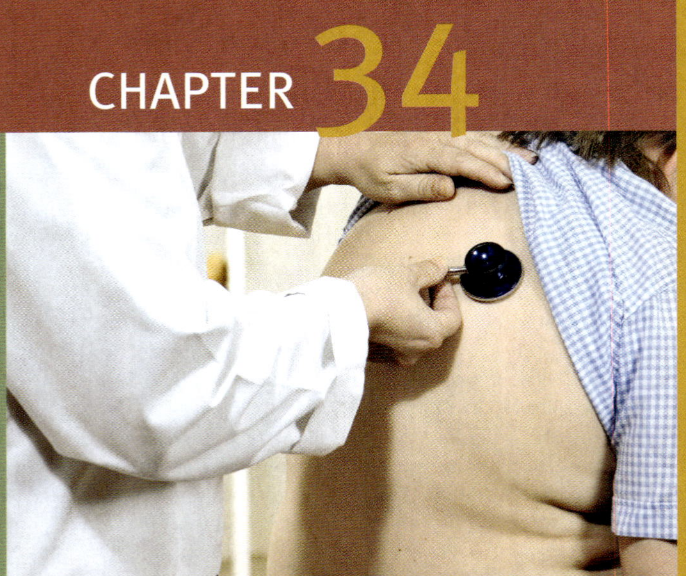

Complicated Pneumonia

Sanjeev Swami, Peter Mattei, and Samir S. Shah

DEFINITION AND EPIDEMIOLOGY

The term complicated pneumonia, in this chapter, will refer to pneumonia complicated by the accumulation of fluid or purulent material in the pleural space; this term includes parapneumonic effusions and empyema. The frequency of complicated pneumonia among all children with community-acquired pneumonia (CAP) is not known. However, complicated pneumonia has been reported to occur in 6–8% of children hospitalized with CAP.[1,2]

Streptococcus pneumoniae and *Staphylococcus aureus* remain the most common bacterial causes of complicated pneumonia (Table 34–1), though the epidemiology of complicated pneumonia appears to be changing. In February 2000, the Food and Drug Administration licensed a heptavalent pneumococcal conjugate vaccine (PCV7), which was subsequently recommended by the Advisory Committee on Immunization Practices and the American Academy of Pediatrics for use in children aged 2 years and younger as well as in older, high-risk children.[3] Vaccine uptake was rapid and substantial declines in rates of invasive pneumococcal disease were documented in children.[4] Randomized clinical trials[5–7] and population-based observational studies[1] suggested that PCV7 use has also decreased the incidence of CAP.

Postlicensure studies have revealed increases in nasopharyngeal carriage and invasive disease caused by pneumococcal serotypes not included in the currently licensed vaccine.[8–10] It is not known whether the changing pneumococcal epidemiology will result in more or less frequent complications among patients with CAP. Investigators in Utah reported a regional increase in the frequency of empyema complicating CAP following PCV7 licensure; 86% of known isolates were pneumococcal serotypes not contained in PCV7.[11] However, the results should be interpreted with caution because fewer than 10% of the isolates were available for serotyping.[11] Furthermore, the investigators reported the absolute number of cases rather than population-based incidence rates.[11] In contrast, adult studies suggest that pneumococcal vaccination reduces pneumonia-associated complication rates. In a large cohort of adults hospitalized with CAP, pneumococcal polysaccharide vaccine recipients were less likely to die of any cause and less likely to develop respiratory failure than individuals with CAP who did not receive the vaccine.[12] Studies of more than 11,000 adults in Spain also found that pneumococcal vaccination reduced the risk of pneumococcal pneumonia (45% reduction), CAP-associated hospitalization, and mortality.[13,14] Vaccination may reduce mortality and metastatic disease by preventing systemic dissemination of the organism during an episode of bacteremia. Whether PCV7 will lead to a similar

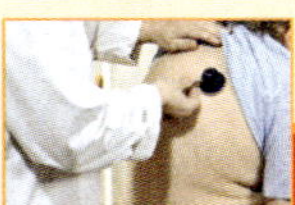

Table 34–1.

Causes of Empyema

Common	Less Common
Streptococcus pneumoniae	*Streptococcus pyogenes*
Staphylococcus aureus	Anaerobes*
Mycobacterium tuberculosis	*Haemophilus influenzae*†
	Group B *Streptococcus*†
	Enteric gram-negative rods†

*Anaerobes include *Fusobacterium* species and *Bacteroides melaninogenicus*.
†*H. influenzae* type b if underimmunized; group B *Streptococcus* and gram-negative rods common in neonates.

decrease in adverse outcomes among children with CAP remains to be determined.

The prevalence of invasive community-acquired infections, including pneumonia, caused by methicillin-resistant *S. aureus* (MRSA) has increased over the past few years.[15,16] Many cases of MRSA pneumonia are associated with empyema and severe necrotizing disease.[17] Several patients with complicated pneumonia caused by MRSA have had a history of recurrent skin infections.[18] Risk factors for MRSA skin and skin structure infections have been identified, however it is not known whether children with CAP and a history of recurrent MRSA skin infections are at increased risk of severe CAP-related complications.

Historically, *Haemophilus influenzae* type B was a leading cause of invasive bacterial infections including complicated pneumonia; however, since the introduction of the *H. influenzae* type B vaccine, it rarely causes infections in immunized children.[19] In neonates, Group B streptococci and enteric Gram-negative rods including *Escherichia coli* are also important causes of complicated pneumonia. Children with severe neurologic impairment are at risk for complicated pneumonia caused by Gram-negative rods following aspiration of gastric contents. In immunocompromised hosts, fungi must also be considered. Although viruses are frequent causes of pneumonia, and can be found in patients with empyema, they are rarely the sole cause of complicated pneumonia; rather, these infections represent a preceding viral infection with subsequent bacterial superinfection.

PATHOGENESIS

In the normal state, the pleural space (the area between the visceral and parietal pleura) contains only a small (<0.3 mL/kg of body weight) amount of thin fluid. There is continuous circulation of this fluid and the lymphatic vessels can cope with several hundred milliliters of extra fluid in a 24-hour period.[20] However, an imbalance between pleural fluid formation and drainage will result in a pleural effusion. Several liters of thick, purulent fluid may accumulate in the pleural space of a child with pneumonia complicated by parapneumonic effusion. The development of an empyema in a child with bacterial pneumonia is a progressive process that can be divided into three stages:

Stage 1 (exudative stage) reflects the host response to infection, which includes recruitment of polymorphonuclear neutrophils (PMNs) to the site of infection. The PMNs release active oxygen metabolites, which lead to increased capillary permeability. This allows protein-rich fluid to enter the pleural spaces, increasing the oncotic pressure in the pleural space and drawing more fluid into that area. During the exudative phase, the fluid remains free-flowing.

Stage 2 (fibropurulent stage) develops as bacterial invasion of the pleural space promotes fibrin deposition, neutrophil migration, and procoagulant activity. Fibroblasts are also recruited into the pleural cavity and begin to deposit collagen. These processes result in the formation of loculations or septations between the visceral and parietal pleura, leading to distinct pockets of pus and fluid.

Stage 3 (organizing stage) occurs with proliferation of fibroblasts. During this stage, the loculations continue to develop and a fibrinous peel is deposited on the pleura, which impedes lung expansion and fluid reabsorption.

CLINICAL PRESENTATION

The clinical presentation of complicated pneumonia is similar to the presentation of uncomplicated pneumonia, but weighted toward the more severe end of the spectrum. The early symptoms of bacterial pneumonia include fever, chills, cough, and dyspnea (Table 34–2). As a parapneumonic effusion develops, children may complain of pleurisy due to irritation of the parietal pleura. As the effusion increases in size, this complaint may lessen as the pleurae become separated. If the effusion becomes large in size, the dyspnea may become much more severe and orthopnea may also develop.

On physical examination, tachypnea is invariably present with the degree depending on a number of factors including the extent of parenchymal consolidation, the size of the pleural effusion, and the degree of fever at the time of the examination. Pulse oximetry often reveals hypoxia, though the extent depends on the degree of consolidation and ventilation/perfusion (V/Q) mismatch. In children with small effusions, it can be difficult to appreciate decreased breath sounds or dullness to percussion. As the size of the effusion increases, these signs become easier to elicit. If the

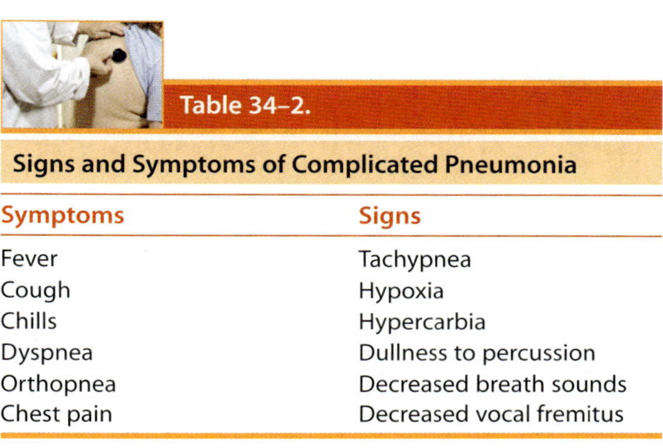

Table 34–2.

Signs and Symptoms of Complicated Pneumonia

Symptoms	Signs
Fever	Tachypnea
Cough	Hypoxia
Chills	Hypercarbia
Dyspnea	Dullness to percussion
Orthopnea	Decreased breath sounds
Chest pain	Decreased vocal fremitus

effusion is small, a pleural rub may be appreciated as the roughened pleurae rub against each other. As the volume of fluid increases, the pleurae become separated and this sign disappears. Depending on the location and degree of parenchymal consolidation relative to the size of the effusion, some patients may also have crackles and egophony. In infants, the physical examination can be challenging as breath sounds from the healthy, uninfected lung may be heard over the infected lung. These children will still have tachypnea unless they are at the point of fatigue in which case they will appear quite ill.

DIFFERENTIAL DIAGNOSIS

There are a number of different causes of pleural effusions in children, and many of them are noninfectious (Table 34–3). Pleural effusion can develop whenever the pleural fluid production exceeds its removal. The production of pleural fluid is governed by the differences in hydrostatic and oncotic pressures in the capillaries and in the pleural space. Processes that increase the hydrostatic pressure in the capillaries (e.g., congestive heart failure) or increase the oncotic pressure in the pleural space (e.g., pulmonary infarction) will lead to increased production of pleural fluid. Additionally, processes that cause decreased capillary oncotic pressure (e.g., nephrotic syndrome, hypoalbuminemia) or decreased hydrostatic pressure in the pleural space will lead to increased pleural fluid. Pleural effusions can also develop if the absorption of pleural fluid is decreased (e.g., thoracic duct obstruction).

DIAGNOSIS

Radiologic Imaging

The diagnosis of complicated pneumonia should be considered in any moderately or severely ill child with CAP and in any patient with CAP who worsens clinically despite antibiotic therapy. If the diagnosis of complicated pneumonia is suspected, the first step is to obtain posterior–anterior (PA) and lateral chest radiographs. Blunting of the costophrenic angles on PA view indicates the presence of a pleural effusion. This finding may not be visible with small effusions; upright posterioanterior radiographs may not show lateral costophrenic angle blunting until 250 mL or more fluid is present.[21] Extensive lower lobe consolidation may also obscure the presence of a pleural effusion on the PA views. In the upright position, small, free-flowing effusions will collect posteriorly and are more readily visualized on lateral radiographs. Lateral radiographs show blunting of the posterior costophrenic angle and the posterior gutter with less fluid than on the PA views; decubitus films with the affected side positioned downward can detect even smaller amounts of pleural fluid.[22] If the effusion is in the exudative stage, the fluid should layer out along the chest wall when the patient is in the decubitus position. If the infection has progressed to the second or third stage, the loculations prevent free movement of the fluid (Figure 34–1).

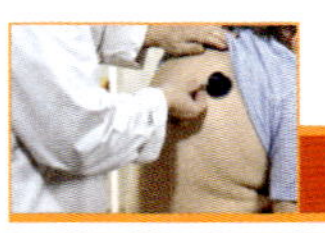

Table 34–3.

Causes of Pleural Effusions

Congestive heart failure	Infection
Systemic lupus erythematosus	Thoracic duct obstruction
Malignancy	Pulmonary lymphangiectasis
Nephrotic syndrome	Capillary leak
Cirrhosis	Pleural irritation
Hypoalbuminemia	Iatrogenic

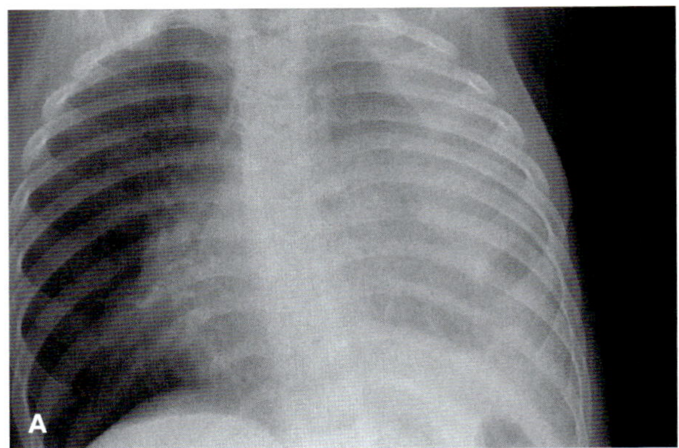

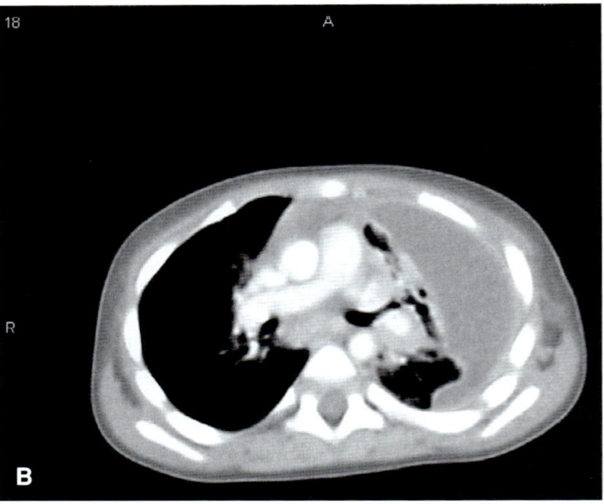

FIGURE 34–1 ■ Radiologic findings in an 18-month-old boy with pneumococcal pneumonia. The upright posterioanterior radiograph **(A)** shows left lung consolidation with a moderately sized pleural effusion. Extensive loculation is likely as the effusion does not layer out in this upright view. Contrast-enhanced computed tomography **(B)** shows a large empyema surrounded by a contrast-enhancing rim.

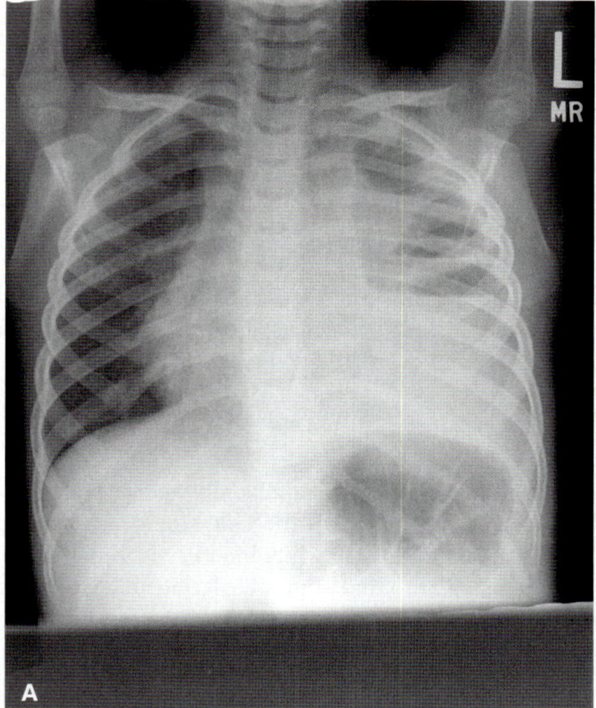

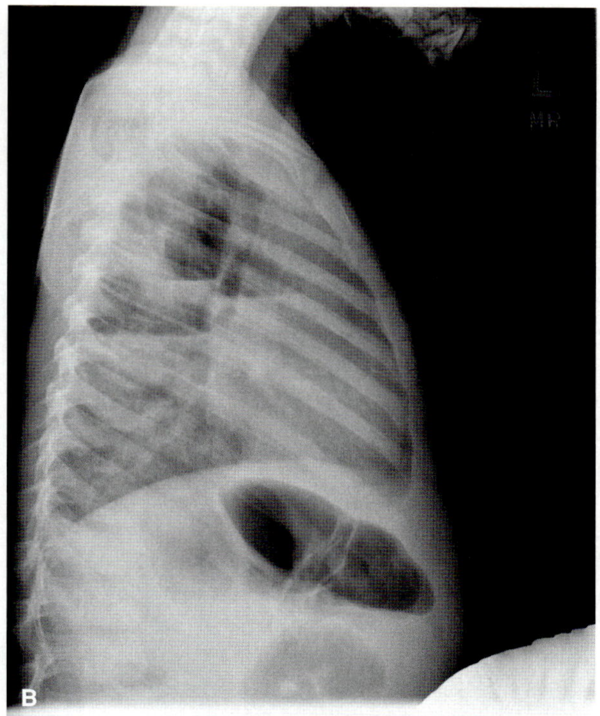

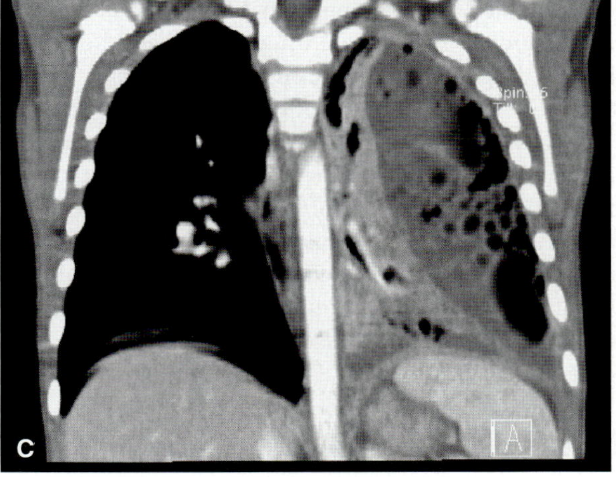

FIGURE 34–2 ■ Radiologic findings in a 4-year-old boy with complicated pneumonia caused by methicillin-resistant *Staphylococcus aureus*. The posterioanterior **(A)** and lateral **(B)** chest radiographs show a moderate left pleural effusion with fluid-filled spaces consistent with necrotizing pneumonia. The large pleural fluid collection has resulted in a rightward shift of the mediastinal structures. Contrast-enhanced computed tomography (coronal view) **(C)** reveals a large and loculated hydropneumothorax that extends 15 cm in the craniocaudal direction and occupies the majority of the left hemithorax. The left lower lob contains multiloculated cavities and numerous air-fluid levels consistent with necrotizing pneumonia. The large amount of air within the pleural space also indicates the presence of a bronchopleural fistula.

Additional evaluation of the chest by computed tomography (CT) or ultrasonography should be performed if there is a significant effusion detected by radiography or if there is concern for loculation based on the decubitus views. Contrast-enhanced CT permits assessment of the extent of consolidation and detection of parenchymal necrosis or abscesses, pleural thickening, and large septations (Figure 34–2). Limitations of CT include the inability to reliably differentiate transudative from exudative effusions in the absence of septations or loculations, and the frequent requirement for sedation in young children. Sedation for radiologic procedures may be difficult in the context of severe respiratory distress. While there may be an increased risk of radiation-induced malignancies in pediatric patients who undergo CT,[23] the seriousness of complicated pneumonia warrants such imaging.

Ultrasonography is also used in the diagnosis and management of complicated pneumonia. It also allows for better visualization of septations than standard radiographs. Since the patient can be repositioned during the procedure, ultrasonography may also allow for better assessment of pleural fluid character, including the extent of pleural fluid loculation, than CT.[24] In addition, ultrasonography does not typically require sedation, does not expose the child to ionizing radiation, and can be performed at the patient's bedside using a portable machine. The major drawbacks of ultrasongraphy are that it is highly operator dependant, requires an experienced radiologist for interpretation, and does not permit adequate assessment of the extent of parenchymal consolidation.

Laboratory Studies

The initial laboratory evaluation includes a complete blood count, blood culture, and inflammatory markers including a C-reactive protein (CRP) and erythrocyte sedimentation rate (ESR). The blood count may reveal leuckocytosis, anemia, and reactive thrombocytosis. Rare complications such as pneumococcal hemolytic–uremic syndrome hemolytic uremic syndrome (HUS) are accompanied by severe anemia and thrombocytopenia. The CRP and ESR are elevated in patients with complicated pneumonia. Establishing a baseline of these values at the time of diagnosis will allow the physician to follow these values over time to assess response to therapy. For example, declining CRP values are reassuring in the context of persistent fevers following pleural drainage. Blood cultures in patients who have not received antibiotics grow the causative organism in 10–25% of cases.[25–27] Testing for *Mycoplasma pneumoniae* may be warranted. One study reported pleural effusions in 20% of patients when lateral decubitus views were obtained.[28] In patients with *M. pneumoniae*, pleural effusions, if present, are usually small and bilateral, though large unilateral effusions have also been described (Figure 34–3).[29,30] A nasopharyngeal or throat swab should be sent for *M. pneumoniae* genome detection by polymerase chain reaction (PCR). Tuberculin skin testing should be performed in children with complicated pneumonia, especially in the context of protracted or indolent symptoms, relevant epidemiologic exposure, or pleural effusion and mediastinal adenopathy out of proportion to the extent of parenchymal consolidation.

Other tests to consider include those for specific diseases or for suspected complications such as autoantibodies (to identify rheumatologic diseases), blood urea nitrogen and creatinine (for HUS), and serum sodium (for syndrome of inappropriate antidiuretic hormone secretion [SIADH]). More commonly, hyponatremia occurs as a consequence of atrial naturetic peptide release from the heart due to lung inflammation and impaired venous return. Many children with complicated pneumonia will have decreased oral intake and decreased urine output, leading to mild or moderate dehydration. However, SIADH should be suspected if there is a history of decreased urine output with evidence of fluid overload on clinical examination.

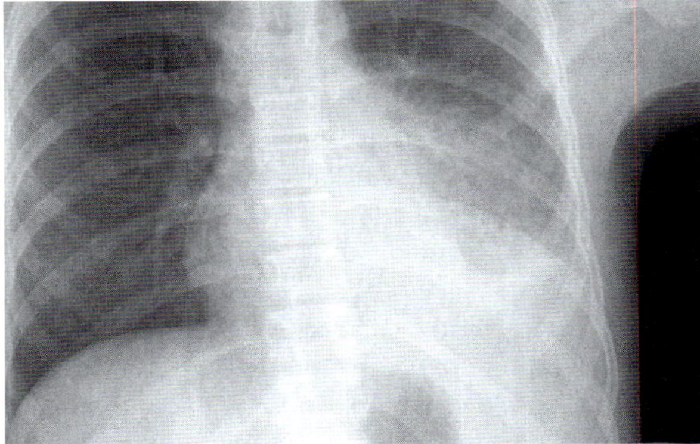

FIGURE 34–3 ■ Posterioanterior view radiograph of a 10-year-old girl with pneumonia caused by *Mycoplasma pneumoniae*. There is consolidation of the left lower lobe with a moderate pleural effusion.

Pleural Drainage

Biochemical analysis of pleural fluid should be performed. Normal pleural fluid has the following characteristics: pH, 7.6; less than 1000 white blood cells/mm^3; glucose content similar to that of plasma; lactate dehydrogenase (LDH) levels less than 50% of plasma; and sodium, potassium, and calcium concentrations similar to interstitial fluid. In 1972, Light et al. published criteria, which classified pleural effusions in adults as exudates or transudates to facilitate differentiation of infection and malignancy, (Table 34–4).[31] The effusion was defined as exudative if it met one of the following criteria: (1) ratio of pleural fluid protein: serum protein >0.5; (2) ratio of pleural fluid LDH: serum LDH >0.6; or (3) pleural fluid LDH greater than two-thirds of the upper limit of normal serum LDH. This classification system had a sensitivity of 98% and a specificity of 83% in identifying exudative effusions and allowed practitioners to quickly narrow their differential diagnosis of pleural effusions. The Light criteria are less useful in children because the incidence of pulmonary malignancy is low and most effusions are caused by infections. Ongoing studies are exploring whether the results of biochemical analysis can be used for prognosis.

Table 34–5 summarizes the tests that should routinely be performed on pleural fluid. The presence of

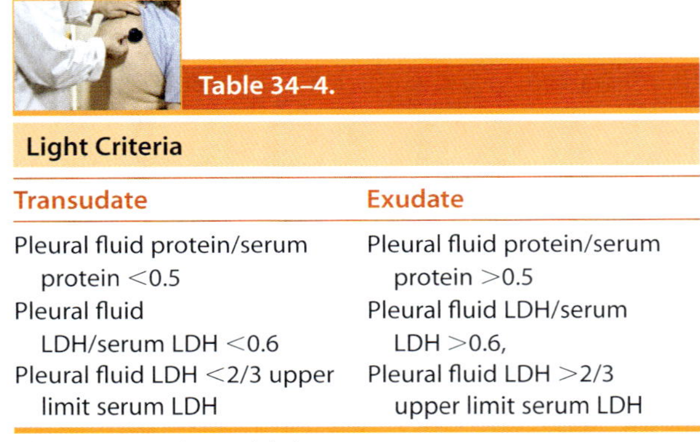

Table 34–4.

Light Criteria

Transudate	Exudate
Pleural fluid protein/serum protein <0.5	Pleural fluid protein/serum protein >0.5
Pleural fluid LDH/serum LDH <0.6	Pleural fluid LDH/serum LDH >0.6,
Pleural fluid LDH <2/3 upper limit serum LDH	Pleural fluid LDH >2/3 upper limit serum LDH

Abbreviation: LDH, lactate dehydrogenase

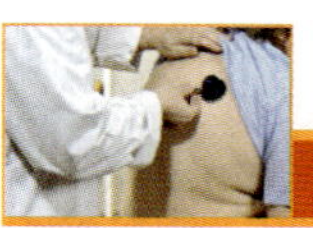

Table 34–5.

Studies to Send from Pleural Fluid*

Routine Pleural Fluid Studies	Situational Pleural Fluid Studies
Cell count with differential	Cytology and flow cytometry
Glucose	*Mycoplasma pneumoniae* PCR
Protein*	Viral antigen immunofluorescence or PCR†
pH	Amylase
Lactate dehydrogenase*	Cholesterol
Gram stain	Triglycerides
Routine bacterial culture (aerobic and anaerobic)	Hematocrit
	Pleural biopsy
Acid fast stain	
Mycobacterial culture	

Also send serum protein and lactate dehydrogenase; may be helpful to compare pleural to serum ratio.

†The number of detectable viruses will increase with time. Most centers currently have testing available for influenza, parainfluenza, adenovirus, respiratory syncytial virus, human metapneumovirus, and human bocavirus. These viruses are infrequent causes of moderate or large pleural effusions.

PCR, polymerase chain reaction.

pleural fluid eosinophilia suggests parasites, fungi, *Mycobacterium tuberculosis*, or *M. pneumoniae* infection, or hypersensitivity disease. Pleural fluid lymphocytosis may indicate *M. tuberculosis* infection or malignancy. While a low pleural glucose usually indicates bacterial infection, other potential causes of low-glucose pleural effusions include hemothorax, *M. tuberculosis*, rheumatoid pleuritis, Churg–Strauss syndrome, paragonimiasis, and lupus pleuritis.

Other pleural fluid tests to identify infectious causes include *M. pneumoniae* PCR and viral detection by PCR or immunofluorescence. Additional pleural fluid testing may also include cytology and flow cytometry (to detect malignancy), amylase, cholesterol, triglycerides, hematocrit, and pleural biopsy. Elevated pleural fluid amylase levels are seen with pancreatitis, pancreatitic pseudocyst, esophageal rupture, and ruptured ectopic pregnancy. Elevated cholesterol ($>$200 mg/dL) and triglyceride ($>$110 mg/dL) levels in the pleural fluid suggest chylothorax from disruption of the thoracic duct or its tributaries (caused by malignancy, sarcoid, amyloidosis, *M. tuberculosis*, or trauma). A hematocrit $>$50% suggests a hemothorax. Pleural biopsy can identify granulomatous changes consistent with *M. tuberculosis* infection.

TREATMENT

Treatment of complicated pneumonia includes antimicrobial therapy and pleural fluid drainage.

Antimicrobial Therapy

Empiric antibiotic therapy should be directed at the most likely pathogens while taking into account the patient's severity of illness and local bacterial resistance patterns. Clindamycin alone or in combination with a third-generation cephalosporin (e.g., cefotaxime, ceftriaxone) is appropriate in most situations. Clindamycin has excellent activity against penicillin-resistant pneumococci[32] as well as group A beta-hemolytic streptococci and many MRSA isolates.[33–35] Cefotaxime or ceftriaxone is added for enhanced coverage against drug-resistant pneumococci. Patients requiring intensive care management (e.g., noninvasive or invasive ventilation, high concentrations of supplemental oxygen) should receive vancomycin or linezolid instead of clindamycin. Both vancomycin and linezolid provide broader Gram-positive coverage since some community-acquired MRSA isolates are intrinsically or inducibly resistant to clindamycin.

There have not been any trials of complicated pneumonia to determine the optimal length of antibiotic therapy. For patients undergoing pleural drainage, a reasonable approach is to continue antibiotics 1 week after resolution of fever. In general, this will mean about 2 weeks of therapy postintervention. A longer course of antibiotics may be required for patients not undergoing pleural drainage. We typically switch from intravenous to oral therapy once the chest tube has been removed. Reasonable oral antibiotic regimens include clindamycin alone or in combination with either amoxicillin or amoxicillin–clavulanate. Oral linezolid is more appropriate for patients who received empiric vancomycin or linezolid therapy. The results of blood or pleural fluid cultures may permit more narrow spectrum therapy.

Pleural Drainage

The size and character of the effusion should guide the pleural drainage decision. Small effusions do not require any intervention, however close monitoring is warranted as the effusion may increase in size. Moderate, large, and loculated collections generally require early pleural fluid drainage. Early pleural drainage may improve outcomes for several reasons: (1) Infections in the fibrinopurulent phase (stage 2) are associated with a worse outcome than infections in the exudative phase (stage 1)[36–39]; (2) The fibrinopurulent stage develops early in the course of infection; (3) Noninvasive methods (e.g., radiologic studies) do not reliably differentiate the fibrinopurulent phase from the exudative phase[37,40,41]; (4) Invasive, nonoperative methods (e.g., needle thoracentesis) using pleural fluid chemistries to classify an effusion as exudative have not been validated in children[31,42]; and (5) Multiple pleural fluid samples from the same patient do not always reveal concordant results.[43,44]

The decision on whether to classify an effusion as small, moderate, or large is more difficult. In adults, the American College of Chest Physicians classifies effusions based on the height of the effusion (for those that are free-flowing) on decubitus radiographs as follows: <10 mm, small; ≥10 mm but <1/2 the hemithorax, moderate; and ≥1/2 the hemithorax, large.[45] While the adult criteria do not directly apply to young children, they can serve as a useful guide. For example, an 8-mm effusion in a 3-year-old could be considered moderate in size since it occupies a much large proportion of the hemithorax than in a 16-year-old.

Options for pleural fluid drainage include thoracentesis, thoracostomy (i.e., chest tube placement) with or without chemical fibrinolysis, video-assisted thoracoscopic surgery (VATS), and open thoracotomy (Table 34–6). At this time, there is considerable controversy over the ideal management strategy for children with complicated pneumonia and a paucity of studies examining this issue.

Historically, standard treatment of complicated pneumonia involved operative debridement and conversion of the closed pleural space to an open drainage with rib resection *only* if there was no definite improvement following tube thoracostomy.[46,47] Several authors, noting the rapid resolution of symptoms in children undergoing earlier open thoracotomy, began to advocate the use of thoracotomy as a definitive therapy rather than a procedure of last resort.[48–51] The advent of less invasive techniques such as VATS in the late 1990s served as an additional impetus to reconsider the strategy of limiting operative intervention only to cases of tube thoracostomy failure.[51–55] The key studies addressing this topic are discussed below.

Avansino et al. systematically reviewed the literature to perform a pooled analysis of observational studies published between 1981 and 2004.[56] Primary operative therapy (VATS or thoracotomy) reduced the length of stay (LOS) by 45% (199 patients from four studies) and the requirement for repeat procedures by 90% (492 patients from nine studies) compared with primary nonoperative therapy (primary thoracostomy or thoracentesis). This review had several limitations. Firstly, the study design did not allow the authors to adjust for important confounding variables such as the timing of the intervention or the choice of empiric antibiotic therapy. Secondly, the included studies had heterogeneous study designs. Finally, the results were biased toward favoring primary operative therapy since

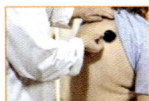

Table 34–6.

Description of Procedures

Procedure	Description	Sedation Requirement
Thoracentesis	Needle inserted between the ribs on the lateral chest wall into the pleural space, usually with ultrasound or computed tomography guidance.	Local anesthesia, minimal (anxiolysis), or moderate sedation
Tube thoracostomy	Large bore, hollow, flexible tube placed between the ribs into pleural space through a 2-cm skin incision on the lateral chest wall. The tube is connected to a canister containing sterile water. Suction is applied to facilitate drainage.	Local anesthesia, moderate or deep sedation
Video-assisted thoracoscopic surgery	Operative technique where a small camera and instruments are inserted into the pleural space through three small (1 cm) incisions of the skin and muscle on the lateral chest wall to mechanically remove purulent material and pleural adhesions. A thoracostomy tube is placed through one of the existing incisions following completion of the procedure.	General anesthesia
Open thoracotomy	Operative technique where instruments are inserted into the pleural space through a single 5–8 cm incision of the skin and muscle on the posterolateral chest wall to mechanically remove purulent material and pleural adhesions. A thoracostomy tube is placed through a second smaller 1–2 cm incision following completion of the procedure.	General anesthesia

patients undergoing primary thoracostomy were grouped together with patients undergoing primary thoracentesis.

Li et al. conducted a retrospective study of 1173 patients using the Kids' Inpatient Database to compare primary operative management (decortication within 2 days of admission) to primary nonoperative management (all other children with complicated pneumonia, including those with initial decortication 3 or more days after admission). The primary endpoint was LOS.[57] Primary operative management was associated with a 4.3-day shorter LOS [95% confidence interval (CI): −6.4 to −2.3 days) compared with primary nonoperative management. However, if the analysis was limited to the subset of patients with empyema as their primary diagnosis, the reduction in LOS was more modest (1.7-day reduction; 95% CI: –0.4 to –3.0 days). The authors also found a significant difference in therapeutic failure between the groups (5.5% for primary operative management vs. 39.3% for nonoperative management).

Shah et al. conducted a study of 961 patients using administrative data from 27 free-standing children's hospitals.[2] In contrast to the study by Li et al., only patients undergoing pleural drainage within 48 hours of hospitalization were included in this study. The primary outcomes were LOS and the requirement for repeat pleural fluid drainage procedures. This study found a 2.7-day reduction (approximately 24% shorter) in LOS for patients undergoing VATS compared with primary tube thoracostomy. In addition, patients in the VATS group had an 84% reduction in need for additional procedures compared with patients initially treated with a thoracostomy (adjusted odds ratio, 0.16; 95% CI: 0.06–0.42).

Kurt et al. conducted a single center randomized trial in the United States comparing VATS with conventional thoracostomy drainage with or without fibrinolysis.[58] The primary endpoints were LOS and days with thoracostomy tube.[58] Secondary endpoints included duration of fever, duration of supplemental oxygen, narcotic use, and number of drainage procedures. Children undergoing VATS (n = 10) had a significantly shorter LOS (mean LOS, 5.8 days) compared with children undergoing primary thoracostomy (n = 8) (mean LOS, 13.3 days; $P < 0.004$). In addition, the duration of chest tube drainage, narcotic use, number of radiographs, and number of procedures were significantly lower in children undergoing VATS compared with children undergoing primary chest tube placement.

Sonnappa et al. conducted a single-center randomized trial in the United Kingdom comparing children undergoing VATS with children undergoing primary thoracostomy with intrapleural urokinase with a primary outcome of LOS after the intervention.[59] The secondary endpoints included total duration of hospitalization, duration of thoracostomy tube, and failure rate. There were no differences in either the primary or secondary outcomes between the two groups. The lack of differences in outcomes stands in stark contrast to studies conducted in the United States where primary VATS has consistently been associated with shorter hospitalizations and fewer repeat pleural drainage procedures than primary thoracostomy.[2,57,58] Differences in causative organisms, timing of presentation for pleural drainage, frequency of chemical fibrinolysis, operative technique, and systems of care could potentially account for such differences in outcomes of children undergoing VATS in the United Kingdom compared with the United States.

The currently available data suggest that early primary VATS is associated with a substantial reduction in the requirement for repeat procedures but a more modest reduction in LOS compared with early primary chest tube placement. While it is tempting to accept early surgical intervention as the new practice standard, we feel that additional data are required. Since some children do remarkably well with chest tube drainage alone, studies should focus on ways to accurately identify this low-risk subgroup of patients. Furthermore, VATS requires specialized surgical training and most community hospitals do not have surgeons with the technical training and expertise to perform this procedure. Therefore, any benefit of primary VATS to patients with complicated pneumonia initially evaluated at community hospitals should be balanced against the delays in pleural drainage that could result from the transfer process. We feel that current guidelines should emphasize the importance of early pleural drainage (within 24–36 hours of hospitalization), regardless of drainage procedure.

Chemical Fibrinolysis

Chemical fibrinolysis (e.g., streptokinase, urokinase, tissue plasminogen activator) does not appear to offer significant benefit though pediatric trials have not had sufficient statistical power to accurately evaluate safety or long-term outcomes. In a randomized trial comparing intrapleural urokinase (n = 29) with intrapleural saline (n = 29), there was no difference between the two groups in the proportion of patients requiring subsequent surgical intervention (9% overall).[60] However, the urokinase group had a 28% shorter LOS (7.5 days vs. 9.5 days; $P = 0.027$).[60] In the randomized trial by Singh et al.,[61] more patients in the saline group (5/21) than in streptokinase group (0/19) required subsequent surgical intervention though this difference did not reach statistical significance; LOS was not assessed. A multicenter randomized trial of 427 adults found that there was no benefit of streptokinase compared with placebo in terms of mortality, requirement for subsequent surgery, radiographic outcomes, or LOS.[62] Adverse events including chest pain, fever, and allergic reaction were more common with streptokinase (7%) than with placebo (3%).[62] We do not currently recommend the use of chemical fibrinolysis in patients with complicated pneumonia.

COURSE AND PROGNOSIS

Studies of short-term outcomes have largely focused on the requirement for repeat procedures and LOS. Persistent fever is common despite early pleural fluid drainage. Among 49 children undergoing VATS within 48 hours of hospitalization, fever was present in 45% and 15% by the 5th and 15th days of hospitalization.[63] Therefore, patients who are clinically improving (e.g., less hypoxia, less chest pain, improved appetite) or have a declining CRP do not necessarily require further intervention after initial pleural drainage. LOS varies substantially by procedure type and illness severity as well as by hospital. The median LOS for children with complicated pneumonia across 27 different tertiary care children's hospitals ranged from 6 to 13 days; 7% of patients overall were hospitalized for 28 days or more.[2] Other potential complications include lung abscess, bronchopleural fistula, and perforation through the chest wall (empyema necessitatis).

Few studies have examined long-term outcomes of children with complicated pneumonia. Scoliosis is uncommon. Abnormalities in lung function are common but no consistent pattern of abnormalities exists and the sample sizes are too small to make meaningful comparisons between drainage procedure and lung function abnormalities. Among 36 patients with complicated pneumonia evaluated by Kohn et al.,[64] 19% of children had mild restrictive lung disease and 16% of children had mild obstructive lung disease. Among 10 patients studied by McLaughlin et al.,[65] five patients had a total lung capacity 1 or more standard deviations below the mean for age; one of these patients was considered to have mild restrictive lung disease (defined as a total lung capacity 2 or more standard deviations below the mean for age). In contrast, seven of the 15 patients studied by Redding et al.[66] had evidence of mild obstructive lung disease while no lung function abnormalities were reported among 13 patients studied by Satish et al.[67] Mortality occurs in less than 1% of children hospitalized with complicated pneumonia.[2]

CLINICAL PEARLS

- Blunting of the costophrenic angle on a posterioanterior radiograph may represent a sizeable pleural effusion.
- Fever may be present for 1–2 weeks after pleural drainage. In a clinically improving patient, additional intervention is not required.
- Tuberculosis should be suspected in patients with pleural effusions in the context of protracted or indolent symptoms.

REFERENCES

1. Grijalva CG, Nuorti JP, Arbogast PG, Martin SW, Edwards KM, Griffin MR. Decline in pneumonia admissions after routine childhood immunisation with pneumococcal conjugate vaccine in the USA: a time-series analysis. *Lancet.* 2007;369:1179-1186.
2. Shah SS, DiCristina CM, Bell LM, Ten Have TR, Metlay JP. Primary early thoracoscopy and reduction in length of stay and procedures among children with complicated pneumonia: results of a multi-center retrospective cohort study. *Arch Pediatr Adolesc Med.* 2008;162(7):675–681.
3. American Academy of Pediatrics. Committee on Infectious Diseases. Policy statement: recommendations for the prevention of pneumococcal infections, including the use of pneumococcal conjugate vaccine (Prevnar), pneumococcal polysaccharide vaccine, and antibiotic prophylaxis. *Pediatrics.* 2000;106:362-366.
4. Shah SS, Ratner AJ. Trends in invasive pneumococcal disease-associated hospitalizations. *Clin Infect Dis.* 2006; 42: e1-e5.
5. Klugman KP, Madhi SA, Huebner RE, Kohberger R, Mbelle N, Pierce N. A trial of a 9-valent pneumococcal conjugate vaccine in children with and those without HIV infection. *N Engl J Med.* 2003;349:1341-1348.
6. Cutts FT, Zaman SM, Enwere G, et al. Efficacy of nine-valent pneumococcal conjugate vaccine against pneumonia and invasive pneumococcal disease in The Gambia: randomised, double-blind, placebo-controlled trial. *Lancet.* 2005;365:1139-1146.
7. Black SB, Shinefield HR, Ling S, et al. Effectiveness of heptavalent pneumococcal conjugate vaccine in children younger than five years of age for prevention of pneumonia. *Pediatr Infect Dis J.* 2002;21:810-815.
8. Steenhoff AJ, Shah, SS, Ratner, AJ, Patil, S, McGowan, KL. Emergence of vaccine-related pneumococcal serotypes as a cause of bacteremia. *Clin Infect Dis.* 2006;42:907-914.
9. Kyaw MH, Lynfield R, Schaffner W, et al. Effect of introduction of the pneumococcal conjugate vaccine on drug-resistant *Streptococcus pneumoniae. N Engl J Med.* 2006; 354:1455-1463.
10. Pichichero ME, Casey JR. Emergence of a multiresistant serotype 19A pneumococcal strain not included in the 7-valent conjugate vaccine as an otopathogen in children. *JAMA.* 2007;298:1772-1778.
11. Byington CL, Korgenski K, Daly J, Ampofo K, Pavia A, Mason EO. Impact of the pneumococcal conjugate vaccine on pneumococcal parapneumonic empyema. *Pediatr Infect Dis J.* 2006;25:250-254.
12. Fisman DN, Abrutyn E, Spaude KA, Kim A, Kirchner C, Daley J. Prior pneumococcal vaccination is associated with reduced death, complications, and length of stay

among hospitalized adults with community-acquired pneumonia. *Clin Infect Dis.* 2006;42:1093-1101.

13. Vila-Corcoles A, Ochoa-Gondar O, Hospital I, et al. Protective effects of the 23-valent pneumococcal polysaccharide vaccine in the elderly population: the EVAN-65 Study. *Clin Infect Dis.* 2006;43:860-868.
14. Vila-Corcoles A, Ochoa-Gondar O, Llor C, Hospital I, Rodriguez T, Gomez A. Protective effect of pneumococcal vaccine against death by pneumonia in elderly subjects. *Eur Respir J.* 2005;26:1086-1091.
15. Klevens RM, Morrison MA, Nadle J, et al. Invasive methicillin-resistant *Staphylococcus aureus* infections in the United States. *JAMA.* 2007;298:1763-1771.
16. Kuehnert MJ, Hill HA, Kupronis BA, Tokars JI, Solomon SL, Jernigan DB. Methicillin-resistant *Staphylococcus aureus* hospitalizations, United States. *Emerg Infect Dis.* 2005;11:868-872.
17. Gonzalez BE, Hulten KG, Dishop MK, et al. Pulmonary manifestations in children with invasive community-acquired *Staphylococcus aureus* infection. *Clin Infect Dis.* 2005;41:583-590.
18. Centers for Disease Control and Prevention, Severe methicillin-resistant *Staphylococcus aureus* community-acquired pneumonia associated with influenza—Louisiana and Georgia, December 2006–January 2007. *MMWR Morb Mortal Wkly Rep.* 2007;56:325-329.
19. Adams WG, Deaver KA, Cochi SL, et al. Decline of childhood *Haemophilus influenzae* type b (Hib) disease in the Hib vaccine era. *JAMA.* 1993;269:221-226.
20. Miserocchi G. Physiology and pathophysiology of pleural fluid turnover. *Eur Respir J.* 1997;10:219-225.
21. Moskowitz H, Platt RT, Schachar R, Mellins H. Roentgen visualization of minute pleural effusion. An experimental study to determine the minimum amount of pleural fluid visible on a radiograph. *Radiology.* 1973;109:33-35.
22. Metersky ML. Is the lateral decubitus radiograph necessary for the management of a parapneumonic pleural effusion? *Chest.* 2003;124:1129-1132.
23. Brenner DJ, Hall EJ. Computed tomography—An increasing source of radiation exposure. *N Engl J Med.* 2007;357: 2277-2284.
24. Yang PC, Luh KT, Chang DB, Wu HD, Yu CJ, Kuo SH. Value of sonography in determining the nature of pleural effusion: analysis of 320 cases. *AJR Am J Roentgenol.* 1992;159:29-33.
25. Hoff SJ, Neblett WW, Edwards KM, et al. Parapneumonic empyema in children: decortication hastens recovery in patients with severe pleural infections. *Pediatr Infect Dis J.* 1991;10:194-199.
26. Freij BJ, Kusmiesz H, Nelson JD, McCracken GH, Jr. Parapneumonic effusions and empyema in hospitalized children: a retrospective review of 227 cases. *Pediatr Infect Dis.* 1984;3:578-591.
27. Byington CL, Spencer LY, Johnson TA, et al. An epidemiological investigation of a sustained high rate of pediatric parapneumonic empyema: risk factors and microbiological associations. *Clin Infect Dis.* 2002;34:434-440.
28. Fine NL, Smith LR, Sheedy PF. Frequency of pleural effusions in mycoplasma and viral pneumonias. *N Engl J Med.* 1970;283:790-793.
29. Narita M, Matsuzono Y, Itakura O, Yamada S, Togashi T. Analysis of mycoplasmal pleural effusion by the polymerase chain reaction. *Arch Dis Child.* 1998;78:67-69.
30. Narita M, Tanaka H. Two distinct patterns of pleural effusions caused by *Mycoplasma pneumoniae* infection. *Pediatr Infect Dis J.* 2004;23:1069 [author reply].
31. Light RW, Macgregor MI, Luchsinger PC, Ball WC, Jr. Pleural effusions: The diagnostic separation of transudates and exudates. *Ann Intern Med.* 1972;77:507-513.
32. Whitney CG, Farley MM, Hadler J, et al. Increasing prevalence of multidrug-resistant *Streptococcus pneumoniae* in the United States. *N Engl J Med.* 2000;343: 1917-1924.
33. Zaoutis TE, Toltzis P, Chu J, et al. Clinical and molecular epidemiology of community-acquired methicillin-resistant *Staphylococcus aureus* infections among children with risk factors for health care-associated infection: 2001–2003. *Pediatr Infect Dis J.* 2006;25:343-348.
34. Chavez-Bueno S, Bozdogan B, Katz K, et al. Inducible clindamycin resistance and molecular epidemiologic trends of pediatric community-acquired methicillin-resistant *Staphylococcus aureus* in Dallas, Texas. *Antimicrob Agents Chemother.* 2005;49:2283-2288.
35. Mishaan AM, Mason EO, Jr, Martinez-Aguilar G, et al. Emergence of a predominant clone of community-acquired *Staphylococcus aureus* among children in Houston, Texas. *Pediatr Infect Dis J.* 2005;24:201-206.
36. Huang HC, Chang HY, Chen CW, Lee CH, Hsiue TR. Predicting factors for outcome of tube thoracostomy in complicated parapneumonic effusion for empyema. *Chest.* 1999;115:751-756.
37. Himelman RB, Callen PW. The prognostic value of loculations in parapneumonic pleural effusions. *Chest.* 1986;90:852-856.
38. Ramnath RR, Heller RM, Ben-Ami T, et al. Implications of early sonographic evaluation of parapneumonic effusions in children with pneumonia. *Pediatrics.* 1998;101:68-71.
39. Donnelly LF, Klosterman LA. CT appearance of parapneumonic effusions in children: findings are not specific for empyema. *AJR Am J Roentgenol.* 1997;169:179-182.
40. Chonmaitree T, Powell KR. Parapneumonic pleural effusion and empyema in children. Review of a 19-year experience, 1962–1980. *Clin Pediatr (Phila).* 1983;22: 414-419.
41. Kearney SE, Davies CW, Davies RJ, Gleeson FV. Computed tomography and ultrasound in parapneumonic effusions and empyema. *Clin Radiol.* 2000;55:542-547.
42. Romero S, Candela A, Martin C, Hernandez L, Trigo C, Gil J. Evaluation of different criteria for the separation of pleural transudates from exudates. *Chest.* 1993;104: 399-404.
43. Read CA, Sporn TA, Yeager H, Jr. Parapneumonic empyema. A pitfall in diagnosis. *Chest.* 1992;101:1712-1713.
44. Conner BD, Lee YC, Branca P, Rogers JT, Rodriguez RM, Light RW. Variations in pleural fluid WBC count and differential counts with different sample containers and different methods. *Chest.* 2003;123:1181-1187.
45. Colice GL, Curtis A, Deslauriers J, et al. Medical and surgical treatment of parapneumonic effusions: an evidence-based guideline. *Chest.* 2000;118:1158-1171.
46. Thomas DF, Glass JL, Baisch BF. Management of streptococcal empyema. *Ann Thorac Surg.* 1966;2:658-664.
47. Stiles QR, Lindesmith GG, Tucker BL, Meyer BW, Jones JC. Pleural empyema in children. *Ann Thorac Surg.* 1970;10:37-44.

48. Kosloske AM, Cartwright KC. The controversial role of decortication in the management of pediatric empyema. *J Thorac Cardiovasc Surg.* 1988;96:166-170.
49. Khakoo GA, Goldstraw P, Hansell DM, Bush A. Surgical treatment of parapneumonic empyema. *Pediatr Pulmonol.* 1996;22:348-356.
50. Rizalar R, Somuncu S, Bernay F, Ariturk E, Gunaydin M, Gurses N. Postpneumonic empyema in children treated by early decortication. *Eur J Pediatr Surg.* 1997;7:135-137.
51. Kern JA, Rodgers BM. Thoracoscopy in the management of empyema in children. *J Pediatr Surg.* 1993;28:1128-1132.
52. Merry CM, Bufo AJ, Shah RS, Schropp KP, Lobe TE. Early definitive intervention by thoracoscopy in pediatric empyema. *J Pediatr Surg.* 1999;34:178-180; discussion 80-1.
53. Gandhi RR, Stringel G. Video-assisted thoracoscopic surgery in the management of pediatric empyema. *JSLS.* 1997;1:251-253.
54. Stovroff M, Teague G, Heiss KF, Parker P, Ricketts RR. Thoracoscopy in the management of pediatric empyema. *J Pediatr Surg.* 1995;30:1211-1215.
55. Grewal H, Jackson RJ, Wagner CW, Smith SD. Early video-assisted thoracic surgery in the management of empyema. *Pediatrics.* 1999;103:e63.
56. Avansino JR, Goldman B, Sawin RS, Flum DR. Primary operative versus nonoperative therapy for pediatric empyema: a meta-analysis. *Pediatrics.* 2005;115:1652-659.
57. Li ST, Gates RL. Primary operative management for pediatric empyema: decreases in hospital length of stay and charges in a national sample. *Arch Pediatr Adolesc Med.* 2008;162:44-48.
58. Kurt BA, Winterhalter KM, Connors RH, Betz BW, Winters JW. Therapy of parapneumonic effusions in children: video-assisted thoracoscopic surgery versus conventional thoracostomy drainage. *Pediatrics.* 2006;118:e547-e553.
59. Sonnappa S, Cohen G, Owens CM, et al. Comparison of urokinase and video-assisted thoracoscopic surgery for treatment of childhood empyema. *Am J Respir Crit Care Med.* 2006;174:221-227.
60. Thomson AH, Hull J, Kumar MR, Wallis C, Balfour Lynn IM. Randomised trial of intrapleural urokinase in the treatment of childhood empyema. *Thorax.* 2002;57:343-347.
61. Singh M, Mathew JL, Chandra S, Katariya S, Kumar L. Randomized controlled trial of intrapleural streptokinase in empyema thoracis in children. *Acta Paediatr.* 2004;93: 1443-1445.
62. Maskell NA, Davies CW, Nunn AJ, et al. U.K. controlled trial of intrapleural streptokinase for pleural infection. *N Engl J Med.* 2005;352:865-874.
63. Schultz KD, Fan LL, Pinsky J, et al. The changing face of pleural empyemas in children: epidemiology and management. *Pediatrics.* 2004;113:1735-1740.
64. Kohn GL, Walston C, Feldstein J, Warner BW, Succop P, Hardie WD. Persistent abnormal lung function after childhood empyema. *Am J Respir Med.* 2002;1:441-1445.
65. McLaughlin FJ, Goldmann DA, Rosenbaum DM, Harris GB, Schuster SR, Strieder DJ. Empyema in children: clinical course and long-term follow-up. *Pediatrics.* 1984;73: 587-593.
66. Redding GJ, Walund L, Walund D, Jones JW, Stamey DC, Gibson RL. Lung function in children following empyema. *Am J Dis Child.* 1990;144:1337-1342.
67. Satish B, Bunker M, Seddon P. Management of thoracic empyema in childhood: does the pleural thickening matter? *Arch Dis Child.* 2003;88:918-921.

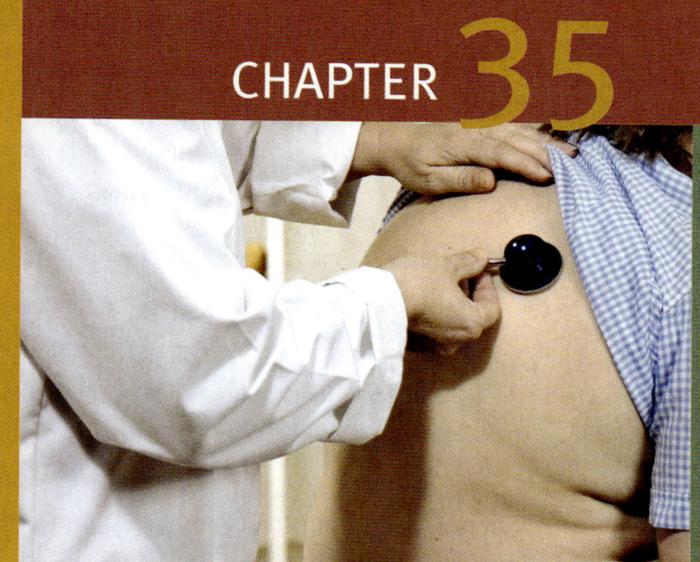

CHAPTER 35

Recurrent Pneumonia

Elizabeth K. Fiorino and Howard B. Panitch

DEFINITIONS AND EPIDEMIOLOGY

A child presenting with recurrent respiratory infections or radiographic abnormalities poses a common diagnostic problem for general pediatricians and pulmonary specialists alike. Pneumonia can be described both in clinical and radiographic terms. The World Health Organization defines pneumonia clinically as cough or dyspnea in association with labored breathing or tachypnea, and radiographically as an opacity occupying at least part of a single lobe and up to the entire lung.[1,2] The incidence of pneumonia in developed countries is approximately 3–3.6 children per 100, whereas in developing countries, it can reach as high as 40 per 100 children.[3] Recurrent pneumonia has been defined as two episodes in 1 year or 3 in a lifetime, with radiographic clearing between episodes.[4] The incidence of recurrent pneumonia among large populations of children is unknown.

Several series have described both the frequency of recurrent pneumonia, as well as the leading causes for such, in various smaller populations of children. These studies demonstrate that the majority of children with recurrent pneumonia have an identifiable cause for their recurrent symptoms. The most common cause, however, varies depending on the characteristics of the population of children studied, whether inpatient or outpatient, referred to a subspecialty or general pediatric service, or from developed or developing countries. In a 10-year review of hospital records at a tertiary care children's hospital, 8% of 2952 children with pneumonia had a recurrent episode.[5] Of those 238 children, 92% had an "underlying illness." The leading diagnosis was oropharyngeal incoordination with aspiration, occurring in 48%, followed by immune disorders. Lodha et al.[6] reviewed all children presenting to a pediatric pulmonary clinic in New Delhi in a 4-year period. Children were included in the analysis, if they met clinical criteria and had radiographic confirmation of pneumonia. Additionally, children with cystic fibrosis and congenital heart disease were excluded. Seventy children of 2264 (3.1%) in a 5-year period met these standards. An underlying illness was diagnosed in 84% of children; the most common diagnosis was recurrent aspiration, in 24.2% of children, followed by immune deficiency and asthma. In contrast, Ciftci et al.[7] reviewed all children admitted to the pediatric infectious disease service of a tertiary care hospital in Turkey. Children without radiographic diagnostic confirmation were excluded from analysis. Nine percent of 288 patients met the criteria. Underlying disease was identified in 85% of patients, with asthma occurring in 32%, and therefore the most common diagnosis. Swallowing dysfunction was present in only 3%. Children with cystic fibrosis and congenital heart disease were included in this analysis.

Eigen et al.[8] found similar results in a population of children referred to a tertiary care pediatric hospital for evaluation of persistent or recurrent pneumonia. Children were divided into two groups—those with apparent causes for persistent or recurrent radiographic densities, and those without. Approximately 50% of those in the group with predisposing causes had either gastroesophageal reflux or oropharyngeal incoordination. Of the group with no apparent condition, nearly half had a family history of atopy, 20% were wheezing at the time of evaluation, and 92% of those old enough (>5 years) to be evaluated by spirometry, demonstrated bronchial hyperresponsiveness. Children in Haiti who were diagnosed with recurrent pneumonia based on World Health Organization clinical criteria were compared with children who had never been diagnosed with pneumonia.[9] Seventy-nine percent of 103 children with recurrent pneumonia had a history of wheezing, and 36% had wheezing with exercise, both higher percentages than in those children without a history of pneumonia.

PATHOGENESIS

Infection of lung parenchyma can occur whenever protective mechanisms are overcome or circumvented. Particles larger than 10 μm are filtered out in the nose, and particles between 2 and 5 μm typically impact on the airway mucosa where they can be removed by the mucus lining layer and mucociliary escalator. Laryngeal structures, including the epiglottis and vocal cords, protect the airway from aspiration of oropharyngeal material during deglutition and from gastric contents if gastroesophageal reflux is present. Cough is a critical mechanism to clear the airways of particles and infecting organisms, and acts as a backup mechanism if the mucociliary escalator or laryngeal defenses are ineffective or overcome. Both the innate and adaptive immune systems operate in the lung to help clear infecting organisms. The former includes a host of molecules like complement, adhesion proteins, collectins, and toll-like receptors. Adaptive immunity includes mast cells, dendritic cells, and macrophages, as well as circulating immunoglobulins. The principal protective immunoglobulin of the upper airway is IgA, while IgG is chiefly responsible for protection of the lower airways and alveoli.

While any of these mechanisms can be overcome by chance, leading to an episode of pneumonia, it is the persistence of an abnormality of some aspect of the lung's defense system that predisposes to recurrent episodes of pneumonia. Thus, impaired cough, structural abnormalities that preclude adequate airway clearance, ineffective physical defense mechanisms to prevent soiling of the lung, an abnormality of mucus or of ciliary function, or a breakdown of host immune function are all possible causes for a child to experience recurrent pneumonia.

CLINICAL PRESENTATION

The clinical presentation of recurrent pneumonia will depend principally on the underlying cause (Table 35–1). Children who have an anatomic defect that predisposes to pneumonia recurrences in a single region will often have no other sign of systemic disease. If bronchiectasis occurs in the region, however, there may be a history of weight loss, or of poor weight gain and of digital clubbing, likely a reflection of a chronic suppurative condition in the chest. Those children who develop recurrent pneumonias in different regions of the lung usually present with other findings beyond fever, cough, and chest crackles. Children with asthma as a cause for recurrent pneumonia typically will be diagnosed during an acute exacerbation of asthma symptoms. Approximately 85% of children with cystic fibrosis also have pancreatic insufficiency, so that symptoms of intestinal malabsorption and growth failure will be present. Infants and children with swallowing dysfunction often have a history of coughing or choking during feedings. While gastroesophageal reflux may be silent, more often there is a history of arching during meals (if esophagitis is present), rumination, frequent effortless regurgitation ("wet burps") or frank emesis. These are frequently accompanied by contemporaneous alterations in the respiratory examination, like tachypnea, cough, or coarse breath sounds. Children with systemic immune deficiencies or primary ciliary dyskinesia will have prominent upper respiratory findings, like recurrent otitis, pansinusitis, and chronic purulent rhinitis. Some immunodeficiency states, like chronic granulomatous disease (CGD) or hyper IgE syndrome also predispose children to recurrent skin infections.

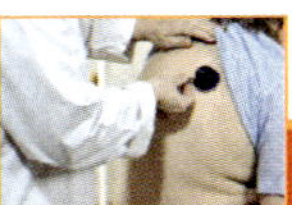

Table 35–1.

Signs and Symptoms
History
Nocturnal cough or cough with activity—asthma
Chronic pansinusitis, purulent rhinitis, recurrent otitis media—immune deficiency, cystic fibrosis, primary ciliary dyskinesia
Choking episode—retained foreign body, aspiration syndromes
Failure to thrive—cystic fibrosis, immune deficiency, bronchiectasis
Malodorous stools—cystic fibrosis
Neurologic impairment—recurrent aspiration, difficulties with airway clearance
Physical examination
Digital clubbing—cystic fibrosis, bronchiectasis, congenital heart disease
Nasal polyps—cystic fibrosis, allergic rhinitis
Dennie's lines, allergic shiners—asthma
Rashes—immune deficiency
Eczema—asthma, hyper IgE syndrome
Dextrocardia—primary ciliary dyskinesia

DIFFERENTIAL DIAGNOSIS

The first important determinant in creating a differential diagnosis is establishing if the disease process has involved the same location or different areas of the lung (Table 35–2). In actual practice, this division depends on

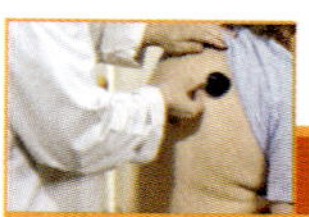

Table 35–2.

Differential Diagnosis

Same Location
- Common
  - Retained foreign body
  - Airway compression
    - Vascular
    - Lymph node
    - Mass
    - Heart
  - Right middle lobe syndrome
  - Bronchiectasis
- Less Common
  - Sequestration
- Rare
  - Endobronchial tumor
  - Congenital malformation
    - Bronchial atresia, stenosis
    - Foregut malformation
    - Cystic adenomatoid malformation

Different Locations
- Common
  - Asthma
  - Aspiration syndromes
- Less Common
  - Cystic fibrosis
  - Sickle hemoglobinopathy
- Rare
  - Primary ciliary dyskinesia
  - Immune deficiency

both a cogent historian and the availability of radiographic data.

Same Location

Pathology affecting a single region can be related to obstruction of the airway lumen that subtends the area by intraluminal obstruction or compression, intrinsic narrowing of the airway, or an abnormality of the involved parenchyma. Causes of intraluminal obstruction include such entities as foreign body, tumor, or mucous plug. Compression of the airway is seen with lymphadenopathy from various causes, including infection—such as tuberculosis, histoplasmosis, and other mycotic infections—and from noninfectious causes, including sarcoidosis and neoplasms. Additionally, external compression can arise from an abnormality of the vasculature, such as a vascular ring, or from mediastinal tumors or duplication cysts.

Structural airway abnormalities that cause retention of secretions can result in chronic or recurrent infection.[10] These include anomalies of airway configuration, such as a tracheal bronchus, which is a right upper lobe bronchus that emanates from the trachea, rather than from the right main bronchus. When its orifice is smaller than normal or the airway takes off from the trachea at an acute angle, the airway is prone to obstruction from secretions. Similarly, a "bridging bronchus," a right lower lobe bronchus that arises from the left bronchial tree, can impair proper drainage. Localized bronchial stricture or stenosis occurs most commonly in a main or middle lobe bronchus,[11] but these lesions can also occur in the distal trachea; especially when acquired as a result of airway intubation and suctioning.[12–14] Bronchial atresia may be asymptomatic, or can result in lobar degeneration distal to the obstruction, leaving a mucus-filled or fluid-filled cystic structure in its place, which can then become infected. Bronchomalacia, or excessive collapsibility of the airway wall, predisposes to retained secretions. Localized bronchiectasis may be congenital, which is rare, or be a result of chronic localized infection or a prior viral illness.[15]

Right middle lobe syndrome is an entity described in both the pediatric and adult literature in which a recurrent radiographic density associated with respiratory symptoms occurs in the right middle lobe region (Figure 35–1). It requires special mention, because of the unique nature of the anatomy of the right middle lobe. The normal anatomy of the right middle lobe—the airway's acute angular take off from the bronchus intermedius, narrower caliber, and longer distance without branching, as well as the lack of collateral ventilation to the lobe itself—predisposes to difficulties with airway clearance and retained secretions. Asthma is the most common underlying disorder associated with the right middle lobe syndrome. Bronchoscopic findings in 52 of 55 children with middle lobe syndrome included airway mucosal edema, retained secretions, and mucus plugging, rather than complete obstruction. Additionally, more than half of these patients had elevated eosinophils in lavage fluid.[16,17]

Congenital lung malformations become infected as a result of either abnormalities in the airways leading to them, or compromised blood flow to them. Bronchogenic cysts, which result from aberrant budding of the tracheobronchial tree during development, are often located centrally and on the right. These unilocular structures do not communicate with the airway, although they may carry their own blood supply. They can become infected, or they may cause symptoms by compressing adjacent airways and impeding airway clearance. Bronchogenic cysts will appear radiodense initially, but become lucent when infected.[18] Congenital cystic adenomatoid malformations (CCAM) are lesions in which varying degrees of cystic and glandular structures replace normal alveolar tissue. A CCAM usually

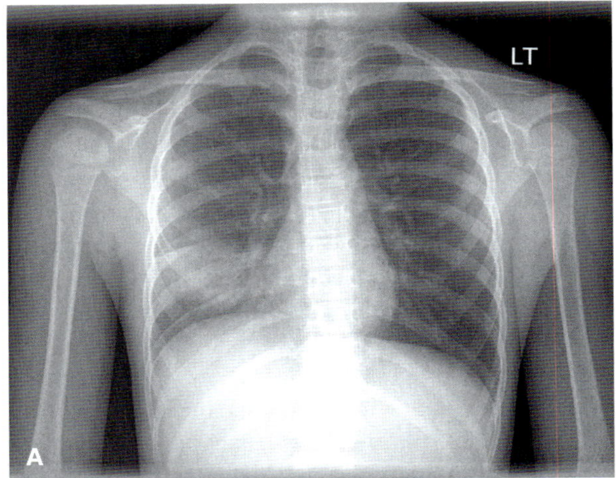

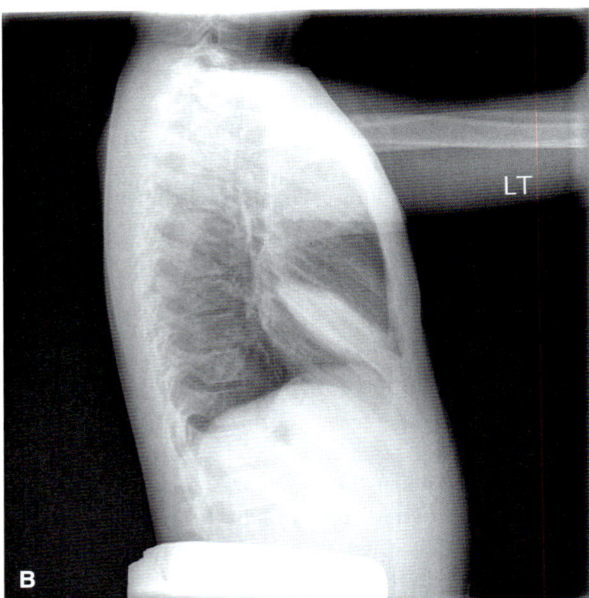

FIGURE 35–1 ■ **(A)** Posterior–anterior and **(B)** lateral radiographs of a 7-year-old girl with asthma and right middle lobe syndrome. There is a density in the right middle lobe that improved following aggressive management of asthma. Subsequent bronchoscopy demonstrated normal anatomy, and bronchoalveolar lavage yielded elevated numbers of eosinophils.

involves a single lobe, unlike bronchogenic cysts, CCAMs communicate with the tracheobronchial tree. On radiographs, CCAMs appear as uni- or multiloculated lucent or dense structures. Pulmonary sequestrations are masses of lung parenchyma usually without connection to the tracheobronchial tree, but with a defined systemic blood supply, usually arising from the aorta. Sequestrations can be intralobar (invested in the pleura of normal lung) or, less commonly, extralobar (covered with their own pleura). Intralobar sequestrations are found most commonly in the left lower lobe and most often present as recurrent pneumonia. Radiographic appearance is initially radiodense, but, with infection, the degree of lucency can increase.

Different Locations

Recurrent pneumonia involving different locations often is associated with a systemic disease process. Aspiration has been described in several case studies as the most common cause of recurrent pneumonia.[5,6] Recurrent pneumonia from aspiration itself can also be associated with several other conditions. Impaired swallowing with inadequate airway protection can result from a variety of neuromuscular disorders, including cranial nerve injury, cerebral palsy, and muscular dystrophy. Anatomic abnormalities of the larynx including vocal cord paralysis or laryngeal cleft compromise airway protection. Esophageal obstruction, from foreign body, foregut malformation, or vascular ring may impair the normal swallow and worsen reflux of gastric contents. Similarly, esophageal dysmotility, from achalasia or tracheoesophageal fistula, also predisposes to aspiration[19] (Figure 35–2).

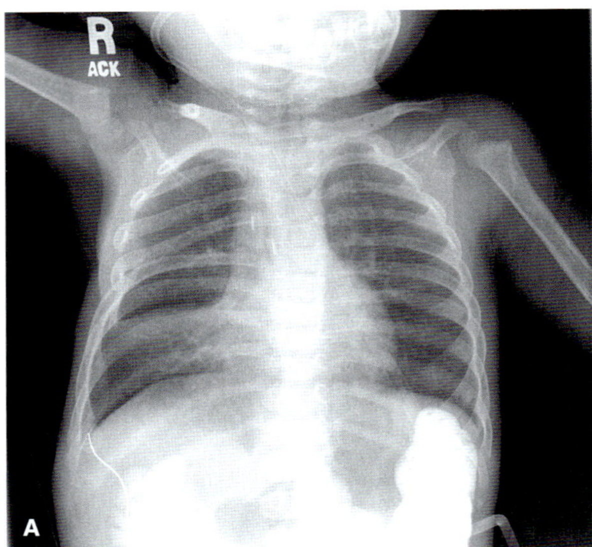

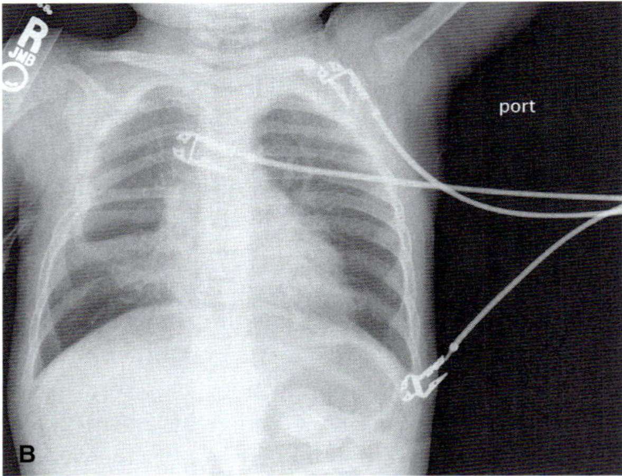

FIGURE 35–2 ■ Anterior–posterior chest radiographs of a child with repaired tracheoesophageal fistula, and history of recurrent aspiration. **(A)** Right middle lobe density at 17 months; **(B)** right middle and left lower lobe densities at 30 months. Interval radiographs demonstrated clearing of the lesions.

Asthma is one of the most common causes of recurrent pneumonia. Undertreated asthma is associated with airway inflammation, increased mucus production, and luminal narrowing from airway wall edema. Whether radiographic densities seen during acute exacerbations represent true areas of infection or atelectasis is often uncertain. Recent data using sensitive detection techniques, however, suggest that acute viral infections account for as much as 85% of asthma exacerbations in school-aged children.[20]

Malfunction or deficiency in any component of the immune system, adaptive or innate, often leads to recurrent pulmonary infections. It is extremely unlikely, however, for a child to have recurrent pneumonia from an immunodeficiency without also having a history of recurrent otitis or sinusitis, and chronic purulent rhinitis. A clear way to classify these defects is into disorders of phagocyte function, B cell function, and T cell function. The most common example of phagocyte dysfunction in children with recurrent pulmonary disease is chronic granulomatous disease (CGD). Children with CGD, with an incidence of 1 in 20,000, experience severe pneumonia and abscesses. Most often, infections are caused by catalase positive organisms like *Staphylococcus aureus*, *Aspergillus* spp., *Burkholderia cepacia*, *Nocardia* spp., and *Serratia* spp. These infections occur as a result of a loss of NADPH oxidative function. Hyper IgE, or Job, syndrome is associated with severe pneumonia, often resulting in pneumatocele formation, eczema, and coarse facial features. The immune defect in hyper IgE syndrome is unclear, but has been hypothesized to relate to neutrophil dysfunction.[21]

Defects in B cells result in problems with formation of antibodies, which are essential for opsonization and clearance of encapsulated organisms, such as *Streptococcus pneumoniae* and *Haemophilus influenzae*. These defects often present in late infancy, after maternal IgG is cleared. X-linked, or Bruton's, agammaglobulinemia, presents with recurrent pneumonias as well as *Pneumocystis carinii* (now *P. jirovecii*) infection. Common variable immune deficiency (CVID), in which there are varying low levels of immune globulins, especially gamma globulin, does not present with opportunistic pathogens, but with recurrent bacterial infections of the sinuses or lungs. If not diagnosed in childhood, individuals with CVID often develop bronchiectasis as adults.[22] IgG subclass deficiencies also can present with recurrent pneumonia. Most is known about IgG2 deficiency, which often presents as asthma. The most common immune globulin defect is IgA deficiency, with an incidence of 1/400–3000. IgA deficiency often coexists with an IgG subclass deficiency. A recent study, however, found that although 50% of a population of IgA-deficient patients presenting to an immunology clinic for evaluation had recurrent respiratory infections, they were not more likely to have an associated IgG2 subclass deficiency or poor responses to the pneumococcal vaccine.[23]

T cells have populations of antigen-presenting or helper cells as well as killer cells. T cells are responsible for the orchestration of the adaptive immune system, as well as direct elimination of viruses and fungi. Severe combined immune deficiency, in which both T cell and B cell function is severely reduced or absent, presents early in infancy. 67% of patients with severe combined immune deficiency have pulmonary disease at diagnosis and are susceptible throughout life to opportunistic pathogens. Other T cell deficiencies can present more subtly. Children with DiGeorge syndrome, associated with 22q11 microdeletion, absent 3rd and 4th pharyngeal pouches, thymic aplasia to hypoplasia, and hypoparathyroidism have a range of immune defects, most commonly pneumonia caused by Gram-negative bacteria and severe respiratory syncytial virus infection. Those with absence of the thymus have more severe defects and are at risk for *pneumocystis* infections. Several conditions present with subtle and combined immune problems, relating to interaction between T and B lymphocytes. Wiskott Aldrich syndrome is an X-linked recessive condition with thrombocytopenia, eczema, and recurrent bacterial infection. Immune defects include lymphopenia and a decreased response to polysaccharide antigens.[24] Ataxia-telangiectasia is a progressive neurologic disorder associated with varying degrees of immune deficiency and recurrent pulmonary involvement.[25]

A local defense mechanism that is critical for clearing the airways of inhaled debris and infecting organisms is the mucociliary escalator. Dysfunction of the mucociliary clearance system occurs in both cystic fibrosis and primary ciliary dyskinesia. In cystic fibrosis, the airway surface liquid is depleted, resulting in increased mucous viscosity and an inability of the cilia to clear airway secretions effectively. Because of the increased mucus viscosity, cough becomes ineffective at clearing secretions. In contrast, primary ciliary dyskinesia affects only the beating action of the cilia, and the mucus itself is normal; cough is effective in this case. In both conditions, however, mucus stasis results in recurrent infections and ultimately leads to bronchiectasis.

Diffuse processes such as hypersensitivity pneumonitis, allergic bronchopulmonary aspergillosis, or eosinophilic pneumonia represent abnormal immunological responses. While these entities do not cause pneumonia per se, recurrent radiographic densities are prominent features in each. Similarly, children with recurrent pulmonary hemorrhage or sickle cell disease can develop diffuse densities and respiratory symptoms with varying degrees of clearing. It is occasionally difficult to distinguish pneumonia in children with sickle cell disease from acute infarction.

DIAGNOSIS

History and Physical Examination

Making the diagnosis of recurrent pneumonia begins with history-taking and physical examination. Symptoms that begin in early infancy point to congenital structural lesions, serious immune deficiency, or other inherited diseases like cystic fibrosis or primary ciliary dyskinesia. Another important historical point is the persistence—or absence—of such symptoms when the patient is well. Most children with immunodeficiency will have persistent upper respiratory evidence of infection, for example, purulent rhinitis, recurrent sinusitis, or otitis, especially when they are not receiving antibiotics. Thus, a history of purulent nasal discharge that recurs whenever the child is taken off antibiotics should prompt a screening of immune function. A recalled episode of choking demands evaluation for foreign body, although one-third of children with a foreign body aspiration will have no such history. Respiratory symptoms that worsen during or shortly after feedings point to possible swallowing dysfunction with or without gastroesophageal reflux. Similarly, when symptoms occur during or soon after an acute viral upper respiratory illness, asthma should be considered as the likely cause of lower respiratory findings. It is helpful to get a history of wheezing during acute episodes, but this is a highly nonspecific finding and other respiratory sounds are often mislabeled by parents as wheezing. In contrast, a history of responsiveness to bronchodilators is once again supportive of a diagnosis of asthma.

Symptoms outside of the respiratory system can also yield important clues to the etiology of recurrent pneumonia. Intestinal malabsorption occurs in 85–90% of children with cystic fibrosis. Recurrent skin infections occur in several immunodeficiency states, and a history of severe eczema can reflect atopy and possible asthma, or immunodeficiency.

Elements in the social history, such as exposure to cigarette smoke and pollutants, or daycare and its exposure to multiple viruses, can point to an etiology such as asthma. Travel history assesses exposure to infectious agents such as tuberculosis, histoplasmosis, and parasites. A family history of early or unexplained death points toward immune deficiency or other systemic diseases like cystic fibrosis.

As with the history, the physical examination should be directed to both sinopulmonary and extrapulmonary findings. Dysmorphic features can be associated with a structural anomaly, or point to an immune deficiency, like DiGeorge syndrome. Growth parameters should be assessed, since failure to thrive suggests a pervasive systemic disease.

The upper respiratory tract yields important clues as to the cause of recurrent chest infections. Dennie's lines, shiners, a transverse crease over the nasal bridge, and scaling of the skin suggest atopy. Otitis media, purulent rhinitis and sinusitis prompt further evaluation for immune deficiency or ciliary dyskinesia. The presence of nasal polyps in children is overwhelmingly associated with either cystic fibrosis or severe allergic rhinitis. Their presence should always be cause to obtain a sweat test. Periodontal disease and candidiasis can point to immune deficiency. Digital clubbing often reflects a pyogenic process in the chest, like bronchiectasis or pulmonary abscess, although it is also present in patients with cyanotic congenital heart disease, inflammatory bowel and liver disease, and bacterial endocarditis. These causes can usually be easily distinguished.

Physical assessment of the respiratory system can point to particular etiologies of recurrent pneumonia, and also will reflect the severity of the underlying condition. Tachypnea, dyspnea with retractions, use of accessory muscles, and oxyhemoglobin desaturation all point to significant and probably widespread disease. Auscultation should include an assessment of air movement, comparison of the right and left sides, and individual regions. Wheezing that is comprised by the same set of sounds transmitted throughout the chest (homophonous wheezing) signifies a central airway obstruction like a retained foreign body, airway compression, or tracheobronchomalacia. Wheezes that contain different sets of sounds regionally reflect peripheral airway obstructions of different degrees, like those that exist in asthma.

Cardiac examination may reveal the presence of situs inversus, associated with 50% of cases of ciliary dyskinesia (Figure 35–3), presence of a cardiac lesion, or heart failure.

Diagnostic Testing

Testing should be guided by the individual situation (Table 35–3 and Figure 35–4). A chest film, both posterior–anterior and lateral, should be a part of the evaluation of every patient with recurrent pneumonia. All prior examinations should be reviewed as well. Ideally, a film should also be taken when the patient is well to differentiate whether the problem is recurrent or chronic. If the patient is acutely ill, adequacy of gas exchange should be established with examination and arterial blood gas analysis. Sputum culture and Gram stain in those who can expectorate aid in establishing the microbiology of an infection—and may refine further the differential diagnosis.

In those with recurrent or persistent focal abnormalities, evaluation is geared to defining abnormalities of the airway—whether internal or external. Bronchoscopy (airway endoscopy) provides direct visualization of airway anatomy and allows assessment for presence of foreign body and extraluminal compression, as well as

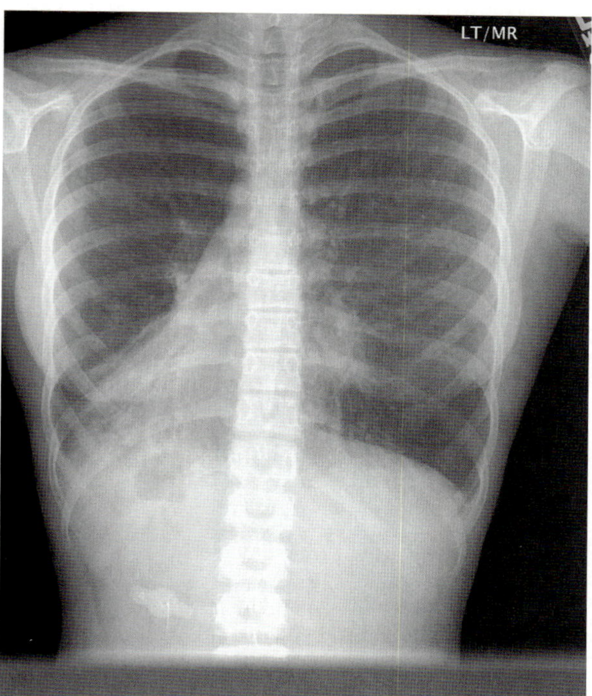

FIGURE 35–3 ■ Posterior–anterior chest radiograph of a 16-year-old girl with Kartagener syndrome. Note dextrocardia along with the right-sided gastric bubble. There is also a density in the right lower lobe that obscures the right hemidiaphragm.

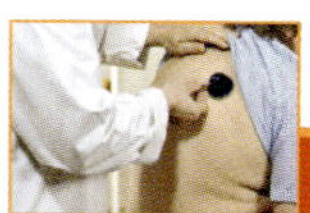

Table 35–3.

Diagnostic Evaluation

In All Patients
Chest radiograph, posterior–anterior and lateral
Review all prior films
Further testing based on history and physical

Same Location
Airway endoscopy
CT scan of the chest
Purified protein derivative
Barium swallow
Magnetic resonance angiography

Different Locations
Sputum culture and Gram stain
CBC with differential
CT scan of the chest
Nuclear scintigraphy
Video swallow study
Sweat chloride analysis
Spirometry with evaluation of response to bronchodilator
Ciliary biopsy
Quantitative immune globulins and subclasses
Lymphocyte panel
Nitroblue tetrazolium or dihydrorhodamine assay

performance of lavage for culture. If a retained foreign body is highly suspected, then the study of choice is rigid (open tube) bronchoscopy under general anesthesia. Otherwise, flexible bronchoscopy, especially under conscious sedation, offers the advantages of more distal airway inspection and an opportunity to see dynamic events, like airway collapse on exhalation. Bronchoalveolar lavage should also be considered in children with recurrent pneumonia in different locations, if they are unable to produce sputum and identification of the infecting organism is desired.

Chest computed tomography (CT) allows for localization of a possible extraluminal airway compression—such as by a lymph node—as well as refinement of the anatomic location of radiographic densities. The CT scan also provides excellent visualization of the involved parenchyma and can be diagnostic for bronchiectasis as well as several congenital lesions. There has been recent interest in multidetector CT scan with virtual tracheobronchoscopy as a less invasive alternative to conventional airway endoscopy.[26]

There are several choices for evaluating the great vessels and the possibility of a vascular ring (Figure 35–5). The choice of which to use will depend on local availability and expertise. A barium esophagram reflects the type of vascular ring from the pattern of compression on the esophagus. More recently, CT angiography and magnetic resonance imaging have been refined to define vascular anomalies with a high degree of accuracy.[27]

Adjunctive testing is aimed at detecting specific diseases. Purified protein derivative should be placed when the history or radiographic findings are suspicious for tuberculosis, and evaluation for fungal infections such as aspergillosis and coccidiomycosis should also be performed. The sweat test, quantitative immunoglobulins with subclasses, complete blood count with differential, antitetanus and diptheria titers, and ciliary biopsy should be performed if the diagnosis is likely to be cystic fibrosis, an immunodeficiency, or primary ciliary dyskinesia. As untreated asthma has been shown to be one of the most common causes for recurrent pneumonia, spirometry, to assess for evidence of airways obstruction and response to bronchodilator, should be performed. In those children who cannot perform spirometry, an alternative is a therapeutic trial of inhaled corticosteroids and bronchodilators for a defined time period.

In those with neurologic dysfunction, evaluation of swallowing function, including a fluoroscopic video swallowing study and scintigraphy to evaluate for both gastroesophageal reflux and abnormal swallow, should be performed.[28] A functional endoscopic swallow study can provide increased information regarding the patient's actual swallow function.

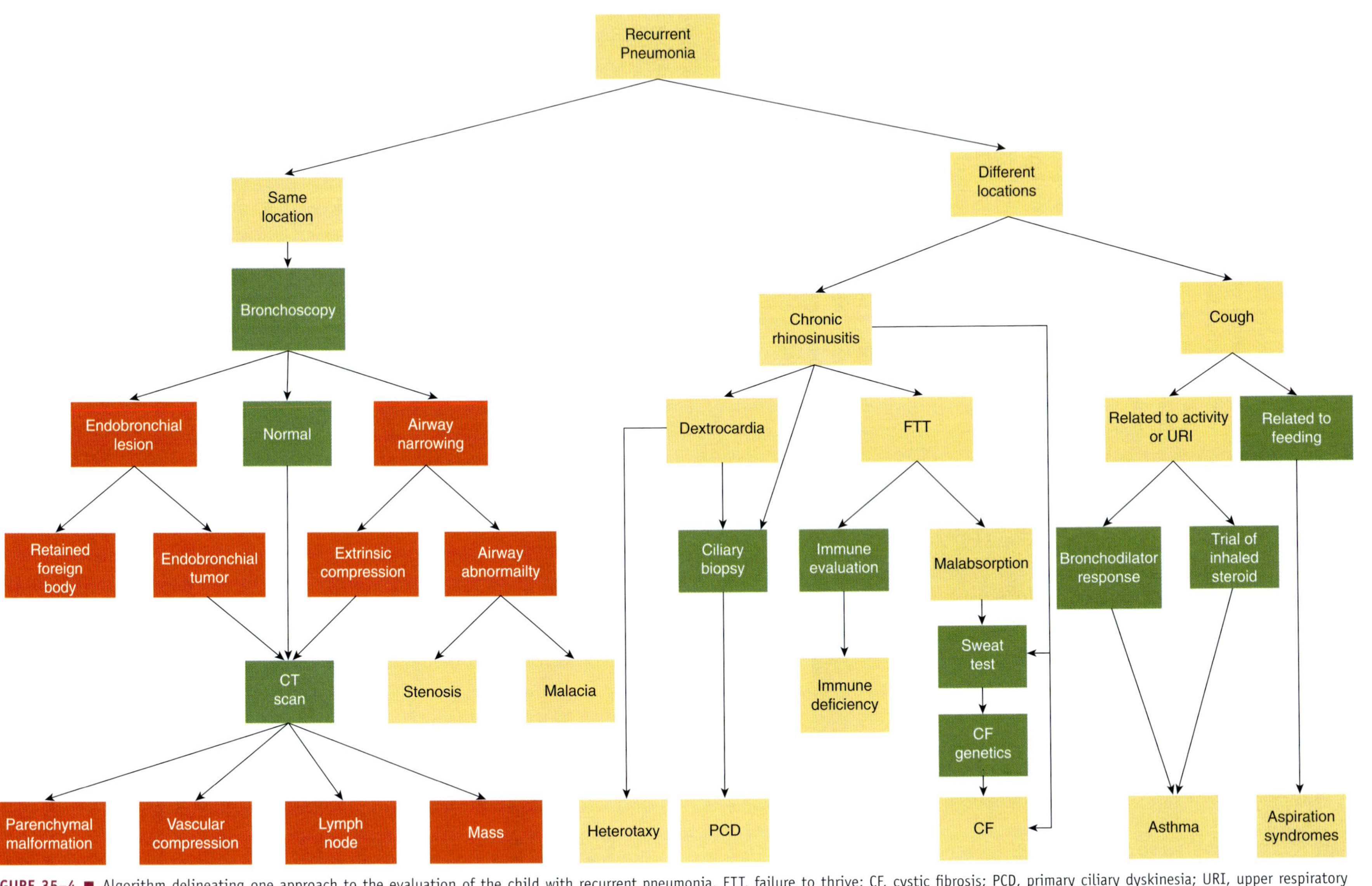

FIGURE 35–4 ■ Algorithm delineating one approach to the evaluation of the child with recurrent pneumonia. FTT, failure to thrive; CF, cystic fibrosis; PCD, primary ciliary dyskinesia; URI, upper respiratory infection.

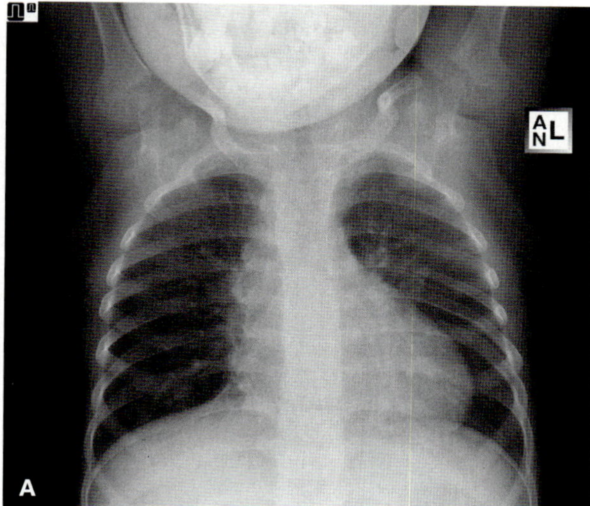

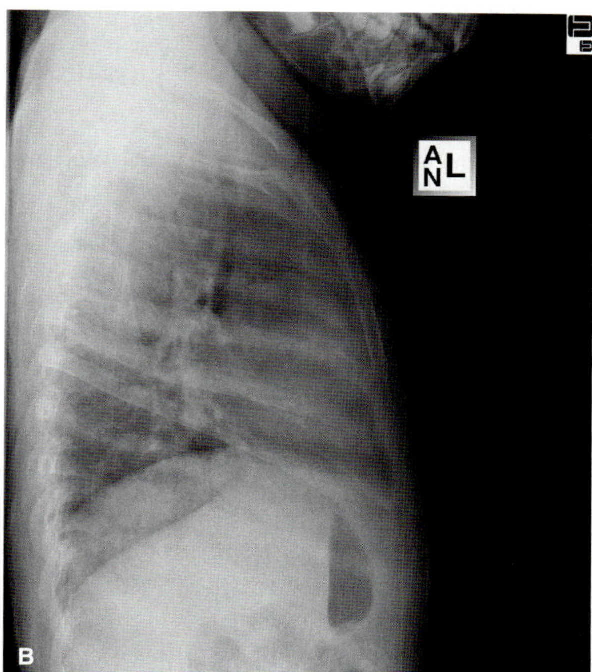

FIGURE 35–5 ■ **(A)** Anterior–posterior and **(B)** lateral chest radiographs of a 5.5-year-old male with a history of right middle lobe pneumonia. Note the leftward deviation of the trachea from a right-sided aortic arch. The child was found to have a vascular ring consisting of a right-sided arch and aberrant subclavian artery.

MANAGEMENT AND TREATMENT

Treatment depends on identifying the underlying cause of recurrent symptoms and whether or not the child is acutely ill. Supplemental oxygen, antibiotics, and ventilatory support should be administered as appropriate. In a patient with recurrent pneumonia, broad-spectrum antibiotic therapy is typically warranted; options include ampicillin-sulbactam, cefotaxime, or piperacillin-tazobactam. Clindamycin or vancomycin should be added to provide coverage against methicillin-resistant *S. aureus* if the patient is severely ill at presentation or if the initial response to therapy is poor.

If there is a problem with retention of secretions, chest physiotherapy or other methods of airway clearance are indicated. When such measures fail and there is a concern for mucous plugs obstructing a central airway, bronchoscopy can be considered to help improve airway clearance. In addition to its role in diagnosis, bronchoscopy has been shown to be therapeutic in aiding resolution of the right middle lobe syndrome.[16] Certain children with underlying diseases, like cystic fibrosis, primary ciliary dyskinesia, and immunodeficiencies, respond well to administration of chronic courses of antibiotics. Often, this is determined on an individual basis, but there are some conditions like X-linked agammaglobulinemia where a role for chronic antibiotic use has been established. In patients with CVID, regular administration of gamma globulin reduces the frequency of pulmonary infections[29] (Figure 35–6).

Surgical treatment for recurrent pneumonia is indicated when congenital malformations of the lung are discovered, or if lesions compress an adjacent bronchus.[30] Vascular rings that compress airways and possibly the esophagus should be divided. Abnormal connections between the airway and digestive tract, for example, H-type tracheoesophageal fistula or laryngotracheoesophageal cleft, must be repaired to halt recurrent soiling of the lung.

COURSE AND PROGNOSIS

For children with recurrent pneumonia relegated to a single region, the outcome is usually excellent. Often, excision of the offending lesion results in complete resolution of the problem.[30] Less commonly, lobectomy is considered when the affected area acts as a nidus for recurrent infections to the remainder of the lung. The course and prognosis for children whose recurrent pneumonia varies regionally usually follows that of the underlying disease and the tools available for treatment. For instance, the prognosis of a child with recurrent pneumonia related to immunoglobulin deficiency can be excellent with replacement therapy and judicious use of antibiotics. For the most common situation that physicians in developed countries will encounter—asthma—the prognosis is good. With adequate therapy with inhaled corticosteroids, asthma (usually) can be effectively managed. Management of recurrent aspiration of oropharyngeal secretions can be somewhat more challenging. With appropriate augmentation of airway clearance therapies, patients with primary ciliary dyskinesia can be expected to have a normal life span. The outcome for those with cystic fibrosis is somewhat more guarded.

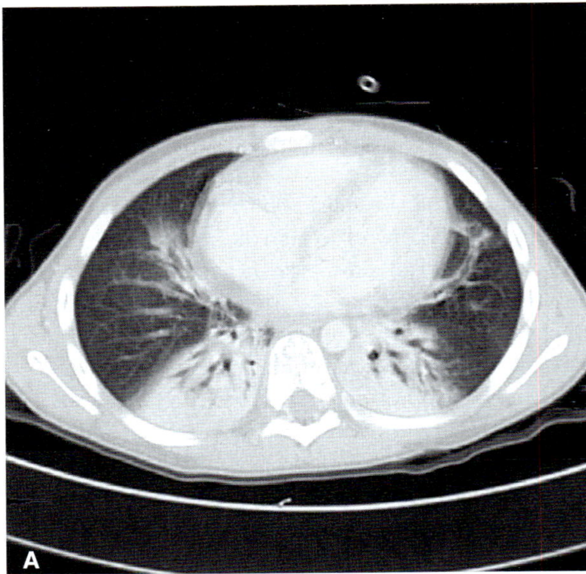

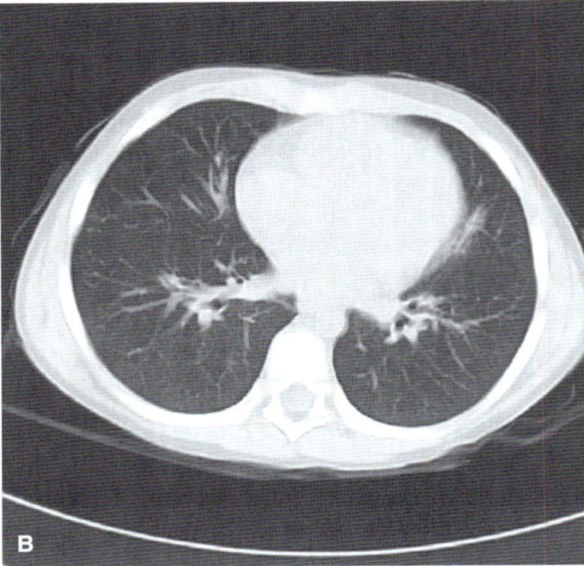

FIGURE 35–6 ■ Initial and follow-up high resolution CTs of the chest of a 10-year-old boy with CVID. **(A)** Initial study demonstrating bilateral densities with areas of early bronchiectasis and tree-in-bud formations; **(B)** following 2 months of intravenous gamma globulin therapy and antibiotics, there is resolution of the parenchymal densities.

PEARLS AND SPECIAL SITUATIONS

- Single or varied regional involvement provides a useful way to guide diagnostic evaluation.
- Always consider undertreated asthma in a child with either uni- or multifocal disease that occurs following common upper respiratory infections.
- The underlying disease predisposing the patient to recurrent pneumonia is often already known.
- However, recurrent pneumonia, especially in children who have growth disturbance, may be the first sign of an immune deficiency.
- If untreated—and sometimes even if treated properly—recurrent pneumonia predisposes to bronchiectasis later in life.

REFERENCES

1. Gove S. Integrated management of childhood illness by outpatient health workers: technical basis and overview. The WHO Working Group on Guidelines for Integrated Management of the Sick Child. *Bull World Health Organ.* 1997;75(suppl 1):7-24.
2. Cherian T, Mulholland EK, Carlin JB, et al. Standardized interpretation of paediatric chest radiographs for the diagnosis of pneumonia in epidemiological studies. *Bull World Health Organ.* 2005;83:353-359.
3. McCracken GH, Jr. Etiology and treatment of pneumonia. *Pediatr Infect Dis J.* 2000; 19:373-377.
4. Wald ER. Recurrent and nonresolving pneumonia in children. *Semin Respir Infect.* 1993;8:46-58.
5. Owayed AF, Campbell DM, Wang EE. Underlying causes of recurrent pneumonia in children. *Arch Pediatr Adolesc Med.* 2000;154:190-194.
6. Lodha R, Puranik M, Natchu UC, Kabra SK. Recurrent pneumonia in children: clinical profile and underlying causes. *Acta Paediatr.* 2002;91:1170-1173.
7. Ciftci E, Gunes M, Koksal Y, Ince E, Dogru U. Underlying causes of recurrent pneumonia in Turkish children in a university hospital. *J Trop Pediatr.* 2003;49:212-215.
8. Eigen H, Laughlin JJ, Homrighausen J. Recurrent pneumonia in children and its relationship to bronchial hyperreactivity. *Pediatrics.* 1982;70:698-704.
9. Heffelfinger JD, Davis TE, Gebrian B, Bordeau R, Schwartz B, Dowell SF. Evaluation of children with recurrent pneumonia diagnosed by World Health Organization criteria. *Pediatr Infect Dis J.* 2002;21:108-112.
10. Sanchez I, Navarro H, Mendez M, Holmgren N, Caussade S. Clinical characteristics of children with tracheobronchial anomalies. *Pediatr Pulmonol.* 2003;35:288-291.
11. Abel RM, Bush A, Chitty L, Harcourt J, Nicholson AG. Congenital lung disease. In: Chernick V, Boat TF, Wilmott RW, Bush A, eds. *Kendig's Disorders of the Respiratory Tract in Children.* Philadelphia, PA: Elsevier Inc; 2006: 280-316.
12. Miller RW, Woo P, Kellman RK, Slagle TS. Tracheobronchial abnormalities in infants with bronchopulmonary dysplasia. *J Pediatr.* 1987;111:779-782.
13. Hauft SM, Perlman JM, Siegel MJ, Muntz HR. Tracheal stenosis in the sick premature infant. Clinical and radiologic features. *Am J Dis Child.* 1988;142:206-209.
14. Brodsky L, Reidy M, Stanievich JF. The effects of suctioning techniques on the distal tracheal mucosa in intubated low birth weight infants. *Int J Pediatr Otorhinolaryngol.* 1987;14:1-14.
15. Valery PC, Torzillo PJ, Mulholland K, Boyce NC, Purdie DM, Chang AB. Hospital-based case-control study of bronchiectasis in indigenous children in Central Australia. *Pediatr Infect Dis J.* 2004;23:902-908.
16. Priftis KN, Mermiri D, Papadopoulou A, Anthracopoulos MB, Vaos G, Nicolaidou P. The role of timely intervention in middle lobe syndrome in children. *Chest.* 2005;128: 2504-2510.

17. Sekerel BE, Nakipoglu F. Middle lobe syndrome in children with asthma: review of 56 cases. *J Asthma.* 2004;41:411-417.
18. Donnelly LF. *Fundamentals of Pediatric Radiology.* Philadelphia, PA: WB Saunders; 2001:23-69.
19. Kovesi T, Rubin S. Long-term complications of congenital esophageal atresia and(or tracheoesophageal fistula. *Chest.* 2004;126:915-925.
20. Johnston SL, Pattemore PK, Sanderson G, et al. Community study of role of viral infections in exacerbations of asthma in 9-11 year old children. *BMJ.* 1995;310:1225-1229.
21. Grimbacher B, Holland SM, Gallin JI, et al. Hyper-IgE syndrome with recurrent infections–an autosomal dominant multisystem disorder. *N Engl J Med.* 1999;340: 692-702.
22. Martinez Garcia MA, de Rojas MD, Nauffal Manzur MD, et al. Respiratory disorders in common variable immunodeficiency. *Respir Med.* 2001;95:191-195.
23. Edwards E, Razvi S, Cunningham-Rundles C. IgA deficiency: clinical correlates and responses to pneumococcal vaccine. *Clin Immunol.* 2004;111:93-97.
24. Ochs HD, Thrasher AJ. The Wiskott-Aldrich syndrome. *J Allergy Clin Immunol.* 2006;117:725-738.
25. Bott L, Lebreton J, Thumerelle C, Cuvellier J, Deschildre A, Sardet A. Lung disease in ataxia-telangiectasia. *Acta Paediatr.* 2007;96:1021-1024.
26. Heyer CM, Nuesslein TG, Jung D, et al. Tracheobronchial anomalies and stenoses: detection with low-dose multidetector CT with virtual tracheobronchoscopy—comparison with flexible tracheobronchoscopy. *Radiology.* 2007; 242: 542-549.
27. Hernanz-Schulman M. Vascular rings: a practical approach to imaging diagnosis. *Pediatr Radiol.* 2005;35:961-979.
28. Ravelli AM, Panarotto MB, Verdoni L, Consolati V, Bolognini S. Pulmonary aspiration shown by scintigraphy in gastroesophageal reflux-related respiratory disease. *Chest.* 2006;130:1520-1526.
29. Orange JS, Hossny EM, Weiler CR, et al. Use of intravenous immunoglobulin in human disease: a review of evidence by members of the Primary Immunodeficiency Committee of the American Academy of Allergy, Asthma and Immunology. *J Allergy Clin Immunol.* 2006;117: S525-S553.
30. Parikh D, Samuel M. Congenital cystic lung lesions: is surgical resection essential? *Pediatr Pulmonol.* 2005;40: 533-537.

CHAPTER 36

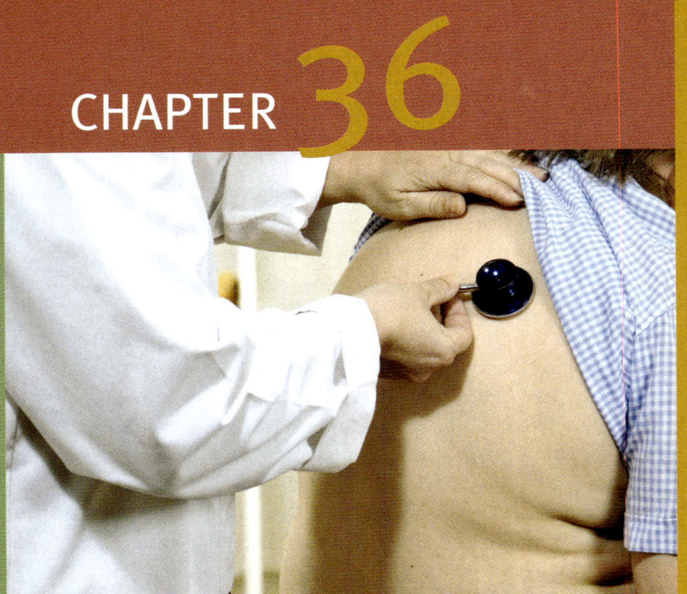

Childhood Tuberculosis

Ben J. Marais

DEFINITIONS AND EPIDEMIOLOGY

Tuberculosis (TB) is an ancient disease; suggestive spinal changes have been described in Neolithic man, and clear evidence of TB bone lesions have been found in mummified remains from Egypt.[1] Hippocrates (460–377 BC) introduced the ancient Greek term for TB, *phthisis*, better known as consumption.[1] Although TB is an ancient disease, it remains one of the major public health challenges of the new millennium. Fuelled mainly by rampant third world poverty and the human immunodeficiency virus (HIV) epidemic, TB affects and kills more people today than ever before. The gravity of the situation is reflected by (1) the fact that the epidemic continues to escalate despite the declaration of a global TB emergency by the World Health Organization (WHO) in 1993 and (2) the increased transmission of drug-resistant TB.

Robert Koch (1843–1910) discovered that *Mycobacterium tuberculosis* causes TB, but it was soon recognized that infection, as indicated by a positive tuberculin skin test (TST), is not at all uncommon. It remains an intriguing and largely unexplained observation that only a small minority of people infected with *M. tuberculosis* ever progress to active disease. In endemic countries, TB control programs focus on the diagnosis and treatment of the most infectious cases (adults with sputum smear-positive TB) in an attempt to control the epidemic. Childhood TB receives little public health emphasis, as children tend to have paucibacillary disease and rarely transmit the organism. However, children in endemic areas carry a huge disease burden and experience considerable TB-related morbidity and mortality.[2,3] In addition, adolescent children frequently develop cavitary disease[4] and contribute to disease transmission within the community, particularly in congregate settings such as schools.[5]

An estimated 8.3 million new TB cases were diagnosed in 2000, of whom 884, 019 (11%) were <15 years of age.[6] Poor countries carry the bulk of the TB disease burden, as exposure to both the organism and the vulnerability to progress to disease following infection are increased in these settings (Figure 36–1).[7] HIV-related immune compromise is the most important factor that increases the vulnerability of individuals to develop TB following exposure and infection, which explains why Sub-Saharan Africa, the region worst affected by HIV, reports the highest TB incidence rates in the world.[8]

The risk to develop active TB following infection is mainly determined by the age and immune status of the child.[9] The highest risk occurs in very young (immune immature) and/or immune-compromised children (Table 36–1).[9] If children do progress to active TB, it usually occurs within 12 months of primary infection.[9] Therefore, the burden of childhood TB provides a valuable epidemiologic perspective, as it reflects ongoing transmission within the community it serves as an important indicator of epidemic control.

PATHOGENESIS

TB is spread via tiny aerosol droplets, predominantly produced by adults with cavitary TB. The risk of infection following TB exposure depends on the infectiousness of the index case, as well as the proximity and duration of contact. In highly endemic areas, the majority of transmission occurs outside the household,[10] but this does not reduce the importance of household exposure, especially in young and vulnerable children. In nonendemic countries like the United States, household exposure remains the most likely source of infection. In general, known household exposure to an adult index case

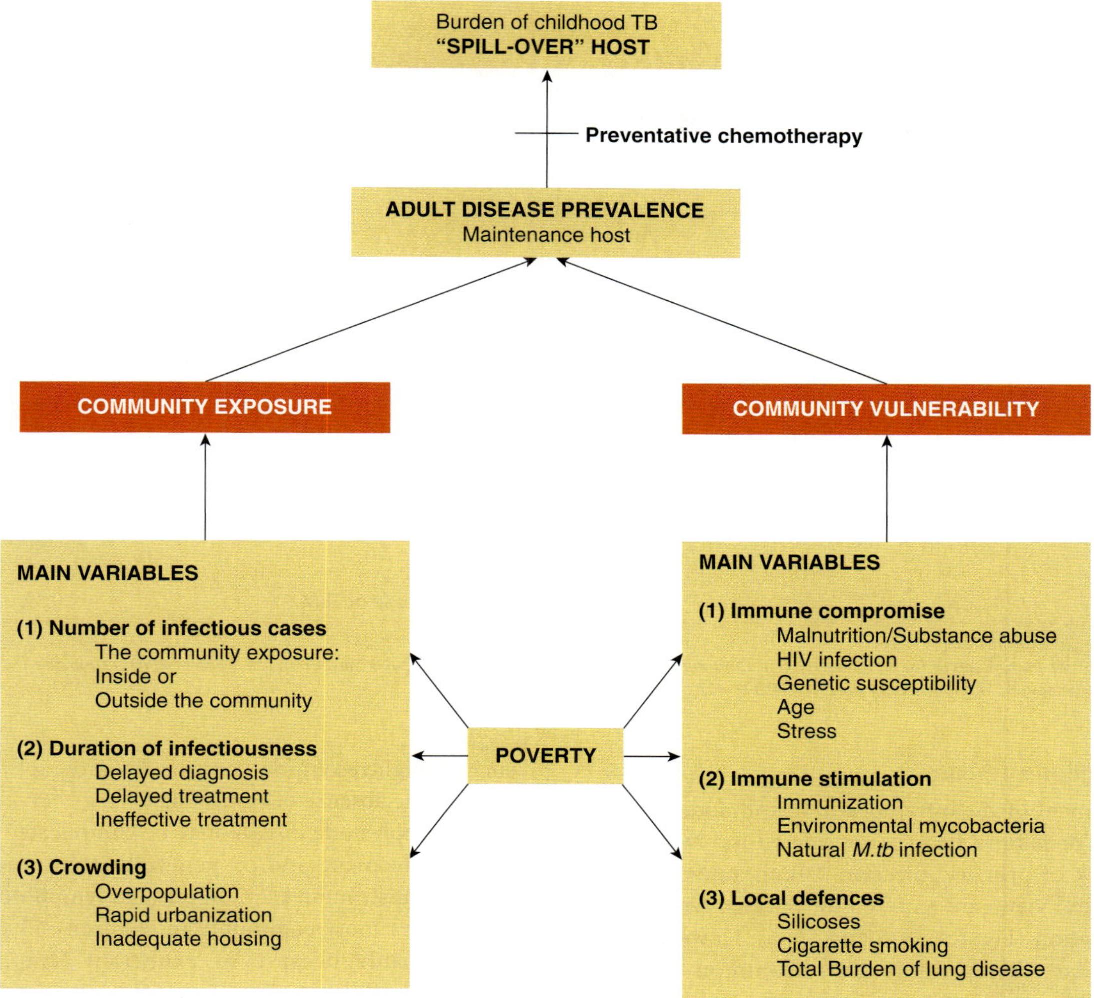

FIGURE 36–1 ■ The main variables that contribute to the prevalence of TB in adults and by extrapolation the burden of childhood TB. (*With permission from Marais BJ, Obihara CC, Warren RM, Schaaf HS, Gie RP, Donald PR. The burden of childhood tuberculosis: A public health perspective. Int J Tuberc Lung Dis. 2005;9(12):1305–13.*)

presents an important opportunity for intervention, providing appropriate health education and preventive chemotherapy.

CLINICAL PRESENTATION

Both intra- and extrathoracic manifestations of TB will be discussed below. Intrathoracic manifestations include mediastinal lymph node disease, pleural and pericardial effusion, disseminated or miliary disease, and adult-type intrathoracic disease. Extrathoracic manifestations include cervical lymphadenitis, tuberculous meningitis, other organ involvement, and, in patients with HIV, immune reconstitution.

Intrathoracic Disease

The TB bacillus usually enters its human host via the lungs; inhalation of an infectious droplet with the right size to penetrate into the periphery of the lung results in a localized area of pneumonic consolidation at the site of organism deposition. This is referred to as the primary (Ghon) focus, from where TB bacilli drain via local lymphatics to the regional lymph nodes. The combination of the Ghon focus and enlarged regional lymph nodes, usually involving the perihilar area, is referred to as the primary complex.[11] Active disease may present with a diverse spectrum of pathology. Figure 36–2 provides a schematic illustration of potential disease progression following primary infection with *M. tuberculosis* and how the various disease manifestations develop.[11] The different disease manifestations show clear patterns related to (1) the time since infection occurred (Figure 36–3)[9] and (2) the age at the time of primary infection (Figure 36–4).[12] The disease manifestations observed in immune-compromised children seem to correlate with those seen in very young (<3 years of age) children.[12,13]

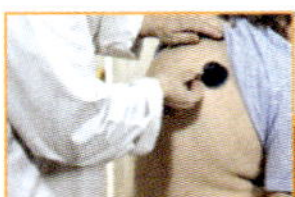

Table 36–1.

Age-Specific Risk to Progress to Disease Following Primary Infection with M. Tuberculosis in Immune-Competent Children

Age at Primary Infection (Yr)	Risk to Progress to Disease	
<1	No disease	50%
	Pulmonary disease	30–40%
	Disseminated (miliary) disease or TBM	10–20%
1–2	No disease	75–80%
	Pulmonary disease	10–20%
	Disseminated (miliary) disease or TBM	2–5%
2–5	No disease	95%
	Pulmonary disease	5%
	Disseminated (miliary) disease or TBM	0.5%
5–10	No disease	98%
	Pulmonary disease	2%
	Disseminated (miliary) disease or TBM	<0.5%
>10	No disease	80–90%
	Pulmonary disease	10–20%
	Disseminated (miliary) disease or TBM	<0.5%

TBM, tuberculous meningitis.
With permission from Marais BJ, Gie RP, Schaaf HS, et al. The natural history of childhood intra-thoracic tuberculosis: a critical review of literature from the pre-chemotherapy era. Int J Tuberc Lung Dis. 2004;8(4):392–402.

Lymph node disease

Involvement of the intrathoracic lymph nodes (perihilar and/or paratracheal) is considered the radiological hallmark of primary infection.[14] Both anteroposterior and lateral views are required for optimal lymph node visualization (Figures 36–5 and 36–6). However, transient hilar adenopathy is not uncommon following recent primary infection, and particular care should be exercised when interpreting results of very sensitive tests such as high-resolution computed tomography of the lung, in the absence of clinical data.[13]

Lymph node disease may be complicated by airway involvement and/or penetration into adjacent anatomical structures.[11] Complicated lymph node disease occurs most commonly in children <5 years of age, probably because of exuberant lymph node responses and the small caliber of their airways. Airway compression results when an airway is surrounded and

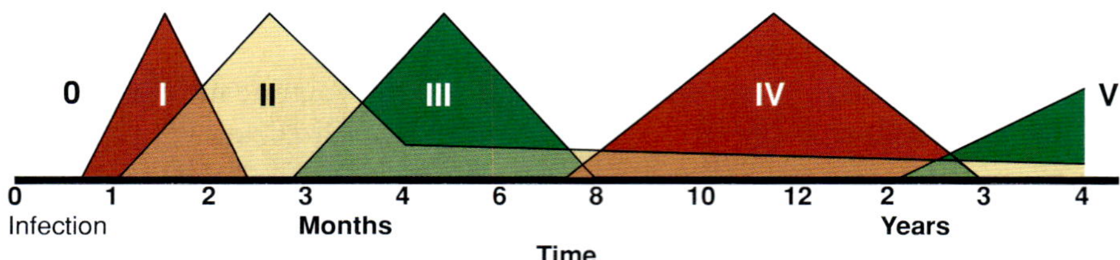

Phase of disease - adapted from the time-table of tuberculosis described by Wallgren[3]

0 Incubation phase
I Hypersensitivity phase
II Phase of miliary tuberculosis and tuberculous meningitis
III Phase of segmental lesions in children < 5 years and pleural effusion in those > 5 years
IV Phase of osteo-articular tuberculosis in children < 5 years and adult-type disease in those > 10 years
V Phase of late manifestations including pulmonary re-activation

Not all these disease manifestations (phases) are equally common and while hypersensitivity is a nearly universal phenomenon following primary infection, the late manifestations are extremely rare. Table 36–6 provide an indication of how common the most important of these disease manifestations are in specific age groups. The vast majority of complications occur in the first 3–12 months following primary infection.

FIGURE 36–2 ■ Schematic timeline of primary intrathoracic tuberculosis. (*With permission from Marais BJ, Gie RP, Schaaf HS, et al. The natural history of childhood intra-thoracic tuberculosis: A critical review of literature from the pre-chemotherapy era. Int J Tuberc Lung Dis. 2004;8(4):392–402.*)

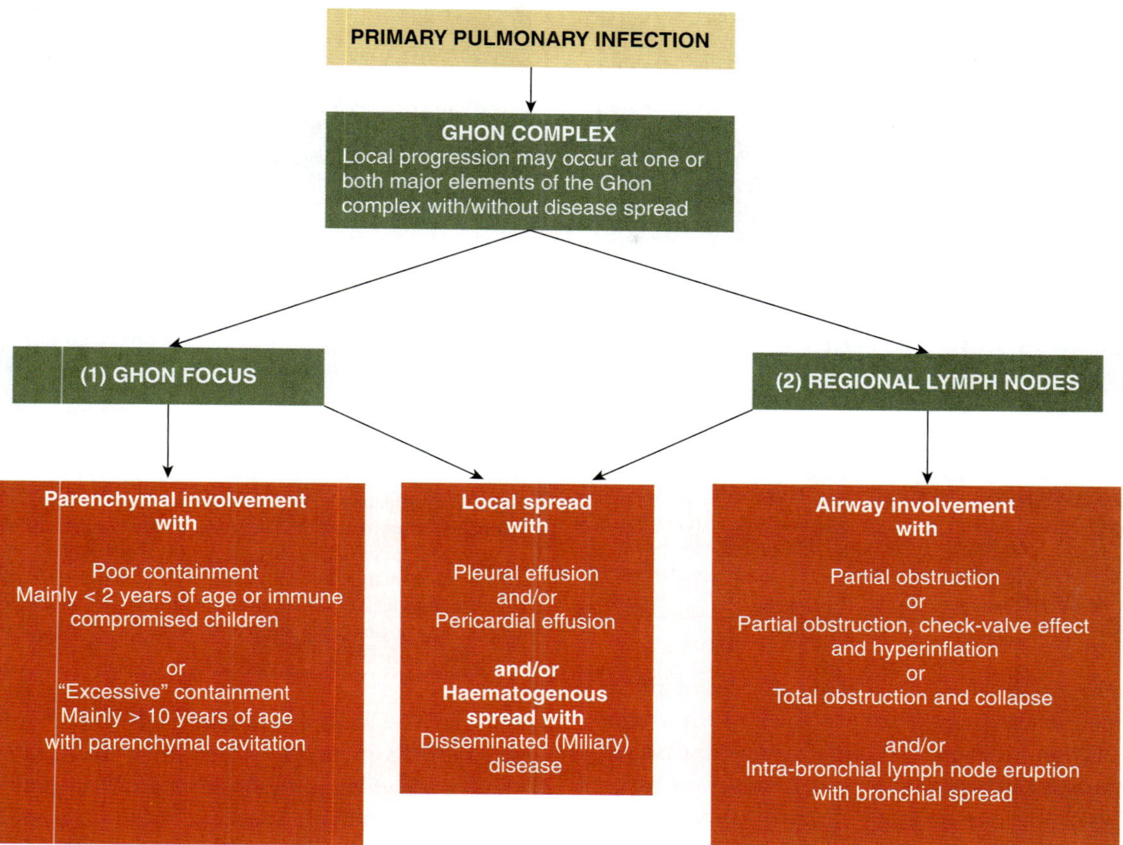

FIGURE 36–3 ■ Schematic illustration of potential disease progression following primary pulmonary infection with *M. tuberculosis*. (*With permission from Marais BJ, Gie RP, Schaaf HS, et al. A proposed radiological classification of childhood intra-thoracic tuberculosis. Pediatr Radiol. 2004;34(11):886–894.*)

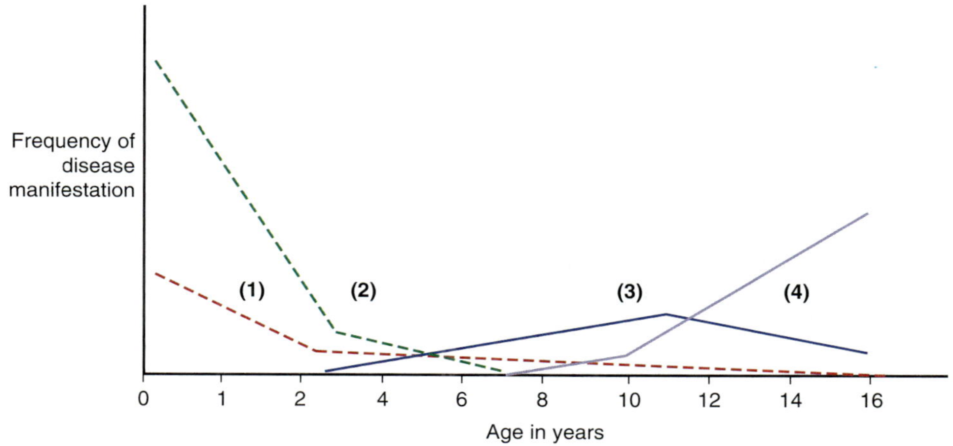

FIGURE 36–4 ■ Age-related manifestations of intrathoracic TB in children, documented during the prechemotherapy era. (*With permission from Marais BJ, Donald PR, Gie RP, Schaaf HS, Beyers N. Diversity of disease in childhood pulmonary tuberculosis. Ann Trop Paediatr. 2005;25(2):79–86.*)

1. Complicated Ghon focus and/or disseminated disease
2. Uncomplicated Ghon focus and/or lymph node disease/Complicated lymph node disease
3. Pleural effusion
4. Adult-type disease

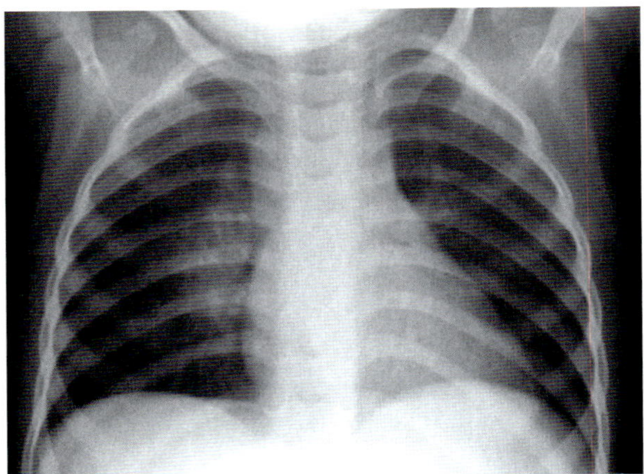

FIGURE 36–5 ■ Lymph node disease (anteroposterior view). (*With permission from Marais BJ, Gie RP, Schaaf HS, et al. A proposed radiological classification of childhood intra-thoracic tuberculosis. Pediatr Radiol. 2004;34(11):886–894.*) (Right hilar lymph node enlargement; note the haziness (flare) that surrounds the lymph node suggesting active inflammation.)

fixated by diseased lymph nodes and associated inflammation, and this may be best visualized on a high-kilovolt chest radiograph (CXR). Various disease presentations include partial airway obstruction with a check-valve effect and alveolar hyperinflation, or total airway obstruction with alveolar collapse. When a diseased lymph node erupts into an airway, caseous

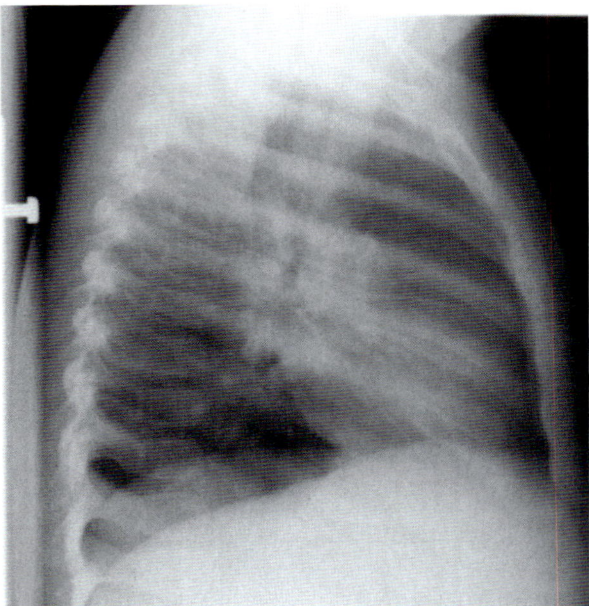

FIGURE 36–6 ■ Lymph node disease (lateral view). (*With permission from Marais BJ, Gie RP, Schaaf HS, et al. A proposed radiological classification of childhood intra-thoracic tuberculosis. Pediatr Radiol. 2004;34(11):886–894.*) (The lateral chest radiograph confirms the existence of enlarged hilar nodes, and the little fluid present in the oblique and transverse fissures suggests an inflammatory response.)

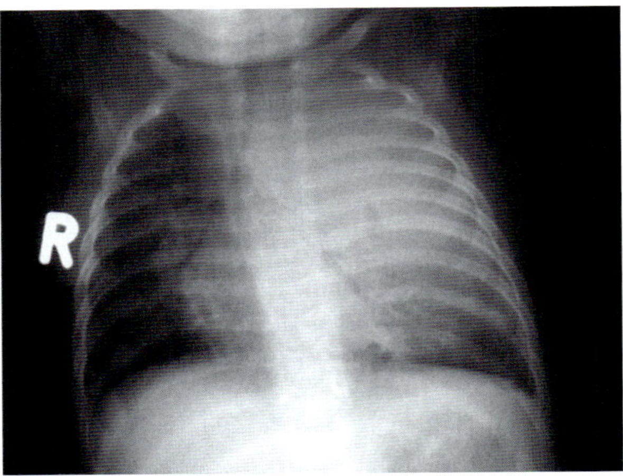

FIGURE 36–7 ■ Lymph node disease with airway compression and caseating pneumonia. (*With permission from Marais BJ, Gie RP, Schaaf HS, et al. A proposed radiological classification of childhood intrathoracic tuberculosis. Pediatr Radiol. 2004;34(11):886–894.*) (Lymph node enlargement with compression of both the trachea and left main bronchus. Expansile alveolar consolidation of the left upper lobe because of caseating pneumonia. A small cavity is visible in the left upper lobe.)

material may be aspirated and the resulting pathology may range from pure hypersensitivity-induced inflammation (dead bacilli and/or "toxins") to destructive caseating pneumonia (virulent bacilli), depending on the bacterial load and viability of the bacilli aspirated. Caseating pneumonia often causes an expansile (bulging against their anatomical boundaries) pneumonic process with visible parenchymal breakdown (Figure 36–7).[15] Penetration into adjacent anatomical structures may involve the phrenic nerve with unilateral diaphragmatic palsy, the esophagus with the formation of a broncho- or tracheoesophageal fistula, and/or the thoracic duct with the formation of a unilateral chylothorax.[11]

Pleural and pericardial effusion

The accumulation of the typical lymphocyte-rich, straw-colored fluid represents a hypersensitivity response. The pleural fluid typically obliterates 30–60% of the affected hemithorax (Figure 36–8), although massive fluid collections may cause mediastinal shift and cardiovascular compromise.[11] In general, isolated pleural effusions are unusual in children <3 years of age and tend to develop soon (within the first 3–9 months) after primary infection.[9]

A loculated fluid collection may indicate TB empyema that results when bacilli actively multiply within the pleural space. This is not common, but immune-compromised individuals seem to be at increased risk.

Pericardial effusion usually develops when a subcarinal lymph node erupts into the pericardial space.[9] On CXR the heart shadow may be enlarged with a

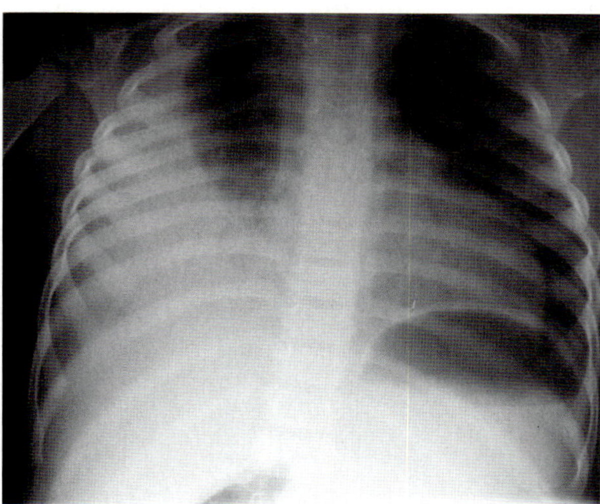

FIGURE 36–8 ■ Unilateral pleural effusion. (*With permission from Marais BJ, Gie RP, Schaaf HS, et al. A proposed radiological classification of childhood intra-thoracic tuberculosis. Pediatr Radiol. 2004;34(11):886–894.*) (Large uncomplicated right-sided pleural effusion. No underlying pathology is visible.)

suggestive globular appearance, but cardiac ultrasound is the most sensitive test to confirm or exclude the presence of a pericardial effusion. Long-term sequelae include constrictive pericarditis, and this is an indication for the use of corticosteroids together with anti-TB treatment.[11]

Disseminated (miliary) disease

Dissemination represents a condition of infinite gradation. Occult dissemination is common following primary infection; however, it rarely progresses to disseminated disease except in very young (<2–3 years of age) and immune-compromised children.[9,13] Typical radiologic signs include the presence of even-sized miliary lesions (<2 mm), which are distributed bilaterally into the very periphery of the lung (Figure 36–9).[11] Diagnostic confusion often exists in HIV-infected children in whom lymphocytic interstitial pneumonitis, malignancies, and opportunistic infections such as *Pneumocystis jeroveci* may present with a similar radiological picture.[16] In these instances, response to treatment and/or bacteriologic confirmation may be the only way to establish a definitive diagnosis.

Adult-type disease

Adult-type disease first appears around puberty (from 8 to 10 years of age) and becomes the dominant disease manifestation during adolescence.[9] As with pulmonary TB in adults, the apical and posterior segments of the upper lobe and the apical segment of the lower lobe are most commonly affected (Figure 36–10). Complications include progressive cavity formation and bronchial spread.[11]

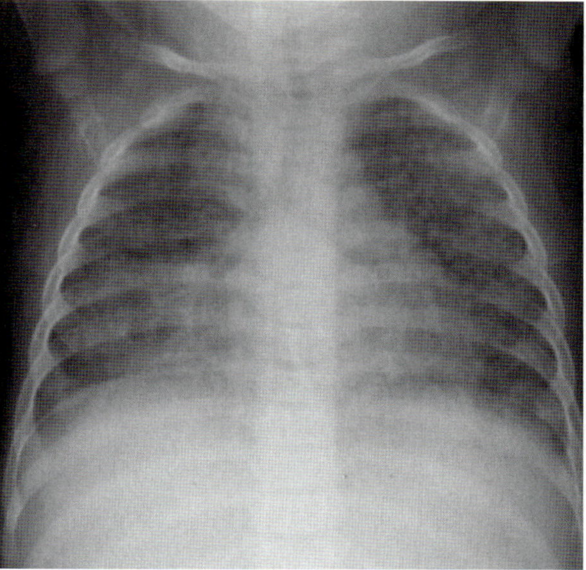

FIGURE 36–9 ■ Disseminated (miliary) disease. (*With permission from Marais BJ, Gie RP, Schaaf HS, et al. A proposed radiological classification of childhood intra-thoracic tuberculosis. Pediatr Radiol. 2004;34(11):886–894.*) (Right-sided paratracheal glands shifting the trachea to the left, with hematogenous dissemination.)

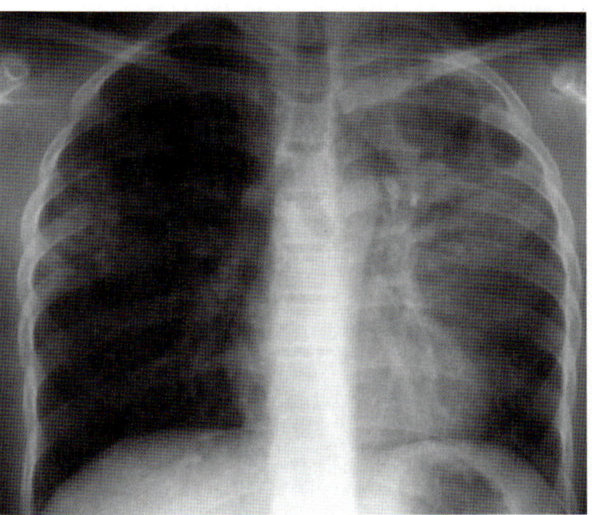

FIGURE 36–10 ■ Adult-type disease. (*With permission from Marais BJ, Gie RP, Schaaf HS, et al. A proposed radiological classification of childhood intra-thoracic tuberculosis. Pediatr Radiol. 2004;34(11): 886–894.*) (Multiple cavities in the left upper lobe with surrounding alveolar consolidation and fibrosis (leading to volume loss) and bronchial spread to the right upper lobe.)

Extrathoracic Disease

Cervical lymphadenitis

The most common extrathoracic manifestation of TB in children is cervical lymphadenitis (Table 36–2). Disease pathology within the lymph node is similar to that seen in other organs, with initial tubercle formation and lymphoid hyperplasia that may progress to caseation and necrosis. Isolated involvement of a single node is rare,

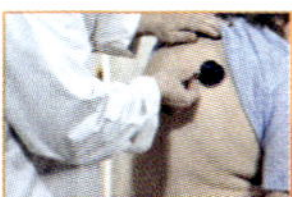

Table 36–2.

Disease Spectrum Documented in a Prospective Community-Based Survey of All Children <13 Years of Age, Treated for TB in a Highly Endemic Area

TB Manifestation	Total (%) (N = 439)
Not TB	85 (19.4)
Intrathoracic TB	307 (69.9)
Ghon focus	
Uncomplicated (with/ without hilar adenopathy)	16/307 (5.2)
Complicated	3/307 (1.0)
Lymph node disease	
Uncomplicated	147/307 (47.9)
Complicated	
Compression	25/307 (8.1)
Consolidation	62/307 (20.6)
Pleurisy	24/307 (7.8)
Pericarditis	1/307 (0.3)
Disseminated (miliary) disease	15/307 (4.9)
Adult-type disease	14/307 (4.6)
Extrathoracic TB	72 (16.4)
Peripheral lymphadenitis	
Cervical	35/72 (48.6)
Other	1/72 (1.4)
Central nervous system TB	
Meningitis	14/72 (19.4)
Tuberculoma	2/72 (2.8
Abdominal TB	1/72 (1.4)
Osteoarticular TB	
Vertebral spondylitis	4/72 (5.6)
Other	7/72 (9.7)
Skin	8/72 (11.1)
Intra- + Extrathoracic TB	25 (5.7)

TB, tuberculosis; not TB, chest radiograph not suggestive of TB (confirmed by two independent child TB experts), no bacteriologic or histologic proof and no extra-thoracic TB recorded; intra- + extrathoracic TB, children with intra- and extrathoracic TB were included in both groups and therefore this number should be deducted to add up to a total of 439 or 100%.
With permission from Marais BJ, Gie RP, Schaaf HS, Hesseling AC, Enarson DA, Beyers N. The spectrum of childhood tuberculosis in a highly endemic area. Int J Tuberc Lung Dis 2006;10:732–738.

and nodes are usually matted because of considerable periadenitis. A cold abscess results when the caseous material liquefies, and this is signified by a soft fluctuant node with violaceous discoloration of the overlying skin; spontaneous drainage and sinus formation may follow. Untreated, the natural course of TB lymphadenitis in an immune-competent host follows a prolonged and relapsing course, often interrupted by transient lymph node enlargement, fluctuation, and/or sinus formation.

Table 36–3 reflects the clinical characteristics of children diagnosed with TB lymphadenitis.[17] A simple clinical algorithm that identifies children with persistent (>4 weeks) cervical adenopathy, without a visible local cause or response to first-line antibiotics, and a cervical mass ≥2 × 2 cm showed excellent diagnostic accuracy in this highly endemic area. However, a clinical diagnostic

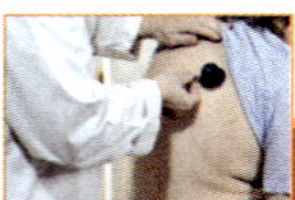

Table 36–3.

Clinical Characteristics of Children with TB Lymphadenitis (n = 35)

Lymph Node Characteristics	Number (%)
Persistence (present for >4weeks, no response to antibiotics)	35 (100)
Size	
<2 × 2 cm	4 (11.4)
(2–4) × (2–4) cm	25 (71.5)
>4 × 4 cm	6 (17.1)
Character	
Single	5 (14.3)
Multiple	
Discreet	14 (40.0)
Matted	16 (45.7)
Solid	28 (80.0)
Fluctuant	
Without secondary bacterial infection	5 (14.3)
With secondary bacterial infection (red and warm)	2 (5.7)
Associated findings	
Tuberculin skin test	
0 mm	2 (5.7)
1–9 mm	0
≥10 mm	33 (94.3)
≥15 mm	32 (91.4)
Mean response 19.1 mm (standard deviation 2.9 mm)	
Constitutional symptoms	
Any symptom	21 (60.0)
Fever	7 (20.0)
Cough	9 (25.7)
Night sweats	8 (22.8)
Fatigue	19 (54.3)
Failure to thrive	10 (28.6)
Chest radiograph	
Suggestive of tuberculosis	13 (37.1)
Lymph node disease	
Uncomplicated	8 (22.8)
With airway compression	1 (2.9)
With parenchymal consolidation	4 (11.4)

Size, transverse diameter of the largest cervical mass; Fatigue, less playful and active since the mass was first noted; failure to thrive, crossing at least one centile line in the preceding 3 months or having lost >10% of bodyweight (minimum 1 kg) over any time interval.
With permission from Marais BJ, Wright C, Gie RP, et al. Etiology of persistent cervical adenopathy in children: a prospective community-based study in an area with a high incidence of tuberculosis. Pediatr Inf Dis J 2006;25:142–146.

approach would be far less accurate in nonendemic areas and in areas where alternative diagnoses, such as Burkitt's lymphoma, are more common. In these settings, a positive TST result may have additional value to indicate mycobacterial disease,[17] although it may not differentiate TB lymph adenitis from disease caused by non-TB mycobacteria.[18] Establishing a definitive tissue and/or culture diagnosis remains preferable, and this can be done in a minimally invasive fashion using fine needle aspiration biopsy.[17]

The mycobacteria that cause cervical lymphadenitis are highly variable in different settings. In areas where the control of bovine TB is poor and milk is not routinely pasteurized, *Mycobacterium bovis* may be a frequent cause, but in areas where TB is endemic and bovine TB is well controlled, *M. tuberculosis* would be the most common causative organism. In developed countries with low rates of TB transmission, non-TB (environmental) mycobacteria and, in particular, *M. avium-intracellulare* are most frequently responsible.[18]

Tuberculous meningitis

Tuberculous meningitis is the most severe manifestation of childhood TB. Bacille Calmette Geurin (BCG) vaccination provides some degree of protection against the severe forms of TB (miliary disease and tuberculous meningitis), but despite universal BCG vaccination severe disease manifestations still occur, mainly affecting very young (immune immature) and/or immunocompromised children in endemic areas.

Other TB manifestations

TB can affect nearly every organ system (Table 36–2), and this is mostly the result of disease progression, which occurs at sites where the TB bacillus was deposited during the initial phase of occult dissemination. In addition, newborn babies may acquire congenital TB via the placenta, in which case the primary (Ghon) focus is usually located in the liver, if the mother develops active TB or *M. tuberculosis* infection with hematogenous dissemination during pregnancy. The experience is that cases of congenital TB are on the rise in countries where TB/HIV coinfection rates among expectant mothers are high.

Immune reconstitution

The clinical syndrome was first documented in the prechemotherapy era, following nutritional rehabilitation and/or the termination of high-dose steroid treatment.[9] Recently, immune reconstitution inflammatory syndrome (IRIS) has emerged as an important complication to consider after the introduction of highly active antiretroviral therapy in HIV-infected, immune-compromised patients.[19] Radiologic signs may include airway compression as a result of increased inflammation surrounding diseased lymph nodes, or dense alveolar consolidation caused by excessive inflammation in areas of previous "subclinical" TB infiltration. This temporary exacerbation of TB symptoms and signs is mainly ascribed to the effects of improved immune function, although a "hypersensitivity" reaction to antigens released by killed TB bacilli may also contribute. It does not indicate treatment failure and should subside spontaneously, although severe cases may require treatment with corticosteroids. In a recent prospective survey of 152 Thai children with low CD4 percentages (<15%), IRIS was documented in 14 (19%), usually within 4 weeks of highly active antiretroviral therapy initiation.[20] The majority of IRIS cases (nine) were caused by atypical mycobacteria, three because of *M. tuberculosis*, and two because of *M. bovis* BCG.

DIAGNOSIS

Establishing a definitive diagnosis of childhood TB remains a challenge. Sputum smear microscopy is positive in <10–15% of children with TB, and culture yields are generally low (30–40%),[21] although it may be considerably higher in children with advanced disease.[22] In low-burden countries the triad of (1) known contact with an infectious source case, (2) a positive TST, and (3) a CXR is frequently used to establish a diagnosis of childhood TB. This provides a reasonably accurate diagnosis in nonendemic settings where exposure to *M. tuberculosis* is rare and usually well documented. However, it has limited value in endemic areas where exposure to, and/or infection with, *M. tuberculosis* is common.[13] Consequently, the diagnosis of TB in endemic areas depends predominantly on the subjective interpretation of the CXR, which provides a fairly accurate diagnosis in experienced hands, despite its many limitations.[23,24] An important concept derived from the natural history of disease is risk stratification, which determines the diagnostic emphasis and guides therapeutic decision making.[13] Exposure and/or infection warrants preventive chemotherapy in all children who are at high risk of developing active TB but are less relevant in low-risk children from endemic areas where infection is a common event.

Symptom-Based Diagnosis

WHO guidelines advise that all children <5 years of age in close contact with a sputum smear-positive index case should be actively traced, screened for TB, and provided preventive chemotherapy once active TB has been excluded.[25] National guidelines frequently regard the TST and CXR as prerequisite tests for adequate screening of household contacts, but these tests are rarely available in endemic areas with limited resources. In these settings, symptom-based screening may have considerable value to improve access to preventive therapy,[26] and this is acknowledged by the most recent WHO guidelines.[25] In low-burden countries where TB eradication is an achievable goal and the risk of reinfection is low, preventive chemotherapy may be provided to everyone with documented TB infection to try and eradicate the pool of latent TB infection, from which future reactivation disease may result.[13]

As a result of the diagnostic limitations mentioned and the difficulty of obtaining a CXR in many endemic areas, a variety of clinical scoring systems have been developed to diagnose active TB. A critical review of these scoring systems concluded that these are severely limited by the absence of standard symptom definitions and inadequate validation.[27] Accurate symptom definition is important to differentiate TB from other common conditions, as poorly defined symptoms (such as a cough of >3 weeks' duration) have poor discriminatory power.[28] However, the diagnostic use of well-defined symptoms with a persistent, nonremitting character holds definite promise in low-risk children (immune-competent children >3 years) in whom TB is usually a slowly progressive disease.[29,30] The most helpful symptoms include (1) persistent, nonremittent coughing or wheezing, (2) documented failure to thrive despite food supplementation (if food security is a concern), and (3) fatigue or reduced playfulness.[29] Clinical follow-up is also a valuable diagnostic tool. In young children (<3 years), who are at greatest risk of developing disseminated (miliary) disease and tuberculous meningitis, persistent or intermittent unexplained fever (>5–7 days) and lethargy are of great importance as well.

In HIV-infected (immune-compromised) children, the diagnostic challenge is most pronounced because of the following factors.[31]

HIV-infected children who live with HIV-infected adults are more likely to be exposed to an adult index case at home. However, HIV-infected adults often have sputum smear-negative TB, and therefore the infection risk posed by this exposure is less appreciated.

The TST has low sensitivity in HIV-infected children and is positive in the minority of HIV-infected children with bacteriologically confirmed TB despite using a reduced induration size cutoff of ≥5 mm.[32]

Chronic pulmonary symptoms from other HIV-related conditions such as gastroesophageal reflux and bronchiectasis are not uncommon, while failure to thrive is a typical feature of both TB and HIV, reducing the specificity of symptom-based diagnostic approaches.

Rapid disease progression may occur, reducing the sensitivity of diagnostic approaches that focus on persistent, nonremitting symptoms.

CXR interpretation is complicated by HIV-related comorbidity such as bacterial pneumonia, lymphocytic interstitial pneumonitis, bronchiectasis, pulmonary Kaposi sarcoma, and the atypical presentation of TB in immune-compromised children.[16]

Immune-Based Diagnosis

Although commercial kits for antibody detection are marketed widely in the developing world, no serological assay is currently accurate enough to replace microscopy and culture.[33] Immune-based diagnosis is complicated by the wide clinical disease spectrum (ranging from subclinical latent infection to various manifestations of active disease) and other factors that influence the immune response such as BCG vaccination, exposure to environmental mycobacteria, and HIV coinfection, all of which are particularly prevalent in endemic areas.[33]

Novel T-cell assays measure interferon-gamma released after stimulation by *M. tuberculosis*-specific antigens. Two assays are currently available as commercial kits: the T-SPOT.*TB*® test (Oxford Immunotec, Oxford, UK), and the QuantiFERON®-TB Gold® assay (Cellestis Ltd, Carnegie, Australia). In general, these tests are regarded as more specific and potentially more sensitive than the traditional TST.[33] However, like the TST, these novel T-cell assays fail to differentiate *M. tuberculosis* infection from active disease.[33] Identifying the correct application of these novel T-cell-based assays in endemic and nonendemic areas remains a priority for future research.

Bacteriology-Based Diagnosis

A positive culture is still regarded as the "gold standard test" to establish a definitive diagnosis of TB in a symptomatic child. Traditional culture methods are limited by suboptimal sensitivity, slow turnaround times, excessive cost (automated liquid broth systems), and the fact that bacteriologic yields in children are low. However, the yield in children with complicated intrathoracic disease is significantly higher than in those with uncomplicated hilar adenopathy (77% vs. 35%),[22] and adolescent children frequently develop sputum smear-positive adult-type disease.[4]

Novel culture-based approaches include TK Medium® (Salubris Inc., Cambridge, MA, USA), a simple colorimetric system that rapidly indicates mycobacterial growth, but its accuracy and robustness in field conditions are still being evaluated.[33] The phage amplification assay uses bacteriophages to infect live *M. tuberculosis* and is commercially available as *FASTPlaque-TB®* (Biotec Laboratories Ltd, Ipswich, Suffolk, UK); a variant (*FASTPlaque-TB Response®*) was designed to rapidly detect rifampin resistance. The test has a turn around time of only 2–3 days but is less sensitive than traditional culture methods, and no information exists on its utility in children.[33] Another novel test is the microscopic observation drug susceptibility assay, which uses an inverted light microscope to rapidly detect mycobacterial growth in liquid growth media. Microscopic observation drug susceptibility is an inexpensive method, which has shown excellent performance under field conditions[34] and may significantly improve the capability to detect pediatric TB in resource-limited settings.[35]

Polymerase chain reaction-based tests amplify nucleic acid regions specific to the *M. tuberculosis* complex but have shown highly variable results and limited utility in children.[33] Detecting antigens instead of antibodies offers another innovative approach, and novel antigen-capture assays that detect lipoarabinomannan in sputum and/or urine samples look promising, but results from field trials are awaited Table 36–4.[36]

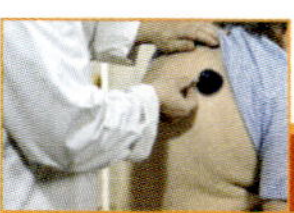

Table 36–4.

Summary of Traditional and Novel Diagnostic Approaches, Their Potential Application and Perceived Problems, and/or Benefits Experienced

Traditional Diagnostic Approaches	Application	Problems/Benefits	Validation
TB culture using solid or liquid broth media	Bacteriologic confirmation of active TB	Slow turnaround time; too expensive for most poor countries; poor sensitivity in children	Accepted gold standard
Chest radiography	Diagnosis of probable active TB	Rarely available in endemic areas with limited resources; accurate disease classification important	Marked inter- and intraobserver variability; reliable in expert hands and in presence of suspicious symptoms
Symptom-based approaches	Diagnosis of probable active TB	Poor symptom definition	Not well validated
Tuberculin skin test (TST)	Diagnosis of *M. tuberculosis* infection	Rarely available in endemic areas with limited resources; does not differentiate latent TB infection (LTBI) from active disease; not sensitive in immune-compromised children; simple to use and less expensive than blood-based tests	Various cutoffs advised in different settings

Novel Diagnostic Approaches	Application	Problems/Benefits	Validation
Symptom Based			
Symptom-based screening	Screening child contacts of adult TB cases	Limited resources required; should improve access to preventive chemotherapy for asymptomatic high-risk contacts in endemic areas	Not well validated
Refined symptom-based diagnosis	Diagnosis of probable active TB	Limited resources required; should improve access to chemotherapy in resource-limited settings; poor performance in HIV-infected children	Additional validation required
Immune Based			
Antibody-based assays	Diagnosis of probable active TB	Simple, point of care testing, variable accuracy, and difficulty in distinguishing LTBI from active TB	Additional validation required
T-cell assays	Diagnosis of LTBI	Limited data in children, inability to differentiate LTBI from active TB; blood volume required (3–5 mL); expensive; may have particular relevance in high-risk children, where LTBI treatment is warranted	Not well validated in children
Bacteriology Based			
Colorimetric culture systems (e.g., TK medium)	Bacteriologic confirmation of active TB	Simple and feasible, limited resources required; potential for contamination in field conditions	Not well validated in children
Phage-based tests (e.g., FASTPlaque-TB)	Diagnosis of probable active TB and detection of rifampin resistance	Requires laboratory infrastructure; performs relatively poorly when used on clinical specimens	Not well validated in children
Microscopic observation drug susceptibility assay	Diagnosis of probable active TB, and detection of drug resistance	Simple and feasible, limited resources required	Not well validated in children
PCR-based tests	Diagnosis of probable active TB and detection of rifampin resistance	■ Rarely available in endemic areas—sensitivity tends to be poor in paucibacillary TB	Extensively evaluated, but evidence not in favor of widespread use at present

(continued)

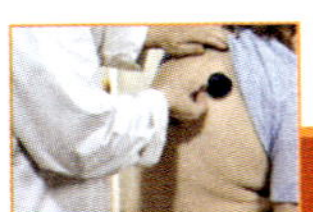

Table 36–4. (continued)

Summary of Traditional and Novel Diagnostic Approaches, Their Potential Application and Perceived Problems, and/or Benefits Experienced

Novel Diagnostic Approaches	Application	Problems/Benefits	Validation
		■ Specificity a concern in endemic areas, where LTBI is common ■ Requires adequate quality control systems	
Antigen-based Assays			
LAM detection assay	Diagnosis of probable active TB	Simple, point of care testing; limited clinical data on accuracy	Not well validated

LAM, lipoarabinomannan; LTBI, latent tuberculosis infection; TB, tuberculosis; TST, tuberculin skin test; PCR, Polymerase chain reaction.
With permission from Marais BJ, Pai M. Recent advances in the diagnosis of childhood tuberculosis. Arch Dis Child. *2007;92:446–452.*

Sample Collection

Even before various bacteriologic detection methods can be applied, sample collection presents a significant challenge, particularly in small children who cannot produce an adequate sputum specimen. Table 36–5 provides an overview of the various sampling methods and the perceived problems and/or benefits of each.

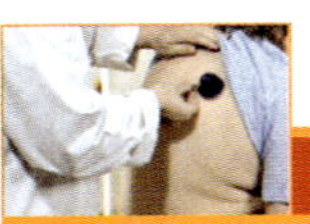

Table 36–5.

Summary of Various Bacteriologic Specimen Collection Methods and Perceived Problems and/or Benefits

Specimen Collection Method	Problems/Benefits	Potential Clinical Application
Sputum	Not feasible in very young children; assistance and supervision may improve the quality of the specimen	Routine sample to be collected in children >7yr of age (all children who can produce a good-quality specimen)
Induced sputum	Increased yield compared to gastric aspirate; no age restriction; specialized technique, which requires nebulization and suction facilities; use outside hospital setting not studied; potential transmission risk	To be considered in the hospital setting on an in- or outpatient basis
Gastric aspirate	Difficult and invasive procedure; not easily performed on an outpatient basis; requires prolonged fasting; sample collection advised on three consecutive days	Routine sample to be collected in hospitalized who cannot produce a good-quality sputum specimen
Nasopharyngeal aspiration	Less invasive than gastric aspirate; no fasting required; comparable yield to gastric aspirate	To be considered in primary health-care clinics or on an outpatient basis
String test	Less invasive than gastric aspirate; tolerated well in children >4 yr; bacteriologic yield and feasibility requires further investigation	Potential to become the routine sample collected in children who can swallow the capsule, but cannot produce a good-quality sputum specimen
Broncho-alveolar lavage	Extremely invasive	Only for use in patients who are intubated or who require diagnostic bronchoscopy
Urine/stool	Not invasive; excretion of *M. tuberculosis* well documented	To be considered with novel sensitive bacteriologic or antigen-based tests
Blood/bone marrow	Good sample sources to consider in the case of probable disseminated TB	To be considered for the confirmation of probable disseminated TB in hospitalized patients
Cerebrospinal fluid (CSF)	Fairly invasive; bacteriologic yield low	To be considered if signs of tuberculous meningitis
Fine needle aspiration	Minimally invasive using a fine 23G needle; excellent bacteriologic yield; minimal side effects	Procedure of choice in children with superficial lymphadenopathy

With permission from Marais BJ, Pai M. Specimen collection methods in the diagnosis of childhood tuberculosis. Indian J Med Microbiol. 2006;24:249-251.

Routine specimen collection includes two to three fasting gastric aspirates, collected on consecutive days and usually requiring hospitalization. The collection of a single specimen using hypertonic-saline-induced sputum collection may provide the same yield as three gastric aspirate specimens.[37] The string test (HDC Corporation, CA, USA) has been used successfully to retrieve *M. tuberculosis* from sputum smear-negative HIV-infected adults and demonstrated superior sensitivity compared to induced sputum[38]; the test is also well tolerated by children as young as 4 years of age.[39] Fine needle aspiration biopsy is a robust and simple technique that provides a rapid and definitive diagnosis in children with superficial TB lymph adenitis; the use of a small 23-gauge needle is well tolerated and associated with minimal side effects.[17] Table 36–5 provides a summary of various bacteriologic specimen collection methods and the perceived problems and/or benefits of each.

TREATMENT

The two principles of anti-TB treatment are to (1) reduce the organism load as rapidly as possible and (2) ensure effective eradication of all persistent bacilli.[13,40] This provides the rationale behind the intensive and continuation phases of current anti-TB treatment regimens. Rapid reduction of the organism load is important to reduce clinical symptoms, limit disease progression, terminate transmission, and reduce the risk of acquired drug resistance. Eradication of persistent (dormant or intermittently metabolizing) bacilli is essential to prevent future disease relapse.[13]

Preventive Chemotherapy

Isoniazid (INH) monotherapy for 6–9 months is the best-studied prophylactic regimen,[40] but poor adherence with unsupervised treatment is a serious concern and alternative prophylactic regimens with improved adherence require consideration.[41] The addition of rifampicin (RMP) to prophylactic regimens has numerous advantages: reducing the risk of INH monoresistance, improving organism eradication, shortening the duration of treatment, and improving adherence.[42] INH and RMP for a duration of 3 months are a well-established prophylactic regimen, which provides equivalent protection to 6–9 months of INH monotherapy, although it is important to remember that RMP interacts with highly active antiretroviral therapy (HAART).[42] In theory, the addition of pyrazinamide (PZA), another drug with strong sterilizing activity, should further improve the sterilizing ability of preventive therapy regimens and shorten the required treatment duration, but this requires further evaluation.[13]

Standard Treatment

The main variables that influence the success of chemotherapy, apart from primary drug resistance, are the bacterial load and the anatomical distribution of bacilli.[13] From a public health perspective, children with TB can be categorized into three groups: (1) sputum smear-negative disease, (2) sputum smear-positive (often cavitary) disease, and 3) disseminated (miliary) disease or TB meningitis.

Sputum smear-negative disease is usually paucibacillary, and therefore the risk of acquired drug resistance is low. Drug penetration into the anatomical sites involved is good, and the successes of three drugs (INH, RMP, and PZA) during the 2-month intensive phase and two drugs (INH and RMP) during the 4-month continuation phase are well established.[13] In the presence of extensive radiographic disease with or without cavitation, and/or suspicion of INH resistance, the use of ethambutol in addition to the three drugs during intensive phase should be contemplated. After completion of the intensive phase, successful organism eradication may be achieved with intermittent (2–3×/week) therapy during the continuation phase.[13]

Sputum smear-positive disease implies a high organism load and an increased risk for random drug resistance.[13] Selecting drug-resistant mutants is a particular concern where INH monoresistance is prevalent, as this increases the likelihood of selecting multi-drug-resistant (MDR) organisms. The use of four drugs (INH, RMP, PZA, and ethambutol) during the 2-month intensive phase should reduce this risk. Once the organism load is sufficiently reduced, intermittent (2–3×/week) therapy with INH and RMP during the 4-month continuation phase is sufficient to ensure organism eradication. However, caution should be exercised when initial treatment response has not been optimal and in patients with HIV.[13]

Disseminated (miliary) disease is frequently associated with central nervous system involvement.[13] It is therefore essential to consider the cerebrospinal fluid (CSF) penetration of drugs used in the treatment of disseminated (miliary) disease. INH and PZA penetrate the CSF well.[43] RMP and streptomycin (S) penetrate the CSF poorly but may achieve therapeutic levels in the presence of meningeal inflammation.[43] The value of streptomycin is limited by poor CSF penetration and intramuscular administration. Ethambutol hardly penetrates the CSF, even in the presence of meningeal inflammation, and has no demonstrated efficacy in the treatment of tuberculous meningitis.[13,43]

A flow diagram has been developed (Figure 36–11) to guide individual patient classification and management.[13] It is based on answering five simple questions: (1) Is the child exposed to or infected with

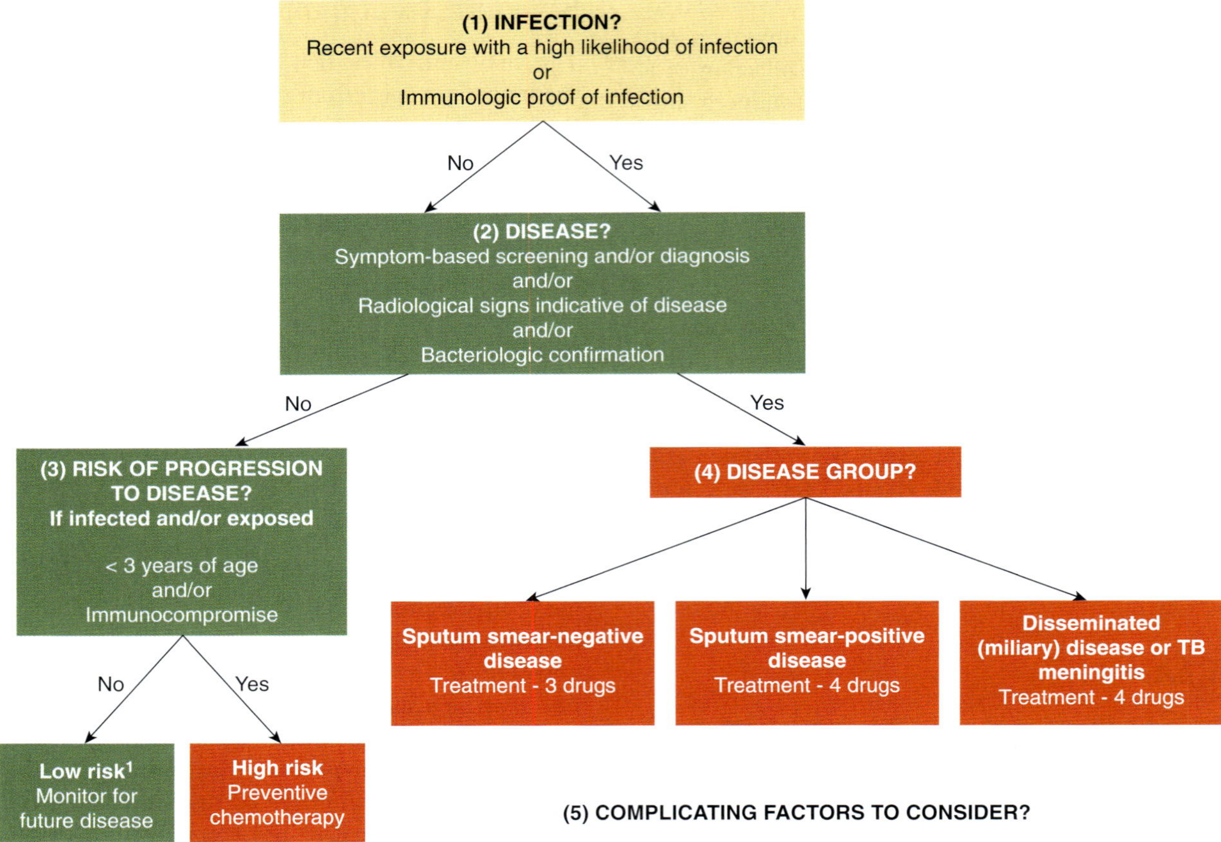

FIGURE 36–11 ■ Flow diagram to guide the diagnosis and appropriate management of children with suspected pulmonary tuberculosis. (*With permission from Marais BJ, Gie RP, Schaaf HS, Beyers N, Donald PR, Starke JR. Childhood pulmonary tuberculosis: Old wisdom and new challenges. Am J Respir Crit Care Med. 2006;173(10):1078–1090.*) (In nonendemic areas where the risk of reinfection is low and where TB eradication is an achievable goal, it would be desirable to provide preventive treatment to all individuals with documented TB infection.)

M. tuberculosis? (2) Does the child have active TB? (3) If the child is exposed or infected but does not have active TB, is preventive chemotherapy indicated? (4) If the child has active TB, what is the appropriate treatment regimen? (5) Are there any special circumstances such as HIV infection, retreatment, or exposure to a drug-resistant source case to consider?

The recommended treatment for intrathoracic TB in children is 6 months of directly observed therapy (DOT) and 2 months of three drugs (INH, RMP, and PZA), followed by 4 months of two drugs (INH and RMP).[26,40] Table 36–6 summarizes current treatment guidelines. RMP-based regimens are effective and cheap, and child-friendly formulations are available; from 2007, child friendly formulations will also be made available via the Global Drug Facility. The cellular immune response assists with organism containment and eradication. Because immune-compromised children lack this important immune contribution, they are at increased risk of disease relapse following standard short-course therapy.[44] It seems prudent to prolong the treatment duration in immune-compromised children, although this has not been verified in placebo-controlled trials. In the absence of sufficient evidence, the current recommendation is to consider prolonging the treatment duration to 9 months.[13,40]

Drug Resistance

The selection of drug-resistant organisms occurs primarily in patients with high organism loads. Because of the paucibacillary nature of childhood TB in general, children contribute little to the creation of the drug resistance problem, but they are severely affected by it. A recent survey from Cape Town recorded INH resistance in 12.4% of child isolates, and MDR (INH and RMP resistance) in 5.3%.[45] This is alarming, as drug resistance patterns among children provide an accurate indication of transmitted drug resistance within the community. The transmission of drug-resistant disease poses a major new challenge to TB control programs globally. However, the principles of diagnosis and treatment remain exactly the same as those outlined for drug-sensitive TB. Following MDR exposure, high-risk children should be protected with appropriate chemoprophylaxis. Table 36–7 provides a list of the first second-line drugs currently

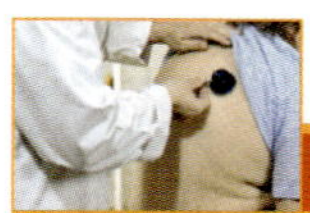

Table 36–6.

Various Childhood TB Disease Groups, Together with the Treatment Rationale and Current ATS Treatment Guidelines Applicable to Each Group

TB Disease Group	Treatment Rationale	ATS Treatment Guideline*
Exposure/latent TB infection (LTBI)	Preventive chemotherapy	6–9H
All children <5 years of age (children <3 years at highest risk)	Relatively high risk of disease progression following infection	
Consider including all HIV-infected children, irrespective of age	Low organism load	
Active disease	Curative treatment	
Sputum smear-negative TB	Low organism load Drug penetration good	2HRZ/4HR
Sputum smear-positive TB	High organism load Drug penetration good	2HRZE/4HR
Disseminated (miliary) TB	High organism load CNS penetration variable	2HRZE/7–10HR†

**Treatment forms part of the DOTS strategy and all curative treatment should be given as directly observed therapy*[41]

†Ethambutol penetrates the CSF poorly, alternative regimens include Ethionamide (which penetrates the CSF well) instead of ethambutol and use double the dose of standard drugs.

H, isoniazid; R, rifampin; Z, pyrazinamide; E, ethambutol; CNS, central nervous system; ATS, American Thoracic Society.

With permission from Marais BJ, Gie RP, Schaaf HS, Beyers N, Donald PR, Starke JR. Childhood pulmonary tuberculosis: Old wisdom and new challenges. Am J Respir Crit Care Med. 2006;173(10):1078–90.

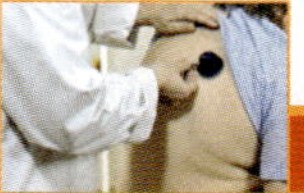

Table 36–7.

First- and Second-Line Anti-TB Drugs and Recommended Dosages in Children

	Mode of Action	Dosage [mg/kg/Dose] (Maximum)*	
		Daily	2–3×/week†
First-line drugs			
Isoniazid	Bactericidal	10–15 (300 mg)	20–30 (900 mg)
Rifampicin	Bactericidal and sterilizing	10–20 (600 mg)	10–20 (600 mg)
Pyrazinamide	Sterilizing	20–40 (2000 mg)	50 (2000 mg)
Ethambutol‡	Bacteriostatic	15–25 (1200 mg)	30–50 (2500 mg)
Second-line drugs			
Ethionamide or prothionamide	Bactericidal	15–20 (1000 mg)	NA
Streptomycin	Bacteriostatic	20–40 (1000 mg)	NA
Fluoroquinolones§	Bactericidal		NA
Ciprofloxacin		20–40 (1500 mg)	
Aminoglycosides	Bacteriostatic		NA
Kanamycin		15–30 (1000 mg)	
Amikacin		15–30 (1000 mg)	
Capreomycin		15–30 (1000 mg)	
Cycloserine or terizidone	Bacteriostatic	10–20 (1000 mg)	NA
Para-aminosalisylic acid (PAS)	Bacteriostatic	200–300 (10 g)	NA

**Recommended dosages are those given in the Red Book (146) unless otherwise specified.*

†2–3×/week intermittent therapy is only advised if directly observed therapy is strictly enforced.

‡Ethambutol should be used with caution in children <7 years of age where visual acuity cannot be evaluated. It seems safe at recommended doses of 15 mg/kg, but doses of 25 mg/kg may be required for the treatment of drug-resistant disease. This is the only drug where the recommended dose for 2× or 3×/week differs (35 mg/kg for 2×/week and 30 mg/kg for 3×/week). A daily maximum dose of 1200 mg (three tablets) is recommended (147).

§Ciprofloxacin is currently the only flouroquinolone that has been recommended for use in children with drug-resistant tuberculosis (148). Reports on the use of levofloxacin, gatifloxacin, and moxafloxacin in children are eagerly awaited; their anti-mycobacterial effect in adults proved to be superior to ciprofloxacin.

With permission from Marais BJ, Gie RP, Schaaf HS, Beyers N, Donald PR, Starke JR. Childhood pulmonary tuberculosis: Old wisdom and new challenges. Am J Respir Crit Care Med. 2006;173(10):1078–90.

available for treatment. The management of drug-resistant TB should be discussed with an expert in the field, as second-line drugs are less potent, have poor sterilizing capability, and are associated with more side effects.

CONCLUSION

Improving the access of (1) high-risk exposed and/or infected children to preventive therapy and (2) all children with active disease to anti-TB treatment will drastically reduce the severe TB-related morbidity and mortality suffered by children in endemic areas. However, the burden of childhood TB is ultimately only a reflection of the level of epidemic control achieved within communities.[7] Current TB control efforts are mainly directed toward reducing transmission by treating sputum smear-positive adults, but little emphasis is placed on reducing the vulnerability of communities. The formulation of the United Nations Millennium Developmental Goals[46] is an important step in this direction, but global political commitment and sufficient funding are required to support this key initiative.

REFERENCES

1. Rubin SA. Tuberculosis. Captain of all these men of death. *Radiol Clin North Am.* 1995;33(4):619-639.
2. Chintu C, Mudenda V, Lucas S, et al. Lung diseases at necropsy in African children dying from respiratory illnesses: a descriptive necropsy study. *Lancet.* 2002;360(9338):985-990.
3. Marais BJ, Hesseling AC, Gie RP, Schaaf HS, Beyers N. The burden of childhood tuberculosis and the accuracy of community-based surveillance data. *Int J Tuberc Lung Dis.* 2006;10(3):259-263.
4. Marais BJ, Gie RP, Hesseling AH, Beyers N. Adult-type pulmonary tuberculosis in children 10–14 years of age. *Pediatr Infect Dis J.* 2005;24(8):743-744.
5. Curtis AB, Ridzon R, Vogel R, et al. Extensive transmission of mycobacterium tuberculosis from a child. *N Engl J Med.* 1999;341(20):1491-1495.
6. Nelson LJ, Wells CD. Global epidemiology of childhood tuberculosis. *Int J Tuberc Lung Dis.* 2004;8(5):636-647.
7. Marais BJ, Obihara CC, Warren RM, Schaaf HS, Gie RP, Donald PR. The burden of childhood tuberculosis: A public health perspective. *Int J Tuberc Lung Dis.* 2005;9(12): 1305-1313.
8. Corbett EL, Watt CJ, Walker N, et al. The growing burden of tuberculosis: global trends and interactions with the HIV epidemic. *Arch Intern Med.* 2003;163(9):1009-1021.
9. Marais BJ, Gie RP, Schaaf HS, et al. The natural history of childhood intra-thoracic tuberculosis: a critical review of literature from the pre-chemotherapy era. *Int J Tuberc Lung Dis.* 2004;8(4):392-402.
10. Schaaf HS, Michaelis IA, Richardson M, et al. Adult-to-child transmission of tuberculosis: household or community contact? *Int J Tuberc Lung Dis.* 2003;7(5):426-431.
11. Marais BJ, Gie RP, Schaaf HS, et al. A proposed radiological classification of childhood intra-thoracic tuberculosis. *Pediatr Radiol.* 2004;34(11):886-894.
12. Marais BJ, Donald PR, Gie RP, Schaaf HS, Beyers N. Diversity of disease in childhood pulmonary tuberculosis. *Ann Trop Paediatr.* 2005;25(2):79-86.
13. Marais BJ, Gie RP, Schaaf HS, Beyers N, Donald PR, Starke JR. Childhood pulmonary tuberculosis: old wisdom and new challenges. *Am J Respir Crit Care Med.* 2006;173(10): 1078-1090.
14. Leung AN, Muller NL, Pineda PR, FitzGerald JM. Primary tuberculosis in childhood: radiographic manifestations. *Radiology.* 1992;182(1):87-91.
15. Goussard P, Gie RP, Kling S, Beyers N. Expansile pneumonia in children caused by *Mycobacterium tuberculosis*: clinical, radiological, and bronchoscopic appearances. *Pediatr Pulmonol.* 2004;38(6):451-455.
16. Graham SM, Coulter JB, Gilks CF. Pulmonary disease in HIV-infected African children. *Int J Tuberc Lung Dis.* 2001;5(1):12-23.
17. Marais BJ, Wright CA, Schaaf HS, et al. Tuberculous lymphadenitis as a cause of persistent cervical lymphadenopathy in children from a tuberculosis-endemic area. *Pediatr Infect Dis J.* 2006;25(2):142-146.
18. Lindeboom JA, Kuijper EJ, Prins JM, Bruijnesteijn van Coppenraet ES, Lindeboom R. Tuberculin skin testing is useful in the screening for nontuberculous mycobacterial cervicofacial lymphadenitis in children. *Clin Infect Dis.* 2006;43(12):1547-1551.
19. Narita M, Ashkin D, Hollender ES, Pitchenik AE. Paradoxical worsening of tuberculosis following antiretroviral therapy in patients with AIDS. *Am J Respir Crit Care Med.* 1998;158(1):157-161.
20. Puthanakit T, Oberdorfer P, Akarathum N, Wannarit P, Sirisanthana T, Sirisanthana V. Immune reconstitution syndrome after highly active antiretroviral therapy in human immunodeficiency virus-infected Thai children. *Pediatr Infect Dis J.* 2006;25(1):53-58.
21. Starke JR. Pediatric tuberculosis: time for a new approach. *Tuberculosis (Edinb).* 2003;83(1–3):208-212.
22. Marais BJ, Hesseling AC, Gie RP, Schaaf HS, Enarson DA, Beyers N. The bacteriologic yield in children with intrathoracic tuberculosis. *Clin Infect Dis.* 2006;42(8): e69-e71.
23. Osborne CM. The challenge of diagnosing childhood tuberculosis in a developing country. *Arch Dis Child.* 1995;72(4):369-374.
24. Theart AC, Marais BJ, Gie RP, Hesseling AC, Beyers N. Criteria used for the diagnosis of childhood tuberculosis at primary health care level in a high-burden, urban setting. *Int J Tuberc Lung Dis.* 2005;9(11):1210-1214.
25. World Health Organization. Guidance for National Tuberculosis Programmes on the Management of Tuberculosis in Children. 2006. (Accessed at http://www.who.int/child-adolescent-health/publications/CHILD_HEALTH/WHO_FCH_CAH_2006.7.htm.)
26. Marais BJ, Gie RP, Hesseling AC, Schaaf HS, Enarson DA, Beyers N. Radiographic signs and symptoms in children treated for tuberculosis: possible implications for symptom-based screening in resource-limited settings. *Pediatr Infect Dis J.* 2006;25(3):237-240.

27. Hesseling AC, Schaaf HS, Gie RP, Starke JR, Beyers N. A critical review of diagnostic approaches used in the diagnosis of childhood tuberculosis. *Int J Tuberc Lung Dis.* 2002;6(12):1038-1045.
28. Marais BJ, Obihara CC, Gie RP, et al. The prevalence of symptoms associated with pulmonary tuberculosis in randomly selected children from a high burden community. *Arch Dis Child.* 2005;90(11):1166-1170.
29. Marais BJ, Gie RP, Hesseling AC, et al. A refined symptom-based approach to diagnose pulmonary tuberculosis in children. *Pediatrics.* 2006;118(5):e1350-e1359.
30. Marais BJ, Gie RP, Obihara CC, Hesseling AC, Schaaf HS, Beyers N. Well defined symptoms are of value in the diagnosis of childhood pulmonary tuberculosis. *Arch Dis Child.* 2005;90(11):1162-1165.
31. Marais BJ, Cotton M, Graham S, Beyers N. Diagnosis and management challenges of childhood TB in the era of HIV. *J Infect Dis.* 2007;196(suppl 1):S76-S85.
32. Madhi SA, Gray GE, Huebner RE, Sherman G, McKinnon D, Pettifor JM. Correlation between $CD4^+$ lymphocyte counts, concurrent antigen skin test and tuberculin skin test reactivity in human immunodeficiency virus type 1-infected and -uninfected children with tuberculosis. *Pediatr Infect Dis J.* 1999;18(9):800-805.
33. Marais BJ, Pai M. Recent advances in the diagnosis of childhood tuberculosis. *Arch Dis Child.* 2007;92:446-452. In press.
34. Moore DA, Evans CA, Gilman RH, et al. Microscopic-observation drug-susceptibility assay for the diagnosis of TB. *N Engl J Med.* 2006;355(15):1539-1550.
35. Oberhelman RA, Soto-Castellares G, Caviedes L, et al. Improved recovery of *Mycobacterium tuberculosis* from children using the microscopic observation drug susceptibility method. *Pediatrics.* 2006;118(1):e100-e106.
36. Boehme C, Molokova E, Minja F, et al. Detection of mycobacterial lipoarabinomannan with an antigen-capture ELISA in unprocessed urine of Tanzanian patients with suspected tuberculosis. *Trans R Soc Trop Med Hyg.* 2005; 99(12):893-900.
37. Zar HJ, Hanslo D, Apolles P, Swingler G, Hussey G. Induced sputum versus gastric lavage for microbiological confirmation of pulmonary tuberculosis in infants and young children: a prospective study. *Lancet.* 2005;365 (9454):130-134.
38. Vargas D, Garcia L, Gilman RH, et al. Diagnosis of sputum-scarce HIV-associated pulmonary tuberculosis in Lima, Peru. *Lancet.* 2005;365(9454):150-152.
39. Chow F, Espiritu N, Gilman RH, et al. La cuerda dulce—a tolerability and acceptability study of a novel approach to specimen collection for diagnosis of paediatric pulmonary tuberculosis. *BMC Infect Dis.* 2006;6:67.
40. Blumberg HM, Burman WJ, Chaisson RE, et al. American thoracic society/centers for disease control and prevention/infectious diseases society of America: treatment of tuberculosis. *Am J Respir Crit Care Med.* 2003;167(4): 603-662.
41. Marais BJ, van Zyl S, Schaaf HS, van Aardt M, Gie RP, Beyers N. Adherence to isoniazid preventive chemotherapy: a prospective community based study. *Arch Dis Child.* 2006;91(9):762-765.
42. Ena J, Valls V. Short-course therapy with rifampin plus isoniazid, compared with standard therapy with isoniazid, for latent tuberculosis infection: a meta-analysis. *Clin Infect Dis.* 2005;40(5):670-676.
43. Ellard GA, Humphries MJ, Allen BW. Cerebrospinal fluid drug concentrations and the treatment of tuberculous meningitis. *Am Rev Respir Dis.* 1993;148(3):650-655.
44. Schaaf HS, Krook S, Hollemans DW, Warren RM, Donald PR, Hesseling AC. Recurrent culture-confirmed tuberculosis in human immunodeficiency virus-infected children. *Pediatr Infect Dis J.* 2005;24(8):685-691.
45. Schaaf HS, Marais BJ, Hesseling AC, Gie RP, Beyers N, Donald PR. Childhood drug-resistant tuberculosis in the western cape province of south Africa. *Acta Paediatr.* 2006;95(5):523-528.
46. United Nations. *The Millennium Development Goals Report 2005.* New York; 2005.

SECTION 8

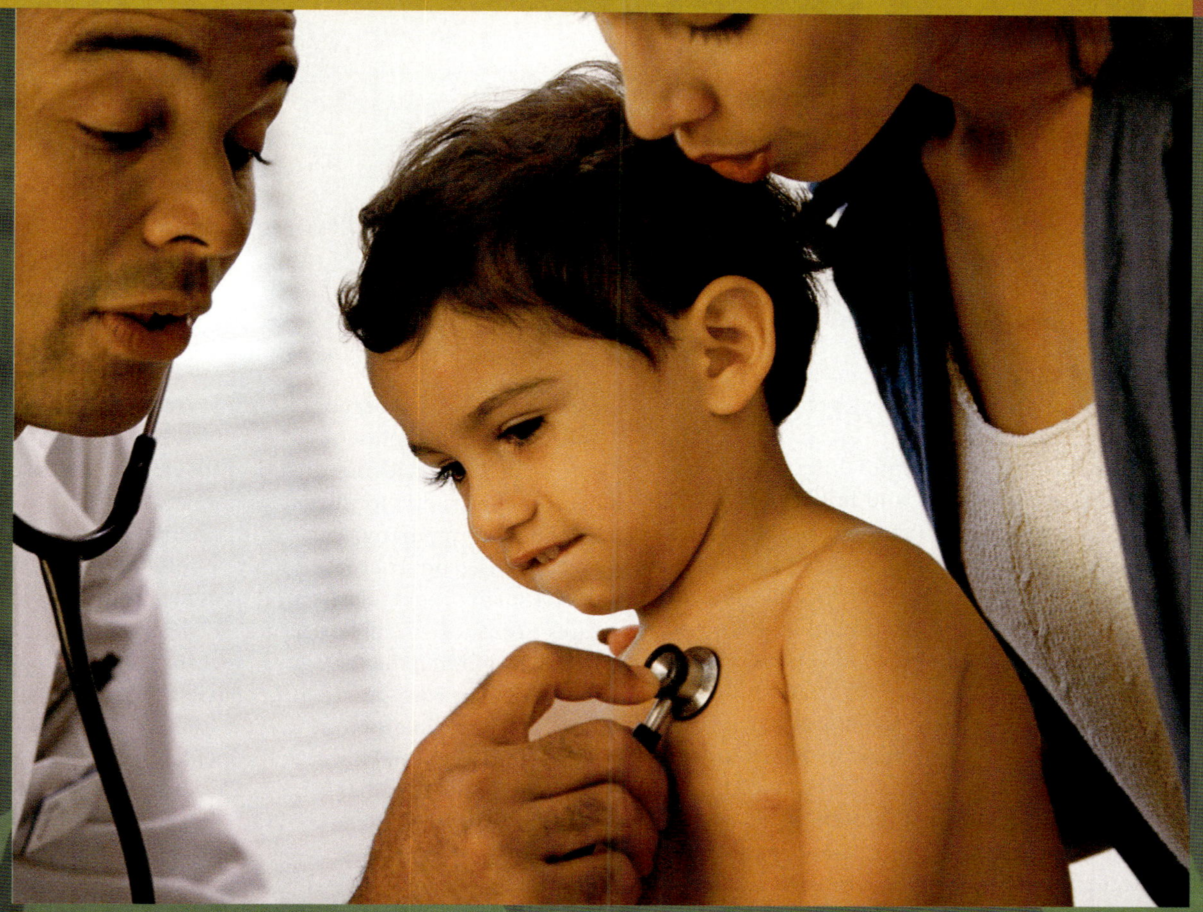

Cardiac Infections

CHAPTER 37

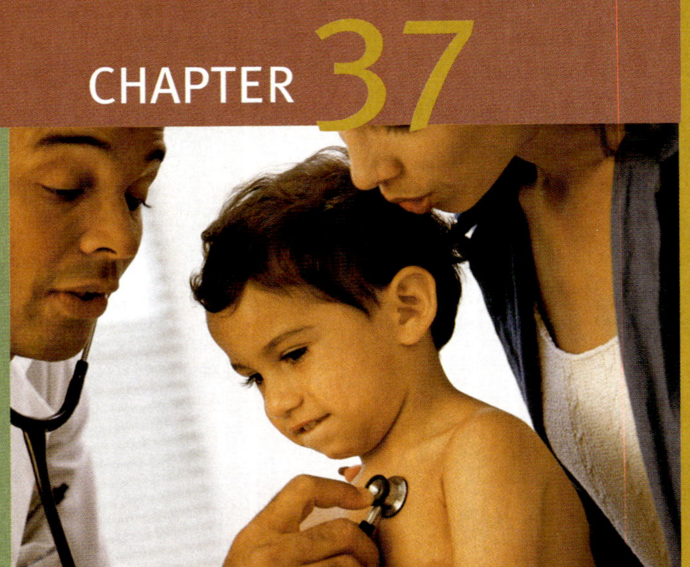

Endocarditis

Michael G. W. Camitta
Joseph W. St. Geme III and
Jennifer S. Li

DEFINITIONS AND EPIDEMIOLOGY

Infective endocarditis (IE) denotes infection of the endocardial surface of the heart and implies the physical presence of microorganisms in the lesion. Although the heart valves are most commonly affected, the disease may also occur within the heart in the location of congenital septal defects or on the endocardial surface in areas of turbulent flow. Extracardiac infections of arteriovenous or arterioarterial shunts (patent ductus arteriosus), infection related to structural aortic arch anomalies, and infections of prosthetic materials such as vascular occluders and stents can also be included in this definition of similar clinical manifestations. Unfortunately, variability in the clinical presentation continues to make the diagnosis of IE clinically challenging. The Duke criteria for the diagnosis of IE have been developed[1] and modified.[2] These criteria have been validated in multiple studies and shown to be superior to other criteria for the diagnosis of IE in the pediatric population.[3–5]

Despite improvements in diagnosis and treatment, IE continues to be associated with high morbidity and mortality. There are several reasons for this persistent morbidity and mortality. Pediatric patients with IE are increasingly complex. In developed countries, the improved survival of children with congenital heart disease has led to a shift in the underlying condition for IE from rheumatic heart disease to congenital heart disease. In addition, there has been an increase in antibiotic-resistant organisms. Targeted antibiotic treatment is the ideal approach to the pharmacologic management of IE. Prevention of IE remains the standard of care, although practices in prophylaxis have been shown to vary widely. Successful management of IE is dependent on the close cooperation of cardiologists, cardiothoracic surgeons, infectious disease specialists, primary-care providers, and the patients themselves.

The true incidence of IE is difficult to determine because the criteria for diagnosis have changed and the methods of reporting vary in different series.[6,7] An analysis based on strict case definitions often reveals that only a small proportion (~20%) of clinically diagnosed cases are categorized as definite. IE occurs less commonly in children than in adults, with an estimated incidence of one case per 1280 pediatric admissions per year[8] vs. approximately one case per 1000 adult hospital admissions per year. However, the incidence of IE in the pediatric population has increased in the past 20 years[9] potentially, in part, because of the improved survival of higher-risk neonates.

While the incidence of IE in pediatric patients has been increasing, the disease remains relatively uncommon in children and infants, in whom it is associated primarily with nosocomial bacteremia in the setting of underlying structural congenital heart disease.[10,11] The incidence of IE in unrepaired congenital heart lesions has become rare because of surgical advances, which have enabled the correction or palliation of nearly all of these defects. The most common repaired congenital heart lesions predisposing to IE in children include aortic valve stenosis, pulmonary atresia, tetralogy of Fallot, complete atrioventricular canal defect, d-transposition of the great arteries, and coarctation of the aorta.[12,13] Unlike most other congenital defects, secundum atrial septal defects and pulmonary valve stenosis are not associated with an increased risk of IE.[12]

Nosocomial IE secondary to therapeutic modalities (intravenous catheters, hyperalimentation lines, pacemakers, dialysis shunts, etc.) is increasingly common. Nosocomial IE is usually a complication of bacteremia induced by an invasive procedure or a vascular device. IE in the absence of underlying congenital heart disease has been reported to be the cause in 8–10% of pediatric cases.[4] There has been an increase in the incidence of fungal endocarditis, which appears to be related to prolonged use of broad-spectrum antibiotics, central venous catheters, and improved survival of sick premature neonates.[14,15] The emerging importance of nosocomial IE in industrialized nations has influenced the microbiology of IE, with an increasing prevalence of *Staphylococcus aureus* and a decreasing prevalence of viridans streptococci among US tertiary-care centers.[16] In children, nosocomial IE in the absence of structural heart disease most often affects the mitral or aortic valve.[9,17,18] *S. aureus* is a unique pathogen because of its virulent properties, its protean manifestations, and its ability to cause IE on architecturally normal cardiac valves.[19]

Presence of a prosthetic valve is an important risk factor for IE in adults, with IE occurring in 1–4% of prosthetic valve recipients in the first year following valve replacement and in approximately 1% of recipients annually thereafter.[20,21] While prosthetic valves are used less frequently in children, mechanical aortic valve replacement is associated with a significant increase in the incidence of IE.[12] Injection drug use is a common predisposing factor for IE in adult patients <40 years of age, with *S. aureus* being the predominant organism. Although less common in children, the yearly prevalence of injection drug use in children aged 12–17 years is 0.11% in comparison to 0.29% for adults between the age of 18 and 25 years.[22] The incidence of IE in adult intravenous drug users may be 30 times higher than the general population.[23] Tricuspid valve involvement is noted in 78%, mitral in 24%, and aortic in 8% of drug abusers with IE.[24] More than one valve is involved in approximately 20% of cases, and some of these infections are polymicrobial.[25,26]

PATHOGENESIS

The endothelial lining of the heart and the cardiac valves is normally resistant to infection with bacteria and fungi. In vitro observations and studies in experimental animals have demonstrated that the development of IE requires the simultaneous occurrence of several independent events, each of which may be influenced by a host of separate factors.[27–30] The valve surface must first be disrupted to produce a suitable site for bacterial attachment. Surface changes may be produced by a variety of local and systemic stresses such as turbulent blood flow in incompletely repaired congenital heart disease or local catheter-induced trauma to the endocardium or valve tissue. These alterations result in the deposition of platelets and fibrin and formation of a so-called sterile vegetation, the lesion of nonbacterial thrombotic endocarditis. Bacteria must then reach this site and adhere to the involved tissue to initiate infection. Transient bacteremia can occur when a mucosal surface heavily colonized with bacteria is traumatized. Certain strains of bacteria appear to have a selective advantage in adhering to platelets and/or fibrin and thus produce IE with a lower inoculum. The ability of these organisms to adhere to nonbacterial thrombotic endocarditis lesions is a crucial early step in the development of IE. Gould and associates showed that organisms frequently associated with IE (*enterococci*, viridans streptococci, *S. aureus*, *S. epidermidis*, and *Pseudomonas aeruginosa*) adhere more avidly to normal canine aortic leaflets in vitro than do organisms uncommon in IE (*Klebsiella pneumoniae*, and *Escherichia coli*).[31] In the rabbit model of IE, *S. aureus* and the viridans streptococci produce IE more readily than do *E. coli*,[32] an observation that correlates with the relative frequency with which these organisms produce IE in humans. Microbial adherence is mediated by several factors, including the presence of surface adhesins such as Fim A, the amount of dextran in the bacterial cell wall, the ability of the organism to bind to fibronectin, and the exposure of extracellular matrix proteins that may support bacterial adherence such as fibrinogen, laminin, and type 4 collagen.[33–36]

Following microbial adherence to damaged endothelium, the surface is rapidly covered with a protective sheath of platelets and fibrin to produce an environment conducive to further bacterial multiplication and vegetation growth. Microbial growth results in the secondary accumulation of more platelets and fibrin until a macroscopic excrescence or vegetation is present. The culmination of this process is mature vegetation consisting of an amorphous collection of fibrin, platelets, leukocytes, red blood cell debris, and dense clusters of bacteria. The surface of most vegetations consists of fibrin and scant numbers of leukocytes. Clumps of bacteria, histiocytes, and monocytes are usually found deep within the vegetation. Giant cells containing ingested bacteria may be found in some vegetations. Extremely high concentrations of bacteria (e.g., 10^9–10^{11} bacteria per gram of tissue) may accumulate deep within vegetations. Some of these bacteria exist in a state of reduced metabolic activity. Following therapy and during the process of healing, capillaries and fibroblasts appear within vegetations, but, without treatment, vegetations are avascular structures.[37]

Vegetations often prevent proper valvular leaflet or cusp coaptation, resulting in valvular incompetence and congestive heart failure. Vegetation growth may result in leaflet perforation, which can manifest as acute congestive heart failure.[38] Patients with mitral or tricuspid valve vegetations may develop chordal rupture when infection progresses beyond the valve orifice. Extension of infection may also occur into surrounding structures such as the valve ring, the adjacent myocardium, the cardiac conduction system, or the mitral-aortic intravalvular fibrosa.[39] Rarely, cavitation of periaortic abscesses may occur into the adjacent aortic wall, resulting in the formation of a diverticulum or aneurysm. Even more rarely such aneurysms may perforate into surrounding structures, resulting in aortic-atrial or aortic-pericardial fistulae.[40]

IE causes the stimulation of both humoral and cellular immunity as manifested by hypergammaglobulinemia, splenomegaly, and the presence of macrophages in the peripheral blood. Rheumatoid factor (anti-IgG IgM antibody) develops in approximately 50% of patients with IE of >6 weeks duration.[41] Antinuclear antibodies also occur in IE and may contribute to the musculoskeletal manifestations, low-grade fever, or pleuritic pain.[42] Opsonic (IgG), agglutinating (IgG and IgM), and complement-fixing (IgG and IgM) antibodies and cryoglobulins (IgG, IgM, IgA, C3, and fibrinogen), various antibodies to bacterial heat-shock proteins, and macroglobulins all have been described in IE.[43–45] Circulating immune complexes have been found in high titers in virtually all patients with IE and may cause a diffuse glomerulonephritis.[46] Some of the peripheral manifestations of IE, such as Osler nodes, may also result from a deposition of circulating immune complexes. Pathologically these lesions resemble an acute Arthus reaction. However, the finding of positive culture aspirates in Osler nodes suggests that these may, in fact, be caused by septic emboli rather than immune complex deposition.[47]

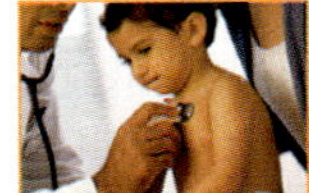

Table 37–1.

Signs and Symptoms of IE in the Pediatric Population

Systemic	Fever
	Fatigue
	Weight loss
	Rigors and diaphoresis
	Cyanosis
Cardiac	New or changing murmur
	Congestive heart failure
	Arrhythmias
	Heart block
	Pericarditis
	Myocarditis
	Myocardial infarction
Pulmonary	Tachypnea
	Pulmonary embolus
	Pulmonary hemorrhage
Gastrointestinal	Abdominal pain
	Hepatomegaly
	Splenomegaly
	Hepatitis
Neurologic	Stroke
	Headache
	Seizure
	Peripheral neuropathy
	Cranial nerve palsy
	Visual changes
Renal	Renal failure
	Hematuria
	Renal infarct
Peripheral	Petechiae
	Osler nodes
	Janeway lesions
	Splinter hemorrhages
	Roth spots
Musculoskeletal	Myalgias
	Arthralgias
	Arthritis
	Osteomyelitis

IE, infective endocarditis.

CLINICAL PRESENTATION

History and Physical

Children with IE typically have an indolent presentation, with generalized symptoms such as prolonged fever with rigors and diaphoresis, fatigue, arthralgias, myalgias, and weight loss.[48] Occasionally, children will present acutely ill with a more fulminant course and require urgent intervention. Although the virulence of the infecting organism can influence the acuity of the presentation, the interval from onset of infection to onset of symptoms is usually short. Symptoms in staphylococcal IE may even begin within a few days of the onset of infection.

The symptoms and signs of IE are protean, and essentially any organ system may be involved (Table 37–1). Four processes contribute to the clinical picture: (1) the infectious process on the valve, including the local intracardiac complications; (2) septic or aseptic embolization to virtually any organ; (3) constant bacteremia, often with metastatic foci of infection; and (4) circulating immune complexes and other immunopathologic factors.[29,49] As a result, the clinical presentation of patients with IE is highly variable and the differential diagnosis is often broad (Table 37–2). The prevalence of nonspecific symptoms may result in a delay in diagnosis or an incorrect diagnosis of another systemic illness.

In recent years, the patient with low-grade fever, malaise, and peripheral stigmata from long-standing IE is not as common a presentation as in the past, reflecting a higher incidence of nosocomial IE and more effective diagnostic modalities nowadays. Fever is usually present in the current era but may be absent (5% of the cases),

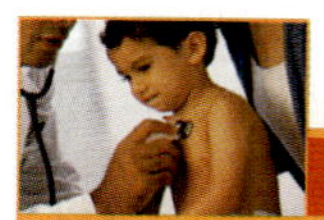

Table 37–2.

Differential Diagnosis of Infective Endocarditis in Children

Fever of unknown origin	Genitourinary infections
	Intra-abdominal infections
	Central venous catheter infections
	Kawasaki disease
	Osteomyelitis
	Rheumatic fever
	Tick-borne infections
	Lyme disease
	Rocky mountain spotted fever
Autoimmune diseases	Juvenile rheumatoid arthritis
	Systemic lupus erythematosis
	Vasculitis
Malignancies	Paraneoplastic syndromes
	Cardiac myxomas
	Carcinoid tumors
	Highly vascular tumors

especially in the setting of congestive heart failure, immunosuppressive therapy, or previous antibiotic therapy.[50,51] Congestive heart failure (CHF) has been reported in 10–20% of pediatric cases of IE.[52–54]

Audible heart murmurs occur in a majority of children with endocarditis related to valve destruction, associated with congenital heart disease, and as nonrelated innocent murmurs. The classic "changing murmur" is less common and has been reported in 21% of pediatric IE cases.[52] Although valvular regurgitation is the most important hemodynamic complication of IE, hemodynamically significant valvular obstruction requiring surgery may occur rarely, even without a prior history of valvular stenosis.[55] IE in patients with congenital heart disease palliated with a systemic to pulmonary shunt can present with cyanosis caused by shunt obstruction, without a change in murmur.

The classic peripheral manifestations of endocarditis are much less common in pediatric patients than in adults. Splinter hemorrhages are linear red to brown streaks in the fingernails or toenails. These are a nonspecific finding and often seen in the elderly or in people experiencing occupation-related trauma. Petechiae from local vasculitis or emboli are found after a prolonged course and usually appear in crops on the conjunctivae, buccal mucosa, palate, and extremities. These lesions are initially red and nonblanching but become brown and barely visible in 2–3 days. Osler nodes are small, painful, nodular lesions usually found in the pads of fingers or toes and occasionally in the thenar eminence. These are 2–15 mm in size and are frequently multiple and evanescent, disappearing in hours to days. Osler nodes are rare in cases of acute IE and are not specific for IE, sometimes occurring in systemic lupus erythematosus, marantic endocarditis, hemolytic anemia, and disseminated gonococcal infection, and in extremities with cannulated radial arteries. Janeway lesions are hemorrhagic, macular, painless plaques with a predilection for the palms or soles. These persist for several days and are thought to be embolic in origin and to occur with greater frequency in staphylococcal IE. Roth spots are oval, pale, retinal lesions surrounded by hemorrhage and are usually located near the optic disk. These may also be found in anemia, leukemia, and connective tissue disorders. Splenomegaly is more common in patients with IE of prolonged duration. Splenic septic emboli are common during IE, but localized signs and symptoms of splenic involvement are absent in approximately 90% of patients with this complication.[56]

Signs and Symptoms of IE

Abscess in or adjacent to the valve annulus is often heralded by the appearance of first- or second-degree heart block and/or fever that persists despite appropriate therapy. Pericarditis is rare but, when present, is usually accompanied by myocardial abscess formation as a complication of staphylococcal infection. Myocarditis may occur as a result of coronary vasculitis or embolic coronary occlusion or from the effects of microbial toxins or immune complex deposition.

Major embolic episodes occur in approximately one-third of cases.[52–54] Splenic artery emboli with infarction may result in left upper quadrant abdominal pain with radiation to the left shoulder, a splenic or pleural rub, or a left pleural effusion. Renal infarctions may be associated with microscopic or gross hematuria, but renal failure, hypertension, and edema are uncommon. Retinal artery embolus is rare with one reported pediatric case[57] and may be manifested by a sudden complete loss of vision. Pulmonary emboli can be a complication of right-sided IE. Coronary artery emboli usually arise from the aortic valve and may cause myocarditis with arrhythmias or myocardial infarction.

Neurologic manifestations occur in 10–15% of pediatric cases, especially in staphylococcal IE.[53,54] Stroke is the most common neurologic complication of IE. Patients with mitral valve IE have a greater risk of stroke than patients with aortic valve IE.[58] The development of clinical neurologic deterioration during IE is associated with a two- to fourfold increase in mortality in adults. Mycotic aneurysms of the cerebral circulation occur in 2–10% of the cases. Other features include seizures, severe headache, visual changes (particularly homonymous hemianopsias), choreoathetoid movements, mononeuropathy, and cranial nerve palsies.

Patients with IE may have symptoms of uremia. In the preantibiotic era, renal failure developed in 25–35% of the patients, but presently fewer than 10% are affected.

Renal disease can present as transient renal insufficiency or glomerulonephritis and is reported to occur in 2–5% of pediatric IE.[53,54] Renal failure is more common with long-standing disease but is usually reversible with appropriate antimicrobial treatment alone.

Septic arthritis has been reported in a small percentage of pediatric cases of IE.[52,53]

DIAGNOSIS

Laboratory Studies

Blood cultures

The blood culture is the single most important laboratory test performed in a diagnostic workup for IE. Bacteremia is usually continuous and low grade; therefore, cultures do not have to be drawn at the time of fever spikes or chills. Based on adult studies, in approximately two-thirds of cases all blood cultures will yield positive results.[59] Two blood specimens will be sufficient to detect the etiologic agent more than 90% of the time. The sensitivity of blood cultures for the detection of *streptococci* is particularly susceptible to prior antibiotic therapy and is also affected by the media employed.[60] Continuous monitoring blood culture systems (e.g., BACTEC and BacT/ALERT) are significantly more sensitive than conventional methods.[61] Blood culture media containing neutralizing resin particles have been especially helpful in improving the detection of *staphylococci* from patients receiving antimicrobial therapy at the time of culture.[62]

On the basis of these studies, the following procedures for culturing blood are recommended. At least three blood culture sets should be obtained in the first 24 hours. More specimens may be necessary if the patient has received antibiotics in the preceding 2 weeks. Blood cultures drawn within 4 hours may yield equal results to those drawn 12–24 hours apart; however, more positive cultures are required for a diagnosis of IE when drawn at shorter intervals. In general, culture of arterial blood offers no advantage over use of venous blood. At least 1–3 mL of blood should be drawn in infants and young children and 5–7 mL in older children.

The interpretation of positive blood cultures requires consideration of the isolated organism and how likely this organism is as a cause of IE. The following organisms are considered to be likely causes of IE when isolated from two or more blood cultures: *S. aureus*, viridans streptococci, *enterococci* (if acquired in the community and not nosocomially), and Group G *streptococci*. False-positive results are likely to be present when organisms such as *Propionibacterium* spp., *Corynebacterium* spp., *Bacillus* spp., and coagulase-negative *staphylococci* are recovered from a single blood culture or a minority of blood culture results. However, since these organisms are also capable of causing IE, it is important to determine if there is persistent bacteremia present as opposed to contamination with skin flora. Persistent bacteremia is likely if (1) positive cultures with organisms likely to cause IE are obtained from two samples collected (12 hours apart or (2) if all of three or a majority of four or more separate blood cultures are positive and if the first and last samples are collected at least 1 hour apart.[1]

Other blood laboratory tests

The utility of other blood tests in the diagnosis of IE is limited. Hematologic parameters are often abnormal in IE, but none is diagnostic. Anemia is frequently present, especially in subacute cases. This anemia usually has the characteristics of anemia of chronic disease, with normochromic, normocytic indices, but can present as hemolytic anemia. Thrombocytopenia and leukocytosis can be seen, sometimes with a high percentage of immature neutrophils (left shift). A significant number of patients have elevation of nonspecific acute-phase reactants such as erythrocyte sedimentation rate, C-reactive protein, procalcitonin, and immunoglobulins. A positive result on assay for rheumatoid factor is found in 40–50% of adult cases, especially when the duration of the illness is >6 weeks.[40] Hematuria can develop with associated proteinuria, red blood cell casts, hypocomplementemia, and renal insufficiency.[48]

Circulating immune complexes and mixed-type cryoglobulins are detectable in most adult patients with IE but also constitute a nonspecific finding.[63]

Culture-negative IE

Blood cultures fail to isolate an etiologic agent in 5–7% of cases.[48,64] Culture-negative IE is most often associated with antibiotic use within the previous 2 weeks. If blood cultures are negative in definite or possible IE, microbiologic considerations include *Bartonella, Coxiella, Brucella, Legionella,* and *Chlamydia* species, and non-*Candida* fungi.[65]

Diagnosis of these organisms requires special culture techniques or measurement of specific antibody titers.

Imaging

Echocardiography

Since its first use in the diagnosis of IE in 1973, echocardiography has become paramount in the process of evaluating IE.[66] It is of crucial importance in detecting vegetations, echogenic distinct masses from the adjacent valve with independent motion from the valve itself. Vegetations have characteristic findings of a shaggy dense band of irregular echoes in a nonuniform distribution on one or more leaflets (Figure 37–1). Echocardiography

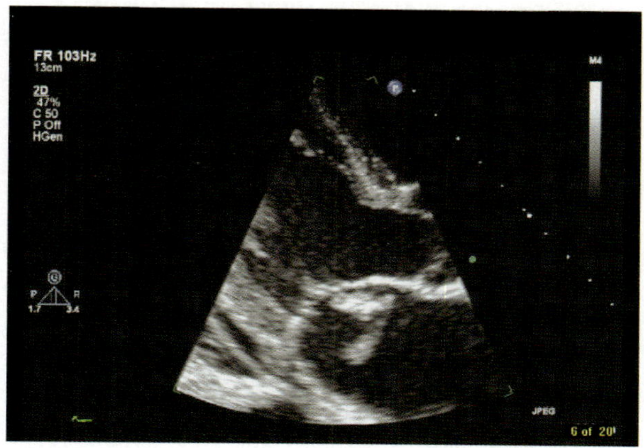

FIGURE 37–1 ■ Mobile vegetation on the mitral valve seen by transthoracic echocardiogram.

may not only confirm the presence of vegetations in the setting of bacteremia, but it also provides important hemodynamic information regarding ventricular function and an estimate of the degree of valvular regurgitation (Figure 37–2). Transthoracic echocardiography (TTE) should be performed in all patients in whom IE appears to be a reasonable diagnosis. TTE is not, however, an appropriate screening test in the evaluation of febrile patients in whom IE is unlikely on clinical grounds or in bacteremic patients with organisms that rarely cause IE, particularly if there is another obvious focus to explain the clinical syndrome.[67] TTE is more reliable in the pediatric population, with a reported sensitivity of 81% for detection of vegetations. One important consideration in children with congenital heart disease is that the echocardiogram be performed in a pediatric echocardiography laboratory and evaluated by a pediatric cardiologist because of the presence of underlying cardiac structural abnormalities. Technically inadequate studies are not of any value in the detection of vegetations. Although still controversial, certain characteristics of vegetations have been suggested to be prognostic of the risk for complications such as embolization or the need for surgery.[68,69] In general, decisions about surgical intervention should be based on findings on the echocardiogram along with clinical parameters.

Transesophageal echocardiography (TEE) has significantly altered the diagnostic approach to patients with suspected IE (Figure 37–3). TEE has been demonstrated to be more sensitive than TTE in adults[70]; however, children often have more clear echocardiographic windows by TTE, generally obviating the need for further imaging. TEE is useful in children with poor TTE imaging, with a negative TTE and a high index of suspicion for IE to more precisely define the site of infection, to evaluate prosthetic valve function, and to evaluate for perivalvular abscess.[71,72]

Electrocardiography

An electrocardiogram should be part of the evaluation of a patient with suspected IE, although it is usually unrevealing. The development of a new arrhythmia has been reported in 5% of cases of endocarditis in congenital heart disease.[54] The presence or new appearance of heart block is important evidence of extension of infection to the valve annulus and conduction system.[73] A new prolongation of the PR interval in a patient with IE is highly diagnostic of the presence of a ring abscess.

Other imaging modalities and tests

Computed tomography and magnetic resonance imaging of the heart have become more prevalent in pediatrics, although the utility of these techniques in detection of IE in this population has not been evaluated. Labeled white blood cell, antibacterial antibody, and platelet studies have shown promise in experimental IE.[74–76] Cardiac catheterization is not used in children, as the anatomic information provided by echocardiography in young patients is usually adequate to establish need for surgical repair or valve replacement.[37]

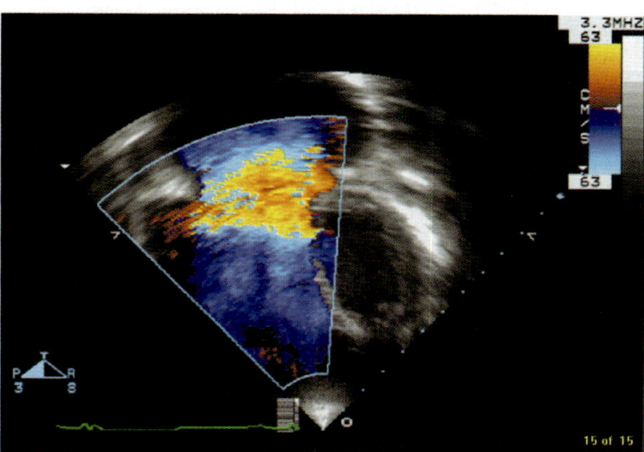

FIGURE 37–2 ■ Free tricuspid insufficiency secondary to damage to the valve leaflets from endocarditis.

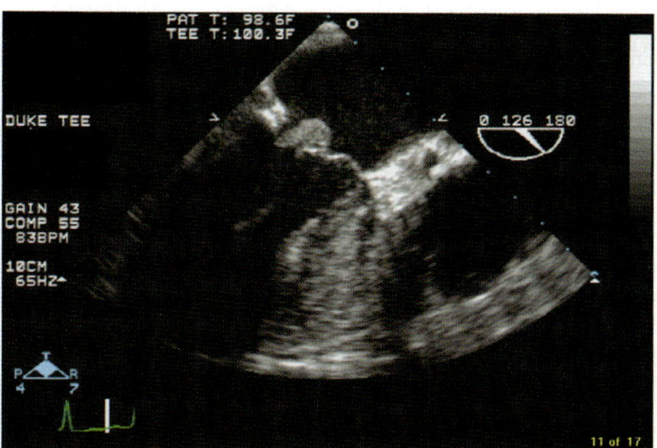

FIGURE 37–3 ■ Vegetation prolapsing through the mitral valve seen by transesophageal echocardiogram.

Diagnostic Criteria for IE

IE is typically a syndrome diagnosis based on the presence of multiple findings rather than a single definitive test result. Practical and logical case definitions for IE are important for both clinicians and researchers who study this complex disease. Accurate identification and classification of patients with IE are important in defining natural history, complications, epidemiology, and treatment outcomes.

Early diagnostic criteria developed by Petersdorf and Pellitier in 1977 and von Reyn and colleagues (Beth Israel criteria) in 1982 have been supplanted by the Duke criteria,[1] which were first proposed in 1994. Direct comparisons of the Duke and Beth Israel criteria have now been carried out in 11 major studies, involving nearly 1400 patients. Multiple studies have demonstrated the superiority of the Duke criteria for the diagnosis of IE in children.[3,4] Modifications of the Duke criteria have recently yielded more specificity to the schema.[2] The modified Duke criteria for the diagnosis of IE are provided in Tables 37–3 and 37–4.

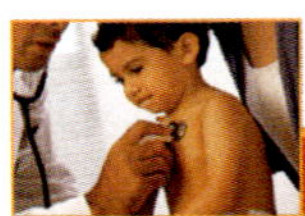

Table 37–3.

Definition of Infective Endocarditis According to the Modified Duke Criteria

Definite infective endocarditis

Pathologic Criteria

1. Microorganisms demonstrated by culture or histologic examination of a vegetation, a vegetation that has embolized, or an intracardiac abscess specimen; or
2. Pathologic lesions; vegetation or intracardiac abscess confirmed by histologic examination showing active endocarditis

Clinical Criteria

1. Two major criteria; or
2. One major criterion and three minor criteria; or
3. Five minor criteria

Possible infective endocarditis

1. One major criterion and one minor criterion
2. Three minor criterion

Rejected

1. Firm alternate diagnosis explaining evidence of infective endocarditis; or
2. Resolution of infective endocarditis syndrome with antibiotic therapy for ≤4 days; or
3. No pathologic evidence of infective endocarditis at surgery or autopsy, with antibiotic therapy for ≤4 days; or
4. Does not meet criteria for possible infective endocarditis, as above

With permission from Li JS, Sexton DJ, Mick N, et al. Proposed modifications to the Duke criteria for the diagnosis of infective endocarditis. Clin Infect Dis. 2000;30(4):633–638.

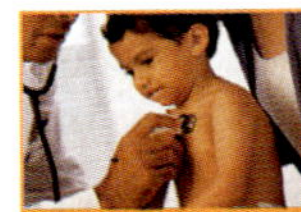

Table 37–4.

Definition of Terms Used in the Modified Duke Criteria for the Diagnosis of Infective Endocarditis

Major Criteria

Blood culture positive for IE
- Typical microorganisms consistent with IE from two separate blood cultures:
  - Viridans streptococci, *Streptococcus bovis*, HACEK group, *S. aureus*; or
  - Community-acquired enterococci, in the absence of a primary focus
- Microorganisms consistent with IE from persistently positive blood cultures, defined as follows:
  - At least two positive cultures or blood samples drawn >12 h apart; or
  - All of three or a majority of ≥4 separate cultures of blood (with first and last sample drawn at least 1 h apart)
  - Single positive blood culture for *Coxiella burnetti* or antiphase I IgG antibody titer >1:800

Evidence of endocardial involvement
- Echocardiogram positive for IE (TEE recommended in patients with prosthetic valves, rated at least "possible IE" by clinical criteria, or complicated IE [paravalvular abscess]; TTE as first test in the other patients, defined as follows:
  - Oscillating intracardiac mass on valve or supporting structures, in the path or regurgitant jets, or in implanted material in the absence of an alternative anatomic explanation; or
  - Abscess; or
  - New partial dehiscence of a prosthetic valve
- New valvular regurgitation (worsening or changing of a preexisting murmur no sufficient)

Minor Criteria

Predisposition, predisposing heart condition, or injection drug use

Fever, temperature >38°C

Vascular phenomena, major arterial emboli, septic pulmonary infarcts, mycotic aneurysm, intracranial hemorrhage, conjunctival hemorrhages, and Janeway lesions

Immunologic phenomena: glomerulonephritis, Osler nodes, Roth spots, and rheumatoid factor

Microbiological evidence: positive blood culture but does not meet a major criterion as noted above or serologic evidence of active infection with organism consistent with IE

IE, infective endocarditis; TEE, transesophageal echocardiography.
With permission from Li JS, Sexton DJ, Mick N, et al. Proposed modifications to the Duke criteria for the diagnosis of infective endocarditis. Clin Infect Dis. 2000;30(4):633–638.

TREATMENT

General Guidelines

Following the establishment of a diagnosis of IE using clinical, microbiological, and echocardiographic methods, antibiotics should be administered in a dose

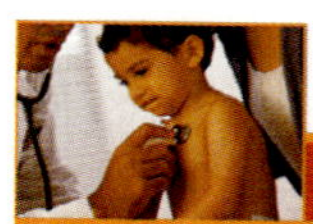

Table 37–5.

Important Considerations for the Antibiotic Treatment of IE

A prolonged course of therapy is necessary in order to eradicate microorganisms growing in valvular vegetations
Bactericidal rather than bacteriostatic antibiotics should be chosen to decrease the possibility of treatment failure or relapses
Parenteral antibiotics give a more sustained level of antibiotic activity and are therefore recommended over oral drugs in most circumstances
Synergistic antibiotic combinations can produce a more rapid bactericidal effect than some single-agent regimens

IE, infective endocarditis.

designed to give sustained bactericidal serum concentrations throughout much of or the entire dosing interval. Certain general principles have been accepted, which provide the framework for the current recommendations for treatment of IE (Table 37–5). Guidelines for outpatient parenteral antibiotic therapy for IE in adults as well as general guidelines for outpatient parenteral antibiotic therapy in all age ranges have been published.[77,78] Pediatric outpatient parenteral antibiotic therapy has been demonstrated to be successful, to have a relatively low risk of complications, and to have a low rehospitalization rate mostly related to issues with vascular access.[79] Patients selected for outpatient therapy should have responded clinically to inpatient therapy, with negative blood cultures, no evidence of intracardiac complications, and stable hemodynamic parameters. Patients' families need to be compliant and capable of managing the technical aspects of intravenous therapy. Such patients require careful, regular monitoring in association with a home health-care service and prompt access to medical care.[48]

The American Heart Association has issued treatment guidelines for children[48] and, more recently, updated specific treatment guidelines based on the microbiologic etiologic agent.[65] General therapeutic considerations are summarized in Tables 37–6 to 37–9.[37,48,65] All dosing is listed as milligram of antimicrobial per kilogram of patient body weight. It is important to remember that the total dose should never exceed the maximum adult dose.

Medical Therapy

Staphylococci

The great majority of *S. aureus* isolates produce a β-lactamase and, therefore, are highly resistant to penicillin G and are termed methicillin-susceptible *S. aureus* (MSSA). The drugs of choice for native valve MSSA are semisynthetic, β-lactamase-resistant penicillins, such as nafcillin or oxacillin (Table 37–6). The addition of gentamicin for the first 3–5 days is optional, as it may increase the killing of the *staphylococci* and facilitate clearance of bacteremia, although it may increase rates of nephrotoxicity and ototoxicity. In patients without a history of type 1 penicillin-allergic reactions, a first-generation cephalosporin such as cefazolin is indicated with or without gentamicin for the first 3–5 days. In patients with MSSA and allergies to β-lactams, vancomycin is the drug of choice with or without gentamicin for the first 3–5 days. However, it must be noted that some evidence suggests than vancomycin is an inferior drug in the treatment of MSSA IE, predominantly because of its slow bactericidal activity and poor tissue penetration.[80]

Coagulase-negative *staphylococci* are usually methicillin resistant (MRSA). Because of cross-resistance, cephalosporins should not be used in these patients. Vancomycin is usually given for at least 6 weeks with or without gentamicin for the first 3–5 days.

Staphylococcal prosthetic valve IE (PVE) is associated with high mortality and requires aggressive management. Treatment for MSSA PVE is with nafcillin or oxacillin, in combination with rifampin for 6–8 weeks and gentamicin during the first 2 weeks. For MRSA PVE, vancomycin is used in combination with rifampin for 6–8 weeks and gentamicin is added during the first 2 weeks. In order to minimize resistance to rifampin, this medication should be added only after antibiotics active against *staphylococci*, such as a β-lactam or vancomycin and an aminoglycoside, have been started and the infection burden of bacteria is significantly reduced. In some cases, MRSA resistant to aminoglycosides (reported to be decreasing in frequency[81]) can be treated with fluoroquinolones, depending on the results of susceptibility testing. Daptomycin is a lipopeptide antibiotic that is bactericidal and has been shown to be effective in treatment of staphylococcal endocarditis in adults.[82] However, experience with daptomycin in children is limited, and thus a safe pediatric dose has not been established.[83] Staphylococcal PVE has been reported to have a very high mortality in adults, even with aggressive medical therapy.[84] For this reason, early surgical valve replacement is often considered. *S. aureus* PVE has been reported to cause a high incidence of intracerebral hemorrhage in adults,[85] and thus the risks of continuing anticoagulation need to be carefully considered.

Viridans Group Streptococci, Streptococcus bovis, and other Nonenterococcal Streptococci

The treatment for endocarditis caused by viridans streptococci is based on the in vitro penicillin minimum

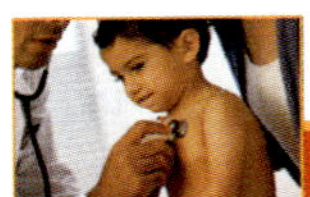

Table 37–6.

Antimicrobial Therapy for Endocarditis Caused by Staphylococci

Organism	Antimicrobial Agent	Dosage per kg per 24 h	Frequency of Administration (h)	Duration (Weeks)
Staphylococcus—methicillin sensitive				
Native valve	Nafcillin or oxacillin	200 mg IV	Q 4–6	6
	Plus optional			
	Gentamicin	3 mg IM or IV	Q 8	3–5 d
Native valve β-lactam allergic	Cefazolin	100 mg IV	Q 8 h	6
	Plus optional			
	Gentamicin	3 mg IM or IV	Q 8	3–5 d
	Or			
	Vancomycin	40 mg IV	Q 6–12	6
Prosthetic valve	Nafcillin or oxacillin	200 mg IV	Q 4–6	6–8
	Or			
	Cefazolin	100 mg IV	Q 8 h	6–8
	Or			
	Vancomycin	40 mg IV	Q 6–12 h	6–8
	Plus			
	Rifampin	20 mg IV or PO	Q 8	6–8
	Plus			
	Gentamicin	3 mg IM or IV	Q 8	2
Staphylococcus—methicillin resistant				
Native valve	Vancomycin	40 mg IV	Q 6–12	6
	Plus optional			
	Gentamicin	3 mg IM or IV	Q 8	3–5 d
Prosthetic valve	Vancomycin	40 mg IV	Q 6–12	6–8
	Plus			
	Rifampin	20 mg IV or PO	Q 8	6–8
	Plus			
	Gentamicin	3 mg IM or IV	Q 8	2

inhibitory concentration (MIC) (Table 37–7). *Streptococci* with a penicillin MIC ≤0.12 μg/mL are considered highly susceptible and are usually treated with penicillin G or ceftriaxone for 4 weeks. Comparable cure rates can be achieved with a combination of penicillin or ceftriaxone with low-dose gentamicin for 2 weeks. A cure rate of 98% has been reported with these regimens in adults,[86,87] but there are no published data on the efficacy of ceftriaxone for the treatment of IE in children. Cefazolin or other first-generation cephalosporins may be substituted for penicillin in patients whose penicillin hypersensitivity is not of the immediate type. Vancomycin is recommended for patients allergic to β-lactams.

When IE is caused by streptococcal strains with a penicillin MIC >0.12 μg/mL and <0.5 μg/mL, combination therapy with penicillin for 4 weeks and low-dose gentamicin for the first 2 weeks of treatment is recommended. In patients allergic to β-lactams, a 4-week course of vancomycin is recommended. When native valve or PVE IE is caused by streptococcal strains with a penicillin MIC >0.5 μg/mL or nutritionally variant streptococci (now classified as *Abiotrophia* species), the regimen for penicillin-resistant enterococcal IE is recommended (Table 37–8).

For highly penicillin-susceptible streptococci PVE (MIC ≤0.12 μg/mL), penicillin G for 6 weeks and gentamicin for 2 weeks are usually indicated. When PVE is caused by relatively penicillin-resistant streptococci (MIC (>0.12–0.5 μg/mL), penicillin G is recommended for 6 weeks and gentamicin for 4 weeks.

Enterococci

IE caused by *enterococci* is usually associated with *Enterococcus faecalis* and occasionally with *Enterococcus faecium*. *Enterococci* are increasingly resistant to most classes of antibiotics, making treatment difficult (Table 37–8). Because of a defective bacterial autolytic enzyme system, cell-wall-active agents are bacteriostatic against *enterococci* and should not be given alone to treat IE. When used in combination with gentamicin, penicillin G and ampicillin facilitate the intracellular uptake of the aminoglycoside, resulting in a bactericidal effect

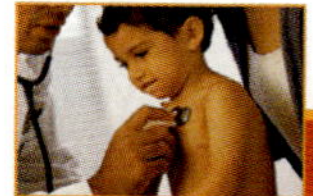

Table 37–7.

Antimicrobial Therapy for Endocarditis Caused by Viridans Group Streptococci, Streptococcus bovis, and Other Nonenterococcal Streptococci

Organism	Antimicrobial Agent	Dosage per kg per 24 h	Frequency of Administration (h)	Duration, (Weeks)
Streptococci—penicillin susceptible (MIC ≤0.12 μg/mL)				
Native valve	Penicillin G	200,000 U IV	Q 4–6	4
	Or			
	Ceftriaxone	100 mg IV	Q 24	4
	OR			
	Penicllin G	200,000 U IV	Q 4–6	2
	Or			
	Ceftriaxone	100 mg IV	Q 24 h	2
	Plus			
	Gentamicin	3 mg IM or IV	Q 8–24	2
Native valve β-lactam allergic	Vancomycin	40 mg IV	Q 6–12	4
Prosthetic valve	Penicillin G	300,000 U IV	Q 4–6	6
	Or			
	Ceftriaxone	100 mg IV	Q 24	6
	OR			
	Vancomycin (β-lactam allergic)	40 mg IV	Q 6–12	6
	Plus			
	Gentamicin	3 mg IM or IV	Q 8–24	2
Streptococci—relatively penicillin resistant (MIC> 0.12–0.5 μg/mL)				
Native valve	Penicillin G	300,000 U IV	Q 4–6	4
	Or			
	Ceftriaxone	100 mg IV	Q 24	4
	Plus			
	Gentamicin	3 mg IM or IV	Q 8–24	2
Native valve β-lactam allergic	Vancomycin	40 mg IV	Q 6–12	4
Prosthetic valve	Penicillin G	300,000 U IV	Q 4–6	6
	Or			
	Ceftriaxone	100 mg IV	Q 24	6
	OR			
	Vancomycin (β-lactam allergic)	40 mg IV	Q 8–12	6
	Plus			
	Gentamicin	3 mg IM or IV	Q 8–24	6

against *enterococci.* Before embarking on therapy, susceptibility of the enterococcal isolate should be determined for penicillins, vancomycin, and aminoglycosides. For strains with intrinsic high-level resistance to penicillin (MIC >16 μg/mL), vancomycin is indicated. Vancomycin is synergistic with aminoglycosides, particularly gentamicin. When high-level resistance to aminoglycosides is detected (500–2000 μg/mL for gentamicin), combination with cell-wall-active agents is no longer synergistic and therefore not recommended. Limited data are available to guide therapy in these difficult cases; however, some experts will attempt high-dose ampicillin combined with imipenem or ceftriaxone for 8–12 weeks.

IE caused by vancomycin-resistant *enterococci* (VRE) is difficult to treat. Most vancomycin-resistant strains of *E. faecalis* and some vancomycin-resistant strains of *E. faecium* are susceptible to achievable concentrations of ampicillin. In such cases, the recommended therapy is ampicillin or penicillin combined with gentamicin. Even when *enterococci* are considered resistant to ampicillin, higher doses can be used in order to achieve sustained plasma levels of >100–150 μg/mL with some treatment efficacy and little toxicity. In 1999,

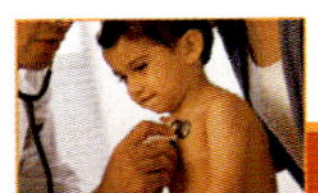

Table 37–8.

Antimicrobial Therapy for Endocarditis Caused by Enterococci on Native or Prosthetic Valves

Organism	Antimicrobial Agent	Dosage per kg per 24 h	Frequency of Administration (h)	Duration (Weeks)
Enterococci—nonresistant				
	Ampicillin	300 mg IV	Q 4–6	4–6
	Or			
	Penicillin G	300,000 U IV	Q 4–6	4–6
	Plus			
	Gentamicin	3 mg IM or IV	Q 8	4–6
	OR			
β-lactam allergic	Vancomycin	40 mg IV	Q 6–12	6
	Plus			
	Gentamicin	3 mg IM or IV	Q 8	6
Enterococci—penicillin resistant				
	Vancomycin	40 mg IV	Q 6–12	6
	Or			
	Ampicillin–sulbactam	300 mg IV	Q 6	6
	Plus			
	Gentamicin	3 mg IM or IV	Q 8	6
Enterococci—aminoglycoside resistant				
	Ampicillin	300 mg IV	Q 4–6	4–6
	Or			
	Penicillin G	300,000 U IV	Q 4–6	4–6
	OR			
	Ampicillin	300 mg IV	Q 4–6	8–12
	Plus			
	Ceftriaxone	100 mg IM or IV	Q 24	8–12
Enterococci—vancomycin resistant				
	Penicillin G	300,000 U IV	Q 4–6	6
	Or			
	Ampicillin	300 mg IV	Q 4–6	6
	Plus			
	Gentamicin	3 mg IM or IV	Q 8	6
Enterococci—penicillin, aminoglycoside, and vancomycin resistant				
	Ampicillin	300 mg IV	Q 4–6	≥8
	Plus			
	Ceftriaxone	100 mg IM or IV	Q 24	≥8
	Or			
	Linezolid	30 mg IV or PO	Q 8 h	≥8
	Or			
	Quinupristin–dalfopristin	22.5 mg IV	Q 8	≥8
	Plus			
	Imipenem/cilastatin	60–100 mg IV	Q 6	≥8

the FDA approved quinupristin/dalfopristin (QD) to treat infections associated with vancomycin-resistant *E. faecium* bacteremia when no alternative treatment is available. However, QD alone is unlikely to be curative in VREF IE because it is not usually bactericidal against *E. faecium*. Endocarditis models suggest that the association of QD with ampicillin may be beneficial. It is important to note that *E. faecalis* is not susceptible to QD. In 2000, the FDA approved linezolid to treat infections associated with vancomycin-resistant *E. faecium*, including cases with bloodstream infection. However, linezolid is bacteriostatic against VRE and therefore cannot be recommended for VRE IE. Newer agents such as daptomycin, telavancin, and dalbavancin may be useful in such cases based on experimental models, but clinical experience is lacking. Unfortunately, case reports of enterococcal resistance to daptomycin are already emerging.[88]

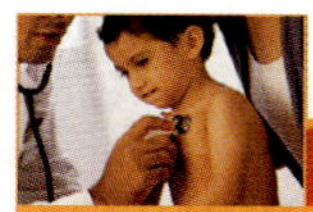

Table 37–9.

Antimicrobial Therapy for HACEK, Gram-Negative, Culture-Negative, and fungal Endocarditis on Native and Prosthetic Valves

Organism	Antimicrobial Agent	Dosage per kg per 24 hr	Frequency of Administration (h)	Duration (Weeks)
HACEK	Ceftriaxone	100 mg IM or IV	Q 24	Four (native) to six (prosthetic)
	Or			
	Ampicillin–sulbactam	300 mg IV	Q 4–6	4–6
	Or			
	Ciprofloxacin	20–30 mg IV or PO	Q 12	4–6
Other Gram negatives				
Empiric therapy	Extended-spectrum penicillin plus β-lactamase inhibitor (piperacillin–tazobactam)	200–300 mg IV	Q 6–8	6
	Or			
	Cephalosporin (ceftazidime)	90–150 mg IV	Q 8	6
	Plus			
	Gentamicin	3 mg IM or IV	Q 8	6
Directed therapy	Tailored to the resistance profile of the individual organisms			
Culture negative				
General approach	Ceftriaxone	100 mg IM or IV	Q 24	6
	Plus			
	Gentamicin	3 mg IM or IV	Q 8	2–6
Suspected Staphylococcal IE	Ampicillin–sulbactam	300 mg IV	Q 4–6	6
Suspected MRSA	Vancomycin	40 mg IV	Q 6–12	6
	Plus			
	Gentamicin	3 mg IM or IV	Q 8	2–6
Suspected fastidious organism	Consider doxycycline and ciprofloxacin with an infectious disease consultation			
Fungal				
Primary therapy	Liposomal amphotericin B	Use with pharmacy and infectious disease consultation		
	Plus optional 5-fluorocytosine	Use with pharmacy and infectious disease consultation		
Suppressive therapy	Fluconazole	6–12 mg IV or PO	Q 24	Indefinite

Gram-Negative IE

HACEK organisms, including *Haemophilus* spp. (*Haemophilus parainfluenzae*, *H. aphrophilus*, and *H. paraphrophilus*), *Actinobacillus actinomycetemcomitans*, *Cardiobacterium hominis*, *Eikenella corrodens*, and *Kingella kingae* are not common in children. These organisms have fastidious growth characteristics, and thus standard culture incubation for 2–3 weeks is recommended for cases in which IE is suspected and the initial blood cultures are negative. Third-generation cephalosporins are recommended for the treatment of HACEK IE (Table 37–9), with a duration of 3–4 weeks for native valves and 6 weeks for PVE.[89] HACEK isolates are typically susceptible in vitro to fluoroquinolones, aztreonam, and trimethoprim–sulfamethoxazole. However, since clinical data are still lacking, these agents should be reserved as an alternative therapy in patients who cannot tolerate β-lactams.

Other Gram-negative bacteria are an infrequent cause of IE in children and are most often nosocomially acquired. Treatment of organisms such as *P. aeruginosa*, *E. coli*, and *Serratia marcescens* should be individualized, based on antimicrobial susceptibility of the specific isolate.[48] Empiric therapy with an extended-spectrum penicillin/β-lactamase inhibitor or cephalosporin together with an aminoglycoside is recommended until final culture testing is completed. Total duration of therapy should be 6 weeks and should be implemented in consultation with an infectious disease specialist.

Fungal IE

The incidence of fungal IE has increased significantly in the past decade, in most cases caused by *Candida* or *Aspergillus* species. Although current recommendations strongly favor a combined medical–surgical approach, the introduction of new fungicidal agents may reduce that need. Any documented or suspected case of fungal IE requires an infectious disease consultation.

A mainstay of antifungal drug therapy is liposomal amphotericin B for at least 6–8 weeks. This agent is much less toxic than routine amphotericin B, which produces multiple side effects, including fever, chills, phlebitis, headache, anorexia, anemia, hypokalemia, renal tubular acidosis, nephrotoxicity, nausea, and vomiting. Depending on the isolate, some experts recommend the addition of 5-fluorocytosine or rifampin to amphotericin B, as these drugs may act synergistically to potentiate fungal killing. In patients who are unable to undergo surgery, after an initial course of amphotericin B, an azole is often used for long-term suppressive therapy. The role of newer antifungals such as posaconazole, micafungin, and capsofungin in the treatment of fungal IE remains unclear, despite their increased use, as reports of efficacy of these agents are limited.

Culture-Negative IE

As a result of the substantial issues in treatment decisions, consultation with an infectious disease specialist is recommended. The primary considerations for therapy are directed against *staphylococci, streptococci,* enterococci, and the HACEK organisms (Table 37–9). An initial approach is to use ceftriaxone and gentamicin. A β-lactamase-resistant penicillin such as ampicillin–sulbactam should be added if there is a high suspicion of staphylococcal IE. Vancomycin should be substituted in patients who are allergic to penicillin and when suspicion of MRSA is high. If clinical improvement occurs, some authorities recommend discontinuation of treatment with the aminoglycoside after 2 weeks. The other agent(s) should be continued for a full 6 weeks of treatment. Patients who are at risk of unusual causes of IE such as *Coxiella, Bartonella, Legionella,* and *Brucella* can be empirically started on doxycycline and ciprofloxacin; however, these pathogens require targeted therapy, which should be undertaken in consultation with an infectious diseases specialist.

Surgical Therapy

Valve replacement has become an important adjunct to medical therapy in the management of IE and is now used in at least 25% of the cases. The generally accepted indications for surgical intervention during active IE are listed in Table 37–10. Of particular importance to pediatric patients with palliated congenital heart disease is development of aortopulmonary shunt obstruction and infected prosthetic material such as in right ventricle to pulmonary artery conduits. The hemodynamic status of the patient, not the activity of the infection, is the critical determining factor in the timing of cardiac valve replacement. Surgery should not be delayed because a full course of antibiotic therapy has not been completed or the patient is still bacteremic. Indeed, the incidence of reinfection of a prosthetic valve after surgery is below 1%. Thus, when CHF is diagnosed in patients with aortic valve IE or persists despite therapy in mitral valve IE, surgery is indicated. Although not systematically studied, most experts recommend continuation of antibiotic therapy postoperatively for 2–6 weeks when surgery is undertaken with active IE.[90]

Most patients with PVE (except those with late disease caused by penicillin-sensitive viridans streptococci)

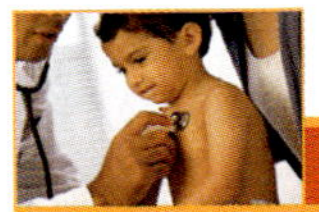

Table 37–10.

Indications for Surgical Intervention in Cases of Endocarditis

Clinical features	Refractory congestive heart failure More than one serious embolic episode Uncontrolled infection Physiologically significant valve dysfunction Ineffective antimicrobial therapy Resection of mycotic aneurysms Most cases of prosthetic valve IE Most cases of IE on prosthetic material in repaired CHD Significant worsening of cyanosis in patients with cyanotic CHD
Echocardiographic features	Valve dehiscence, rupture, perforation, or fistula Perivalvular or myocardial abscesses Persistent large vegetations after a systemic embolic episode An increase in vegetation size after 4 weeks of antimicrobial therapy New heart block Large (>10 mm) anterior mitral valve vegetations Acute aortic or mitral insufficiency with signs of ventricular failure Shunt or conduit obstruction in repaired or palliated CHD

CHD, congenital heart disease.

require valve replacement. Similarly, valve replacement is necessary in a significant proportion of patients with IE on native valves after a medical cure, particularly with aortic valve involvement, which is more likely to be hemodynamically significant.

Medical therapy alone can be considered even in the face of the listed risk factors if there are significant comorbid conditions such as central nervous system bleeding. The morbidity and mortality of surgery must be carefully considered when patients are at high risk of bypass complication.

Prevention of IE

Antimicrobial prophylaxis before selected dental and invasive surgical and diagnostic procedures has become standard and routine in most countries, despite the fact that no prospective study has been performed that proves that such therapy is clearly beneficial. Studies have shown that amoxicillin prophylaxis results in a decrease in procedure-related bacteremia in a general population of pediatric patients.[91] However, only one-half of all patients who develop IE have a cardiac disorder that would have prompted IE prophylaxis in the first place.[37] Maintenance of meticulous dental hygiene is of equal importance to antibiotic prophylaxis in the prevention of IE, and compliance with dental hygiene is difficult in the pediatric population. In addition, it is advisable to instruct all patients to avoid gingival trauma with toothpicks and high-pressure water irrigation devices.

The guidelines for antimicrobial prophylaxis for IE formulated by an expert committee of the American Heart Association are the regimens most widely used by clinicians in the United States. The guidelines were significantly revised in 2007 as the committee concluded that (1) IE is much more likely to result from frequent exposure to random bacteremia than to medical procedures, (2) only an extremely small number of cases of IE might be prevented by antibiotic prophylaxis even if 100% effective, (3) the risk of antibiotic-associated events exceeds the benefit or prophylaxis, and (4) proper maintenance of oral health and hygiene is more important than antibiotic prophylaxis for dental procedure in reducing the risk of IE. The procedures with the highest risk of bacteremia were refined, and prophylaxis is now recommended only for patients with the highest risk of an adverse outcome after an episode of IE.[92]

Table 37–11 outlines the conditions associated with the highest risk for IE based on the new American Heart Association guidelines. Certain procedures and conditions are known to present the highest risk of bacteremia, and therefore antibiotic prophylaxis is recommended. This encompasses all dental procedures that involve manipulation of gingival or periapical region of teeth or perforation of oral mucosa. This also includes surgical procedures in the setting of an active infection, invasive respiratory tract procedures, and procedures where antibiotics would be given to prevent wound infections (Table 37–12). However, there is no evidence of the effectiveness of prophylaxis during these procedures to prevent IE. Routine prophylaxis solely to prevent IE is no longer recommended for GI or GU procedures. For example, clinicians must often use judgment in selecting dose and

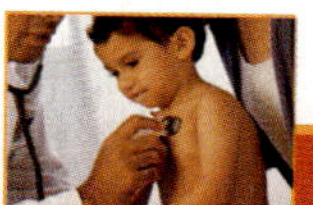

Table 37–11.

Cardiac Conditions Associated with the Highest Risk of Adverse Outcome from IE

Prosthetic cardiac valve
Previous IE
Congenital heart disease (CHD)
Unrepaired cyanotic CHD, including palliative shunts and conduits
Completely repaired congenital heart defect with prosthetic material or device, whether placed by surgery or by catheter intervention, during the first 6 months after the procedure
Repaired CHD with residual defects at the site or adjacent to the site of a prosthetic patch or prosthetic device (which inhibits endothelialization)
Cardiac transplant patients who develop cardiac valvulopathy

IE, infective endocarditis.

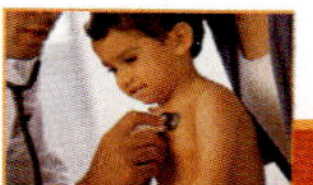

Table 37–12.

Situations Where Antibiotic Prophylaxis Is Recommended in High-Risk Patients

Dental procedures with manipulation of gingival tissues or periapical region of teeth or perforation of oral mucosa
Respiratory tract procedures involving incision or biopsy of respiratory mucosa (various microorganisms)
Invasive respiratory tract procedures to treat an established infection (viridans group streptococci if unknown infectious agent, otherwise targeted therapy)
Gastrointestinal (GI) or genitourinary (GU) procedures in the face of an established infection (*Enterococcus*)
Gastrointestinal (GI) or genitourinary (GU) procedures receiving prophylaxis to avoid wound infection or sepsis (*Enterococcus*)
Urinary tract manipulation with enterococcal urinary tract infection (UTI) or colonization
Procedures involving infected skin, skin structure, or muscle (*staphylococci* and β-hemolytic *streptococci*)

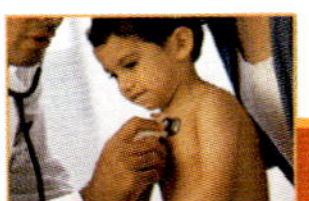

Table 37–13.

Recommended Regimens for Endocarditis Prophylaxis

Patient Situation	Antimicrobial Agent	Dosage 30–60 min Before Procedure
Dental procedures		
No allergy to penicillins		
Oral	Amoxicillin	50 mg/kg PO
Unable to take oral medication	Ampicillin	50 mg/kg IM or IV
	Or	
	Cefazolin or ceftriaxone	50 mg/kg IM or IV
Allergy to penicillins or ampicillin		
Oral	Cephalexin*	50 mg/kg PO
	Or	
	Clindamycin	20 mg/kg PO
	Or	
	Azithromycin or clarithromycin	15 mg/kg PO
Unable to take oral medication	Cefazolin or ceftriaxone	50 mg/kg IM or IV
	Or	
	Clindamycin	20 mg/kg IM or IV
Surgical procedures in the presence of an active infection	Chosen with respect to the known or likely infectious agent(s)	

**Cephalosporins should not be used in an individual with a history of anaphylaxis, angioedema, or urticaria with penicillins or ampicillin.*

duration of antimicrobial therapy in elderly or obese patients or in those with underlying renal disease. Furthermore, there are sometimes instances in which the risk of prophylactic therapy may actually outweigh the risk of postprocedure endocarditis. Patients in such circumstances often have cardiac lesions of questionable or little hemodynamic consequence, have a documented or possible drug allergy, or are undergoing procedures in which the risk of bacteremia is extremely low.

The antimicrobial regimens suggested by the American Heart Association for IE prophylaxis are listed in Table 37–13.

Pearls/Special Situations

1. Antibiotic doses in children are calculated per kg but should never exceed the maximum published adult dosage.
2. Obtain an infectious disease consult in any complex case of IE or when there is any uncertainty in the diagnosis or therapy. The complications of IE can be devastating, so it is better to be overly careful.

REFERENCES

1. Durack DT, Lukes AS, Bright DK. New criteria for diagnosis of infective endocarditis: utilization of specific echocardiographic findings. Duke Endocarditis Service. *Am J Med.* 1994;96(3):200-209.
2. Li JS, Sexton DJ, Mick N, et al. Proposed modifications to the Duke criteria for the diagnosis of infective endocarditis. *Clin Infect Dis.* 2000;30(4):633-638.
3. Tissieres P, Gervaix A, Beghetti M, Jaeggi ET. Value and limitations of the von Reyn, Duke, and modified Duke criteria for the diagnosis of infective endocarditis in children. *Pediatrics.* 2003;112(6, pt 1):e467.
4. Stockheim JA, Chadwick EG, Kessler S, et al. Are the Duke criteria superior to the Beth Israel criteria for the diagnosis of infective endocarditis in children? *Clin Infect Dis.* 1998;27(6):1451-1456.
5. Del Pont JM, De Cicco LT, Vartalitis C, et al. Infective endocarditis in children: clinical analyses and evaluation of two diagnostic criteria. *Pediatr Infect Dis J.* 1995;14(12):1079-1086.
6. Steckelberg JM, Melton LJ, III, Ilstrup DM, Rouse MS, Wilson WR. Influence of referral bias on the apparent clinical spectrum of infective endocarditis. *Am J Med.* 1990;88(6):582-588.
7. Von Reyn CF, Levy BS, Arbeit RD, Friedland G, Crumpacker CS. Infective endocarditis: an analysis based on strict case definitions. *Ann Intern Med.* 1981;94(4, pt 1):505-518.
8. Van Hare GF, Ben-Shachar G, Liebman J, Boxerbaum B, Riemenschneider TA. Infective endocarditis in infants and children during the past 10 years: a decade of change. *Am Heart J.* 1984;107(6):1235-1240.
9. Stull TL, LiPuma JJ. Endocarditis in children. In: Kaye D, ed. *Infective Endocarditis.* 2nd ed. New York: Raven Press; 1992:313-327.
10. Baltimore RS. Infective endocarditis in children. *Pediatr Infect Dis J.* 1992;11(11):907-912.

11. Valente AM, Jain R, Scheurer M, et al. Frequency of infective endocarditis among infants and children with *Staphylococcus aureus* bacteremia. *Pediatrics.* 2005;115(1):e15-e9.
12. Morris CD, Reller MD, Menashe VD. Thirty-year incidence of infective endocarditis after surgery for congenital heart defect. *JAMA.* 1998;279(8):599-603.
13. Di Filippo S, Delahaye F, Semiond B, et al. Current patterns of infective endocarditis in congenital heart disease. *Heart.* 2006;92(10):1490-1495.
14. Tissieres P, Jaeggi ET, Beghetti M, Gervaix A. Increase of fungal endocarditis in children. *Infection.* 2005;33(4): 267-272.
15. Millar BC, Jugo J, Moore JE. Fungal endocarditis in neonates and children. *Pediatr Cardiol.* 2005;26(5):517-536.
16. Cabell CH, Jollis JG, Peterson GE, et al. Changing patient characteristics and the effect on mortality in endocarditis. *Arch Intern Med.* 2002;162(1):90-94.
17. Baltimore RS. Infective endocarditis. In: Jenson HB, Baltimore RS, eds. *Pediatric Infectious Diseases: Principles and Practice.* Norwalk, CT: Appleton & Lange; 2002:845-856.
18. Saiman L, Prince A, Gersony WM. Pediatric infective endocarditis in the modern era. *J Pediatr.* 1993;122(6): 847-853.
19. Petti CA, Fowler VG, Jr. *Staphylococcus aureus* bacteremia and endocarditis. *Cardiol Clin.* 2003;21(2):219-233, vii.
20. Grover FL, Cohen DJ, Oprian C, Henderson WG, Sethi G, Hammermeister KE. Determinants of the occurrence of and survival from prosthetic valve endocarditis. Experience of the veterans affairs cooperative study on valvular heart disease. *J Thorac Cardiovasc Surg.* 1994;108(2):207-214.
21. Kassai B, Gueyffier F, Cucherat M, Boissel JP. Comparison of bioprosthesis and mechanical valves, a meta-analysis of randomised clinical trials. *Cardiovasc Surg.* 2000;8(6):477-483.
22. Substance Abuse and Mental Health Services Administration. (2006). *Results from the 2005 National Survey on Drug Use and Health: National Findings* (Office of Applied Studies, NSDUH Series H-30, DHHS Publication No. SMA 06-4194). Rockville, MD.
23. Cerubin CE, Baden M, Favaler F, et al. Infectious endocarditis in narcotic addicts. *Ann Intern Med.* 1968;69: 1091.
24. Levine DP, Crane LR, Zervos MJ. Bacteremia in narcotic addicts at the Detroit medical center. II. Infectious endocarditis: a prospective comparative study. *Rev Infect Dis.* 1986;8(3):374-396.
25. Mathew J, Addai T, Anand A, Morrobel A, Maheshwari P, Freels S. Clinical features, site of involvement, bacteriologic findings, and outcome of infective endocarditis in intravenous drug users. *Arch Intern Med.* 1995;155(15): 1641-1648.
26. Saravolatz LD, Burch KH, Quinn EL, Cox F, Madhavan T, Fisher E. Polymicrobial infective endocarditis: an increasing clinical entity. *Am Heart J.* 1978;95(2):163-168.
27. Scheld WM. Pathogenesis and pathophysiology of infective endocarditis. In: Sande MAKD, Root RK, eds. *Endocarditis, Contemporary Issues in Infectious Diseases.* Vol 1. London: Churchill Livingstone; 1984:1-32.
28. Freedman LR. The pathogenesis of infective endocarditis. *J Antimicrob Chemother.* 1987;20(suppl A):1-6.
29. Livornese LL, Jr., Korzeniowski OM. Pathogenesis of infective endocarditis. In: Kaye D, ed. *Infective Endocarditis.* New York: Raven Press; 1992:19-35.
30. Tunkel AR, Scheld WM. Experimental models of endocarditis. In: Kaye D, ed. *Infective Endocarditis.* New York: Raven Press; 1992:37-56.
31. Gould K, Ramirez-Ronda CH, Holmes RK, Sanford JP. Adherence of bacteria to heart valves in vitro. *J Clin Invest.* 1975;56(6):1364-1370.
32. Freedman LR, Valone J, Jr. Experimental infective endocarditis. *Prog Cardiovasc Dis.* 1979;22(3):169-180.
33. Ramirez-Ronda CH. Effects of molecular weight of dextran on the adherence of *Streptococcus sanguis* to damaged heart valves. *Infect Immun.* 1980;29(1):1-7.
34. Lowrance JH, Baddour LM, Simpson WA. The role of fibronectin binding in the rat model of experimental endocarditis caused by *Streptococcus sanguis. J Clin Invest.* 1990;86(1):7-13.
35. Becker RC, DiBello PM, Lucas FV. Bacterial tissue tropism: an in vitro model for infective endocarditis. *Cardiovasc Res.* 1987;21(11):813-820.
36. Fenno JC, LeBlanc DJ, Fives-Taylor P. Nucleotide sequence analysis of a type 1 fimbrial gene of *Streptococcus sanguis* FW213. *Infect Immun.* 1989;57(11):3527-3533.
37. Li J, Corey GR, Fowler VG. Infective Endocarditis. In: Topol EJ, ed. *The Textbook of Cardiovascular Medicine. 3rd ed.* Philadelphia, PA: Lippincott, Williams, & Wilkins; 2006:402-419.
38. Weinstein L. Life-threatening complications of infective endocarditis and their management. *Arch Intern Med.* 1986;146(5):953-957.
39. Karalis DG, Bansal RC, Hauck AJ, et al. Transesophageal echocardiographic recognition of subaortic complications in aortic valve endocarditis. Clinical and surgical implications. *Circulation.* 1992;86(2):353-362.
40. Anguera I, Miro JM, Vilacosta I, et al. Aorto-cavitary fistulous tract formation in infective endocarditis: clinical and echocardiographic features of 76 cases and risk factors for mortality. *Eur Heart J.* 2005;26(3):288-297.
41. Williams RC, Kunkel HG. Rheumatoid factors and their disappearance following therapy in patients with SBE. *Arthritis Rheum.* 1962;5:126.
42. Bacon PA, Davidson C, Smith B. Antibodies to *Candida* and autoantibodies in sub-acute bacterial endocarditis. *Q J Med.* 1974;43(172):537-550.
43. Qoronfleh MW, Weraarchakul W, Wilkinson BJ. Antibodies to a range of *Staphylococcus aureus* and *Escherichia coli* heat shock proteins in sera from patients with *S. aureus* endocarditis. *Infect Immun.* 1993;61(4):1567-1570.
44. Hurwitz D, Quismorio FP, Friou GJ. Cryoglobulinaemia in patients with infectious endocarditis. *Clin Exp Immunol.* 1975;19(1):131-141.
45. Laxdal T, Messner RP, Williams RC, Jr., Quie PG. Opsonic, agglutinating, and complement-fixing antibodies in patients with subacute bacterial endocarditis. *J Lab Clin Med.* 1968;71(4):638-653.
46. Bayer AS, Theofilopoulos AN, Eisenberg R, Dixon FJ, Guze LB. Circulating immune complexes in infective endocarditis. *N Engl J Med.* 1976;295(27):1500-1505.
47. Alpert JS, Krous HF, Dalen JE, O'Rourke RA, Bloor CM. Pathogenesis of Osler's nodes. *Ann Intern Med.* 1976;85(4):471-473.
48. Ferrieri P, Gewitz MH, Gerber MA, et al. Unique features of infective endocarditis in childhood. *Circulation.* 2002;105(17):2115-2126.

49. Freedman LR. Infective endocarditis and other intravascular infections. In: Braude AI, David CE, Fierer J, eds. *Medical Microbiology and Infectious Diseases.* Philadelphia, PA: WB Saunders; 1981:1511.
50. Terpenning MS, Buggy BP, Kauffman CA. Infective endocarditis: clinical features in young and elderly patients. *Am J Med.* 1987;83(4):626-634.
51. Bradley SF. *Staphylococcus aureus* infections and antibiotic resistance in older adults. *Clin Infect Dis.* 2002;34(2): 211-216.
52. Martin JM, Neches WH, Wald ER. Infective endocarditis: 35 years of experience at a children's hospital. *Clin Infect Dis.* 1997;24(4):669-675.
53. Knirsch W, Haas NA, Uhlemann F, Dietz K, Lange PE. Clinical course and complications of infective endocarditis in patients growing up with congenital heart disease. *Int J Cardiol.* 2005;101(2):285-291.
54. Niwa K, Nakazawa M, Tateno S, Yoshinaga M, Terai M. Infective endocarditis in congenital heart disease: Japanese National Collaboration Study. *Heart.* 2005;91(6):795-800.
55. Charney R, Keltz TN, Attai L, Merav A, Schwinger ME. Acute valvular obstruction from streptococcal endocarditis. *Am Heart J.* 1993;125(2, pt 1):544-547.
56. Ting W, Silverman NA, Arzouman DA, Levitsky S. Splenic septic emboli in endocarditis. *Circulation.* 1990;82 (5 suppl):IV105-IV109.
57. Sakata K, Misawa Y, Kato M, Take A, Takahashi T, Hasegawa T. A case of infective endocarditis with multiple embolic complications. *Nippon Kyobu Geka Gakkai Zasshi.* 1992;40(9):1759-1763.
58. Anderson DJ, Goldstein LB, Wilkinson WE, et al. Stroke location, characterization, severity, and outcome in mitral vs aortic valve endocarditis. *Neurology.* 2003;61(10): 1341-1346.
59. Pelletier LL, Jr., Petersdorf RG. Infective endocarditis: A review of 125 cases from the University of Washington Hospitals, 1963-72. *Medicine (Baltimore).* 1977;56(4): 287-313.
60. McKenzie R, Reimer LG. Effect of antimicrobials on blood cultures in endocarditis. *Diagn Microbiol Infect Dis.* 1987;8(3):165-172.
61. Wilson ML, Harrell LJ, Mirrett S, Weinstein MP, Stratton CW, Reller LB. Controlled evaluation of BACTEC PLUS 27 and roche septi-chek anaerobic blood culture bottles. *J Clin Microbiol.* 1992;30(1):63-66.
62. Doern GV, Gantz NM. Detection of bacteremia in patients receiving antimicrobial therapy: an evaluation of the antimicrobial removal device and 16B medium. *J Clin Microbiol.* 1983;18(1):43-48.
63. Mueller C, Huber P, Laifer G, Mueller B, Perruchoud AP. Procalcitonin and the early diagnosis of infective endocarditis. *Circulation.* 2004;109(14):1707-1710.
64. Lamas CC, Eykyn SJ. Blood culture negative endocarditis: analysis of 63 cases presenting over 25 years. *Heart.* 2003;89(3):258-262.
65. Baddour LM, Wilson WR, Bayer AS, et al. Infective endocarditis: diagnosis, antimicrobial therapy, and management of complications: a statement for healthcare professionals from the Committee on Rheumatic Fever, Endocarditis, and Kawasaki Disease, Council on Cardiovascular Disease in the Young, and the Councils on Clinical Cardiology, Stroke, and Cardiovascular Surgery and Anesthesia, American Heart Association: endorsed by the Infectious Diseases Society of America. *Circulation.* 2005;111(23):e394-e434.
66. Dillon JC, Feigenbaum H, Konecke LL, Davis RH, Chang S. Echocardiographic manifestations of valvular vegetations. *Am Heart J.* 1973;86(5):698-704.
67. Kuruppu JC, Corretti M, Mackowiak P, Roghmann MC. Overuse of transthoracic echocardiography in the diagnosis of native valve endocarditis. *Arch Intern Med.* 2002;162(15):1715-1720.
68. Vuille C, Nidorf M, Weyman AE, Picard MH. Natural history of vegetations during successful medical treatment of endocarditis. *Am Heart J.* 1994;128(6, pt 1):1200-1209.
69. Tischler MD, Vaitkus PT. The ability of vegetation size on echocardiography to predict clinical complications: a meta-analysis. *J Am Soc Echocardiogr.* 1997;10(5):562-568.
70. Erbel R, Rohmann S, Drexler M, et al. Improved diagnostic value of echocardiography in patients with infective endocarditis by transoesophageal approach. A prospective study. *Eur Heart J.* 1988;9(1):43-53.
71. Daniel WG, Mugge A, Martin RP, et al. Improvement in the diagnosis of abscesses associated with endocarditis by transesophageal echocardiography. *N Engl J Med.* 1991;324(12):795-800.
72. Ayres NA, Miller-Hance W, Fyfe DA, et al. Indications and guidelines for performance of transesophageal echocardiography in the patient with pediatric acquired or congenital heart disease: report from the task force of the Pediatric Council of the American Society of Echocardiography. *J Am Soc Echocardiogr.* 2005;18(1):91-98.
73. Meine TJ, Nettles RE, Anderson DJ, et al. Cardiac conduction abnormalities in endocarditis defined by the duke criteria. *Am Heart J.* 2001;142(2):280-285.
74. Wiseman J, Rouleau J, Rigo P, Strauss HW, Pitt B. Gallium-67 myocardial imaging for the detection of bacterial endocarditis. *Radiology.* 1976;120(1):135-138.
75. Wong DW, Dhawan VK, Tanaka T, Mishkin FS, Reese IC, Thadepalli H. Imaging endocarditis with Tc-99m-labeled antibody—an experimental study: concise communication. *J Nucl Med.* 1982;23(3):229-234.
76. Riba AL, Thakur ML, Gottschalk A, Andriole VT, Zaret BL. Imaging experimental infective endocarditis with indium-111-labeled blood cellular components. *Circulation.* 1979;59(2):336-343.
77. Andrews MM, von Reyn CF. Patient selection criteria and management guidelines for outpatient parenteral antibiotic therapy for native valve infective endocarditis. *Clin Infect Dis.* 2001;33(2):203-209.
78. Tice AD, Rehm SJ, Dalovisio JR, et al. Practice guidelines for outpatient parenteral antimicrobial therapy. IDSA guidelines. *Clin Infect Dis.* 2004;38(12):1651-1672.
79. Gomez M, Maraqa N, Alvarez A, Rathore M. Complications of outpatient parenteral antibiotic therapy in childhood. *Pediatr Infect Dis J.* 2001;20(5):541-543.
80. Levine DP, Fromm BS, Reddy BR. Slow response to vancomycin or vancomycin plus rifampin in methicillin-resistant *Staphylococcus aureus* endocarditis. *Ann Intern Med.* 1991;115(9):674-680.
81. Barada K, Hanaki H, Ikeda S, et al. Trends in the gentamicin and arbekacin susceptibility of methicillin-resistant *Staphylococcus*

aureus and the genes encoding aminoglycoside-modifying enzymes. *J Infect Chemother.* 2007;13(2):74-78.

82. Fowler VG, Jr., Boucher HW, Corey GR, et al. Daptomycin versus standard therapy for bacteremia and endocarditis caused by *Staphylococcus aureus. N Engl J Med.* 2006; 355(7):653-665.
83. Akins RL, Haase MR, Levy EN. Pharmacokinetics of daptomycin in a critically ill adolescent with vancomycin-resistant enterococcal endocarditis. *Pharmacotherapy.* 2006;26(5):694-698.
84. John MD, Hibberd PL, Karchmer AW, Sleeper LA, Calderwood SB. *Staphylococcus aureus* prosthetic valve endocarditis: optimal management and risk factors for death. *Clin Infect Dis.* 1998;26(6):1302-1309.
85. Stryjewski ME, Corey GR. Treatment protocols for bacterial endocarditis and infection of electrophysiologic cardiac devices. In: Pace JL, Rupp ME, Finch RG, eds. *Biofilms, Infections, and Antimicrobial Therapy.* Boca Raton, FL: CRC Press; 2005: 427-448.
86. Francioli P, Etienne J, Hoigne R, Thys JP, Gerber A. Treatment of streptococcal endocarditis with a single daily dose of ceftriaxone sodium for 4 weeks. Efficacy and outpatient treatment feasibility. *JAMA.* 1992;267(2):264-267.
87. Wilson WR, Thompson RL, Wilkowske CJ, Washington JA, II, Giuliani ER, Geraci JE. Short-term therapy for streptococcal infective endocarditis. Combined intramuscular administration of penicillin and streptomycin. *JAMA.* 1981;245(4):360-363.
88. Kanafani ZA, Federspiel JJ, Fowler VG, Jr. Infective endocarditis caused by daptomycin-resistant *Enterococcus faecalis*: a case report. *Scand J Infect Dis.* 2007;39(1):75-77.
89. Le T, Bayer AS. Combination antibiotic therapy for infective endocarditis. *Clin Infect Dis.* 2003;36(5):615-621.
90. Fowler VG, Jr., Scheld WM, Bayer AS. Cardiovascular infections: endocarditis and intravascular infections. In: Mandell GL, Bennett JE, Dolin R, eds. *Principles and Practice of Infectious Diseases.* 6th ed. Philadelphia: Churchill Livingstone; 2004:975-1002.
91. Lockhart PB, Brennan MT, Kent ML, Norton HJ, Weinrib DA. Impact of amoxicillin prophylaxis on the incidence, nature, and duration of bacteremia in children after intubation and dental procedures. *Circulation.* 2004;109(23): 2878-2884.
92. Wilson W, Taubert KA, Gewitz M, et al. Prevention of infective endocarditis. Guidelines from the American Heart Association. A guideline from the American Heart Association Rheumatic Fever, Endocarditis, and Kawasaki Disease Committee, Council on Cardiovascular Disease in the Young, and the Council on Clinical Cardiology, Council on Cardiovascular Surgery and Anesthesia, and the Quality of Care and Outcomes Research Interdisciplinary Working Group. *Circulation.* 2007; 116(15):1736-1754.

CHAPTER 38

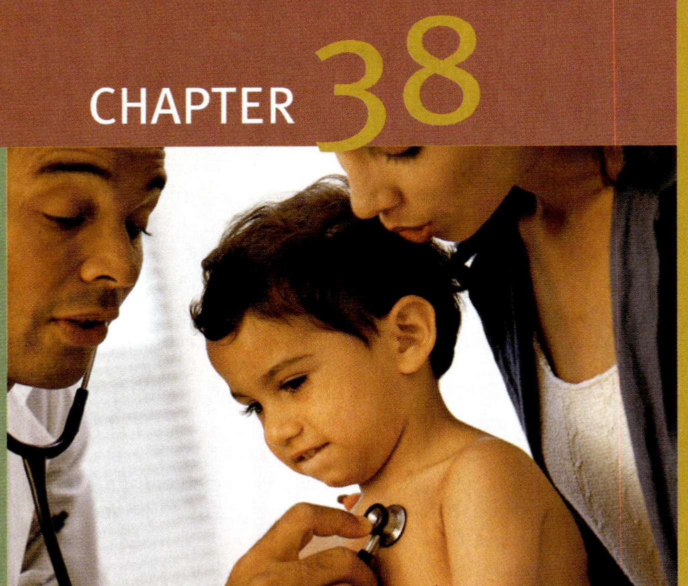

Myocarditis and Pericarditis

Sarah C. McBride and Joshua W. Salvin

DEFINITIONS AND EPIDEMIOLOGY

Myocarditis is a term used to describe an inflammatory infiltrative process within the muscular walls of the heart leading to degeneration and necrosis of cardiac myocytes. It is now understood that a spectrum of disease with overlapping clinical and histological characteristics exists, beginning with myocarditis and progressing to dilated cardiomyopathy. The clinical presentation ranges from the asymptomatic patient with mild ventricular dysfunction, ECG changes, and a self-resolving process to the patient with fulminant heart failure leading to dilated cardiomyopathy. Pericarditis, inflammation of the pericardium, may occur in isolation or with myocarditis and often presents in a similar fashion.

The most common causes of myocarditis and pericarditis are infectious diseases, specifically viral etiologies, though specific diagnosis is achieved in less than half of cases.[1] Therefore, myocarditis is most often deemed idiopathic. While the majority of cases are sporadic, there are reports of epidemics. Other causes of myocardial or pericardial inflammation include immune-mediated conditions, toxins, and medication side effects. This chapter focuses on the infectious etiologies of myocarditis and pericarditis, diagnosis, and disease management.

MYOCARDITIS

Pathogenesis

Current understanding of disease pathogenesis in myocarditis has come in large part from murine models. Three overlapping stages of disease have been described: (1) direct myocardial invasion by a cardiotropic triggering agent (usually thought to be viral); (2) immunologic activation; and (3) ongoing inflammation, circulation of antiheart antibodies and abnormal ventricular remodeling.[2]

In acute viral myocarditis, data suggest that cardiotropic viral RNA (ribonucleic acid) enters the myocytes through endocytosis and produces viral protein that activates an immune cascade in the host. Inflammatory cellular infiltration with macrophages and natural killer cells enhances expression of inflammatory cytokines, specifically interleukin IL-1, IL-2, tumor necrosis factor (TNF), and interferon-γ,[3,4] resulting in further inflammatory cell recruitment. Cytokines activate inducible nitric oxide synthase in cardiac myocytes.[5] Nitric oxide has been shown to play an important role both in inhibiting viral replication and in producing intense myocardial inflammation.[6,7] In addition, circulating autoantibodies directed against cardiac contractile, structural, and mitochondrial proteins have been detected in cardiac biopsy specimens in both humans and mice with myocarditis.[8] Removal of autoantibodies by immunoabsorption techniques seems to improve cardiac function and decrease inflammation.[9–11]

It is therefore deduced that a normal host immune response facilitates clearance of infectious agents. However, with immunologic imbalance, infectious agents may persist in the myocardium leading to ongoing immune-mediated myocyte destruction and myocardial injury. Detection of viral RNA in autopsy specimens of patients with dilated cardiomyopathy has supported the theory that persistence of viruses in the myocardium is capable of inducing ongoing myocardial injury resulting in acute or chronic dilated cardiomyopathy.

Clinical Presentation

History and physical examination

With differences in age and overall immune status, pediatric myocarditis may have variable clinical presentations. Many cases of myocarditis are suspected to be subclinical without apparent illness. The ability of most pediatric patients to compensate for decreased cardiac function can cause cardiovascular symptoms to be minimal in myocarditis until acute collapse or sudden death occurs.

Infants often present with poor feeding, vomiting, fever, irritability, and cardiorespiratory symptoms. Pallor and cyanosis may be evident on physical examination with mottled skin when depressed cardiac output causes poor perfusion. Respirations may be rapid and labored. Cardiovascular examination findings relate to congestive heart failure and include tachycardia, a prominent third heart sound ("gallop") with muffled heart sounds on auscultation. A systolic murmur at the cardiac apex may be appreciated when mitral regurgitation is present. Lung auscultation may reveal diffuse rales. The liver is often enlarged. Infants with injury related to intrauterine myocarditis may present with more chronic signs and symptoms.

Older children and adolescents may complain of palpitations and chest pain in addition to lethargy and abdominal pain. Low-grade fever is common and a history of recent viral illness is often reported, usually 1–2 weeks prior to presentation. As disease progresses and cardiac output is affected, diaphoresis, exercise intolerance, and respiratory symptoms become more prominent. Syncope or even sudden death may result from either myocardial dysfunction or cardiac arrhythmias. Examination findings suggest congestive heart failure, and in contrast to infants may include jugular venous distention and rales on pulmonary examination. Resting tachycardia is a prominent feature of myocarditis. Because myocarditis can occur in the setting of more systemic illness, additional examination findings related to other organ system dysfunction may be present.

A complete medication history should be obtained, as well as an account of other exposures that can cause toxin-mediated myocarditis. Preexisting rheumatologic or autoimmune disease accompanied by a history and examination suggestive of cardiac disturbance should raise concern for myocardial inflammation.

Signs and symptoms

Tachycardia almost always accompanies fever in the pediatric patient, and, therefore, extra diligence is required for recognizing tachycardia out of proportion to the degree of fever. Persistent tachycardia is often the only initial suggestion of myocarditis. If tachycardia does not improve appropriately after competing causative factors (such as fever, pain, and dehydration) are

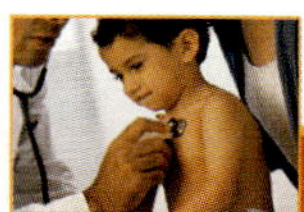

Table 38–1.

Signs and Symptoms Associated with Myocarditis

Signs and Symptoms Associated with Myocarditis
Infants
Poor feeding
Fever
Irritability
Periodic pallor
Diaphoresis
Mild cyanosis
Tachypnea
Tachycardia
Hepatomegaly
Children and Adolescents
Lethargy
Malaise
Low-grade fever
Rash
Pallor
Poor appetite
Abdominal pain
Diaphoresis
Palpitations
Exercise intolerance
Respiratory distress
Resting tachycardia
Jugular venous distention
Hepatomegaly
Pulmonary rales
Arrhythmias
Syncope
Sudden death

addressed, further cardiac evaluation is warranted. Signs and symptoms of myocarditis are listed in Table 38–1 and may include fever, tachycardia, pallor, cyanosis, respiratory distress if pulmonary edema ensues, a gallop, and hepatosplenomegaly caused by venous congestion. Evidence of an upper respiratory illness is common in viral myocarditis.

In noninfectious cases of myocarditis, signs, and symptoms related to the underlying cause should be elicited. With autoimmune and rheumatologic illnesses, a rash or joint findings may also be evident. More chronic symptoms may be present in these diseases.

Differential Diagnosis

Table 38–2 summarizes the differential diagnosis of myocarditis. Although infectious causes of myocarditis are most common (Tables 38–3 and 38–4), noninfectious etiologies (Table 38–5) should be considered when evaluating a patient with signs and symptoms of myocarditis. The most common viral pathogens include enteroviruses, particularly coxsackievirus B, as well as

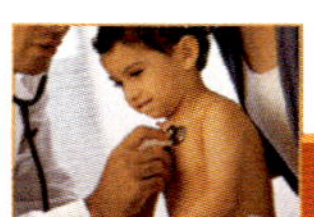

Table 38–2.

Differential Diagnosis of Myocarditis
Newborn/Infant
Sepsis
Hypoxia
Hypoglycemia
Hypocalcemia
Anatomic heart disease
Idiopathic dilated cardiomyopathy
Barth's syndrome
Endocardial fibroelastosis
Anomalous left coronary artery from the pulmonary artery
Cerebral arterial venous malformation
Child/Adolescent
Idiopathic dilated cardiomyopathy
X-linked dilated cardiomyopathy
Autosomal-dominant dilated cardiomyopathy
Anomalous left coronary artery from the pulmonary artery
Endocardial fibroelastosis
Chronic tachyarrhythmia
Pericarditis

adenovirus serotypes 2 and 5, and influenza. Other infectious etiologies include Rickettsiae, other bacteria, parasites, fungi, protozoa, and yeast.

Drugs may cause myocarditis, in particular, some antimicrobials and antifungals. Underlying autoimmune diseases, such as juvenile rheumatoid arthritis and ulcerative colitis as well as collagen vascular diseases, are known to be associated with myocarditis.

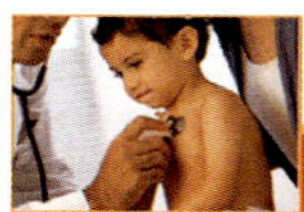

Table 38–3.

Viral Causes of Myocarditis
Common
Adenovirus
Enteroviruses
Cocksackievirus A, B
Echoviruses
Less Common
Parvovirus
Influenza A/B
Epstein–Barr virus
Cytomegalovirus
Herpes simplex
Varicella
HIV
Rhinoviruses
Rare
Arboviruses
Rubella
Hepatitis B, C
Measles
Mumps
Polio
Rabies

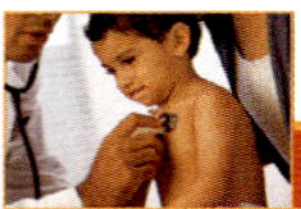

Table 38–4.

Nonviral Infectious Causes of Myocarditis
Bacterial
Rickettsiae
Meningococcus
Klebsiella
Leptospira
Mycoplasma
Salmonella
Clostridia
Mycobacteria
Brucella
Legionella
Streptococcus
Listeria
Smallpox
Treponema pallidum
Protozoal
Trypanosoma cruzi
Toxoplasmosis
Amebiasis
Other Parasitic
Toxocara canis
Schistosomiasis
Heterophyiasis
Cysticercosis
Echinococcus
Visceral larva migrans
Trichinosis
Fungi and Yeasts
Actinomycosis
Coccidioidomycosis
Histoplasmosis
Candida

Diagnosis

The diagnosis of myocarditis can be difficult to confirm, but should be suspected when a patient presents with unexplained congestive heart failure or ventricular tachycardia (Figure 38–1). Table 38–6 summarizes the laboratory and radiologic evaluation of the patient with suspected myocarditis.

Chest radiograph findings

Chest radiograph may be normal early in disease progression. Cardiomegaly and prominent pulmonary vasculature markings consistent with pulmonary edema and congestive heart failure occur in more advanced disease (Figure 38–2).

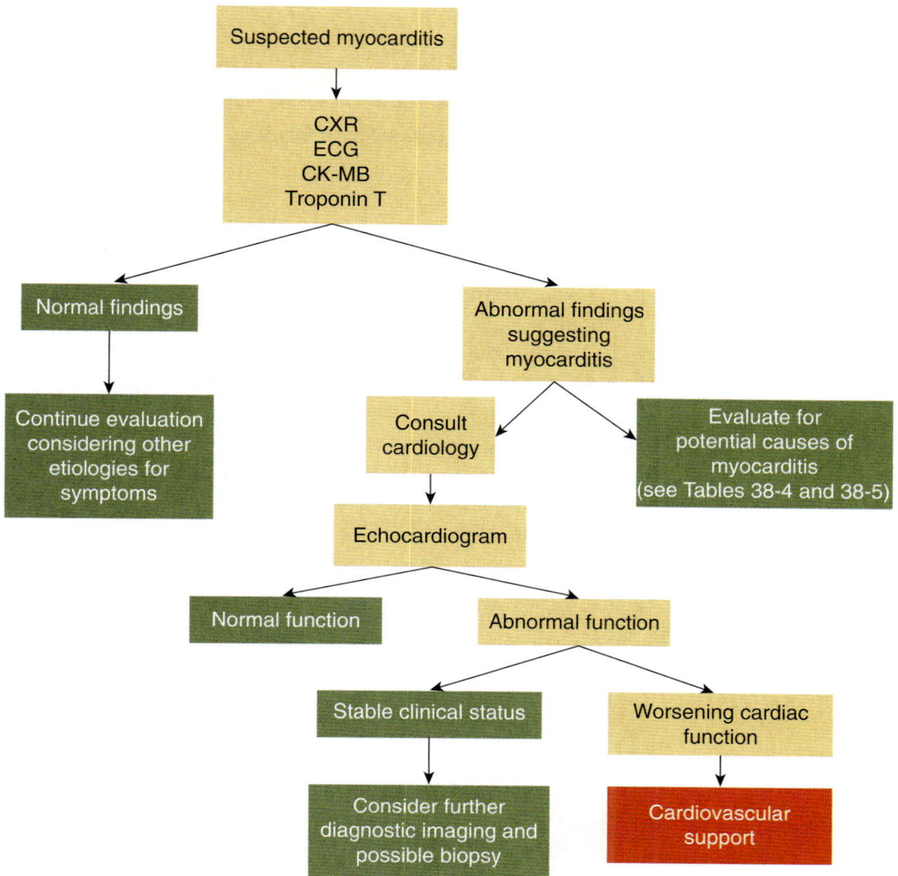

FIGURE 38–1 ■ Algorithm for evaluation of suspected myocarditis in the pediatric patient.

Electrocardiographic findings

ECG findings in acute myocarditis are generally nonspecific and may include sinus tachycardia. Low voltages in the QRS complexes (generally less than 5 mm total amplitude in all limb leads) may be seen, although prominent left-sided forces may be seen when a patient presents with left ventricular dilation. Low-voltage or inverted T waves may also be present. Evidence of myocardial ischemia with widened Q waves (>35 ms) and S–T changes may be seen. Arrhythmias may occur and include supraventricular tachycardia, ventricular tachycardia, as well as A-V block and atrial fibrillation (Figure 38–3).

Echocardiographic findings

A dilated left ventricle with depressed function may be seen, evident by global hypokinesis as well as increased left ventricular end-diastolic and end-systolic dimensions and decreased shortening and ejection fractions. Pericardial effusion is not uncommon in association with myocarditis. Coronary artery abnormalities (e.g., anomalous left coronary artery from the pulmonary artery) or other structural variants should be excluded as alternate causes of dilated cardiomyopathy when performing echocardiography (Figure 38–4).

Serum markers for myocardial injury

Myocardial muscle creatinine kinase isoenzyme (CK-MB) and cardiac troponin T are both serum markers that may be elevated in acute myocarditis. However, data to support their utility in diagnosis and following clinical course among patients with myocarditis is limited.[12,13] CK-MB and cardiac troponin T levels tend to be higher among patients with acute viral myocarditis compared with dilated cardiomyopathy patients with congestive heart failure. There is recently reported data to support the use of cardiac troponin T levels of 0.052 ng/mL or greater as a reliable noninvasive indicator of acute myocarditis in children.[14,15]

Magnetic resonance imaging

Advanced noninvasive imaging methods are now used to assess the extent of inflammation in patients with acute myocarditis, including contrast-enhanced cardiovascular magnetic resonance imaging.[16,17] Adult studies of advanced cardiovascular magnetic resonance technology have further demonstrated its use as a tool for noninvasive diagnosis with the ability to detect small, often patchy areas of myocardial injury and inflammation.[18]

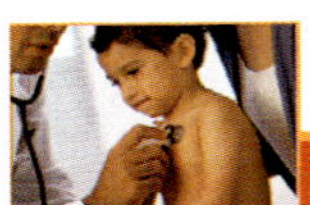

Table 38–5.

Noninfectious Causes of Myocarditis

Toxins
Cocaine
Ecstacy (3,4-methylenedioxy-N-methylamphetamine)
Anthracyclines
Interleukins-2, 4
Scorpion

Drug Hypersensitivity
Sulfonamides
Cephalosporins
Penicillins
Tetracycline
Amphotericin B
Isoniazid
Phenylbutazone
Methyldopa
Phenytoin
Hydrochlorothiazide
Furosemide
Digoxin
Tricyclic antidepressants
Dobutamine

Immune-mediated Conditions
Kawasaki disease
Inflammatory bowel disease
Rheumatoid arthritis
Systemic lupus erythematosus
Thyrotoxicosis
Diabetes mellitus
Rheumatic fever
Churg–Strauss
Sarcoidosis
Scleroderma
Wegener's granulomatosis
Takayasu's arteritis

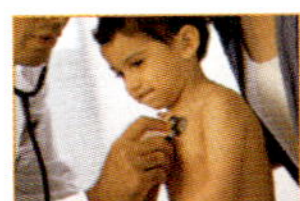

Table 38–6.

Evaluation of Patient with Suspected Myocarditis

Cardiac Evaluation
ECG
CXR
ECHO
Cardiac MRI
Cardiac catheterization (for biopsy and hemodynamic evaluation)
CT scan of head and abdomen (for transplant evaluation)

Blood Tests
Electrolytes, BUN, CR, Uric acid
Liver function tests, total serum albumin
Thyroid function tests
CBC with differential
ESR
CRP
Coagulation profile
CK-MB
Troponin C
ANA
Toxicology screen
For newborns and infants:
Metabolic evaluation: Lactate, ammonia, pyruvate, carnitine level (total and free), acylcarnitine, serum organic acids and amino acids, chromosomal analysis
Prior to blood product transfusion or IVIG:
Serologies for enterovirus, adenovirus, coxsackie A and B, echovirus, influenza, HIV, CMV, RSV, EBV, hepatitis, and Lyme.
Transplant serologies

Other Tests
Urine organic acids
Nasopharyngeal aspirate or endotracheal tube aspirate
Rapid viral panel

Endomyocardial biopsy

Endomyocardial biopsy should be strongly considered in consultation with a pediatric cardiologist after competing etiologies of dilated cardiomyopathy have been excluded and refractory symptoms of heart failure persist despite standard medical management. Significant and life-threatening arrhythmias, symptoms suggestive of a systemic immune-mediated process, such as rash, fever, or eosinophilia, or other evidence of collagen vascular disease, give further reason to perform a biopsy for tissue analysis.

Biopsy of endomyocardial tissue has historically been the gold standard method for diagnosing acute myocarditis. However, its ability to demonstrate myocardial inflammation by histology is limited by the patchy nature of inflammatory infiltrate present in this disease. The "Dallas criteria" were developed in 1986 for diagnostic standardization in adult patients and require "a process characterized by an inflammatory infiltrate of the myocardium with necrosis and/or degeneration of adjacent myocytes not typical of ischemic damage" to definitively diagnose myocarditis.[19] The Dallas criteria have historically been applied to pediatric patients. Because of the patchy nature of myocardial injury, at least five tissue samples for histologic analysis should be obtained from the right ventricular free wall during cardiac catheterization. However, among patients who died of postmortem-confirmed myocarditis, Dallas criteria were met in only about 50% of cases.[20,21] Other studies report similarly limited results using biopsy for diagnosis.[22–24] Furthermore, a virus has been identified in tissue samples that did not meet Dallas criteria for myocarditis.[25] Finally, the presence of Dallas criteria myocarditis has not been shown to identify patients who will respond to immune modulation therapy and does not predict prognosis.[26]

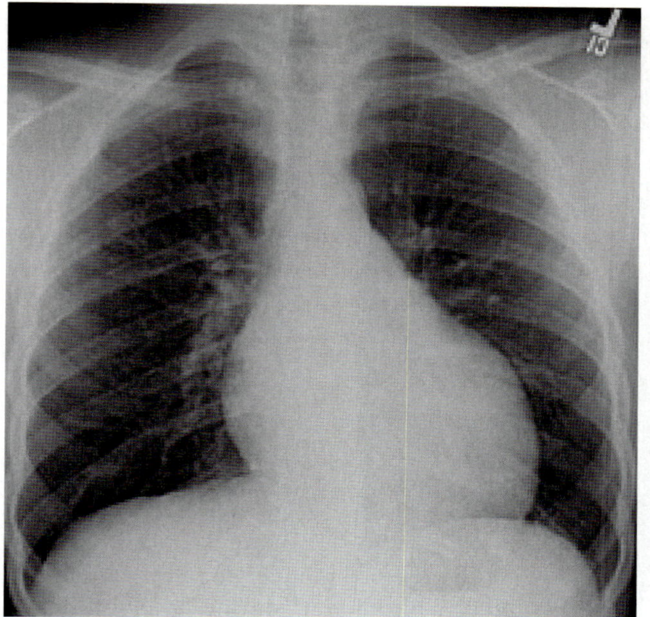

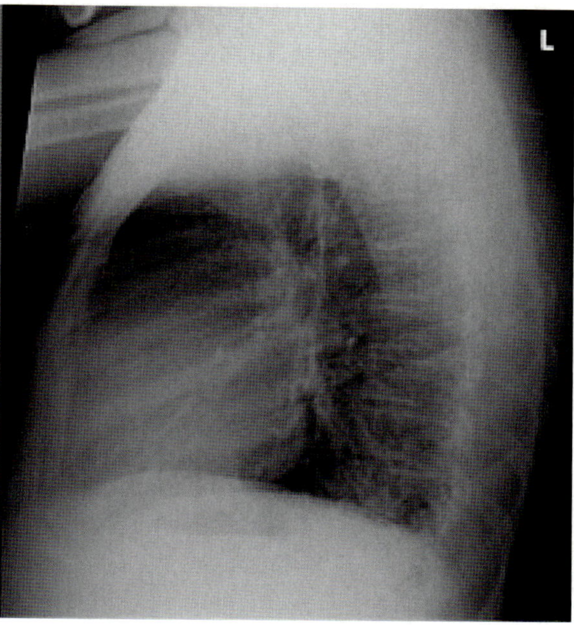

FIGURE 38–2 ■ The chest radiograph reveals an enlarged cardiac silhouette with prominent pulmonary vascular markings on both anterior–posterior and lateral views. (*With permission from Geggel R, ed. Multimedia Library of Congenital Heart Disease. Boston, MA: Children's Hospital. http://www.childrenshospital.org/mml/cvp.*)

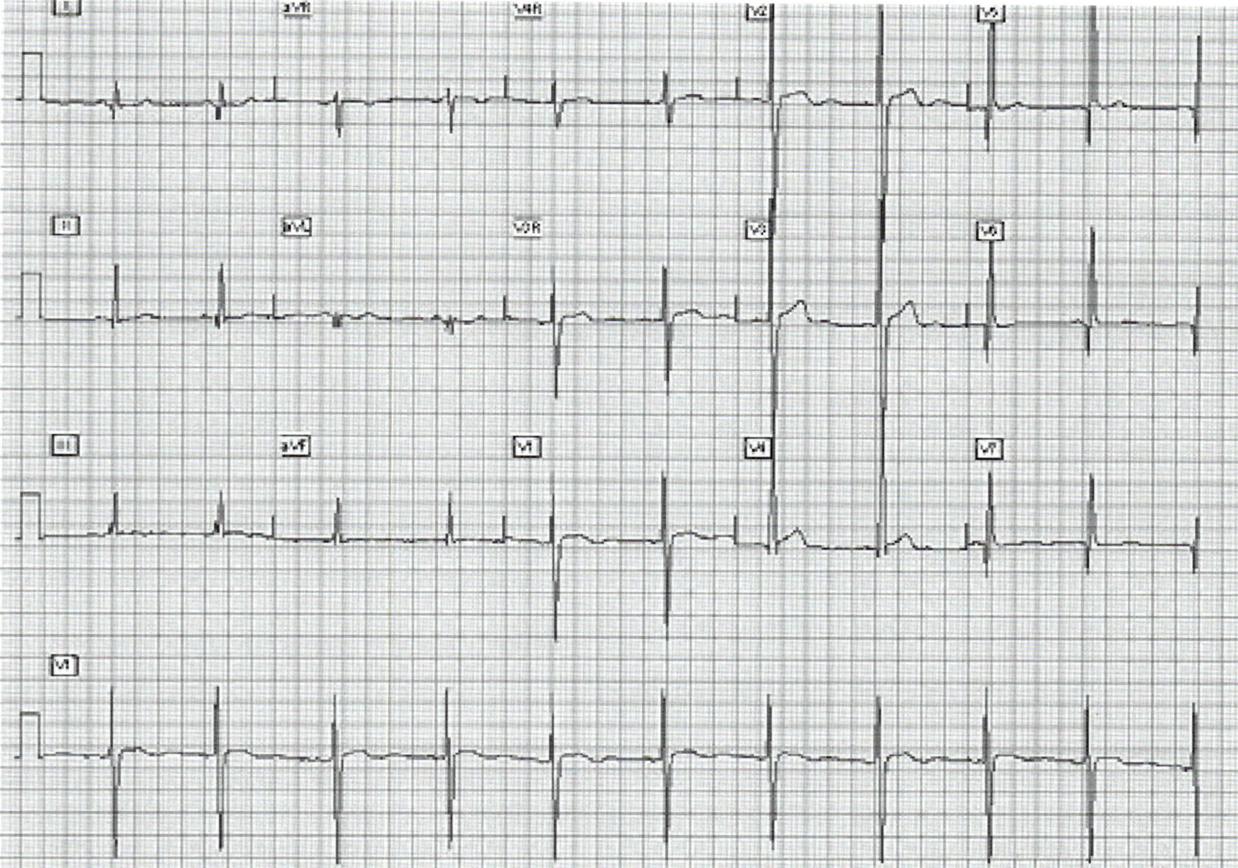

FIGURE 38–3 ■ The electrocardiogram tracing shows left ventricular forces at the upper limits of normal (S wave in V2 30 mm, 95% for age) and nonspecific T-wave flattening in the inferior and lateral leads). T-wave abnormalities are common in patients with myocarditis. (*With permission from Geggel R, ed. Multimedia Library of Congenital Heart Disease. Boston, MA: Children's Hospital. http://www.childrenshospital.org/mml/cvp.*)

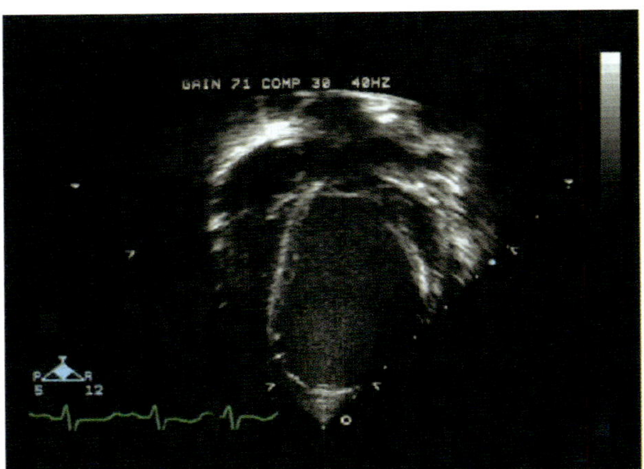

FIGURE 38–4 ■ Shown is a still frame from an apical four chamber echocardiographic view of a child with myocarditis. The left ventricle is markedly dilated and poorly functioning. (*With permission from Geggel R, ed. Multimedia Library of Congenital Heart Disease. Boston, MA: Children's Hospital. http://www.childrenshospital.org/mml/cvp.*)

Recognizing that the incidence of myocarditis has been underrepresented using traditional biopsy diagnosis, broader clinical–pathological criteria that incorporate newer diagnostic techniques are used for more accurate identification of patients with myocarditis. In patients in whom biopsy is indicated, MRI may be used to target areas of myocardial inflammation, which are most likely to yield tissue samples representative of disease.

In an effort to identify viral presence in myocarditis patients for diagnosis, treatment, and prognosis, biopsy specimens are now routinely tested using polymerase chain reaction (PCR) and ribonucleic acid hybridization for rapid and specific viral detection.

Detection of viruses in myocardial tissue

Viruses are considered the most common cause of myocarditis, but confirmation relies on identification of a viral pathogen in the myocardial tissue. In the past, this has depended on successful viral isolation using peripheral culture methods and or serial serology. Endomyocardial biopsy samples of myocardium were routinely culture-negative in cases of suspected acute viral myocarditis. With the advent of PCR, viral detection is becoming more common from cardiac tissue and body fluids. Using PCR in 38 myocardial tissue samples from patients with suspected myocarditis and 17 control samples, Martin et al. detected virus in 68% of myocarditis patients and none from the controls.[25] A study by Bowles et al.[27] sampled myocardial tissue from 624 patients with myocarditis and 149 patients with dilated cardiomyopathy, and used PCR analysis for viral diagnosis. Viral genome was detected from 38% of myocarditis patients (142 with adenovirus, 85 with enterovirus, 18 with cytomegalovirus), as well as a few cases with influenza, herpes simplex virus, Epstein–Barr virus, parvovirus, respiratory syncytial virus, and influenza A. Importantly, viral material was also detected among 20% of the dilated cardiomyopathy patients (18 with adenovirus and 12 with enterovirus), supporting persistent viral infection as an etiologic factor in the development of dilated cardiomyopathy. Pauschinger et al. found 24 of 94 patients with idiopathic dilated cardiomyopathy had adenoviral or enteroviral positive PCR testing from cardiac tissue samples.[28]

Treatment

Immunotherapies

Variable success has been reported using immunotherapies in the early treatment of acute myocarditis, including the use of immune globulin, prednisone, methylprednisolone, azathioprine, and OKT3.[29–32] The goal in using these agents has been to reduce the inflammatory response that is thought to lead to myocardial injury. However, there is a debate whether suppressing the body's initial systemic immune response to a viral illness, as in acute viral myocarditis, leads to delayed or insufficient viral clearance. Unfortunately, clear evidence of efficacy and improved clinical outcome in pediatric patients with acute myocarditis, who receive immunosuppressive therapies, remains controversial.[33–35] However, significant benefit has been reported in adults with acute myocarditis who have evidence of cardiac autoantibodies on biopsy compared to a lack of benefit among patients without autoantibodies.[36]

Cardiovascular support

For patients with severely compromised ventricular function and in whom symptoms of decreased oxygen delivery are present, support with inotropic agents, phosphodiesterase inhibitors, and diuretics is necessary. Cardiogenic shock with circulatory collapse may require mechanical support of the circulation with extracorporeal membrane oxygenation or ventricular assist device. Extracorporeal membrane oxygenation and ventricular assist device therapies are often used as a "bridge" to cardiac transplantation.

Outcome

The overall survival rate without cardiac transplant among pediatric patients with biopsy-proven myocarditis has been estimated at 75–80%, with no significant difference using immunosuppressive therapies.[31,37] Interestingly, adult data show an improved long-term survival rate at 5 years after biopsy-proven myocarditis among patients with fulminant myocarditis when compared to those with acute (nonfulminant) myocarditis.[38]

PERICARDITIS

Pericardial disease describes pathology related to the pericardial membranes and potential fluid space surrounding the heart. Pericarditis may be associated with congenital causes, inflammatory conditions, infection, and other chronic disease processes. An approach to the patient with suspected pericarditis is shown in Figure 38–5.

Pathogenesis

Acute pericarditis comprises an inflammatory infiltration of the pericardial membranes, often with excessive pericardial fluid accumulation. The pericardial sac normally contains approximately 15–35 mL of serous fluid in the average adult, and exists because of a space between the inner visceral pericardium (epicardium) and outer parietal pericardium. Inflammatory fluid causing pericarditis can be either effusive (constrictive hemodynamics persist after the pericardial effusion is removed) or noneffusive, and can cause tamponade physiology in extreme cases.

Clinical Presentation

Chest pain is present in many cases of acute pericarditis, but may be absent when disease has been more indolent. The quality of the pain tends to be sharp and precordial in nature, often worse upon inspiration or with coughing. Pain is usually most severe in the recumbent position, can radiate to the left shoulder or arm, and may be partially relieved by leaning forward or upon sitting upright. Fever is a common symptom, particularly with infectious etiologies. Cardiac auscultation often reveals a pericardial friction rub. Patients may present with evidence of sepsis, particularly in bacterial pericarditis.

Constrictive pericarditis, which can occur with chronic fibrosis of the pericardium, may present with signs and symptoms of heart failure (including dyspnea, orthopnea, and hepatomegaly) caused by restricted ventricular filling and an increase in diastolic pressures among all four cardiac chambers.

Pericardial effusion and tamponade

Acute pericarditis is often associated with the accumulation of excess pericardial fluid, which may be transudative or exudative in nature. These pericardial effusions, depending on their overall size and rate of

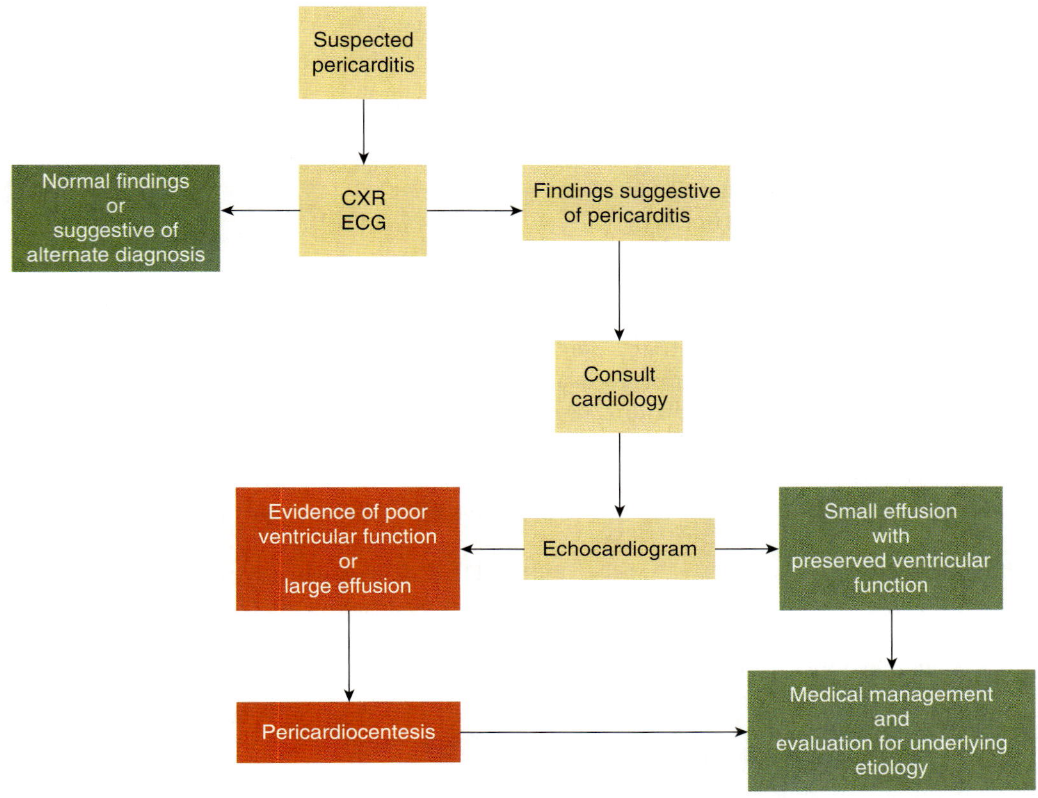

FIGURE 38–5 ■ Algorithm for evaluation of suspected pericarditis in the pediatric patient.

accumulation, have a varying effect on cardiac function. In cases where fluid accumulates slowly and the pericardium is compliant enough to avoid elevation in intrapericardial pressure, cardiac function is preserved. However, cardiac tamponade or cardiac failure can occur in small or large effusions when they accumulate rapidly, causing increased intrapericardial pressure and limited venous return to the heart. This ultimately causes decreased diastolic filling and resultant compromised cardiac output. The classic finding in tamponade physiology is pulsus paradoxus, defined as a decrease in systolic blood pressure greater than or equal to 10mm Hg with inspiration. This can be detected by Korotkoff sounds with manual blood pressure measurement or by a change in the pulse-oximetry waveform during inspiration.[39] ECG in tamponade demonstrates diffusely low QRS voltages.

Differential Diagnosis

Etiologies of pericarditis are listed in Table 38–7 and include infectious as well as noninfectious causes. Both viral and bacterial infections can cause acute pericarditis with significant pericardial effusions. Noninfectious causes include autoimmune conditions, connective tissue disease, malignancy, postpericardiotomy syndrome, and trauma.

Diagnosis

Chest radiograph findings

On chest radiograph, the cardiac silhouette may be enlarged in cases where a sizeable effusion is present. Associated pleural fluid may be visible as well, commonly on the left side of the diaphragm. Potential etiologies may be suggested by additional findings, such as pneumonia or evidence of malignancy.

Electrocardiographic findings

ECG findings early in disease, may demonstrate J-point and S–T elevation in the inferior and anterior leads, as well as PR segments that are deflected in a direction opposite to the P wave in each lead. With progression of disease, J-points may return to baseline with T wave flattening and eventual inversion.

Echocardiographic findings

Echocardiography is considered the primary imaging modality for the evaluation of pericardial effusion. However, loculated effusions are often difficult to detect using echocardiography and can be better visualized using CT or MRI (Figure 38–6). Another advantage to echocardiography is its ability to assess ventricular function and Doppler evidence for tamponade physiology.

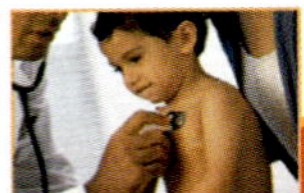

Table 38–7.

Etiologies of Pediatric Acute Pericarditis

- Idiopathic
- Bacterial
  - *Neisseria meningitidis*
  - *Hemophilus influenza*
  - *Staphylococcus aureus*
  - *Mycobacterium tuberculosis*
  - *Borrelia burgdorferi*
- Viral
  - Coxsackie virus
  - Cytomegalovirus
  - Human immunodeficiency virus
  - Other viruses
- Fungal
  - *Candida*
  - Other fungi
- Parasitic
  - *Toxoplasma gondii*
- Vasculitis
- Systemic lupus erythematosus
- Rheumatoid arthritis
- Dermatomyositis
- Scleroderma
- Rheumatic fever
- Inflammatory bowel disease
- Kawasaki disease
- Malignancy
- Graft versus host disease
- Pneumonia
- Uremia
- Drugs
- Chest wall irradiation
- Trauma
- Postpericardiotomy

Laboratory evaluation

The value of blood tests is limited in screening for acute pericarditis. Cardiac troponin may be elevated, but may be more representative of adjacent myocardial inflammation. Other systemic markers of inflammation may be elevated, such as peripheral white blood cell count and erythrocyte sedimentation rate. Testing for specific diseases known to cause pericardial disease are indicated when suggested by history and examination features. Fluid analysis, when obtained during pericardiocentesis, may be diagnostic in cases because of bacterial or malignant etiologies. In general, pericardial biopsy is not considered helpful in diagnosis.

Treatment

Nonsteroidal anti-inflammatory medications, such as ibuprofen, are the first-line treatment for pericarditis. In

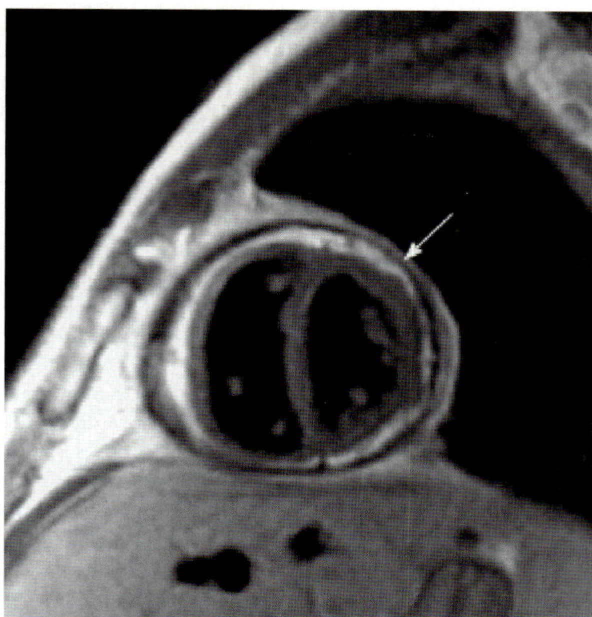

FIGURE 38–6 ■ Magnetic resonance imaging fast spin echo image with blood suppression in a ventricular short-axis plane showing circumferential thickening of the pericardium (black rim between the epicardial and pericardial fat) consistent with pericarditis (arrow). (*With permission from Geggel R, ed. Multimedia Library of Congenital Heart Disease. Boston, MA: Children's Hospital. http://www.childrenshospital.org/mml/cvp.*)

cases that do not respond adequately to this intervention, corticosteroids may be given. Pericardiocentesis is reserved for cases in which tamponade physiology is present or when particularly large fluid volumes are present. This procedure is generally performed using percutaneous needle aspiration in the subxiphoid region, ideally with the guidance of ultrasound or fluoroscopy. Acutely while awaiting drainage, intravascular volume expansion may aid in cardiac filling. Inotropes and vasoconstrictors are generally ineffective in tamponade physiology. Recurrent effusions that do not respond to medical management often require surgical pericardotomy.

REFERENCES

1. Bowles NE, Ni J, Kearney DL, et al. Detection of viruses in myocardial tissues by polymerase chain reaction: evidence of adenovirus as a common cause of myocarditis in children and adults. *J Am Coll Cardiol.* 2003;42:466-472.
2. Liu P, Mason J. Advances in the understanding of myocarditis. *Circulation.* 2001;104:1076-1082.
3. Kawai C. From myocarditis to cardiomyopathy: mechanisms of inflammation and cell death: learning from the past for the future. *Circulation.* 1999;99:1091-1100.
4. Matsumori A, Yamada T, Suzuki H, Matoba Y, Sasayama S. Increased circulating cytokines in patients with myocarditis and cardiomyopathy. *Br Heart J.* 1994;72:561-566.
5. Zaragoza C, Ocampo C, Saura M, et al. The role of inducible nitric oxide synthase in the host response to coxsackie myocarditis. *Proc Natl Acad Sci U S A.* 1998;95:2469-2474.
6. Zaragoza C, Ocampo CJ, Saura M, McMillan A, Lowenstein CJ. Nitric oxide inhibition of Coxsackie replication in vivo. *J Clin Invest.* 1997;100:1760-1767.
7. Mikami S, Kawashima S, Kanazawa K, et al. Low-dose N omega-nitro-L-arginine methyl ester treatment improves survival rate and decreases myocardial injury in a murine model of viral myocarditis induced by Coxsackievirus B3. *Circ Res.* 1997;81:504-511.
8. Pankuweit S, Portig I, Lottspeich F, Maisch B. Autoantibodies in sera of patients with myocarditis: characterization of the corresponding proteins by isoelectric focusing and N-terminal sequence analysis. *J Mol cell Cardiol.* 1997; 29:77-84.
9. Felix SB, Stuaudt A, Dorffel WV, et al. Hemodynamic effects of immunoadsorption and subsequent immunoglobulin substitution in dilated cardiomyopathy: Three-month results from a randomized study. *Am J Cardiol.* 2000;35: 1590-1598.
10. Felix SB, Staudt A, Landsberger M, et al. Removal of cardiodepressant antibodies in dilated cardiomyopathy by immunoadsorption. *J Am Coll Cardiol.* 2002;39:646-652.
11. Staudt A, Schaper F, Stangl V, et al. Immunohistological changes in dilated cardiomyopathy induced by immunoadsorption therapy and immunoglobulin substitution. *Circulation.* 2001;103:2681-2686.
12. Smith SC, Ladenson JH, Mason JW, Jaffe AS. Elevations of cardiac troponin I associated with myocarditis: experimental and clinical correlates. *Circulation.* 1997;95: 163-168.
13. Lauer B, Niederau C, Kuhl U, et al. Cardiac troponin T in patients with clinically suspected myocarditis. *J Am Coll Cardiol.* 1997;30:1354-1359.
14. Soongswang J, Durongpisitkul K, Ratanarapee S, et al. Cardiac troponin T: its role in the diagnosis of clinically suspected acute myocarditis and chronic dilated cardiomyopathy in children. *Pediatr Cardiol.* 2002;23: 531-535.
15. Soongswang J, Durongpisitkul K, Nana A, et al. Cardiac troponin T: a marker in the diagnosis of acute myocarditis in children. *Pediatr Cardiol.* 2005;26:45-49.
16. Gagliardi MG, Bevilacqua M, Di Renzi P, et al. Usefullness of magnetic resonance imaging for diagnosis of acute myocarditis in infants and children, and comparison with endomyocardial biopsy. *Am J Cardiol.* 1991;68:1089-1091.
17. Abdel-Ary H, Boye P, Zagrosek A, et al. Diagnostic performance of cardiovascular magnetic resonance in patients with suspected myocarditis: comparison of different approaches. *J Am Coll Cardiol.* 2005;45:1812-1822.
18. Mahrholdt H, Goedecke C, Wagner A, et al. Cardiovascular magnetic resonance assessment of human myocarditis: a comparison to histology and molecular pathology. *Circulation.* 2004;109:1250-1258.
19. Aretz HT, Billingham ME, Edwards WD, et al. Myocarditis: a histopathologic definition and classification. *Am J Cardiovasc Pathol.* 1987;1:3-14.
20. Chow LH, Radio SJ, Sears TD, McManus BM. Insensitivity of right ventricular endomyocardial biopsy in the diagnosis of myocarditis. *J Am Coll Cardiol.* 1989;14:915-920.
21. Hauck AJ, Kearney DL, Edwards WD. Evaluation of postmortem endomyocardial biopsy specimens from

38 patients with lymphocytic myocarditis: implications for role of sampling error. *Mayo Clin Proc.* 1989;64:1235-1245.

22. Schmaltz AA, Apitz J, Hort W, Maisch B. Endomyocardial biopsy in infants and children: experience in 60 patients. *Pediatr Cardiol.* 1990;11:15-21.
23. Nugent AW, Davis AM, Kleinert S, et al. Clinical, electrocardiographic, and histologic correlations in children with dilated cardiomyopathy. *J Heart Lung Transplant.* 2001;20: 1152-1157.
24. Chandra RS. The role of endomyocardial biopsy in the diagnosis of cardiac disorders in infants and children. *Am J Cardiovasc Pathol.* 1987;1:157-172.
25. Martin AB, Webber S, Fricker J, et al. Acute myocarditis: rapid diagnosis by PCR in children. *Circulation.* 1994;90:330-339.
26. Mason JW, O'Connell JB, Herskowitz A, et al. A Clinical trial of immunosuppressive therapy for myocarditis. The Myocarditis Treatment Trial Investigators. *N Engl J Med.* 1995;333:269-275.
27. Bowles NE, Ni J, Kearney DL, et al. Detection of viruses in myocardial tissues by polymerase chain reaction: evidence of adenovirus as a common cause of myocarditis in children and adults. *J Am Coll Cardiol.* 2003;42:466-472.
28. Pauschinger M, Bowles NE, Fuentes-Garcia FJ, et al. Detection of adenoviral genome in the myocardium of adult patients with idiopathic left ventricular dysfunction. *Circulation.*1999:1348-1354.
29. Drucker NA, Colan SD, Lewis AB, et al. y-Globulin treatment of acute myocarditis in the pediatric population. *Circulation.* 1994;89:252-257.
30. English RF, Janosky JE, Ettedgui JA, Webber SA. Outcomes for children with acute myocarditis. *Cardiol Young.* 2004;14:448-493.
31. Feltes TF, Adatia I. Immunotherapies for acute viral myocarditis in the pediatric patient. *Pediatr Crit Care Med.* 2006;7(6):S17-S20.
32. Robinson J, Hartling L, Vandermeer B, Crumley E, Klassen TP. Intravenous immunoglobulin for presumed viral myocarditis in children and adults. *Cochrane Database Syst Rev.* 2005;(1):CD004370. doi:10.1002/14651858.
33. Chen H, Liu J, Yang M. Corticosteroids for viral myocarditis. *Cochrane Database Syst Rev.* 2006;(4):CD004471. doi:10.1002/14651858.
34. Frustaci A, Chimenti C, Calabrese F, et al. Immunosuppressive therapy for active lymphocytic myocarditis virological and immunologic profile of responders versus nonresponders. *Circulation.* 2003;107:857-863.
35. Lee KJ, McCrindle BW, Bohn DJ, et al. Clinical outcomes of acute myocarditis in childhood. *Heart.* 1999;82: 226-233.
36. McCarthy RE, Boehmer JP, Hruban RH, et al. Long-term outcome of fulminant myocarditis as compared with acute (nonfulminant) myocarditis. *N Engl J Med.* 2000;342:690-695.
37. Tamburro RF, Ring JC, Womback K. Detection of pulsus paradoxus associated with large pericardial effusions in pediatric patients by analysis of the pulse-oximetry waveform. *Pediatrics.* 2002;109:673.

SECTION 9

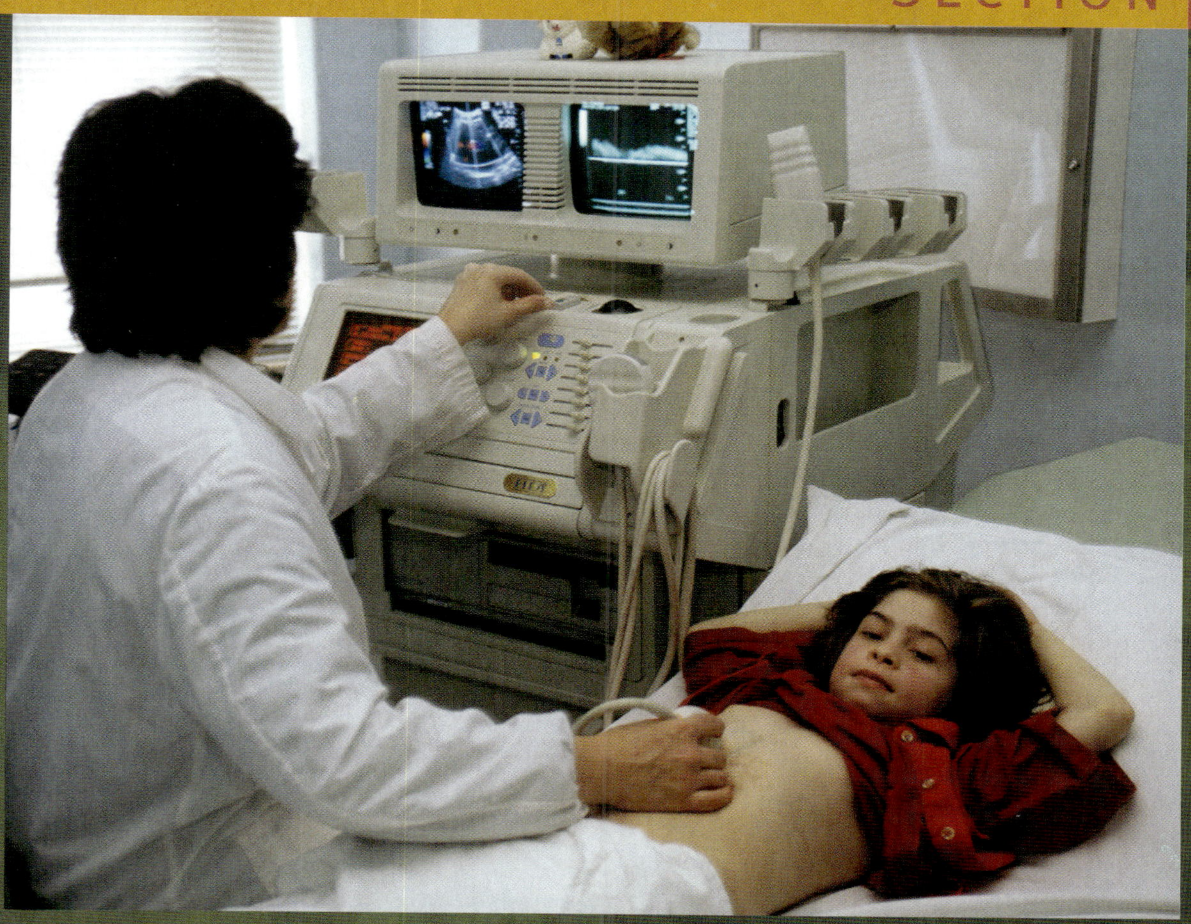

Gastrointestinal Infections

CHAPTER 39

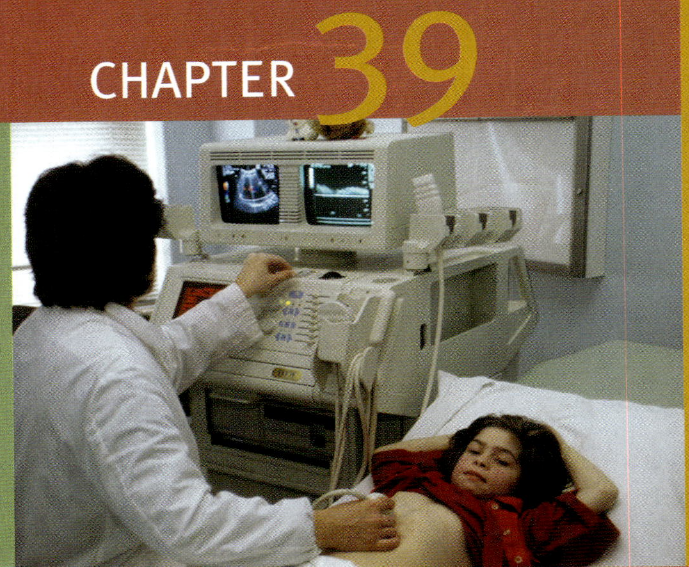

Gastroenteritis

Philip R. Spandorfer

DEFINITIONS AND EPIDEMIOLOGY

Gastroenteritis is commonly defined as either the acute onset of vomiting or the acute onset of diarrhea with or without vomiting. Vomiting is defined as the acute onset of forceful expulsion of gastric secretions through the oral cavity and should be differentiated from posttussive emesis and gastroesophageal reflux. Diarrhea is defined as loose or watery stools. When bloody diarrhea and fever are present, the illness is referred to as dysentery. The majority of gastroenteritis in the developed countries occurs due to a viral etiology, predominantly rotavirus, whereas bacteria are responsible for the majority of cases in less developed nations. Relatively common causes of gastroenteritis are listed in Table 39–1.

In the United States, children develop between one and three episodes of gastroenteritis per year. This disease burden results in 3.5 million physician visits, 200,000 hospitalizations, 900,000 hospital days, and approximately 300 deaths annually.[1] Children will invariably have had an episode of rotavirus gastroenteritis by the age of 5 years.[2] Furthermore, rotavirus has been found to cause a more serious illness than other pathogens; children with rotavirus gastroenteritis are five times more likely to become dehydrated than children with other causes of acute gastroenteritis.[3]

Internationally, there are over 1 billion cases of gastroenteritis and 1 to 3 million deaths attributed to dehydration annually.[4] Most deaths occur in regions that have poor access to health care. Although the number of deaths due to dehydration seems high, this number represents an 80% decrease from the 1980s when there were approximately 5 million deaths per year.[5]

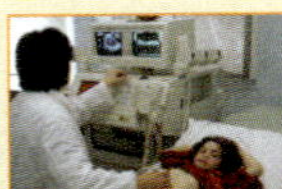

Table 39–1.

Causes of Gastroenteritis

Viral
Rotavirus
Astrovirus
Norovirus and other calicviruses
Adenovirus (types 40 and 41)
Picornavirus
Norwalk virus
Bacterial
Campylobacter species (particularly jejuni)
Clostridium difficle
Escherichia coli
Salmonella species (e.g., typhi)
Shigella species
Mycobacteria avium complex
Vibrio cholera
Yersinia enterocolitica
Aeromonas species
Parasite
Giardia
Cryptosporidium spp.

PATHOGENESIS

The intestinal tract is constantly secreting and absorbing fluids. In fact, it secretes and absorbs approximately 6 L of fluid in a day from saliva, gastric secretions, pancreatic secretions, and intestinal secretions. When the reabsorption process is disrupted, children can sustain large volume losses and become dehydrated.[6]

Gastroenteritis, whether viral, bacterial, or parasitic in origin, is transmitted primarily via the fecal oral route; some viruses may also be transmitted by the airborne route. Once ingested, viral particles enter the enterocytes of the small intestinal villi and induce villus shortening and cell destruction. Cell destruction generates cytokines and chemokines, which cause inflammation. The inflammation impairs absorption of nutrients, particularly carbohydrates, and potentiates the diarrhea. Villus cells are temporarily replaced with immature crypt-like cells that cause the intestine to secrete water and electrolytes. Some viral proteins also act as entertoxins directly. Recovery occurs when the villi regenerate and the villus epithelium matures.[7]

Bacteria, on the other hand, utilize three mechanisms to induce illness; adhesion, toxin production, and mucosal invasion. The bacteria need to adhere to the intestinal mucosa in order to multiply and cause disease. Adhesion occurs through hair-like fimbria that bind to receptors on the intestinal cell wall. The mucosal adherence may interfere with absorption or even cause fluid secretion, both of which ultimately lead to increased diarrhea. They may secrete enterotoxins that alter small intestine function. This alteration may stimulate secretion and cause watery diarrhea. The toxins can block sodium absorption, which also increases water and electrolyte losses. They may also trigger inflammation that also increases diarrhea. Cytotoxins can cause cell death of the distal small intestine or colon and lead to bloody mucousy stools. They may be invasive bacteria and cause ulceration or abscess formation, which also causes white blood cells and visible blood in the stool. Dehydration from diarrhea tends to result more from watery diarrhea as the volume tends to be greater than that seen with bloody mucousy stools.[7]

Vomiting is controlled by the emetic center in the medulla. The emetic center receives input primarily from four areas: the gastrointestinal tract, the chemoreceptor trigger zone, the vestibular apparatus, and the cerebral cortex. The gastrointestinal tract and the chemoreceptor trigger zone activate the emetic process during gastroenteritis whereas the vestibular apparatus and cerebral cortex tend not to be involved. Chemoreceptors in the intestine can stimulate the emetic center via vagal afferent nerves and afferent fibers associated with the sympathetic nervous system. The chemoreceptor trigger zone senses chemicals in the blood. If there is a potentially toxic substance detected, the emetic center is triggered and the vomiting process begins. When the emetic center is triggered to induce emesis, the normal peristaltic activity of the gastrointestinal tract (GI) stops and reverses direction, such that a peristaltic wave starts near the ileum and pushes contents in a reverse direction towards the duodenum. Duodenal distention is one of the factors that stimulates the actual act of emesis.[8]

Once the process of gastroenteritis has started, clinical concern focuses on dehydration. Under normal conditions, water comprises 70% of lean body mass, with two-thirds intracellular and one-third extracellular. Of the extracellular water component, 25% is circulating in plasma and 75% is interstitial. When patients have fluid losses from gastroenteritis, most of the fluid comes from the extracellular component. With time, usually days, fluid will shift from the intracellular compartment to the extracellular compartment to compensate for the fluid losses. Fluid that is lost from the body during gastroenteritis tends to have an electrolyte composition similar to plasma with a few exceptions; gastric fluid has higher hydrogen and chloride concentrations whereas fluid losses from the pancreas have a high bicarbonate concentration.[9] The different etiologic agents tend to cause different electrolyte losses as well. Cholera tends to have a high sodium loss, other bacterial agents are intermediate in the sodium lost, and viral agents tend to cause a diarrhea with a lower sodium loss (Figure 39–1).[10] These sodium losses will affect treatment recommendations.

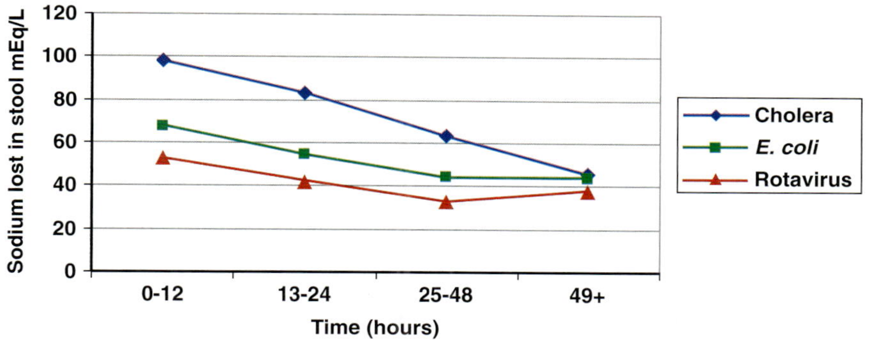

FIGURE 39–1 ■ Sodium losses from cholera, bacterial GE, VGE. Decreasing amount of sodium lost in the stool over time from various etiologies of gastroenteritis. Notice that there is a larger amount of sodium lost with cholera as compared to rotavirus.

CLINICAL PRESENTATION

Patients typically report nausea, anorexia, abdominal pain, vomiting, and diarrhea. Some patients have fever. In viral gastroenteritis, vomiting often precedes the diarrhea by several days. It is during the vomiting-only phase of the illness that making the correct diagnosis could be difficult. For the typical course of illness, symptoms last for 3–7 days. If the patient has carbohydrate malabsorption from damage to the brush border, then drinking fluids with high concentrations of simple carbohydrates (i.e., juice) or dairy products with lactose tends to exacerbate the diarrhea. Caliciviruses (e.g., Norwalk agent) often present with isolated vomiting though diarrhea, fever, headache, malaise, and myalgias are frequently reported. Bloody diarrhea is more common in bacterial gastroenteritis, particularly shigella, salmonella, and invasive strains of *Escherichia coli.*

The physical examination should first focus on determining the degree of dehydration. There are several guidelines and scoring systems that assist in determining the degree of dehydration. A recent metanalysis evaluated signs and symptoms of dehydration (Table 39–2).[11] Perhaps the most clinically useful system is a four-point dehydration score (Table 39–3). This system assesses general appearance, presence of sunken eyes, dry mucous membranes, and delayed capillary refill. Each feature present scores one point. The system is interpreted as a score of zero is not dehydrated, a score of one is mild dehydration, a score of two is moderate dehydration, and a score of three to four is severe dehydration.[12]

DIFFERENTIAL DIAGNOSIS

Acute gastroenteritis remains a clinical diagnosis and there are numerous etiologies that can present with vomiting or diarrhea and should be considered prior to making the diagnosis of gastroenteritis. Causes of vomiting and diarrhea are summarized in Tables 39–4 and 39–5.

DIAGNOSIS

The diagnosis of gastroenteritis remains a clinical diagnosis based on the presence of acute forceful vomiting or three or more loose or watery stools in a 24-hour period in the absence of other clinical features that suggest an alternate cause (e.g., peritoneal signs). Testing of stool for the presence of viral antigens (e.g., rotavirus) or stool cultures may be helpful in situations where there is confusion as to the correct diagnosis, but is unnecessary for routine cases of gastroenteritis.

Laboratory Evaluation

Much discussion has occurred about the need for laboratory evaluation in dehydrated patients. The use of laboratory values does not aid in the diagnosis or in determining the degree of dehydration. However, laboratories may assist in directing treatment.[13–15] Approximately one-third of moderately dehydrated patients will also be hypoglycemic.[16] Hence, an important laboratory value to check in a dehydrated patient would be serum glucose. Serum electrolyte measurements should be considered in the following situations: (1) History or

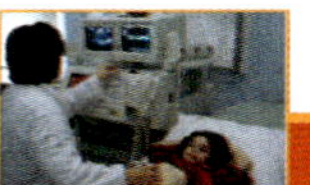

Table 39–2.

Signs and Symptoms of the Presence of At Least 5% Dehydration

Finding	LR if Present	LR if Absent	Sensitivity	Specificity
Prolonged capillary refill	4.1 (1.7–9.8)†	0.57 (0.39–0.82)	0.6 (0.29–0.91)	0.85 (0.72–0.98)
Abnormal skin turgor	2.5 (1.5–4.2)†	0.66 (0.57–0.75)	0.58 (0.40–0.75)	0.76 (0.59–0.93)
Abnormal respiratory pattern	2.0 (1.5–2.7)†	0.76 (0.62–0.88)	0.43 (0.31–0.55)	0.79 (0.72–0.86)
Sunken eyes	1.7 (1.1–2.5)	0.49 (0.38–0.63)†	0.75 (0.62–0.88)	0.52 (0.22–0.81)
Dry mucous membranes	1.7 (1.1–2.6)	0.41 (0.21–0.79)†	0.86 (0.80–0.92)	0.44 (0.13–0.74)
Cool extremity*	1.5, 18.8	0.89, 0.97	0.10, 0.11	0.93, 1.00
Weak pulse*	3.1, 7.2	0.66, 0.96	0.04, 0.25	0.86, 1.00
Absent tears	2.3 (0.9–5.8)	0.54 (0.26–1.13)	0.63 (0.42–0.84)	0.68 (0.43–0.94)
Increased heart rate	1.3 (0.8–2.0)	0.82 (0.64–1.05)	0.52 (0.44–0.60)	0.58 (0.33–0.82)
Sunken fontanelle	0.9 (0.6–1.3)	1.1 (0.82–1.54)	0.49 (0.37–0.60)	0.54 (0.22–0.87)
Poor overall appearance	1.9 (0.97–3.8)	0.46 (0.34–0.61)†	0.80 (0.57–1.04)	0.45 (−0.1 to1.02)

**These findings were evaluated only in two studies and a pooled value was not obtained; the range of the point estimates is presented.*

†The likelihood ratio is interpreted such that the likelihood of dehydration would increase if the LR if present is greater than 1.0. Clinically useful values have an LR positive value of 2 or more with a 95% CI that does not cross 1.0. Furthermore, the LR if absent would be interpreted such that the likelihood of dehydration would decrease if the sign was absent. Clinically useful values have an LR negative value of 0.5 or less and have 95% CI that does not cross 1.0. Values indicated by symbol † are the clinically helpful values.

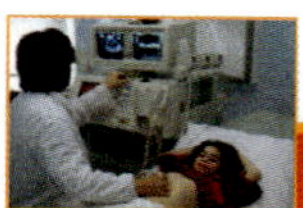

Table 39–3.

Four-Point Dehydration Scoring System*

Ill appearance (tired, washed-out appearing)
Capillary refill greater than 2 seconds
Dry mucous membranes
Absent tears

**The interpretation of the scoring system is that the patient receives 1 point for each sign or symptom present. The maximum score is 4 points. A score of 0 points indicates no dehydration present, 1 point indicates mild dehydration, 2 points indicates moderate dehydration, and 3–4 points indicates severe dehydration.*

suspicion of improper formula preparation; (2) excessive water administration; (3) age younger than 6 months; and (4) clinical suspicion of an electrolyte abnormality. Low serum bicarbonate levels indicate more significant dehydration.

Stool cultures are helpful when there is bloody diarrhea. *Salmonella*, *Shigella*, and *Camplyobacter* can be detected by routine stool bacterial culture; special cultures are required for *Yersinia enterocolitica*, *Vibrio cholerae*, *Vibrio parahaemolyticus*, and *E. coli* O157:H7. Fecal leukocytes are often present with invasive or cytotoxin-producing bacteria (usually polymorphonuclear; if mononuclear, consider *Salmonella typhi*). However, negative tests do not reliably exclude the diagnosis of bacterial gastroenteritis. In the developed world, fecal leukocyte testing results rarely alter clinical management. If there is a clinical suspicion for *Clostridium difficile* or a parasitic infection, appropriate studies should be performed.

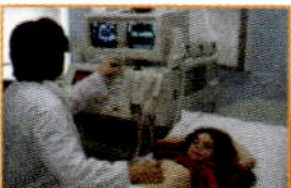

Table 39–4.

Differential Diagnosis of Vomiting

Common Causes
Pneumonia
Urinary tract infection/pyleonephritis
Appendicitis
Other surgical abdomen*
Gastroesophageal reflux in infants
Posttussive emesis

Uncommon Causes
Increased intracranial pressure/brain tumor
Hepatitis
Central nervous system infection
Poisoning
Diabetic ketoacidosis
Pregnancy
Metabolic disorders

**Includes pyloric stenosis, intussusception, volvulus, and small bowel obstruction.*

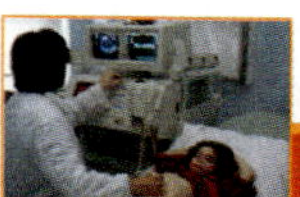

Table 39–5.

Differential Diagnosis of Diarrhea

Common Causes
Toddler's diarrhea (nonspecific diarrhea of childhood)
Diarrhea associated with antibiotic use
Fecal incontinence associated with constipation
Malabsorption (carbohydrate primarily)

Uncommon Causes
Inflammatory bowel disease
Cystic fibrosis
Celiac disease
Primary immunodeficiencies*

**Includes IgA deficiency, X-linked agammaglobulinemia, and severe combined immune deficiency.*

TREATMENT

The immediate treatment of gastroenteritis focuses on identifying the degree of dehydration present and addressing shock if present (Figure 39–2).[17] If shock is present, then immediate intravenous or intraosseous access should be obtained and aggressive fluid resuscitation instituted with 20 mL per kg boluses of isotonic saline. Frequent reevaluation is required for the severely dehydrated patient who presents in shock. However, since many families seek medical care at the early onset of vomiting, the patient may be found not to be dehydrated. The nondehydrated patient with gastroenteritis should receive supportive care, consideration of an appropriate antiemetic to abate the emesis, and instructions on oral rehydration therapy (ORT). ORT is the recommended initial treatment of choice for patients with mild to moderate dehydration.[1,18] Intravenous fluid therapy should be the primary treatment of choice for severely dehydrated patients.

Oral Rehydration Therapy

ORT is the frequent administration of small volumes of an appropriate oral rehydration solution. ORT should be differentiated from an oral challenge as ORT utilizes the glucose sodium cotransport mechanism in the intestinal tract to absorb water (Figure 39–3). It has been shown to be as effective as intravenous fluid therapy for mild-to-moderately dehydrated patients and was successful as first-line therapy in over 80% of dehydrated patients treated in an emergency department.[19–21] This finding was shown prior to the widespread use of the antiemetic 5-HT_3 receptor antagonist, ondansetron, which has improved the success rate of ORT.[22–24] If the patient is not in shock, then it is prudent to administer an antiemetic that has minimal side effects such as

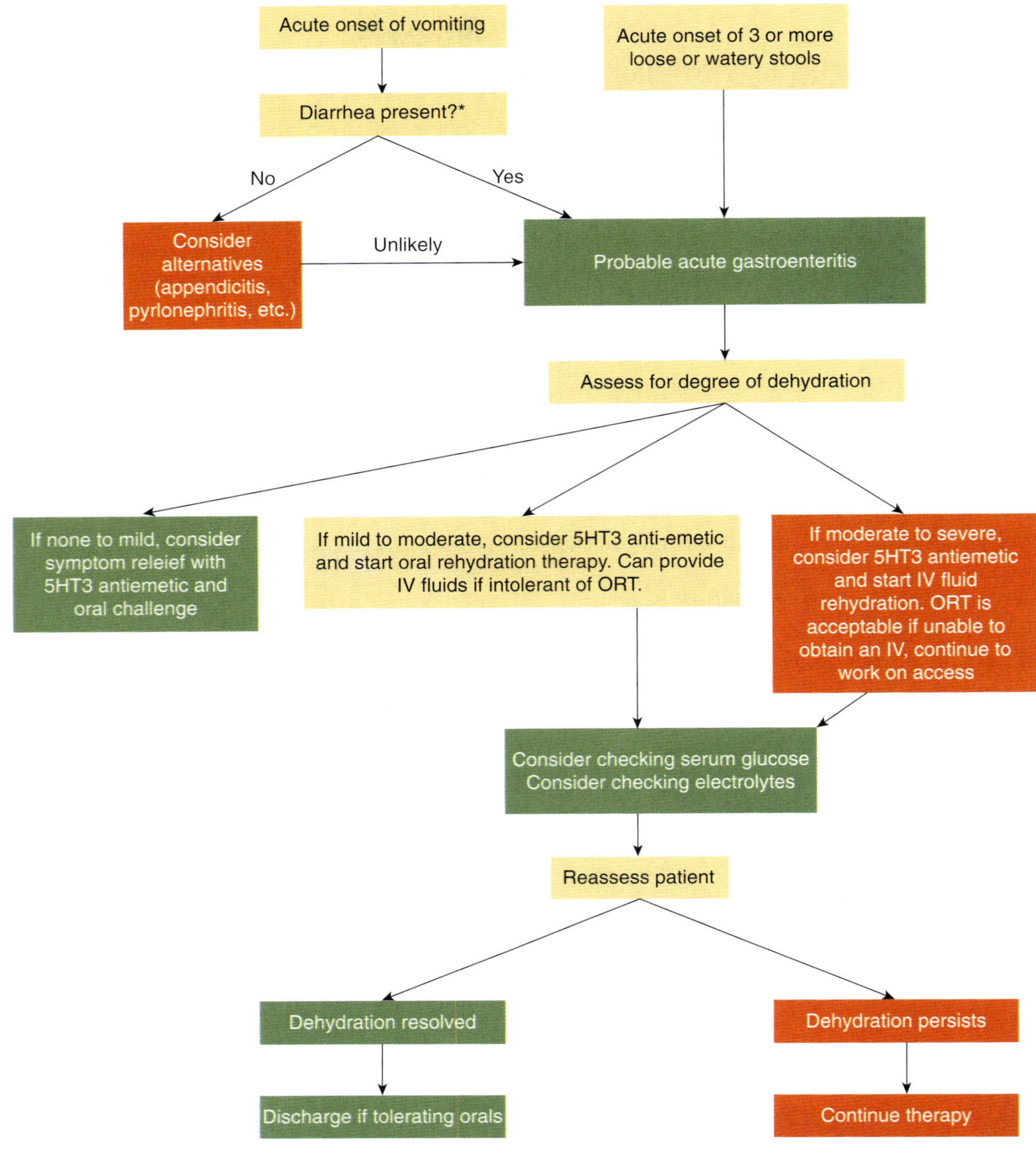

FIGURE 39–2 ■ Management of acute gastroenteritis.
*Bloody diarrhea—send bacterial culture and C. Difficile tests, if relevent antibiotic exposure.

ondansetron. The orally disintegrating tablet (ODT) can be placed on the tongue a few minutes prior to initiation of ORT. Although there are not clear dosing guidelines for gastroenteritis, 1-mg ondansetron solution is effective for children weighing up to 10 kg, 2 mg ondansetron ODT is effective for children weighing 10–20 kg, and 4 mg ondansetron ODT can be used for children weighing over 20 kg. It is emphasized that ORT should be differentiated from much more commonly used oral challenge. Simply giving a child something to drink, whether it is an oral rehydration solution or juice, is an oral challenge and may be sufficient treatment in many cases. However, ORT is the use of an appropriate rehydration solution administered in small volumes frequently. A reasonable ORT protocol is the administration of 5–10 mL of an unflavored electrolyte solution (such as pedialyte) via a syringe or small cup every 5 minutes. This fluid aliquot can be administered slowly over the 5-minute interval if the child is nauseated or all at once if the child is tolerating ORT well. The volume administered can be increased as the child tolerates. The actual amount of fluid the child requires for correction of the dehydration is based on the degree of dehydration present. If the child is mildly dehydrated, they are considered to

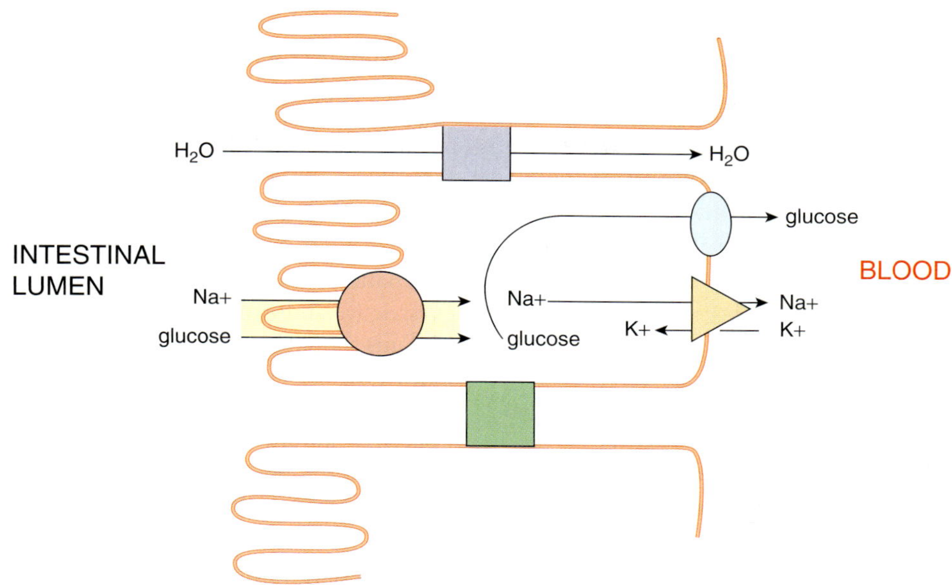

FIGURE 39–3 ■ Physiology of oral rehydration therapy. (Oral rehydration therapy utilizes passive transport mechanisms to absorb water from the intestinal lumen into the circulating plasma. The sodium glucose cotransport mechanism is one of the most common passive cotransport systems and is depicted in this schematic. For every molecule of sodium absorbed, there is a molecule of glucose (or amino acid) absorbed. There is a sodium gradient maintained by the sodium potassium ATPase system. Water is passively absorbed via the sodium gradient. This system is maintained even in severe cases of diarrhea.)

have a 5% total body water loss with a 50 mL/kg deficit, whereas moderately dehydrated children are considered to have a 5–10% water loss and a 50–100 mL/kg fluid deficit, and severely dehydrated patients are considered to have greater than 10% dehydration with more than 100 mL/kg fluid deficit. The total fluid deficit can be calculated by multiplying the percentage dehydration by the present weight. The result of that calculation is the amount of fluid required to completely correct the fluid losses. However, patients who are tolerating ORT well and are less dehydrated can be sent home to continue the therapy and finish the complete correction of their dehydration. If the patient is not tolerating ORT, then the child should be rehydrated with intravenous fluids. The reasons for children not tolerating ORT include oral refusals, persistent severe vomiting, ongoing losses that exceed intake, somnolence, and parental noncompliance with ORT instructions. The child who did not tolerate ORT initially may tolerate it if attempted again.[25,26]

On occasion, there may be difficulty in obtaining intravenous access in a dehydrated patient. ORT can be instituted if the child can cooperate with the treatment. If not, then nasogastric tube administration of oral rehydration solutions would be appropriate.[27]

It is important to select an oral rehydration solution for use in ORT. The World Health Organization has two oral rehydration solutions with varying concentrations of sodium. The higher sodium concentration fluid (90 mEq/L) is appropriate for cholera as there is a very high loss of sodium in the stool with cholera. The lower sodium concentration (75 mEq/L) is appropriate for bacterial etiologies as there is an intermediate stool sodium loss due to the bacterial organisms. The oral maintenance solutions, such as pedialyte, have an even lower sodium concentration of 45 mEq/L and are appropriate for most cases of viral gastroenteritis in previously well-hydrated, well-nourished children.[28,29] An explanation as to why each solution is appropriate for the respective etiologies relates to the amount of sodium lost in the stool. As can be seen in Figure 39–1, there is a greater amount of sodium lost in the stool from cholera and hence a greater amount of sodium needs to be replaced. Bacterial etiologies have an intermediate amount of sodium loss in the stool and viral etiologies have the lowest amount of stool sodium losses.[10]

Intravenous Fluid Rehydration

Intravenous fluid rehydration should be utilized for patients who are severely dehydrated or for mild-to-moderately dehydrated patients who failed ORT. After venous access has been obtained, isotonic saline is administered in 20 mL per kg aliquots. Frequent re-evaluations will assist the clinician in determining the duration of therapy. Glucose-containing solutions should be avoided for bolus rehydration as 20 mL per kg will deliver a glucose load that is greater than the recommended dose for documented hypoglycemia.[17] It has been clearly shown that rapid intravenous rehydration is effective and deficit replacement over a 24-hour period is no longer necessary.[30,31]

Ongoing Care

Once the patient has been rehydrated as demonstrated by the resolution or improvement of the signs and symptoms initially present, outpatient management of the ongoing illness is appropriate. However, children, younger than 36 months or so, may need to demonstrate tolerance of oral fluids prior to discharge. If the patient needs hospitalization for ongoing treatment, it has been shown that these patients do well in short stay units.[32,33]

Aftercare Instructions

Parents should be instructed on appropriate rehydration techniques to manage any ongoing illness at home, particularly syringe administration of oral rehydration fluids. The use of ondansetron is appropriate to assist in the reduction of episodes of emesis at home. Currently, there is no medication that is recommended to reduce the severity of diarrhea. The American Academy of Pediatrics and the World Health Organization recommend the resumption of a normal diet as soon as rehydration has been completed. In general, foods with large amounts of simple carbohydrates or fat will be less well tolerated than complex carbohydrates, yogurt, unseasoned meats, etc. On occasion, lactose may not be well tolerated and avoidance of dairy products with lactose may improve the diarrhea. The commonly taught BRAT diet (bananas, rice, apple sauce, toast) is unnecessarily restrictive and is no longer recommended.[34] Breast-fed infants should resume breast feeding as soon as possible and formula-fed infants should resume full-strength feeds. There is no need for dilution of the formula.[15] The parents should follow up with the primary care provider. If there is concern that the child is worsening, then the patient requires reevaluation.

Bacterial Gastroenteritis

Bacterial causes of gastroenteritis require antibiotic therapy in certain situations (Table 39–6).

Table 39–6.

Indications for Antibiotic Therapy for Bacterial Gastroenteritis

Bacteria	Indication	Agent	Comment
Aeromonas spp.	Prolonged disease	TMP/SMX, ciprofloxacin	
Camplyobacter jejuni	Severe or systemic infection or immunodeficiency	Azithromycin, fluoroquinolones, erythromycin	Associated with postinfectious syndromes including Guillain–Barré and Reiter's syndromes
Clostridium difficile	Symptomatic and not improving	Metronidazole (IV or PO), oral vancomycin, or cholestyramine	Classically associated with prolonged antibiotic exposure but sporadic cases may occur
Cryptosporidium parvum	Immunocompromised or severe and protracted diarrhea	Nitozoxanide	Usually occurs in immunocompromised hosts; outbreaks among immunocompetent individuals linked to contaminated city water supplies, swimming pools, and daycares
Escherichia coli (Travelers diarrhea)	Severe or systemic infection	TMP/SMX, fluoroquinolones	
Salmonella spp.	Age <3 months, immunodeficiency, or disseminated disease	Ampicillin, cefotaxime, ciprofloxacin, azithromycin	Nontyphii Salmonella infections are associated with exposure to reptiles, raw eggs, and undercooked poultry
Shigella spp.	Dysentery or epidemic setting (e.g., daycare)	Ceftriaxone, azithromycin, fluoroquinolones, TMP/SMX	Neurologic findings (e.g., seizures, encephalopathy) may precede bloody diarrhea; high peripheral band count is a characteristic laboratory feature
Vibrio cholerae	Treatment decreases illness duration	Ciprofloxacin, TMP/SMX, tetracyclines	
Yersinia enterocolitica	Sepsis, immunedeficiency	Cefotaxime, TMP/SMX, fluoroquinolones	Pain mimics appendicitis; associated with chitterlings exposure and iron overload syndromes

REFERENCES

1. American Academy of Pediatrics, Provisional Committee on Quality Improvement, Subcommittee on Acute Gastroenteritis. Practice parameter: the management of acute gastroenteritis in young children. *Pediatrics.* 1996; 97:424-436.
2. Grimwood K, Buttery JP. Clinical update: rotavirus gastroenteritis and its prevention. *Lancet.* 2007;370(9584): 302-304.
3. Giaquinto C, Van Damme P, Huet F, et al. Clinical consequences of rotavirus acute gastroenteritis in Europe, 2004–2005: the REVEAL Study. *J Infect Dis.* 2007;195 (suppl 1):S26-S35.
4. Linhanes AC, Bresee JS. Rotavirus vaccine and vaccination in Latin America. *Pan Am J Public Health.* 2000;8:305-331.
5. Black RE, Morris SS, Byrce J. Where and why are 10 million children dying every year? *Lancet.* 2003;361:2226-2234.
6. Despopoulos A, Silbernagl S. Nutrition and digestion. In: Despopoulos A, Silbernagl S, eds. *Color Atlas of Physiology.* 4th ed. New York: Thieme Medical Publishers; 1991:228.
7. World Health Organization. The Epidemiology and Etiology of Diarrhoea. *Readings on Diarrhoea: Student Manual.* Geneva, Switzerland: World Health Organization; 1992:9.
8. Alhashimi D, Alhashimi H, Fedorowicz Z. Antiemetics for reducing vomiting related to acute gastroenteritis in children and adolescents. Cochrane Database of Systematic Reviews 2006, Issue 4. Art. No.: CD005506. DOI: 10.1002/14651858.CD005506.pub3.
9. Finberg L. Therapy of dehydration resulting from gastrointestinal fluid loss. In: Finberg, L, Kravath, RE, Hellerstein, S, eds. *Water and Electrolytes in Pediatrics: Physiology, Pathophysiology, and Treatment.* 2nd ed. Philadelphia: W.B. Saunders Company; 1993:141-147.
10. Molla MA, Rahman M, Sarker SA, Sack DA, Molla A. Stool electrolyte content and purging rates in diarrhea caused by rotavirus, enterotoxigenic *E. coli* and *V. cholerae* in children. *J Pediatr.* 1981;98(5):835-838.
11. Steiner MJ, DeWalt DA, Byerley JS. Is this child dehydrated? *JAMA.* 2004;291(22):2746-2754.
12. Gorelick MH, Shaw KN, Murphy KO. Validity and reliability of clinical signs in the diagnosis of dehydration in children. *Pediatrics.* 1997;99(5):e6.
13. Wathen JE, MacKenzie T, Bothner JP. Usefulness of the serum electrolyte panel in the management of pediatric dehydration treated with intravenously administered fluids. *Pediatrics.* 2004;114:1227-1234.
14. Teach SJ, Yates EW, Feld LG. Laboratory predictors of fluid deficit in acutely dehydrated children. *Clin Pediatr.* July, 1997;395-400.
15. King CK, Glass R, Bresee JS, Duggan C. Managing acute gastroenteritis among children: oral rehydration, maintenance, and nutritional therapy. *MMWR.* 2003;52:1-16.
16. Hirschhorn N, Lindenbaum JL, Greenough WB, Alam SM. Hypoglycemia in children with acute diarrhea. *Lancet.* July, 1966;128-133.
17. Shaw KN, Spandorfer PR. Dehydration. In: Fleisher, GR, Ludwig, S, Henretig, FM, Ruddy, RM, Silverman, BK, eds. *Textbook of Pediatric Emergency Medicine.* 5th ed. Philadelphia: Lippincott Williams & Wilkins; 2006:233-238.
18. World Health Organization. *The Treatment of Diarrhea: A Manual for Physicians and Other Senior Health Workers.* Geneva: World Health Organization; 1995. WHO/CDD/SER/80.2 Rev.3.
19. Atherly-John YC, Cunningham SJ, Crain EF. A randomized trial of oral vs. intravenous rehydration in a pediatric emergency department. *Arch Pediatr Adolesc Med.* 2002;156:1240-1243.
20. Spandorfer PR, Alessandrini EA, Joffe MD, Localio R, Shaw KN. Oral versus intravenous rehydration of moderately dehydrated children: a randomized, controlled trial. *Pediatrics.* 2005;115:295-301.
21. Fonseca BK, Holdgate A, Craig JC. Enteral vs. Intravenous rehydration therapy for children with gastroenteritis: a meta-analysis of randomized controlled trials. *Arch Pediatr Adolesc Med.* 2004;158:483-490.
22. Ramsook C, Sahagun-Carreon I, Kozinetz CA, Moro-Sutherland D. A randomized trial comparing oral ondansetron with placebo in children with acute gastroenteritis. *Ann Emerg Med.* 2002;39(4):397-403.
23. Reeves JJ, Shannon MW, Fleisher GR. Ondansetron decreases vomiting associated with acute gastroenteritis: a randomized, controlled trial. *Pediatrics.* 2002;109(4):e62.
24. Freedman SB, Adler M, Seshadri R, Powell EC. Oral Ondansetron for gastroenteritis in a pediatric emergency department. *N Engl J Med.* 2006;354(16):1698-1705.
25. Spandorfer PR, Upham BD. Oral rehydration. In: Henretig, FM, King, C, eds. *Textbook of Pediatric Emergency Medicine Procedures.* 2nd ed. Philadelphia: Lippincott Williams & Wilkins; 2008:853-858.
26. Goepp JG, Santosham M. Oral rehydration therapy. In: Oski FA, DeAngelis CD, Feigin RD, McMillan JA, Warshaw JB, eds. *Principles and Practice of Pediatrics.* 2nd ed. Philadelphia: JB Lippincott Co.; 1994:849-859.
27. Nager AL, Wang VJ. Comparison of nasogastric and intravenous methods of rehydration in pediatric patients with acute dehydration. *Pediatrics.* 2002;109(4):566-572.
28. Gavin, N, Merrick, N, Davidson, B. Efficacy of glucose-based oral rehydration therapy. *Pediatrics.* 1996;98(1): 45-51.
29. Choice Study Group. Multicenter, randomized, double-blind clinical trial to evaluate the efficacy and safety of a reduced osmolarity oral rehydration salts solution in children with acute watery diarrhea. *Pediatrics.* 2001;101:613-618.
30. Reid SR, Bonadio WA. Outpatient rapid intravenous rehydration to correct dehydration and resolve vomiting in children with acute gastroenteritis. *Ann Emerg Med.* 1996;28(3):318-323.
31. Kanaan U, Dell K, Hoagland J, O'Riordan MA, Furman L. Accelerated intravenous rehydration. *Clin Pediatr.* 2003;42:421-426.
32. McConnochie KM, Conners GP, Lu E, Wilson C. How commonly are children hospitalized for dehydration eligible for care in alternative settings? *Arch Pediatr Adolesc Med.* 1999;153:1233-1241.
33. Mallory MD, Kadish H, Zebrack M, Nelson D. Use of a pediatric observation unit for treatment of children with dehydration caused by gastroenteritis. *Pediat Emerg Care.* 2006;22(1):1-6.
34. Duggan C, Nurko S. "Feeding the gut": the scientific basis for continued enteral nutrition during acute diarrhea. *J Pediatr.* 1997;131(6):801-808.

CHAPTER 40

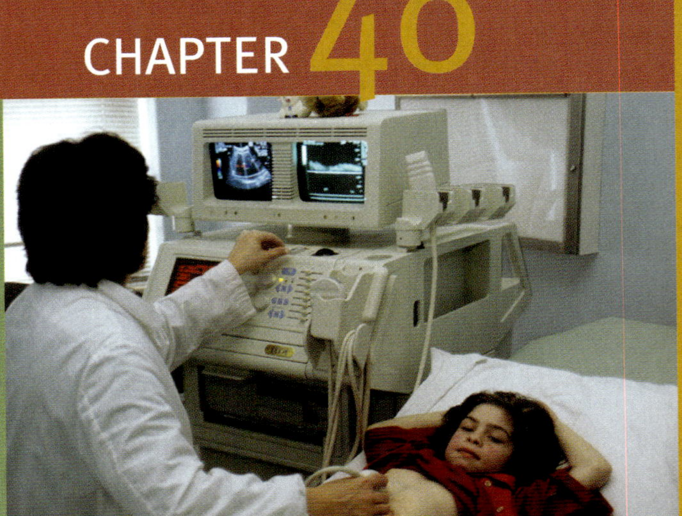

Hepatitis

Binita M. Kamath and Barbara A. Haber

Numerous pathogens can directly or indirectly cause hepatitis. However, primary viral infection of the liver is most commonly caused by several specific hepatotropic viruses. Several such viruses have been identified, in particular A, B, C, D, E, and G (Table 40–1). The characteristics, epidemiology, clinical features, and management of these viruses differ significantly. The discussion here will focus largely on viral hepatitis caused by hepatitis A, B, and C.

DEFINITIONS AND EPIDEMIOLOGY

Hepatitis A

Hepatitis A virus (HAV) is a common infection in the United States and worldwide. The incidence in the United States has declined significantly with the introduction of the vaccination.[1,2] The incidence of reported acute HAV has declined to 1.5 cases per 100,000 people.

Table 40–1.

Clinical Characteristics of Hepatotropic Viruses

	Hepatitis A	Hepatitis B	Hepatitis C	Hepatitis D	Hepatitis E	Hepatitis G
Transmission	Fecal–oral	Vertical, infected needles, sexual contact, and close bodily contact	Vertical, infected needles, sexual contact, and transfusion prior to 1992	Infected needles and sexual contact (coinfection with HBV)	Fecal–oral	Vertical, blood transfusion, and sexual contact
Fulminant hepatitis	Rare	Rare	Rare	Yes, with HBV	Yes, in pregnant women	No
Chronicity	No	Yes*	Yes†	Yes	No	No
Treatment of chronic disease	N/A	IFN or lamivudine	IFN and ribavarin	IFN	N/A	N/A
Vaccine	Two doses, universally recommended for children more than 12 months	Three doses, universally recommended in children	None	HBV vaccine	None	None

**Risk for chronicity is inversely related to age at acquisition; 90% of patients infected during the perinatal period develop chronic infection.*

†80% develop chronic infection.

IFN, interferon; HBV, hepatitis B virus.

Some of this decline may also be attributable to an improvement in hygiene and sanitation practices. HAV is spread by the fecal–oral route, from person to person, and is highly contagious. A typical setting for an outbreak of HAV infection is a childcare center, especially one that includes children who are not yet toilet trained. International travelers to developing countries are also at particular risk of contracting HAV. Parenteral transmission of HAV, although uncommon, has been reported.[3]

Hepatitis B

Hepatitis B virus (HBV) remains a global health problem, despite the availability of an effective vaccine. Approximately 1 million individuals die from HBV-related liver disease each year.[4] The prevalence of HBV carriers varies from 0.1% to 2% in Western countries to 10–20% in southeast Asia and sub-Saharan Africa.[4–7] With the implementation of universal vaccination in 1991 within the United States, acute HBV incidence has declined significantly, to the lowest rate ever recorded: 1.8 cases per 100,000 people in 2005.[2] Declines occurred among all age groups but were greatest among children aged younger than 15 years. In Western countries, the majority of children with newly acquired HBV are immigrants, the children of immigrants, and adoptees.

HBV is found in all body fluids, and its epidemiology is similar to human immunodeficiency virus (HIV). The prevalence of chronic HBV infection and the mode of transmission vary by geography. In countries where HBV is endemic, perinatal transmission is the most important cause of chronic infection, although this also occurs in the United States in children of HBV-infected mothers who do not receive appropriate immunoprophylaxis at birth. The infants of all women who are hepatitis B surface antigen (HBsAg)-positive are at risk; vertical transmission occurs in 5–20% of infants born to HBsAg-positive mothers. However, mothers who are hepatitis B e antigen (HBeAg)-positive are more likely to transmit the virus with vertical transmission occurring in 70–90% of infants born to HBsAg-positive mothers who are also HBeAg positive. Postnatal infection is also possible from household contacts in endemic countries, where the HBsAg carrier rates are high and vaccination is not common. In low-prevalence areas, unprotected sexual intercourse and intravenous drug use are the major routes of spread. Horizontal transmission may also occur via minor breaks in the skin or close bodily contact in households where children are living with HBV-infected individuals or in communities of immigrants. Posttransfusion HBV infection should rarely occur with current screening protocols.

Hepatitis C

Hepatitis C virus (HCV) is a staggering global health problem, with approximately 250,000 children and more than 3 million adults being chronically infected in the United States.[2,8,9] HCV is particularly prevalent in Egypt.[10] It is the most common indication for liver transplantation in this country. The incidence of acute HCV infection has decreased since the implementation of blood bank screening in 1990, and the most common risk factor for acquisition of infection in adults is now injection-drug use. Sexual transmission can also occur, although with less efficiency than HBV or HIV. Vertical transmission is the most important route for childhood infection and occurs with a transmission rate of approximately 4%, which increases to 22% in women with concomitant HIV infection.[11] The risk of maternal–fetal transmission is also increased by the level of maternal HCV viremia. Household contact rarely leads to horizontal transmission.

PATHOGENESIS

Hepatitis A

HAV is a small RNA hepatovirus, belonging to the picornavirus group. It is remarkably resistant to heat, cold, and acidity and can remain stable in the environment for long periods. An outbreak of HAV has even been associated with frozen strawberries imported from Mexico and served in the Michigan school district. HAV is ingested and replicates in the small bowel. It migrates to the liver via the portal vein and enters the hepatocytes. HAV infection occurs in two phases. In the first noncytopathic phase, viral replication occurs within the cytoplasm of the hepatocyte. Notably, as an RNA virus, it does not integrate in the host chromosome. In the second cytopathic stage, there is hepatocellular damage and destruction, mediated by HAV-specific T cells.[12,13] Newly synthesized HAV is excreted in bile and shed in the stool. Fecal excretion of viral particles correlates with maximum infectivity in the early phase of illness and continues until the onset of hepatitis.

Hepatitis B

HBV is a hepadnavirus. The HBV genome consists of circular DNA, which encodes for the envelope (HBsAg) and core proteins (hepatitis B core antigen—HBcAg) and HBV DNA polymerase. HBV has a specific tropism for hepatocytes. The virus attaches to the hepatocyte and replicates within the nucleus,[14] generating large quantities of HBsAg, which can be detected in the circulation in acute or chronic infection. During the replication, the viral genome is converted into a covalently closed circular DNA and this is very resistant to antiviral therapy, thereby accounting for the difficulty in clearing the virus in chronic HBV treatment. The pathogenesis of HBV disease is related to cytotoxic T-cell-mediated lysis of infected hepatocytes.

There are eight genotypes of HBV: A–G. There is geographic variability in the prevalence of these genotypes. Recent data suggest that the genotype is associated with outcomes of HBV disease. Genotype A is more likely to respond to therapy with interferon (IFN).[15] Genotype C has been associated with the development of hepatocellular carcinoma.[16]

Mutations in the HBV genome are common, although the significance of only some of these is understood. The most common mutation identified is the "precore variant" caused by a single point mutation in the region encoding the precore. This mutation is associated with absence of HBeAg, the presence of hepatitis B e antibody (anti-HBe) but high levels of viremia. This mutant is stable and although it cannot secrete HBeAg, HBV replication is unaffected. HBeAg is an important target for the body's immune responses, and this therefore helps this mutant evade the host's defense.

Hepatitis C

HCV is a single-stranded RNA virus with its own unique genus, hepacivirus. The HCV genome encodes structural and nonstructural peptides.[17] The structural peptides comprise nucleocapsid and envelope proteins. The portion of the genome encoding for the envelope protein displays hypervariable regions, which results in the rapid accumulation of mutations. Many genetic variants can coexist in an individual, thus allowing the virus to evade the host defense mechanisms.[18] The pathogenesis of HCV infection in children is poorly understood but evidence from adults implicates immune-mediated hepatocyte damage.

There are six major HCV genotypes (1–6) with different subtypes and geographic variability.[19] Genotypes 1, 2, and 3 are the most common in the United States, with genotype 1 being the most common amongst these. HCV genotype is one of the strongest predictors of response to current therapies, and therefore genotyping must be ascertained prior to the initiation of treatment. Response to treatment is significantly lower in patients with genotype 1 as compared to those with genotype 2 or 3 (see Section "Treatment").[20]

CLINICAL PRESENTATION

All the hepatotropic viruses can result in acute and chronic infection (with the exception of HAV), although these differ significantly in the propensity to develop chronicity. Typical manifestations of acute viral hepatitis include malaise, fever, abdominal pain, and jaundice. However, these symptoms are not specific and may even be missed altogether.

Hepatitis A

The incubation period for HAV is 15–50 days. Most children with HAV infection are asymptomatic. Approximately one-third of infected children have the abrupt onset of nonspecific findings such as fever, nausea, diarrhea, emesis, and abdominal pain. Mild hepatomegaly and splenomegaly are common in the symptomatic group. Most preschool-aged children do not develop jaundice, so this illness may be dismissed as an intercurrent viral illness. The illness is generally self-limited, and the severity of symptoms is worse with older age. Over the age of 14 years approximately 70% of individuals will present with jaundice. In children <6 years, jaundice, when it does occur, usually resolves in 2 weeks, but adolescents and adults may be symptomatic for weeks to months.

Fulminant hepatic failure associated with acute HAV is very rare, occurring in <1% of cases. It is more common in individuals with other underlying chronic liver disease. On occasion, HAV may present atypically with a relapsing hepatitis, or with extrahepatic manifestations (vasculitis, arthritis, transverse myelitis, and aplastic anemia). HAV does not progress to chronic infection.

Although HAV is never a chronic infection, the disease burden is real. Illness can be severe and protracted. Furthermore, people can remain reservoirs of infection long after the symptoms of infection have passed.

Hepatitis B

The incubation period for HBV is 50–180 days. Acute HBV infection in children varies from asymptomatic infection to fulminant illness. The typical course of acute HBV infection has three phases, namely prodromal, symptomatic, and convalescence. The prodromal phase is rarely associated with immune-mediated features such as membranous glomerulonephropathy and vasculitis. The symptomatic phase, which begins 2–3 weeks later, is characterized by fatigue, fever, nausea, jaundice, and abdominal pain. Fatigue may be prolonged, but most of the symptoms resolve after 1–3 months. In infants and young children, acute HBV infection may be associated with Gianotti–Crosti syndrome, which is manifested by papular acrodermatitis on the face, buttocks, and limbs and lymphadenopathy (this condition can also occur with infection by viruses other than HBV). Fulminant HBV infection occurs more often in older children and adolescents.

The likelihood of progressing to chronic HBV infection is inversely related to the age at which the infection is acquired. Up to 90% of neonates will progress to chronic infection compared with 25–50% of children infected between the ages of 1 and 5 years, 6–10% of school-age children, and 1–5% of adults.[21] Most children with chronic HBV infection are asymptomatic and diagnosed during routine screening. Chronic HBV infection is rarely associated with membranous glomerulonephropathy and polyarteritis nodosa.

The natural history of chronic HBV in children is variable and also depends on age at acquisition. Perinatally acquired HBV infection is typically characterized by immunotolerance. These children remain HBeAg and HBsAg positive with very high serum HBV DNA; however, histologic injury is typically mild and they have minimally elevated serum aminotransferases. Few of these children spontaneously seroconvert (Table 40–2): only 2% per year of children younger than 3 years, and 4–5% per year of children older than 3 years.[22,23] This group of children with perinatally acquired immunotolerant HBV infection are typically Asian and comprise approximately half the pediatric population with chronic HBV infection.[24]

Individuals who acquire HBV infection during childhood usually have lower HBV DNA but more evidence of hepatitis with elevated alanine transferase (ALT) levels. These children commonly seroconvert to anti-HBe during the second decade of life.[25] After spontaneous HBeAg seroconversion, carriers have minimal HBV DNA, normal ALT, and minimal histologic changes on liver biopsy. Most children who achieve this inactive carrier state remain in this condition for years to decades.[24,26] Lifelong follow-up is required to ascertain that the inactive carrier state is maintained.[25]

Hepatocellular carcinoma is a feared complication of chronic HBV infection and is reported in children.[27,28] It is most likely to occur in the second decade of life. Many pediatric hepatologists perform annual serum alpha fetoprotein levels and surveillance abdominal ultrasonography for hepatocellular carcinoma; there are little data to support this practice.[24]

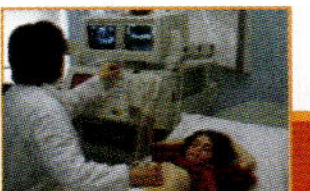

Table 40–2.

Hepatitis B: Definitions and Serology

Hepatitis B Disease State	Serologic Findings: Present	Serologic Findings: Absent
Acute hepatitis B	HBsAg IgM anti-HBc HBeAg	Anti-HBe Anti-HBs
HBV immune	Anti-HBs Anti-HBc positive if immune as a result of resolved infection	HbsAg
Chronic HBV	HBsAg (>6 months duration) Anti-HBc HbeAg	Anti-HBe Anti-HBs
Immunotolerant HBV	HbsAg HbeAg High HBV DNA Minimally elevated aminotransferases	Anti-HBe
Seroconversion	HBsAg Anti-HBc	HbeAg Anti-HBs

HBV, hepatitis B virus; HBsAg, hepatitis B surface antigen; HBeAg, hepatitis B e antigen; anti-HBe, hepatitis B e antibody.

Hepatitis C

The incubation period for HCV is 2 weeks to 6 months but averages 6–7 weeks. Acute HCV infection largely goes undetected in the pediatric setting and is indistinguishable from acute HAV or HBV. The acute illness usually passes unnoticed, but if symptoms are present these usually occur approximately 2 months after exposure. Only 10% of cases of acute illness are associated with jaundice.

HCV has a high propensity to develop chronic infection, occurring in 80% or more of cases.[29] The natural progression of chronic HCV infection in adults is somewhat defined—an adverse outcome in terms of risk of cirrhosis and hepatocellular carcinoma is associated with older age at acquisition of infection, presence of coinfection, alcoholic liver disease, and male gender. However, there is a paucity of data in children exploring the natural history of chronic HCV in the pediatric population. Chronic hepatitis and cirrhosis do occur in children with chronic HCV, although the disease is clearly more benign as compared to adults. There are very few reported cases of hepatocellular carcinoma in adolescents and young adults with childhood-acquired HCV.[30] It should be noted that, like adults, children with normal biochemistry can have advanced liver histology. Liver disease in children with HCV also does not correlate with specific genotypes or HCV RNA levels.[31]

Studies reporting the rates of spontaneous clearance of HCV infection in children are contradictory.[31–33] It appears that children with transfusion-acquired HCV have a higher chance of clearing the virus than those with vertical transmission.[34] Infants with perinatally acquired infection who do clear HCV will likely do so in the first 2 years of life.[9]

DIFFERENTIAL DIAGNOSIS

The differential diagnosis of viral hepatitis varies according to the clinical presentation (Table 40–3). Most

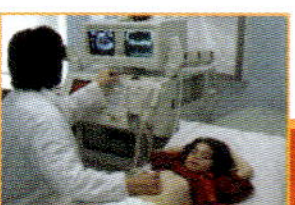

Table 40–3.

Differential Diagnosis of Hepatitis

Acute Hepatitis*	Hepatitis A virus
	Hepatitis B virus
	Hepatitis C virus
	Other viruses (adenovirus, Epstein–Barr virus, and coxsackie)
	Drugs or toxins
	Wilson disease
	Autoimmune hepatitis
Chronic Hepatitis†	Hepatitis B virus
	Hepatitis C virus
	Autoimmune hepatitis
	Wilson disease
	Alpha-1-antitrypsin deficiency

*Key features include fever, nausea, abdominal pain, and jaundice.
†May be asymptomatic but key features, if present, include fatigue, malaise, jaundice, and bruising.

young children with acute HAV will be asymptomatic, and others with acute HBV or HCV will have a nonspecific illness with fever, nausea, and malaise. These symptoms may be easily missed, and liver disease may never be considered. If jaundice is present then a hepatic cause is sought. An approach to the evaluation of a child with acute hepatitis is presented in Figure 40–1. In the acute

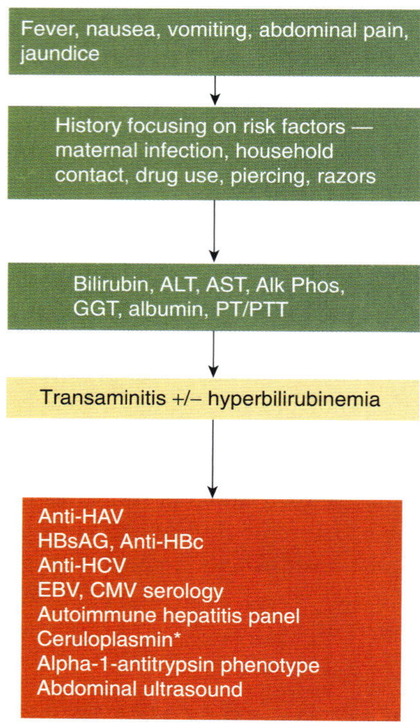

FIGURE 40–1 ■ Diagnostic algorithm for hepatitis.
*Screen for Wilson disease.

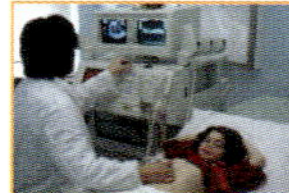

Table 40–4.

Patients to Screen for HBV

Patients to screen for HBV:
1. Child born to a woman with HBV infection
2. All internationally adopted children
3. Immigrant from high-prevalence areas
4. Household contacts of individuals with HBV
5. Patient with high-risk behaviors (injection drug use)
6. Patient with any evidence of liver disease

HBV, hepatitis B virus.

setting, it is important to evaluate the child for any synthetic dysfunction (coagulopathy), which may indicate fulminant hepatic failure (synthetic dysfunction with mental status changes). HAV, HBV, and HCV may rarely present with fulminant disease. Wilson disease (a disorder of copper metabolism) may certainly present in older children with these symptoms and the rapid onset of fulminant hepatic failure. Other viral infections such as Epstein–Barr virus, cytomegalovirus, or adenovirus may also be causative agents.

In children, chronic HBV or HCV is most likely to be asymptomatic and identified on routine screening (Tables 40–4 and 40–5). They may even have normal or minimally elevated serum transaminases. If a child has evidence of synthetic impairment as manifested clinically by ascites, jaundice, splenomegaly, bruising, or bleeding, this may be more indicative of another chronic liver disease such as autoimmune hepatitis or alpha-1-antitrypsin deficiency. These conditions are more likely to cause endstage liver disease in childhood than chronic HBV or HCV. It is worth noting, of course, that HBV and HCV may coexist with any other chronic liver disease of childhood.

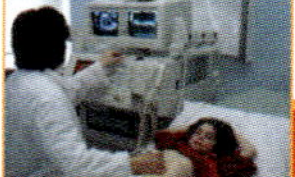

Table 40–5.

Patients to Screen for HCV

Patients to screen for HCV:
1. Child born to a woman with HCV infection
2. Child adopted from a country with high incidence of HCV
3. Patient with high-risk behaviors (injection drug use and multiple sexual partners)
4. Individual with needlestick injury
5. Patient with HIV infection
6. Patient with any evidence of liver disease
7. Patient who received transfusion or transplantation prior to 1992
8. Individual in corrections facility

HCV: hepatitis C virus.

DIAGNOSIS

A diagnostic approach to hepatitis is displayed in Figure 40–1.

Hepatitis A

Acute or recent HAV infection is detected by the presence of anti-HAV immune globulin (Ig) M in serum, and this is the gold standard for diagnosis. The antibody is positive from the onset of symptoms and remains positive for 4–6 months afterward. Anti-HAV IgG in serum indicates previous infection and lifelong immunity.

Hepatitis B

Screening for HBV infection should begin with HBsAg and anti-HBs. The presence of HBsAg denotes acute or chronic infection (Table 40–6), although HBsAg is occasionally detected within 3 weeks of immunization of healthy individuals. Anti-HBs identifies individuals who are immune, either by virtue of a resolved infection or by immunization. Certain patient populations should be screened routinely (Table 40–4).

IgM antibody to HBcAg (IgM anti-HBc) is the only marker that is specific to acute or recent HBV infection (except in infants) and as such has limited use. Anti-HBc is present with acute, resolved, or chronic infection although is not present after immunization. HBeAg is present in infected people with high infectivity, and anti-HBe is also present in infected people but these individuals are at lower risk of transmitting HBV. These serologies are summarized in Table 40–4. Quantitative HBV DNA measures are useful for determining treatment strategies. Children who are being considered for treatment should also undergo a liver biopsy.

Hepatitis C

Anti-HCV IgG antibody assays are the most useful screening tool in HCV infection, but there is no antibody pattern that distinguishes between past or present infection. There are no IgM HCV assays. The presence of HCV RNA, anti-HCV, and elevated aminotransferases may denote acute or chronic infection, and it may not be possible to distinguish these.

The presence of anti-HCV antibody denotes ongoing infection; up to 80% of patients who are infected have detectable antibody within 15 weeks of infection and within 5–6 weeks of hepatitis onset. HCV RNA can be detected in plasma by reverse transcription polymerase chain reaction (PCR) within 1–2 weeks of infection. A positive immunoassay for HCV should be followed up by a qualitative HCV RNA assay. If the initial qualitative RNA assay is negative, infection is not completely ruled out and a follow-up qualitative assay should be performed 4 weeks after the initial test. A quantitative HCV PCR is performed to determine viral load prior to making decisions regarding therapy. Chronic HCV infection is defined as the persistence of HCV RNA for at least 6 months.

Neither serum ALT nor HCV genotype nor viral load correlates with histologic severity. Therefore, liver biopsy is necessary to detect fibrosis and progression to cirrhosis. Liver biopsy is usually, but not always, performed prior to initiating therapy. HCV genotyping is mandatory, as it helps predict likelihood of response to therapy and duration of therapy.

The diagnosis of perinatal HCV transmission is confused by the passive transfer of maternal antibody, which may persist for up to 18 months of age, and by the ability of some infants to clear HCV spontaneously. Infants of women with chronic HCV should be tested by PCR every 6 months until the age of 2 years to determine if they have chronic infection.

High-risk populations who should be screened for HCV infection are summarized in Table 40–5.

TREATMENT

Hepatitis A

The management of acute HAV infection is supportive only, if required at all. Children diagnosed with acute HAV should be excluded from day care or school until

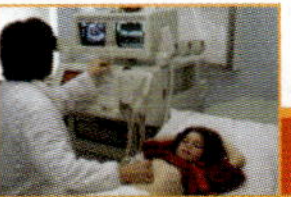

Table 40–6.

Interpretation of Hepatitis B Testing

HBsAg	Hepatitis B surface antigen	Detection of acute or chronic infection
Anti-HBs	Antibody to HBsAg	Immunity after vaccination or resolved infection
HBeAg	Hepatitis B e antigen	Infected, with high infectivity
Anti-HBe	Antibody to HBeAg	Infected, with low infectivity
Anti-HBc	Antibody to hepatitis B core antigen	Acute, resolved, or chronic infection
IgM anti-HBc	IgM antibody to HBcAg	Acute or recent infection

HBsAg, hepatitis B surface antigen; anti-HBe, hepatitis B e antibody; HBeAg, hepatitis B e antigen; HBcAg, hepatitis B core antigen.

1 week after the onset of symptoms to limit transmission when fecal excretion is high.[35] Even after they return to school it is crucial to adhere to universal precautions, as HAV may be present in stool for several months.

Hepatitis B

There is no specific therapy for acute HBV infection. Lamivudine and IFN-α are both licensed as single agents for use in the pediatric population with chronic HBV. The main treatment challenge in chronic HBV infection is selecting which children to treat. After the age of 3 years, children will undergo spontaneous seroconversion at a rate of 4–5% per year.[24] Therefore, currently treatment is offered to children with biochemically and histologically active disease who are considered at risk of developing cirrhosis. Specifically this includes children who are HBeAg positive and have elevated ALT values (two times the upper limit of normal). Current therapies are ineffective unless the ALT is elevated.

IFN-α has a beneficial and durable response (defined as a loss of HBV DNA or HBeAg seroconversion) in 30–50% of patients.[36,37] It is administered as a three-times-a-week subcutaneous injection for 24 weeks and has significant side effects including flu-like symptoms (fever, myalgia, and headache), neutropenia, depression, and weight loss. Treatment is contraindicated in children with significant neuropsychiatric disease because of the associated mood disturbance. Lamivudine, an oral nucleoside analog, inhibits HBV replication by competing with the natural nucleoside triphosphates for incorporation into viral DNA. Lamivudine has a more benign side-effect profile than IFN-α. However, there is no defined optimal duration of treatment for lamivudine, and its prolonged use is associated with the selection of resistant mutants. There does not appear to be any benefit in combination therapy. Adefovir, another oral nucleotide analog, has good efficacy in adults whilst inducing less viral resistance than lamivudine. This agent is currently undergoing a clinical trial in children. Many new medications, such as pegylated IFN (peginterferon) and other oral agents, are under investigation for pediatric chronic HBV infection.

General recommendations for a child with chronic HBV infection include not sharing toothbrushes with household members and hepatitis A vaccination. Adolescents should not share razors and needles, should avoid heavy alcohol use, and should be advised regarding prevention of sexual transmission. All household contacts should receive hepatitis B immunization. Children with chronic HBV infection should also undergo periodic screening for hepatocellular carcinoma with measurement of serum transaminases, alpha-fetoprotein, and abdominal ultrasound. There are no standard guidelines for the frequency of screening, although laboratory studies twice a year and ultrasound annually is reasonable.

Hepatitis C

The high likelihood of chronic infection with HCV makes treatment of acute HCV an attractive option. However, in contrast to HBV, immunoglobulin is ineffective against HCV caused by the rapid mutation rate. Although IFN-α has been used in study populations with some success, it is not yet standard of care.

The aim of treatment in chronic HCV infection is to achieve a sustained viral response, which is defined as the absence of HCV RNA in serum 6 months after the completion of therapy. IFN-α is Food and Drug Administration approved for chronic HCV infection in this country for children aged 2 years or older (it is contraindicated in younger than this because of neurotoxicity). Ribavarin is also approved for children aged 3 years or older. Peginterferon, which only requires once a week dosing, is available for children by participation in clinical trials. The current treatment options for chronic HCV in children are IFN-α or peginterferon monotherapy, or in combination with ribavarin. Combination therapy with IFN-α and ribavarin has proven safety and efficacy in children.[20] Peginterferon with ribavarin is even more effective in adults and is likely to be approved for use in children in the near future.

Since the natural history of chronic HCV is not well defined in children, there is controversy over which children to select for treatment. Children certainly should not be excluded from therapy, and, in fact, a meta-analysis of reported pediatric trials suggested that children actually have higher response rates than adults.[38] The decision to treat children with chronic HCV is made based on genotype, viral count, and histology; although the need for liver biopsy is controversial. Children with HCV genotypes 2 or 3 have a high (>70%) probability of achieving a sustained viral response.[24] Viral load, benign histology, and young age are also factors that predict a favorable response to treatment. Unlike chronic HBV infection, serum ALT does not predict response to therapy. The decision to treating children with genotypes 2 or 3 and children with progressive histology is relatively clear. However, children with genotype 1 and minimal histologic involvement pose a therapeutic challenge, as the benefit of therapy is unclear.

All patients with chronic HCV infection should receive hepatitis A and B vaccinations. General recommendations include not sharing toothbrushes and razors, and adolescents should be cautioned about sexual transmission, alcohol ingestion, and sharing needles. Maternal HCV infection is not a contraindication to breastfeeding.

Other Hepatotropic Viruses

Hepatitis D (Delta Agent)

Hepatitis D (HDV) is a defective virus, which consists of a single strand of RNA and its envelope consists of HBsAg. Therefore, it is only a pathogen in the presence of coinfection with HBV. Serologic tests are available to test for HDV; however, testing is only indicated in known HBV carriers. Coinfection with HDV is associated with fulminant hepatitis or a more aggressive course of chronic hepatitis. Treatment and prevention of HDV are the same as for HBV.

Hepatitis E

Hepatitis E virus is a single-stranded virus without an envelope, which is associated with outbreaks of acute hepatitis in Asia, the Middle East, and Mexico. The mode of transmission is fecal–oral, often via contaminated water. Hepatitis E virus is a significant cause of fulminant hepatitis in endemic areas, and most particularly affects pregnant women with increased mortality and fetal loss. There is no risk of chronic infection. Treatment is supportive only.

Hepatitis G

Hepatitis G virus is a single-strand RNA virus. It is efficiently transmitted via blood transfusion and sexual contact. Vertical transmission is also high. It often coexists with HCV, HBV, and HIV. Despite the efficiency of transmission of this virus, there is no evidence that it causes any significant liver disease, and therefore testing is not routinely performed for this agent.

PREVENTION

Postexposure prophylaxis with Ig is effective in preventing symptomatic HAV infection when given within 2 weeks of exposure. It is recommended for unvaccinated household contacts and to all unvaccinated staff and attendees of day-care centers. Ig is not routinely recommended in the school setting.

Two inactivated HAV vaccines are available in the United States, and vaccination has been incorporated into the routine childhood immunization schedule since 2006. The vaccine is recommended at 1 year of age, and the two doses in the series should be given at least 6 months apart. The vaccine may be administered concomitantly with Ig, if indicated. In most states, adolescents are required to have evidence of HAV immunization in middle school or on entrance to high school.

Hepatitis B vaccine is recommended universally to all infants beginning at birth. The series (of three or four doses, depending on if a birth dose is given) should be completed by 6–18 months of age. In most states, adolescents are required to provide proof of HBV immunization in middle school or on entrance to high school. Perinatal HBV transmission can be largely prevented with the concomitant use of hepatitis B Ig and vaccine at birth. All pregnant women are screened with HBsAg testing to identify newborns at risk, since infants should receive hepatitis B Ig within 12 hours of birth. Hepatitis B immune globulin post-exposure prophylaxis is also used in combination with hepatitis B vaccine in unvaccinated older individuals.

There is no immunoprophylaxis or vaccine currently available for HCV.

REFERENCES

1. Fiore AE, Wasley A, Bell BP. Prevention of hepatitis A through active or passive immunization: recommendations of the Advisory Committee on Immunization Practices (ACIP). *MMWR Recomm Rep.* 2006;55(RR-7):1-23.
2. Wasley A, Miller JT, Finelli L. Surveillance for acute viral hepatitis—United States, 2005. *MMWR Surveill Summ.* 2007;56(3):1-24.
3. Rosenblum LS, Villarino ME, Nainan OV, et al. Hepatitis A outbreak in a neonatal intensive care unit: risk factors for transmission and evidence of prolonged viral excretion among preterm infants. *J Infect Dis.* 1991;164(3):476-482.
4. Maynard JE. Hepatitis B: global importance and need for control. *Vaccine.* 1990;8(suppl):S18-S20; discussion S1-S3.
5. Gish RG, Gadano AC. Chronic hepatitis B: current epidemiology in the Americas and implications for management. *J Viral Hepat.* 2006;13(12):787-798.
6. Lavanchy D. Hepatitis B virus epidemiology, disease burden, treatment, and current and emerging prevention and control measures. *J Viral Hepat.* 2004;11(2):97-107.
7. McMahon BJ. Epidemiology and natural history of hepatitis B. *Semin Liver Dis.* 2005;25(suppl 1):3-8.
8. Armstrong GL, Wasley A, Simard EP, McQuillan GM, Kuhnert WL, Alter MJ. The prevalence of hepatitis C virus infection in the United States, 1999 through 2002. *Ann Intern Med.* 2006;144(10):705-714.
9. Jonas MM. Children with hepatitis C. *Hepatology.* 2002;36(5 suppl 1):S173-S178.
10. Frank C, Mohamed MK, Strickland GT, et al. The role of parenteral antischistosomal therapy in the spread of hepatitis C virus in Egypt. *Lancet.* 2000;355(9207):887-891.
11. Yeung LT, King SM, Roberts EA. Mother-to-infant transmission of hepatitis C virus. *Hepatology.* 2001;34(2):223-229.
12. Baba M, Hasegawa H, Nakayabu M, Fukai K, Suzuki S. Cytolytic activity of natural killer cells and lymphokine activated killer cells against hepatitis A virus infected fibroblasts. *J Clin Lab Immunol.* 1993;40(2):47-60.
13. Fleischer B, Fleischer S, Maier K, et al. Clonal analysis of infiltrating T lymphocytes in liver tissue in viral hepatitis A. *Immunology.* 1990;69(1):14-19.
14. Scaglioni PP, Melegari M, Wands JR. Recent advances in the molecular biology of hepatitis B virus. *Baillieres Clin Gastroenterol.* 1996;10(2):207-225.
15. Tillmann HL. Antiviral therapy and resistance with hepatitis B virus infection. *World J Gastroenterol.* 2007;13(1):125-140.
16. Chan HL, Sung JJ. Hepatocellular carcinoma and hepatitis B virus. *Semin Liver Dis.* 2006;26(2):153-161.

17. Major ME, Feinstone SM. The molecular virology of hepatitis C. *Hepatology.* 1997;25(6):1527-1538.
18. Lauer GM, Walker BD. Hepatitis C virus infection. *N Engl J Med.* 2001;345(1):41-52.
19. Simmonds P, Holmes EC, Cha TA, et al. Classification of hepatitis C virus into six major genotypes and a series of subtypes by phylogenetic analysis of the NS-5 region. *J Gen Virol.* 1993;74(pt 11):2391-2399.
20. Gonzalez-Peralta RP, Kelly DA, Haber B, et al. Interferon alfa-2b in combination with ribavirin for the treatment of chronic hepatitis C in children: efficacy, safety, and pharmacokinetics. *Hepatology.* 2005;42(5):1010-1018.
21. Elisofon SA, Jonas MM. Hepatitis B and C in children: current treatment and future strategies. *Clin Liver Dis.* 2006;10(1):133-148, vii.
22. Chang MH, Hsu HY, Hsu HC, Ni YH, Chen JS, Chen DS. The significance of spontaneous hepatitis B e antigen seroconversion in childhood: with special emphasis on the clearance of hepatitis B e antigen before 3 years of age. *Hepatology.* 1995;22(5):1387-1392.
23. Hsu HY, Chang MH, Chen DS, Lee CY, Sung JL. Baseline seroepidemiology of hepatitis B virus infection in children in Taipei, 1984: a study just before mass hepatitis B vaccination program in Taiwan. *J Med Virol.* 1986;18(4): 301-307.
24. Shneider BL, Gonzalez-Peralta R, Roberts EA. Controversies in the management of pediatric liver disease: hepatitis B, C and NAFLD: summary of a single topic conference. *Hepatology.* 2006;44(5):1344-1354.
25. Lok AS, McMahon BJ. Chronic hepatitis B. *Hepatology.* 2007;45(2):507-539.
26. Bortolotti F, Guido M, Bartolacci S, et al. Chronic hepatitis B in children after e antigen seroclearance: final report of a 29-year longitudinal study. *Hepatology.* 2006; 43(3):556-562.
27. Hsu HC, Wu MZ, Chang MH, Su IJ, Chen DS. Childhood hepatocellular carcinoma develops exclusively in hepatitis B surface antigen carriers in three decades in Taiwan. Report of 51 cases strongly associated with rapid development of liver cirrhosis. *J Hepatol.* 1987;5(3):260-267.
28. Hsu HY, Chang MH, Ni YH, Chen HL. Survey of hepatitis B surface variant infection in children 15 years after a nationwide vaccination programme in Taiwan. *Gut.* 2004;53(10):1499-1503.
29. Barrera JM, Bruguera M, Ercilla MG, et al. Persistent hepatitis C viremia after acute self-limiting posttransfusion hepatitis C. *Hepatology.* 1995;21(3):639-644.
30. Strickland DK, Jenkins JJ, Hudson MM. Hepatitis C infection and hepatocellular carcinoma after treatment of childhood cancer. *J Pediatr Hematol Oncol.* 2001;23(8): 527-529.
31. Bortolotti F, Resti M, Marcellini M, et al. Hepatitis C virus (HCV) genotypes in 373 Italian children with HCV infection: changing distribution and correlation with clinical features and outcome. *Gut.* 2005;54(6):852-857.
32. Jara P, Resti M, Hierro L, et al. Chronic hepatitis C virus infection in childhood: Clinical patterns and evolution in 224 white children. *Clin Infect Dis.* 2003;36(3):275-280.
33. Ceci O, Margiotta M, Marello F, et al. Vertical transmission of hepatitis C virus in a cohort of 2,447 HIV-seronegative pregnant women: a 24-month prospective study. *J Pediatr Gastroenterol Nutr.* 2001;33(5):570-575.
34. Davison SM, Mieli-Vergani G, Sira J, Kelly DA. Perinatal hepatitis C virus infection: diagnosis and management. *Arch Dis Child.* 2006;91(9):781-785.
35. American Academy of Pediatrics. Hepatitis A. In: Pickering LK, ed. *Red Book: 2006. Report of the Committee on Infectious Diseases.* 27th ed. Elk Grove Village, IL: American Academy of Pediatrics; 2006:328.
36. Ruiz-Moreno M, Rua MJ, Molina J, et al. Prospective, randomized controlled trial of interferon-alpha in children with chronic hepatitis B. *Hepatology.* 1991;13(6):1035-1039.
37. Sokal EM, Conjeevaram HS, Roberts EA, et al. Interferon alfa therapy for chronic hepatitis B in children: a multinational randomized controlled trial. *Gastroenterology.* 1998;114(5):988-995.
38. Jacobson KR, Murray K, Zellos A, Schwarz KB. An analysis of published trials of interferon monotherapy in children with chronic hepatitis C. *J Pediatr Gastroenterol Nutr.* 2002;34(1):52-58.

CHAPTER 41

Antibiotic-Associated Diarrhea and *Clostridium difficile*-Associated Disease

Louis Valiquette and Jacques Pépin

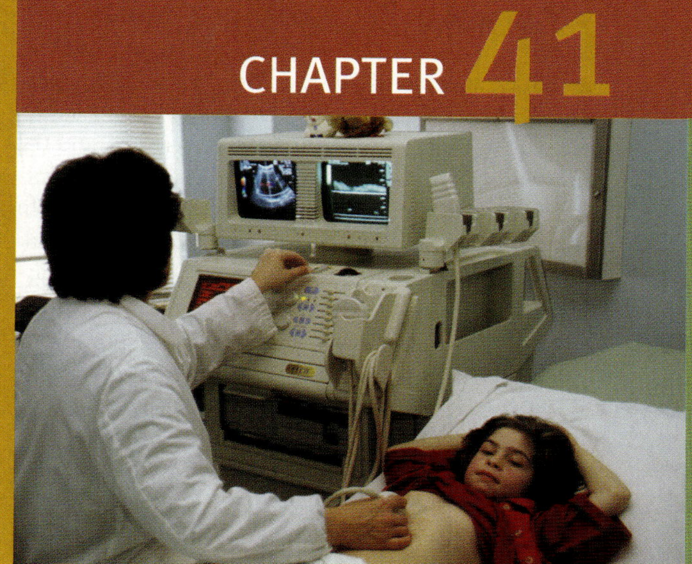

DEFINITIONS AND EPIDEMIOLOGY

Antibiotic-associated diarrhea (AAD) or unexplained diarrhea occurring with the administration of antibiotics is a common complication of antimicrobial therapy, for which several underlying mechanisms have been proposed: (1) disturbance of the normal intestinal flora, (2) allergic and/or toxic effects of the drug on the intestinal mucosa, (3) pharmacologic effects on motility, and (4) overgrowth of toxin-producing *Clostridium difficile. C. difficile*–associated disease (CDAD) is an infection of the colon that develops almost exclusively in the setting of antimicrobial use and is associated with a wide spectrum of symptoms, from mild diarrhea to pseudomembranous colitis, and in some cases toxic megacolon and death. Pseudomembranous colitis, characterized by severe inflammation of the inner lining of the colon with the formation of pseudomembranous material, is usually caused by *C. difficile* infection. Other toxin-producing pathogens have been associated with AAD, like *Staphylococcus aureus,*[1] *Clostridium perfringens,*[1] and *Klebsiella oxytoca,*[2] but they remain infrequent.

C. difficile is found in various natural habitats and in feces of mammals. Patients acquire *C. difficile* from the hospital environment or from stools of colonized or infected patients, via the hands of medical or nursing staff. In the first days after birth, neonates rarely exhibit *C. difficile* in their stools.[3,4] However, during the first few weeks of life they rapidly become colonized. In a study of preterm infants, colonization rate was 15% at 7 days, increasing to 33% at 14–21 days; toxin B was detected in 90% of stool specimens of those colonized.[5] Other researchers reported colonization rates of 31% at 10 days, 71% between 10 and 19 days, 85% between 20 and 29 days, and 100% after 30 days of life.[4] Between 25% and 100% of infants aged 6–12 months are colonized[3,4,6,7]; in this older population, a lower proportion (15–38%) of those colonized have toxigenic strains.[7–9] The duration of the carrier state is unknown. Caesarean section, duration of hospitalization, exposure to anti-infectives, underlying comorbidities and exclusive formula-feeding are risk factors for *C. difficile* colonization.[7,9,10]

In the general population, AAD occurs in 5–32% of patients between initiation of therapy and up to 2 months after the end of treatment.[11–14] Among 650 outpatient children receiving oral antibiotics, 11% developed AAD, beginning a mean of 5.3 (±3.5) days after the start of antimicrobial treatment and lasting a mean of 4.0 (±3.0) days. Younger children (<2 years; 18%) are more likely to experience AAD than their older counterparts (≥2 years; 3%). Certain classes of antibiotics are associated with an increased risk of AAD, the most frequent culprit being amoxicillin/clavulanate (which causes diarrhea in 23% of recipients).[15]

In adults, toxigenic *C. difficile* is the most frequent cause of nosocomial AAD and is implicated in 10–30% of cases.[16] In children, this relationship is much weaker. Young children, who often are asymptomatic carriers of toxigenic *C. difficile* strains, are also highly sensitive to the nonspecific diarrheal effects of some antibiotics. Consequently, reports of *C. difficile* toxin-positive stools in young children with AAD (found in 9–13% of such cases[17,18]) might overestimate the number of genuine CDAD cases. In a case-control study comparing age-matched toxigenic *C. difficile* positive and negative patients with diarrhea, no difference was found in symptoms, risk factors, or outcomes (albeit most CDAD cases were treated with oral metronidazole). Alternative etiologies were found in 50% of toxigenic *C. difficile* patients (viral enteric pathogens in 39%).[19] Consequently, confirmed outbreaks of pediatric nosocomial CDAD (n-CDAD) have been rarely documented.[20]

Since the end of 2002, outbreaks due to a hypervirulent clone have been reported in the United States, Canada, the United Kingdom, France, Belgium, and the Netherlands.[21] This has completely changed the epidemiology and clinical impacts of CDAD in adults. In the province of Quebec, Canada, more than 30 hospitals have been struggling with an epidemic of CDAD characterized by a high case-fatality rate (16.7%) and increased risk of recurrence following metronidazole or vancomycin treatment, mostly in patients aged 65 years and older.[22–24] These outbreaks have been associated with an emerging toxinotype III ribotype NAP1/027 strain characterized by massive toxins A and B hyperproduction.[25] However, little information is available on the impact of NAP1/027 on children. In a retrospective analysis of 200 CDAD cases diagnosed in a university-affiliated pediatric hospital in 2000–2003 (no characterization of strains was performed, but this analysis has taken place in a city plagued by NAP1/027 outbreaks during that period), a majority were outpatients at onset, but 23% needed to be hospitalized for the care of CDAD. Out of 110 patients treated for CDAD, 31% experienced at least 1 recurrence, none required a colectomy and only 2 died.[26] The frequent need for hospitalization may reflect the higher virulence of the predominant strain within this pediatric population. In a well-defined population of Canada where NAP1/027 emerged at the end of 2002, the incidence of CDAD increased from 36 per 100,000 in 1991–1992 to 156 per 100,000 in 2003; while the incidence among people aged ≥65 years increased 10-fold, to 866 per 100,000 in 2003, the annual incidence in children remained stable, between 20 and 40 per 100,000.[23] This suggests that children are much less prone than the elderly to develop symptomatic infections when exposed to NAP1/027.

Community-acquired CDAD (c-CDAD) incidence is difficult to appraise, since several reports are based on retrospective databases within which past exposure to health care services is not always clear. In 1995, a prospective nationwide study in Sweden reported an annual population incidence of 58 cases per 100,000 inhabitants, combining nosocomial and community-acquired cases. In inhabitants aged 0–19 years, the population incidence rate was 20 per 100,000. To assess the proportion of c-CDAD, they specifically searched for prior contact with health care facilities. An absence of prior hospitalization was reported in 28% of cases, and this proportion increased to 52% in children younger than 4 years.[27]

Antibiotics exposure within the previous 8 weeks is the strongest risk factor for CDAD, and all types of antibiotics have been implicated. In children, one outbreak was associated with lincomycin usage.[20] Among adults, some antibiotic classes are more likely to cause normal flora disruption and CDAD than others, as shown in Table 41–1. Similar data are not available for children. The emergent, hypervirulent, NAP1/027 strain has been consistently associated with the use of fluoroquinolones,[22,28,29] which would have limited consequences for children among whom quinolones are rarely used. Host factors associated with CDAD in children include acquired or congenital causes of colonic stasis (e.g., infant botulism, Hirschprung's disease)[30–33] and imunosuppression (e.g., cancer, organ transplantation, etc.).[34–36]

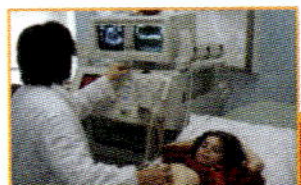

Table 41–1.

Antibiotics Associated with C. difficile-Associated Disease

High Risk	Moderate Risk	Low Risk
Clindamycin	Doxycycline	Trimethoprim
Cephalosporins (second and third generations)	Macrolides first-generation cephalosporins	Sulfonamides Aminoglycosides
Ampicillin/ amoxicillin	Piperacillin/ tazobactam	Metronidazole
Fluoroquinolones	Ticarcillin/ clavulanic acid	Vancomycin
	Carbapenems	

Cystic fibrosis patients are frequently colonized with toxigenic *C. difficile* strains,[37] presumably a consequence of frequent hospitalizations and repeated use of broad-spectrum antibiotics. However, CDAD is unusual in this population, with one case report and a case series of four patients with fulminant CDAD.[38,39] Several hypotheses have been raised to explain the scarcity of CDAD in cystic fibrosis patients: unique intestinal environment due to pancreatic insufficiency, higher rate of colonization by bacteria having an inhibiting effect on *C. difficile* growth, and lack of mucosal receptors for *C. difficile* toxins.

PATHOGENESIS

C. difficile is a gram-positive, obligate anaerobic, endospore-forming bacillus. The ability of *C. difficile* to form spores under unfavorable growth conditions is the key to its transmissibility and resistance to eradication. Spores have thick walls and are metabolically inactive; thus, they withstand extremes of temperature, drying, atmospheric oxygen, and other unfavorable conditions. Sporulation allows *C. difficile* to resist the low-level disinfectants used for routine surface cleaning in health care facilities and at home,[1] and may also be a key factor promoting endogenous relapses of CDAD after treatment. Spores survive the low pH of the stomach and germinate in the small bowel and colon. *C. difficile* is harmless in many individuals because its proliferation is limited by competition from the normal colonic flora. Once a patient has been exposed, the risk of developing

CDAD is driven by the disruption of normal intestinal flora and host factors (impaired immune response).

In patients with abnormal colonic flora, usually due to antibiotic consumption but also due to antineoplastic agents (some of which have antimicrobial properties), both toxigenic and nontoxigenic strains can proliferate. Only toxigenic isolates cause disease. *C. difficile* may produce at least three different toxins: toxin A, toxin B, and binary toxin. Toxins A and B disrupt the cytoskeleton of colonic epithelial cells and destroy the epithelial layer. They also induce production of proinflammatory cytokines resulting in marked colonic mucosal inflammation. Binary toxin (actin-specific ADP-ribosyl-transferase), which is similar to the *C. perfringens* iota toxin, also disrupts the cytoskeleton of cells in tissue culture,[40] but its effects in animal models of *C. difficile* infection have been equivocal.[41] Binary toxin was recently identified in 6% of strains in a single center,[41] but its gene is present in virtually all isolates of NAP1/027. The NAP1/027 hypervirulent clone has deletions in the *tcdC* gene, a putative negative regulator of toxin A and B expression, this in turn resulting in increased production of toxins A and B (16–22 times higher than with other strains) and more severe disease.[25,42] The contribution of binary toxin to NAP1/027 pathogenesis remains unclear.[25]

There are several theories to explain why neonates do not exhibit symptoms, despite high colonization rates: immaturity of toxin receptors,[43] neutralizing effects of maternal antibodies[7,43] and immaturity of neonatal immune system.[43,44] Serum antibodies against *C. difficile* toxins A and B are found in 60–70% of children older than 3 years. In a cohort of infants and children with diarrhea and *C. difficile* in their stools, 35% had serum IgA below normal range and 16% had low-serum IgG. They were classified as transient hypogammaglobulinemia of infancy, because they all increased their Ig levels over the following 12 months. Patients with hypogammaglobulinemia are more likely to experience a recurrence.[45] A specific immune response persists throughout life and may have a protective role against disease occurrence and relapses in adults.[46,47]

CLINICAL PRESENTATION

Colonization by *C. difficile* may result in different clinical presentations: (1) asymptomatic carriage; (2) nonspecific colitis; (3) pseudomembranous colitis (fulminant or not); and (4) recurrent disease. Most patients present with watery diarrhea, albeit 10–15% have bloody stools. Diarrhea usually starts 3–21 days after the use of antibiotics and, prior to the emergence of NAP1/027, was frequently self-limited. Fever and colicky abdominal pains often accompany watery stools. In the most severe cases, a toxic megacolon may develop and lead to perforation and peritonitis. Leukemoid reactions are more common in patients infected with NAP1/027, and a patient with diarrhea and a leukocytosis higher than 25,000 per μL should be considered to have CDAD until proven otherwise. Among elderly adults with NAP1/027 infection, septic shock can develop in the absence of peritonitis. Complicated CDAD (defined by one or more of: toxic megacolon, perforation, shock-necessitating vasopressors, other indication for an emergency colectomy, death within 30 days of diagnosis) has been reported repeatedly in recent outbreaks associated with NAP1/027 in adults but rarely in children.[23] In most cases, diarrhea improves within a few days of treatment, but recurrences are frequent and can be difficult to treat.

DIFFERENTIAL DIAGNOSIS

Differential diagnosis of diarrhea in children is broad and addressed in other sections of this book. Infectious causes of diarrhea are frequently linked to specific exposures, and can be classified as nosocomial or community-acquired, the latter with or without recent travel history (Table 41–2). Nosocomial diarrhea is a frequent nosocomial infection in children. Viral pathogens

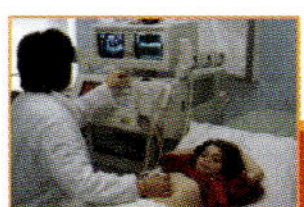

Table 41–2.

Differential Diagnosis of Acute Infectious Diarrhea in Children

Nosocomial diarrhea
Rotavirus
Adenovirus
C. difficile
Other viruses (norovirus, astrovirus, echovirus, etc.)
Outpatient setting with no recent travel history
Virus
Rotavirus
Adenovirus
Astrovirus
Norovirus
Bacterial pathogens
C. jejuni
EHEC
Salmonella
Shigella
Outpatient setting with a recent travel history
Bacterial pathogens
ETEC
Salmonella sp.
Shigella sp.
C. jejuni
Yersinia sp.
Parasites
E. histolytica
G. lamblia

(rotavirus, adenovirus, etc.) are the primary causes of nosocomial diarrhea, and *C. difficile* is the most frequent bacterial etiology in industrialized countries. In the developing world, enteropathogens associated with acute diarrhea (*Salmonella, Shigella,* etc.) are more frequently reported. In the outpatient setting, *C. difficile* is an infrequent pathogen. When found, it can correspond to CDAD or merely reflect asymptomatic carriage with a concomitant coinfection causing the diarrhea.

DIAGNOSIS

In practice, when a patient exposed to antibiotics develops diarrhea, the diagnostic algorithm merely attempts to sort out those with CDAD from all others. In adults, diagnosis of CDAD is usually confirmed by toxin detection in stools, or in selected cases by endoscopy. In the pediatric population, diagnosis is more difficult. First, as endoscopy is more invasive and usually requires anesthesia, it is infrequently performed. Second, asymptomatic carriage of toxigenic *C. difficile* strains limits the clinical utility of toxin testing in infants.

Culture of *C. difficile* followed by toxin detection would be the most sensitive test but is cumbersome and used only in research settings. Culture is essential for strain-typing studies that are essential to identify outbreak strains and cross infections. In clinical practice, the cell culture cytotoxicity assay (CTA) is generally considered as the gold standard because of its high specificity and biologic sensitivity (5 pg of toxin B). The main drawbacks are that it is labor-intensive, has a slow turnaround time (≥48 hours), and requires tissue culture facilities and expertise.[8] Therefore, an enzyme immuno-assay (EIA) for toxins A and/or B of *C. difficile* is frequently used for routine testing. When compared to CTA, sensitivity of EIA ranges between 65% and 85%, but its specificity ranges between 94% and 100%.[8,16,48] The EIA has a rapid turnaround time (<24 hours), is technically easy-to-perform, and is cheaper than CTA. Although most toxigenic strains (~97%) produce both toxins A and B, outbreaks associated with strains that produce toxin B only were recently reported.[49,50] These toxin A negative strains have been identified in children and can represent as much as 22–48% of toxigenic strains.[8,51,52] To circumvent this problem, we recommend selection of A + B EIA tests or CTA. Clinicians must be aware that false-negative results occur and should repeat the test and/or seek diagnosis by endoscopy or CT scan when the clinical suspicion of CDAD is high.

Endoscopy reveals inflamed and edematous mucosa with multiple discrete, nodular, and polypoid lesions covered with yellowish exudates (pseudomembranes) with skip areas of normal mucosa (Figure 41–1). In severe cases, the mucosa may be completely covered by pseudomembranes. Some cases show nonspecific mucosal inflammation without pseudomembrane formation. Usually the findings are so characteristic for experienced endoscopists that a biopsy is not needed. Endoscopy can be useful when stools are not available because of ileus, when a rapid diagnosis is necessary, or when the stool toxin test is negative but clinical suspicion remains.

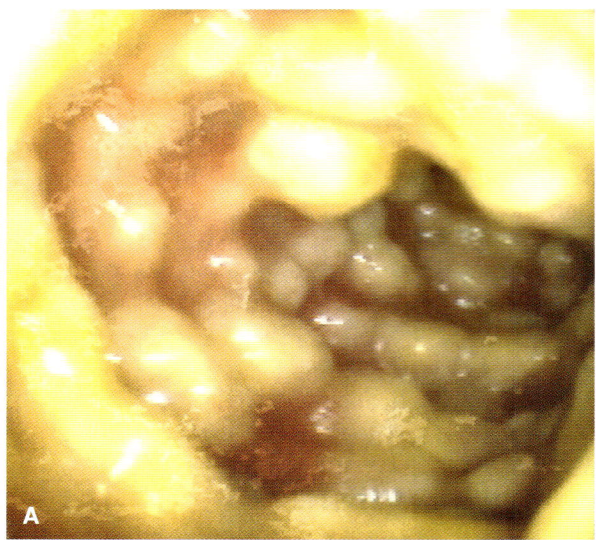

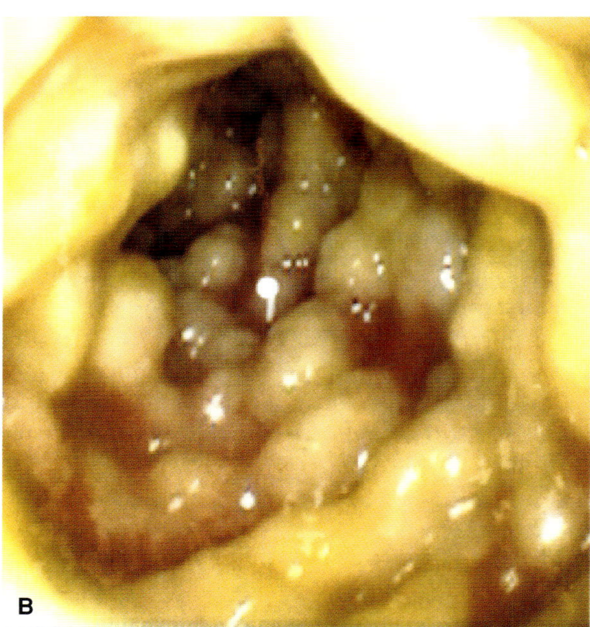

FIGURES 41–1 ■ (A) and **(B)**. Photos taken during endoscopic evaluation of a patient with severe *C. difficile* colitis. Both figures show inflamed and edematous mucosa with numerous discrete nodular and polypoid lesions overlying an erythematous and edematous mucosa.

CT scanning should not normally be needed for diagnosis and probably has a low sensitivity in mild to moderate disease. However, it can be extremely useful in severe cases. Using the criteria of colonic wall thickening >4 mm, pericolic stranding, unexplained ascites, nodularity of the colonic wall, and the accordion sign, a retrospective review of 110 patients reported a sensitivity of

52%, a specificity of 93%, a positive predictive value of 88%, and a negative predictive value of 67%.[53] CT findings in children are similar to those in adults.[54,55]

MANAGEMENT

The first steps in managing CDAD are to discontinue, whenever possible, the inciting antibiotics, and to implement rehydration. Physicians should avoid antiperistaltic agents as they may increase the risk of toxic megacolon (Figure 41–2).[56] Sometimes, the diarrhea has spontaneously subsided by the time results of the toxin assay become available, and no antibiotic treatment is needed. In centers where the NAP1/027 hypervirulent clone is present, empirical treatment is started when clinical suspicion is high, pending results of the toxin assay; clinicians should follow closely patients with rapidly progressing symptoms to identify potentially life-threatening complications. In patients with very severe and protracted disease, a surgeon should be consulted to evaluate the need for an emergency colectomy, which can be life-saving.[57]

TREATMENT

A treatment algorithm is shown in Figure 41–3. Traditionally, metronidazole and oral vancomycin have been the main agents used for CDAD treatment.

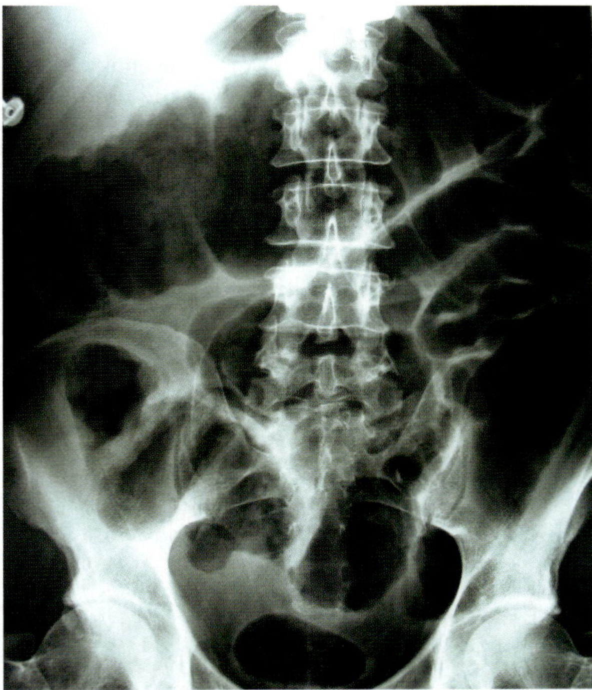

FIGURE 41–2 ■ Plain abdominal radiograph showing a patient with toxic megacolon caused by *C. difficile* colitis.

The equivalence of these two drugs is based on two randomized controlled trials that showed no difference in outcomes but included small numbers of patients (<50 per arm).[58,59] However, vancomycin is the only FDA-approved drug for treating CDAD and has favourable pharmacokinetics, with faecal levels generally exceeding 1000 mg/L.[60,61] For that reason, some authorities recommend that vancomycin be used as the initial treatment of very severe cases of CDAD.[62] Its use as initial treatment for CDAD markedly decreased in the mid-1990s following recommendations by the Hospital Infection Control Practices Advisory Committee to avoid using vancomycin in hospitals, to reduce the selection pressure for the emergence of vancomycin-resistant enterococci.[63] Since then, metronidazole (20–40 mg/kg per day, in three to four doses, for 10–14 days) has been recommended as the first-line treatment of CDAD, with oral vancomycin (40–50 mg/kg per day, in four doses) to be used mainly if metronidazole is found to be ineffective, contraindicated or poorly tolerated.[62] In a retrospective observational study that covered the period 1991–2003, after adjustment for confounding factors reflecting severity of disease and host characteristics, patients who received vancomycin as their initial treatment were less likely to develop a complicated outcome than those treated with metronidazole.[23] However, after the emergence of NAP1/027 in the same hospital, vancomycin was no longer superior to metronidazole, perhaps because toxin production is so rapid that the disease follows its natural course.[24] Intravenous metronidazole is an alternative for patients in whom an oral treatment is not possible, or in combination with oral vancomycin in complicated CDAD. Intravenous vancomycin is not excreted in the bowel and should never be used to treat CDAD.

Bacitracin is generally considered inferior to metronidazole and vancomycin and is no longer used. Several bacteria and yeasts (*Bifidobacterium* sp., *Lactobacilli* GG, *Saccharomyces boulardii*) have been proposed for prevention of AAD. A recent meta-analysis of randomized placebo-controlled trials of probiotics for AAD prevention demonstrated a lack of effect when analyzing data based on intention-to-treat analysis[64] There is no evidence that probiotics reduce the risk of CDAD among patients receiving high-risk antibiotics, nor that they reduce the risk of recurrences. Administration of *S. boulardii* can cause fungemia, especially in immunosuppresed patients.[65] Therefore, we do not recommend probiotics for CDAD treatment or prevention.

Several novel treatments for CDAD are currently investigated in phase III trials, including nitazoxanide (an agent approved for the treatment of cryptosporidiosis and giardiasis),[66] rifaximin (a poorly absorbed rifamycin), and tolevamer—a toxin-binding polymer.

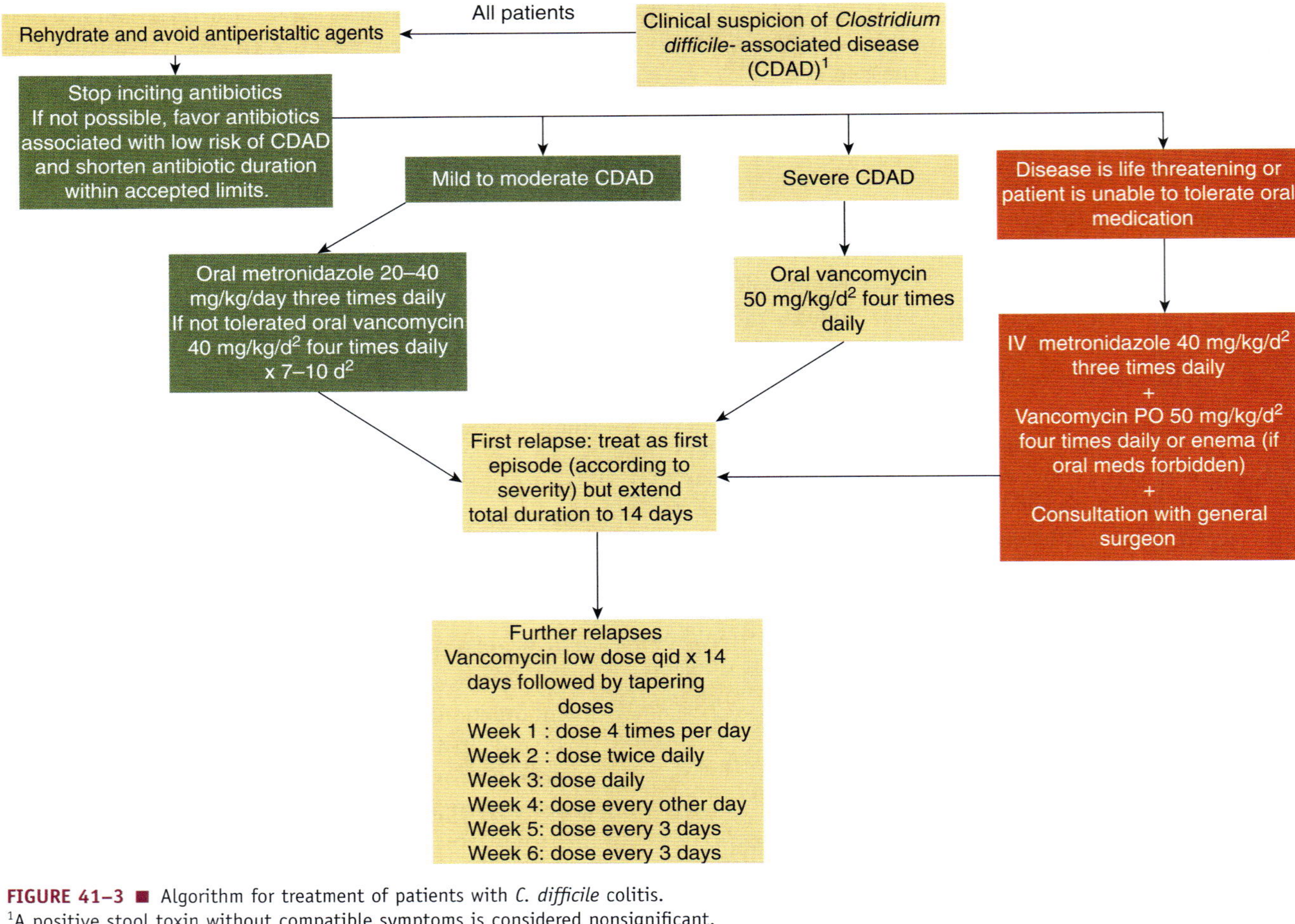

All patients
Rehydrate and avoid antiperistaltic agents
Clinical suspicion of Clostridium difficile- associated disease (CDAD)[1]
Stop inciting antibiotics
If not possible, favor antibiotics associated with low risk of CDAD and shorten antibiotic duration within accepted limits.
Mild to moderate CDAD
Severe CDAD
Disease is life threatening or patient is unable to tolerate oral medication
Oral metronidazole 20–40 mg/kg/day three times daily
If not tolerated oral vancomycin 40 mg/kg/d[2] four times daily x 7–10 d[2]
Oral vancomycin 50 mg/kg/d[2] four times daily
IV metronidazole 40 mg/kg/d[2] three times daily
+
Vancomycin PO 50 mg/kg/d[2] four times daily or enema (if oral meds forbidden)
+
Consultation with general surgeon
First relapse: treat as first episode (according to severity) but extend total duration to 14 days
Further relapses
Vancomycin low dose qid x 14 days followed by tapering doses
Week 1 : dose 4 times per day
Week 2 : dose twice daily
Week 3: dose daily
Week 4: dose every other day
Week 5: dose every 3 days
Week 6: dose every 3 days

FIGURE 41–3 ■ Algorithm for treatment of patients with *C. difficile* colitis.
[1]A positive stool toxin without compatible symptoms is considered nonsignificant.
[2]Maximal adult dose is 500 mg four times daily.

COURSE AND PROGNOSIS

In most children, CDAD is a self-limited disease with diarrhea lasting for 4–5 days. Complications associated with CDAD in children are unusual but include dehydration, electrolyte imbalance, shock, hypoalbuminemia, toxic megacolon, and colon perforation. In a 13-year retrospective review of CDAD, 301 cases were identified in patients less than 18 years of age, only 4 of whom (1.3%) developed complicated CDAD (as defined above). Several unusual complications of CDAD have been reported in children: reactive arthritis,[67,68] rectal prolapse,[69] Henoch–Shonlein purpura,[70] and hemolytic–uremic syndrome.[71,72] Rare cases of extraintestinal *C. difficile* infections have been reported in children: bacteremia,[73,74] chronic osteomyelitis in a patient with sickle cell disease, and appendicitis with a *C. difficile* peritonitis.[75]

Recurrences occur in 20–31% of cases, but are less common in children than in the elderly.[26,76,77] About one fourth of children with one recurrence experience a second recurrence within 60 days.[77] The first recurrence of CDAD is generally treated with the same antibiotic that was used for the initial episode. For the unfortunate patients who experience more than one recurrence, the most effective strategy is probably the administration of tapered/pulsed oral vancomycin, given qid for 10–14 days, tid for a week, bid for a week, daily for a week, and then every other day for several weeks. It is thought that this provides rapid killing of vegetative forms as the spores germinate, while allowing the normal flora to build up and eventually compete with *C. difficile.*[78] Cholestyramine is poorly effective in patients with multiple relapses.

REFERENCES

1. Asha NJ, Tompkins D, Wilcox MH. Comparative analysis of prevalence, risk factors, and molecular epidemiology of antibiotic-associated diarrhea due to *Clostridium difficile*, *Clostridium perfringens*, and *Staphylococcus aureus*. *J Clin Microbiol*. 2006;44(8):2785-2791.
2. Hogenauer C, Langner C, Beubler E, et al. *Klebsiella oxytoca* as a causative organism of antibiotic-associated hemorrhagic colitis. *N Engl J Med*. 2006;355(23):2418-2426.

3. Matsuki S, Ozaki E, Shozu M, et al. Colonization by *Clostridium difficile* of neonates in a hospital, and infants and children in three day-care facilities of Kanazawa, Japan. *Int Microbiol.* 2005;8(1):43-48.
4. Miyazaki S, Matsunaga T, Kawasaki K, et al. Separate isolation of *Clostridium difficile* spores and vegetative cells from the feces of newborn infants. *Microbiol Immunol.* 1992;36(2):131-138.
5. El-Mohandes AE, Keiser JF, Refat M, Jackson BJ. Prevalence and toxigenicity of *Clostridium difficile* isolates in fecal microflora of preterm infants in the intensive care nursery. *Biol Neonate.* 1993;63(4):225-229.
6. Penders J, Vink C, Driessen C, London N, Thijs C, Stobberingh EE. Quantification of Bifidobacterium spp. Escherichia coli and *Clostridium difficile* in faecal samples of breast-fed and formula-fed infants by real-time PCR. *FEMS Microbiol Lett.* 2005;243(1):141-147.
7. Tullus K, Aronsson B, Marcus S, Mollby R. Intestinal colonization with *Clostridium difficile* in infants up to 18 months of age. *Eur J Clin Microbiol Infect Dis.* 1989;8(5): 390-393.
8. Collignon A, Ticchi L, Depitre C, Gaudelus J, Delmee M, Corthier G. Heterogeneity of *Clostridium difficile* isolates from infants. *Eur J Pediatr.* 1993;152(4):319-322.
9. Rexach CE, Tang-Feldman YJ, Cantrell MC, Cohen SH. Epidemiologic surveillance of *Clostridium difficile* diarrhea in a freestanding pediatric hospital and a pediatric hospital at a university medical center. *Diagn Microbiol Infect Dis.* 2006;56(2):109-114.
10. Penders J, Thijs C, Vink C, et al. Factors influencing the composition of the intestinal microbiota in early infancy. *Pediatrics.* 2006;118(2):511-521.
11. Wistrom J, Norrby SR, Myhre EB, et al. Frequency of antibiotic-associated diarrhoea in 2462 antibiotic-treated hospitalized patients: a prospective study. *J Antimicrob Chemother.* 2001;47(1):43-50.
12. Elstner CL, Lindsay AN, Book LS, Matsen JM. Lack of relationship of *Clostridium difficile* to antibiotic-associated diarrhea in children. *Pediatr Infect Dis.* 1983;2(5): 364-366.
13. McFarland LV. Epidemiology, risk factors and treatments for antibiotic-associated diarrhea. *Dig Dis.* 1998;16(5): 292-307.
14. Talbot-Smith A, Heyworth J. Antibiotic use, gastroenteritis and respiratory illness in South Australian children. *Epidemiol Infect.* 2002;129(3):507-513.
15. Turck D, Bernet JP, Marx J, et al. Incidence and risk factors of oral antibiotic-associated diarrhea in an outpatient pediatric population. *J Pediatr Gastroenterol Nutr.* 2003;37(1):22-26.
16. Poutanen SM, Simor AE. *Clostridium difficile*-associated diarrhea in adults. *CMAJ.* 2004;171(1):51-58.
17. Thompson CM, Jr., Gilligan PH, Fisher MC, Long SS. Clostridium difficile cytotoxin in a pediatric population. *Am J Dis Child.* 1983;137(3):271-274.
18. Mitchell DK, Van R, Mason EH, Norris DM, Pickering LK. Prospective study of toxigenic *Clostridium difficile* in children given amoxicillin/clavulanate for otitis media. *Pediatr Infect Dis J.* 1996;15(6):514-519.
19. Tang P, Roscoe M, Richardson SE. Limited clinical utility of *Clostridium difficile* toxin testing in infants in a pediatric hospital. *Diagn Microbiol Infect Dis.* 2005;52(2):91-94.
20. Ferroni A, Merckx J, Ancelle T, et al. Nosocomial outbreak of *Clostridium difficile* diarrhea in a pediatric service. *Eur J Clin Microbiol Infect Dis.* 1997;16(12):928-933.
21. Kuijper EJ, van den Berg RJ, Debast S, et al. Clostridium difficile ribotype 027, toxinotype III, the Netherlands. *Emerg Infect Dis.* 2006;12(5):827-830.
22. Loo VG, Poirier L, Miller MA, et al. A predominantly clonal multi-institutional outbreak of *Clostridium difficile*-associated diarrhea with high morbidity and mortality. *N Engl J Med.* 2005;353(23):2442-2449.
23. Pepin J, Valiquette L, Alary ME, et al. *Clostridium difficile*-associated diarrhea in a region of quebec from 1991 to 2003: A changing pattern of disease severity. *CMAJ.* 2004; 171(5):466-472.
24. Pepin J, Valiquette L, Gagnon S, et al. Outcomes of patients with *Clostridium difficile*-associated disease treated with metronidazole, vancomycin or both, before and after the emergence of a hypervirulent strain. *Am J Gastroenterol.* 2007;102:2781-2788.
25. Warny M, Pepin J, Fang A, et al. Toxin production by an emerging strain of *Clostridium difficile* associated with outbreaks of severe disease in North America and Europe. *Lancet.* 2005;366(9491):1079-1084.
26. Morinville V, McDonald J. *Clostridium difficile*-associated diarrhea in 200 Canadian children. *Can J Gastroenterol.* 2005;19(8):497-501.
27. Karlstrom O, Fryklund B, Tullus K, Burman LG. A prospective nationwide study of *Clostridium difficile*-associated diarrhea in Sweden. The Swedish *C. Difficile* Study Group. *Clin Infect Dis.* 1998;26(1):141-145.
28. Muto CA, Pokrywka M, Shutt K, et al. A large outbreak of *Clostridium difficile*-associated disease with an unexpected proportion of deaths and colectomies at a teaching hospital following increased fluoroquinolone use. *Infect Control Hosp Epidemiol.* 2005;26(3):273-280.
29. Pepin J, Saheb N, Coulombe MA, et al. Emergence of fluoroquinolones as the predominant risk factor for *Clostridium difficile*-associated diarrhea: a cohort study during an epidemic in Quebec. *Clin Infect Dis.* 2005; 41(9):1254-1260.
30. Pozo F, Soler P, Ladron de Guevara C. Pseudomembranous colitis associated with Hirschsprung's disease. *Clin Infect Dis.* 1994;19(6):1160-1161.
31. Fenicia L, Da Dalt L, Anniballi F, Franciosa G, Zanconato S, Aureli P. A case if infant botulism due to neurotoxigenic Clostridium butyricum type E associated with *Clostridium difficile* colitis. *Eur J Clin Microbiol Infect Dis.* 2002; 21(10):736-738.
32. Parsons SJ, Fenton E, Dargaville P. *Clostridium difficile* associated severe enterocolitis: a feature of Hirschsprung's disease in a neonate presenting late. *J Paediatr Child Health.* 2005;41(12):689-690.
33. Schechter R, Peterson B, McGee J, Idowu O, Bradley J. *Clostridium difficile* colitis associated with infant botulism: Near-fatal case analogous to Hirschsprung's enterocolitis. *Clin Infect Dis.* 1999;29(2):367-374.
34. Pituch H, vavn Belkum A, van den Braak N, et al. Clindamycin-resistant, toxin A-negative, toxin B-positive *Clostridium difficile* strains cause antibiotic-associated diarrhea among children hospitalized in a hematology unit. *Clin Microbiol Infect.* 2003;9(8):903-904.

35. Schuller I, Saha V, Lin L, Kingston J, Eden T, Tabaqchali S. Investigation and management of *Clostridium difficile* colonisation in a paediatric oncology unit. *Arch Dis Child.* 1995;72(3):219-222.
36. West M, Pirenne J, Chavers B, et al. *Clostridium difficile* colitis after kidney and kidney–pancreas transplantation. *Clin Transplant.* 1999;13(4):318-323.
37. Yahav J, Samra Z, Blau H, Dinari G, Chodick G, Shmuely H. Helicobacter pylori and *Clostridium difficile* in cystic fibrosis patients. *Dig Dis Sci.* 2006;51(12):2274-2279.
38. Hussain SZ, Chu C, Greenberg DP, Orenstein D, Khan S. *Clostridium difficile* colitis in children with cystic fibrosis. *Dig Dis Sci.* 2004;49(1):116-121.
39. Rivlin J, Lerner A, Augarten A, Wilschanski M, Kerem E, Ephros MA. Severe *Clostridium difficile*-associated colitis in young patients with cystic fibrosis. *J Pediatr.* 1998; 132(1):177-179.
40. Perelle S, Gibert M, Bourlioux P, Corthier G, Popoff MR. Production of a complete binary toxin (actin-specific ADP-ribosyltransferase) by *Clostridium difficile* CD196. *Infect Immun.* 1997;65(4):1402-1407.
41. Geric B, Carman RJ, Rupnik M, et al. Binary toxin-producing, large clostridial toxin-negative *Clostridium difficile* strains are enterotoxic but do not cause disease in hamsters. *J Infect Dis.* 2006;193(8):1143-1150.
42. Spigaglia P, Mastrantonio P. Molecular analysis of the pathogenicity locus and polymorphism in the putative negative regulator of toxin production (TcdC) among *Clostridium difficile* clinical isolates. *J Clin Microbiol.* 2002;40(9):3470-3475.
43. Eglow R, Pothoulakis C, Itzkowitz S, et al. Diminished *Clostridium difficile* toxin A sensitivity in newborn rabbit ileum is associated with decreased toxin A receptor. *J Clin Invest.* 1992;90(3):822-829.
44. Leung DY, Kelly CP, Boguniewicz M, Pothoulakis C, LaMont JT, Flores A. Treatment with intravenously administered gamma globulin of chronic relapsing colitis induced by *Clostridium difficile* toxin. *J Pediatr.* 1991;118(4, pt 1): 633-637.
45. Gryboski JD, Pellerano R, Young N, Edberg S. Positive role of *Clostridium difficile* infection in diarrhea in infants and children. *Am J Gastroenterol.* 1991;86(6):685-689.
46. Kyne L, Warny M, Qamar A, Kelly CP. Association between antibody response to toxin A and protection against recurrent *Clostridium difficile* diarrhoea. *Lancet.* 2001;357(9251):189-193.
47. Kyne L, Warny M, Qamar A, Kelly CP. Asymptomatic carriage of *Clostridium difficile* and serum levels of IgG antibody against toxin A. *N Engl J Med.* 2000;342(6): 390-397.
48. Wilkins TD, Lyerly DM. *Clostridium difficile* testing: after 20 Years, still challenging. *J Clin Microbiol.* 2003;41(2): 531-534.
49. Al-Barrak A, Embil J, Dyck B, et al. An outbreak of toxin A negative, toxin B positive *Clostridium difficile*-associated diarrhea in a Canadian tertiary-care hospital. *Can Commun Dis Rep.* 1999;25(7):65-69.
50. Kuijper EJ, de Weerdt J, Kato H, et al. Nosocomial outbreak of *Clostridium difficile*-associated diarrhoea due to a clindamycin-resistant enterotoxin A-negative strain. *Eur J Clin Microbiol Infect Dis.* 2001;20(8):528-534.
51. Kader HA, Piccoli DA, Jawad AF, McGowan KL, Maller ES. Single toxin detection is inadequate to diagnose *Clostridium difficile* diarrhea in pediatric patients. *Gastroenterology.* 1998;115(6):1329-1334.
52. Markowitz JE, Brown KA, Mamula P, Drott HR, Piccoli DA, Baldassano RN. Failure of single-toxin assays to detect *Clostridium difficile* infection in pediatric inflammatory bowel disease. *Am J Gastroenterol.* 2001;96(9): 2688-2690.
53. Kirkpatrick ID, Greenberg HM. Evaluating the CT diagnosis of *Clostridium difficile* colitis: should CT guide therapy? *Am J Roentgenol.* 2001;176(3):635-639.
54. Zamora S, Coppes MJ, Scott RB, Mueller DL. *Clostridium difficile*, pseudomembranous enterocolitis: striking CT and sonographic features in a pediatric patient. *Eur J Radiol.* 1996;23(2):104-106.
55. Blickman JG, Boland GW, Cleveland RH, Bramson RT, Lee MJ. Pseudomembranous colitis: CT findings in children. *Pediatr Radiol.* 1995;25(suppl 1):S157-S159.
56. Walley T, Milson D. Loperamide related toxic megacolon in *Clostridium difficile* colitis. *Postgrad Med J.* 1990; 66(777):582.
57. Lamontagne F, Labbe AC, Haeck O, et al. Impact of emergency colectomy on survival of patients with fulminant *Clostridium difficile* colitis during an epidemic caused by a hypervirulent strain. *Ann Surg.* 2007;245(2):267-272.
58. Teasley DG, Gerding DN, Olson MM, et al. Prospective randomised trial of metronidazole versus vancomycin for *Clostridium difficile*-associated diarrhoea and colitis. *Lancet.* 1983;2(8358):1043-1046.
59. Wenisch C, Parschalk B, Hasenhundl M, Hirschl AM, Graninger W. Comparison of vancomycin, teicoplanin, metronidazole, and fusidic acid for the treatment of *Clostridium difficile*-associated diarrhea. *Clin Infect Dis.* 1996;22(5):813-818.
60. Baird DR. Comparison of two oral formulations of vancomycin for treatment of diarrhoea associated with *Clostridium difficile. J Antimicrob Chemother.* 1989;23(1): 167-169.
61. Keighley MR, Burdon DW, Arabi Y, et al. Randomised controlled trial of vancomycin for pseudomembranous colitis and postoperative diarrhoea. *Br Med J.* 1978;2(6153): 1667-1669.
62. Fekety R. Guidelines for the diagnosis and management of *Clostridium difficile*-associated diarrhea and colitis. American college of gastroenterology, practice parameters committee. *Am J Gastroenterol.* 1997;92(5):739-750.
63. Recommendations for preventing the spread of vancomycin resistance. Hospital infection control practices advisory committee. *Emerg Infect Dis.* 1995;1(2):66.
64. Johnston BC, Supina AL, Vohra S. Probiotics for pediatric antibiotic-associated diarrhea: a meta-analysis of randomized placebo-controlled trials. *CMAJ.* 2006;175(4): 377-383.
65. Herbrecht R, Nivoix Y. *Saccharomyces cerevisiae* fungemia: an adverse effect of *Saccharomyces boulardii* probiotic administration. *Clin Infect Dis.* 2005;40(11): 1635-1637.
66. Cohen SA. Use of nitazoxanide as a new therapeutic option for persistent diarrhea: a pediatric perspective. *Curr Med Res Opin.* 2005;21(7):999-1004.

67. Loffler HA, Pron B, Mouy R, Wulffraat NM, Prieur AM. *Clostridium difficile*-associated reactive arthritis in two children. *Joint Bone Spine.* 2004;71(1):60-62.
68. Cron RQ, Gordon PV. Reactive arthritis to *Clostridium difficile* in a child. *West J Med.* 1997;166(6):419-421.
69. Harris PR, Figueroa-Colon R. Rectal prolapse in children associated with *Clostridium difficile* infection. *Pediatr Infect Dis J.* 1995;14(1):78-80.
70. Boey CC, Ramanujam TM, Looi LM. *Clostridium difficile*-related necrotizing pseudomembranous enteritis in association with Henoch-Schonlein purpura. *J Pediatr Gastroenterol Nutr.* 1997;24(4):426-429.
71. Butani L. Hemolytic uremic syndrome associated with *Clostridium difficile* colitis. *Pediatr Nephrol.* 2004;19 (12):1430.
72. Rooney N, Variend S, Taitz LS. Haemolytic uraemic syndrome and pseudomembranous colitis. *Pediatr Nephrol.* 1988;2(4):415-418.
73. Byl B, Jacobs F, Struelens MJ, Thys JP. Extraintestinal *Clostridium difficile* infections. *Clin Infect Dis.* 1996;22 (4):712.
74. Cid A, Juncal AR, Aguilera A, Regueiro BJ, Gonzalez V. *Clostridium difficile* bacteremia in an immunocompetent child. *J Clin Microbiol.* 1998;36(4):1167-1168.
75. Garcia-Lechuz JM, Hernangomez S, Juan RS, Pelaez T, Alcala L, Bouza E. Extra-intestinal infections caused by *Clostridium difficile. Clin Microbiol Infect.* 2001;7(8): 453-457.
76. Pepin J, Alary ME, Valiquette L, et al. Increasing risk of relapse after treatment of *Clostridium difficile* colitis in Quebec, Canada. *Clin Infect Dis.* 2005;40 (11):1591-1597.
77. Pepin J, Routhier S, Gagnon S, Brazeau I. Management and outcomes of a first recurrence of *Clostridium difficile*-associated disease in Quebec, Canada. *Clin Infect Dis.* 2006;42(6):758-764.
78. McFarland LV, Elmer GW, Surawicz CM. Breaking the cycle: treatment strategies for 163 cases of recurrent *Clostridium difficile* disease. *Am J Gastroenterol.* 2002; 97(7):1769-1775.

SECTION 10

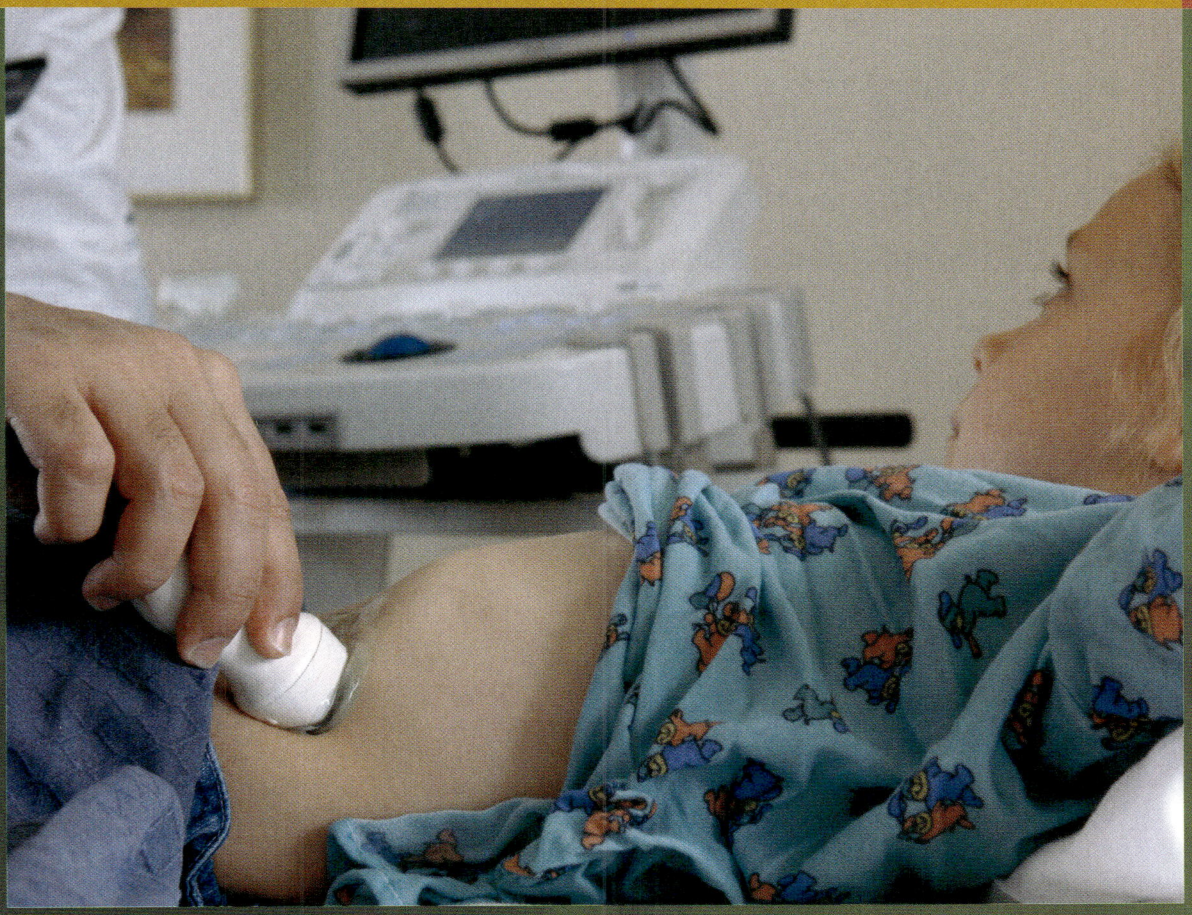

Genitourinary Infections

CHAPTER 42

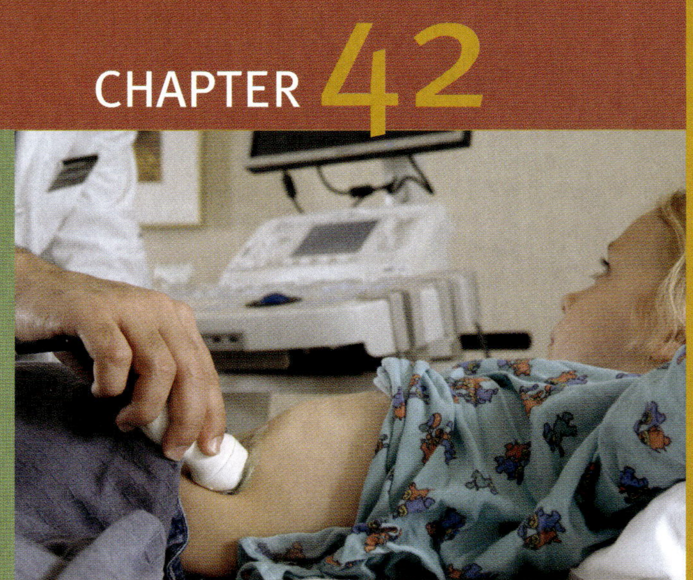

Urinary Tract Infections

Mercedes M. Blackstone and Joseph J. Zorc

DEFINITIONS AND EPIDEMIOLOGY

Urinary tract infection (UTI) is defined by the presence of microorganisms within the urinary tract, which is usually sterile. Since asymptomatic colonization of the urinary tract can occur, definitive diagnosis often relies upon a constellation of features that might include history and examination findings, elevated inflammatory markers, and repeat urine cultures. UTIs are typically divided into lower tract disease, where infection is localized to the bladder and urethra (cystitis and urethritis), and upper tract disease, where it extends to the ureter and kidney (pyelonephritis). Although both upper and lower tract disease may result in significant morbidity, pyelonephritis in particular is associated with renal scarring and subsequent hypertension, chronic renal disease, and preeclampsia.[1,2]

UTIs are the most common serious bacterial infections affecting infants and young children. In recent decades, UTI has been increasingly recognized as an important occult cause of fever in young children. Rates of UTI vary widely with respect to age, gender, race, and other factors. Screening studies performed in emergency departments suggest an overall prevalence of UTI of up to 5% in febrile children younger than 2 years.[3,4] Peak incidence of UTI occurs in the first year of life for all children, with a second peak occurring among female adolescents. After infancy, females are far more likely than males to have a UTI. A population-based European study reported a cumulative UTI incidence of 7.8% for girls by age 7 years.[5] One factor influencing the relatively higher rates of UTI in male infants is circumcision status; uncircumcised males younger than a year are approximately 10 times more likely to develop UTI than their circumcised counterparts.[6] In young children, race appears to be an independent risk factor for UTI. In an emergency department study, Caucasian females younger than 2 years with fever ≥39°C have a UTI prevalence of 16% compared to a 2.7% prevalence among nonwhite girls.[4]

PATHOGENESIS

Bacterial pathogens cause the vast majority of UTIs, but viruses, fungi, and parasites can cause infection as well. UTI occurs when enteric stool pathogens or skin flora ascend through the urethra, infecting the bladder or spreading further into the upper urinary tract. The shorter urethra in females has been implicated in their predisposition to UTI. Similarly, uncircumcised infants harbor increased numbers of uropathogenic bacteria in the periurethral area.[7] Bacterial invasion is the result of the interaction between bacteriologic properties such as adhesion, virulence, and motility as well as anatomic and genetic properties that influence host response.[8] Some racial and genetic differences may be explained by differences in blood group antigens on the surface of uroepithelial cells, which affect bacterial adherence. An association of certain Lewis blood group phenotypes has been found in children with UTIs[9] and in women with recurrent UTIs.[10] Studies suggest that there may be a genetic predisposition to acute pyelonephritis caused by an inherited defect in neutrophil migration and activation.[11] Rarely, in young infants, infection may be caused by hematogenous spread rather than ascending infection.

The etiologic agents associated with UTI are shown in Table 42–1. Almost all clinically significant urinary infections are monomicrobial rather than polymicrobial. Most uncomplicated UTIs are caused by the gram-negative Enterobacteriaceae family. *Escherichia coli*

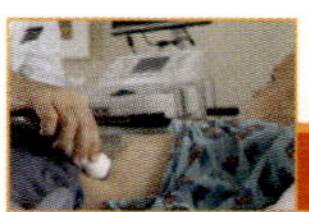

Table 42–1.

Etiology of Urinary Tract Infections

Common
Gram-negative organisms
- *Escherichia coli*
- *Klebsiella* spp.
- *Proteus mirabilis*
- *Enterobacter* spp.
- *Serratia* spp.

Gram-positive organisms
- *Staphylococcus saprophyticus*
- Group B streptococci
- *Enterococcus* spp.

Less Common
Pseudomonas spp.
Citrobacter spp.
Staphylococcus aureus
Coagulase-negative staphylococci

Rare
Corynebacterium urealyticum
U. urealyticum
M. hominis

Nonbacterial
Candida spp.
Adenovirus

causes the vast majority of acute infections.[12] Organisms such as *Proteus*, *Enterobacter*, *Citrobacter*, and *Klebsiella* spp. are more commonly encountered in cases of recurrent UTI, particularly in cases of urinary anomalies. *Pseudomonas* sp., while not usually a cause of UTI in healthy children, is a significant pathogen for hospitalized children, immunocompromised children, and children with indwelling catheters or frequent bladder instrumentation. Gram-positive organisms account for a minority of uncomplicated UTIs (approximately 5–10%); those most commonly encountered include *Enterococcus* sp., *Staphylococcus saprophyticus*, and group B streptococci. *S. saprophyticus* tends to infect sexually active adolescent females. Candidal UTIs typically occur in children with indwelling catheters who are receiving broad-spectrum antibiotics or in children in the neonatal intensive care unit.[13] *Ureaplasma urealyticum* and *Mycoplasma hominis* may also be associated with pathogenic infection.[14] Adenovirus is a relatively common nonbacterial cause of hemorrhagic cystitis.

CLINICAL PRESENTATION

The clinical manifestations of UTI are protean and vary based on the child's age and the location of the infection.

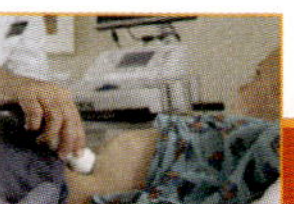

Table 42–2.

Clinical Features Associated with UTI

Infants
Common Signs and Symptoms
- Fever
- Irritability
- Lethargy
- Poor feeding
- Vomiting
- Dehydration

Possible Associated Findings
- Jaundice
- Failure to thrive
- Abdominal or flank mass
- Labial adhesions
- Vaginal discharge or foreign body
- Phimosis
- Diarrhea or constipation

Older Children and Adolescents
Common Signs and Symptoms
- Fever
- Abdominal pain
- Urinary frequency
- Urinary urgency
- Dysuria
- Hematuria
- Vomiting
- Suprapubic pain and tenderness
- Flank pain and tenderness
- Constipation
- Incontinence
- Secondary enuresis

See Table 42–2 for a summary of important findings on history and physical examination. School-aged children and adolescents with cystitis may present with the classic findings seen in adults such as dysuria, hematuria, urinary frequency and urgency, and suprapubic abdominal discomfort. Upper tract infections may present with flank pain, fevers, chills, nausea, and vomiting. Secondary enuresis can also suggest UTI in a child. Families should be asked about chronic constipation, dysfunctional elimination habits, prior UTIs, recent antibiotic use, history of vesicoureteral reflux, or urinary abnormalities, previous undiagnosed febrile illnesses, and family history of UTI.

Infants and young children pose a much greater diagnostic challenge than older children, since they most often present with isolated fever or nonspecific symptoms. In a prospective prevalence study of more than 2000 febrile children younger than 2 years, signs and symptoms localizing to the urinary tract such as malodorous urine, hematuria, or tenderness on examination were rare. Children with UTI were somewhat more likely to have no source of fever on examination and to be ill appearing, but half of the infants with UTI were described as well appearing and more than half had another potential source of fever on examination.[4,15] Therefore, even in the presence of another potential fever source such as upper respiratory infection, gastroenteritis, or otitis media, clinicians must consider the diagnosis of UTI. Although nonspecific symptoms such as vomiting, diarrhea, and poor feeding were initially reported to be present in approximately one-third of patients with UTI,[16] two large prevalence studies of young febrile children found that infants with and without UTI were equally likely to have these symptoms.[3,4]

Jaundice has been associated with UTI in young infants as well. A study of 160 asymptomatic jaundiced infants younger than 8 weeks found an incidence of UTI of 7.5%. Infants with conjugated hyperbilirubinemia and onset of jaundice after 8 days of age were more likely to have positive urine cultures.[17]

Physical examination in the older child and adolescent may demonstrate classic findings such as suprapubic and flank tenderness. Infants will often have an unremarkable examination with the exception of fever. Clinicians should pay close attention to the abdominal and perineal examinations in children when UTI is suspected. A distended bladder may be palpable, and since constipation can predispose to urinary stasis and infection, hard stool may be palpable as well. While less common, it is important to check for an abdominal or flank mass in infants, since this could be consistent with ureteropelvic junction obstruction or massive renal hydrocephalus. The perineum should be inspected for signs of trauma, labial adhesions, or evidence of vulvovaginitis in females. In males, the penis should be examined and particular care should be taken to make sure that the foreskin can be easily retracted in uncircumcised males.

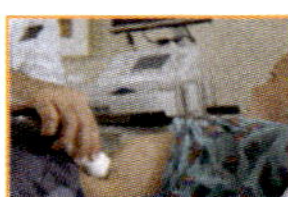

Table 42–3.

Differential Diagnosis of UTI

Infants

Common Conditions
- Viral infection such as gastroenteritis

Less Common Conditions
- Occult bacteremia
- Occult pneumonia
- Meningitis

Toddler and School-Aged Children

Common conditions
- Vaginal foreign body
- Vulvovaginitis
- Behavioral problems
- Gastroenteritis

Less Common Conditions
- Group A streptococcal infection
- Kawasaki disease
- Appendicitis
- Diabetes
- Sexually-transmitted infection from child abuse
- Rare Conditions
- Spinal cord process (tumor, abscess)
- Hypercalcemia

Adolescents

Common Conditions
- Urethritis
- Vaginitis
- Cervicitis
- Pelvic inflammatory disease
- Gastroenteritis

Less Common Conditions
- Urinary calculi
- Gallbladder disease
- Appendicitis
- Diabetes

Rare Conditions
- Spinal cord process (tumor, abscess)
- Hypercalcemia

DIFFERENTIAL DIAGNOSIS

The differential diagnosis of UTI differs depending on the child's age (see Table 42–3). In the febrile infant without a source, the clinician is most often faced with the differential diagnosis of occult fever and should recognize that UTI is the most likely serious bacterial infection in this scenario. In the older child, the differential diagnosis may include causes of dysuria or urinary frequency, including vaginal processes or diabetes as well as causes of fever and abdominal pain such as appendicitis. Kawasaki disease has been described to cause sterile pyuria in association with prolonged fever and other symptoms such as rash and conjunctivitis.

DIAGNOSIS

Screening for UTI

Clearly, symptoms localizing to the urinary tract should prompt screening for UTI. The far more difficult problem is when to screen young children who present with isolated fever or nonspecific symptoms. The American Academy of Pediatrics (AAP) has addressed this question in its practice parameter on UTI. Since infants and young children are at highest risk for renal scarring with UTI, they focus on children younger than 2 years and recommend that clinicians consider UTI in any case of unexplained fever.[2] To help narrow this scope

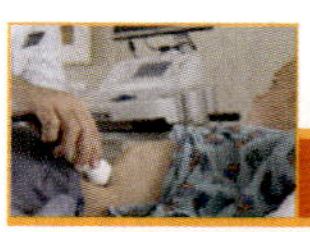

Table 42-4.

Clinical Factors to Determine Risk of UTI and Need for Further Screening in Girls 2–24 months of Age with Fever

Parameter	Relative Risk of UTI (95% Confidence Interval)
Age less than 1 year	2.8 (1.6–5.1)
Fever for 2 days or more	1.5 (0.9–2.6)
White race	6.0 (3.7–9.5)
Absence of a source of fever	1.9 (1.1–3.2)
Temperature ≥39°C	1.7 (0.9–3.1)

Table from Zorc JJ, Kiddoo DA, Shaw KN. Diagnosis and management of pediatric urinary tract infections. Clin Microbiol Rev. 2005;18(2):417–422; data adapted from Gorelick MH, Shaw KN. Clinical decision rule to identify febrile young girls at risk for urinary tract infection. Arch Pediatr Adolesc Med. 2000;154(4):386–390.

somewhat, several authors developed and validated a clinical decision rule to identify febrile young girls (ages 2–24 months) at risk for UTI (Table 42–4).[18] They recommended screening for UTI when two or more of these factors were present based on a 95% sensitivity to detect UTI with this strategy. Although there is currently no validated clinical decision rule for males, risk factors such as age younger than 6 months, being uncircumcised, and lack of alternative source of fever should prompt UTI screening.[4,6,19,20]

Collection Methods

Once the decision to obtain urine has been made, based either on history or on these epidemiologic risk factors, several collection options are available. Proper collection of the urine specimen is extremely important since contaminated specimens can lead to a missed diagnosis or unnecessary antibiotics. In toilet-trained children, a midstream clean-catch specimen can be obtained after cleansing of the urethral meatus. After some earlier pediatric studies suggested that there was no difference in contamination rates among toilet-trained children with and without perineal cleaning prior to voiding,[21–23] a randomized trial[24] of 350 children found that cleaning significantly lowers contamination rates (7.8% in cleaning group versus 23.9% in noncleaning group). Positioning girls backward on the toilet can also prevent vaginal contamination by helping to spread the labia.

Suprapubic aspiration is a viable option for young children, particularly since it bypasses the distal urethra, a common site of contamination. Ultrasound assessment of the bladder can increase the success rate of this procedure. The most commonly utilized technique in young children is bladder catheterization. As with the clean-catch method, it is important to discard the first few drops of urine since these are likely to be contaminated with flora from the distal urethra. The use of a sterile bag affixed to the perineum results in unacceptably high false-positive cultures and is therefore not recommended as a collection technique for urine culture. In certain settings or in low-risk patients, however, it may be appropriate to screen urine using a bag specimen and to have a selective approach to catheterization. A study comparing this technique and bladder catheterization in the same children found that bag specimens were very sensitive for UTI but lacked specificity [specificity, 0.62; 95% confidence interval (CI): 0.56–0.69] compared with catheterized specimens (specificity, 0.97–95% CI 0.95–0.99).[25]

Rapid Tests

Urine culture is the gold standard for diagnosis of UTI, but results are unavailable for 24–48 hours. As such, several rapid diagnostic tests are available for faster UTI detection. These include: Urine dipstick testing for leukocyte esterase (LE) and nitrites; traditional urinalysis, which is typically done by microscopy on a *centrifuged* specimen; and enhanced urinalysis, using a hemocytometer cell count and Gram stain of *unspun* urine. Multiple studies have compared the performance of these tests and these results have been combined in two recent meta-analyses (see Table 42–5). Gorelick and Shaw found that a positive Gram stain on uncentrifuged urine had the best combination of sensitivity and specificity as indicated by the likelihood ratios [positive likelihood ratio (LR), 18.5; negative LR, 0.07] and that the presence of both LE and nitrites on urine dipstick performed nearly as well.[26] Interpretation of likelihood ratios is discussed in Chapter 6 (Infectious Diseases Epidemiology). Huicho et al. concluded instead that pyuria of at least 10 wbc/hpf or at least 10 wbc/mm^3 on microscopy *and* a positive Gram stain are the best screening tests for UTI.[27] Urine dipstick may be the most affordable and readily available option in the majority of office settings and is fairly sensitive and specific. Enhanced urinalysis has superior sensitivity to standard urinalysis (approximately 95%) and has been recommended for children younger than 60 days who are at high risk for serious bacterial illness.[28] In summary, all of the following are suggestive but not diagnostic of UTI: ≥10 wbc on a spun or unspun specimen, a positive Gram stain, or positive LE or nitrites. Since the only way to definitively diagnose UTI is by culture, a urine culture should be sent on all patients with suspected UTI. Failure to do so will result in missing the approximately 10–30% of UTIs that will not be picked up on most screening tests.

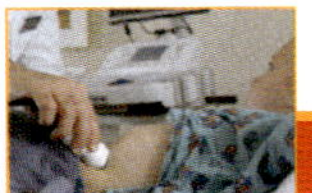

Table 42–5.

Predictive Value of Laboratory Tests in the Diagnosis of UTI in Young Children*

Test	Sensitivity (Range in %)	Specificity (Range in %)	Neg. Likelihood Ratio
Dipsticks			
Nitrites	50 (16–72)	98 (95–100)	0.51
LE	83 (64–89)	84 (71–95)	0.20
Either LE or nit.	88 (71–100)	93 (76–98)	0.13
Standard UA micro (≥5 wbcs/hpf)	67 (55–88)	79 (77–84)	0.42
Hemocytometer cell count (≥10 bcs/mm^3)	77 (57–92)	89 (37–95)	0.26
Gram stain (any organisms)	93 (80–98)	95 (87–100)	0.07
Enhanced UA (cell count *and* GS$^+$)	85 (75–88)	99 (99)	0.15
Enhanced UA (cell count *or* GS$^+$)	95 (94–96)	89 (84–93)	0.06

**Summary estimates are provided in addition to the range reported among studies reviewed in a meta-analysis.*
Table from Zorc JJ, Kiddoo DA, Shaw KN. Diagnosis and management of pediatric urinary tract infections. Clin Microbiol Rev. 2005;18(2):417-422. Data adapted from Gorelick MH, Shaw KN. Screening tests for urinary tract infection in children: A meta-analysis. Pediatrics. 1999;104(5):e54.
LE, leukocyte esterase; UA micro, microscopic urinalysis; wbcs/hpf, white blood cells per high-powered field; GS, Gram stain.

Urine Culture

Although growth of pathogenic bacteria from the normally sterile urine is the gold standard for diagnosis of UTI, what constitutes a significant colony count varies by collection method. Children who are toilet trained can use the clean-catch method, which is susceptible to urethral contamination. Using this modality, UTI is often defined as $\geq 10^5$ colony-forming units (CFU) of a single pathogen. Since this mode of collection is relatively easy, and since contamination results in many false-positive results, obtaining a second clean-catch specimen prior to treatment may be prudent.[2] In young children, urine cultures are most commonly obtained via transurethral catheterization. Using this technique, one can generally assume that growth of $\geq 10^4$ CFU of a single pathogen represents a UTI. Suprapubic aspiration is the most specific method of collection since the risk of contamination is extremely small. Therefore, the presence of any bacteria in a urine sample obtained in this manner is significant.

Asymptomatic Bacteriuria

Even in cases where suprapubic aspiration is performed, growth of bacteria may not necessarily indicate UTI given the potential for benign colonization of the urinary tract with bacteria, an entity known as asymptomatic bacteriuria. The topic of asymptomatic bacteriuria has been somewhat controversial since its discovery by Kunin and colleagues in the 1950s.[29,30] Several Scandinavian long-term screening studies have helped to elucidate this complex issue.[31] In the 1970s, Lindberg et al. identified 117 schoolgirls of age 7–15 years who had asymptomatic bacteriuria detected by screening urine culture.[32] They were randomized to antibiotic treatment or observation, and at 3-year follow-up, renal growth was similar in both groups and no benefit from antibiotic treatment was demonstrated. None of the girls who were left untreated went on to develop symptomatic infection. Asymptomatic bacteriuria has been examined among infants as well. Among a cohort of 3581 infants who were screened during the first year of life, 2.5% of boys and 0.9% of girls were found to have asymptomatic bacteriuria confirmed on suprapubic aspiration.[33,34] Only 2 of 45 infants went on to develop symptomatic infection; in the majority of infants, the bacteriuria cleared spontaneously within a few months. There were an additional 42 infants in the study population who developed symptomatic UTI during the first year of life; none of these had screened positive for asymptomatic bacteriuria previously. Therefore, asymptomatic bacteriuria does not appear to be a precursor to symptomatic infection. In fact, it is hypothesized that colonization may provide some degree of protection from invasive bacteria that potentially may be disrupted by antibiotic treatment.[31]

Laboratory Testing

A few laboratory parameters have been examined to help determine not only whether bacteriuria is consistent with acute infection, but also the location of the infection within the urinary tract. Commonly used markers of inflammation such as white blood cell count, erythrocyte sedimentation rate (ESR), and C-reactive protein (CRP) cannot reliably distinguish pyelonephritis and cystitis. While CRP is the best among these and has a sensitivity of greater than 92% for pyelonephritis, it has a low specificity, which limits its applicability.[35,36] Although not as widely available (although a rapid test exists in some centers), multiple studies[35–38] have found that an elevated serum procalcitonin level appears to be more highly correlated with renal involvement than an elevated CRP. If made more available, this test could potentially alter the management and disposition of febrile patients with UTI.

A blood culture should be performed in young infants with UTI since they are at higher risk of bacteremia.[39,40] Febrile infants older than 2 months with UTI do not routinely require lumbar puncture. Concomitant invasive meningitis appears to be rare; an association of UTI with aseptic meningitis has been reported[41] but is controversial and may represent coincidental CSF infection and bacteruria.

Radiological Studies

Ultrasound

Imaging of the urinary collection system has become the standard of care for young children with a first UTI, although this is not entirely evidence-based.[42] The purpose of this is to detect and treat urinary abnormalities such as obstructive lesions or vesicoureteral reflux (VUR), thereby potentially reducing renal scarring and long-term sequelae. Several imaging modalities are available. Renal ultrasound has the advantages of being noninvasive, easy-to-obtain, and affordable, and has therefore largely replaced the intravenous pyelogram as the anatomical study of choice. It demonstrates abnormalities such as hydronephrosis, duplications of the collecting system, ureteroceles, and infectious complications such as renal abscesses. However, ultrasound is neither sensitive nor specific for detection of vesicoureteral reflux[43,44] and does not identify pyelonephritis or scarring as well as other techniques.[45–47]

The utility of routine ultrasound has recently been called into question, particularly since many renal anomalies are now detected on prenatal ultrasounds.[48] In a prospective trial of 309 young children with first febrile UTI, 88% of children had normal ultrasounds; abnormalities that were detected did not alter management.[49] In a similar prospective study from Israel, renal ultrasound results failed to change the management of any of the 255 children enrolled.[43] At present, the American Academy of Pediatrics continues to recommend ultrasound for all patients younger than 2 years.[2]

Voiding cystourethrogram

The voiding cystourethrogram (VCUG) has been in use consistently since the 1960s and is an excellent test for the detection of VUR, which has a prevalence in young children of 30–40%.[50] This test involves catheterizing the bladder and filling it with contrast material; VU reflux may be detected during the voiding phase as intravesical pressure increases. VCUG can be performed using standard contrast or a radionuclide (the latter is also known as radionuclide cystography or RNC). Both types have advantages: The contrast study is thought to show greater anatomic detail, but the radionuclide study appears to have higher sensitivity.[51,52] Since the traditional contrast VCUG is better at demonstrating urethral and bladder anomalies, the AAP recommends this study for young boys who are at risk for posterior urethral valves or girls with dysfunctional voiding.[2]

The question of whether to perform a VCUG is somewhat controversial. Although VUR is common, and VCUG is accurate in diagnosing VUR, the utility of this diagnosis remains unclear. Often, the reflux is low grade and does not require surgical repair (see Figure 42–1 for grades of VUR). A recent meta-analysis cautioned against using VUR identified on VCUG as a proxy for renal damage; their results showed that VUR was a weak predictor for evidence of renal damage on nuclear scan in hospitalized children with UTI.[53] Furthermore, reflux appears to occur intermittently. In a retrospective study of 306 children with first UTIs who had both initial and follow-up radionuclide VCUGs, with a mean interval between scans of 465 days (SD 258 days), the presence and grade of reflux varied greatly with time.[54] Some patients who initially had no reflux were found to have reflux (up to Grade III) on the follow-up study. The reverse was also true: Of 275 children with Grade I reflux on the initial examination, 39% had no reflux on the subsequent study. A common current practice involves treating children with significant VUR with prophylactic antibiotics to prevent renal scarring. Multiple authors have called for well-designed placebo-controlled trials in order to support or refute this practice.[49,55,56] Until such

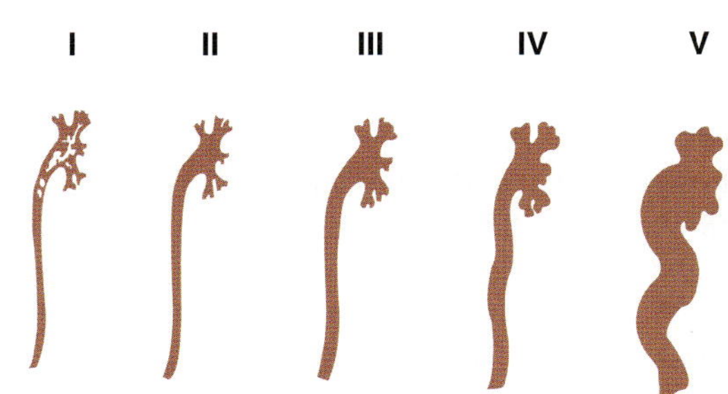

FIGURE 42–1 ■ Grades of vesicoureteral reflux. Urine refluxes progressively further towards the kidney, and the ureter and renal pelvis become increasingly tortuous and dilated.

evidence exists, the true value of VCUG is somewhat indeterminate.

Although longitudinal data are lacking, current AAP guidelines recommend a VCUG in young children with UTI.[2] If a VCUG is ordered, it can be obtained at any time after diagnosis of UTI. The concern that VCUG performed early after diagnosis will falsely elevate the incidence of VUR has not been substantiated by studies; in fact, early VCUG has a benefit in terms of improving patient compliance.[57,58]

Renal scan

Although reflux has been associated with scarring, scars are seen in the absence of reflux as well. The renal scan involves the injection of dimercaptosuccinic acid (DMSA), which is labeled with the radionuclide Technetium-99m, and has become the gold standard for the detection of renal scarring. Scanning is performed 2–4 hours after injection, and areas of decreased cortical uptake of the radiotracer indicate old scars or acute pyelonephritis. The sensitivity and specificity of DMSA scan for pyelonephritis is well supported in animal studies.[59,60] Renal scans detect pyelonephritis in many children without reflux. Studies of febrile UTIs report initial defects and subsequent scarring detected by renal scan in 34–70% and 9.5–38%, respectively.[61] Despite the ample evidence that these scans are very sensitive for the detection of scarring, the clinical importance of these scars remains unknown.[62]

Moreover, the optimal timing of these studies is unclear, since it can be difficult to distinguish true scars from transient defects on renal scan up to 6 months after acute infection caused by the presence of residual inflammatory changes.[63] In a prospective cohort study of 150 children with first UTI who had follow-up renal scans 2 years after diagnosis, 75 children had initially abnormal scintigrams and 20 children had persistent defects on the follow-up study. No new defects were found on the follow-up scan. The likelihood of persistent scars, however, did not correlate with clinical parameters such as a history of recurrent infections or grade of VUR.[64] This study and others suggest that in the setting of a normal renal scan at the time of UTI, it may be appropriate to omit a further anatomic evaluation since these children do not appear to be at risk for subsequent scar formation.[64–66] Although some authors have advocated including DMSA scans in the initial evaluation of children with UTI and have suggested that they could modify treatment,[65,67] the most recent AAP practice parameter concludes that the role of DMSA scans in clinical care is unclear and does not recommend their routine use.[2] Figure 42–2 provides a proposed summary algorithm for the diagnosis and evaluation of UTI in children older than 2 months.

TREATMENT

Inpatient Versus Outpatient Therapy

Children with UTIs require prompt recognition and treatment, not only to eradicate the acute infection and prevent urosepsis, but also to prevent the long-term renal sequelae (See Figure 42–2 for an empiric treatment approach). This treatment has traditionally included hospital admission for young children with pyelonephritis. Several studies have challenged this convention. Hoberman et al. conducted a large randomized controlled trial comparing a 14-day course of oral cefixime versus 11 days of oral cefixime after 3 days of inpatient IV cefotaxime in children aged 1–24 months with febrile UTI.[40] Clinical outcomes including time to defervescence, symptomatic UTI recurrence, and renal scarring at 6 months were similar between groups. The authors acknowledge that the study was underpowered to compare small subgroups of children, so caution may be warranted in applying these results to high-risk subgroups such as the youngest children. A subsequent study similarly found that the addition of one dose of IM ceftriaxone did not improve outcomes at 48 hours among children with febrile UTIs who were given 10 days of oral antibiotic therapy.[68] This study did not perform long-term follow-up beyond 6 months and therefore could not compare later outcomes. A Canadian study suggests that a third alternative—daily IV antibiotics at an outpatient treatment center until defervescence—may be another feasible option for select patients, and allows for close medical supervision.[69] The current AAP Practice Parameter recommends initial inpatient IV antibiotics for young children who are toxic-appearing, dehydrated, unable to tolerate oral intake, or when the clinician has concerns about patient compliance.[2]

Antibiotic Selection

Common uropathogens associated with first UTI are typically sensitive to many antimicrobials. In immunosuppressed children, children with indwelling catheters, and children with recurrent UTIs, initial antibiotics should be broad spectrum and should cover the pathogens involved in prior infections. Empiric therapy should be guided by local resistance patterns as well as factors affecting compliance such as taste and dosing frequency.

For hospitalized patients, commonly used empiric IV antibiotics include cefotaxime, ceftriaxone, or the combination of ampicillin and gentamicin. Amoxicillin is commonly used as empiric therapy in the outpatient setting, although *E. coli* resistance to amoxicillin has been increasing. The impact of such resistance on clinical cure rates is unclear. Comparative studies have found higher cure rates

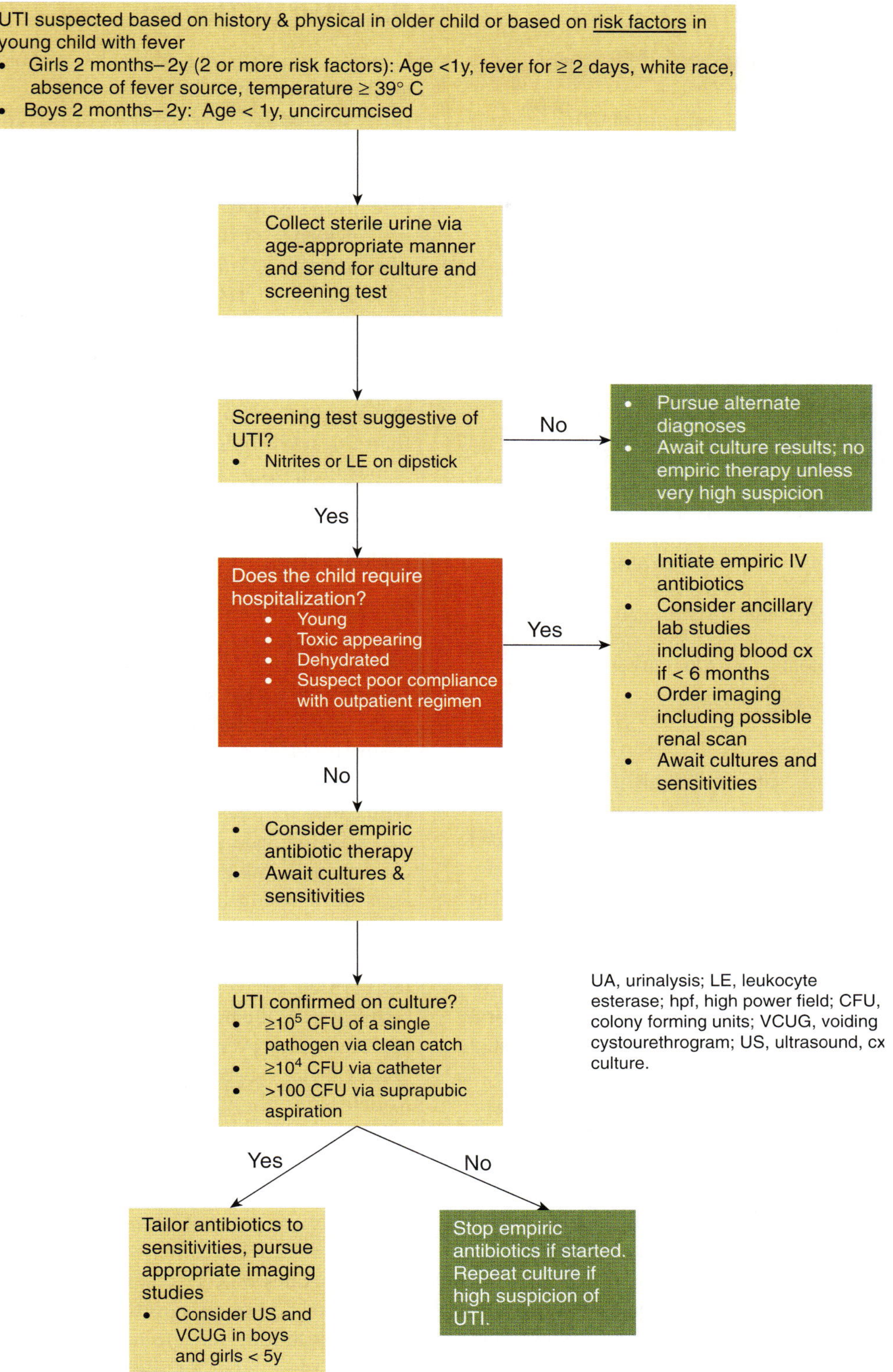

UTI suspected based on history & physical in older child or based on risk factors in young child with fever
• Girls 2 months–2y (2 or more risk factors): Age <1y, fever for ≥ 2 days, white race, absence of fever source, temperature ≥ 39° C
• Boys 2 months–2y: Age < 1y, uncircumcised
Collect sterile urine via age-appropriate manner and send for culture and screening test
Screening test suggestive of UTI?
• Nitrites or LE on dipstick
No
• Pursue alternate diagnoses
• Await culture results; no empiric therapy unless very high suspicion
Yes
Does the child require hospitalization?
• Young
• Toxic appearing
• Dehydrated
• Suspect poor compliance with outpatient regimen
Yes
• Initiate empiric IV antibiotics
• Consider ancillary lab studies including blood cx if < 6 months
• Order imaging including possible renal scan
• Await cultures and sensitivities
No
• Consider empiric antibiotic therapy
• Await cultures & sensitivities
UTI confirmed on culture?
• ≥10^5 CFU of a single pathogen via clean catch
• ≥10^4 CFU via catheter
• >100 CFU via suprapubic aspiration
Yes
No
Tailor antibiotics to sensitivities, pursue appropriate imaging studies
• Consider US and VCUG in boys and girls < 5y
Stop empiric antibiotics if started. Repeat culture if high suspicion of UTI.
UA, urinalysis; LE, leukocyte esterase; hpf, high power field; CFU, colony forming units; VCUG, voiding cystourethrogram; US, ultrasound, cx culture.

FIGURE 42–2 ■ Algorithm for diagnosis and treatment of first UTI in children >2 months.

with trimethoprim–sulfamethoxazole,[2] although resistance to this drug may also be rising in some areas.[70,71] Nonetheless, because of high urine concentrations of many antibiotics like amoxicillin, clinical response is often observed despite in vitro resistance. Oral third-generation cephalosporins such as cefixime and ceftibuten are also reasonable empiric therapeutic options in the young infant with UTI; they provide excellent activity

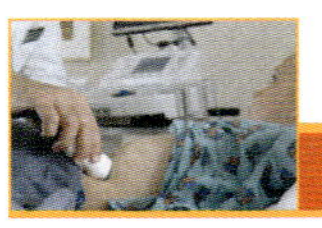

Table 42–6.

Common Antimicrobials for Treatment of UTI

Antimicrobial	Dosage (mg/kg per day)
Parenteral	
Ampicillin	100 divided qid
Gentamicin	7.5 divided tid
Cefazolin	100 divided tid
Ceftriaxone (Rocephin)	75 qd
Cefotaxime (Claforan)	120 divided tid
Oral	
Amoxicillin	20–40 divided tid
Amoxicillin-clavulanate (Augmentin)	45 of amoxicillin component divided bid
Cotrimoxazole (Bactrim, Septra)	6–12 of trimethoprim component divided bid
Cephalexin (Keflex)	50–100 divided qid
Cefixime (Suprax)	8 divided bid
Nitrofurantoin (Macrodantin)	5–7 divided qid
Cefdinir (Omnicef)	14 qd
Sulfisoxazole (Gantrisin)	120–150 divided qid

against enteric gram-negative rods with once daily dosing (Table 42–6).

While fluoroquinolones are very widely prescribed for adults with UTI, their use in children has historically been restricted as a result of early animal studies that found an effect on musculoskeletal development. Although data are limited, fluoroquinolones may be an alternative for outpatient UTI management in high-risk or complicated UTIs.[72] Commonly used empiric oral and parenteral antimicrobials and their doses are listed in Table 42–6.

Defervescence typically occurs within approximately 48 hours of initiation of treatment, but prolonged fever may occur in a minority of cases. Because of the discrepancy between in vivo and in vitro sensitivities, it is not necessary to empirically change antibiotics in children who are clinically improving or to perform a "test of cure" urine culture. Hospitalized children receiving multiple or broad-spectrum IV antibiotics should be switched to more directed therapy, if possible, once urine culture results and antibiotic susceptibility patterns are known. For patients with enterococcal UTI, amoxicillin, ciprofloxacin, and linezolid are reasonable options for oral therapy. For highly resistant enterococcal isolates, the cost of linezolid in this situation must be weighed against the benefits and risks of continued hospitalization or peripherally inserted central venous catheterization and home antibiotic administration.

Duration of Therapy

Controversy exists regarding the optimal duration of antibiotic therapy. Adults with simple cystitis are routinely treated for short courses of therapy (1–3 days), whereas children have typically received 7–14 days of therapy. The rationale for the longer treatment course in children is that the majority of children with UTI have evidence of upper tract disease. A meta-analysis of randomized, controlled trials found that there was a 74% increased risk of treatment failure for those receiving short-course therapy (3 days or less) compared with those receiving long-course antibiotic therapy (7–14 days).[73] As such, the AAP Practice Parameter continues to recommend that children younger than 2 years complete 7–14 days of antibiotic therapy.[2] It may be appropriate to apply the adult data supporting short courses of antibiotics to adolescent patients, in whom it is easier to distinguish simple cystitis from pyelonephritis.

Antibiotic Prophylaxis

Children with VUR are at risk for subsequent infections and renal scarring. Young children with low-grade reflux are likely to experience spontaneous resolution, while older children and those with Grades IV and V reflux may require surgical management. Despite limited scientific evidence, it has been recommended that children with low-grade VUR receive antibiotic prophylaxis until resolution of the reflux. Generally, either trimethoprim–sulfamethoxazole or nitrofurantoin at half the therapeutic dose are recommended for prophylaxis. In recent years, this practice has come under scrutiny since the health benefits of chronic prophylaxis are largely unproven. A recent Cochrane review of available evidence called for large, blinded randomized trials to determine the efficacy of antibiotic prophylaxis in children susceptible to UTI.[74] One recent trial evaluated 236 children of all ages with acute pyelonephritis, with or without VUR, and randomized them to either receive prophylaxis or not. At 1 year of follow-up, there was no significant difference between the two groups with regard to rates of UTI recurrence or development of renal scars.[73] More prospective studies that are double blinded with long-term follow-up are required to further elucidate whether the current practice is truly beneficial. The existing AAP recommendation states that young children should continue to receive prophylactic antibiotics at least until the completion of imaging studies.[2] Children with recurrent UTIs, severe VUR, and anatomical abnormalities of the urinary tract may merit referral to a pediatric urologist (see Table 42–7) for the determination of duration of antibiotic prophylaxis.

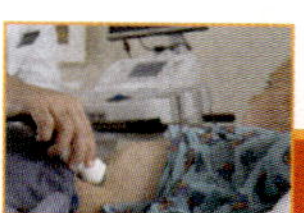

Table 42–7.

Indications for Urology Referral in UTI Patients

Abnormal anatomy seen on imaging
Vesicoureteral reflux grade III or above
Neurogenic bladder
Dysfunctional voiding seen on imaging
Recurrent or refractory UTIs
Indwelling catheters or stents

SUMMARY

In summary, increased vigilance on the part of practitioners and screening for UTI in febrile young children has dramatically reduced the morbidity associated with this diagnosis. Although there are several areas that remain ripe for further study, there is good evidence about the epidemiology, diagnosis, and treatment of UTI in children. Key principles of improving outcomes for pediatric UTI include maintaining a high index of suspicion, particularly in young children with fever; understanding the strengths and limitations of screening tests for UTI; and using evidence-based guidelines to approach further anatomic work-up of UTI, while recognizing the limitations of current knowledge in this area.

REFERENCES

1. Jacobson SH, Eklof O, Eriksson CG, Lins LE, Tidgren B, Winberg J. Development of hypertension and uraemia after pyelonephritis in childhood: 27 Year follow up. *BMJ.* 1989;299(6701):703-706.
2. Practice parameter: the diagnosis, treatment, and evaluation of the initial urinary tract infection in febrile infants and young children. American Academy of Pediatrics. Committee on Quality Improvement. Subcommittee on Urinary Tract Infection. *Pediatrics.* 1999;103(4, pt 1):843-852.
3. Hoberman A, Chao HP, Keller DM, Hickey R, Davis HW, Ellis D. Prevalence of urinary tract infection in febrile infants. *J Pediatr.* 1993;123(1):17-23.
4. Shaw KN, Gorelick M, McGowan KL, Yakscoe NM, Schwartz JS. Prevalence of urinary tract infection in febrile young children in the emergency department. *Pediatrics.* 1998;102(2):e16.
5. Hellstrom A, Hanson E, Hansson S, Hjalmas K, Jodal U. Association between urinary symptoms at 7 years old and previous urinary tract infection. *Arch Dis Child.* 1991; 66(2):232-234.
6. Wiswell TE, Roscelli JD. Corroborative evidence for the decreased incidence of urinary tract infections in circumcised male infants. *Pediatrics.* 1986;78(1):96-99.
7. Wiswell TE, Miller GM, Gelston HM, Jr., Jones SK, Clemmings AF. Effect of circumcision status on periurethral bacterial flora during the first year of life. *J Pediatr.* 1988;113(3):442-446.
8. Bergsten G, Wullt B, Svanborg C. *Escherichia coli*, fimbriae, bacterial persistence and host response induction in the human urinary tract. *Int J Med Microbiol.* 2005;295 (6-7):487-502.
9. Jantausch BA, Criss VR, O'Donnell R, et al. Association of Lewis blood group phenotypes with urinary tract infection in children. *J Pediatr.* 1994;124(6):863-868.
10. Sheinfeld J, Schaeffer AJ, Cordon-Cardo C, Rogatko A, Fair WR. Association of the Lewis blood-group phenotype with recurrent urinary tract infections in women. *N Engl J Med.* 1989;320(12):773-777.
11. Lundstedt AC, Leijonhufvud I, Ragnarsdottir B, Karpman D, Andersson B, Svanborg C. Inherited susceptibility to acute pyelonephritis: a family study of urinary tract infection. *J Infect Dis.* 2007;195(8):1227-1234.
12. Jellheden B, Norrby RS, Sandberg T. Symptomatic urinary tract infection in women in primary health care. Bacteriological, clinical and diagnostic aspects in relation to host response to infection. *Scand J Prim Health Care.* 1996;14(2):122-128.
13. Phillips JR, Karlowicz MG. Prevalence of Candida species in hospital-acquired urinary tract infections in a neonatal intensive care unit. *Pediatr Infect Dis J.* 1997;16(2):190-194.
14. Lilla L, Edit S, Eva K. Detection of *Mycoplasma* species in urinary tract infections in children. *Bacteriol Virusol Parazitol Epidemiol.* 2004;49(1-2):33-36.
15. Shaw KN, Gorelick MH. Fever as a sign of urinary tract infection. *Clin Pediatr Emerg Med.* 2000;1(2):117-123.
16. McCracken GH, Jr. Diagnosis and management of acute urinary tract infections in infants and children. *Pediatr Infect Dis J.* 1987;6(1):107-112.
17. Garcia FJ, Nager AL. Jaundice as an early diagnostic sign of urinary tract infection in infancy. *Pediatrics.* 2002;109(5):846-851.
18. Gorelick MH, Shaw KN. Clinical decision rule to identify febrile young girls at risk for urinary tract infection. *Arch Pediatr Adolesc Med.* 2000;154(4):386-390.
19. To T, Agha M, Dick PT, Feldman W. Cohort study on circumcision of newborn boys and subsequent risk of urinary-tract infection. *Lancet.* 1998;352(9143):1813-1816.
20. Hoberman A, Wald ER, Reynolds EA, Penchansky L, Charron M. Pyuria and bacteriuria in urine specimens obtained by catheter from young children with fever. *J Pediatr.* 1994;124(4):513-519.
21. Lohr JA, Donowitz LG, Dudley SM. Bacterial contamination rates for non-clean-catch and clean-catch midstream urine collections in boys. *J Pediatr.* 1986;109(4):659-660.
22. Lohr JA, Donowitz LG, Dudley SM. Bacterial contamination rates in voided urine collections in girls. *J Pediatr.* 1989;114(1):91-93.
23. Saez-Llorens X, Umana MA, Odio CM, Lohr JA. Bacterial contamination rates for non-clean-catch and clean-catch midstream urine collections in uncircumcised boys. *J Pediatr.* 1989;114(1):93-95.
24. Vaillancourt S, McGillivray D, Zhang X, Kramer MS. To clean or not to clean: effect on contamination rates in midstream urine collections in toilet-trained children. *Pediatrics.* 2007:119(6):e1288-1293.
25. McGillivray D, Mok E, Mulrooney E, Kramer MS. A head-to-head comparison: "Clean-void" bag versus catheter urinalysis in the diagnosis of urinary tract infection in young children. *J Pediatr.* 2005;147(4):451-456.

26. Gorelick MH, Shaw KN. Screening tests for urinary tract infection in children: a meta-analysis. *Pediatrics.* 1999; 104(5):e54.
27. Huicho L, Campos-Sanchez M, Alamo C. Meta-analysis of urine screening tests for determining the risk of urinary tract infection in children. *Pediatr Infect Dis J.* 2002; 21(1):1-11, 88.
28. Herr SM, Wald ER, Pitetti RD, Choi SS. Enhanced urinalysis improves identification of febrile infants ages 60 days and younger at low risk for serious bacterial illness. *Pediatrics.* 2001;108(4):866-871.
29. Kunin CM. A ten-year study of bacteriuria in schoolgirls: final report of bacteriologic, urologic, and epidemiologic findings. *J Infect Dis.* 1970;122(5):382-393.
30. Kunin CM. The natural history of recurrent bacteriuria in schoolgirls. *N Engl J Med.* 1970;282(26):1443-1448.
31. Hansson S, Martinell J, Stokland E, Jodal U. The natural history of bacteriuria in childhood. *Infect Dis Clin North Am.* 1997;11(3):499-512.
32. Lindberg U, Claesson I, Hanson LA, Jodal U. Asymptomatic bacteriuria in schoolgirls. VIII. Clinical course during a 3-year follow-up. *J Pediatr.* 1978;92(2):194-199.
33. Wettergren B, Jodal U, Jonasson G. Epidemiology of bacteriuria during the first year of life. *Acta Paediatr Scand.* 1985;74(6):925-933.
34. Wennerstrom M, Hansson S, Jodal U, Stokland E. Primary and acquired renal scarring in boys and girls with urinary tract infection. *J Pediatr.* 2000;136(1):30-34.
35. Smolkin V, Koren A, Raz R, Colodner R, Sakran W, Halevy R. Procalcitonin as a marker of acute pyelonephritis in infants and children. *Pediatr Nephrol.* 2002;17(6): 409-412.
36. Prat C, Dominguez J, Rodrigo C, et al. Elevated serum procalcitonin values correlate with renal scarring in children with urinary tract infection. *Pediatr Infect Dis J.* 2003;22(5):438-442.
37. Gervaix A, Galetto-Lacour A, Gueron T, et al. Usefulness of procalcitonin and C-reactive protein rapid tests for the management of children with urinary tract infection. *Pediatr Infect Dis J.* 2001;20(5):507-511.
38. Pecile P, Miorin E, Romanello C, et al. Procalcitonin: a marker of severity of acute pyelonephritis among children. *Pediatrics.* 2004;114(2):e249-e254.
39. Bachur R, Caputo GL. Bacteremia and meningitis among infants with urinary tract infections. *Pediatr Emerg Care.* 1995;11(5):280-284.
40. Hoberman A, Wald ER, Hickey RW, et al. Oral versus initial IV therapy for urinary tract infections in young febrile children. *Pediatrics.* 1999;104(1, pt 1):79-86.
41. Adler-Shohet FC, Cheung MM, Hill M, Lieberman JM. Aseptic meningitis in infants younger than six months of age hospitalized with urinary tract infections. *Pediatr Infect Dis J.* 2003;22(12):1039-1042.
42. Dick PT, Feldman W. Routine diagnostic imaging for childhood urinary tract infections: a systematic overview. *J Pediatr.* 1996;128(1):15-22.
43. Zamir G, Sakran W, Horowitz Y, Koren A, Miron D. Urinary tract infection: is there a need for routine renal ultrasonography? *Arch Dis Child.* 2004;89(5):466-468.
44. Mahant S, Friedman J, MacArthur C. Renal ultrasound findings and vesicoureteral reflux in children hospitalised with urinary tract infection. *Arch Dis Child.* 2002; 86(6):419-420.
45. Shanon A, Feldman W, McDonald P, et al. Evaluation of renal scars by technetium-labeled dimercaptosuccinic acid scan, IV urography, and ultrasonography: a comparative study. *J Pediatr.* 1992;120(3):399-403.
46. Andrich MP, Majd M. Diagnostic imaging in the evaluation of the first urinary tract infection in infants and young children. *Pediatrics.* 1992;90(3):436-441.
47. Moorthy I, Wheat D, Gordon I. Ultrasonography in the evaluation of renal scarring using DMSA scan as the gold standard. *Pediatr Nephrol.* 2004;19(2):153-156.
48. Calisti A, Perrotta ML, Oriolo L, Ingianna D, Sciortino R. Diagnostic workup of urinary tract infections within the first 24 months of life, in the era of prenatal diagnosis. The contribution of different imaging techniques to clinical management. *Minerva Pediatr.* 2005;57(5):269-273.
49. Hoberman A, Charron M, Hickey RW, Baskin M, Kearney DH, Wald ER. Imaging studies after a first febrile urinary tract infection in young children. *N Engl J Med.* 2003;348(3):195-202.
50. Downs SM. Technical report: urinary tract infections in febrile infants and young children. The Urinary Tract Subcommittee of the American Academy of Pediatrics Committee on Quality Improvement. *Pediatrics.* 1999;103 (4):e54.
51. McLaren CJ, Simpson ET. Direct comparison of radiology and nuclear medicine cystograms in young infants with vesico-ureteric reflux. *BJU Int.* 2001;87(1):93-97.
52. Polito C, Rambaldi PF, La Manna A, Mansi L, Di Toro R. Enhanced detection of vesicoureteric reflux with isotopic cystography. *Pediatr Nephrol.* 2000;14(8–9):827-830.
53. Gordon I, Barkovics M, Pindoria S, Cole TJ, Woolf AS. Primary vesicoureteric reflux as a predictor of renal damage in children hospitalized with urinary tract infection: a systematic review and meta-analysis. *J Am Soc Nephrol.* 2003;14(3):739-744.
54. Grmek M, Fettich J. The importance of follow-up of children with vesicoureteral reflux grade 1. *Acta Paediatr.* 2003;92(4):435-438.
55. Williams GJ, Lee A, Craig JC. Long-term antibiotics for preventing recurrent urinary tract infection in children. *Cochrane Database Syst Rev.* 2001(4):CD001534.
56. Williams G, Lee A, Craig J. Antibiotics for the prevention of urinary tract infection in children: a systematic review of randomized controlled trials. *J Pediatr.* 2001;138(6): 868-874.
57. Mahant S, To T, Friedman J. Timing of voiding cystourethrogram in the investigation of urinary tract infections in children. *J Pediatr.* 2001;139(4):568-571.
58. McDonald A, Scranton M, Gillespie R, Mahajan V, Edwards GA. Voiding cystourethrograms and urinary tract infections: how long to wait? *Pediatrics.* 2000;105(4):E50.
59. Rushton HG, Majd M, Chandra R, Yim D. Evaluation of 99mtechnetium-dimercapto-succinic acid renal scans in experimental acute pyelonephritis in piglets. *J Urol.* 1988;140(5, pt 2):1169-1174.
60. Craig JC, Wheeler DM, Irwig L, Howman-Giles RB. How accurate is dimercaptosuccinic acid scintigraphy for the diagnosis of acute pyelonephritis? A meta-analysis of experimental studies. *J Nucl Med.* 2000; 41(6):986-993.

61. Zorc JJ, Kiddoo DA, Shaw KN. Diagnosis and management of pediatric urinary tract infections. *Clin Microbiol Rev.* 2005;18(2):417-422.
62. Stokland E, Hellstrom M, Jacobsson B, Jodal U, Sixt R. Evaluation of DMSA scintigraphy and urography in assessing both acute and permanent renal damage in children. *Acta Radiol.* 1998;39(4):447-452.
63. Ditchfield MR, Summerville D, Grimwood K, et al. Time course of transient cortical scintigraphic defects associated with acute pyelonephritis. *Pediatr Radiol.* 2002; 32(12):849-852.
64. Ditchfield MR, Grimwood K, Cook DJ, et al. Persistent renal cortical scintigram defects in children 2 years after urinary tract infection. *Pediatr Radiol.* 2004;34(6): 465-471.
65. Biggi A, Dardanelli L, Pomero G, et al. Acute renal cortical scintigraphy in children with a first urinary tract infection. *Pediatr Nephrol.* 2001;16(9):733-738.
66. Rushton HG, Majd M, Jantausch B, Wiedermann BL, Belman AB. Renal scarring following reflux and nonreflux pyelonephritis in children: evaluation with 99mtechnetium-dimercaptosuccinic acid scintigraphy. *J Urol.* 1992;147(5): 1327-1332.
67. Biggi A, Dardanelli L, Cussino P, et al. Prognostic value of the acute DMSA scan in children with first urinary tract infection. *Pediatr Nephrol.* 2001;16(10):800-804.
68. Baker PC, Nelson DS, Schunk JE. The addition of ceftriaxone to oral therapy does not improve outcome in febrile children with urinary tract infections. *Arch Pediatr Adolesc Med.* 2001;155(2):135-139.
69. Gauthier M, Chevalier I, Sterescu A, Bergeron S, Brunet S, Taddeo D. Treatment of urinary tract infections among febrile young children with daily IV antibiotic therapy at a day treatment center. *Pediatrics.* 2004;114(4):e469-e476.
70. Ladhani S, Gransden W. Increasing antibiotic resistance among urinary tract isolates. *Arch Dis Child.* 2003;88(5):444-445.
71. Allen UD, MacDonald N, Fuite L, Chan F, Stephens D. Risk factors for resistance to "first-line" antimicrobials among urinary tract isolates of *Escherichia coli* in children. *CMAJ.* 1999;160(10):1436-1440.
72. Koyle MA, Barqawi A, Wild J, Passamaneck M, Furness PD, III. Pediatric urinary tract infections: The role of fluoroquinolones. *Pediatr Infect Dis J.* 2003;22(12):1133-1137.
73. Garin EH, Olavarria F, Garcia Nieto V, et al. Clinical significance of primary vesicoureteral reflux and urinary antibiotic prophylaxis after acute pyelonephritis: a multicenter, randomized, controlled study. *Pediatrics.* 2006; 117(3):626-632.
74. Williams GJ, Wei L, Lee A, Craig JC. Long-term antibiotics for preventing recurrent urinary tract infection in children. *Cochrane Database Syst Rev.* 2006;3:CD001534.

CHAPTER 43

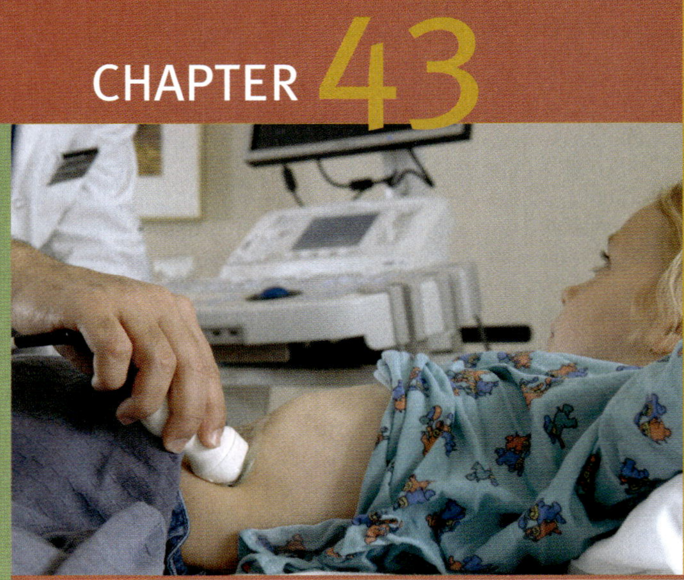

Pelvic Inflammatory Disease

Oana Tomescu and Nadja G. Peter

DEFINITION AND EPIDEMIOLOGY

Pelvic inflammatory disease (PID) is a complex inflammatory disorder of the female upper genital tract that usually develops as a result of an initiating sexually transmitted infection, but can also be caused by iatrogenic uterine instrumentation.[1–6] The term denotes a wide spectrum of histopathologic entities including endometritis, salpingitis, oophoritis, peritonitis, and abscess formation. Clinically, PID can manifest in a wide range of symptoms, from subtle pelvic discomfort to frank peritonitis and hemodynamic shock. A distinct entity called subclinical PID has been recognized as an asymptomatic infection with evidence of upper genital tract inflammation; despite lack of symptoms, subclinical PID is suspected to result in the same long-term reproductive sequelae as its symptomatic counterpart.[7–10]

Burden of Disease

Surveillance data suggest that lifetime prevalence of PID for women in the United States is 8%,[1] with 20% of cases affecting adolescent females.[11,12] Estimates of the true burden of this disease, though, are likely inaccurate because this syndrome is not reportable and is substantially underdiagnosed because of atypical presentations. Incidence is decreasing from a peak of 1 million cases annually in the early 1980s to 420,000 cases in the year 2001.[6,11,13] Similarly, hospitalization rates have substantially decreased since 1980s, reflecting a shift to outpatient management. Total medical cost of PID was estimated at $2.7 billion for the year 1990,[14] but because of the decreased incidence and hospitalization rates, total expenditure in 1998 was $1.88 billion, with long-term reproductive sequelae representing 40% of that sum.[15]

Risk Factors

Demographic, behavioral, and contraceptive practices have been evaluated in cross-sectional studies as risk factors for PID (Table 43–1). Among demographic risk factors, age younger than 19 years,[16–18] lower socioeconomic group,[16,19] non-Caucasian race,[16,17,20] lack of married status,[16,21] and less education[17,22] have been associated with increased risk of PID. Behavioral risk factors overlap with those for acquiring STIs. High-risk behaviors include early sexual debut,[16,18,19,23] having multiple sexual partners,[23–25] and having a current or past STI.[16,18–21,26] A history of PID is reported by some[19] but not all[17,18] authors as an independent risk factor for

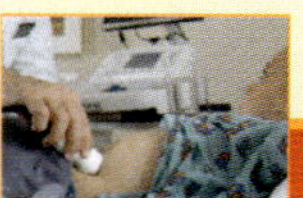

Table 43–1.

Risk Factors for PID

Risk Factors for PID
Demographic
Age younger than 19 years
Low socioeconomic group
Non-Caucasian Race
Nonmarried status
Lower education
Behavioral
Early sexual debut (age younger than 15 years)
New or multiple sexual partners
Current or past STI
Substance abuse
Contraceptive
Lack of any contraception
Inconsistent condom use

recurrence. Use of substances like alcohol,[18,27] tobacco,[17,19,22,28] and cocaine[17] may also increase PID risk. Additionally, engaging in sex during menses[19,24] and douching[29–31] are behaviors that remain controversially associated with PID.

Contraceptive practices also alter the risk of PID. Lack of any contraception is associated with 7.6-fold increased PID risk,[24] while inconsistent condom use increases risk by three-fold.[17] Intrauterine devices (IUDs) have traditionally been associated with the development of PID,[32,33] but recent data demonstrate that the risk is limited to the first 20 days following IUD insertion[34] and possibly if the IUD is inserted during concurrent cervicitis.[35] IUD placement otherwise, perhaps even in populations with high prevalence of STIs, appears safe.[32] Whether hormonal contraception alters PID risk remains unresolved. Both combination oral and progesterone-only injectable forms are associated with increased risk of *Chlamydia trachomatis* cervicitis.[36–38] Oral contraceptive use by a large cohort of women resulted in a nonsignificant reduction in PID risk.[36] Use of depot medroxyprogesterone significantly decreased PID risk by 60% among this cohort,[36] but was associated with increased risk in a different study.[19] Interestingly, case-control data showed that women with subclinical PID diagnosed by endometrial biopsy were 4.3 times more likely to be on oral contraceptives than women with recognized PID,[39] whereas use of oral contraception by a large cohort of women with acute PID was associated with a nonsignificant trend toward a reduced pain score.[18] These data indicate that the decreased risk associated with hormonal contraceptives may be attributable to a decrease in presenting symptomatology, rather than to an absolute reduction in PID incidence.

PATHOGENESIS

Pathogenesis of PID involves a complex interaction between host immune defenses, genetic factors, and bacterial and/or viral virulence factors.[5,40] Ascending infection into the upper genital tract occurs either by direct extension from the cervix or by lymphatic spread.[41] Any decrease in host immune factors, such as loss of the cervical mucous plug during menses, decreased immunologic endometrial and oviductal secretions detected in adolescence and during the proliferative phase of the menstrual cycle,[12,42] and changes in vaginal pH caused by bacterial vaginosis (BV) infection, can enhance the ascension of primary and secondary invaders. Factors that facilitate upward migration of pathogens, such as retrograde menstrual flow and adherence to and transport by sperm, also increase susceptibility to infection.[5,12,40] Furthermore, the presence of certain human leukocyte antigen class II alleles can modulate PID risk, indicating that genetic factors contribute to pathogenesis as well.[43]

PID is a polymicrobial process. *C. trachomatis* and *Neisseria gonorrhoeae* are the iniating infection in 40–70% of cases of acute PID.[41,44–46] Approximately 25% of women with asymptomatic *C. trachomatis* or *N. gonorrhoeae* cervicitis have evidence of endometritis on biopsy and, therefore, are classified as having subclinical PID.[7] Other organisms that have been isolated from the upper genital tracts of women with PID include *Ureaplasma urealyticum, Mycoplasma hominis, Haemophilus influenzae, Escherichia coli,* various streptococci, and HSV-2.[44,45,47–49] Recently *Mycoplasma genitalium*, a causative agent of urethritis in men, is being evaluated as a possible etiologic agent of PID.[50–53] BV likely contributes to PID pathogenesis as well. For example, BV-associated organisms are commonly isolated from the upper genital tracts of women with acute PID,[27,47,54,55] and 15% of women with BV have endometritis on biopsy.[7]

CLINICAL PRESENTATION

The clinical presentation of PID varies greatly, with symptoms ranging from severe, debilitating abdominal or pelvic pain to a more subtle syndrome for which many females may not even seek medical attention. Important components of the patient's history of present illness include description of the pain and associated genitourinary, gastrointestinal, and systemic symptoms. The clinician should also elicit the patient's sexual history, which includes the patient's age at sexual debut, number of lifetime as well as recent partners, frequency of coitus, date of last sexual encounter, history of STIs or prior PID, and the type and frequency of contraceptive use. Furthermore, a thorough menstrual history should be obtained, including information about age at menarche, the date of the last menstrual period, and any atypical symptoms during and since the last menstrual period.

Numerous symptoms can be associated with infection of the upper genital tract in females, but no single symptom is sensitive and specific enough to accurately predict the diagnosis of PID (Table 43–2).[56–60] Abdominal or pelvic pain is the most common symptom reported. The pain is often bilateral, dull, and achy in character, classically occurs with or immediately after menses, and can be exacerbated by jarring movements, such as walking or intercourse. Symptoms of lower genital tract infection are often present, including vaginal discharge, burning, or an abnormal odor. Fewer than 50% of all women with PID report fever. Irregular uterine bleeding, either spotting between menses or abnormally heavy and/or painful menses, is a symptom of

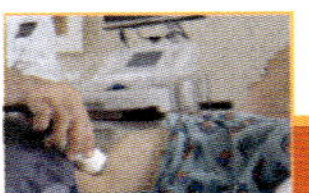

Table 43–2.

Test Characteristics of Symptoms in PID

Symptom	Prevalence (%)	Sensitivity (%)	Specificity (%)
Abdominal or pelvic pain	>95	80	50
Abnormal vaginal discharge	55–75	74	24
Reported fevers	35–45	35–40	75
Irregular bleeding	30–35	38–50	57–85
Urinary symptoms	15–20	20–35	60–82
Nausea and vomiting	10	14	88
Anorectal symptoms	5–10	10	92–95

Adapted from References 56–60.

endometritis. Urinary symptoms occur in approximately 20% of females with PID, while gastrointestinal symptoms, such as decreased appetite, nausea, and vomiting, are less common. Lastly, right upper quadrant pain suggests possible perihepatitis, which is present in 5–10% of adults, but may be more prevalent in adolescents with PID.[61]

The physical examination should focus on vital signs and on detailed examination of the abdomen and pelvis. Abdominal examination may show diffuse tenderness that is often bilateral, usually greatest in the lower quadrants, and may be accompanied by rebound, guarding, and decreased bowel sounds. On pelvic examination, the presence of a strong odor or vaginal discharge suggests concomitant *Trichomonas vaginalis* or BV infection. A mucopurulent cervical discharge indicates possible cervicitis, and tenderness of the pelvic organs on bimanual examination signifies upper genital tract involvement. The presence of occult or frank blood on rectal examination, though, makes an alternate diagnosis more likely. Physical examination findings tend to have better sensitivity and specificity profiles than clinical symptoms, but no one sign is pathognomonic for PID (Table 43–3).[56–60,62] Adnexal tenderness has the highest sensitivity (95%) of all physical examination findings, but has only intermediate specificity; therefore, its absence can help rule out PID, but its presence does not guarantee the diagnosis. Cervical motion tenderness, a sign classically thought of in association with PID, has even lower sensitivity (82–92%) and just as low specificity as adnexal tenderness for this complex infection. Both mucopurulent cervical discharge and bilateral abdominal tenderness, though, have higher specificities and, thus, are better predictors of PID.[59] The other physical examination findings are not as helpful given their limited positive and negative predictive values.

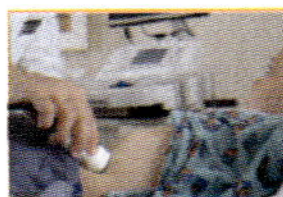

Table 43–3.

Sensitivity and Specificity of Physical Examination Signs in PID

Sign	Sensitivity (%)	Specificity (%)
Adnexal tenderness	95	4–74
Cervical motion tenderness	82–92	12–72
Mucopurulent cervical discharge	75	93
Bilateral tenderness	58	92
Abdominal guarding and/or rebound	64	63
Palpable adnexal mass	48–52	70–75
Vaginal discharge	74–80	24–30
Elevated temperature	11–47	64–95

Adapted from References 56–60, 62.

DIFFERENTIAL DIAGNOSIS

Because the signs and symptoms of PID are so diverse, the differential diagnosis of this syndrome is extensive (Table 43–4). Gynecologic emergencies that can mimic the spectrum of symptoms of PID include ectopic pregnancy,

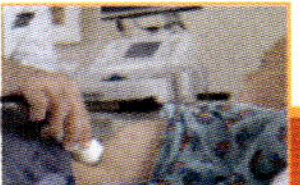

Table 43–4.

Differential Diagnosis of PID

Gynecologic
Ectopic pregnancy
Spontaneous or threatened abortion
Ovarian torsion
Ruptured corpus luteum cyst
Endometriosis
Uterine fibroids
Pelvic adhesions
Dysmenorrhea

Gastrointestinal
Hepatitis
Peritonitis
Appendicitis
Diverticulitis
Gastroenteritis
Inflammatory bowel disease
Obstipation
Cholecystitis

Urinary Tract
Cystitis
Pyelonephritis
Ureteral calculi

Other
Pneumonia
Sickle cell crisis
Abdominal or pelvic trauma

spontaneous or threatened abortion, and ovarian torsion. Other gynecologic conditions include ruptured ovarian cysts, endometriosis, uterine fibroids, pelvic adhesions, and even dysmenorrhea. Gastrointestinal illnesses that share overlapping symptoms with PID are peritonitis, appendicitis, diverticulitis, gastroenteritis, inflammatory bowel disease, and even obstipation. The presence of right upper quadrant pain with PID further broadens the differential to include cholecystitis and hepatitis. Lastly, urinary tract disorders, such as cystitis, pyelonephritis, and ureteral calculi, and miscellaneous causes of abdominal pain, such as pneumonia, sickle cell crisis, and abdominal and/or pelvic trauma, can mimic this infection as well.

CLINICAL SEQUELAE

Acute Complications: Tubo-Ovarian Abscess and Fitz–Hugh–Curtis Syndrome

Tubo-ovarian abscess (TOA), a serious complication of PID, is characterized as an inflammatory mass involving fallopian tube, ovary, and adjacent structures such as bowel and pelvic peritoneum.[4,63] The prevalence of TOA among hospitalized women with PID is estimated to be as high as 17–30%[64,65]; among outpatients with PID, rates seem to be less than 5%,[66,67] although screening for TOA is not universally undertaken and may affect the accuracy of these data. Patients with TOA are not always more toxic appearing than patients with uncomplicated PID[64,66] and fewer than 30% have a palpable adnexal mass on examination.[4,12,64,66] Acute phase reactants are sometimes, but not always, elevated to a greater extent than in uncomplicated PID.[68] If TOA is suspected, an emergent ultrasound is required since the presence of this complication changes PID management.

Fitz–Hugh–Curtis (FHC) syndrome[61] denotes acute inflammation of the liver capsule, and occurs in 5–10% of adults[58] and in approximately 25% of adolescents[69] with PID. Most often associated with *N. gonorrhoeae* and *C. trachomatis,* perihepatitis usually results from either direct extension of organisms from the fallopian tubes along the paracolic gutters, or in the case of *C. trachomatis,* through an exaggerated immune response.[70] Clinically, FHC syndrome is characterized by right upper quadrant pain that is typically pleuritic and usually referred to the right shoulder or arm; importantly, the pain is not always temporally associated with concomitant PID pain or symptoms of a lower genital tract infection.[71] Liver associated enzymes are either normal or mildly elevated, thus helping differentiate this disorder from hepatitis and gall stone disease. Adjunctive tests, such as CBC, ESR, or CRP are inconsistently elevated, while ultrasonography and tests for *N. gonorrhoeae* and *C. trachomatis* can help establish the diagnosis.[61] Perihepatitis makes the diagnosis of concurrent PID even more enigmatic, but it should be considerd in the differential diagnosis in sexually active females, especially adolescents, who have right upper quadrant pain with or without concurrent pelvic symptoms.

Long-term Complications: Infertility, Ectopic Pregnancy, Chronic Pelvic Pain

Infertility, ectopic pregnancy, and chronic pelvic pain (CPP) are long-term complications of PID and account for a significant portion of the economic burden of this syndrome.[14] Case-control studies have shown that women who delay treatment longer than 3 days have a 2–3.5-fold higher rate of infertility and/or ectopic pregnancy compared to women with PID who seek care early.[72] After one episode of PID, the risk of infertility and ectopic pregnancy increases ten-fold and seven-fold, respectively[73]; furthermore, this risk doubles with each successive episode.[73,74] CPP afflicts approximately 20–35% of women who have had PID[75,76] and leads to substantial morbidity. Retrospective chart reviews indicate that CPP is the main indication of 12% of the 590,000 hysterectomies performed in the United States each year,[1] while prospective cohort data show that women who develop CPP after PID have significantly reduced physical and mental health scores.[77]

DIAGNOSIS

The diagnosis of PID is challenging because the syndrome can encompass variable combinations of a wide spectrum of clinical entities. Thus, the presentation of PID can vary greatly: symptoms are protean and no physical examination finding is pathognomonic for the disease. Furthermore, no single diagnostic gold standard exists, thus clinical diagnosis retains central importance. Not surprisingly then, because of the complex nature of this syndrome, PID is diagnosed correctly by clinical findings alone only 65% of the time.[78] Combinations of diagnostic criteria that seek to improve the sensitivity or specificity of the clinical diagnosis do so at the expense of the other.

CDC Criteria for Diagnosis of PID

In the past, CDC diagnostic criteria for PID required the presence of *three* mandatory components: abdominal pain, adnexal tenderness, and cervical motion tenderness.[79] The sensitivity of all three criteria, though, was shown to be only 83%,[62] indicating that many cases of true PID were misclassified. In order to maximize the sensitivity of the clinical criteria, reduce the number of missed or delayed diagnoses, and decrease reproductive sequelae, the current CDC guidelines[48] recommend

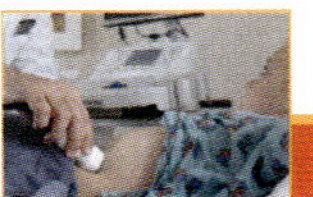

Table 43–5.

2006 CDC Diagnostic Criteria for PID

Minimum Criteria
Cervical motion tenderness
OR
Uterine tenderness
OR
Adnexal tenderness

Adjunctive Clinical Criteria
Temperature > 101°F (>38.3°C)
Abnormal cervical or vaginal purulent discharge
Presence of abundant WBC on saline microscopy
Elevated ESR or CRP
Documentation of cervical infection with *Neisseria gonorrhoeae* or *Chlamydia trachomatis*

Adapted from Centers for Disease Control and Prevention: Sexually transmitted diseases treatment guidelines, 2006. http://www.cdc.gov/std/treatment/2006/pid.htm.

suspecting PID in any sexually active female at risk for STIs who has experienced pelvic or abdominal pain, if at least *one* of the minimum criteria is present on pelvic examination: cervical motion *or* uterine *or* adnexal tenderness (Table 43–5). The presence of any of the adjunctive clinical criteria, such as temperature > 101°F, abnormal vaginal discharge, positive saline microscopy of vaginal secretions, elevated ESR or CRP, or documented infection with *N. gonorrhoeae* or *C. trachomatis*, can be used to enhance the specificity of the minimum criteria, but are not required to make the diagnosis of PID.

Proposed Diagnostic Approach

Every clinician should have a low threshold for suspecting PID in any sexually active female with current or recent abdominal or pelvic pain. In order to improve the accuracy of this diagnosis, though, providers should utilize a systematic approach (Table 43–6). Important historical components include information about the patient's pain and other associated symptoms, a complete sexual, contraceptive and menstrual history, and a screen for PID risk factors. The physical examination should focus on vital signs and a detailed examination of the abdomen and pelvis. The minimum laboratory evaluation for every patient suspected of having PID includes a urine pregnancy test, saline microscopy of vaginal secretions, and PCR tests for *N. gonorrhoeae* and *C. trachomatis*. A normal wet mount has 94.5% negative predictive value for the presence of PID,[80] while positive *N. gonorrhoeae* and *C. trachomatis*. PCR tests are highly predictive of endometritis in the right clinical setting.[60,62] Adjunctive tests such as a CBC, ESR, and CRP

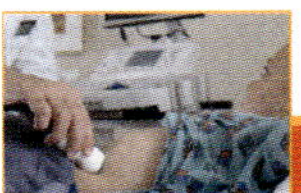

Table 43–6.

Diagnostic Approach for PID

History
Description of pain
Associated symptoms
Sexual history
Contraceptive history
Menstrual history
Screen for risk factors of PID

Physical Examination
Complete vital signs
Focused cardiopulmonary examination
Detailed abdominal and pelvic examination

Minimum Evaluation
Urine pregnancy test
Saline microscopy of vaginal secretions
Tests for *Neisseria gonorrhoeae* and *Chlamydia trachomatis*
Offer HIV testing

Adjunctive Tests
ESR, CRP, CBC

Additional Diagnostic Modalities
US with Doppler
MRI
Endometrial biopsy
Laparoscopy

can be obtained, but should not delay the diagnosis, since these values are not uniformly elevated in all cases of PID.[58,59,81] Normal results of all three tests, though, have been shown to have a negative predictive value of 100%.[82] Finally, every female diagnosed with this infection should be offered HIV testing.[48]

Adjuvant modalities, such as ultrasound, MRI, endometrial biopsy, and laparoscopy, play a minor role in the initial diagnosis of PID given their costs, risks, and limited availability. None of these entities have perfect sensitivity and specificity profiles. Transvaginal ultrasonography has only 81% sensitivity and 78% specificity when compared to laparoscopy,[83] but the addition of color flow Doppler greatly improves the positive and negative predictive value of this imaging modality.[84] MRI has 95% sensitivity and 89% specificity in diagnosing PID,[83] while the sensitivity of endometrial biopsy is 92% and its specificity is 87% when compared to laparoscopy.[85] Laparoscopy itself, once considered the gold standard for the diagnosis of PID, has low accuracy in early or mild disease,[86–89] and when compared to fimbrial biopsy, has only 27% sensitivity and 92% specificity.[87] The CDC recommends that use of these diagnostic techniques be limited to patients not responding to initial therapy or to those in whom an alternate emergent diagnosis cannot be excluded.[48] Furthermore, because endometritis and salpingitis can occur concomitantly or in exclusion of one other, the CDC recommends that an endometrial biopsy be performed in every woman with negative laparoscopic findings.[48]

MANAGEMENT

Outpatient Versus Inpatient Treatment of PID

In recent years there has been a shift to outpatient management of PID. A recent large multicenter randomized controlled trial, called the PID Evaluation and Clinical Health (PEACH) Study, has provided evidence to substantiate this change in management.[75] The study randomized 831 women with mild to moderate PID to either initial inpatient treatment with intravenous cefoxitin and doxycycline or outpatient treatment consisting of a single IM dose of cefoxitin and oral doxycycline.[90] There were no significant differences between the inpatient and outpatient groups in terms of long-term outcomes, such as infertility (17.9% versus 18.4%), frequency of PID recurrence (16.6% versus 12.4%), CPP (29.8% versus 33.7%), and ectopic pregnancy (0.3 versus 1%).[75] There was, however, a trend toward improved eradication of endometritis at 30 days in the inpatient group (45.9% versus 37.6%, $p = 0.09$).[75] Interestingly, a large portion of both treatment groups experienced clinical sequelae, which raises questions about the accuracy of the initial diagnosis and clinical cure rates of the antibiotic regimens utilized in this study. The equivalent outcomes between both groups, though, demonstrate that hospitalization of every female with PID is not warranted.

The CDC suggests hospitalization if a surgical emergency (such as appendicitis) cannot be excluded by the initial workup, or if the patient is pregnant, has not responded to oral antibiotics, is unable to follow or tolerate an outpatient oral regimen, has severe illness, nausea, vomiting, or high fever, or if the patient has a TOA.[48] An implicit yet critically important part of outpatient management is the ability and volition of the patient to engage in close 72-hour follow-up in order to evaluate treatment response. This factor is especially salient to the care of adolescents who may have limited resources to coordinate appropriate follow-up. No current data exist, however, that demonstrate superiority of outcomes for hospitalized adolescents; thus the decision to hospitalize teens with PID should be based on the above criteria. Additionally, no definitive recommendation exists to hospitalize women in their later reproductive years either, despite data from a small cross-sectional study of hospitalized women with PID showing that women older than 35 years had a more complicated course than their younger counterparts.[91]

CDC-Recommended Regimens

The CDC currently recommends several parenteral and oral regimens for the treatment of PID (Table 43–7).[48,92] Total treatment duration is 14 days. Parenteral therapy,

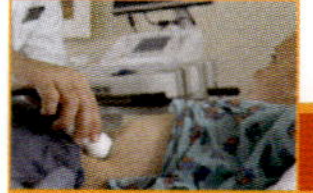

Table 43–7.

CDC Recommended Antibiotic Regimens for PID

	Inpatient Regimens*,†	Outpatient Regimens†#
A.	Cefotetan 2 g or Cefoxitin 2 g IV q12h IV q6h plus Doxycycline 100 mg po or IV‡ q12h	Ceftriaxone 250 mg IM once plus Doxycycline 100 mg po bid
B.	Clindamycin 900 mg IV q8h plus Gentamicin loading dose at 2 mg/kg IM or IV then maintenance at 1.5 mg/kg IV q8h (single daily dosing may be substituted)	Cefoxitin with Probenecid 2 g IM once 1 g po once plus Doxycycline 100 mg po bid
C.	Ampicillin/Sulbactam 3 g IV q6h plus Doxycycline 100 mg po or IV q12h	Third-generation cephalosporin IM (e.g., ceftizoxime or cefotaxime) plus Doxycycline 100 mg po bid

**Parenteral antibiotics can be discontinued 24 hours after clinical improvement and should be followed by a course of doxycycline 100 mg po bid or clindamycin 450 mg po qid for a total of 14 days of treatment.*

†Quinolones are no longer recommended in the treatment of PID or for any N. gonorrhea infection.[92,95] In case of penicillin allergy, patients should be hospitalized and treated with regimen B, or if suspicion for N. gonorrhoeae is low and close follow-up can be established, an oral azithromycin regimen can be used.

‡Oral doxycycline is preferred to parenteral because of phlebitis associated with intravenous infusion.

Adapted from Centers for Disease Control and Prevention: Sexually transmitted diseases treatment guidelines, 2006. http://www.cdc.gov/std/treatment/2006/pid.htm; Centers for Disease Control and Prevention. Update to CDC's Sexually transmitted diseases treatment guidelines, 2006: Fluoroquinolones no longer recommended for treatment of gonococcal infections. MMWR Morb Mortal Wkly Rep. 2007;56;332–336.

#Consider addition of metronidazole, see text for details.

if initiated, can be discontinued 24 hours after clinical improvement, and oral doxycycline or clindamycin should be instituted for the remainder of treatment. Intravenous doxycycline is associated with painful phlebitis and should be avoided whenever possible.[48,75] Outpatient regimens include a single IM dose of a third-generation cephalosporin plus a 14-day course of doxycycline, with or without metronidazole. Coverage of anaerobes is suggested but not mandated by the CDC[48,92] because conflicting data show that while anaerobic gram-negative rods can result in endometritis,[20] many of the antibiotic regimens that do not cover anaerobes have good clinical and microbial cure rates.[25] Regimens utilizing either a single dose[93] or a 7-day course[94] of azithromycin have shown equivalent clinical cure rates compared to current oral regimens but are not yet endorsed by the CDC because of growing concern for emerging macrolide resistance.

Because of increasing prevalence of quinolone-resistant *N. gonorrhoeae* (QRNG), the CDC no longer recommends the use of fluoroquinolones for treatment of gonococcal infections, including associated conditions such as PID. [92,95] Currently, therefore, cephalosporins are the only class of antibiotics that is approved for outpatient management of PID, which significantly complicates treatment of this infection in patients with severe allergic reactions to penicillin or other beta-lactam antibiotics. Spectinomycin is an alternate choice in this situation, but is not available in the United States. Therefore, patients allergic to penicillin should either be hospitalized and treated with clindamycin and gentamycin, or if there is low suspicion for *N. gonorrhoeae*, can be managed as outpatients with azithromycin, as long as cultures, antimicrobial-sensitivity testing, and close follow-up are undertaken.

While management of FHC Syndrome is similar to that of uncomplicated PID,[61] treatment of TOA differs significantly. CDC guidelines mandate that all females with TOA be hospitalized and that parenteral regimens include anaerobic coverage.[48,92] Length of treatment is generally for 14–21 days. No evidence exists that parenteral therapy for the entire duration of treatment results in superior outcomes. Most clinicians use clindamycin instead of doxycycline for oral therapy in order to achieve improved anaerobic coverage.[48,92] Drainage or surgery is indicated if medical therapy does not attain clinical improvement.[48,63,65]

Management of PID in Special Populations: HIV-Positive Females and Adolescents

There is conflicting data on whether HIV-positive females suffer more severe manifestations of PID,[96–99] thus, the CDC does not currently mandate more aggressive management or hospitalization of all HIV-positive patients with PID.[48,92] Old retrospective studies showed slower response rates to treatments, increased rates of surgery, and longer hospitalization stays for HIV-positive women with PID,[98,100] but more current data support similar outcomes between HIV-positive and HIV-negative women, except possibly for those with a low-CD4 count.[96,97,101]

Treatment of youth also deserves special consideration. Incidence of PID is 5–10-fold greater in adolescents than in adults,[11,12] a finding that may be partially related to increased risk-taking behavior among this population.[102] Adolescents, though, also have decreased secretion of cervical immunoglobulins, lower overall serologic immunity and increased cervical ectopy, all of which allow pathogens to adhere more readily to the columnar cells of the endocervix and initiate an ascending infection.[11,12,40,42] Additional risk factors for PID among adolescents include having older sexual partners, a history of involvement with protective services, and a history of suicide attempts.[18] Clinicians who care for adolescents should also realize that teens have decreased access to health care, which makes them less likely to initiate care or engage in necessary follow-up.[103,104] Health care providers should use increased sensitivity when treating adolescents with PID: offering compassionate and honest care,[105] seeing the patient alone for at least part of the visit, and ensuring confidentiality[103] are factors that can make a difference in outcomes among adolescents with this infection.

Primary and Secondary Prevention of PID

Central to primary prevention of PID is universal screening for *C. trachomatis* and, in some US cities, for *N. gonorrhoeae* as well. Unequivocal data exist that universal screening decreases the prevalence of STIs, PID, and ectopic pregnancy.[106,107] Promotion of barrier methods is another strategy to decrease the incidence of PID. Inconsistent condom use has been shown to increase risk of PID threefold,[17] and there is some evidence from the PEACH trial that consistent use can decrease recurrence of this complex infection and its long-term sequelae.[108]

Recurrent PID is estimated to comprise up to 47% of all cases.[109] Secondary prevention strategies seek to improve not only eradication of the primary episode, but also patient adherence and partner treatment rates as well. Evidence shows that clinicians manage PID correctly only 35–60% of the time.[110–112] Most antibiotic errors involve the duration of doxycycline, the choice of azithromycin or cefixime as first-line therapy, or inadequate ceftriaxone dose.[110] Furthermore, adequate follow-up instructions are given less than 30% of the time.[110,111] A subset of the PEACH trial evaluated treatment adherence using pill bottle electronic monitoring devices: results showed that patients took only 70% of the total prescribed doses of doxycycline, 17% of which were taken within the optimal time period.[113] Retrospective data indicate that 25% of adolescents being treated for recurrent PID reported noncompliance with their initial regimen, while 70% did not tell their partners to get treated.[109] Different partner treatment initiatives have been studied and show equivalent outcomes.[114] In sum, in order to decrease recurrence of this complex infection and its devastating repercussions, health care providers absolutely need to ensure that every patient treated for PID is prescribed the correct antibiotic regimen, is given careful instructions for treatment adherence, and has both appropriate follow-up as well as a concrete plan for getting her partner treated.

PEARLS

- Right upper quadrant pain should raise suspicion for Perihepatitis associated with PID.
- Tubo-ovarian abscess occurs in up to one-third of women hospitalized for treatment of PID; <30% of women with a TOA will have a pulpable adneral mass.

REFERENCES

1. Haggerty C, Ness RB. Epidemiology, pathogenesis, and treatment of pelvic inflammatory disease. *Expert Rev Anti Infect Ther.* 2006;4(2):235-247.
2. Crossman SH. The challenge of pelvic inflammatory disease. *Am Fam Physician.* 2006;73:859-864.
3. Barrett S, Taylor C. A review on pelvic inflammatory disease. *Int J STD AIDS.* 2005;16:715-721.
4. Beigi RH, Wiesenfeld HC. Pelvic inflammatory disease: new diagnostic criteria and treatment. *Obstet Gynecol Clin N Am.* 2003;30:777-793.
5. Simms I, Stephenson JM. Pelvic inflammatory disease epidemiology: what do we know and what do we need to know? *Sex Transm Infect.* 2000;76:80-87.
6. Sweet RL. Pelvic inflammatory disease. In: Sweet RL, Gibbs RS, ed. *Infectious Diseases of the Female Genital Tract.* 4th ed. Philadelphia: Lippincott Williams Wilkins; 2001:368-412.
7. Wiesenfeld HC, Hillier SL, Krohn MA, et al. Lower genital tract infection and endometritis: insight into subclinical pelvic inflammatory disease. *Obstet Gynecol.* 2002;100:456-463.
8. Achilles SL, Amortegui AJ, Wiesenfeld HC. Endometrial plasma cells: do they indicate subclinical pelvic inflammatory disease? *Sex Transm Dis.* 2005;32:185-188.
9. Wiesenfeld HC, Sweet RL, Ness RB, et al. Comparison of acute and subacute pelvic inflammatory disease. *Sex Transm Dis.* 2005;32:400-405.
10. Eckert LO, Hawes SE, Wolner-Hanssen PK, et al. Endometritis: the clinical-pathologic syndrome. *Am J Obstet Gynecol.* 2002;186:690-695.
11. Banikarim C, Chacko MR. Pelvic inflammatory disease in adolescents. *Adolesc Med Clin.* 2004;15:273-285.
12. Igra V. Pelvic inflammatory disease in adolescents. *AIDS Patient Care STDS.* 1998;12:109-124.
13. Department of Health and Human Services Centers for Disease Control and Prevention: Sexually Transmitted Disease Surveillance, 2004. http://www.cdc.gov/std/stats/default.htm. Accessed August 01, 2008.
14. Washington AE, Katz P. Cost and payment source for pelvic inflammatory: trends and projections, 1983 through 2000. *JAMA.* 1991;266:2565-2569.
15. Rein DB, Kassler WJ, Irwin KL, Rabiee L. Direct medical cost of pelvic inflammatory disease and its sequelae: decreasing but still substantial. *Obstet Gynecol.* 2000;95:397-402.
16. Simms I, Stephenson JM, Mallinson H, et al. Risk factors associated with pelvic inflammatory disease. *Sex Transm Dis.* 2006;82:452-457.
17. Ness RB, Soper DE, Holley RL, et al. Hormonal and barrier contraception and risk of upper genital tract disease in the PID Evaluation and Clinical Health (PEACH) Study. *Am J Obstet Gynecol.* 2001;185:121-127.
18. Suss AL, Homel P, Hammerschlag M, Bromberg K. Risk factors for pelvic inflammatory disease in inner-city adolescents. *Sex Transm Dis.* 2000;27:289-291.
19. Ness RB, Smith KJ, Chang CH, Schisterman EF, Bass DC. Prediction of pelvic inflammatory disease among young, single, sexually active women. *Sex Transm Dis.* 2006;33:137-142.
20. Hillier SL, Kiviat NB, Hawes SE, et al. Role of bacterial vaginosis-associated organisms in endometritis. *Am J Obstet Gynecol.* 1996;175:435-441.
21. Gogate A, Brabin L, Gogate S, et al. Risk factors for laparoscopically confirmed pelvic inflammatory disease: findings from Mumbai (Bombay), India. *Sex Transm Infect.* 1998;74:426-432.
22. Viberga I, Odlind V, Lazdane G. Characteristics of women at low risk of STI presenting with pelvic inflammatory disease. *Eur J Contracept Reprod Health Care.* 2006;11:60-68.
23. Chandra A, Martinez GM, Mosher WD, Abra JC, Jones J. Fertility, family planning and reproductive health of US women: data from the 2002 National Survey of Family Growth. *Vital Health Stat.* 2005;25:1-160.
24. Jossens MO, Eskenazi B, Schachter J, Sweet RL. Risk factors for pelvic inflammatory disease: a case-control study. *Sex Transm Dis.* 1996;23:239-247.
25. Walker CK, Workowski KA, Washington AE, Soper D, Sweet RL. Anaerobes in pelvic inflammatory disease: implications for the Centers for Disease Control and Prevention's guidelines for treatment of sexually transmitted diseases. *Clin Infect Dis.* 1999:28(suppl 1):S29-S36.
26. Ness RB, Hillier SL, Kip KE, et al. Bacterial vaginosis and risk of pelvic inflammatory disease. *Obstet Gynecol.* 2004;104:761-769.
27. Jonsson M, Karlsson R, Rylander E, Gustavsson A, Wadell G. The associations between risk behavior and reported history of sexually transmitted diseases among

young women: a population based study. *Int J STD AIDS.* 1997;8:501-505.
28. Scholes D, Daling J, Stergachis A. Current cigarette smoking and risk of acute pelvic inflammatory disease. *Am J Public Health.* 1992;82:1352-1355.
29. Ness RB, Soper DE, Holley RL, et al. Douching and endometritis: results from the PID Evaluation and Clinical Health (PEACH) Study. *Sex Transm Dis.* 2001; 28:240-245.
30. Scholes D, Daling JR, Sterlgachis A, et al. Vaginal douching as a risk factor for acute pelvic inflammatory disease. *Obstet Gynecol.* 1993;81:601-606.
31. Rothman KJ, Funch DP, Alfredson T, et al. Randomised field trial of vaginal douching, pelvic inflammatory disease, and pregnancy. *Epidemiology.* 2003;14:340-348.
32. Grimes DA. Intrauterine device and upper-genital-tract infection. *Lancet.* 2000;356:1013-1019.
33. Gareen IF, Greenland S, Morgenstern H. IUD and pelvic inflammatory disease: meta-analysis of published studies, 1974-1990. *Epidemiol.* 2000;11:589-597.
34. Farley TM, Rosenberg MJ, Rowe PJ, Chen JH, Meirik O. Intrauterine devices and pelvic inflammatory disease: an international perspective. *Lancet.* 1992;339:785-788.
35. Faunders A, Telles E, Cristofoletti ML, et al. The risk of inadvertent intrauterine device insertion in women carries of endocervical *Chlamydia trachomatis. Contraception.* 1998;58:105-109.
36. Baeten JM, Nyange PM, Richardson BA, et al. Hormonal contraception and risk of sexually transmitted disease acquisition: results from a prospective study. *Am J Obstet Gynecol.* 2001;185:380-385.
37. Cottingham J, Hunter D. Chalmydia trachomatis and oral contraceptive use: a quantitative review. *Genitourin Med.* 1992;68:209-216.
38. Stuart GS, Castano PM. Sexually transmitted infections and contraceptives: Selective issues. *Obstet Gynecol Clin N Am.* 2003;30:795-808.
39. Ness RB, Keder LM, Soper DE, et al. Oral contraception and the recognition of endometritis. *Am J Obstet Gynecol.* 1997;176:580-585.
40. Rice PA, Schachter J. Pathogenesis of pelvic inflammatory disease: what are the questions? *JAMA.* 1991; 266:2587-2593.
41. Brook I. Microbiology and management of polymicrobial female genital tract infections in adolescents. *J Pediatr Adolesc Gynecol.* 2002;15:217-226.
42. Shrier LA, Bowman FP, Lin M, Crowley-Nowick PA. Mucosal immunity of the adolescent female genital tract. *J Adolesc Health.* 2003;32:183-186.
43. Ness RB, Brunham RC, Shen C, Bass DC for the PID Evaluation and Clinical Health (PEACH) Study Investigators. Associations among human leukocyte antigen (HLA) class II DQ variants, bacterial sexually transmitted diseases, endometritis, and fertility among women with clinical pelvic inflammatory disease. *Sex Transm Dis.* 2004;31:301-304.
44. Audu BM, Kudi AA. Microbial isolates and antibiogram from endocervical swabs of patients with pelvic inflammatory disease. *J Obstet Gynecol.* 2004;24:161-164.
45. Heinonen PK, Miettinen A. Laparoscopic study on the microbiology and severity of acute pelvic inflammatory disease. *Eur J Obstet Gynecol Reprod Biol.* 1994;57:85-89.
46. Jossens MO, Schacter J, Sweet RL. Risk factors associated with pelvic inflammatory disease of differing microbial etiologies. *Obstet Gynecol.* 1994;83:989-997.
47. Soper DE, Brockwell NJ, Dalton HP, Johnson D. Observations concerning the microbial etiology of acute salpingitis. *Am J Obstet Gynecol.* 1994;170:1008-1014.
48. Centers for Disease Control and Prevention: sexually transmitted diseases treatment guidelines, 2006. http://www.cdc.gov/std/treatment/2006/pid.htm.
49. Cherpes TL, Wiesenfeld HC, Melan MA, et al. The associations between pelvic inflammatory disease, *Trichomonas vaginalis* infection, and positive herpes simplex virus type 2 serology. *Sex Transm Dis.* 2006;33: 747-752.
50. Ross JDC. Is *Mycoplasma genitalium* a cause of pelvic inflammatory disease? *Infect Dis Clin North Am.* 2005;19:407-413.
51. Cohen CR, Manhart LE, Bukusi EA, et al. Association between *Mycoplasma genitalium* and acute endometritis. *Lancet.* 2002;359:765-766.
52. Cohen CR, Mugo NR, Astete SG, et al. Detection of *Mycoplasma genitalium* in women with laparoscopically diagnosed acute salpingitis. *Sex Transm Dis.* 2005;81:463-466.
53. Simms I, Eastick K, Malinson H, et al. Associations between *Mycoplasma genitalium, Chlamydia trachomatis* and pelvic inflammatory disease. *J Clin Pathol.* 2003;56:616-618.
54. Ness RB, Kip KE, Hillier SL, et al. A cluster analysis of bacterial vaginosis-associated microflora and pelvic inflammatory disease. *Am J Epidemiol.* 2005;162:585-590.
55. Haggerty CL, Hillier SL, Bass DC, Ness RB for the PID Evaluation and Clinical Health Study Investigators. Bacterial vaginosis and anaerobic bacteria are associated with endometritis. *Clin Infect Dis.* 2004;39:990-995.
56. Simms I, Warbuton F, Westrom L. Diagnosis of pelvic inflammatory disease: time for a rethink. *Sex Transm Infect.* 2003;79:491-494.
57. Blake DR, Fletcher K, Joshi N, Emans SJ. Identification of symptoms that indicate a pelvic examination is necessary to exclude PID in adolescent women. *J Pediatr Adolesc Gynecol.* 2003;16:25-30.
58. Peifert JF, Soper DE. Diagnositic evaluation of pelvic inflammatory disease. *Infect Dis Obstet Gynecol.* 1994;2:38-48.
59. Kahn JG, Walker C, Washington AE, Landers DV, Sweet R. Diagnosing pelvic inflammatory disease. A comprehensive analysis and consideration for developing a new model. *JAMA.* 1991;266:2594-2604.
60. Hagdu A, Westrom L, Brooks C, et al. Multivariate analysis of prognostic variables in patients with acute pelvic inflammatory disease. *Am J Obstet Gynecol.* 1986;155: 954-960.
61. Peter NG, Clark LR, Jaeger JR. Fitz-Hugh-Curtis syndrome: a diagnosis to consider in women with right upper quadrant pain. *Cleve Clin J Med.* 2004;71:233-239.
62. Peipert JF, Ness RB, Blume J, et al. Clinical predictors of endometritis in women with symptoms and signs of pelvic inflammatory disease. *Am J Obstet Gynecol.* 2001;184:856-864.
63. Krivak TC, Cooksey C, Propst AM. Tubo-ovarian abscess: diagnosis, medical and surgical management. *Compr Ther.* 2004;30:93-100.

64. Slap G, Forke CM, Cnaan A, et al. Recognition of tubo-ovarian abscess in adolescents with pelvic inflammatory disease. *J Adolesc Health.* 1996;18:397-403.
65. Wiesenfeld HC, Sweet RL. Progress in management of tubo-ovarian abscess. *Clin Obstet Gynecol.* 1993;36:433-444.
66. Mollen CJ, Pletcher JR, Bellah RD, Lavelle JM. Prevalence of tubo-ovarian abscess in adolescents diagnosed with pelvic inflammatory disease in a pediatric emergency department. *Pediatr Emerg Care.* 2006;22:621-625.
67. Shrier LA, Moszczenski SA, Emans SJ, et al. Three years of a clinical practice guideline for uncomplicated pelvic inflammatory disease in adolescents. *J Adolesc Health.* 2000;27:57-62.
68. Reljic M, Gorisek B. C-reactive protein and the treatment of pelvic inflammatory disease. *Int J Gynaecol Obstet.* 1998;60:143-150.
69. Litt IF, Cohen MI. Perihepatitis associated with salpingitis in adolescents. *JAMA.* 1978;240:1253-1254.
70. Money DM, Hawes SE, Eschenbach DA, et al. Antibodies to the chlamydial 60 kd heat-shock protein are associated with laparoscopically confirmed perihepatitis. *Am J Obstet Gynecol.* 1997;176:870-877.
71. Counselman FL. An unusual presentation of Fitz-Hugh-Curtis syndrome. *J Emerg Med.* 1994;12;167-170.
72. Hillis S, Joesoef R, Marchbanks P, et al. Delayed care of pelvic inflammatory disease as a risk factor for impaired fertility. *Am J Obstet Gynecol.* 1993;86:321-325.
73. Westrom LV. Sexually transmitted diseases and infertility. *Sex Transm Dis.* 1994;21(2 suppl):S32-S37.
74. Westrom L, Joesoef MJ, Reynolds G, Hagdu A, Thompson SE. Pelvic inflammatory disease and fertility: a cohort study of 1844 women with laparoscopically verified disease and 657 control women with normal laparascopic results. *Sex Transm Dis.* 1992;19:185-192.
75. Ness RB, Soper DE, Holley RL, et al. Effectiveness of inpatient and outpatient treatment strategies for women with pelvic inflammatory disease: results from the pelvic inflammatory disease evaluation and clinical health (PEACH) randomized trial. *Am J Obstet Gynecol.* 2002;186:929-937.
76. Haggerty CL, Peipert JF, Weitzen S, et al. Predictors of chronic pelvic pain in an urban population of women with symptoms and signs of pelvic inflammatory disease. *Sex Transm Dis.* 2005;32:293-299.
77. Haggerty CL, Schulz R, Ness RB for the PID Evaluation and Clinical Health (PEACH) Study Investigators. Lower quality of life among women with chronic pelvic pain after pelvic inflammatory disease. *Obstet Gynecol.* 2003;102:934-939.
78. Sellors J, Mahony J, Goldsmith C, et al. The accuracy of clinical findings and laparoscopy in pelvic inflammatory disease. *Am J Obstet Gynecol.* 1991;164:113-120.
79. Centers for Disease Control and Prevention. Sexually transmitted diseases treatment guidelines, 1998. *MMWR Recomm Rep.* 1998;47:1-111.
80. Yudin MH, Hillier SL, Woesenfeld HC, et al. Vaginal polymorphonuclear leukocytes and bacterial vaginosis as markers for histologic endometritis among women without symptoms of pelvic inflammatory disease. *Am J Obstet Gynecol.* 2003;188:318-323.
81. Cibula D, Kuzel D, Fucikova Z, Svabik K, Zivny J. Acute exacerbation of recurrent pelvic inflammatory disease. Laparoscopic findings in 141 women with a clinical diagnosis. *J Reprod Med.* 2001;46:49-53.
82. Peipert JF, Boardman L, Hogan JW, Sung J, Mayer KH. Laboratory evaluation of acute upper genital tract infection. *Obstet Gynecol.* 1996;87:730-736.
83. Tukeva TA, Aronen HJ, Karjalainen P, et al. MR imaging in pelvic inflammatory disease: comparison with laparoscopy and US. *Radiology.* 1999;210:209-216.
84. Molander P, Sjoberg J, Paavonen J, Cacciatore B. Transvaginal power Doppler findings in laparoscopically proven acute pelvic inflammatory disease. *Ultrasound Obstet Gynecol.* 2001;17:233-237.
85. Kiviat NB, Wolner-Hanssen P, Eschenbach DA, et al. Endometrial histopathology in patients with culture-proved upper genital tract infection and laparoscopically diagnosed acute salpingitis. *Am J Surg Pathol.* 1990;14:167-175.
86. Peifert JF, Boardman LA, Sung CJ. Performance of clinical and laparoscopic criteria for the diagnosis of upper genital tract infection. *Infect Dis Obstet Gynecol.* 1997;5:291-296.
87. Molander P, Finne P, Sjoberg J, Sellors J, Paavonene J. Observer agreement with laparoscopic diagnosis of pelvic inflammatory disease using photographs. *Obstet Gynecol.* 2003;101:875-880.
88. Eckert LO, Hawes SE, Wolner-Hanssen PK, et al. Endometritis: the clinical-pathologic syndrome. *Am J Obstet Gynecol.* 2002;186:690-695.
89. Gaitan H, Angel E, Diaz R, et al. Accuracy of five different diagnostic techniques in mild-to-moderate pelvic inflammatory disease. *Infect Dis Obstet Gynecol.* 2002;10:171-180.
90. Ness RB, Soper DE, Peipert J, et al. Design of the PID evaluation and clinical health (PEACH) study. *Control Clin Trials.* 1998;19:499-514.
91. Jamieson DJ, Duerr A, Macasaet MA, Peterson HB, Hillis SD. Risk factors for a complicated clinical course among women hospitalized with pelvic inflammatory disease. *Infect Dis Obstet Gynecol.* 2000;8:88-93.
92. Centers for Disease Control and Prevention. Update to CDC's sexually transmitted diseases treatment guidelines, 2006: Fluoroquinolones no longer recommended for treatment of gonococcal infections. *MMWR Morb Mortal Wkly Rep.* 2007;56;332-336.
93. Rustomjee R, Kharsany AB, Connolly CA, Karim SS. A randomized controlled trial of azithromycin versus doxycycline/ciprofloxacin for the syndromic management of sexually transmitted infections in a resource-poor setting. *J Antimicrob Chemother.* 2002;49:875-878.
94. Bevan CD, Ridgeway GL, Rothermel CD. Efficacy and safety of azithromycin as montherapy or combined with metronidazole compared with two standard mulidrug regimens for the treatment of acute pelvic inflammatory disease. *J Int Med Res.* 2003;31:45-54.
95. Centers for Disease Control and Prevention: updated recommended treatment regimens for gonococcal infections and associated conditions. http://www.cdc.gov/std/treatment/2006/updated-regimens.htm.
96. Mugo NR, Kiehlbauch JA, Nguti R, et al. Effect of human immunodeficiency virus-1 infection on treatment

outcome of acute salpingitis. *Obstet Gynecol.* 2006;107:807-812.

97. Cohen CR, Sinei S, Reilly M, et al. Effect of human immunodeficiency virus infection upon acute salpingitis: a laparoscopic study. *J Infect Dis.* 1998;178:1352-1358.
98. Barbosa C, Macasaet M, Brockmann S, et al. Pelvic inflammatory disease and human immunodeficiency virus infection. *Obstet Gynecol.* 1997;89:65-70.
99. Irwin KL, Moorman AC, O'Sullivan MJ, et al. Influence of human immunodeficiency virus infection on pelvic inflammatory disease. *Obstet Gynecol.* 2000;95:525-534.
100. Korn AP, Landers DV, Green JR, Sweet RL. Pelvic inflammatory disease in human immunodeficiency virus-infected women. *Obstet Gynecol.* 1993;82:765-768.
101. Bukusi EA, Cohen CR, Stevens CE, et al. Effects of human immunodeficiency virus 1 infection on microbial origins of pelvic inflammatory disease and on efficacy of ambulatory oral therapy. *Am J Obstet Gynecol.* 1999;181:1374-1381.
102. Centers for Disease Control and Prevention. Youth risk behavior surveillance- United States, 2003. *MMWR Morb Mort Wkly Rep.* 2004;53:19-22;S4.
103. Cheng TL, Savageau JA, Sattler AL, Dewitt TG. Confidentiality in health care: a survey of knowledge, perception and attitudes among high school students. *JAMA.* 1993;269:1404-1407.
104. Klein JD, Slap GB, Elster B, Schonberg SK. Access to health care for adolescents: a position paper of the Society for Adolescent Medicine. *J Adolesc Health.* 1992;13: 162-170.
105. Ginsburg KR, Slap GB, Cnaan A, et al. Adolescents' perceptions of factors affecting their decisions to seek health care. *JAMA.* 1995;273:1913-1918.
106. Scholes D, Stergachis A, Heidrich FE, et al. Prevention of pelvic inflammatory disease by screening for cervical chlamydial infection. *NEJM.* 1996;334:1362-1366.
107. Hillis S, Nakashima A, Amsterdam L, et al. The impact of a comprehensive Chlamydia prevention program in Wisconsin. *Fam Plan Perspect.* 1995;27:108-111.
108. Ness, RB, Randall H, Richter HE, et al. Condom use and the risk of recurrent pelvic inflammatory disease, chronic pelvic pain, or infertility following an episode of pelvic inflammatory disease. *Am J Public Health.* 2004;94:1327-1329.
109. Kelly AM, Ireland M, Aughey D. Pelvic inflammatory disease in adolescents: high incidence and recurrence rates in an urban teen clinic. *J Pediatr Adolesc Gynecol.* 2004;17:383-388.
110. Trent M, Ellen JM, Walker A. Pelvic inflammatory disease in adolescents: care delivery in prediatric ambulatory settings. *Pediatr Emerg Care.* 2005;21:431-436.
111. Bechmann KR, Melzer-Lange MD, Gorelick MH. Emergency department management of sexually transmitted infections in US adolescents: results from the National Hospital Ambulatory Medical Care Survey. *Ann Emerg Med.* 2004;43:333-338.
112. Hessol NA, Priddy FH, Bolan G, et al. Management of pelvic inflammatory disease by primary care physicians: a comparison with Centers for Disease Control and Prevention guidelines. *Sex Transm Dis.* 1996;23: 157-163.
113. Dunbar-Jacob J, Sereika SM, Foley SM, et al. Adherence to oral therapies in pelvic inflammatory disease. *J Womens Health.* 2004;13:285-291.
114. Schillinger JA, Kissinger P, Calvet H, et al. Patient-delivered partner treatment with azithromycin to prevent repeat Chlamydia trachomatis infection among women: a randomized, controlled trial. *Sex Transm Dis.* 2003;30:49-56.

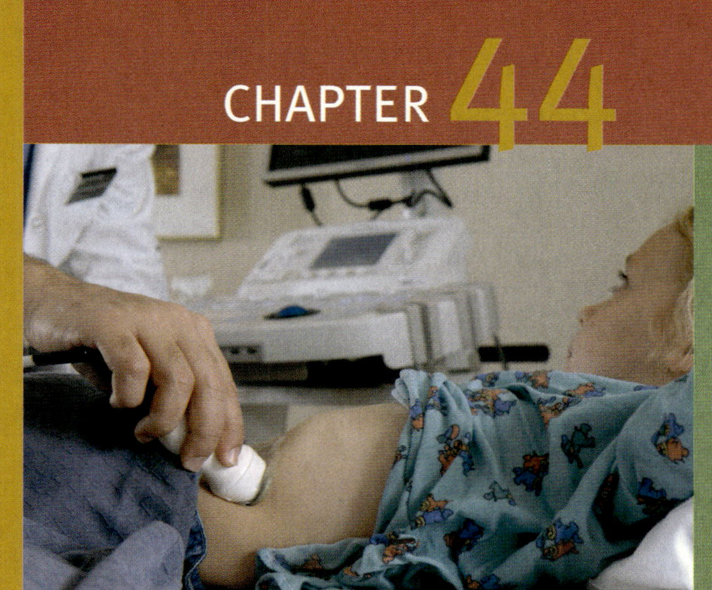

CHAPTER 44

Sexually Transmitted Infections in Adolescents

Leonard J. Levine and Sarah M. Taub

INTRODUCTION

According to the Centers for Disease Control and Prevention's (CDC) 2005 Youth Risk Behavior Surveillance survey, nearly one-half of US high school students report ever having had sexual intercourse.[1] Over 60% of high school seniors report a history of sexual intercourse, while 20% of seniors report having had at least four sexual partners. Even higher numbers of adolescents engage in other, noncoital sexual behaviors, including oral sex.[2–4] Young people age 15–24 years old make up one-fourth of sexually active individuals in the United States, yet acquire nearly one-half of all new sexually transmitted infections (STIs) each year.[5] Sexually active adolescents are at high risk for contracting STIs for a variety of reasons. While many adolescents report the use of condoms, they are not necessarily using them consistently or correctly.[6,7] They are more likely than adults to experiment with multiple sexual partners,[8–10] to engage in riskier sex while under the influence of alcohol or drugs,[8,11] to have a poor understanding of STI transmission and consequences of infection,[12] and to face barriers to accessing confidential health care.[13,14] In addition, the presence of columnar epithelial cells in the cervical ectropion of female adolescents increases susceptibility to infection with certain sexually transmitted organisms.

This chapter will focus on four sexually transmitted genital infections commonly found in the adolescent population. Three of these infections—chlamydia, trichomoniasis, and human papillomavirus (HPV)—together account for nearly 90% of new STIs among 15–24-years-old youth.[15] Gonorrhea, the second most common infection reported to the CDC and a significant risk factor for chronic reproductive health problems, will be discussed in the section with chlamydia as a major cause of cervicitis and urethritis in teenagers.

CHLAMYDIA AND GONORRHEA: CERVICITIS AND URETHRITIS

Epidemiology

Chlamydia is the most frequently reported STI in the United States, with an estimated 3 million cases annually. At least 70% of genital chlamydia infections are in adolescents and young adults, 15–24 years old.[5] CDC surveillance data has repeatedly shown infection rates to be highest in 15–19-years-old females. In 2005, the rate of chlamydia infection in adolescent females (15–19 years old) was nearly 2,800 per 100,000 population.[16] Rates in males are highest for 20- to 24-year olds, with 805 per 100,000 population, followed next by males 15- to 19-year olds (505 per 100,000 population). This reflects common patterns of partnering, in which adolescent women are more commonly engaging in sex with slightly older males.

Gonorrhea, the second most common reportable disease, has infection rates similar in distribution to those of chlamydia infections. In 2005, adolescents aged 15–19 years had the highest reported rates of gonorrhea among women, with reported rates of 625 per 100,000 population.[16] Rates in males are highest for 20- to 24-year olds, with 437 per 100,000 population, followed next by 15- to 19-year-old males, with 261 per 100,000 population.

Pathogenesis

Chlamydia trachomatis is an obligate intracellular bacterium that infects mucosal columnar epithelial cells, particularly of the cervix and urethra. The organism, transmitted through secretions, attaches to these epithelial cells, enters them, and begins to replicate. The replication process induces an immune response and cell wall rupture. The bursting of the epithelial cell contributes to cell death and the release of more infectious particles, which infect nearby cells and are transmitted to other hosts through sexual contact.[17] Symptoms may develop after a 1–3-week incubation period, but mucosal damage may go undetected by infected individuals.

Neisseria gonorrhoeae is a gram-negative intracellular diplococcus. Several of its outer membrane proteins facilitate attachment to mucosal epithelial cells found in the genitourinary tract and other mucous membranes. Host defenses can be evaded through adaptation and alteration of these surface structures. Cytotoxicity and inflammation contribute to mucosal damage and its accompanying symptomatology.[18] As with chlamydia, patients with genital infections caused by *N. gonorrhoeae* may be asymptomatic for months.

The asymptomatic nature of these infections in many patients poses increased risk for transmission, especially when considering adolescent cognitive development. Teenagers who have not progressed from concrete to abstract thinking are likely to equate the absence of symptoms with the absence of infection. Combining this thinking with an adolescent's perceived sense of invincibility makes him or her less likely to take precautions (e.g., condom use) when engaging in sexual activity.

Female adolescents are particularly at risk for chlamydia and gonorrhea infections because of the presence of cervical ectopy, or the ectropion.[19] As girls progress through puberty, columnar epithelium on the ectocervix undergoes transformation to squamous epithelial cells. The persistence of columnar cells on the ectocervix of adolescent females forms a ring around the os known as the ectropion. Its presence increases the risk for acquiring a cervicitis, as columnar cells are particularly susceptible to invasion by *N. gonorrhoeae* and *C. trachomatis*.[20]

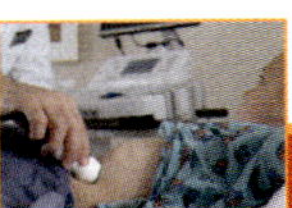

Table 44–1.

Signs and Symptoms of Genital Infections with Neisseria gonorrhoeae and Chlamydia trachomatis

Symptoms	Signs
Females (Cervicitis and Urethritis)	
May have no symptoms	Mucopurulent discharge at os
Vaginal discharge	Erythematous cervix
Dyspareunia	Edema of cervix
Postcoital bleeding	Cervical friability
Intermenstrual bleeding	Microscopy of vaginal fluid:
Dysuria	Leukorrhea (10 wbc/hpf)
Males (Urethritis)	
May have no symptoms	May have no examination findings
Dysuria	Discharge expressed from urethra
Urethral discharge	Positive leukocyte esterase test on first void urine
Urethral meatus pruritis	

Clinical Presentation

Cervicitis

The majority of adolescent females with cervicitis are asymptomatic.[17] When symptoms are present, they can include a purulent vaginal discharge, vaginal spotting, dyspareunia, and irregular vaginal bleeding (see Table 44–1). A speculum examination in these patients may reveal an erythematous, edematous cervix with a mucopurulent discharge at the cervical os. Touching the cervix with a cotton-tipped swab can induce bleeding. This phenomenon, known as friability, is likely the underlying etiology of the bleeding these patients may experience after sexual intercourse. Saline microscopy of a vaginal swab may demonstrate a preponderance of white blood cells, usually >10 wbc/hpf.

Untreated cervicitis can lead to more complicated infections. *N. gonorrhoeae* or *C. trachomatis*, accompanied by a variety of vaginal microorganisms, can ascend into the upper reproductive tract, leading to pelvic inflammatory disease (PID) in 10–40% of untreated women.[21] PID and its associated complications (tuboovarian abscess and perihepatitis, or Fitz–Hugh–Curtis syndrome) can lead to serious sequelae, such as infertility, ectopic pregnancy, and chronic pelvic pain.[22,23] PID is discussed in depth in Chapter 43. *N. gonorrhoeae* can also infect Bartholin's and Skene's glands in the vulvar region, leading to painful abscesses, as well as spread hematogenously to cause a disseminated gonococcal infection (see Table 44–2).

Urethritis

The urethritis seen in men with chlamydia or gonorrhea is usually asymptomatic. Clinical manifestations are absent in over 90% of chlamydia infections and over 60% of gonorrhea urethral infections in males.[24] When present, dysuria and urethral discharge are the more common symptoms experienced. The physical examination is usually unremarkable, although a clear to purulent discharge may be expressed from the urethral

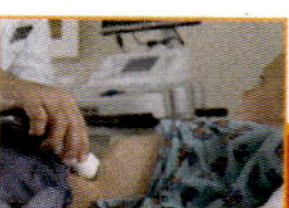

Table 44–2.

Clinical Syndromes Seen in Sexually Active Adolescents with Gonorrhea and Chlamydia Infections

Gonorrhea		Chlamydia	
Males	**Females**	**Males**	**Females**
Asymptomatic	Asymptomatic	Asymptomatic	Asymptomatic
Urethritis	Urethritis	Urethritis	Urethritis
Epididymitis	Cervicitis	Epididymitis	Cervicitis
Proctitis	Salpingitis	Proctitis	Salpingitis
Pharyngitis	Perihepatitis	Conjunctivitis	Perihepatitis
Conjunctivitis	Proctitis	Reiter syndrome†	Proctitis
DGI*	Pharyngitis		Conjunctivitis
	Conjunctivitis		Reiter syndrome†
	Bartholin gland abscess		
	DGI*		

**DGI = Disseminated Gonococcal Infection (arthritis, tenosynovitis, dermatitis; less frequently, pericarditis, endocarditis, osteomyelitis, meningitis)*
†Reiter syndrome = A postinfectious syndrome consisting of conjunctivitis, dermatitis, urethritis, and arthritis.

meatus. If the urethral infection spreads in a retrograde manner, infection of the epididymis can ensue. Patients with epididymitis present with scrotal pain and swelling, with clinical examination findings consistent with an enlarged, tender epididymis palpable in the scrotum. Urethritis may also accompany cervical infection in females. If the possibility of sexual activity is not considered in an adolescent female with dysuria and urinary frequency, health care providers may jump to presumptively treat such patients for a simple cystitis, thereby missing the opportunity to diagnose and treat an STI.

Although this discussion of chlamydia and gonorrhea is limited to cervical and urethral infections, other nongenital clinical syndromes resulting from sexual transmission of these organisms are listed in Table 44–2. These presentations may result as complications of genital infection, or as the result of noncoital behaviors, such as oral and anal sex.

Differential Diagnosis

The differential diagnosis of chlamydia and gonorrhea lower genital infection ranges from other STIs to noninfectious etiologies. Table 44–3 lists the common causes of vaginal discharge in adolescent females and urethritis in males. In addition to *C. trachomatis* and *Trichomonas vaginalis* (discussed below), *Mycoplasma hominis*, and *Ureaplasma urealyticum* have been implicated as less common causes of nongonococcal urethritis in males.

Diagnosis

Diagnostic tests include both culture and nonculture tests, such as nucleic acid amplification tests (NAATs), DNA hybridization (nonamplified DNA probe), and direct fluorescent antibody. Table 44–4 lists the relative sensitivities and specificities for each test. Culture tests, which are performed on cervical and urethral swab specimens, offer the advantage of high specificity (>99%). This makes it the preferred method for criminal

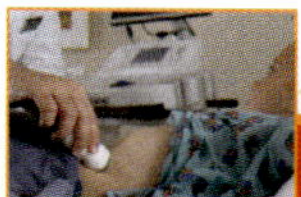

Table 44–3.

Differential Diagnosis for Vaginal Discharge (Females) and Urethritis (Males)

Vaginal discharge
- Physiologic discharge (normal)
- Infections
  - Gonorrhea cervicitis
  - Chlamydia cervicitis
  - *Mycoplasma genitalium* cervicitis
  - *Trichomonas vaginitis*
  - *Candida vaginitis*
  - Bacterial vaginosis
  - Herpes simpex virus
- Foreign body (e.g., condom or tampon)
- Nonspecific vulvovaginitis caused by hygiene habits (e.g., wiping technique, aggressive cleansing with washcloths)
- Local irritation caused by use of feminine hygiene products (e.g., douching)
- Intravaginal hormonal contraception (e.g., Nuva Ring)
- Allergic or contact dermatitis
- Dermatoses
  - Seborrhea
  - Psoriasis
  - Lichen simplex chronicus
  - Lichen sclerosis

Urethritis
- Gonorrhea
- Chlamydia
- Trichomoniasis
- *Mycoplasma genitalium*
- *Ureaplasma urealyticum*

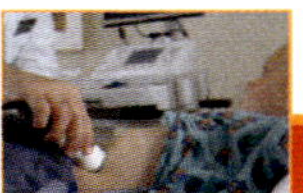

Table 44-4.

Diagnostic Tests for Neisseria gonorrhoeae and Chlamydia trachomatis: Sensitivities and Specificities

	C. trachomatis		N. gonorrhoeae	
Diagnostic Test	Sensitivity (%)	Specificity (%)	Sensitivity (%)	Specificity (%)
Culture	70–85	100	80–95	100
NAATs				
PCR	89–90	98–99	92–94	99–100
TMA	94–97	98–99	91–99	98–99
SDA	92–95	91–98	85–98	97–100
DNA hybridization	65–83	99	92–96	98–99
DFA	80–85	99	N/A	N/A
EIA	53–76	95	N/A	N/A
Gram stain				
Symptomatic male			90–95	95–100
Asymptomatic male/female			50–70	95–100

NAATs, Nucleic acid amplification tests; PCR, Polymerase chain reaction; TMA, Transcription-mediated amplification; SDA, Strand displacement amplification; DFA, Direct fluorescent antibody; EIA, Enzyme immunoassay

Adapted from Gaydos CA. Nucleic acid amplification tests for gonorrhea and chlamydia: practice and applications. Infect Dis Clin North Am. 2005;19(2):367–386.

investigations, such as cases of rape or sexual abuse. Culture for *N. gonorrhoeae* can also be used to determine antimicrobial susceptibility, which is increasingly important as antibiotic resistance continues to rise with this organism. The disadvantages of culture include relatively low sensitivity, problems maintaining organism viability in transport, and a longer turnaround time for results compared to nonculture tests.[25] In addition, cultures are more invasive than some nonculture tests, given that females require a speculum examination to swab the cervix, while males require urethral swabs.

NAATs are an important addition to STI testing in adolescents. NAATs detect and amplify organism-specific DNA or RNA from both *N. gonorrhoeae* and *C. trachomatis*. Technologies used include polymerase chain reaction (PCR), strand displacement amplification, and transcription-mediated amplification. NAATs are advantageous because of their high sensitivity and specificity. In general, sensitivities are superior to culture, reaching as high as 98–99%.[25,26] This is largely because of the fact that these tests can produce a signal from a single copy of target DNA or RNA, which also obviates the need to adequately collect and transport a viable organism (as is the case with culture). NAATs are advantageous in adolescents because of the potential for less invasive collection methods. Not only can they be performed on cervical and urethral swabs, but they can also be performed on first-void urine specimens, with no significant difference in sensitivity.[25,26] This decreases the need to rely on speculum examinations and urethral swabs, which may be difficult or undesirable in certain patients or clinical settings. It also allows for routine asymptomatic screening programs targeting larger numbers of adolescents, a practice that is recommended by the CDC and the U.S. Preventive Services Task Force.[27–29] Although they have the advantage of urine-based testing, NAATs cannot be used for pharyngeal or rectal specimens, an important consideration for adolescents engaging in oral and anal sex. These sites still require the use of culture.

Other nonculture tests include direct fluorescent antibody, nucleic acid hybridization (DNA probe), enzyme immunoassay for chlamydia, and Gram stain for gonorrhea. These tests, while cheaper, are used less frequently because of a lower sensitivity than NAATs and an inability to use them with urine specimens.[25] Like NAATs, they cannot be used on other nongenital specimens (e.g., pharynx and rectum). Detection of intracellular gram-negative diplococci in polymorphonuclear leukocytes by Gram stain has a sensitivity of 90–95% for the diagnosis of gonorrhea in men; in women, endocervical samples may be colonized with other gram-negative coccobacillary organisms, thus resulting in a lower sensitivity (range, 50–70%).[26]

Treatment

The management of genital gonorrhea and chlamydia in adolescents involves prompt treatment with antimicrobial agents not only to eliminate symptoms and transmission risk, but also to prevent complications that occur when these organisms ascend to the upper reproductive tract as seen with PID or epididymitis (e.g., tubo-ovarian abscess, infertility, and ectopic pregnancy risks). In addition, management includes the prompt treatment of sexual partners and extensive patient education and risk-reduction counseling.

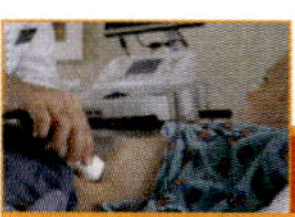

Table 44–5.

Pharmacologic Treatment of Lower Genital Infections with Gonorrhea and Chlamydia

Chlamydia	Gonorrhea
*Recommended Regimens**	*Recommended Regimens*
Azithromycin 1 g po × 1 dose	Ceftriaxone 125 mg IM × 1 dose
Doxycycline 100 mg po bid × 7 d	Cefixime 400 mg po × 1 dose[†]
Alternative Regimens	*Listed in 2006 Guidelines but no longer recommended[‡]*
Erythromycin base 500 mg po qid × 7 d	Ciprofloxacin 500 mg po × 1 dose
Erythromycin ethylsuccinate 800 mg po qid × 7 d	Ofloxacin 400 mg po × 1 dose
Ofloxacin 300 mg po bid × 7 d	Levofloxacin 250 mg po × 1 dose
Levofloxacin 500 mg po daily × 7 d	

**For pregnant adolescents, use only the azithromycin regimen.*
†Limited availability of cefixime in the United States.
‡Quinolone-resistant N. gonorrhoeae has led to the retraction of these recommendations from the 2006 CDC guidelines.

Current antibiotic regimens for treating uncomplicated *C. trachomatis* and *N. gonorrhoeae* genital infections are presented in Table 44–5. These are based on recommendations published by the CDC in its 2006 Sexually Transmitted Diseases (STD) Treatment Guidelines.[27] It is important to remember that these are guidelines for infections of the lower reproductive tract. Antibiotic regimens for infections ascending to the upper tract (e.g., uterus, fallopian tubes, epididymis) are different. The management strategies for PID are discussed in Chapter 43.

Chlamydia trachomatis

A 7-day course of doxycycline is a relatively inexpensive and highly effective form of therapy for chlamydia cervicitis and urethritis (>95% cure rate).[17] However, the single-dose treatment with azithromycin allows for on-site or in-office treatment. This can be particularly helpful when treating adolescents, for whom patient compliance or confidentiality issues may prevent successful completion of a longer antibiotic course at home. In addition, azithromycin is the preferred antibiotic when treating pregnant adolescents, given the risks of doxycycline to a developing fetus.

Neisseria gonorrhoeae

For cervical and urethral infections with *N. gonorrhoeae*, the CDC's 2006 STD Treatment Guidelines recommend the single-dose treatment options found in Table 44–5. However, the treatment of gonorrhea has become more complicated since the guidelines were published because of increasing resistance of *N. gonorrhoeae* to fluoroquinolones. Quinolone-resistant *N. gonorrhoeae*, previously a concern primarily outside the United States,[30,31] has become more common in the United States. and higher rates were initially found in Hawaii and California, as well as among men having sex with men.[32,33] However, data from the CDC-sponsored Gonococcal Isolate Surveillance Project[34] has demonstrated increasing resistance patterns in other geographical areas and demographics across the United States. As a result, the 2006 Treatment Guidelines included a statement that "quinolones should not be used for the treatment of gonorrhea among men having sex with men or in areas with increased Quinolone-resistant *N. gonorrhoeae* prevalence in the United States or for infections acquired while traveling abroad." This recommendation was most recently updated in April 2007 based on additional Gonococcal Isolate Surveillance Project data demonstrating even higher rates of Quinolone-resistant *N. gonorrhoeae* in heterosexual and homosexual populations in the United States. Currently, the CDC "no longer recommends the use of fluoroquinolones for the treatment of gonococcal infections and associated conditions" such as PID.[35] This leaves the cephalosporins as the mainstay of gonorrhea treatment. Because cefixime is not readily available in the United States at this time,[36] intramuscular administration of ceftriaxone is now the primary management option.

Because of the high frequency of concomitant chlamydia infection, it is often recommended that gonorrhea (GC) treatment also include empiric antibiotic coverage for Chlamydia unless testing shows no coinfection.[37,38]

Other management strategies

Patients should notify any sexual partner from the preceding 60–90 days (or the most recent partner if >60 days) of their infection and encourage them to seek evaluation and treatment as well. Patients should be advised to avoid sex until treatment (of themselves and their partner) is complete. The risk of coinfection with other STIs such as human immunodeficiency virus (HIV) should be discussed with adolescents. In addition, health care providers should help teenagers develop strategies (such as use of barrier contraceptives, routine screening, or abstinence) to prevent future exposure to these infections. It is recommended that treated patients be rescreened in 3 months to check for reinfection. NAATs can remain positive for either of these organisms for 3 weeks following treatment so retesting should be delayed for at least a month with this method.

TRICHOMONIASIS

Epidemiology

Over 170 million new cases of trichomoniasis occur annually worldwide.[39] Nearly 8 million of those cases are in the United States, with approximately 2 million cases annually in the adolescent population.[5] Manifesting as vaginitis in women and urethritis in men, prevalence estimates range from 2% to 3% in the general adolescent and young adult population[40] to 17–54% among attendees of STI clinics.[41–43] Much of the available data on trichomoniasis comes from female populations. Because of problems with detection methods, diagnosis can be difficult, particularly in males, and is, therefore, likely underestimated in both sexes.

Pathogenesis

Trichomoniasis results from infection with the organism, *T. vaginalis. T. vaginalis*, an anaerobic parasitic protozoan transmitted through genitourinary secretions, adheres to mucosal surfaces in the urogenital tract. It is classically described as a pear-shaped eukaryotic organism approximately 7 × 9 μm in size.[44] Four anterior flagella, along with an undulating membrane with an embedded fifth flagellum, give the parasite mobility and may contribute to host cell damage. Adhesion to vaginal and urethral epithelial cells, damaging effects of hydrolases, local cellular immune responses, and production of cytotoxic molecules are other mechanisms of pathogenesis contributing to the mucosal inflammation caused by infection.[44,45] Infection can be detected within 2 days of sexual contact, with a typical incubation period of 4–28 days. Infections can go undetected for a long time, sometimes persisting in women for months to years in epithelial crypts and periurethral glands.[46] Infections with *T. vaginalis* have been associated with preterm rupture of membranes, preterm delivery, low birth weight, pelvic inflammatory disease, and an increased risk of acquiring HIV (facilitated by local inflammation and breakdown of the genital mucosal barrier).[42,47–51]

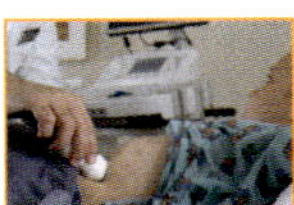

Table 44–6.

Symptoms, Signs, and Wet Prep Findings of Genital Infection with Trichomonas vaginalis

Females (Vaginitis and Urethritis)	Males (Urethritis)
Symptoms	Symptoms
May not have symptoms	May not have symptoms
Vaginal discharge	Dysuria
Vaginal odor	Urethral discharge
Vulvar itch	Urethral meatus pruritis
Dysuria	
Signs	Signs
Vulvar erythema/excoriation/edema	May have no examination findings
Erythematous vaginal mucosa	Discharge expressed from urethra
Colpis macularis (infrequent)	Positive leukocyte esterase test (on first-void urine)
Vaginal microscopy (wet prep) findings	
Motile trichomonads	
White blood cells	
Positive amine odor ("whiff") test	
pH of vaginal fluid >4.5	

Clinical Presentation

Approximately one-half of women with trichomoniasis are symptomatic, while most infected men (>90%) have no symptoms at all.[39,44] When symptoms are present in adolescent females, they are consistent with the vaginitis and urethritis caused by *T. vaginalis* (see Table 44–6). These include a vaginal discharge, vulvar itching, and dysuria. The discharge is typically characterized as yellow–green, watery, and malodorous. Because vulvar pruritus may be the patient's only complaint, many health care providers may miss the diagnosis of trichomoniasis by assuming the presence of a candidal infection (a common cause of vaginal itch) and treating empirically with an antifungal agent. Symptoms encountered by infected males usually reflect a urethritis, with dysuria being the most common complaint. It is thought that 11–19% of nongonococcal urethritis in males can be attributed to infection with *T. vaginalis*.[41,44,52]

Physical and speculum examination findings in women may include vulvar erythema and a frothy yellow–green vaginal discharge. A rarely seen but often described finding is colpis macularis, which represents punctuate hemorrhages in cervical epithelium that give the appearance of a "strawberry cervix."[53] Little has been described for physical findings in men, as they are rarely present.

Differential Diagnosis

When a genital infection with *T. vaginalis* is suspected, it is important to also consider the diagnoses listed in Table 44–3. In addition to trichomoniasis, non-STIs, such as candida and bacterial vaginosis (overgrowth of *Gardnerella vaginalis* and other anaerobes) also involve a shift in vaginal flora resulting in discharge and irritation. A nonspecific vaginitis can result from chemical irritants (such as perfumed soaps, bubble baths, and douching), poor hygiene, retained foreign body (e.g., tampon, condom), tight-fitting clothes, aggressive scrubbing of the vagina or vulva with washcloths, or the use of intravaginal contraception (e.g., Nuva Ring).[54,55] If symptoms are present in an adolescent male, other causes of urethritis should be considered (see Table 44–3).

Diagnosis

The most commonly used diagnostic tool to detect trichomoniasis is microscopic examination of vaginal fluid. Diagnosis is made upon visualization of motile trichomonads on saline wet mount, as can be seen in Figure 44–1. A cotton-tipped swab is used to sample the posterior fornix of the vagina during a speculum examination. If a speculum examination is difficult to perform or not otherwise indicated, a blind vaginal swab (by the provider or the patient herself) will also suffice.[56,57] To maintain the viability of the protozoa, the swab should be placed immediately into a test tube with a few drops of saline and then spread onto a glass slide for microscopic evaluation as soon as possible (preferably within 10 minutes).[44] The active movement of the organisms or their beating flagella helps distinguish trichomonads from the many white blood cells likely to populate the microscopic field. Unfortunately, the sensitivity of saline wet prep is low, with reports in symptomatic women varying from 42% to 70% (and even lower if no symptoms).[43,44,58,59] Therefore, the absence of visible trichomonads does not exclude the diagnosis and very often leads to undertreatment of this STI. Additional diagnostic findings when examining vaginal fluid include an elevated pH (>4.5), white blood cells on wet prep, and, occasionally a fishy odor after mixing with 10% KOH (the positive "whiff test" resulting from release of amines and more commonly seen with bacterial vaginosis). Although examining a concentrated first-void urine for motile trichomonads in males is possible, this is an extremely insensitive test to use and therefore not recommended. The same holds true for microscopic evaluation of male urethral swabs. Diagnosis of trichomoniasis in males is, therefore, usually made presumptively based on symptoms or by having sexual contact with a partner known to be infected.

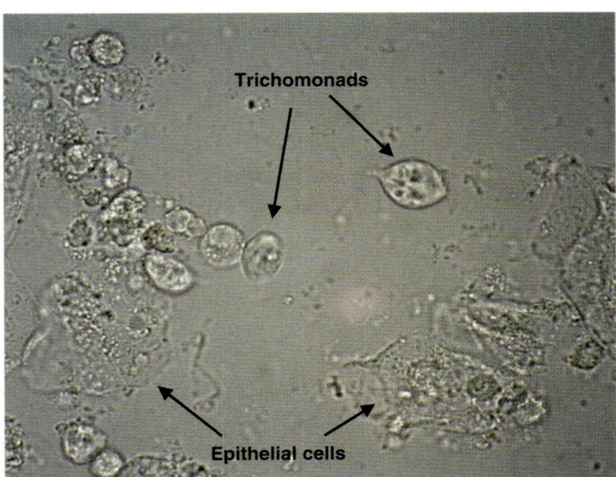

FIGURE 44–1 ■ *T. vaginalis* on vaginal microscopy (wet prep) from an adolescent female. (*Photo courtesy of Jean-Pierre de Chadarevian, MD and Leonard Levine, MD.*)

Other point-of-care tests for *T. vaginalis* include a rapid antigen detection test (OSOM Trichomonas Rapid Test [Genzyme Diagnostics, Cambridge, MA]) and a nucleic acid probe test (Affirm VP III [Becton Dickenson, Sparks, MD]), which produce in-office results in 10 and 45 minutes, respectively. These tests are useful if a microscope is not available. They have a higher sensitivity (over 80% on vaginal specimens) than saline microscopy, with a slightly lower specificity (95–98% vs. 100%), but are less readily available.[43,44,60–62]

Trichomonas culture is considered the current "gold standard" for diagnosis of trichomoniasis. A commercially available culture method (InPouch TV test; BioMed Diagnostics, San Jose, CA) involves the inoculation of liquid growth medium in a prepackaged clear pouch that is examined under direct microscopy serially over 5 days. Vaginal swabs and male urethral swabs and first-void urine can be used with this technique. While more sensitive than the aforementioned tests (~95%, with >95% specificity),[58,63,64] results are not available for a few days, thereby delaying diagnosis.

With sensitivity >95% and specificity of 99%, newer PCR technologies to identify *T. vaginalis* in urine and vaginal fluid may help increase identification and treatment of this often underdiagnosed STI, especially in asymptomatic adolescents.[65,66] However, no FDA-approved PCR test for trichomoniasis is currently available in the United States.

Treatment

The only class of drugs deemed useful for the treatment of trichomoniasis is the nitroimidazoles. Metronidazole 2 g in a single oral dose is the preferred regimen. Alternative regimens using metronidazole or tinidazole can be found in Table 44–7. Metronidazole is 90–95% effective in treating the infection.[27] Patients should be forewarned of metronidazole's metallic taste and potential for GI upset, and should be discouraged from taking the medication on an empty stomach. Although adolescents are below the legal drinking age, they are known to experiment or use alcohol. Patients should, therefore, be warned of the disulfiram-like effects of metronidazole and advised to avoid alcohol for 24–72 hours posttreatment.[27] Although intravaginal metronidazole gel is used for the management of bacterial vaginosis, it is far inferior to oral regimens in the treatment of trichomoniasis, especially when the urethra or paravaginal glands are infected.[27] Topical therapies are therefore not recommended.

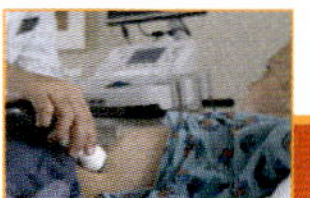

Table 44–7.

Medical Management of Trichomoniasis

Trichomoniasis
Recommended Regimens
Metronidazole 2 g po × 1 dose
Tinidazole 2 g po × 1 dose
Alternative Regimen
Metronidazole 500 mg po bid × 7 d

Adapted from Centers for Disease Control and Prevention. Sexually Transmitted Diseases Treatment Guidelines, 2006. MMWR. 2006;55(No. RR-11):1–94.

As discussed in the previous section on gonorrhea and chlamydia, the treatment of trichomoniasis should also include extensive counseling of adolescents about partner notification and treatment, avoidance of sex until treated, risks of coinfection with other STIs, and future prevention strategies.

GENITAL HUMAN PAPILLOMAVIRUS

Epidemiology

Over 100 genotypes of HPV have been identified by PCR analysis, of which over 30 types are transmitted sexually.[67] Generally, HPV types can be subdivided into those that cause genital and mucosal lesions (e.g., condyloma acuminata) and those that cause nongenital cutaneous lesions (e.g., palmar and plantar warts).[68] Genital lesions include anogenital warts, mild to high-grade changes in cervical epithelium, and (much less commonly) cancers of the cervix, vulva, anus, and penis.

HPV is the most common STI in the United States, affecting up to 20 million Americans aged 15–49.[5] Recent estimates show prevalence rates of 24.5% among females aged 14–19 years and 44.8% among women aged 20–24 years. Similar numbers have been found in males, although prevalence rates of symptom-free genital HPV infection among males is not well established.[69] Approximately, 9.2 million sexually active youth aged 15–24 years are currently infected with genital HPV, with over 4 million new infections detected in 2000.[5] Risk of acquisition increases with the number of lifetime sexual partners and with earlier age at first sexual intercourse.[70]

Pathogenesis

HPV is most commonly acquired during penetrative intercourse (vaginal or anal sexual contact) by direct inoculation of the virus into the epidermal layers through microdefects in the epithelial layer. Other types of genital contact (i.e., oral–genital) can lead to transmission but are much less common. Sexual activity is the best predictor of acquiring HPV. The greater the number of sexual partners and the sexual activity of that partner, the higher is the risk of HPV infection.[71] Another important risk factor is related to the large area of active immature metaplasia at the cervical transformation zone. In addition, genital infections can be transmitted vertically from mothers to newborns via passage through the birth canal producing respiratory papillomas, though this is rare.

Most genital HPV infections are transient in immunocompetent patients, as they are spontaneously cleared by the body's host defenses. It has been elucidated that cell-mediated immunity is the key component in clearing HPV infections.[72] Patients with cell-mediated immunodeficiencies such as HIV have more frequent and severe HPV disease.

HPV types are characterized by their oncogenic potential. The major clinical conditions associated with HPV types involved in genital infections are listed in Table 44–8. Low-risk HPV types cause genital warts and benign or low-grade cervical epithelium changes, but

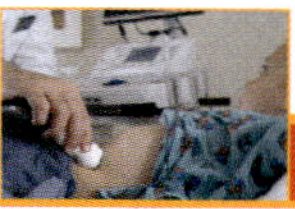

Table 44–8.

Common Genital HPV Infections and Major Clinical Associations

Disease	HPV Types	Transmission
Condylomata acuminata (anogenital warts)	6, 11	Skin to skin, sexual contact
Cervical dysplasia with high risk for carcinoma	16, 18, 31, 33, 35, 39, 45, 51, 52, 56, 58, 59, 68, 73, 82	Vaginal intercourse
Cervical dysplasia with low risk for carcinoma	6, 11, 40, 42, and others	Vaginal intercourse
Anal carcinoma	16, 18, 31, 33	Anal intercourse
Recurrent respiratory papillomatosis	6, 11	Mother to child at birth

Adapted from Partridge JM, Koutsky LA. Genital human papillomavirus infection in men. Lancet Infect Dis. 2006; 6:21–31.

are rarely found in association with invasive cancers. High-risk HPV types are associated with a range of changes in cervical epithelium that range from mild to high-grade dysplasia, as well as anogenital cancers. Based on the evidence from 11 case-control studies by the International Agency for Research on Cancer, 15 HPV types have been identified as high-risk types, and 12 categorized as low-risk types.[73]

Clinical Presentation

Condyloma acuminata (anogenital warts) is the most common presentation of genital HPV infection. The majority is benign and most commonly attributable to infection with HPV type 6 or 11. Condyloma acuminata can present as exophytic, papillomatous growths, but may also be small, discrete, sessile, smooth-topped papules or nodules. Color ranges from flesh-colored to reddish brown in appearance. Patients are most often asymptomatic, but they can experience pruritus, pain, and bleeding. Multiple sites are often involved, so it is necessary to inspect the entire lower genital tract, perineum, and anus. Common locations include the introitus, vulva, perineum, penis, and perianal areas. These warts may regress spontaneously or persist on the skin.

Differential Diagnosis

Other diagnoses that may be confused with genital warts include molluscum contagiosum (which often has central umbilication), syphilitic condyloma lata (distinguished by dark-field microscopy and positive syphilis serology), benign skin tags, verrucous carcinoma, and benign penile pearly papules.[68]

Diagnosis

The diagnosis of genital warts is primarily clinical, made by visual inspection. For lesions harder to detect, such as those on the cervix, diagnosis can be aided by the application of 5% acetic acid solution. Within minutes, condylomata appear as white patches. However, this technique has high false-negative and false-positive results.[74] Biopsy is reserved for unclear circumstances.

Treatment

Although benign, genital warts are often cosmetically unacceptable to the patient and may enlarge if left untreated. An extensive assortment of pharmacologic and nonpharmacologic treatments is available, with no definitive first-line therapy. Treatments can remove warts in most patients, but recurrences are frequent.

Patient- and provider-administered therapies are presented in Table 44–9. Patient-administered therapies include podofilox 0.5% solution or gel (an antimitotic agent that disrupts cell division) and imiquimod 5% cream (which stimulates the innate cell-mediated immune response). Both of these applications require a several-week application, and can induce local reactions, such as erythema and swelling.

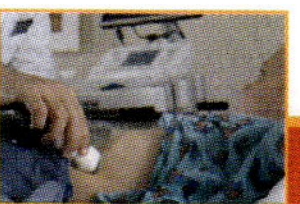

Table 44–9.

Treatment of External Genital Warts

Patient-Applied Topical Therapies	Provide-Administered Therapies
Podofilox 0.5% solution or gel bid × 3 d	Cryotherapy (liquid nitrogen)
Repeat regimen for 4 wk	Repeat weekly as needed
Imiquimod 5% cream QHS three times a wk × 16 wk	Trichloroacetic acid 80–90%
	Repeat weekly as needed
	Surgical removal
	Intralesional interferon
	Laser surgery

Adapted from Centers for Disease Control and Prevention. Sexually Transmitted Diseases Treatment Guidelines, 2006. MMWR. 2006;55(No. RR-11):1–94.

Common provider-administered therapies include trichloroacetic acid or bichloroacetic acid, which cause coagulation of proteins and may require weekly administration until resolution. Cryotherapy with liquid nitrogen, surgical excision, CO_2 laser treatment, and electrocautery are other destructive therapies utilized. Most of these treatments have been associated with clearance or significant reduction in lesions, with roughly equivalent recurrence rates.[27] Choice of primary therapy is dependent on location and size of lesions, patient preferences, provider skill and experience, and cost.

Cervical cell abnormalities

Although the primary focus of the HPV discussion in this chapter is on genital warts, it is important to recognize the cervical implications of this virus for adolescents. Although infection of the cervix with high-risk HPV is common in young sexually active patients, the infection is usually transient. The virus is undetectable in 70% of patients within 1 year of infection and in 91% within 2 years of infection. Persistence of high-risk HPV is necessary for progression of disease to invasive carcinoma.[75] The American College of Obstetricians and Gynecologists (ACOG) recommends starting annual cervical cytology screening (i.e., Papanicolaou smear) 3 years after initiating sexual intercourse, but no later than age 21. The recommendation to wait 3 years after initiating sexual intercourse is to provide opportunity for clearance of transient HPV infections and prevent overtreatment of low-grade lesions.

While cervical cancer is exceedingly rare in the immunocompetent adolescent population, the main goal of screening is to detect, follow, and treat high-risk type HPV. According to the recent ACOG published guidelines, aggressive management of benign lesions in adolescents should be avoided because most cervical intraepithelial neoplasia (CIN grades 1 and 2) regress spontaneously.[76] Refer to the ACOG guidelines for further details.

Prevention

In June 2006, a new quadrivalent HPV vaccine, Gardasil® (Merck & Co., Inc., Whitehouse Station, NJ), was approved by the Food and Drug Administration.[77] This vaccine protects against the four HPV types primarily responsible for genital warts (types 6 and 11) and cervical cancer (types 16 and 18). The vaccine is administered through a series of three intramuscular injections over a 6-month period (0, 2, and 6 months). The Advisory Committee on Immunization Practices (ACIP) recommends use of the vaccine in females aged 9- to 26-year old.[78] A bivalent vaccine that protects against HPV types 16 and 18 is expected in the near future.[79]

Ideally, the HPV vaccine should be administered prior to sexual activity, as it will only protect against those HPV types not yet acquired by the patient. However, sexually active women should also be offered this vaccine, since we do not know to which individual strains a women has been previously exposed. Currently, there is not enough data in men to support use of vaccine, but studies are ongoing. Duration of vaccine prevention is unclear, but current studies show effectiveness for at least 5 years.[78] Although this vaccine could dramatically reduce the morbidity and mortality of HPV-associated diseases, it does not replace other prevention strategies, such as cervical cancer screening or protective sexual behaviors.

REFERENCES

1. Eaton DK, Kann L, Kinchen S, et al. Youth risk behavior surveillance–United States, 2005. *MMWR Surveill Summ.* 2006;55(5):1-108.
2. Mosher WD, Chandra A, Jones J. Sexual behavior and selected health measures: men and women 15-44 years of age, United States, 2002. *Adv Data.* 2005(362):1-55.
3. Stone N, Hatherall B, Ingham R, McEachran J. Oral sex and condom use among young people in the United Kingdom. *Perspect Sex Reprod Health.* 2006;38(1):6-12.
4. So DW, Wong FY, DeLeon JM. Sex, HIV risks, and substance use among Asian American college students. *AIDS Educ Prev.* 2005;17(5):457-468.
5. Weinstock H, Berman S, Cates W, Jr. Sexually transmitted diseases among American youth: incidence and prevalence estimates, 2000. *Perspect Sex Reprod Health.* 2004;36(1): 6-10.
6. Hatherall B, Ingham R, Stone N, McEachran J. How, not just if, condoms are used: the timing of condom application and removal during vaginal sex among young people in England. *Sex Transm Infect.* 2007;83(1):68-70.
7. Shrier LA, Goodman E, Emans SJ. Partner condom use among adolescent girls with sexually transmitted diseases. *J Adolesc Health.* 1999;24(5):357-361.
8. Diclemente RJ, Wingood GM, Sionean C, et al. Association of adolescents' history of sexually transmitted disease (STD) and their current high-risk behavior and STD status: a case for intensifying clinic-based prevention efforts. *Sex Transm Infect.* 2002;29(9):503-509.
9. Finer LB, Darroch JE, Singh S. Sexual partnership patterns as a behavioral risk factor for sexually transmitted diseases. *Fam Plann Perspect.* 1999;31(5):228-236.
10. Kelley SS, Borawski EA, Flocke SA, Keen KJ. The role of sequential and concurrent sexual relationships in the risk of sexually transmitted diseases among adolescents. *J Adolesc Health.* 2003;32(4):296-305.
11. Millstein SG, Moscicki AB. Sexually-transmitted disease in female adolescents: effects of psychosocial factors and high risk behaviors. *J Adolesc Health.* 1995;17(2):83-90.
12. Ethier KA, Kershaw T, Niccolai L, Lewis JB, Ickovics JR. Adolescent women underestimate their susceptibility to sexually transmitted infections. *Sex Transm Infect.* 2003;79(5):408-411.
13. Klein JD, McNulty M, Flatau CN. Adolescents' access to care: teenagers' self-reported use of services and perceived access to confidential care. *Arch Pediatr Adolesc Med.* 1998;152(7):676-682.
14. Klein JD, Wilson KM, McNulty M, Kapphahn C, Collins KS. Access to medical care for adolescents: results from the 1997 commonwealth fund survey of the health of adolescent girls. *J Adolesc Health.* 1999;25(2):120-130.
15. Boonstra H. Comprehensive approach needed to combat sexually transmitted infections among youth. The Guttmacher Report on Public Policy, March 2004:3-4,13.
16. Centers for Disease Control and Prevention. Sexually Transmitted Disease Surveillance, 2005. Atlanta, GA: Department of Health and Human Services; 2006.
17. Shafer M, Countouriotis A. Chlamydia trachomatis. In: Neinstein L, ed. *Adolescent Health Care: A Practical Guide.* 4th ed. Philadelphia, PA: Lippincott Williams & Wilkins; 2002:1138-1160.
18. Cohen MS, Sparling PF. Mucosal infection with *Neisseria gonorrhoeae.* Bacterial adaptation and mucosal defenses. *J Clin Invest.* 1992;89(6):1699-1705.
19. Chacko MR, Lovchik JC. Chlamydia trachomatis infection in sexually active adolescents: prevalence and risk factors. *Pediatrics.* 1984;73(6):836-840.
20. Shrier LA. Sexually transmitted diseases in adolescents: biologic, cognitive, psychologic, behavioral, and social issues. *Adolesc Med Clin.* 2004;15(2):215-234.
21. Sheeder J, Stevens-Simon C, Lezotte D, Glazner J, Scott S. Cervicitis: to treat or not to treat? The role of patient preferences and decision analysis. *J Adolesc Health.* 2006;39(6):887-892.
22. Karaer A, Avsar FA, Batioglu S. Risk factors for ectopic pregnancy: a case-control study. *Aust N Z J Obstet Gynaecol.* 2006;46(6):521-527.

23. Gray-Swain MR, Peipert JF. Pelvic inflammatory disease in adolescents. *Curr Opin Obstet Gynecol.* 2006;18(5):503-510.
24. Simpson T, Oh MK. Urethritis and cervicitis in adolescents. *Adolesc Med Clin.* 2004;15(2):253-271.
25. Johnson RE, Newhall WJ, Papp JR, et al. Screening tests to detect Chlamydia trachomatis and *Neisseria gonorrhoeae* infections–2002. *MMWR Recomm Rep.* 2002;51(RR-15):1-38; quiz CE1-4.
26. Gaydos CA. Nucleic acid amplification tests for gonorrhea and chlamydia: practice and applications. *Infect Dis Clin North Am.* 2005;19(2):367-386, ix.
27. Centers for Disease Control and Prevention. Sexually transmitted diseases treatment guidelines, 2006. *MMWR.* 2006;55(No. RR-11):1-94.
28. Screening for chlamydial infection: recommendations and rationale. *Am J Prev Med.* 2001;20(3 suppl):90-94.
29. Screening for gonorrhea: recommendation statement. *Ann Fam Med.* 2005;3(3):263-267.
30. Surveillance of antibiotic resistance in *Neisseria gonorrhoeae* in the WHO Western Pacific Region, 2005. *Commun Dis Intell.* 2006;30(4):430-433.
31. Martin IM, Hoffmann S, Ison CA. European surveillance of sexually transmitted infections (ESSTI): the first combined antimicrobial susceptibility data for *Neisseria gonorrhoeae* in Western Europe. *J Antimicrob Chemother.* 2006;58(3):587-593.
32. Iverson CJ, Wang SA, Lee MV, et al. Fluoroquinolone resistance among *Neisseria gonorrhoeae* isolates in Hawaii, 1990-2000: role of foreign importation and increasing endemic spread. *Sex Transm Dis.* 2004;31(12):702-708.
33. Increases in fluoroquinolone-resistant *Neisseria gonorrhoeae* among men who have sex with men–United States, 2003, and revised recommendations for gonorrhea treatment, 2004. *MMWR Morb Mortal Wkly Rep.* 2004;53(16):335-338.
34. CDC. Sexually Transmitted Disease Sureveillance 2004 Supplement: Gonococcal Isolate Surveillance Project (GISP) Annual Report 2004. Atlanta, GA: U.S. Department of Health and Human Services, 2005.
35. Update to CDC's sexually transmitted diseases treatment guidelines, 2006: Fluoroquinolones no longer recommended for treatment of gonococcal infections. *MMWR Morb Mortal Wkly Rep.* 2007;56(14):332-336.
36. Discontinuation of cefixime tablets–United States. *MMWR Morb Mortal Wkly Rep.* 2002;51(46):1052.
37. Lyss SB, Kamb ML, Peterman TA, et al. Chlamydia trachomatis among patients infected with and treated for *Neisseria gonorrhoeae* in sexually transmitted disease clinics in the United States. *Ann Intern Med.* 2003;139(3):178-185.
38. Miller WC, Ford CA, Morris M, et al. Prevalence of chlamydial and gonococcal infections among young adults in the United States. *JAMA.* 2004;291(18):2229-2236.
39. Sena AC, Miller WC, Hobbs MM, et al. *Trichomonas vaginalis* infection in male sexual partners: implications for diagnosis, treatment, and prevention. *Clin Infect Dis.* 2007;44(1):13-22.
40. Miller WC, Swygard H, Hobbs MM, et al. The prevalence of trichomoniasis in young adults in the United States. *Sex Transm Dis.* 2005;32(10):593-598.
41. Schwebke JR, Hook EW, III. High rates of *Trichomonas vaginalis* among men attending a sexually transmitted diseases clinic: implications for screening and urethritis management. *J Infect Dis.* 2003;188(3):465-468.
42. Van Der Pol B, Williams JA, Orr DP, Batteiger BE, Fortenberry JD. Prevalence, incidence, natural history, and response to treatment of *Trichomonas vaginalis* infection among adolescent women. *J Infect Dis.* 2005;192(12):2039-2044.
43. Wendel KA, Workowski KA. Trichomoniasis: challenges to appropriate management. *Clin Infect Dis.* 2007;44(suppl 3):S123-S129.
44. Schwebke JR, Burgess D. Trichomoniasis. *Clin Microbiol Rev.* 2004;17(4):794-803.
45. Syed TS, Braverman PK. Vaginitis in adolescents. *Adolesc Med Clin.* 2004;15(2):235-251.
46. Haward M, Shafer M. Vaginitis and cervicitis. *Adolescent Health Care: A Practical Guide.* 4th ed. Philadelphia, PA: Lippincott Williams & Wilkins, 2002:1011-1028.
47. Hardy PH, Hardy JB, Nell EE, Graham DA, Spence MR, Rosenbaum RC. Prevalence of six sexually transmitted disease agents among pregnant inner-city adolescents and pregnancy outcome. *Lancet.* 1984;2(8398):333-337.
48. Cotch MF, Pastorek JG, II, Nugent RP, et al. *Trichomonas vaginalis* associated with low birth weight and preterm delivery. The vaginal infections and prematurity study group. *Sex Trans Dis.* 1997;24(6):353-360.
49. Laga M, Manoka A, Kivuvu M, et al. Non-ulcerative sexually transmitted diseases as risk factors for HIV-1 transmission in women: results from a cohort study. *AIDS* (London, England). 1993;7(1):95-102.
50. Sorvillo F, Kerndt P. *Trichomonas vaginalis* and amplification of HIV-1 transmission. *Lancet.* 1998;351(9097):213-214.
51. Minkoff H, Grunebaum AN, Schwarz RH, et al. Risk factors for prematurity and premature rupture of membranes: a prospective study of the vaginal flora in pregnancy. *Am J Obstetr Gynecol.* 1984;150(8):965-972.
52. Joyner JL, Douglas JM, Jr., Ragsdale S, Foster M, Judson FN. Comparative prevalence of infection with *Trichomonas vaginalis* among men attending a sexually transmitted diseases clinic. *Sex Trans Dis.* 2000;27(4):236-240.
53. Petrin D, Delgaty K, Bhatt R, Garber G. Clinical and microbiological aspects of *Trichomonas vaginalis. Clin Microbiol Rev.* 1998;11(2):300-317.
54. Freeto JP, Jay MS. "What's really going on down there?" A practical approach to the adolescent who has gynecologic complaints. *Pediatr Clin North Am.* 2006;53(3):529-545, viii.
55. Hatcher R, Nelson, AL. Combined hormonal contraceptive methods. In: Hatcher R, Trussell J, Stewart F, et al. ed. *Contraceptive Technology.* 18th ed. New York, NY: Ardent Media, Inc; 2004:391-460.
56. Holland-Hall CM, Wiesenfeld HC, Murray PJ. Self-collected vaginal swabs for the detection of multiple sexually transmitted infections in adolescent girls. *J Pediatr Adolesc Gynecol.* 2002;15(5):307-313.
57. Smith K, Harrington K, Wingood G, Oh MK, Hook EW, III, DiClemente RJ. Self-obtained vaginal swabs for diagnosis of treatable sexually transmitted diseases in adolescent girls. *Arch Pediatr Adolesc Med.* 2001;155(6):676-679.

58. Sobel JD. What's new in bacterial vaginosis and trichomoniasis? *Infect Dis Clin North Am.* 2005;19(2):387-406.
59. Wiese W, Patel SR, Patel SC, Ohl CA, Estrada CA. A meta-analysis of the Papanicolaou smear and wet mount for the diagnosis of vaginal trichomoniasis. *Am J Med.* 2000;108(4):301-308.
60. Briselden AM, Hillier SL. Evaluation of affirm VP microbial identification test for gardnerella vaginalis and *Trichomonas vaginalis. J Clin Microbiol.* 1994;32(1):148-152.
61. DeMeo LR, Draper DL, McGregor JA, et al. Evaluation of a deoxyribonucleic acid probe for the detection of *Trichomonas vaginalis* in vaginal secretions. *Am J Obstetr Gynecol.* 1996;174(4):1339-1342.
62. Huppert JS, Batteiger BE, Braslins P, et al. Use of an immunochromatographic assay for rapid detection of *Trichomonas vaginalis* in vaginal specimens. *J Clin Microbiol.* 2005;43(2):684-687.
63. Patel SR, Wiese W, Patel SC, Ohl C, Byrd JC, Estrada CA. Systematic review of diagnostic tests for vaginal trichomoniasis. *Infect Dis Obstetr Gynecol.* 2000;8(5-6):248-257.
64. Ohlemeyer CL, Hornberger LL, Lynch DA, Swierkosz EM. Diagnosis of *Trichomonas vaginalis* in adolescent females: InPouch TV culture versus wet-mount microscopy. *J Adolesc Health.* 1998;22(3):205-208.
65. Wendel KA, Erbelding EJ, Gaydos CA, Rompalo AM. *Trichomonas vaginalis* polymerase chain reaction compared with standard diagnostic and therapeutic protocols for detection and treatment of vaginal trichomoniasis. *Clin Infect Dis.* 2002;35(5):576-580.
66. Caliendo AM, Jordan JA, Green AM, Ingersoll J, Diclemente RJ, Wingood GM. Real-time PCR improves detection of *Trichomonas vaginalis* infection compared with culture using self-collected vaginal swabs. *Infect Dis Obstetr Gynecol.* 2005;13(3):145-150.
67. Genital HPV Infection—CDC fact sheet. May 2004. http://www.cdc.gov/std/HPV/STDFact-HPV.htm#common. Accessed March 17, 2007.
68. Ahmed AM, Madkan V, Tyring SK. Human papillomaviruses and genital disease. *Dermatol Clin.* 2006;24(2):157-165, vi.
69. Partridge JM, Koutsky LA. Genital human papillomavirus infection in men. *Lancet Infect Dis.* 2006;6(1):21-31.
70. Dunne EF, Unger ER, Sternberg M, et al. Prevalence of HPV infection among females in the United States. *JAMA.* 2007;297(8):813-819.
71. Moscicki AB, Hills N, Shiboski S, et al. Risks for incident human papillomavirus infection and low-grade squamous intraepithelial lesion development in young females. *JAMA.* 2001;285(23):2995-3002.
72. Nicholls PK, Moore PF, Anderson DM, et al. Regression of canine oral papillomas is associated with infiltration of CD4+ and CD8+ lymphocytes. *Virology.* 2001;283(1):31-39.
73. Munoz N, Bosch FX, de Sanjose S, et al. Epidemiologic classification of human papillomavirus types associated with cervical cancer. *N Engl J Med.* 2003;348(6):518-527.
74. Mansur C. Human papillomaviruses. In: Tyring SK, ed. *Mucocutaneous Manifestations of Viral Diseases.* New York, NY: Marcel Dekker, Inc; 2002:247-294.
75. Bartholomew DA. Human papillomavirus infection in adolescents: a rational approach. *Adolesc Med Clin.* 2004;15(3):569-595.
76. ACOG Committee Opinion. Evaluation and management of abnormal cervical cytology and histology in the adolescent. Number 330, April 2006. *Obstet Gynecol.* 2006;107(4):963-968.
77. FDA licenses new vaccine for prevention of cervical cancer and other diseases in females caused by human papillomavirus. June 2006. http://www.fda.gov/bbs/topics/NEWS/2006/NEW01385.html. Accessed March 17, 2007.
78. Markowitz LE, Dunne EF, Saraiya M, Lawson HW, Chesson H, Unger ER. Quadrivalent human papillomavirus vaccine: recommendations of the advisory committee on immunization practices (ACIP). *MMWR Recomm Rep.* 2007;56(RR-2):1-24.
79. Speck LM, Tyring SK. Vaccines for the prevention of human papillomavirus infections. *Skin Therapy Lett.* 2006;11(6):1-3.

SECTION 11

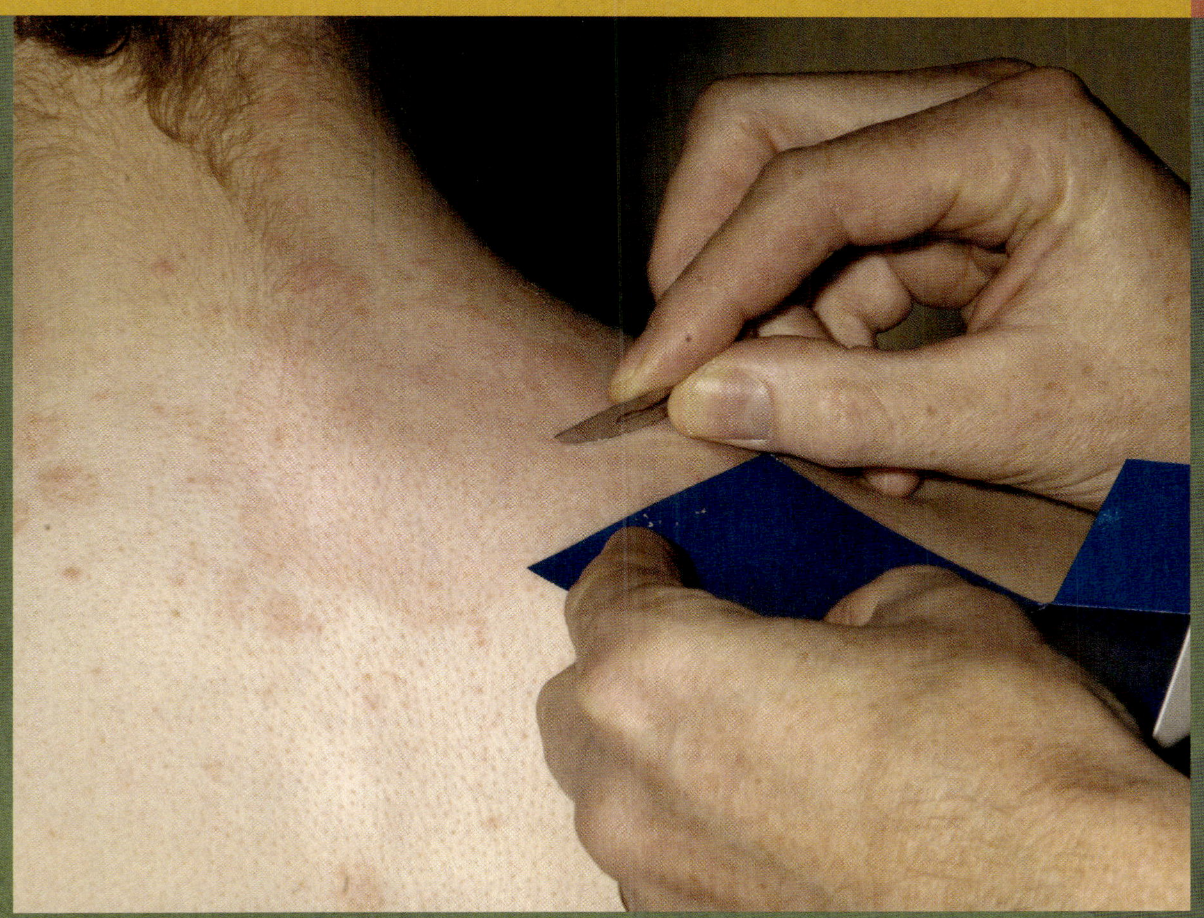

Skin Infections

CHAPTER 45

Skin and Skin Structure Infections

Matthew Kronman

DEFINITIONS AND EPIDEMIOLOGY

Skin is composed of an outermost, avascular layer of epidermis with an inner layer of dermis made up of elastic tissue, collagen, and reticular fibers. Subcutaneous tissue includes fat cells, connective tissue, and muscle. Blood vessels pass through subcutaneous tissues to reach the dermis (Figure 45–1).

Bacterial skin and skin structure infections (SSIs) can be subdivided into two groups: superficial and deep (Figure 45–1). Superficial infections tend to evolve from local spread of organisms, but can also represent circulating toxin-mediated disease. Common superficial infections include impetigo, folliculitis, carbuncles, furuncles, paronychia, cellulitis, and erysipelas (Table 45–1). Deeper infections include abscess and pyomyositis and instead tend to arise by the hematogenous spread of organisms from a distant site. This chapter will review cellulitis, cutaneous abscess, and pyomyositis (Table 45–2).

Cellulitis is an indistinctly bordered infection of subcutaneous tissue and dermis (Figure 45–2). Periorbital and orbital cellulitis are discussed elsewhere (Chapter 22). Skin compromise caused by abrasions, lacerations, insect bites, trauma, or underlying dermatitis is the most common predisposing risk factor for the development of cellulitis and is identified in approximately two-thirds of cases.[1] The most common causes of cellulitis in healthy children are *Staphylococcus aureus* and Group A β-hemolytic streptococci (GABHS). Group B streptococci should be considered as a potential cause of cellulitis in patients younger than 3 months.[2] Rare causes of cellulitis include nonserotype-b *Hemophilus influenzae*,[3] *Nocardia* species,[4] and *Mycobacterium* species.[5] *Pasteurella* species are common causes of cellulitis after animal bites, and anaerobic organisms should be considered after human bites (see Chapter 46, Bite Wound Infections). Immunocompromised patients are at higher risk of cellulitis due to other organisms such as *Pseudomonas aeruginosa*,[6] and children with reptile exposures and bites are at risk for cellulitis caused by *Salmonella* or *Serratia* species.[7]

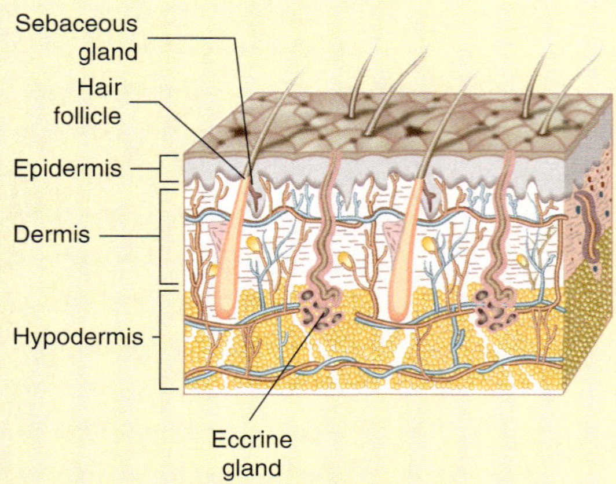

FIGURE 45–1 ■ Basic skin anatomy.

An abscess is a discrete collection of pus and cellular debris separated from its surroundings by a fibrinoid wall. *S. aureus* and GABHS predominate as causes. Less common causes include *Escherichia coli*, anaerobes,[8] *Enterobacter* spp., *Klebsiella* spp., *P. aeruginosa*, and nontuberculous mycobacteria.[9,10] In the last 15 years, community-acquired methicillin-resistant *S. aureus* (CA-MRSA) infections have increased dramatically throughout the United States, frequently causing cellulitis or cutaneous abscesses in children.[11–18] Outbreaks of CA-MRSA disease and carriage have been associated with athletic teams[19–21] and daycare attendance;[22,23] intrafamilial spread of CA-MRSA has been described,[24,25] and

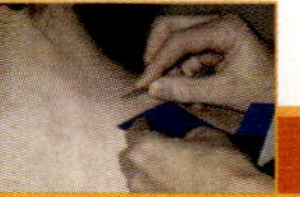

Table 45–1.

Common Superficial Skin and Skin Structure Infections

Disease	Definition	Most Common Causes	Less Common Causes to Consider	Treatment
Impetigo	Well-localized superficial skin infection with or without bulla formation	MSSA, GABHS		Topical mupirocin or retapamulin; Oral clindamycin, cephalexin, erythromycin, or amoxicillin plus clavulanic acid for 7–10 d
Folliculitis	Collection of superficial infections in hair follicles without deeper involvement	MSSA	*Pseudomonas*, coagulase-negative staphylococci	Warm compresses, topical mupirocin, retapamulin or chlorhexidine; oral cephalexin or dicloxacillin for severe cases for 7–10 d
Furuncle	Microabscess arising at a hair follicle in slightly deeper tissue than folliculitis	MSSA, MRSA		Hot, wet compresses; surgical drainage; oral clindamycin (if MRSA suspected) or cephalexin for 7–10 d
Carbuncle	Organized collection of adjacent furuncles; may have multiple areas of drainage	MSSA, MRSA		Hot, wet compresses; surgical drainage; oral clindamycin (if MRSA suspected) or cephalexin for 7–10 d
Paronychia	Infection of the skin surrounding the nail bed	MSSA, GABHS	Candida, Anaerobes, *Streptococcus viridans*, *Pseudomonas*, *Proteus*, *Moraxella*, *Klebsiella*, *Eikenella*	Warm compresses; surgical drainage (for deeper lesions); oral clindamycin or amoxicillin–clavulanate for 7–10 d
Erysipelas	Superficial form of cellulitis with distinct margins and involving lymphatics	GABHS	MSSA, *S. pneumoniae*, *Klebsiella pneumoniae*, *Yersinia enterocolitica*	Local skin care; parenteral penicillin initially, oral cephalexin or clindamycin (if staphylococci suspected) for a total length of 10 d

MSSA, methicillin-sensitive Staphylococcus aureus; *MRSA, methicillin-resistant* Staphylococcus aureus; *GABHS, group A β-hemolytic streptococci.*

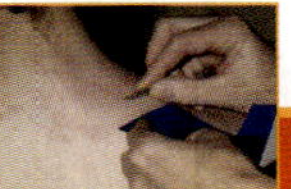

Table 45–2.

Etiology of Skin and Skin Structure Infections

Disease	Definition	Most Common Causes	Less Common Causes to Consider
Cellulitis	Indistinctly bordered infection of subcutaneous tissue and dermis	MSSA, MRSA, GABHS	GBS (patients $<$3 months old), *H. influenzae*, *Pseudomonas*, *Serratia*, *Salmonella*, *Nocardia*, *Mycobacteria*, *Pasteurella*
Abscess	Discrete collection of pus and cellular debris separated from its surroundings by a fibrinoid wall	MSSA, MRSA, GABHS	*E. coli*, anaerobes, *Enterobacter*, *Klebsiella*, *Pseudomonas*, and *Mycobacteria*
Pyomyositis	Acute infection of muscle and surrounding connective tissue, usually with abscess formation	MSSA, MRSA, GABHS	*Clostridium*, *Salmonella*, Group C streptococci, *Mycobacteria*, anaerobes

MSSA, methicillin-sensitive Staphylococcus aureus; *MRSA, methicillin-resistant* Staphylococcus aureus; *GABHS, group A β-hemolytic streptococci; GBS, group B streptococci.*

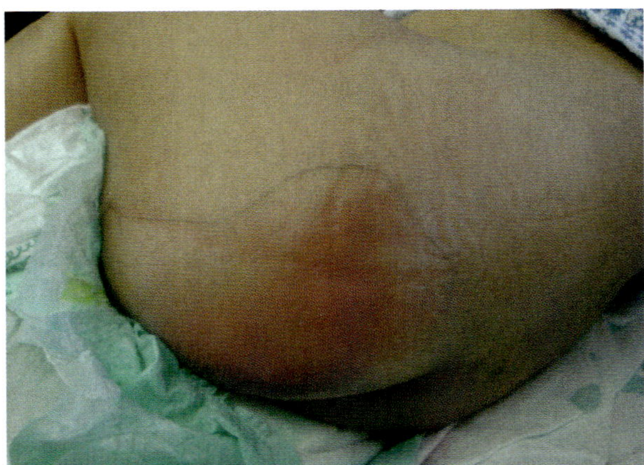

FIGURE 45–2 ■ Cellulitis with superficial abscess formation in the left buttock of a 6-month-old infant. Note the indistinct margins and the appearance of fluctuance coming to a head inferiorly and medially. (*Courtesy of Dr. Samir S. Shah.*)

there are even reports of family members transmitting CA-MRSA to their hospitalized children.[26,27] The majority of these community-acquired infections are clonally related, suggesting that community spread and acquisition of MRSA has become commonplace.[28] The prevalence of MRSA varies dramatically by location; 61% of nasal *S. aureus* isolates were MRSA in a pediatric population in Texas in 2005, while a 2007 study of more than 1300 children in Switzerland found only 0.18% of nasal *S. aureus* isolates to be MRSA.[29,30] However, the asymptomatic nasal carriage of CA-MRSA appears to be increasing in the United States. Asymptomatic CA-MRSA nasal colonization of children in Nashville increased from 0.8% in 2001 to 9.2% in 2004.[31]

A prospective study of risk factors associated with pediatric CA-MRSA infections (89% of which represented skin and SSIs) noted an increased rate of CA-MRSA infections in African American patients compared to Hispanic or white patients.[13] Native Americans and Pacific Islanders are other racial groups reported to be at increased risk for CA-MRSA infection.[32,33] Eczema and asthma were the most common underlying illnesses in one study; patients with atopic dermatitis have long been known to have a markedly increased carriage rate of *S. aureus,* even on clinically unaffected skin, ranging from 70% to 90%.[13,34,35] The prevalence of MRSA-infected skin lesions in children with atopic dermatitis has been shown to increase with age.[36] Another study of CA-MRSA in the United States noted an increased incidence of all CA-MRSA disease (approximately three-quarters of which were SSIs) in children younger than 2 years.[37] The same study noted an increased CA-MRSA disease incidence in African American patients relative to white patients, though only in one of two communities studied.[37] It is currently unclear whether certain races have a genetic basis for increased susceptibility to CA-MRSA infection, or whether the increased incidence of CA-MRSA disease in certain groups merely reflects socioeconomic status. However, one study investigating risks for CA-MRSA disease found no difference between groups with different insurance types (used as a proxy for socioeconomic status).[13] Other factors predisposing people to SSIs in general include immunodeficiency, skin trauma or surgical wounds, and vascular compromise.

Pyomyositis (also known as tropical myositis or myositis tropicans) is an acute infection of muscle and surrounding connective tissue, usually with abscess formation, seen most commonly after trauma, varicella, or vigorous exercise.[38–40] A 2:1 male predominance has been described.[41] Pyomyositis occurs more frequently in tropical climates and during warm seasons, and is caused most often by *S. aureus* and GABHS.[41] As with more superficial infections, MRSA is becoming an increasingly common causative organism and patients with MRSA pyomyositis tend to be younger than those with methicillin-sensitive *Staphylococcus aureus* (MSSA) pyomyositis.[42] Anaerobes such as *Clostridium* species and polymicrobial infections are rarer causes of pyomyositis.[43] Other rare causes include *Salmonella* species,[44] Group C streptococci,[45] and *Mycobacterium* species.[46] Human immunodeficiency virus (HIV) infection is thought to be a risk factor for pyomyositis due to the underlying host defense abnormalities as well as HIV myopathy, which occurs in patients with late-stage disease.[47]

PATHOGENESIS

Most SSIs are caused by bacteria that transiently colonize the skin such as GABHS and *S. aureus.* Persistent nasopharyngeal colonization with *S. aureus* occurs in 20–40% of all patients[48,49]; other less commonly colonized body sites include the axilla, vagina, and the perineum.[50] Patients colonized with *S. aureus* are more likely to develop skin infections and postoperative wound infections, most of which are caused by the colonizing strain rather than an exogenous souce.[51,52]

Normal resident skin flora include micrococci, coagulase-negative staphylococci, *Propionibacterium* spp. (on head and upper trunk), *Corynebacterium* spp., and *Acinetobacter* spp. (in intertriginous areas), and yeasts such as *Candida* spp. and *Malassezia furfur* (on the head, mucosae, and nail folds).[53] While some of these species can cause infections, micrococci and coagulase-negative staphylococci rarely do. *Propionibacterium* spp. (such as *P. acnes*) are anaerobic Gram-positive bacilli with affinity for sebaceous glands; *P. acnes* causes acne and folliculitis of the head and neck.

For skin infections to develop, host defense mechanisms must be compromised and the balance between resident skin flora and transient flora must shift to favor transient flora. Host defense mechanisms include an intact stratum corneum, epidermal Langerhans and dendritic cells, keratinocyte secretions, neutrophils, and epidermal T lymphocytes.[54] Various lipids and breakdown products of the stratum corneum layer of skin have innate antimicrobial activity.[55] Factors favoring transient bacteria include increased skin temperature, increased humidity, cutaneous disease, young age or prematurity, and recent use of antibiotics.

Local trauma, surgery, chronic disease, and immunodeficiency can compromise host defense mechanisms and are implicated in many skin infections. Breakdown of the stratum corneum exposes new cell surface receptors that allow adherence and translocation of skin bacteria. Diseases that increase the risk for staphylococcal infection include renal failure requiring dialysis, chronic granulomatous disease, hyperimmunoglobulin E syndrome, Chediak–Higashi syndrome, leukemia, neutropenia secondary to chemotherapy, and solid organ and hematopoietic stem cell transplantation.[50]

Deeper infections can arise by three distinct mechanisms: (1) direct spread of more superficial infections such as folliculitis, furuncles, or carbuncles; (2) metastatic spread of organisms from a more distant source via a hematogenous or lymphatic route; and (3) penetrating trauma, in which organisms are carried into deep tissue by the penetrating object.

CA-MRSA has been recognized as an increasingly common cause of subcutaneous abscesses. Many CA-MRSA isolates harbor a gene encoding the virulence factor Panton–Valentine leukocidin (PVL), a pore-forming cytotoxin that damages membranes of neutrophils, monocytes, and macrophages and thereby allows the organism to create abscesses more easily.[56] PVL appears to be a virulence factor for skin and SSIs; in a study that screened 172 *S. aureus* strains for PVL but not for antibiotic resistance patterns, PVL was isolated from 93% of strains causing furunculosis, 55% of those causing cellulitis, and 50% of those causing cutaneous abscesses.[57] A study of adults presenting with SSIs to an emergency department in 2004 noted that 98% of the CA-MRSA isolates contained the PVL gene, and 97% had an identical genotype, called USA300.[58] The USA300 genotype appears to be quite common among CA-MRSA isolates. It has been found in 87% of isolates from an emergency department in one study, in more than 90% of all CA-MRSA isolates in one Houston center, the majority of those in a Dallas center, and has been highly conserved among infections in one study of professional football players.[59–63]

The exact pathogenesis of pyomyositis is unclear. Experimental animal models show that pyomyositis may develop as a consequence of hematogenous seeding of traumatized muscle.[38] Invasive Group A streptococcal infections such as pyomyositis occur after varicella infection, suggesting that pyomyositis may also develop by local extension of infection after skin damage without antecedent bacteremia.[64,65] Group A streptococci isolates causing myositis and myonecrosis demonstrate protease and exotoxin activity that may impair local host defenses to allow rapid spread of infection through host tissues.[66]

CLINICAL PRESENTATION

Cellulitis presents as an indistinctly bordered area of erythema, warmth, edema, and tenderness on the skin. Systemic symptoms such as fever and malaise may or may not be present. Patients are almost never toxic-appearing, and approximately three-quarters of cases are uncomplicated.[1] Two-thirds of cases appear on an extremity, with the remainder on the face, neck, and trunk. Approximately 25% of cellulitis cases are associated with abscess and approximately 1% are associated with osteomyelitis or septic arthritis.[1]

Subcutaneous abscesses present similarly to cellulitis, with indistinct borders, erythema, warmth, edema, and tenderness. The skin overlying an abscess may be taut and shiny. Early in the course of an abscess, most patients will have a focal area of tender induration and, as the abscess progresses, this area becomes fluctuant, indicating the presence of a discrete abscess pocket amenable to surgical drainage. As with cases of cellulitis, systemic symptoms may or may not be present though systemic symptoms are more likely with larger lesions. Some subcutaneous abscesses will spontaneously drain purulent or serosanguinous material.

Pyomyositis typically evolves through three stages. In the first, or invasive, stage, clinical findings are insidious and somewhat nonspecific, with dull muscle cramping, anorexia and occasional low-grade fevers, and may last up to 3 weeks.[38,41] Fewer than 2% of patients present at this stage.[67] The second, or suppurative stage, evolves with increasing systemic symptoms such as fever and physical findings become more focal with localized muscle pain. Overlying skin may or may not be erythematous. Approximately half of patients will have focal muscle swelling.[42] Most patients present during this suppurative stage. Patients presenting in the third, or late, stage will have profound systemic symptoms such as septic shock, requiring urgent treatment. Large proximal muscle groups are the most commonly affected, including the quadriceps, hamstring, iliopsoas, and pelvic muscles.[38,41] Less commonly affected muscle groups include the back, neck, distal lower extremity, and shoulder girdle muscles.[42]

Children may present with limp or refusal to bear weight, and the clinical presentation can often mimic that of a septic arthritis of the hip when the psoas muscle is involved. Children with septic arthritis of the hip typically have significant pain with passive hip range of motion and tend to keep the hip in a position of flexion and external rotation (see Chapter 48, Septic Arthritis). Children with isolated pyomyositis of hip muscles should have normal hip range of motion and children with psoas pyomyositis may have slightly decreased hip range of motion. Examining full active and passive range of motion of the hip, particularly hip abduction and extension, can therefore help distinguish between hip septic arthritis and localized pyomyositis.

In one study, children with pyomyositis frequently had concomitant osteomyelitis (41%) or septic arthritis (7%).[42] Inflammatory markers tend to be elevated, with mean C-reactive protein being 16.3 mg/dL, mean erythrocyte sedimentation rate 62 mm/h, and white blood cell count >15,000/mm^3.[42] Creatine kinase (CK) and other muscle enzyme levels tend to be normal or trivially elevated.[42] Care should be taken to distinguish pyomyositis from necrotizing fasciitis, which evolves rapidly over hours, and whose hallmarks include pain out of proportion to visible physical findings, pain on palpation outside areas of erythema, and crepitus.

DIFFERENTIAL DIAGNOSIS

The differential diagnosis of bacterial SSIs is extensive (Table 45–3). Other infectious causes of superficial skin

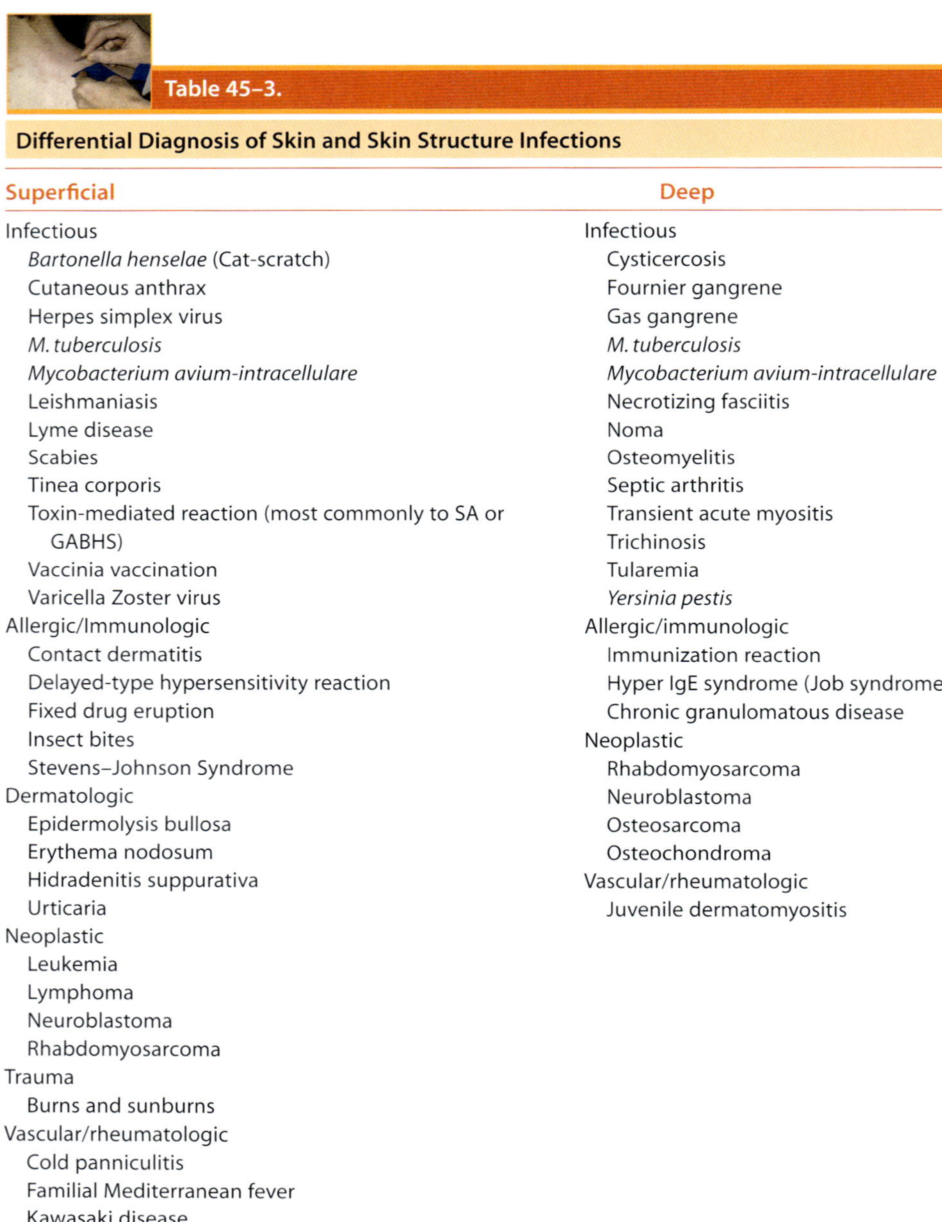

Table 45–3.

Differential Diagnosis of Skin and Skin Structure Infections

Superficial	Deep
Infectious	Infectious
Bartonella henselae (Cat-scratch)	Cysticercosis
Cutaneous anthrax	Fournier gangrene
Herpes simplex virus	Gas gangrene
M. tuberculosis	*M. tuberculosis*
Mycobacterium avium-intracellulare	*Mycobacterium avium-intracellulare*
Leishmaniasis	Necrotizing fasciitis
Lyme disease	Noma
Scabies	Osteomyelitis
Tinea corporis	Septic arthritis
Toxin-mediated reaction (most commonly to SA or GABHS)	Transient acute myositis
Vaccinia vaccination	Trichinosis
Varicella Zoster virus	Tularemia
Allergic/Immunologic	*Yersinia pestis*
Contact dermatitis	Allergic/immunologic
Delayed-type hypersensitivity reaction	Immunization reaction
Fixed drug eruption	Hyper IgE syndrome (Job syndrome)
Insect bites	Chronic granulomatous disease
Stevens–Johnson Syndrome	Neoplastic
Dermatologic	Rhabdomyosarcoma
Epidermolysis bullosa	Neuroblastoma
Erythema nodosum	Osteosarcoma
Hidradenitis suppurativa	Osteochondroma
Urticaria	Vascular/rheumatologic
Neoplastic	Juvenile dermatomyositis
Leukemia	
Lymphoma	
Neuroblastoma	
Rhabdomyosarcoma	
Trauma	
Burns and sunburns	
Vascular/rheumatologic	
Cold panniculitis	
Familial Mediterranean fever	
Kawasaki disease	
Pyoderma gangrenosum	
Reflex sympathetic dystrophy	

SA, S. aureus; *GABHS, group A β-hemolytic streptococci.*

infections include viruses (herpes simplex virus, varicella zoster virus), bacteria (mycobacteria, *Bartonella henselae*), yeasts (i.e., tinea corporis), parasites (scabies, leishmaniasis), and rickettsiae (Lyme disease). Toxin-mediated reactions to staphylococcal or streptococcal infections can also cause diffuse erythroderma and can mimic superficial skin infections.

Deep SSIs also have a broad differential diagnosis (Table 45–3). The most common infectious conditions associated with deep SSIs are osteomyelitis and septic arthritis. Pyomyositis should be differentiated from transient acute myositis, which is often occurs as an autoimmune reaction to a viral infection. Gas gangrene is a fulminant form of pyomyositis with myonecrosis, often occurring in the setting of contaminated surgical wounds, caused by *Clostridium* species. The most important clinical entity to distinguish from routine deeper SSIs is necrotizing fasciitis. Necrotizing fasciitis is a rapidly progressive and potentially life-threatening infection that spreads along the fascial planes of subcutaneous tissues. Necrotizing fasciitis often follows other local infections, such as varicella, is most common in children younger than 5 years, and is commonly caused by GABHS.[68] Development of necrotizing fasciitis following primary varicella infection has been associated with ibuprofen use.[69] Other disease categories to consider in the differential diagnosis of both superficial and deep SSIs include allergic, primary dermatologic, neoplastic, traumatic, and vascular.

DIAGNOSIS

Cellulitis and Abscess

Diagnosis of superficial bacterial skin infections is largely clinical and microbiologic; radiographic evaluation is seldom necessary. Gram stain and culture of purulent material expressed from the site of folliculitis, carbuncles, and furuncles frequently reveals a causative organism. Potassium hydroxide preparation of skin cells may sometimes be warranted in cases of paronychia and folliculitis to diagnose infections caused by *Candida* spp. or *M. furfur*.

While aspirates from the point of maximal inflammation may yield causal organisms more often than those from the leading edge of a cellulitis, the overall yield is low, ranging from 10% to 30%, and is therefore not routinely indicated.[70–73] Full septic workup including blood and cerebrospinal fluid cultures should be performed on patients younger than 3 months of age suspected of having cellulitis, because up to 90% of patients in this age group with Group B streptococcal infections (GBS) have concomitant bacteremia.[2,74] In older children, blood cultures are seldom useful in the diagnosis of superficial skin infections. Blood cultures isolate organisms in approximately 5% of erysipelas cases[75] and 2% of cellulitis cases and more commonly yield contaminants in areas where *H. influenzae* serotype b (Hib) is no longer prevalent.[1]

The increasing prevalence of MRSA in skin and SSIs has dramatically altered our diagnostic approach to superficial SSIs and abscesses.[11–18] Community-acquired MRSA isolates causing skin and SSI also tend to carry the staphylococcal cassette chromosome (SCC) *mecIV*, which confers resistance to β-lactam antibiotics.[76,77] Cultures of purulent material are being performed more frequently and antibiotic susceptibility should be performed on all isolates obtained.

MRSA isolates should be examined for inducible clindamycin resistance. Acquisition by isolates of *S. aureus* of erythromycin-resistance methylase (*erm*) genes can cause either constitutive or inducible resistance to macrolide (e.g., erythromycin or azithromycin), lincosamide (e.g., clindamycin), or streptogramin-B (e.g., quinupristin-dalfopristin) antibiotics. Resistance is conferred by methylation of bacterial 23S ribosomal RNA.[78] Constitutive resistance to these antibiotics is readily apparent using routine antibiotic susceptibility determination methods (see Chapter 1, Diagnostic Microbiology). Erythromycin is a rapid inducer of resistance when the *erm* gene is present, while clindamycin induces resistance slowly.

Inducible clindamycin resistance in *S. aureus* isolates varies geographically, from less than 1% of pediatric isolates in Houston,[60] to 3% of previously healthy children in Philadelphia between 2001 and 2003,[79] to 7% of children in Dallas in 2002.[61] Thirteen percent of pediatric CA-MRSA isolates in a study in the northeast United States in 2003–2004 were clindamycin-resistant (both constitutive and inducible),[80] and 43% of pediatric CA-MRSA isolates in a small study in Baltimore showed inducible clindamycin resistance.[81] There is concern that the proportion of isolates inducibly resistant to clindamycin is growing.[80] Some populations may have up to 60% inducible clindamycin resistance in MSSA and up to 33% in CA-MRSA.[82] A report in a population of Texas children, however, showed that inducible clindamycin resistance decreased from 93% to 7% of CA-MRSA isolates between 1999 and 2002.[61]

Testing for inducible clindamycin resistance is called the D-test and is performed as follows: Antibiotic-impregnated wafers are placed on the culture medium in the routine disk diffusion (Kirby–Bauer) manner and a disk containing erythromycin is placed within 15–20 mm of a disk containing clindamycin.[78] If the *S. aureus* isolate is susceptible to both antibiotics, full, circular zones of inhibition will be seen around each of the antibiotic disks. Some *S. aureus* strains will contain genes for erythromycin resistance without clindamycin resistance (such as the *msr*(A) gene, which encodes for an erythromycin efflux mechanism for which clindamycin is not a substrate[83]), and so a full, circular zone of inhibition will form around the clindamycin disk while the organism will be resistant to erythromycin and therefore able to grow right up to the erythromycin disk. If the isolate contains the inducible *erm* gene, the zone of inhibition around the clindamycin disk will be a distorted D-shape, with the flat side closest to the erythromycin disk (Figure 45–3). This shape develops because erythromycin is a potent inducer of resistance, so the organisms close to the erythromycin disk gain clindamycin resistance and can therefore grow closer to the clindamycin disk on the culture medium. If the D-test is not performed, *S. aureus* isolates can appear to be clindamycin susceptible when they in fact have inducible clindamycin resistance. In vitro studies have demonstrated rapid development of clindamycin resistance by *S. aureus* isolates containing the *erm* gene for inducible clindamycin resistance.[78] While there has been debate as to the clinical importance of inducible clindamycin resistance, currently clinicians avoid the use of clindamycin for treatment of *S. aureus* isolates exhibiting such resistance.[84,85]

Pyomyositis

Blood cultures are more commonly useful in deeper skin structure and muscular infections; a combination of blood and wound cultures are positive in approximately 60% of pediatric pyomyositis cases.[42] Blood cultures alone yield the organism in approximately 20% of cases. Computed tomography (CT) scanning can identify fluid collections and rim enhancement of abscesses,[86] and soft tissue magnetic resonance imaging (MRI) can show enlargement of the affected muscle group with increased T1-weighted signal, hyperintense fluid collections on T2 imaging, and rim-enhanced lesions with administration of gadolinium (Figures 45–4 and 45–5).[86,87] While MRI has largely become the imaging modality of choice for diagnosing deep SSIs, ultrasound can also be used when MRI or CT are unavailable

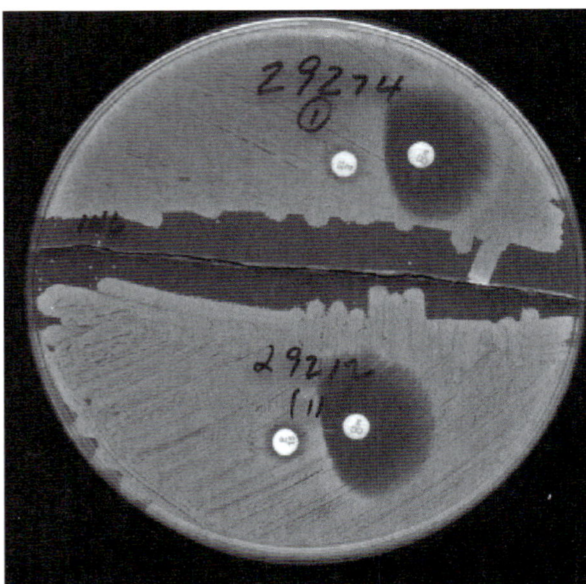

FIGURE 45–3 ■ A positive D-test for inducible clindamycin resistance in an isolate of *S. aureus*. (*Adapted from Buescher, Curr Opin Pediatr, 2005.*)

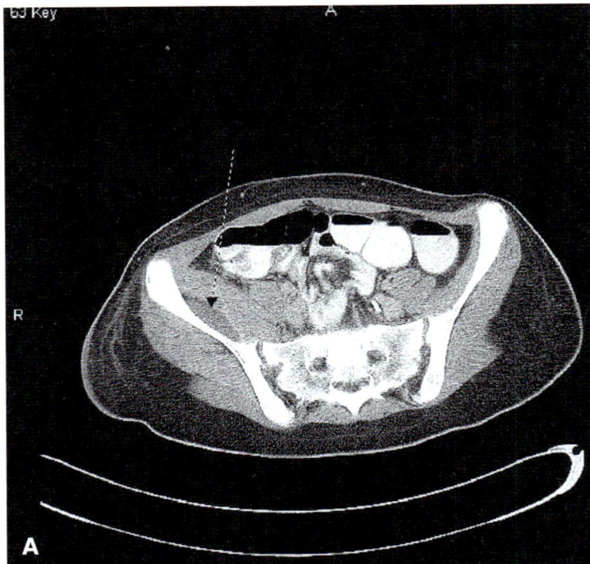

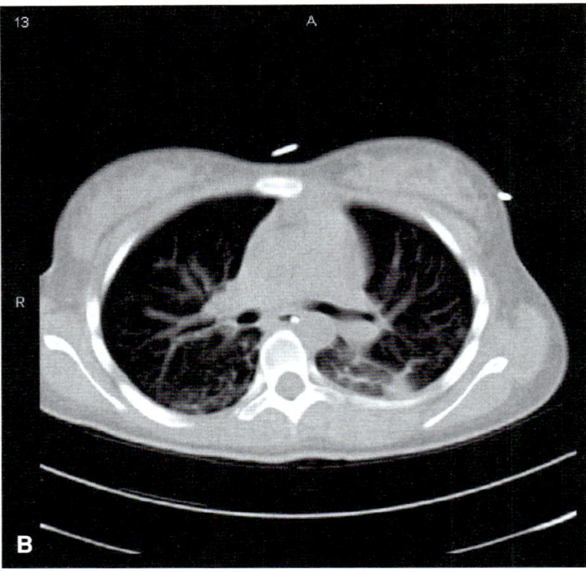

FIGURE 45–4 ■ Contrast-enhanced computed tomography of the pelvis and chest of a 14-year-old girl with **(A)** a fluid collection in the right iliopsoas with a peripherally enhancing rim to suggest abscess formation (arrow) and associated thrombosis extending from the right common femoral vein to the right common iliac vein resulting in **(B)** pulmonary septic emboli. (*Courtesy of Dr. Samir S. Shah.*)

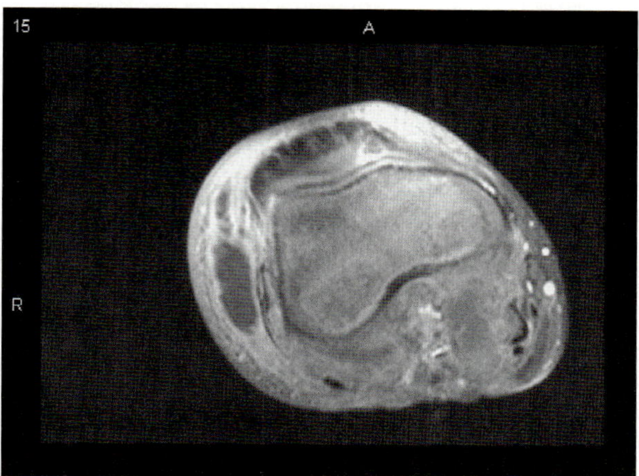

FIGURE 45–5 ■ Magnetic resonance imaging (MRI) scan of a 9-year-old boy with a 5.1 × 4.4 × 1.1 cm peripherally enhancing, loculated fluid collection in the subcutaneous tissues lateral to the distal femur.

or when an effort is being made to avoid radiation exposure to the patient.[88] Ultrasound may even be preferable for lesions in the extremities, while lesions in the pelvis are better examined using MRI.[89] Ultrasound can also be used to guide needle aspiration of fluid to facilitate microbiologic diagnosis. MRI is the most useful imaging modality for differentiating pyomyositis alone from those cases that occur with concomitant septic arthritis or osteomyelitis. Necrotizing fasciitis is distinguished from pyomyositis primarily by its rapid clinical progression and clinical context.

TREATMENT

Because the diagnosis of superficial infections will be clinical in the majority of patients, therapy always needs to be tailored to the most likely organisms and the regional antibiotic resistance patterns. Empiric choice of antimicrobials for superficial skin infections has been changing as the prevalence of CA-MRSA has risen. Epidemiologic evidence suggests that younger age, African American race (in some communities), and lower socioeconomic status are risk factors for CA-MRSA infection versus CA-MSSA infection; however, no clinical features reliably distinguish with certainty SSIs caused by methicillin-resistant *S. aureus* from those caused by methicillin-sensitive *S. aureus.* Small, open lesions may be amenable to topical antimicrobial therapy alone, either with mupirocin three times daily or with the newer agent retapamulin twice daily for 5–7 days.[90] If human or animal bites have preceded the development of cellulitis, treatment consists of amoxicillin–clavulanate orally (25–40 mg/kg/d divided every 8–12 hours) as an outpatient or ampicillin–sulbactam parenterally (100–200 mg/kg/d divided every 6 hours) as an inpatient for more significant infections (see Chapter 46, Bite Wound Infections).

In patients with larger abscesses, nonpurulent cellulitis, or systemic toxicity, oral or intravenous therapy is required. Clindamycin has become the most common empiric antimicrobial in many centers for treatment of cellulitis and abscess because of its tissue penetration, oral bioavailability, and current low levels of resistance.[12,15,16] Use of clindamycin is not without its disadvantages, however. The incidence of pseudomembranous colitis after clindamycin is estimated at 1% and there are concerns that clindamycin resistance is increasing.[80,91] Trimethoprim-sulfamethoxazole (TMP-SMX) also has good activity against CA-MRSA and low levels of resistance, but has poor activity against streptococci.[37] Dermatologic side effects such as urticaria and exfoliative dermatitis are common with TMP-SMX at a rate between 2% and 3%, with serious drug reactions (such as erythema multiforme or Stevens–Johnson syndrome) estimated at 0.06%.[92] In areas of increasing CA-MRSA prevalence and increasing clindamycin resistance, TMP-SMX may be a reasonable first-line agent for superficial SSIs. Few data are available to support the use of doxycycline and minocycline though cure rates for SSIs treated with these tetracyclines in one retrospective case series were similar to those reported for clindamycin.[93]

Other antibiotics previously used for SSIs may no longer be ideal for treatment of these infections. Erythromycin resistance is common among CA-MRSA isolates, and many cutaneous infections are polymicrobial and include GABHS as a causative organism.[37] Resistance to macrolides appears to be increasing among skin GABHS isolates and is currently estimated at more than 12% and increases with age.[36,94] A Centers for Disease Control report of four children with fatal invasive CA-MRSA disease notes that all four were initially treated with a cephalosporin, and routine use of cephalosporins alone for deeper SSIs has decreased since that time.[95] Rifampin is often highly active against CA-MRSA, but a high rate of mutations conferring rifampin resistance precludes its use alone.

Vancomycin should be used for severe or life-threatening SSIs to cover for the possibility of CA-MRSA. Because clindamycin has no Gram-negative activity and some SSIs are polymicrobial, the addition of a third-generation cephalosporin should also be considered in severe infections or toxic-appearing patients until culture results are available. Linezolid (30 mg/kg/d in three divided doses either orally or parenterally) and quinupristin–dalfopristin (7.5 mg/kg given every 8–12 hours) are alternate, second-line agents that can be considered if resistance patterns, side effects, or allergies make first-line antimicrobials unsuitable.[96] Neither is an ideal treatment option, since linezolid can cause myelosuppression and has a high cost, and quinupristin–dalfopristin can cause drug–drug interactions, hyperbilirubinemia, arthralgias, and myalgias. Two additional antibiotics, tigecycline and daptomycin, have also been approved by the Food and Drug Administration for intravenous treatment of SSIs caused by MRSA in adults; both have cure rates similar to vancomycin. Tigecycline is a minocycline derivative and thus cannot be administered to children younger than 8 years of age. Daptomycin has rapid bactericidal activity by a novel mechanism of action; this cyclic lipopeptide disrupts the bacterial membrane through formation of transmembrane channels that lead to leakage of intracellular ions and subsequent depolarization of the cellular membrane. Neither tigecycline nor daptomycin should be routinely used in children until additional data is available. See Figure 45–6 for an approach to selecting empiric therapy for skin and SSIs and appropriate dosing.

Cutaneous abscesses more than 5 cm in diameter are more likely to require inpatient treatment.[97] A small study of children presenting to the emergency department noted that patients who had received ineffective antibiotics but also incision and drainage did as well as those who had received effective antibiotics and drainage, suggesting that in many children incision and drainage alone may provide sufficient treatment.[97] There are no randomized, controlled trials, however, to prove that incision and drainage alone may be curative. Larger abscesses may require placement of gauze packing or a drain (such as a Penrose) to facilitate debridement of necrotic tissue and wound drainage (Figure 45–7). In our experience, some parents prefer Penrose drain placement with resorbable sutures because home gauze packing changes can be uncomfortable and difficult in the pediatric population.

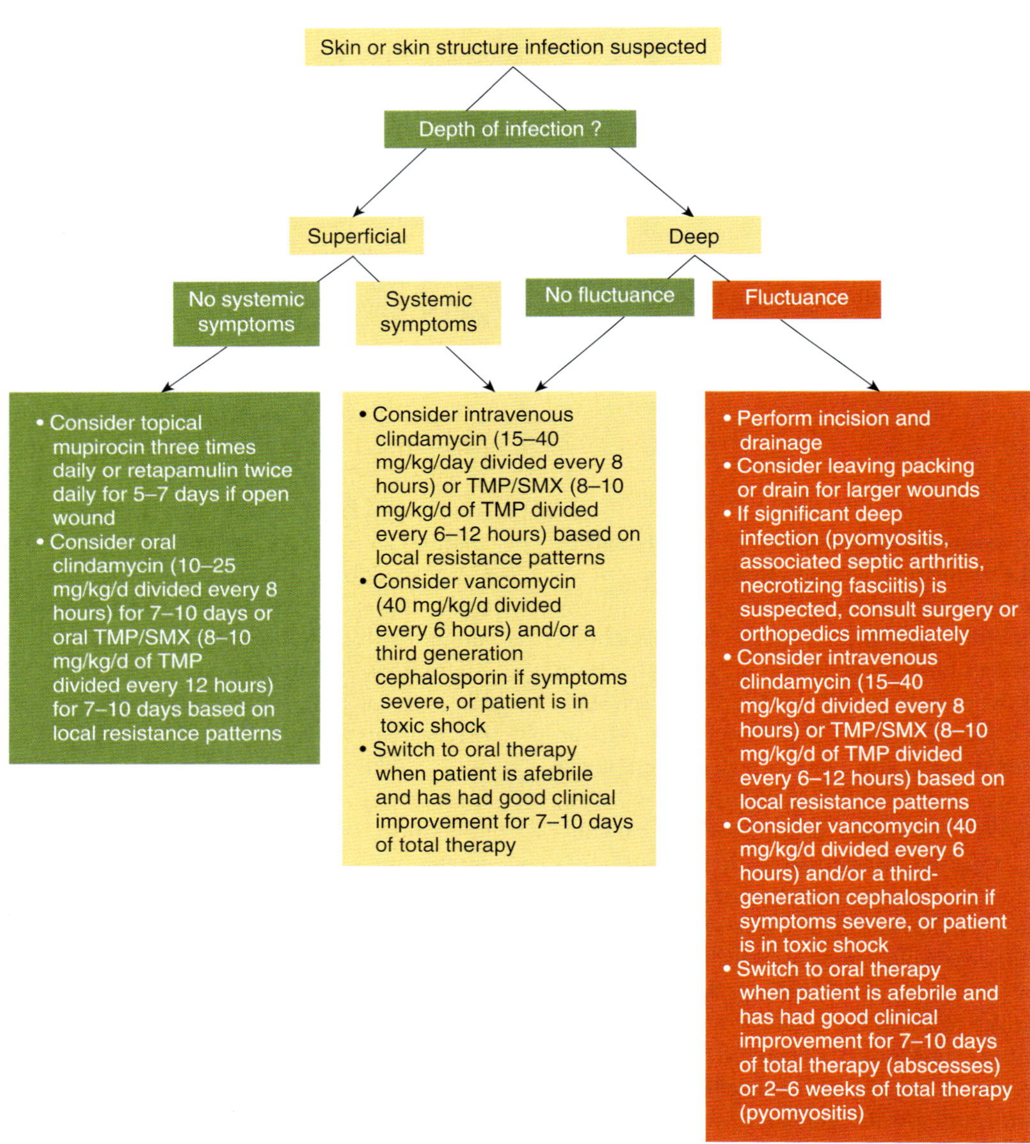

FIGURE 45–6 ■ An approach to empiric therapy for skin and skin structure infections.

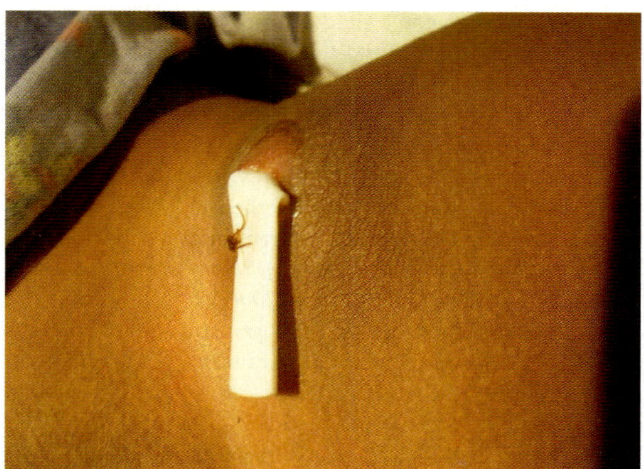

FIGURE 45–7 ■ A community-acquired MRSA abscess in the left inguinal region of a 17-month-old African American girl. Note the Penrose drain sutured in place with resorbable sutures and the local erythema and swelling.

Treatment of pyomyositis often requires surgical drainage, which can be performed percutaneously, using ultrasound or CT guidance, or via an open incision.[38,41] Some patients will require placement of a drain to facilitate wound healing. Intravenous clindamycin is a good first-line choice for empiric treatment; vancomycin and/or a third-generation cephalosporin should be considered for patients with severe or life-threatening infections. There are not good data to guide the overall length of antibiotic therapy for pyomyositis; most patients will receive 2–6 weeks of total therapy, beginning with parenteral antibiotics and switching to oral antibiotics when inflammatory markers have reached near normal, fevers have abated, and clinical response has been adequate.[38] The typical total length of antibiotic therapy is 3 weeks.[42]

OTHER CONSIDERATIONS

Given the increasing prevalence of CA-MRSA and the fact that more than one in four children are persistently colonized by *S. aureus*, many have considered strategies for eradication of MRSA colonization to prevent future infections. To date, a Cochrane database systematic review has shown that there is insufficient evidence to recommend any treatment strategy for continued MRSA eradication.[98] Most randomized trials to investigate MRSA eradication have enrolled small numbers of adult patients and have had limited follow-up.[99,100] However, a randomized, controlled study from 2000 to 2003 comparing a 7-day course of 2% chlorhexidine gluconate daily washes, 2% mupirocin ointment applied to the anterior nares three times daily, rifampin (300 mg twice daily), and doxycycline (100 mg twice daily) compared to no treatment noted a 74% clearance rate of MRSA in the treatment group versus a 32% clearance rate in the no-treatment group at 3 months after treatment or randomization.[101] These results persisted for 8 months in 54% of patients in the treatment group. Intranasal mupirocin and a similar decolonization regimen with chlorhexidine gluconate or hexachlorophene washes (with and without oral antibiotics) have also been used to curtail nosocomial outbreaks and spread of MRSA in adult settings and in a neonatal intensive care unit.[102–104] The common USA300 genotype of CA-MRSA was sequenced in 2006 and identified a plasmid conferring resistance to mupirocin, however, so future decolonization regimens may need to be altered to prevent the emergence of mupirocin resistance.[105]

Though there are not data to support the ability of in-home decolonization regimens to create long-term and persistent MRSA eradication, many families that have experienced significant or recurrent MRSA infections are interested in attempting to decolonize the members of the family. One example of a possible regimen to suggest to families follows:

- Intranasal mupirocin three times a day, for 7 days.
- Showers with either 2% chlorhexidine gluconate or 3% hexachlorophene on days 1, 3, and 7 of the regimen, with special attention paid to the ears, neck, axillae, and groin.
- Wash and change towels and linens on days 1 and 7 of the regimen; towels and linens should not be shared among family members.

Oral rifampin or clindamycin is occasionally prescribed, though the added benefit of systemic therapy is unclear. This regimen is not ideal for patients younger than 3 months or patients with significant areas of skin breakdown.

REFERENCES

1. Sadow KB, Chamberlain JM. Blood cultures in the evaluation of children with cellulitis. *Pediatrics.* 1998;101:E4.
2. Mittal MK, Shah SS, Friedlaender EY. Group B streptococcal cellulitis in infancy. *Pediatr Emerg Care.* 2007; 23:324-325.
3. Campos J, Roman F, Perez-Vazquez M, Oteo J, Aracil B, Cercenado E. Infections due to *Haemophilus influenzae* serotype E: microbiological, clinical, and epidemiological features. *Clin Infect Dis.* 2003;37:841-845.
4. Fergie JE, Purcell K. Nocardiosis in South Texas children. *Pediatr Infect Dis J.* 2001;20:711-714.
5. Chadha R, Grover M, Sharma A, et al. An outbreak of post-surgical wound infections due to *Mycobacterium* abscessus. *Pediatr Surg Int.* 1998;13:406-410.
6. Milstone AM, Ruff AJ, Yeamans C, Higman MA. *Pseudomonas aeruginosa* pre-septal cellulitis and bacteremia in a pediatric oncology patient. *Pediatr Blood Cancer.* 2005;45:353; discussion 4.
7. Hsieh S, Babl FE. *Serratia marcescens* cellulitis following an iguana bite. *Clin Infect Dis.* 1999;28:1181-1182.

8. Brook I, Frazier EH. Aerobic and anaerobic bacteriology of wounds and cutaneous abscesses. *Arch Surg.* 1990; 125:1445-1451.
9. Brantley JS, Readinger AL, Morris ES. Cutaneous infection with *Mycobacterium* abscessus in a child. *Pediatr Dermatol.* 2006;23:128-131.
10. Steenhoff AP, Wood SM, Shah SS, Rutstein RM. Cutaneous *Mycobacterium avium* complex infection as a manifestation of the immune reconstitution syndrome in a human immunodeficiency virus-infected child. *Pediatr Infect Dis J.* 2007;26:755-757.
11. Gorak EJ, Yamada SM, Brown JD. Community-acquired methicillin-resistant *Staphylococcus aureus* in hospitalized adults and children without known risk factors. *Clin Infect Dis.* 1999;29:797-800.
12. Herold BC, Immergluck LC, Maranan MC, et al. Community-acquired methicillin-resistant *Staphylococcus aureus* in children with no identified predisposing risk. *JAMA.* 1998;279:593-598.
13. Sattler CA, Mason EO, Jr., Kaplan SL. Prospective comparison of risk factors and demographic and clinical characteristics of community-acquired, methicillin-resistant versus methicillin-susceptible *Staphylococcus aureus* infection in children. *Pediatr Infect Dis J.* 2002;21: 910-917.
14. Frank AL, Marcinak JF, Mangat PD, Schreckenberger PC. Community-acquired and clindamycin-susceptible methicillin-resistant *Staphylococcus aureus* in children. *Pediatr Infect Dis J.* 1999;18:993-1000.
15. Hussain FM, Boyle-Vavra S, Bethel CD, Daum RS. Current trends in community-acquired methicillin-resistant *Staphylococcus aureus* at a tertiary care pediatric facility. *Pediatr Infect Dis J.* 2000;19:1163-1166.
16. Fergie JE, Purcell K. Community-acquired methicillin-resistant *Staphylococcus aureus* infections in south Texas children. *Pediatr Infect Dis J.* 2001;20:860-863.
17. Purcell K, Fergie JE. Exponential increase in community-acquired methicillin-resistant *Staphylococcus aureus* infections in South Texas children. *Pediatr Infect Dis J.* 2002;21:988-989.
18. Purcell K, Fergie J. Epidemic of community-acquired methicillin-resistant *Staphylococcus aureus* infections: a 14-year study at Driscoll Children's Hospital. *Arch Pediatr Adolesc Med.* 2005;159:980-985.
19. Lindenmayer JM, Schoenfeld S, O'Grady R, Carney JK. Methicillin-resistant *Staphylococcus aureus* in a high school wrestling team and the surrounding community. *Arch Intern Med.* 1998;158:895-899.
20. Begier EM, Frenette K, Barrett NL, et al. A high-morbidity outbreak of methicillin-resistant *Staphylococcus aureus* among players on a college football team, facilitated by cosmetic body shaving and turf burns. *Clin Infect Dis.* 2004;39:1446-1453.
21. Stacey AR, Endersby KE, Chan PC, Marples RR. An outbreak of methicillin resistant *Staphylococcus aureus* infection in a rugby football team. *Br J Sports Med.* 1998;32:153-154.
22. Adcock PM, Pastor P, Medley F, Patterson JE, Murphy TV. Methicillin-resistant *Staphylococcus aureus* in two child care centers. *J Infect Dis.* 1998;178:577-580.
23. Shahin R, Johnson IL, Jamieson F, McGeer A, Tolkin J, Ford-Jones EL. Methicillin-resistant *Staphylococcus aureus* carriage in a child care center following a case of disease. Toronto Child Care Center Study Group. *Arch Pediatr Adolesc Med.* 1999;153:864-868.
24. Faden H, Ferguson S. Community-acquired methicillin-resistant *Staphylococcus aureus* and intrafamily spread of pustular disease. *Pediatr Infect Dis J.* 2001;20:554-555.
25. Huijsdens XW, van Santen-Verheuvel MG, Spalburg E, et al. Multiple cases of familial transmission of community-acquired methicillin-resistant *Staphylococcus aureus. J Clin Microbiol.* 2006;44:2994-2996.
26. Al-Tawfiq JA. Father-to-infant transmission of community-acquired methicillin-resistant *Staphylococcus aureus* in a neonatal intensive care unit. *Infect Control Hosp Epidemiol.* 2006;27:636-637.
27. Gastelum DT, Dassey D, Mascola L, Yasuda LM. Transmission of community-associated methicillin-resistant *Staphylococcus aureus* from breast milk in the neonatal intensive care unit. *Pediatr Infect Dis J.* 2005;24: 1122-1124.
28. Naimi TS, LeDell KH, Boxrud DJ, et al. Epidemiology and clonality of community-acquired methicillin-resistant *Staphylococcus aureus* in Minnesota, 1996-1998. *Clin Infect Dis.* 2001;33:990-996.
29. Alfaro C, Mascher-Denen M, Fergie J, Purcell K. Prevalence of methicillin-resistant *Staphylococcus aureus* nasal carriage in patients admitted to Driscoll Children's Hospital. *Pediatr Infect Dis J.* 2006;25:459-461.
30. Heininger U, Datta F, Gervaix A, et al. Prevalence of nasal colonization with methicillin-resistant *Staphylococcus aureus* (MRSA) in children a multicenter cross-sectional study. *Pediatr Infect Dis J.* 2007;26: 544-546.
31. Creech CB, II, Kernodle DS, Alsentzer A, Wilson C, Edwards KM. Increasing rates of nasal carriage of methicillin-resistant *Staphylococcus aureus* in healthy children. *Pediatr Infect Dis J.* 2005;24:617-621.
32. Groom AV, Wolsey DH, Naimi TS, et al. Community-acquired methicillin-resistant *Staphylococcus aureus* in a rural American Indian community. *JAMA.* 2001;286: 1201-1205.
33. Castrodale LJ, Beller M, Gessner BD. Over-representation of Samoan/Pacific Islanders among patients with methicillin-resistant *Staphylococcus aureus* (MRSA) infections at a large family practice clinic in Anchorage, Alaska, 1996-2000. *Alaska Med.* 2004;46:88-91.
34. Leyden JJ, Marples RR, Kligman AM. *Staphylococcus aureus* in the lesions of atopic dermatitis. *Br J Dermatol.* 1974;90:525-530.
35. Aly R, Maibach HI, Shinefield HR. Microbial flora of atopic dermatitis. *Arch Dermatol.* 1977;113:780-782.
36. Arkwright PD, Daniel TO, Sanyal D, David TJ, Patel L. Age-related prevalence and antibiotic resistance of pathogenic staphylococci and streptococci in children with infected atopic dermatitis at a single-specialty center. *Arch Dermatol.* 2002;138:939-941.
37. Fridkin SK, Hageman JC, Morrison M, et al. Methicillin-resistant *Staphylococcus aureus* disease in three communities. *N Engl J Med.* 2005;352:1436-1444.
38. Spiegel DA, Meyer JS, Dormans JP, Flynn JM, Drummond DS. Pyomyositis in children and adolescents: report of 12 cases and review of the literature. *J Pediatr Orthop.* 1999;19:143-150.

39. Jayoussi R, Bialik V, Eyal A, Shehadeh N, Etzioni A. Pyomyositis caused by vigorous exercise in a boy. *Acta Paediatr.* 1995;84:226-227.
40. Meehan J, Grose C, Soper RT, Kimura K. Pyomyositis in an adolescent female athlete. *J Pediatr Surg.* 1995;30:127-128.
41. Gubbay AJ, Isaacs D. Pyomyositis in children. *Pediatr Infect Dis J.* 2000;19:1009-1012; quiz 13.
42. Pannaraj PS, Hulten KG, Gonzalez BE, Mason EO, Jr, Kaplan SL. Infective pyomyositis and myositis in children in the era of community-acquired, methicillin-resistant *Staphylococcus aureus* infection. *Clin Infect Dis.* 2006;43:953-960.
43. Brook I. Pyomyositis in children, caused by anaerobic bacteria. *J Pediatr Surg.* 1996;31:394-396.
44. Sharieff GQ, Lee DM, Anshus JS. A rare case of Salmonella-mediated sacroiliitis, adjacent subperiosteal abscess, and myositis. *Pediatr Emerg Care.* 2003;19:252-254.
45. Pong A, Chartrand SA, Huurman W. Pyomyositis and septic arthritis caused by group C Streptococcus. *Pediatr Infect Dis J.* 1998;17:1052-1054.
46. Rajapakse CD, Shingadia D. Tuberculous pyomyositis of the left quadratus lumborum. *Arch Dis Child.* 2006; 91:512.
47. Widrow CA, Kellie SM, Saltzman BR, Mathur-Wagh U. Pyomyositis in patients with the human immunodeficiency virus: an unusual form of disseminated bacterial infection. *Am J Med.* 1991;91:129-136.
48. Kluytmans J, van Belkum A, Verbrugh H. Nasal carriage of *Staphylococcus aureus*: Epidemiology, underlying mechanisms, and associated risks. *Clin Microbiol Rev.* 1997;10:505-520.
49. Peacock SJ, de Silva I, Lowy FD. What determines nasal carriage of *Staphylococcus aureus*? *Trends Microbiol.* 2001;9:605-610.
50. Jain A, Daum RS. Staphylococcal infections in children: Part 1. *Pediatr Rev.* 1999;20:183-191.
51. Wenzel RP, Perl TM. The significance of nasal carriage of *Staphylococcus aureus* and the incidence of postoperative wound infection. *J Hosp Infect.* 1995;31:13-24.
52. Yu VL, Goetz A, Wagener M, et al. *Staphylococcus aureus* nasal carriage and infection in patients on hemodialysis. Efficacy of antibiotic prophylaxis. *N Engl J Med.* 1986; 315:91-96.
53. Lubbe J. Secondary infections in patients with atopic dermatitis. *Am J Clin Dermatol.* 2003;4:641-654.
54. Wagner DK, Sohnle PG. Cutaneous defenses against dermatophytes and yeasts. *Clin Microbiol Rev.* 1995;8:317-335.
55. Miller SJ, Aly R, Shinefeld HR, Elias PM. In vitro and in vivo antistaphylococcal activity of human stratum corneum lipids. *Arch Dermatol.* 1988;124:209-215.
56. Tristan A, Ferry T, Durand G, et al. Virulence determinants in community and hospital meticillin-resistant *Staphylococcus aureus*. *J Hosp Infect.* 2007;65 (suppl 2):105-109.
57. Lina G, Piemont Y, Godail-Gamot F, et al. Involvement of Panton–Valentine leukocidin-producing *Staphylococcus aureus* in primary skin infections and pneumonia. *Clin Infect Dis.* 1999;29:1128-1132.
58. Moran GJ, Krishnadasan A, Gorwitz RJ, et al. Methicillin-resistant *S. aureus* infections among patients in the emergency department. *N Engl J Med.* 2006;355:666-674.
59. Frazee BW, Lynn J, Charlebois ED, Lambert L, Lowery D, Perdreau-Remington F. High prevalence of methicillin-resistant *Staphylococcus aureus* in emergency department skin and soft tissue infections. *Ann Emerg Med.* 2005;45:311-320.
60. Mishaan AM, Mason EO, Jr., Martinez-Aguilar G, et al. Emergence of a predominant clone of community-acquired *Staphylococcus aureus* among children in Houston, Texas. *Pediatr Infect Dis J.* 2005;24:201-206.
61. Chavez-Bueno S, Bozdogan B, Katz K, et al. Inducible clindamycin resistance and molecular epidemiologic trends of pediatric community-acquired methicillin-resistant *Staphylococcus aureus* in Dallas, Texas. *Antimicrob Agents Chemother.* 2005;49:2283-2288.
62. Kazakova SV, Hageman JC, Matava M, et al. A clone of methicillin-resistant *Staphylococcus aureus* among professional football players. *N Engl J Med.* 2005;352: 468-475.
63. McDougal LK, Steward CD, Killgore GE, Chaitram JM, McAllister SK, Tenover FC. Pulsed-field gel electrophoresis typing of oxacillin-resistant *Staphylococcus aureus* isolates from the United States: establishing a national database. *J Clin Microbiol.* 2003;41:5113-5120.
64. Brogan TV, Nizet V, Waldhausen JH, Rubens CE, Clarke WR. Group A streptococcal necrotizing fasciitis complicating primary varicella: a series of fourteen patients. *Pediatr Infect Dis J.* 1995;14:588-594.
65. Vugia DJ, Peterson CL, Meyers HB, et al. Invasive group A streptococcal infections in children with varicella in Southern California. *Pediatr Infect Dis J.* 1996;15:146-150.
66. Talkington DF, Schwartz B, Black CM, et al. Association of phenotypic and genotypic characteristics of invasive Streptococcus pyogenes isolates with clinical components of streptococcal toxic shock syndrome. *Infect Immun.* 1993;61:3369-3374.
67. Chiedozi LC. Pyomyositis. Review of 205 cases in 112 patients. *Am J Surg.* 1979;137:255-259.
68. Eneli I, Davies HD. Epidemiology and outcome of necrotizing fasciitis in children: an active surveillance study of the Canadian Paediatric Surveillance Program. *J Pediatr.* 2007;151:79-84,e1.
69. Zerr DM, Alexander ER, Duchin JS, Koutsky LA, Rubens CE. A case–control study of necrotizing fasciitis during primary varicella. *Pediatrics.* 1999;103:783-790.
70. Howe PM, Eduardo Fajardo J, Orcutt MA. Etiologic diagnosis of cellulitis: comparison of aspirates obtained from the leading edge and the point of maximal inflammation. *Pediatr Infect Dis J.* 1987;6:685-686.
71. Newell PM, Norden CW. Value of needle aspiration in bacteriologic diagnosis of cellulitis in adults. *J Clin Microbiol.* 1988;26:401-404.
72. Sigurdsson AF, Gudmundsson S. The etiology of bacterial cellulitis as determined by fine-needle aspiration. *Scand J Infect Dis.* 1989;21:537-542.
73. Swartz MN. Clinical practice. Cellulitis. *N Engl J Med.* 2004;350:904-912.
74. Albanyan EA, Baker CJ. Is lumbar puncture necessary to exclude meningitis in neonates and young infants: lessons from the group B streptococcus cellulitis–adenitis syndrome. *Pediatrics.* 1998;102:985-986.
75. Bisno AL, Stevens DL. Streptococcal infections of skin and soft tissues. *N Engl J Med.* 1996;334:240-245.
76. Bhattacharya D, Carleton H, Tsai CJ, Baron EJ, Perdreau-Remington F. Differences in clinical and molecular

characteristics of skin and soft tissue methicillin-resistant *Staphylococcus aureus* isolates between two hospitals in Northern California. *J Clin Microbiol.* 2007;45:1798-1803.

77. LaPlante KL, Rybak MJ, Amjad M, Kaatz GW. Antimicrobial susceptibility and staphylococcal chromosomal cassette mec type in community- and hospital-associated methicillin-resistant *Staphylococcus aureus. Pharmacotherapy.* 2007;27:3-10.
78. Panagea S, Perry JD, Gould FK. Should clindamycin be used as treatment of patients with infections caused by erythromycin-resistant staphylococci? *J Antimicrob Chemother.* 1999;44:581-582.
79. Zaoutis TE, Toltzis P, Chu J, et al. Clinical and molecular epidemiology of community-acquired methicillin-resistant *Staphylococcus aureus* infections among children with risk factors for health care-associated infection: 2001-2003. *Pediatr Infect Dis J.* 2006;25:343-348.
80. Braun L, Craft D, Williams R, Tuamokumo F, Ottolini M. Increasing clindamycin resistance among methicillin-resistant *Staphylococcus aureus* in 57 northeast United States military treatment facilities. *Pediatr Infect Dis J.* 2005;24:622-626.
81. Siberry GK, Tekle T, Carroll K, Dick J. Failure of clindamycin treatment of methicillin-resistant *Staphylococcus aureus* expressing inducible clindamycin resistance in vitro. *Clin Infect Dis.* 2003;37:1257-1260.
82. Patel M, Waites KB, Moser SA, Cloud GA, Hoesley CJ. Prevalence of inducible clindamycin resistance among community- and hospital-associated *Staphylococcus aureus* isolates. *J Clin Microbiol.* 2006;44:2481-2484.
83. Leclercq R. Mechanisms of resistance to macrolides and lincosamides: nature of the resistance elements and their clinical implications. *Clin Infect Dis.* 2002;34:482-492.
84. Rao GG. Should clindamycin be used in treatment of patients with infections caused by erythromycin-resistant staphylococci? *J Antimicrob Chemother.* 2000;45:715.
85. Drinkovic D, Fuller ER, Shore KP, Holland DJ, Ellis-Pegler R. Clindamycin treatment of *Staphylococcus aureus* expressing inducible clindamycin resistance. *J Antimicrob Chemother.* 2001;48:315-316.
86. Gordon BA, Martinez S, Collins AJ. Pyomyositis: characteristics at CT and MR imaging. *Radiology.* 1995;197:279-286.
87. Soler R, Rodriguez E, Aguilera C, Fernandez R. Magnetic resonance imaging of pyomyositis in 43 cases. *Eur J Radiol.* 2000;35:59-64.
88. Chau CL, Griffith JF. Musculoskeletal infections: Ultrasound appearances. *Clin Radiol.* 2005;60:149-159.
89. Trusen A, Beissert M, Schultz G, Chittka B, Darge K. Ultrasound and MRI features of pyomyositis in children. *Eur Radiol.* 2003;13:1050-1055.
90. Pankuch GA, Lin G, Hoellman DB, Good CE, Jacobs MR, Appelbaum PC. Activity of retapamulin against *Streptococcus pyogenes* and *Staphylococcus aureus* evaluated by agar dilution, microdilution, E-test, and disk diffusion methodologies. *Antimicrob Agents Chemother.* 2006;50:1727-1730.
91. Kelly CP, Pothoulakis C, LaMont JT. *Clostridium difficile* colitis. *N Engl J Med.* 1994;330:257-262.
92. Bigby M, Jick S, Jick H, Arndt K. Drug-induced cutaneous reactions. A report from the Boston Collaborative Drug Surveillance Program on 15,438 consecutive inpatients, 1975 to 1982. *JAMA.* 1986;256:3358-3363.
93. Ruhe JJ, Monson T, Bradsher RW, Menon A. Use of long-acting tetracyclines for methicillin-resistant *Staphylococcus aureus* infections: Case series and review of the literature. *Clin Infect Dis.* 2005;40:1429-1434.
94. Critchley IA, Sahm DF, Thornsberry C, Blosser-Middleton RS, Jones ME, Karlowsky JA. Antimicrobial susceptibilities of *Streptococcus pyogenes* isolated from respiratory and skin and soft tissue infections: United States LIBRA surveillance data from 1999. *Diagn Microbiol Infect Dis.* 2002;42:129-135.
95. From the Centers for Disease Control and Prevention. Four pediatric deaths from community-acquired methicillin-resistant *Staphylococcus aureus*—Minnesota and North Dakota, 1997-1999. *JAMA.* 1999;282:1123-1125.
96. Daum RS. Clinical practice. Skin and soft-tissue infections caused by methicillin-resistant *Staphylococcus aureus. N Engl J Med.* 2007;357:380-390.
97. Lee MC, Rios AM, Aten MF, et al. Management and outcome of children with skin and soft tissue abscesses caused by community-acquired methicillin-resistant *Staphylococcus aureus. Pediatr Infect Dis J.* 2004;23:123-127.
98. Loeb M, Main C, Walker-Dilks C, Eady A. Antimicrobial drugs for treating methicillin-resistant *Staphylococcus aureus* colonization. *Cochrane Database Syst Rev.* 2003;CD003340.
99. Harbarth S, Dharan S, Liassine N, Herrault P, Auckenthaler R, Pittet D. Randomized, placebo-controlled, double-blind trial to evaluate the efficacy of mupirocin for eradicating carriage of methicillin-resistant Staphylococcus aureus. *Antimicrob Agents Chemother.* 1999;43:1412-1416.
100. Chang SC, Hsieh SM, Chen ML, Sheng WH, Chen YC. Oral fusidic acid fails to eradicate methicillin-resistant Staphylococcus aureus colonization and results in emergence of fusidic acid-resistant strains. *Diagn Microbiol Infect Dis.* 2000;36:131-136.
101. Simor AE, Phillips E, McGeer A, et al. Randomized controlled trial of chlorhexidine gluconate for washing, intranasal mupirocin, and rifampin and doxycycline versus no treatment for the eradication of methicillin-resistant Staphylococcus aureus colonization. *Clin Infect Dis.* 2007;44:178-185.
102. Hill RL, Duckworth GJ, Casewell MW. Elimination of nasal carriage of methicillin-resistant *Staphylococcus aureus* with mupirocin during a hospital outbreak. *J Antimicrob Chemother.* 1988;22:377-384.
103. Tomic V, Svetina Sorli P, Trinkaus D, Sorli J, Widmer AF, Trampuz A. Comprehensive strategy to prevent nosocomial spread of methicillin-resistant *Staphylococcus aureus* in a highly endemic setting. *Arch Intern Med.* 2004;164:2038-2043.
104. Khoury J, Jones M, Grim A, Dunne WM, Jr., Fraser V. Eradication of methicillin-resistant *Staphylococcus aureus* from a neonatal intensive care unit by active surveillance and aggressive infection control measures. *Infect Control Hosp Epidemiol.* 2005;26:616-621.
105. Diep BA, Gill SR, Chang RF, et al. Complete genome sequence of USA300, an epidemic clone of community-acquired methicillin-resistant *Staphylococcus aureus. Lancet.* 2006;367:731-739.

CHAPTER 46

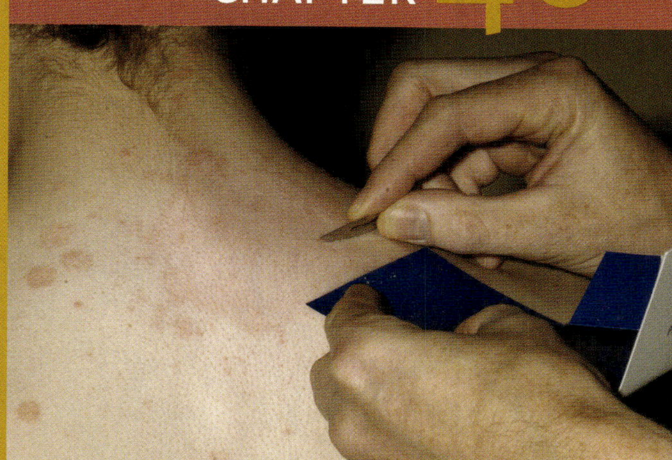

Bite Wound Infections

Toni Gross and Jill M. Baren

DEFINITIONS AND EPIDEMIOLOGY

This chapter focuses on the clinical evaluation and management of wounds caused by bites from a variety of species, predominantly mammals. Treatment of infected bite wounds, as well as prophylaxis of selected uninfected bite wounds, will be covered.

Animal bites occur frequently in the United States, accounting for at least 1% of all visits to hospital emergency departments each year.[1,2] Approximately, 80% of all bite wounds are minor in nature and do not require medical attention.[3] Five to ten percent of bite wounds warrant suturing, and 2% require hospital admission. The overall morbidity of bite wounds, however, includes infectious complications, cosmetic complications, disability, psychological trauma, and medical expenses. Annual health care expenditure for the treatment of bite wounds is estimated to be between $30 million and $100 million.[2–4]

It is widely accepted that bite wounds are more common in children, especially those of age 5–9 years, and are more common in boys. School-aged children comprise 30–50% of all mammalian bite victims, while accounting for only 15% of the population.[5] The number of reported bite wounds grossly underestimates the actual number of bites that occur each year. A survey of children aged 4–18 years revealed that 45% had been bitten by a dog during their lifetime, despite annual reported bite rates of 0.5% for children 5–14 years of age.[6]

The vast majority of mammalian bite wounds (80–90%) are inflicted by dogs. In 1994, an estimated 4.7 million dog bites occurred in the United States, necessitating close to 800,000 medical visits.[7] Cat bites are second in frequency (5–10%) with an estimated 400,000 per year,[8] followed by human bites (2–3% of mammalian bites). More than 70% of bites are caused by the victim's own pet or an animal known to them.[2]

Wounds caused by bites, or through accidental contact with teeth or fangs, can cause different types of tissue injury, most commonly abrasions and lacerations. Bite wounds that result in medical attention also include punctures, avulsion of soft tissue, crushing of tissue, fractures, and violation of normally sterile sites, such as joint spaces. The amount of pressure generated by dog bites is likely to produce localized crush injuries, with devitalized tissue that is prone to infection. Sixty percent of dog bite wounds are punctures, 10% are lacerations, and 30% are a combination of both. In contrast, 85% of cat bite wounds are punctures, 3% are lacerations, and 12% are a combination of both.[9] Puncture wounds are harder to cleanse and irrigate, and thus have a high infection rate. Human bites are equally likely to produce lacerations, punctures, or a combination of both.[10]

Most mammalian bite wounds occur on the extremities, especially the hands and arms.[1,7] In children younger than 5 years, a larger proportion (50–70%) of bite injuries occur to the face and head, especially those caused by dogs.[1,11] This is because of the child's small stature, disproportionate head size relative to the body size, willingness to bring the face close to the animal, and a lack of motor skills to protect themselves.[12] The middle third of the face, comprising the lips, nose, and cheeks, has been referred to as the "central target area."[13] Human bite wounds occur predominantly on the hands (86%). Approximately half of these are clenched-fist injuries, caused by the patient's hand forcefully striking another individual in the mouth. Fourteen percent of human bite wounds involve deep structures (e.g., tendons, muscles, and nerves), likely accounted for by the predominance of wounds to the hands.[10]

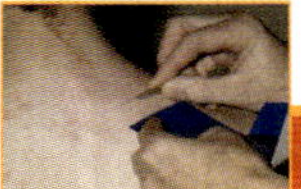

Table 46–1.

Infection Rate by Source of Bite and Wound Site

Factor	Infection Rate 9(%)
Source of bite	
Dog	3–18
Cat	~50
Human	10–50
Rodent	2–10
Wound Site	
Head/neck	2–12
Hand	9–30
Arm	2–27
Trunk	0
Lower extremity	4–18

Sequelae of bite wounds include scarring, disability, and infection. Ten to twenty deaths per year are caused by dog bites.[14] The potential for untoward sequelae directly correlates with delay in appropriate medical attention and improper wound care.[15,16] Infection complicates approximately 16% of mammalian bite wounds, with individual studies reporting rates as low as 3% and as high as 67%.[2,4,11,17–32] The incidence of infection is highest for cat bites (~50%), followed by human bites (15–50%), and dog bites (3–18%).[7,9,13] Infection rates for wounds exposed to seawater are higher than those for terrestrial wounds.[33] Facial and head wounds, even when closed primarily, have the lowest infection rates.[34] Hand wounds have the highest infection rate[2,16,19,21,23,24,29,30] (Table 46–1). A retrospective review of 322 pediatric patients with human bite wounds showed an infection rate of 9.3%. Bite wounds resulting in abrasions rather than lacerations did not become infected.[22]

Most bite wound infections are polymicrobial. The median number of microorganisms isolated from infected mammalian bite wounds is four to five. *Pasteurella* spp. are the most common isolates from both dog (50%) and cat (75%) bites.[9] *Streptococcus* spp., *Staphylococcus* spp., *Moraxella* spp., and *Neisseria* spp. are common aerobic pathogens in dog and cat bite infections. Anaerobes are found in 30–40% of dog bite wound infections.[35] Anaerobic organisms most frequently isolated from dog and cat bite infections are *Bacteroides* spp., *Fusobacterium* spp., *Peptostreptococcus* spp., *Prevotella* spp., *Porphyromonas gingivalis*, and *Capnocytophaga canimorsus*[35] (Table 46–2). Infected human bite wounds are most likely to contain *Streptococcus* spp. and *Staphylococcus* spp. *Eikenella corrodens*, a facultative anaerobe, is the third most frequent isolate. Common anaerobic pathogens in human bite wound infections include *Prevotella* spp., *Fusobacterium* spp., *Veillonella* spp., and *Peptostreptococcus* spp.[10] (Table 46–3).

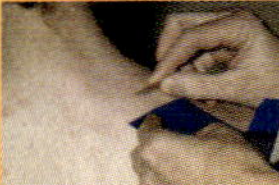

Table 46–2.

Predominant Microorganisms Isolated from Infected Dog and Cat Bite Injuries

Aerobes	Dog Bite (%)	Cat Bite (%)
Pasteurella	50	75
P. canis	26	2
P. multocida		
P. multocida	12	54
P. septica	10	28
P. gallicida	2	0
Streptococcus	46	46
S. mitis	22	23
S. mutans	12	11
S. pyogenes	12	0
S. sanguis II	8	12
Staphylococcus	46	35
S. aureus	20	4
S. epidermidis	18	18
Neisseria	16	19
Moraxella	10	35
Anaerobes		
Fusobacterium	32	33
Bacteroides	30	28
Porphyromonas	28	30
Prevotella	28	19

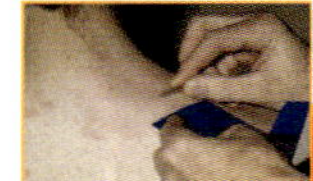

Table 46–3.

Predominant Microorganisms Isolated from Infected Human Bite Injuries

Aerobes	
Streptococcus	84%
S. anginosus	52%
S. pyogenes	14%
Staphylococcus	54%
S. aureus	30%
S. epidermidis	22%
E. corrodens	30%
Haemophilus	22%
Corynebacterium	12%
Gemella	12%
Anaerobes	
Prevotella	36%
Fusobacterium	34%
Veillonella species	24%
Peptostreptococcus	22%
Campylobacter	16%
Eubacterium	16%

Aquatic environments harbor large numbers of bacteria. *Vibrio* spp. are the most prevalent. Other microorganisms include *Aeromonas hydrophila*, *Plesiomonas* spp., *Mycobacterium marinum*, and *Erysipelothrix rhusiopathiae*. The most common pathogens in bite wound infections occurring in the aquatic environment, however, remain *Staphylococcus aureus* and *Streptococcus pyogenes*, representing the individual's skin flora.

PATHOGENESIS

All bite wounds should be considered contaminated with bacteria. In general, the microorganisms that inoculate bite wounds are the bacteria present either in the oral cavity of the biting animal, on the skin of the victim, or in the environment where the bite occurred (e.g., aquatic vs. terrestrial environment). Pathogens in or on the wound may cause local infection via direct inoculation.

Other potential complications include osteomyelitis, septic arthritis, tenosynovitis, local abscesses, and more rarely, endocarditis, meningitis, brain abscess, and sepsis. Asplenic patients are particularly susceptible to septic complications caused by *C. canimorsus* infection following dog bites.[36] Reported cases of intracranial abscesses have followed animal bites, including bird pecking, to the head.

The risk of infection is greatest for crush injuries, puncture wounds, and wounds to the hand[8] (Table 46–4). Crush injuries cause tissue devitalization, hindering wound healing. Puncture wounds prove to be problematic because they are difficult to adequately cleanse, irrigate, and debride. Puncture wounds have been shown to become infected 1.5–3 times as often as lacerations.[30] The increased propensity for cats to cause puncture wounds likely accounts for the increased rate of infection of cat bites compared to other mammalian bites. The hand's closed anatomic compartments and close proximity of bones and joint cavities to the skin surface cause decreased resistance to infection. Dog bites to the hand are approximately three times more likely to become infected than those elsewhere in the body.[37] The increased infection rate reported for human bites is at least partially accounted for by the increased likelihood for human bites to occur on the hands.

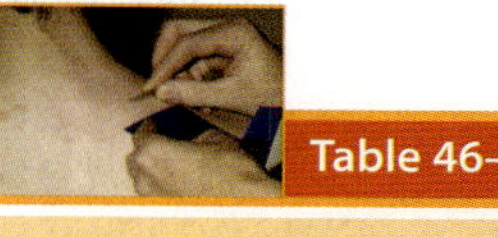

Table 46–4.

Infection Rate by Wound Type and Delay in Treatment

Factor	Infection Rate (%)
Type of Wound	
Abrasion	0–4
Laceration	6–15
Puncture	17–22
Avulsion	0–10
Treatment Delay	
8 h	1
>24 h	6–66

Wound infections associated with dog and cat bites are abscesses in 16%, purulent open wounds in 48%, and nonpurulent cellulitis, lymphangitis, or both in 36%.[9] Wound infections associated with human bites are abscesses in 48%, purulent wounds in 46%, and nonpurulent cellulitis, lymphangitis, or both in 6%[10] (Figure 46–1).

Clinical Presentation

Victims of bite wounds can be divided into two categories: those that present within 8–12 hours of the injury, and those that seek attention more than 12 hours after the incident. The former group usually does not have evidence of infection, but are seeking medical care secondary to concerns for rabies and other infections or disfigurement. The latter group more often presents with signs and symptoms of infection.[13]

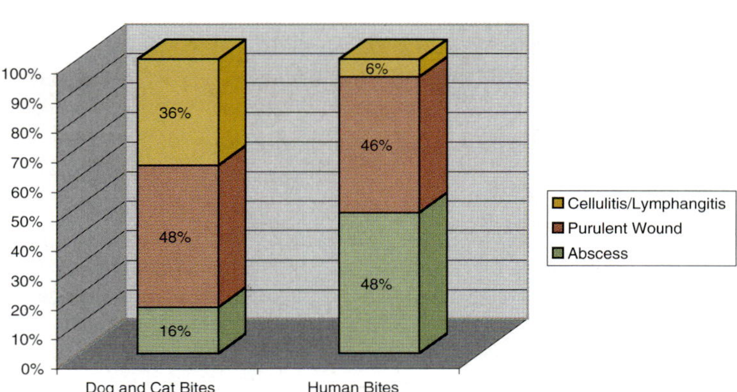

FIGURE 46–1 ■ Types of bite wound infections.

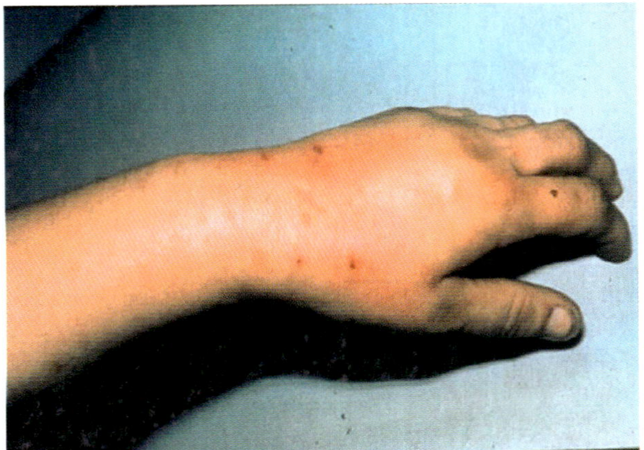

FIGURE 46–2 ■ Cellulitis caused by cat bite.

It is important to distinguish a contaminated but uninfected bite wound from a bite wound infection. Uninfected bite wounds may show a normal inflammatory response of swelling and mild redness, without the frank erythema and warmth of infection. One small series showed that wound site swelling without other signs of infection was present 2–3 days after the bite in 9% of patients.[28] The radius of hyperemia surrounding an uninfected wound should not exceed 2 mm.[4] Infected bite wounds may present several ways. Wounds may show cellulitis (erythema, warmth, pain), swelling, induration, lymphangitis, adenopathy, frank abscess formation, or purulent discharge (Figure 46–2). Fever is present in less than 10% of patients.[37]

The latency period between injury and first symptoms of infection varies depending on the source of the bite. The median time to first symptoms is shorter for cat bites (12 hours) than for human bites (22 hours) or dog bites (24 hours).[9,10] *Pasteurella* is known for causing a rapidly developing infection.

Bites that occur in the aquatic environment have characteristic appearances, depending upon the infecting agent. Wounds infected by *Vibrio* spp. present as vesicles with surrounding edema and erythema that rapidly develop into hemorrhagic bullae. Wounds infected with *Aeromonas* present similarly to staphylococcal cellulitis, but can develop bullae with purulent discharge. Fever and regional lymphadenopathy are associated signs. The lesions are very painful. If inadequately treated, gas within the soft tissues, necrotizing fasciitis, or osteomyelitis can develop. *E. rhusiopathiae*, seen often in fish-handlers, causes erysipeloid, a self-limited illness that presents as pain or pruritis at the wound site, and a characteristic ring-shaped lesion with a sharply demarcated purplish–red border.

Differential Diagnosis

Differentiating an infected wound from an uninfected wound is an important first step. The practitioner should then evaluate the extent of injury diligently, including a thorough examination of the affected area, testing of nerve and tendon function, roentograms and laboratory studies as indicated, and consultation with a specialist when warranted. For hand wounds, if there is pain with active or passive motion, a more serious infection of deep structures should be suspected.

Rapid onset of symptoms from the time of bite (<12 hours) is associated with *Pasteurella multocida* infection. *Pasteurella* spp. are common in both nonpurulent infections and abscesses. *Staphylococci* and *streptococci* have been isolated more frequently from nonpurulent infections, although both are seen commonly in abscesses.[9,10] Anaerobic organisms are more commonly associated with abscesses than other types of infections in mammalian bites. *E. corrodens* is also more frequently associated with abscesses. Abscesses associated with human bite wounds are likely to be associated with *Streptococcus* (83%), *Staphylococcus* (54%), *Eikenella* (42%), *Fusobacterium* (42%), and *Prevotella* (42%).[10]

Diagnosis

Physical examination should determine the status of a bite wound as infected or uninfected. Diagnostic criteria are shown in Table 46–5. A wound should be considered infected if it meets one of three major criteria or four of five minor criteria.[9,10]

Uninfected bite wounds should not be cultured, as Gram stain and culture have not been shown to reliably predict which wounds will become infected and which organisms will be pathologically responsible.[29,38] If infected wounds are cultured, a Gram stain and cultures for aerobic and anaerobic bacteria should be sent. The recommended method for obtaining wound culture is closed-needle aspiration for abscesses and standard swabs of the base of open lacerations. Puncture wounds large enough for insertion of a swab may be cultured after cleansing the edges of the wound with a povidone–iodine solution. Practitioners should be mindful that most routine laboratories will not employ techniques adequate for

Table 46–5.

Wound Infection Diagnostic Criteria

One of Three Major Criteria	or	Four of Five Minor Criteria
Fever		Erythema extending >3 cm from the wound edge
Abscess		Tenderness
Lymphangitis		Swelling
		Purulent drainage
		Peripheral white blood cell count >12,000 cells/mm[3]

isolation of all pathogenic organisms from bite wounds. For this reason, negative cultures do not exclude infection being present in a wound. Cultures instead should be used to expand coverage for organisms recovered in culture that are not adequately covered by empiric antibiotic therapy. Some authors recommend reserving cultures for wounds showing mixed organisms on Gram stain or in cases not responding to previous antibiotic treatment.[29]

Management

Adequate cleansing of the wound, along with prevention of tetanus and rabies, are universally accepted measures for the management of uninfected bite wounds. The use of prophylactic antibiotics and wound closure are controversial. An algorithm for the management of bite wounds is presented in Figure 46–3.

GENERAL MEASURES

All wounds, even if apparently minor, deserve careful exploration to evaluate for underlying fractures, lacerated tendons or nerves, or penetration of joint spaces. All of these deeper injuries may likely require hospitalization or surgical repair. Hand bites in particular require very careful exploration. Any wound overlying a joint capsule or tendon, with suspected violation of either, necessitates consultation with a hand surgeon. Roentograms may be helpful in delineating the extent of injury and excluding the presence of a foreign body. (Figure 46–4) Consider ordering an X-ray when a fracture is possible, when a foreign body may be present, when the bone or joint may have been penetrated, or when infection is documented in proximity to a bone or joint. Once serious injury is ruled out, the practitioner should evaluate the wound for possible functional and cosmetic consequences, and the likelihood of local or systemic infectious complications. Documentation should include a diagram of the location and extent of injuries, the presence or absence of swelling or devitalized tissue, range of motion, status of nerve and tendon function, and presence or absence of signs of infection, including regional adenopathy.

The history should include the circumstances of injury (whether the animal was provoked or not), as well as ownership of the animal. It is important to note the patient's allergies, current medications, and immunization status. Underlying medical conditions, such as diabetes, steroid use, or other immune-modulating disorders should be noted. Consultation with local public health authorities may be necessary for rabies prophylaxis recommendations and reporting of animal bites.

Wound irrigation and careful debridement significantly reduces the incidence of infection.[29] All lacerations should be irrigated using high pressure, by using a 20-mL syringe attached to an 18- or 20-gauge intravenous catheter. A minimum of 250 mL of sterile saline should be used for irrigation of the wound, but an increased volume is often necessary. Puncture wounds are more difficult to irrigate, and should be done with careful consideration to prevent subcutaneous tissue damage caused by high-pressure irrigation. Eschars should be removed in order to eliminate all contamination from the wound. Necrotic skin tags and devitalized tissue should be sharply debrided, with careful consideration of the resultant wound edges and their approximation. Puncture wounds should not be debrided. Any foreign material should be removed from the wound during irrigation and debridement.[8] In the pediatric patient, the practitioner should strongly consider sedation, anxiolysis, and analgesia, in consultation with a specialist if warranted, to facilitate complete irrigation, debridement, and potential wound repair.

Bite wounds should be immobilized, especially if located in an area of significant movement, like the hand. Patients should be instructed to keep the wounded extremity elevated. Hand and wrist wounds should be treated with a splint and sling. Lower extremity wounds should be treated with bed rest. Immobilization and elevation should be continued for several days.[8]

POSTEXPOSURE PROPHYLAXIS OF TETANUS AND RABIES

Patients who have not completed the primary series of tetanus immunization (<three doses) should receive tetanus toxoid and tetanus immunoglobulin. Patients who have completed the primary series, but have not had a booster within the last 5 years should receive tetanus toxoid[39] (Table 46–6). It is recommended that adolescents and adults receive tetanus toxoid as the newer Tdap vaccine. Rabies prophylaxis should be given to patients who are bitten by dogs, cats, or ferrets known or suspected to be rabid; and to patients bitten by bats, skunks, raccoons, foxes, and woodchucks caused by the high incidence of rabies in these species. Public health officials should be consulted for bites caused by livestock, rodents, lagomorphs (rabbits, hares, pikas), and escaped dogs, cats, and ferrets[40] (Table 46–7).

WOUND CLOSURE

Wound closure is especially important for improved cosmetic outcomes, especially in large gaping lacerations or bites to prominent sites, such as the face (Figure 46–5). A prospective evaluation of 145 patients with mammalian bite wounds presenting to an emergency department within 0–7 hours of injury, all treated with skin sutures, showed an infection rate of 5.5%. In comparison, reported infection rates for

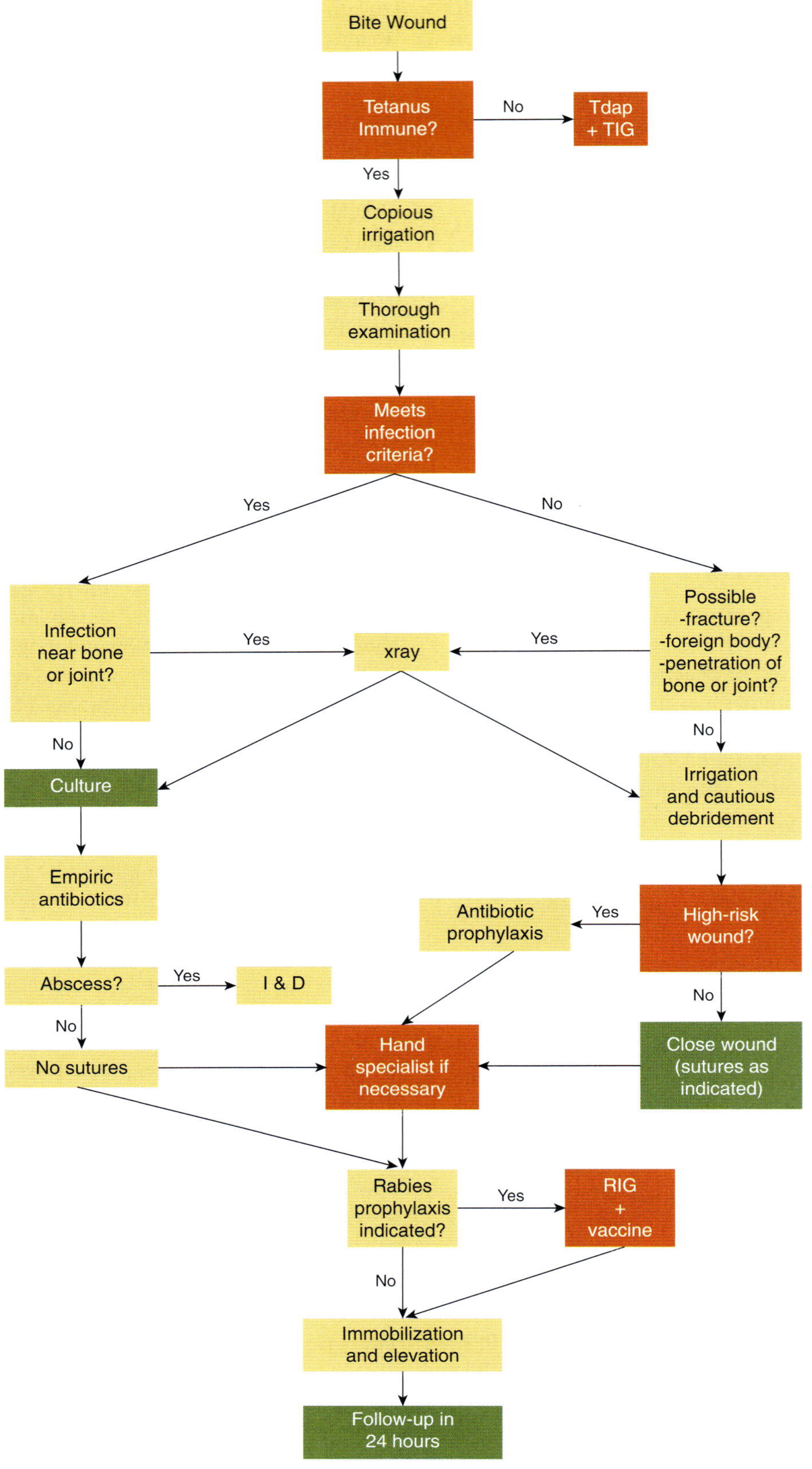

FIGURE 46–3 ■ Algorithm for management of bite wound.

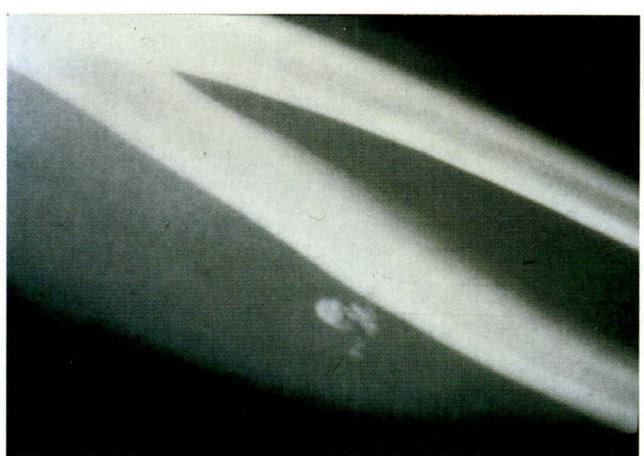

FIGURE 46–4 ■ Subcutaneous foreign body following dog bite.

Table 46–6.

Guide to Tetanus Prophylaxis

History of Absorbed Tetanus Toxoid (Doses)	Tdap	TIG
<3 or unknown	Yes	Yes
≥3 (last dose <5 years ago)	No	No
≥3 (last dose ≥5 years ago)	Yes	No

Adapted from Red Book 2006.

sutured nonbite wounds range from 3% to 7%.[34] A prospective study of 759 dog bite wounds, exclusive of hand, foot, and puncture wounds, found no statistically significant difference in the infection rate between wounds that were sutured and those that were not.[14] A smaller study of dog bite wounds, comparing those treated with sutures to those left to heal by secondary intention, showed an overall infection rate of 7.7%, with no significant difference between the treatment groups. None of these patients received prophylactic antibiotics, and a significant proportion of infected wounds were on the hands.[21]

Bite wounds that pose a risk for poor cosmesis should be sutured after thorough irrigation and debridement. Wounds seen more than 24 hours after injury should *not* be sutured. Because foreign bodies may serve as an additional risk for infection, deep layer sutures should be avoided. Hand wounds should be evaluated by a specialist before deciding to close with skin sutures. In the absence of an available specialist, hand wounds are best left to heal by secondary intention.

PROPHYLACTIC ANTIBIOTICS

Several studies have attempted to elucidate the role of prophylactic antibiotics, but have suffered from small numbers of enrolled patients and a low incidence of infection. In a recent Cochrane Collaboration review of antibiotic prophylaxis for mammalian bites, analysis of eight randomized controlled trials showed no statistically significant reduction in the infection rate of mammalian bite wounds after administration of prophylactic antibiotics.[2] These results are to be interpreted cautiously, because of the small number of patients and heterogeneity of studies. When human bites and hand bites were analyzed independently, infection rates for patients treated with prophylactic antibiotics were

Table 46–7.

Guide to Rabies Prophylaxis

Animal Type	Evaluation and Disposition of Animal	Postexposure Prophylaxis Recommendations
Dogs, cats, and ferrets	Healthy and available for 10 days of observation	Prophylaxis only if animal develops signs of rabies
	Rabid or suspected of being rabid	Immediate immunization and rabies immune globulin
	Unknown (escaped)	Consult public health officials
Bats, skunks, raccoons, foxes, and most other carnivores; woodchucks	Regarded as rabid unless geographic area is known to be free of rabies or until animal proven negative by laboratory tests	Immediate immunization and rabies immune globulin
Livestock, rodents, and lagomorphs (rabbits, hares, and pikas)	Consider individually	Consult public health officials

Adapted from Red Book 2006.

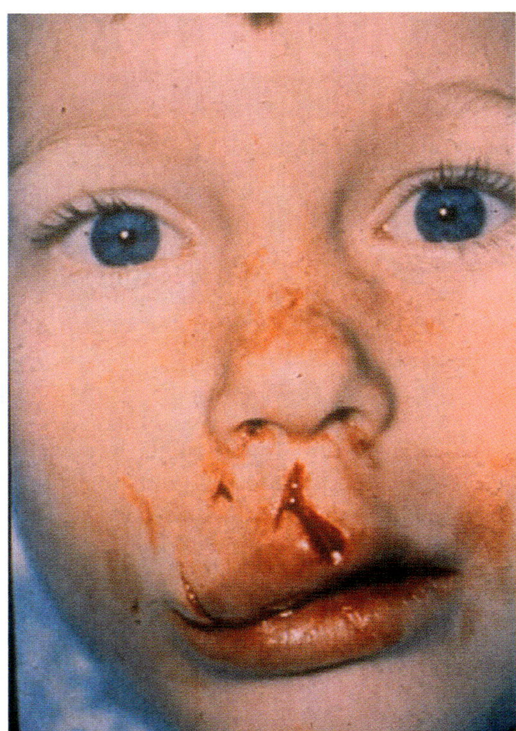

FIGURE 46–5 ■ Lacerations to the face should undergo primary closure.

significantly lower than the infection rate in the control groups (0% vs. 47% in human bite wounds, and 2% vs. 28% for hand bites).[2] Several researchers have found a significant reduction in infection for bite wounds to the hands treated with prophylactic antibiotics.[19,24]

Bite wounds can be stratified in terms of risk for infection. Patients with low risk wounds do not require prophylactic antibiotics, while those with high-risk wounds should be treated prophylactically with antibiotics. All hand and wrist wounds are high risk, including those that are less than 24 hours old and those that do not penetrate a joint capsule or tendon, and should be treated prophylactically with antibiotics. Other high-risk bite wounds are listed in Table 46–8.[8] Low-risk human bites include those that occur at sites other than the hands or feet, are not over cartilaginous structures, present within 24 hours of injury, and are not puncture wounds.[4] Patients who present >24 hours following injury, with no signs of wound infection, may not require prophylactic antibiotics, as most wounds that are going to become infected will have done so by this time. Prophylactic antibiotics are not recommended in the routine treatment of patients with snakebites who show no signs of tissue necrosis.

Certain patients should always receive prophylactic antibiotics, regardless of type or site of bite. Any patient with immune compromise, such as patients with hematologic malignancies or diabetes, patients on corticosteroid therapy, and patients with prior splenectomy or functional asplenia, should receive wound prophylaxis.

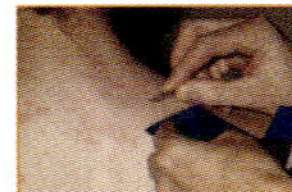

Table 46–8.

High-Risk Bite Wounds
Bites to hands or wrists
Crush injuries
Puncture wounds
Cat bites
Bites that occur in aquatic environment
Injuries that involve bone or joint
Injuries adjacent to a prosthetic joint
Injury in immune-compromised individual

INFECTED WOUNDS

Patients whose bite wounds are infected at initial presentation should also receive tetanus and rabies prophylaxis, as indicated, as well as empiric antibiotics while awaiting wound cultures. Abscesses should be incised and drained using standard techniques. Most infected wounds can be treated in the outpatient setting. Inpatient treatment of bite wound infections is required in several situations. Severe cellulitis, the presence of fever and/or chills, or rapidly spreading infection should be managed in an inpatient setting. Any infection that has advanced past one joint or involves bone, joint, tendon, or nerve should be treated with parenteral antibiotics. Finally, any patient who has failed outpatient therapy or who may not reliably complete outpatient therapy should be hospitalized.

FOLLOW-UP

Patients with bite wounds should be seen in follow-up within 24 hours of initial treatment. Any increase in pain, swelling, or cellulitis should prompt hospitalization.

Treatment

Empiric and prophylactic antibiotic therapy should be directed against the microorganisms found most frequently in bite wound infections. The most common bacteria vary according to the biting animal, the environment of the bite, and the type of wound infection, if present. Empiric therapy for dog and cat bite wounds should be directed against *Pasteurella*, *Streptococci*, *Staphylococci*, and anaerobes, while empiric therapy for human bite wounds should include coverage against *Streptococci*, *Staphylococci*, *E. corrodens*, and anaerobes[41] (Table 46–9).

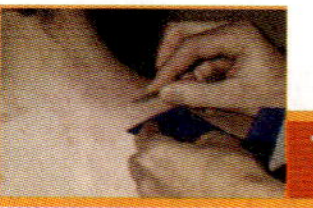

Table 46–9.

Recommended Empiric Antibiotic Therapy

Source of Bite	Oral Route	Oral Alternatives for Penicillin-Allergic Patients	Intravenous Route	Intravenous Alternatives for Penicillin-Allergic Patients
Dog, cat, mammal	Amoxicillin–clavulanate (30–50 mg/kg/d)	Second- or third-generation cephalosporin or trimethoprim–sulfamethoxazole (8–10 mg/kg/d) plus Clindamycin (25–40 mg/kg/d)	Ampicillin–sulbactam (100–200 mg/kg/d)	Second- or third-generation cephalosporin or trimethoprim–sulfamethoxazole (8–10 mg/kg/d) plus Clindamycin (25–40 mg/kg/d)
Reptile	Amoxicillin-clavulanate (30–50 mg/kg/d)	Second- or third-generation cephalosporin or trimethoprim–sulfamethoxazole (8–10 mg/kg/d) plus Clindamycin (25–40 mg/kg/d)	Ampicillin-sulbactam (100–200 mg/kg/d) plus Gentamicin (7.5 mg/kg/d)	Clindamycin (25–40 mg/kg/d) plus Gentamicin (7.5 mg/kg/d)
Human	Amoxicillin–clavulanate (30–50 mg/kg/d)	Second- or third-generation cephalosporin or trimethoprim–sulfamethoxazole (8–10 mg/kg/d) plus Clindamycin (25–40 mg/kg/d)	Ampicillin–sulbactam (100–200 mg/kg/d)	Second- or third-generation cephalosporin or trimethoprim–sulfamethoxazole (8–10 mg/kg/d) plus Clindamycin (25–40 mg/kg/d)

Adapted from Red Book 2006.

Bite wounds that occur in the aquatic environment require additional empiric antibiotics to cover microorganisms present in the water, regardless of the type of biting animal. The choice of antibiotic used for aquatic bite wounds is determined by the type of water in which the bite occurred. Injuries that occur in saltwater should receive antibiotic coverage for *Vibrio* spp. such as ceftazidime or cefotaxime plus doxycycline or ciprofloxacin. Freshwater wounds should be treated with antibiotics that cover *A. hydrophila* and *Pseudomonas aeruginosa*; ceftazidime, imipenem, or ciprofloxacin are reasonable options.

Many microorganisms isolated from infected dog and cat bite wounds are beta-lactamase producers. Optimal empiric therapy should include either a combination of a beta-lactam antibiotic and a beta-lactamase inhibitor, a second-generation cephalosporin with anaerobic activity (e.g., cefoxitin), or combination therapy with either penicillin and a first-generation cephalosporin or clindamycin and a fluoroquinolone. Antimicrobial agents of choice for dog bite wound infections are amoxicillin/clavulanic acid and ampicillin/sulbactam. Metronidazole plus ampicillin offers another good choice.[35] One study has evaluated the efficacy of prophylactic trimethoprim–sulfamethoxazole for dog bites, and demonstrated a nearly significant reduction in the incidence of hand infections.[23] The role of clindamycin, increasingly used for coverage of community-acquired methicillin-resistant *S. aureus*, has not been examined in bite wound infections.

Recent surveillance data of *Pasteurella* strains isolated from infected bite wounds in humans indicate that amoxicillin, cefotaxime, azithromycin, and clarithromycin are all effective as single agents.[42] Trimethoprim–sulfamethoxazole usually offers good coverage for *Pasteurella*. In addition, doxycycline, minocycline, and several fluoroquinolones are effective, but may not be appropriate drugs for pediatric patients.

Amoxicillin–clavulanic acid and moxifloxacin demonstrate the best activity against the most frequently isolated strains of bacteria from human bite wounds. *E. corrodens* has a peculiar susceptibility pattern, being susceptible to penicillin, but resistant to penicillinase-resistant penicillins, such as dicloxicillin.[43] *E. corrodens* has been found to be uniformly resistant to clindamycin.[43] Erythromycin, antistaphylococcal penicillins, first-generation cephalosporins, metronidazole, and most aminoglycosides also have poor activity against *E. corrodens*. In vitro susceptibility testing of 151 clinical strains of *E. corrodens* found all isolates to be sensitive to ampicillin/sulbactam, amoxicillin/clavulanic acid, and cefoxitin. Relative resistance to doxycycline was found in 17.8%.[43] For penicillin-allergic pediatric patients, a combination of antibiotics may be necessary for empiric coverage of human bite wounds, including clindamycin plus a second- or third-generation cephalosporin.[10]

Marine environment wounds should be treated with doxycycline and a third- or fourth-generation cephalosporin or a fluoroquinolone. Patients with bite wounds occurring in freshwater should receive a third- or fourth-generation cephalosporin.

Ciprofloxacin, like other fluoroquinolones, is associated with arthropathy and histopathologic changes in weight-bearing joints of juvenile animals. The American Academy of Pediatrics states that the use of fluoroquinolones (e.g., ciprofloxacin, gatifloxacin, levofloxacin, moxifloxacin) in children younger than 18 years of age may be justified. The most recent recommendations for the use of fluoroquinolones in children state two circumstances in which they may be useful: (1) infection is caused by multidrug-resistant pathogens, and (2) parenteral therapy is not feasible and no other effective oral agent is available. The drugs should be used only after careful assessment of the risks and benefits for the individual patient and after these benefits and risks have been explained to the parents or caregivers.[44] Doxycycline and minocycline are generally not recommended for use in children younger than 8 years owing to risk for tooth enamel hypoplasia and discoloration.

Course and Prognosis

Patients with infected bite wounds should be reevaluated 24 hours after initial treatment. If the wound appears clinically worse, inpatient therapy is required. If the condition is better, further follow-up can be dictated by the return of signs or symptoms of infection. With initial adequate wound care, most bite wound infections will resolve after 5–7 days of antibiotics. High-risk wounds that are initially left open should be considered for delayed closure in 3–5 days. The results of cultures should guide treatment of refractory infections.

Pearls

1. Wounds evaluated more than 24 hours after the injury should not be sutured, when possible.
2. Rabies prophylaxis should be administered to patients bitten by dogs, cats, or ferrets with known or suspected rabies and to all patients with bites from bats, skunks, raccoons, foxes, or woodchucks.
3. While not all otherwise healthy patients with bite wounds require antibiotic prophylaxis, patients with immunocompromising conditions such as hematologic malignancies, diabetes, splenectomy, or functional asplenia should always receive antibiotic prophylaxis regardless of the type or site of the bite.

REFERENCES

1. Hodge D, Tecklenburg FW. Bites and stings. In: Fleisher GR, Ludwig S, Henretig FM, eds. *Textbook of Pediatric Emergency Medicine*. 5th ed. Philadelphia: Lippincott Williams & Wilkins; 2006:1061-1064.
2. Medeiros I, Saconato H. Antibiotic prophylaxis for mammalian bites. *Cochrane Database Syst Rev*. 2001;2: CD001738.
3. Weiss HB, Friedman DI, Coben JH. Incidence of dog bite injuries treated in emergency departments. *JAMA*. 1998;279(1):51-53.
4. Broder J, Jerrard D, Olshaker J, Witting M. Low risk of infection in selected human bites treated without antibiotics. *Am J Emerg Med*. 2004;22(1):10-13.
5. Wiley JF. Mammalian bites: review of evaluation and management. *Clin Pediatr*. 1990;29(5):283-287.
6. Beck AM, Jones BA. Unreported dog bites in children. *Public Health Rep*. 1985;100(3):315-321.
7. Centers for Disease Control and Prevention. Nonfatal dog bite-related injuries treated in hospital emergency departments–United States, 2001. *MMWR*. 2003;52(26): 605-610.
8. Goldstein EJC. Bite wounds and infection. *Clin Infect Dis*. 1992;14:633-638.
9. Talan DA, Citron DM, Abrahamian FM, Moran GJ, Goldstein EJC. Bacteriologic analysis of infected dog and cat bites. *N Engl J Med*. 1999;340(2):85-92.
10. Talan DA, Abrahamian FM, Moran GJ, et al. Clinical presentation and bacteriologic analysis of infected human bites in patients presenting to emergency departments. *Clin Infect Dis*. 2003;37:1481-1489.
11. Avner JR, Baker DM. Dog bites in urban children. *Pediatrics*. 1991;88(1):55-57.

12. Overall KL, Love M. Dog bites to humans–demography, epidemiology, injury, and risk. *JAMA*. 2001;218(12): 1923-1934.
13. Palmer J, Rees M. Dog bites of the face: a 15 year review. *Br J Plast Surg*. 1983;36:315-318.
14. Dire DJ. Emergency management of dog and cat bite wounds. *Emerg Med Clin N Am*. 1992;10(4):719-735.
15. Smith PF, Meadowcroft AM, May DB. Treating mammalian bite wounds. *J Clin Pharm Ther*. 2000;25:85-89.
16. Dire DJ, Hogan DE, Walker JS. Prophylactic oral antibiotics for low-risk dog bite wounds. *Pediatr Emerg Care*. 1991;8(4):194-199.
17. Akhtar N, Smith MJ, McKirdy S, Page RE. Surgical delay in the management of dog bite injuries in children, does it increase the risk of infection? *J Plast Reconstr Aesthet Surg*. 2006;59:80-85.
18. Donkor P, Bankas DO. A study of primary closure of human bite injuries to the face. *J Oral Maxillofac Surg*. 1997;55:479-481.
19. Cummings P. Antibiotics to prevent infection in patients with dog bite wounds: a meta-analysis of randomized trials. *Ann Emerg Med*. 1994;23(3):535-540.
20. Dire DJ, Hogan DE, Riggs MW. A prospective evaluation of risk factors for infections from dog-bite wounds. *Acad Emerg Med*. 1994;1(3):258-266.
21. Maimaris C, Quinton DN. Dog-bite lacerations: a controlled trial of primary wound closure. *Arch Emerg Med*. 1988;5(3):156-161.
22. Baker DM, Moore SE. Human bites in children. *Am J Dis Child*. 1987;141:1285-1290.
23. Jones DA, Stanbridge TN. A clinical trial using co-trimoxazole in an attempt to reduce wound infection rates in dog bite wounds. *Postgrad Med J*. 1985;61:593-594.
24. Rosen RA. The use of antibiotics in the initial management of recent dog-bite wounds. *Am J Emerg Med*. 1985;3(1):19-23.
25. Schweich P, Fleisher G. Human bites in children. *Pediatr Emerg Care*. 1985;1(2):51-53.
26. Elenbaas RM, McNabney WK, Robinson WA. Evaluation of prophylactic oxacillin in cat bite wounds. *Ann Emerg Med*. 1984;13(3):155-157.
27. Elenbaas RM, McNabney WK, Robinson WA. Prophylactic oxacillin in dog bite wounds. *Ann Emerg Med*. 1982;11(5):248-251.
28. Boenning DA, Fleisher GR, Campos JM. Dog bites in children: epidemiology, microbiology, and penicillin prophylactic therapy. *Am J Emerg Med*. 1983;1:17-21.
29. Callaham M. Prophylactic antibiotics in common dog bite wounds: a controlled study. *Ann Emerg Med*. 1980;9(8): 410-414.
30. Callaham ML. Treatment of common dog bites: Infection risk factors. *JACEP*. 1978;7(3):83-87.
31. Skurka J, Willert C, Yogev R. Wound infection following dog bite despite prophylactic penicillin. *Infection*. 1986;14(3):134-135.
32. Brakenbury PH, Muwanga C. A comparative double blind study of amoxicillin/clavulanate vs placebo in the prevention of infection after animal bites. *Arch Emerg Med*. 1989;6(4):251-256.
33. Noonburg GE. Management of extremity trauma and related infections occurring in the aquatic environment. *J Am Acad Orthop Surg*. 2005;13(4):243-253.
34. Chen E, Hornig S. Shepherd SM, Hollander JE. Primary closure of mammalian bites. *Acad Emerg Med*. 2000;7(2):157-161.
35. Rodriguez AJ, Barbella R, Castaneda L. Anaerobic dog bite wound infection. *Ann N Y Acad Sci*. 2000;916:665-667.
36. Weber DJ, Hansen AR. Infections resulting from animal bites. *Infect Dis Clin N Am*. 1991;5(3):663-679.
37. Stefanopoulos PK, Tarantzopoulou. Facial bite wounds: Management update. *Int J Oral Maxillofac Surg*. 2005;34: 464-472.
38. Goldstein EJC, Sutter VL, Finegold SM. Susceptibility of *Eikenella corrodens* to ten cephalosporins. *Antimicrob Agents Chemother*. 1978;14(4):639-641.
39. American Academy of Pediatrics. Tetanus. In: Pickering LK, Baker CJ, Long SS, McMillan JA, ed. *Red Book: 2006 Report of the Committee on Infectious Diseases*. 27th ed. Elk Grove Village, IL: American Academy of Pediatrics; 2006:648-653.
40. American Academy of Pediatrics. Rabies. In: Pickering LK, Baker CJ, Long SS, McMillan JA, ed. *Red Book: 2006 Report of the Committee on Infectious Diseases*. 27th ed. Elk Grove Village, IL: American Academy of Pediatrics; 2006:552-559.
41. American Academy of Pediatrics. Bite wounds. In: Pickering LK, Baker CJ, Long SS, McMillan JA, ed. *Red Book: 2006 Report of the Committee on Infectious* Diseases. 27th ed. Elk Grove Village, IL: American Academy of Pediatrics; 2006:191-195.
42. Lion C, Conroy MC, Carpentier AM, Lozniewski A. Antimicrobial susceptibilities of pasteurella strains isolated from humans. *Int J Antimicrob Agents*. 2006;27: 290-293.
43. Goldstein EJC, Citron DM, Merriam CV, Warren YA, Tyrrell KL, Fernandez H. In vitro activities of a new desfluoroquinolone, BMS 284756, and seven other antimicrobial agents against 151 isolates of *Eikenella corrodens*. *Antimicrob Agents Chemother*. 2002;46:1141-1143.
44. American Academy of Pediatrics. The use of systemic fluoroquinolones. *Pediatrics*. 2006;118(3):1287-1292.

SECTION 12

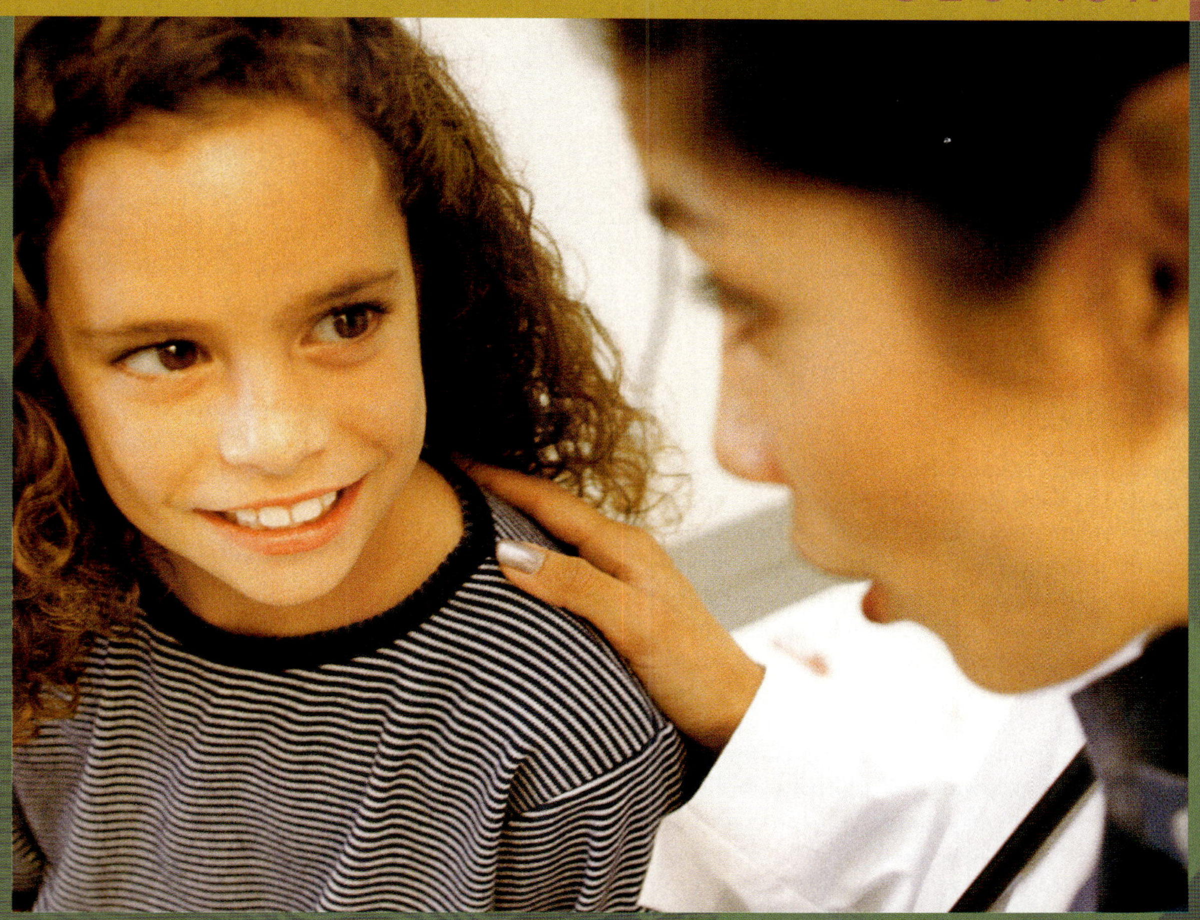

Bone and Joint Infections

CHAPTER 47

Osteomyelitis

Sandra Arnold

DEFINITIONS

Osteomyelitis is an inflammatory condition of bones usually caused by bacterial, or more rarely, fungal infection. Acute hematogenous osteomyelitis (AHO) is the most common form of osteomyelitis in children.[1] It occurs as a result of hematogenous deposition of bacteria within bone following symptomatic or asymptomatic bacteremia. The time from onset of symptoms to diagnosis is usually rapid, within 14 days, although certain sites of infection (particularly vertebral and calcaneal) may have a more insidious course and present subacutely.[2] Chronic osteomyelitis presents with either chronic, persistent, low-grade symptoms or an exacerbation of symptoms after a period of relative disease quiescence.[3] The reported duration of symptoms required to establish a diagnosis of chronic osteomyelitis is quite varied, ranging from 6 weeks to 6 months. The distinction between acute and chronic osteomyelitis is important as it helps define the necessary treatment modalities given that a longer duration of symptoms before treatment may allow for the development of necrotic bone and soft tissues. Nonhematogenous osteomyelitis occurs with direct contamination of bone from trauma, surgery, or spread of infection from an adjacent soft tissue infection.[4] This may present as acute or chronic infection. The primary focus of this chapter will be AHO as it is the form of disease that will be seen most commonly in primary care.

The reported incidence of AHO has ranged from 0.1 per 1000 children younger than 12 years to 8.7 per 1000 children younger than 13 years.[5–7] In regions where community-associated methicillin resistant *Staphylococcus aureus* (CA-MRSA) is common, the incidence may be increasing but there are no population-based studies.[8] Approximately 50–60% of children with AHO are younger than 5 years with approximately half of those being younger than 2 years.[1,5–10] Most studies have documented a male predominance of AHO of approximately 1.5–2:1.[1,6,7,9–11]

PATHOGENESIS

AHO results from the interplay of host and microbial factors.[12] The vascular anatomy of bone in infants and children uniquely presdisposes to bacterial infection in the metaphyseal region of long bones or the "metaphyseal-equivalent" portions of irregular or flat bones (e.g., apophyseal growth plates, such as the tibial tubercle, or greater trochanter).[13] Bacteria enter the bone through the nutrient artery and travel to the metaphyseal arterioles. These arterioles form sharp loops adjacent to the epiphyseal growth plate and empty into venous sinusoids in the metaphysis of long bones and metaphyseal-equivalent areas. Sluggish blood flow through these sinusoids and endothelial gaps in the tips of growing metaphyseal vessels are thought to predispose to bacterial deposition in these sites.[14]

Once infection is initiated, pus spreads through vascular canals leading to vascular compression and compromise, ischemia, and bone necrosis. Perforation of the cortex of bone results in periosteal elevation and subperiosteal abscess.[12] Capillaries that cross the physis, present in children younger than 18 months, allow spread of metaphyseal infection into the epiphysis[15] although older children may also develop epiphyseal infection.[15] Septic arthritis of an adjacent joint may result from spread across these transphyseal vessels and/or via direct spread from the subperiosteal space in those joints in which the metaphysis is contained within the joint capsule (hip, knee, shoulder).[16]

MICROBIOLOGY

S. aureus is the most common organism isolated from children with culture-confirmed AHO. It accounts for between 40% and 80% of all cases.[1,5–11,17–21] CA-MRSA infections have become very common in some regions and are becoming the predominant etiologic agent of AHO.[8,22–24] *S. aureus* is uniquely suited to infect bone as it expresses multiple virulence factors that promote attachment to bone in addition to evasion of host defenses.[12] It is also able to evade the immune response and antibiotics by forming a biofilm in which the bacteria are embedded[25] and by surviving for prolonged periods within osteoblasts, neutrophils, and endothelial cells.[26]

Streptococcus pyogenes (group A *Streptococcus*) is the most common streptococcal species isolated from AHO,[1,5–8,20,27] occurring more frequently in children with varicella infection.[27] *Streptococcus agalactiae* (group B *Streptococcus*) causes osteomyelitis in neonates and rarely in older children.[8,20,28,29] *Streptococcus pneumoniae* is most common among children younger than 2 years and usually causes with septic arthritis alone or with concomitant AHO.[8,30] *Haemophilus influenzae* type B[1,5,6,9,19,21] has virtually disappeared with routine infant immunization.[7,8,10,11,31] *Salmonella* is a pathogen most frequently associated with osteomyelitis in children with sickle cell disease,[32] although it may be occasionally isolated in AHO from otherwise healthy children.[1,8–10] Other enteric gram-negative organisms, such as *Escherichia coli* and *Enterobacter* spp., are encountered in neonates[28,29] and children with sickle cell disease.[32] Coagulase-negative staphylococci and other low pathogenicity organisms, reported in some case series, are unlikely pathogens except in the setting of nonhematogenous osteomyelitis.

Anywhere from 15% to 68% of cases of osteoarticular infections are culture negative when blood culture and bone/joint aspirates are used in combination.[1,5–11,33] It is assumed that the majority of these cases are staphylococcal.[10] *Kingella kingae*, a fastidious, gram-negative, is also implicated in culture negative infections, particularly septic arthrits.[10,20,34,35] Isolation of this fastidious organism is improved with inoculation of specimens into automated blood culture systems and with the use of a *Kingella*-specific polymerase chain reaction test.[34,36] Unusual organisms causing osteomyelitis and associated with negative conventional cultures include *Mycobacterium tuberculosis, Blastomyces dermatidis, Coccidioides immitis, Bartonella henselae* (agent of cat-scratch disease) and *Coxiella burnettii* (agent of Q fever). Opportunistic fungi, such as *Aspergillus* spp., may be seen in immunocompromised patients.

CLINICAL PRESENTATION

Common clinical findings on presentation with AHO include fever (40–90%[1,5,10,11]) and focal bone pain and/or tenderness (56–91%[1,5,9,11]). Patients with fever are more likely to present within a few days of symptom onset.[5] If the infection is in a weight-bearing bone, the patient may present with limp. Failure to walk or crawl or pseudoparalysis may be present in young infants who are unable to verbalize focal pain.[29] Other signs and symptoms that may be seen are localized swelling, erythema, and warmth and decreased range of motion of an adjacent joint.[1,5,11] Table 47–1 presents the most common signs and symptoms of AHO.

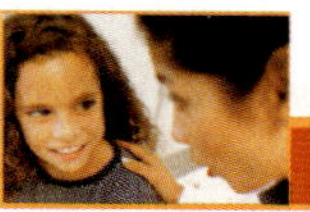

Table 47–1.

Signs and Symptoms of Osteomyelitis at Clinical Presentation

Fever
Bone pain or tenderness
Limp or reduced use of extremity (pseudoparalysis)
Erythema
Swelling
Toxic appearance
Shock*
Pneumonia*

**Some children will have signs of shock or pulmonary involvement, usually with S. aureus, particularly with CA-MRSA.*

Children may present with a clinical picture of severe infection or pneumonia as well. It is important to consider musculoskeletal infection in the differential diagnosis of any patient presenting with severe infection, especially in young children who cannot verbalize pain and the primary site of infection in the bone may be overlooked.

AHO disproportionately affects the long bones of the lower extremities (55% of all bones infected). Table 47–2 shows the relative proportions of the bones

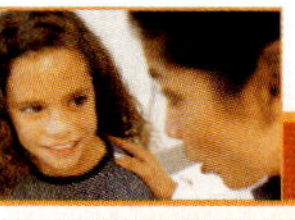

Table 47–2.

Proportion of Osteomyelitis Cases Affecting Various Bones*

Bone/Region	Proportion (%)
Femur	28
Tibia	22
Fibula	5
Humerus	10
Radius	4
Ulna	2
Calcaneus	5
Pelvis	10
Vertebra	2
Hand	4
Foot	6
Clavicle	2

**Excludes unusual miscellaneous bones (scapula, ribs) as only 1 or 2 cases across all series, intervertebral disk infections and infections of facial and skull bones (usually dues to contiguous focus or trauma).*

most frequently involved in osteomyelitis.[1,5,8,10,11,37] Multifocal bone infections occur in 4–9% of children with AHO.[1,37,38]

DIFFERENTIAL DIAGNOSIS

The differential diagnosis of AHO includes soft tissue infections such as cellulitis, myositis, and fasciitis (Table 47–3). Patients with osteomyelitis of bones with minimal overlying muscle or subcutaneous tissue (e.g., tibia, fibula, distal radius, and ulna) may present with erythema and induration of the skin mimicking cellulitis. Osteomyelitis should be suspected in cases where the degree of pain is disproportionate to the clinical findings of dermal inflammation. Myositis and fasciitis may occur concomitantly with AHO and are generally distinguished with imaging or surgical exploration. Hematologic malignancies may present with fever and bone pain or limp as well. In indolent cases where fever is low grade or absent, the differential diagnosis includes trauma and benign or malignant bone tumors.

AHO must be distinguished from acute inflammatory or infectious arthritis. Joint swelling, erythema, reduced mobility and joint effusion are present in these latter conditions. In 10–20% of patients with AHO, reduced range of motion of an adjacent joint may be caused by septic arthritis of the affected joint.[1,8,10]

Children with osteoarticular infections caused by CA-MRSA appear to have more severe disease at clinical presentation compared with those with MSSA infection.[22,39–45] This enhanced virulence does not appear to be related to its antibiotic resistance pattern and failure to initiate prompt appropriate therapy but because of other genetic features of this organism, the precise mechanisms of which remain elusive.[46,47] These children have an increased risk of subperiosteal abscess necessitating repeated surgical procedures,[22,43,44] septic thrombophlebitis[24,43,48] and severe sepsis with shock and death.[23] The risk of overwhelming infection is higher in older children and adolescents.[23] In this era of conjugate vaccines, invasive bacterial infections secondary to *S. pneumoniae*, *H. influenzae* type B and *Neisseria menigitidis* are becoming increasingly rare. *S. aureus* in general and MRSA in particular must be considered as the primary differential diagnosis of sepsis in an otherwise healthy patient. Frequently, the musculoskeletal system will be the primary site of infection in these patients; thus, a bone, joint or deep muscle focus of infection should be sought in any patient presenting with signs and symptoms of sepsis.[23]

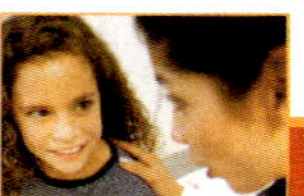

Table 47–3.

Differential Diagnosis of Acute Hematogenous Osteomyelitis

Common conditions
Cellulitis
Septic arthritis
Toxic synovitis
Leukemia
Sickle cell bone crisis
Uncommon conditions
Myositis
Fasciitis
Bone tumor (benign or malignant)
Juvenile idiopathic arthritis
Chronic recurrent multifocal osteomyelitis

DIAGNOSIS

Laboratory Testing

The diagnosis of AHO is made with a combination of clinical findings and supportive laboratory and imaging studies. Laboratory findings that are suggestive of AHO include elevations in acute phase reactants, such as the white blood cell count, C-reactive protein (CRP) and erythrocyte sedimentation rate (ESR). None of these tests is sufficiently specific or sensitive to be used to rule in or out the diagnosis of AHO.[1,10,23,37,49,50] The ESR is elevated in 70–90% of patients with a median value of 50–60 mm/h; however, values vary greatly from normal (<10–20 mm/h) to >140 mm/h. CRP values show a similar pattern with close to 100% patients having elevated values spanning a broad range. Children with AHO with an adjacent septic arthritis tend to have higher CRP values.[51,52] The greatest utility for the ESR and CRP appears to be in monitoring disease progression and resolution. ESR usually reaches a peak by day 3–5 of admission with a gradual decline to normal by the end of therapy (approximately 3–5 weeks).[49–51] The CRP peaks by the second day of admission and normalizes within 7–10 days of effective therapy.[49–51]

Pathogenic bacteria are isolated from 50–85% of children with AHO.[1,8,10,37,38] The blood culture alone is positive in 30–55% of cases.[1,8,37,38] Culture of aspirates of bone or subperiosteal abscess and from joint fluid from adjacent infected joints may enhance isolation of pathogens; however, in practice, the willingness of surgeons to obtain a bone aspirate from a patient who does not have a clinical requirement for surgery (i.e., for drainage of a subperiosteal abscess or debridement of necrotic bone) varies among institutions. The rate of isolation of bacteria from subperiosteal pus is high and, thus, should be attempted where possible.[8,9]

Radiographic Diagnosis

Plain radiography

The role of plain radiographs in early infection is to exclude other pathologic conditions. A frequently made error is using plain radiographs to exclude the possibility of AHO early in disease. It is extremely important to remember that bone pain or limp in a child with fever is an acute osteoarticular infection until proven otherwise. The earliest findings are soft tissue swelling with blurring of soft tissue planes.[53] Bone destruction (osteolysis) may not be seen for 7–10 days after the onset of infection because loss of approximately 50% of bone mineralization is required for changes to be apparent on plain films (Figure 47–1); early treatment with antibiotics may arrest bone loss and typical radiographic changes may never appear.[54,55] Periosteal reaction or elevation associated with abscess is seen later as infection extends through and erodes the cortex. One may also see widening of the adjacent joint space because of effusion from a concurrent septic arthritis.

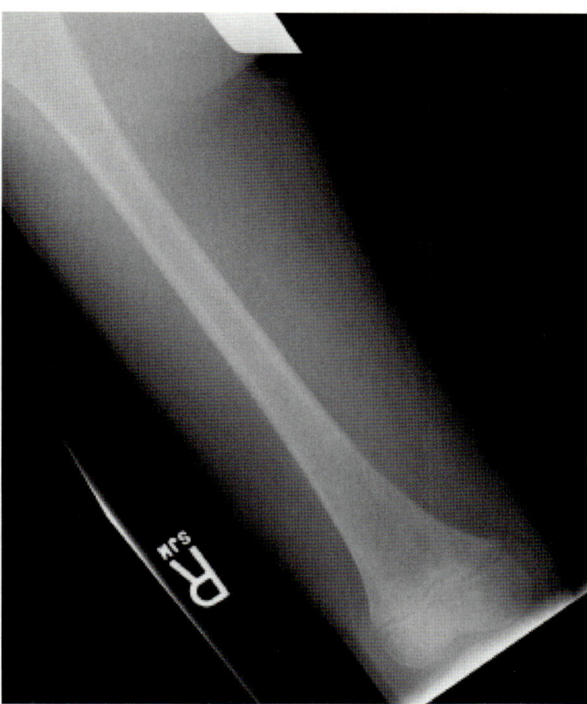

FIGURE 47–1 ■ Acute osteomyelitis of the distal femur with osteolysis.

Scintigraphy

Bone scintigraphy may be positive as soon as 24–48 hours after onset of symptoms.[54] Technetium-99m-methylene diphosponate localizes in areas of inflammation secondary to hyperemia and early bone resorption. A three-phase bone scan suggested in diagnosing AHO.[54,56] The first phase is the angiographic or flow phase which consists of serial images of the suspected area of infection during infusion of the isotope. The second phase, or blood-pool image, is obtained within 5 minutes of injection when isotope has pooled in tissues because of the increased blood flow associated with inflammation. The third phase, or bone phase, is obtained approximately 3 hours later after the isotope has washed out of the soft tissues (Figure 47–2). Osteomyelitis causes a focal increase in uptake in all three phases, whereas, cellulitis results in diffuse increased uptake in the first two phases and either no or diffusely increased uptake in the third. The sensitivity of the three-phase bone scan is 90–95%[54,56–58] making this a very useful test in clinical practice. Specificity is lower as bone scintigraphy cannot distinguish among infection, neoplasm, and trauma. False negative (either normal or "cold" spots) bone scans result from limitation of

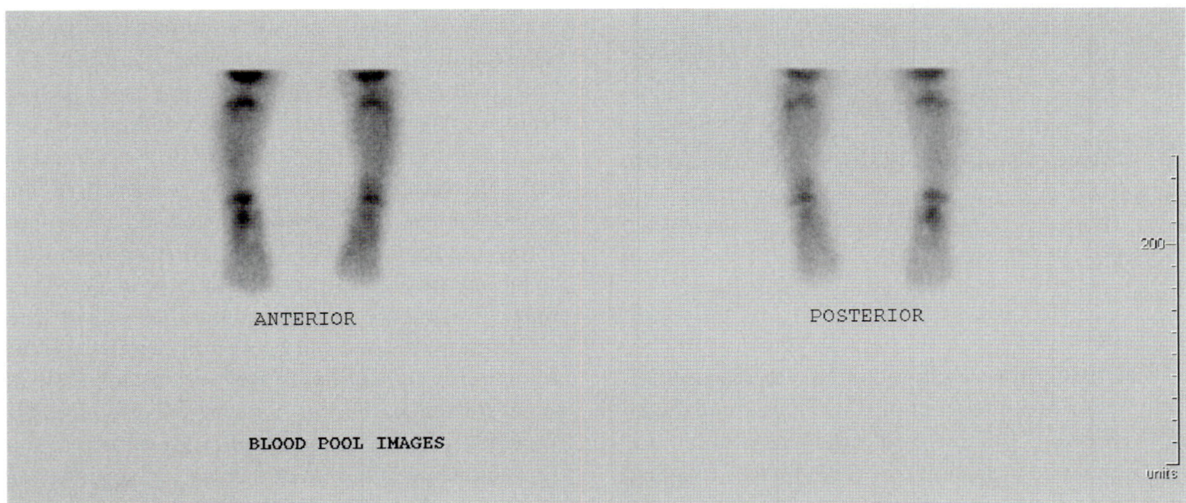

FIGURE 47–2 ■ Blood-pool images of the lower extremities from a bone scan of a patient with osteomyelitis of the right calcaneus.

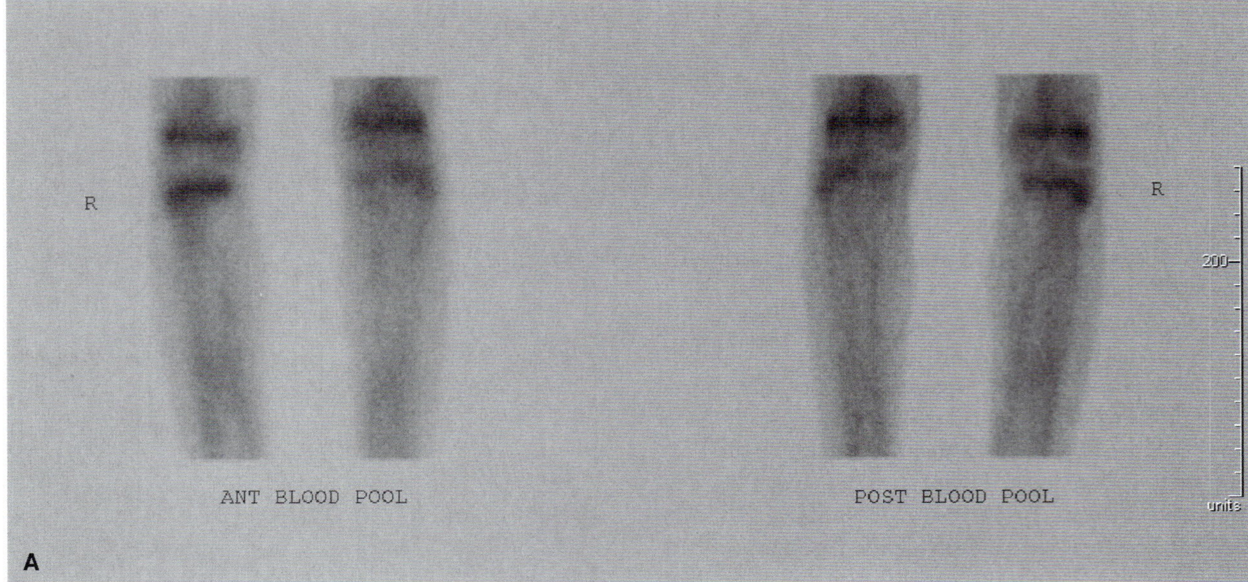

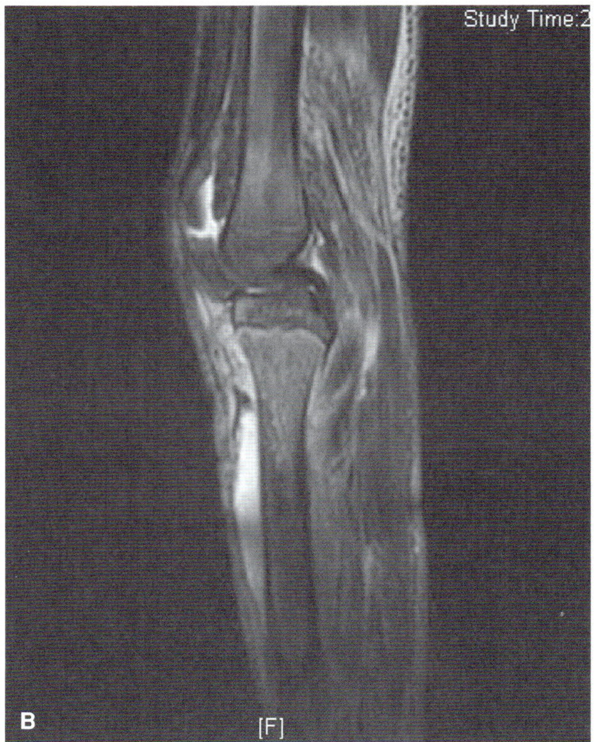

FIGURE 47–3 ■ Bone scan **(A)** and MRI **(B)** of a patient with extensive osteomyelitis of the right tibia with large subperiosteal abscess. Falsely negative bone scan demonstrates no abnormality.

the usual tissue hyperemia secondary to sinsusoidal thrombosis or pressure from pus in the vascular channels[59–62] (Figure 47–3); thus, in a patient for whom there is a high index of suspicion for AHO, further imaging should be undertaken in the face of a negative bone scan. Use of other isotopes, such as Gallium-67 or Indium-111-labeled leukocyte, are not routinely recommended.[63]

Ultrasound

Ultrasound can detect a variety of abnormalities including edema of muscle and subcutaneous tissues which may be maximal near bone, thickening of periosteum and elevation of the periosteum greater than 2 mm including subperiosteal abscess.[64] It is sensitive and specific for the diagnosis of AHO (both 90%) and is useful where access to nuclear medicine or magnetic resonance imaging is limited.

Computed tomography (CT) and magnetic resonance imaging (MRI)

These studies are sensitive tools in the diagnosis of AHO. The most useful property of CT scanning is the detection of intraosseus gas, sequestra, and involucra (see section "Chronic Osteomyelitis")[65] (Figure 47–4). The greatest utility of MRI is its ability to provide a detailed image of the infected area with superb delineation of the extent of the disease of both bone and adjacent soft tissues. The earliest change seen is edema of bone marrow, demonstrating low-signal intensity (dark) on spin echo T1-weighted images and high-signal intensity (bright) on fast spin echo T2-weighted images[65–67] (Figure 47–5). Such findings are not specific for osteomyelitis and can be seen in neoplasia, trauma, or bone infarct. MRI has proved very useful in identifying abscesses in children with pelvic osteomyelitis or those who did not have prompt improvement in symptoms following initiation of therapy.[67] A suggested algorithm to guide diagnostic imaging of children with suspected AHO is provided in Figure 47–6.

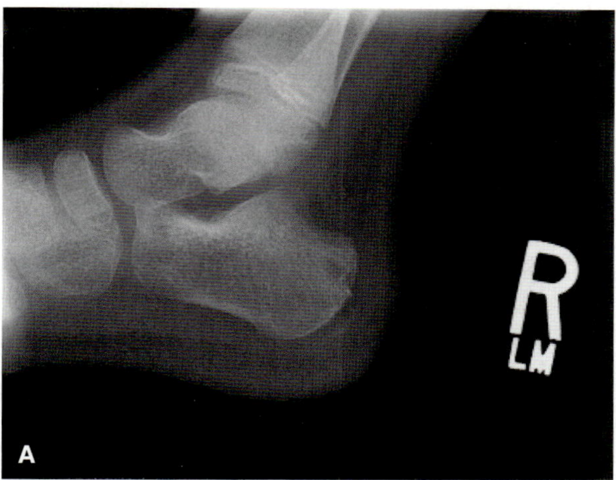

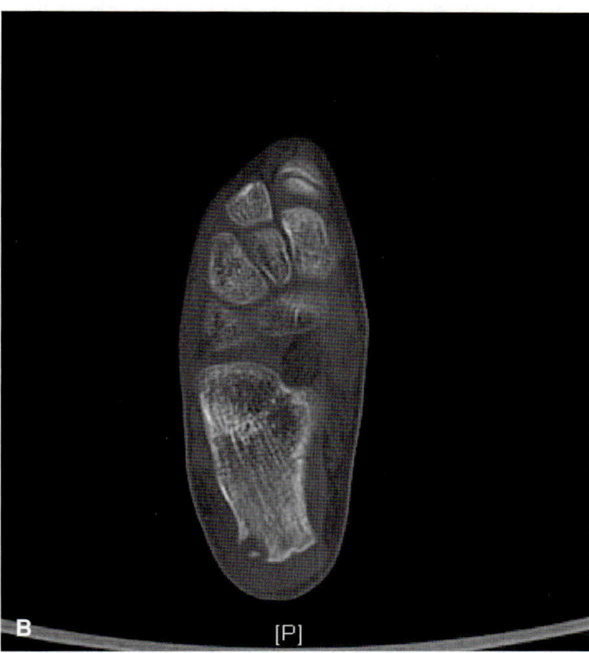

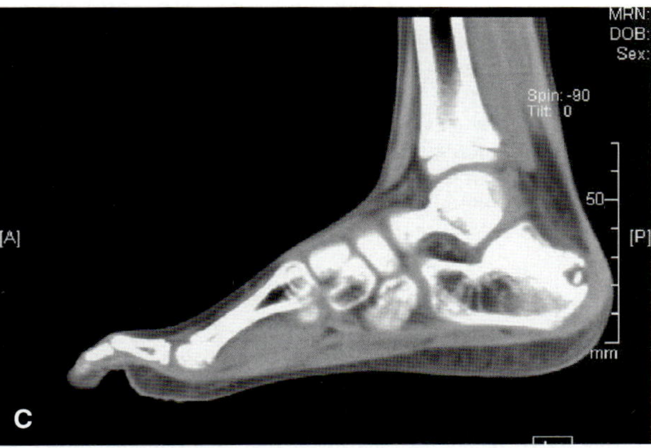

FIGURE 47–4 ■ Chronic osteomyelitis of the calcaneus with formation of a sequestrum. Radiograph **(A)** and CT (**B** and **C**) images demonstrate a large cortical defect in the posterior calcaneus with a hyperdensitiy seen in the overlying soft tissues compatible with sequestrum.

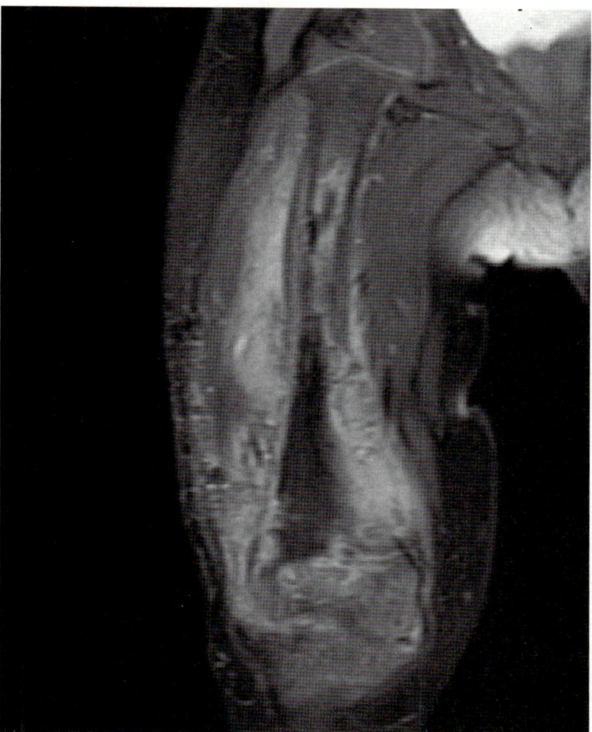

FIGURE 47–5 ■ MRI of severe osteomyelitis of the femur with diffuse osteomyelitis and surround subperiosteal abscess.

MANAGEMENT

Surgical Management

Surgery with aspiration of bone and cortical window creation used to be a routine part of care; however, studies have not demonstrated an advantage to routine surgical intervention in addition to antibiotics. Surgical intervention should be reserved for clinically significant subperiosteal or muscle abscess or cases in which the diagnosis is in doubt. Some surgeons will perform bone aspirates for culture.

Medical Management

Several points of controversy persist regarding the antimicrobial management of AHO: Total duration of therapy and the use of oral stepdown to oral therapy following a period of parenteral therapy. The lack of large prospective randomized trials of treatment duration or oral stepdown therapy fuel ongoing debate on these issues.

Duration of therapy

Early retrospective case series demonstrated a greater risk of relapse in children with staphylococcal osteomyelitis who received fewer than 3 weeks of therapy[1]; thus, it

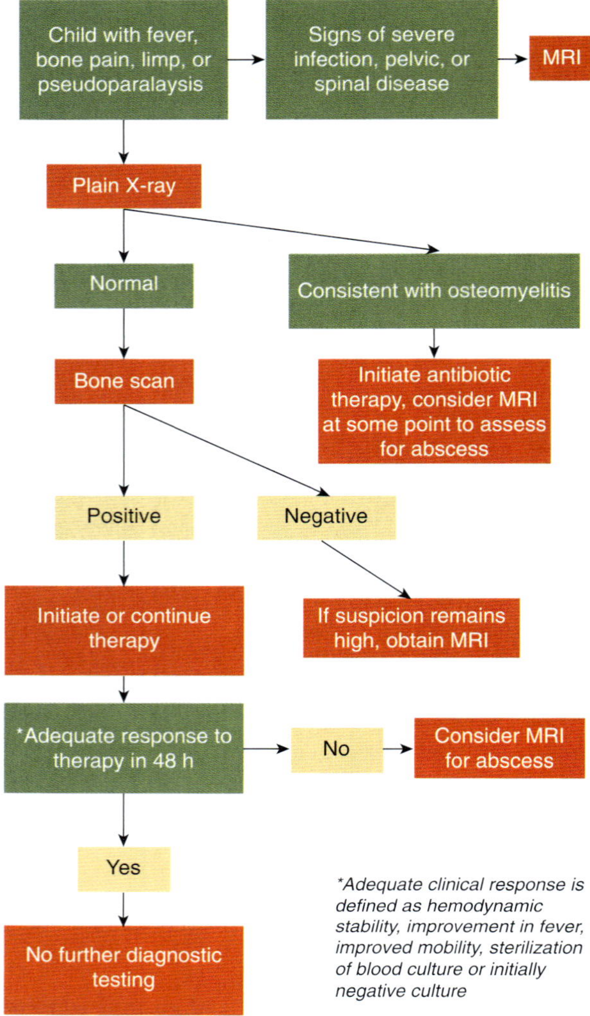

FIGURE 47–6 ■ Recommended diagnostic imaging algorithm for diagnosis of acute hematogenous osteomyelitis.

became accepted that 4–6 weeks of therapy were required to minimize the risk of relapse and development of chronic osteomyelitis. More recent studies have demonstrated that the duration of therapy may be safely reduced by monitoring the CRP and the ESR until both have normalized, usually within 3–4 weeks.[51,68] In patients with complicated disease, as is being seen more frequently with CA-MRSA, longer courses of therapy seem prudent and are required to achieve normalization of the ESR.

Oral stepdown therapy

Although unacceptably high treatment failure rates were seen initially with shorter courses of parenteral therapy, greater understanding of bone and synovial fluid penetration of antibiotics[69] and routine use of higher doses led many to attempt oral therapy again to obviate the need for maintaining prolonged intravenous access.[21] For some time, it was recommended that this oral stepdown therapy only be used when monitoring of serum bactericidal titers (SBTs) could be guaranteed. SBTs measure the bactericidal power of the patient's serum against the infecting organism.[70] However, treatment failure is rare among patients given high doses of oral antibiotics (2–3 times the usual dose).[21,51,68,71,72] Some clinicians will obtain drug levels in place of SBTs to detect the occasional patient in whom oral bioavailability is poor. While many centers continue to use oral stepdown therapy, many others have been using peripherally inserted central catheters which are often easily inserted at the bedside to provide home parenteral therapy. Each route of therapy has its own set of advantages and disadvantages. The primary disadvantage of prolonged intravenous therapy is the risk of complications from a central venous catheter, primarily infection and thrombosis both of which may require emergency department visits or hospital readmission.[73] The benefits include lack of reliance on gastric absorption of oral antibiotics and possible better compliance. Oral stepdown therapy does not put patients at risk for central venous catheter infection or upper extremity thrombosis; however, compliance may be more of an issue and there may be the occasional patient who has poor oral bioavailability. A systematic review and meta-analysis of 12 prospective cohort studies, little difference was demonstrated in the cure rate at least 6 months later between short- (≤7 days, pooled cure rate 95.2%) and long-course intravenous therapy (>7 days, pooled cure rate 98.8%)[74] (Figure 47–7).

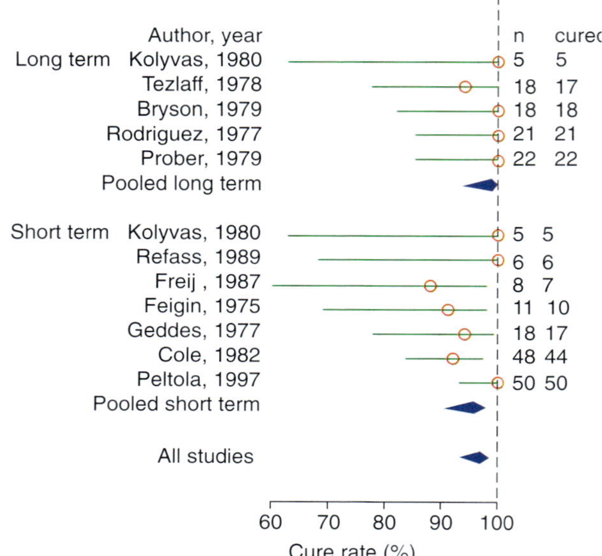

FIGURE 47–7 ■ Cure rate versus duration of parenteral antimicrobial therapy. Long-term parenteral antimicrobials is defined as ≥7 days. Short-term parenteral antimicrobials is defined as <7 days. *(From Le Saux N, Howard A, Barrowman NJ, Gaboury I, Sampson M, Moher D. Shorter courses of parenteral antibiotic therapy do not appear to influence response rates for children with acute hematogenous osteomyelitis: a systematic review. BMC Infect Dis. 2002;2:16.)*

Antibiotic selection

The choice of empiric therapy is based upon the age of the child and any predisposing conditions (Table 47–4); however, empiric therapy should include coverage for *Staph. aureus* in all cases. For example, children with sickle cell disease also require coverage for *Salmonella*, those with varicella also require coverage for group A *Streptococcus*, and neonates also require coverage for group B *Streptococcus* and enteric gram-negative bacteria. Therapeutic agents used in MSSA osteomyelitis include the penicillinase-resistant penicillins (nafcillin, oxacillin, cloxacillin), first and second generation cephalosporins (cefazolin, cephalexin, cefuroxime) and clindamycin. For MRSA, clindamycin, vancomycin, and trimethoprim-sulfamethoxazole are used. It is reasonable to empirically treat patients for CA-MRSA when 10–15% of staphylococcal isolates are CA-MRSA, although there is no data to support any particular threshold.[75] In those areas where most CA-MRSA isolates are clindamycin susceptible, clindamycin is reasonable empiric coverage. For those areas where more isolates express constitutive or inducible resistance to clindamycin (inducible resistance as determined by the D-test), empiric therapy with vancomycin is recommended. Vancomycin should also be included in empiric therapy in critically ill children with musculoskeletal sepsis. Recommended doses of these antibiotics are found in Table 47–5.

There are little systematic data on the use of newer anti–gram-positive agents in osteomyelitis. Linezolid is an oxazolidinone antibiotic that is approved in children for the therapy of pneumonia and skin and soft tissue infections including those caused by MRSA.[76–78] There is limited experience, in adults, in its use in acute and chronic osteomyelitis.[79,80] It has the benefit of being available in an oral preparation for stepdown therapy. Daptomycin is another new agent with extremely limited experience in osteomyelitis[81,82] and no currently approved indications in children. Given the increasing incidence of CA-MRSA infections, however, there will be greater pressure for use of these agents in children in the future.

The final therapy chosen depends upon the organism isolated. Many cases of AHO are culture-negative (up to 50%) and empiric therapy must be continued. It is generally believed that most patients with culture negative disease have staphylococcal infection and patients with culture negative disease have been demonstrated to be cured with antistaphylococcal therapy (for MSSA or MRSA depending on the prevalence). Treatment of MSSA with first or second generation cephalosporins also provides empiric coverage for *Kingella*; however, the use of clindamycin and vancomycin for MRSA leaves potential *Kingella* infections untreated. In children with negative cultures, who have not improved adequately on empiric therapy, therapy should be changed to include coverage for MRSA, *Salmonella* or *Kingella* and additional imaging obtained (if not already done) to assess for subperiosteal or deep soft tissue abscess.

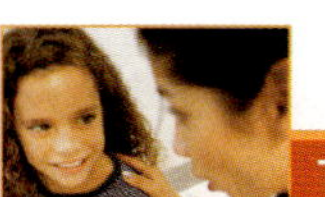

Table 47–4.

Likely Pathogens and Empiric Coverage for Osteomyelitis by Age

Age	Pathogens	Empiric Antibiotic Choices
Neonates	Group B *Streptococcus* *Staphylococcus aureus* Gram-negative rods Group A *Streptococcus*	Nafcillin or cefazolin or clindamycin or vancomycin and cefotaxime or gentamicin
≤2 years	*Staphylococcus aureus** *Kingella kingae* Group A *Streptococcus* *Streptococcus pneumoniae* *Salmonella* spp.	Nafcillin or cefazolin or clindamycin and vancomycin and ceftriaxone
>2 years	*Staphylococcus aureus** *Kingella kingae* Group A *Streptococcus* Salmonella spp.	Nafcillin or cefazolin or clindamycin or vancomycin and possibly ceftriaxone

**For methicillin-resistant* Staphylococcus. aureus, *additional options include linezolid or trimethoprim-sulfamethoxazole either alone or in combination with rifampin.*

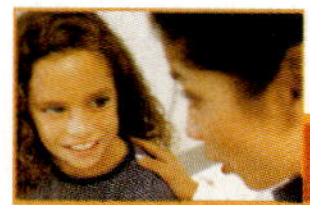

Table 47–5.

Recommended Antibiotic Doses for Osteomyelitis (Including Doses for Oral Stepdown Therapy)

Antibiotic	Recommended Dose (mg/kg/d)	Divided Daily Doses
Nafcillin	150	4
Cefazolin	150	3
Ceftriaxone	100	1–2
Cefotaxime	150	3
Clindamycin	30–40 IV or oral	3–4
Vancomycin	40–60	4
Gentamicin	5–7.5	3
Cephalexin	100–150	4
Cefuroxime	100	2
Linezolid	20–30	2–3

COMPLICATIONS

Subperiosteal and deep soft tissue abscess[8,22] and septic thrombophlebitis[24,83,84] are among the most common complications of AHO. Septic shock and necrotizing

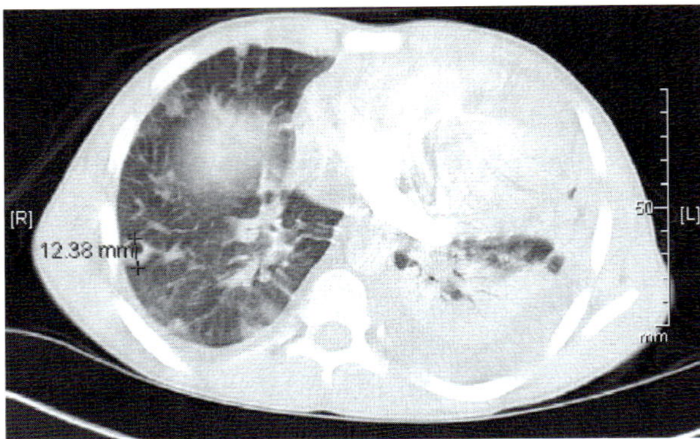

FIGURE 47–8 ■ CT scan of the chest of a patient with CA-MRSA osteomyelitis of the femur and occlusive clot (septic thrombophlebitis) of the right femoral vein. Extensive pneumonia of the left lung with pleural effusion. Patchy opacities with cavity formation on right consistent with septic emboli.

pneumonia are less common[8,23] (Figure 47–8). These complications are being identified more frequently with the emergence of CA-MRSA. Patients with CA-MRSA infection require a thorough evaluation for complications and multisystem infection. Chest tube or surgical drainage of complicated pleural effusion may be required. In addition, patients with septic thrombophlebitis may require anticoagulation and/or thrombolysis depending on the severity of the clot.[24,84]

SPECIAL CLINICAL SITUATIONS

Sickle Cell Disease

Children with sickle cell disease are at increased risk of serious bacterial infection including osteomyelitis. *Salmonella* infection is twice as common as *S. aureus* in this group of patients compared with otherwise healthy children with AHO.[32] Other gram-negative bacilli are overrepresented in this group as well. Painful, bony crises and osteomyelitis may be indistinguishable by history and clinical examination.[85] Unfortunately, there is no way to definitively distinguish infarct from osteomyelitis by imaging with plain film, bone scan, or MRI. Some advocate MRI with gadolinium[86] while others have used combined technetium bone scanning and sulfur colloid bone marrow scanning to distinguish between these conditions.[87] One should have a low threshold for biopsy or bone aspirate in the setting of a slow to resolve pain crisis. Patients require an empiric course of antibiotic therapy (including coverage for *Salmonella* spp.) when osteomyelitis cannot be ruled out. The optimal duration of therapy in this setting is unknown; a longer course (up to 6 weeks) with oral stepdown therapy is reasonable.

Neonatal Osteomyelitis

Osteomyelitis is an important infection among healthy term infants as well as sick and/or preterm infants requiring intensive care. Among healthy and sick newborns, osteomyelitis is one of the common manifestations of late-onset group B *Streptococcus* infection.[28,88] *S. aureus*, *S. pneumoniae* and enteric gram-negative bacilli comprise the majority of the remaining cases.[28,29] Children with group B *Streptococcus* osteomyelitis tend to have an uncomplicated clinical course with very little in the way of systemic inflammation.[28,88]

Osteomyelitis in the NICU setting may be hematogenous[89] or by direct inoculation heel puncture.[90,91] A multitude of pathogens may cause osteomyelitis in this setting including *S. aureus* (including CA-MRSA), enteric gram-negatives, coagulase-negative *Staphylococcus*, group B *Streptococcus* and *Candida* spp.[29,92–94]

Pelvic Osteomyelitis

Approximately 10% of AHO cases involve the bony pelvis with the ilium and ischium the most commonly affected.[1,37,95,96] Pelvic osteomyelitis may be misdiagnosed early in the course of infection as a septic hip or intra-abdominal infection/inflammation as a result of the poor localization of signs and symptoms; thus, it should be considered in the differential diagnosis of a febrile child with a limp or range of motion limitations of the hip.[94,95] The most useful clinical indicator of the site of infection is point tenderness. Diagnosis of this condition may be made promptly with scintigraphy, MRI or CT (which may be done to assess for intra-abdominal abscess, appendicitis, or deep muscle abscesss).

Vertebral Osteomyelitis and Diskitis

Vertebral osteomyelitis is much less common in children than in adults. It accounts for approximately 2% of all cases of AHO.[1,37] Like pelvic osteomyelitis, it may present in an insidious manner without back pain with nonspecific or constitutional symptoms only.[97,98] Typically, there will be no abnormality on plain X-ray early in the course of disease. The earliest sign of infection is narrowing of the disk space followed by loss of bone density in the aspect of the vertebral body closest to the cartilaginous plate. One may see involvement of two adjacent vertebrae. Index of suspicion is crucial for obtaining the appropriate imaging (bone scan or MRI). The advantage of MRI is the ability to detect epidural abscess which may complicate vertebral osteomyelitis.

Diskitis is a rare condition but an important differential diagnosis of vertebral osteomyelitis.[97,99,100] It is most common in the toddler age group. Diskitis and vertebral osteomyelitis may represent extremes of the same condition with differential clinical presentation between affected age groups secondary to developmental changes in the blood supply to the intervertebral disks and vertebrae. The clinical presentation is typically insidious with generalized fussiness progressing to limp or refusal to walk, crawl, or sit. Older children may complain of back pain. Constitutional symptoms and laboratory signs of inflammation may be mild or absent. Diagnosis is made by demonstrating a narrowed intervertebral disk space on plain X-ray, most commonly in the lumbar region, after about 2–3 weeks of symptoms. There may be associated erosion of adjacent vertebral end plates. MRI will demonstrate abnormalities in the disk and adjacent vertebrae if present and will assess for the presence of alternate diagnoses including spinal tumors and epidural abscess. An infectious etiology is hypothesized but many cultures are sterile and patients may recover without therapy. In children with positive cultures, *S. aureus* is the most common agent but *Kingella* and *Salmonella* are also reported. Diskitis is discussed in more detail in Chapter 49.

Nonhematogenous Osteomyelitis

Osteomyelitis may occur as a result of nonhematogenous infection of bone. This most commonly occurs following trauma, such as compound fractures,[101,102] puncture and bite wounds,[103] and surgery (orthopedic procedures or sternotomy), with or without prosthetic material.[4,104] It may also occur by spread from a contiguous focus of infection, for example infected decubitus[4,104] or neuropathic skin ulcers[4,104] or facial and skull base osteomyelitis from contiguous sinusitis, mastoiditis, or dental infection.[105]

Many patients present with indolent low-grade fever and pain.[4,104] Some will have more acute presentations with erythema and swelling of the site. There may be purulent drainage from a sinus tract or a poorly healing wound overlying the site of infection. Peripheral white blood cell count and ESR are not reliably elevated. Radiographic appearance is highly variable with chronic infections being more likely to demonstrate abnormalities on plain films. It may be difficult to distinguish overlying soft tissue inflammation from infected bone on technetium bone scanning. CT and MRI are useful for defining the extent of disease and associated soft tissue infection particularly in skull and facial osteomyelitis where infection may have spread intracranially.[105]

Cultures of sinus tract drainage are unreliable and bone or deep soft tissue biopsy is frequently required to determine the etiologic agent(s).[106,107] *S. aureus* is still among the most common pathogens, especially for sites contaminated during surgery, but the microbiology is defined by the location of the disease and its origin.[4] Polymicrobial infection is not uncommon. Treatment includes surgical debridement of infected bone and soft tissue along with prolonged antibiotic therapy up to 4–6 months for chronic infections. Most patients receive initial intravenous therapy with stepdown to oral antibiotics if appropriate agents are available.

Osteochondritis of the foot resulting from a puncture wound is a unique clinical syndrome. Infection occurs in a minority of individuals with puncture wounds, usually those occurring through a sneaker.[108] Onset of symptoms may be acute to subacute (up to 21 days). *Pseudomonas aeruginosa* is the most common pathogen in this condition although other gram-negative bacteria, such as *E. coli* and *Proteus* have been reported.[109–111] *S. aureus* is an occasional pathogen as well. This condition responds well to thorough surgical debridement and drainage of pus. Following this, 2 weeks of appropriate antibiotic therapy has been demonstrated to be sufficient. Parenteral antipseudomonal antibiotics including piperacillin, ticarcillin, and ceftazidime are appropriate initial agents. Step down therapy with ciprofloxacin should be considered.

Unusual organisms

A variety of unusual bacterial pathogens may cause osteomyelitis. Osteomyelitis is an atypical manifestation of cat-scratch disease, caused by *B. henselae.*[112,113] Sacroiliitis and spondylitis are common complications of brucellosis, a zoonosis acquired by the consumption of unpasteurized animal milk products.[114] *C. burnettii*, the agent of Q fever, is a rare cause of granulomatous osteomyelitis.[115]

Fungi may cause osteomyelitis in immunocompromised and competent hosts. Osteomyelitis caused by *Aspergillus* spp. is described in patients with chronic granulomatous disease[116,117] and hematologic malignancy.[118] Individuals with T-cell defects may develop osteomyelitis caused by *Cryptococcus* neoformans.[119,120] Osteomyelitis caused by *Candida* spp. occurs as a complication of candidemia.[121] In immunocompetent individuals, the endemic mycoses, geographically distinct, thermally dimorphic fungi, may cause osteomyelitis, with or without apparent pulmonary disease. This is significantly more common with blastomycosis[122,123] and coccidioidomycosis[124] than with histoplasmosis.[125]

Tuberculosis is a major cause of osteoarticular infections worldwide, although it is an uncommon manifestation in children.[126] The most frequently encountered musculoskeletal presentations of tuberculosis are vertebral (Pott's disease) and synovial. Solitary and multifocal bone lesions are uncommon in children but may involve almost any bone in the body, but the metaphyses of long bones are the most commonly involved. PPD and chest X-ray should be performed, although a negative PPD should not be used to rule out tuberculosis. Patients will have associated pulmonary disease only 50% of the time.

An unusual organism should be suspected in the setting of a subacute osteomyelitis not responding to antimicrobial therapy for typical pathogens. A high index of suspicion and knowledge of the epidemiology of these pathogens will lead to the diagnosis. Clues to the diagnosis will come from radiographs but pathologic examination of biopsies will be required in most cases. Definitive diagnosis is made by special stains and/or culture of the organism (fungal, tuberculous) or with serology (*Bartonella, Brucella, Coxiella, Coccidioides*).

Chronic Osteomyelitis

Chronic osteomyelitis occurs when there is vascular compromise as a result of infection in the vascular channels and bone necrosis occurs. The fragments of bone with pus are called sequestra while involucrum is the periosteal new bone that forms around the sequestrum. Bone necrosis may begin as early as 10 days into acute osteomyelitis and sequestrum and involucrum as early as 3 weeks. Infection of surrounding soft tissues ensues with the eventual formation of a sinus tract. These areas form a nidus for ongoing infection as necrotic bone is relatively impervious to antibiotic therapy.[3,12,127]

The diagnosis of chronic osteomyelitis is made with a typical history and with imaging.[2,104,128] Chronic osteomyelitis may occur after a recognized but incompletely treated episode of acute osteomyelitis or may result from the relentless progression of a low-grade, insidious infection with intermittent flares. The clinical presentation may be indistinguishable from benign and malignant bone tumors.[129] Radiologic imaging is helpful. Plain radiography, CT, and MRI may reveal the features of sequestrum, involucrum, and/or abscess that indicate the presence of infection.[12,104,127–130] Definitive diagnosis rests with biopsy and culture of bone. Sinus tract cultures are unreliable and reveal a different organism from bone approximately 60–70% of the time.[106,107,131] Only the presence of *S. aureus* in a sinus tract culture appears to be reasonably predictive of the bone culture result.[107,131]

S. aureus is the most common organism isolated from chronic osteomyelitis; however, many other organisms may be identified including streptococci, gram-negatives, including *Pseudomonas* and anaerobic organisms such as *Bacteroides*. Polymicrobial infection, especially trauma-related, is not uncommon.[3,104,128,131,132]

Treatment of chronic osteomyelitis often requires a combination of surgical and medical therapy. Many orthopedic experts advocated extensive debridement of bone and soft tissue, leaving behind only bleeding healthy tissue. The dead space is filled with a muscle flap, bone graft, or antibiotic impregnated polymethyl methacrylate beads.[127,129,133,134] This is accompanied by antibiotic therapy targeting the isolated organism (or the organism known to have caused the primary infection) or empiric therapy to cover the most likely organisms in the event of sterile cultures. With the broad array of potential pathogens, reasonable empiric coverage for situation where polymicrobial disease is likely is clindamycin and ciprofloxacin as it provides broad spectrum gram-positive, gram-negative, and anaerobic coverage. The appropriate duration of antimicrobial therapy for chronic osteomyelitis is unknown. Six weeks of antibiotics is felt to be sufficient when surgery has been extensive and necrotic bone fully debrided.[3,132] The data in children is limited but medical therapy alone has been used to successfully treat chronic osteomyelitis without radiographic evidence of sequestrum or pus.[3,104,130,132,135] Longer courses of treatment, up to 4–6 months, may be used when surgical debridement is limited or absent. It is reasonable to use oral stepdown therapy in this setting, provided appropriate oral agents are available for the isolated organisms.

Chronic recurrent multifocal osteomyelitis (CRMO)

CRMO is an inflammatory bone disease that resembles infectious osteomyelitis but no infectious agent can be identified in cultures of biopsies.[136,137] It is characterized by recurrent and remittent pain and swelling in the affected bones. There may be single or multiple, symmetric, or asymmetric sites of involvement at any time. Flares may be associated with fever and elevated acute phase reactants. The most common sites of involvement are the metaphyses of long bones as in AHO; the presence of lesions on the clavicle or vertebral bodies should raise the suspicion of CRMO. Radiographic abnormalities consist of radiolucent lesions with sclerosis consistent with acute and chronic osteomyelitis. The etiology is unknown and pathologic examination reveals acute and chronic inflammatory changes. It is frequently associated with other inflammatory conditions including psoriasis, palmoplantar pustulosis, pyoderma gangrenosum, and inflammatory bowel disease.[138,139] There are no randomized controlled trials of treatment modalities but steroids and nonsteroidal antiinflammatories have been used with success to control symptoms. Gamma interferon has been used with favorable outcomes in a few patients.[140] While the outcome of CRMO is generally good, some patients have a prolonged disease course with a significant impact on quality of life.[141]

REFERENCES

1. Dich VQ, Nelson JD, Haltalin KC. Osteomyelitis in infants and children: a review of 163 cases. *Am J Dis Child.* 1975;129:1273-1278.

2. Gonzalez-Lopez JL, Sleto-Martin FJ, Cubillo-Martin A, et al. Subactue osteomyelitis in children. *J Pediatr Orthop.* 2001;120:101-104.
3. Cole WG. The management of chronic osteomyelitis. *Clin Orthop Relat Res.* 1991:84-89.
4. Dubey L, Krasinski K, Hernana-Schulman M. Osteomyelitis secondary to trauma or infected contiguous soft tissue. *Pediatr Infect Dis J.* 1988;7:26-34.
5. Dahl LB, Høyland A-L, Dramsdahl H, Kaaresen PI. Acute osteomyelitis in children: a population-based retrospective study 1965-1994. *Scand J Infect Dis.* 1998;30: 573-577.
6. Craigen MAC, Watters J, Hackett JS. The changing epidemiology of osteomyelitis in children. *J Bone Joint Surg Br.* 1992;74:541-545.
7. Blyth MJG, Kincaid R, Craigen MAC, Bennet GC. The changing epidemiology of acute and subacute haematogenous osteomyelitis in children. *J Bone Joint Surg Br.* 2001;83(1):99-102.
8. Arnold SR, Elias D, Buckingham SC, et al. Changing patterns of acute hematogenous osteomyelitis and septic arthitis: emergence of community associated methicillin resistant *Staphylococcus aureus. J Pediatr Orthop.* 2006; I26:703-708.
9. Scott RJ, Christofersen MR, Robertson WW, Davidson RS, Rankin L, Drummond DS. Acute osteomyelitis in children: a review of 116 cases. *J Pediatr Orthop.* 1990;10:649-652.
10. Floyed RL, Steele RW. Culture-negative osteomyelitis. *Pediatr Infect Dis J.* 2003;22:731-735.
11. Karwowska A, Davies HD, Jadavji T. Epidemiology and outcome of osteomyelitis in the era of sequential intravenous-oral therapy. *Pediatr Infect Dis J.* 1998;17: 1021-1026.
12. Lew DP, Waldvogel FA. Osteomyelitis. *Lancet.* 2004; 364:369-379.
13. Nixon GW. Hematogenous osteomyelitis of metaphyseal-equivalent locations. *Am J Roentgenol.* 1978;130: 123-129.
14. Norden CW. Lessons learned from animal models of osteomyelitis. *Rev Infect Dis.* 1988;10:103-110.
15. Rosenbaum DM, Blumhagen JD. Acute epiphyseal osteomyelitis in children. *Radiology.* 1985;156:89-92.
16. Perlman MH, Patzakis MJ, Kumar JP, Holtom PD. The incidence of joint involvement with adjacent osteomyelitis in pediatric patients. *J Pediatr Orthop.* 2000;20:40-43.
17. Feigin RD, Pickering LK, Anderson D, Keeney RE, Shackleford PG. Clindamycin treatment of osteomyelitis and septic arthritis in children. *Pediatrics.* 1975;55: 213-223.
18. Cole WG, Dalziel RE, Leitl S. Treatment of acute osteomyelitis in childhood. *J Bone Joint Surg Br.* 1982;64:218-223.
19. Gillespie WJ, Mayo KM. The management of acute haematogenous osteomyelitis in the antibiotic era. A study of the outcome. *J Bone Joint Surg Br.* 1981;63: 126-131.
20. Moumile K, Merckx J, Glorion C, Pouliquen JC, Berche P, Ferroni A. Bacterial aetiology of acute osteoarticular infections in children. *Acta Paediatr.* 2005;94:419-422.
21. Nelson JD, Bucholz RW, Kunmiesz H, Shelton S. Benefits and risks of sequential parenteral-oral cephalosporin therapy for suppurative bone and joint infections. *J Pediatr Orthop.* 1982;2:255-262.
22. Martinez-Aguilar G, Avalos-Mishaan A, Hulten K, Hammerman W, Mason EO, Kaplan SL. Community-acquired, methicillin-resistant and methicillin-susceptible *Staphylococcus aureus* musculoskeletal infections in children. *Pediatr Infect Dis J.* 2004;23:701-706.
23. Gonzalez BE, Martinez-Aguilar G, Hulten KG, et al. Severe staphylococcal sepsis in adolescents in the era of community-acquired methicillin-resistant *Staphylococcus aureus. Pediatrics.* 2005;115:642-648.
24. Crary SE, Buchanan GR, Drake CE, Journeycake JM. Venous thrombosis and thromboembolism in children with osteomyelitis. *J Pediatr.* 2006;149:537-541.
25. Costerton W, Veeh R, Shirtliff M, Pasmore M, Post C, Ehrlich G. The application of biofilm science to the study and control of chronic bacterial infections. *J Clin Invest.* 2003;112:1466-1477.
26. Gresham HD, Lowrance JH, Caver TE, Wilson BS, Cheung AL, Lindberg FP. Survival of *Staphylococcus aureus* inside neutrophils contributes to infection. *J Immunol.* 2000;164:3713-3722.
27. Ibia EO, Imoisili M, Pikis A. Group A β-hemolytic streptococcal osteomyelitis in children. *Pediatrics.* 2003;112: e22-e26.
28. Edwards MS, Baker CJ, Wagner ML, Taber LH, Barrett FF. An etiologic shift in infantile osteomyelitis: the emergence of the group B Streptococcus. *J Pediatr.* 1978;93:578-583.
29. Wong M, Isaacs D, Howman-Giles R, Uren R. Clinical and diagnostic features of osteomyelitis occurring in the first three months of life. *Pediatr Infect Dis J.* 1995;14: 1047-1053.
30. Bradley JS, Kaplan SL, Tan TQ, et al. Pediatric pneumococcal bone and joint infections. *Pediatrics.* 1998;102: 1376-1382.
31. Bowerman SG, Green NE, Mencio GA. Decline of bone and joint infections attributable to *Haemophilus influenzae* type b. *Clin Orthop Relat Res.* 1997:128-133.
32. Burnett MW, Bass JW, Cook BA. Etiology of osteomyelitis complicating sickle cell disease. *Pediatrics.* 1998;101: 296-297.
33. Jaberi FM, Shahcheraghi GH, Ahadzadeh M. Short-term intravenous antibiotic treatment of acute hematogenous bone and joint infection in children: a prospective randomized trial. *J Pediatr Orthop.* 2002;22:317-320.
34. Verdier I, Gayet-Ageron A, Ploton C, et al. Contribution of a broad range polymerase chain reaction to the diagnosis of osteoarticular infecitons caused by *Kingella kingae. Pediatr Infect Dis J.* 2005;24:692-696.
35. Yagupsky P, Dagan R, Howard CB, Einhorn M, Kassis I, Simu A. Clinical features and epidemiology of invasive *Kingella kingae* infections in Southern Israel. *Pediatrics.* 1993;92:800-804.
36. Chometon S, Benito Y, Chaker M, et al. Specific real-time polymerase chain reaction places *Kingella kingae* as the most common cause of osteoarticular infections in young children. *Pediatr Infect Dis J.* 2007;26: 377-381.
37. Faden H, Grossi M. Acute osteomyelitis in children. Reassessment of etiologic agents and their clinical characteristics. *Am J Dis Child.* 1991;145:65-69.

38. Dahl LB, Høyland A-L, Dramshahl H, Kaaresen PI. Acute osteomyelitis in children: a population-based retrospective study 1965-1994. *Scand J Infect Dis.* 1998;30:573-577.
39. Diep BA, Sensabaugh GF, Somboona NS, Carleton HA, Perdreau-Remington F. Widespread skin and soft-tissue infections due to two methicillin-resistant *Staphylococcus aureus* strains harboring the genes for Panton-Valentine leucocidin. *J Clin Microbiol.* 2004;42:2080-2084.
40. Dietrich DW, Auld DB, Mermel LA. Community-acquired methicillin-resistant *Staphylococcus aureus* in southern New England children. *Pediatrics.* 2004;113:e347-e352.
41. Fergie JE, Purcell K. Community-acquired methicillin-resistant *Staphylococcus aureus* infections in South Texas children. *Pediatr Infect Dis J.* 2001;20:860-863.
42. Fridkin SK, Hageman JC, Morrison M, et al. Methicillin-resistant *Staphylococcus aureus* disease in three communities. *N Engl J Med.* 2005;352:1436-1444.
43. Gonzalez BE, Martinez-Aguilar G, Hulten KG, et al. Severe staphylococcal sepsis in adolescents in the era of community-acquired methicillin-resistant *Staphylococcus aureus. Pediatrics.* 2005;115:642-648.
44. Arnold SR, Elias D, Buckingham SC, et al. Changing patterns of acute hematogenous osteomyelitis and septic arthritis emergence of community-associated methicillin-resistant *Staphylococcus aureus. J Pediatr Orthop.* 2006;26:703-708.
45. Naimi TS, LeDell KH, Como-Sabetti K, et al. Comparison of community- and health care-associated methicillin-resistant *Staphylococcus aureus* infection. *JAMA.* 2003;290:2976-2984.
46. Vandenesch F, Naimi T, Enright MC, et al. Community-acquired methicillin-resistant *Staphylococcus aureus* carrying Panton-Valentine leukocidin genes: worldwide emergence. *Emerg Infect Dis.* 2003;9:978-984.
47. Voyich JM, Otto M, Mathema B, et al. Is Panton-Valentine leukocidin the major virulence determinant in community-associated methicillin-resistant *Staphylococcus aureus* disease? *J Infect Dis.* 2006;194:1761-1770.
48. Martinez-Aguilar G, Hammerman WA, Mason EOJ, Kaplan SL. Clindamycin treatment of invasive infections caused by community-acquired, methicillin-resistant and methicillin-susceptible *Staphylococcus aureus* in children. *Pediatr Infect Dis J.* 2003;22:593-598.
49. Unkila-Kallio L, Kallio MJT, Eskola J, Peltola H. Serum C-reactive protein, erythrocyte sedimentation rate, and white blood cell count in acute hematogenous osteomyelitis of children. *Pediatrics.* 1994;93:59-62.
50. Khachatourians AG, Patzakis MJ, Roidis N, Holtom PD. Laboratory minotoring in pediatric acute osteomyelitis and septic arthritis. *Clin Orthop Relat Res.* 2003:186-194.
51. Peltola H, Unkila Kallio L, Kallio MT, Aalto K, Anttolainen I, Fagerholm R. Simplified treatment of acute staphylococcal osteomyelitis of childhood. *Pediatrics.* 1997;99:846-850.
52. Unkila Kallio L, Kallio MJT, Peltola H. The usefulness of c-reactive protein levles in the identification of concurrent septic arthritis in children who have acute hematogenou osteomeelitis. A comparison with the usefulness of the erythrocyte sedimentation rate and the white blood-cell count. *J Bone Joint Surg Am.* 1994;76-A:848-853.
53. Capitanio MA, Kirkpatrick JA. Early roentgen observations in acute osteomyelitis. *Am J Roentgenol.* 1970;108:488-496.
54. Majd M, Frankel RS. Radionclide imaging in skeletal inflammatory and ischemic disease in children. *Am J Roentgenol.* 1976;126:832-841.
55. Treves S, Khettry J, Broker FH, Wilkinson RH, Watts H. Osteomyelitis: early scintigraphic detection in children. *Pediatrics.* 1976;57:173-186.
56. Gilday DL, Paul DJ, Paterson J. Diagnosis of osteomyelitis in children by combined blood pool and bone imaging. *Radiology.* 1975;117:331-335.
57. Tuson CE, Hoffman EB, Mann MD. Isotope bone scanning for acute osteomyelitis and septic arthritis in children. *J Bone Joint Surg Br.* 1994;76(2):306-310.
58. Howie DW, Savage JP, Wilson TG, Paterson D. The technetium phosphate bone scan in the diagnosis of osteomyelitis in childhood. *J Bone Joint Surg Am.* 1983;65:431-437.
59. Handmaker H. Acute hematogenous osteomyelitis: has the bone scan betrayed us? *Radiology.* 1979;135:787-789.
60. Hamdan J, Asha M, Mallouh A, Usta H, Talab Y, Ahmad M. Technetium bone scintigraphy in the diagnosis of osteomyelitis in children. *Pediatr Infect Dis J.* 1987;6:529-532.
61. Jones DC, Cady RB. "Cold" bone scans in acute osteomyelitis. *J Bone Joint Surg Br.* 1981;63-B(3):376-378.
62. Wald ER, Mirro R, Gartner JC. Pitfalls in the diagnosis of acute osteomyelitis by bone scan. *Clin Pediatr (Phila).* 1980;19:597-601.
63. Schauwecker DS. The scintigraphic diagnosis of osteomyelitis. *Am J Roentgenol.* 1992;158:9-18.
64. Howard CB, Einhorn M, Dagan R, Nyska M. Ultrasound in diagnosis and management of acute haematogenous osteomyelitis in children. *J Bone Joint Surg Br.* 1993;75(1):79-82.
65. Gold RH, Hawkins RA, Katz RD. Bacterial osteomyelitis: findings on plain radiography, CT, MR, and scintigraphy. *Am J Roentgenol.* 1991;157:365-370.
66. Mazur JM, Ross G, Cummings RJ, Hahn GA, McCluskey WP. Usefulness of magnetic resonance imaging for the diagnosis of acute msuculoskeletal infections in children. *J Pediatr Orthop.* 1995;15:144-147.
67. Connolly LP, Connolly SA, Drubach LA, Jaramillo D, Treves ST. Acute Hematogenous Osteomyelitis of Children: assessment of skeletal scintigraphy-based diagnosis in the era of MRI. *J Nucl Med.* 2002;43:1310-1316.
68. Syrogiannopoulos GA, Nelson JD. Duration of antimicrobial therapy for acute suppurative osteoarticular infections. *Lancet.* 1988;1(8575-8576):37-40.
69. Tetzlaff TR, Howard JB, McCracken GH, Calderon E, Larrondo J. Antibiotic concentrations in pus and bone of children with osteomyelitis. *J Pediatr.* 1978;92:135-140.
70. Prober CG, Yeager AS. Use of the serum bactericidal titer to assess the adequacy of oral antibiotic therapy in the treatment of acute hematogenous osteomyelitis. *J Pediatr.* 1979;95:131-135.
71. Bachur R, Pagon Z. Success of short-course parenteral antibiotic therapy for acute osteomyelitis of childhood. *Clin Pediatr (Phila).* 2007;46:30-35.

72. Daver NG, Shelburne SA, Atmar RL, et al. Oral step-down therapy is comparable to intravenous therapy for *Staphylococcus aureus* osteomyelitis. *J Infect.* 2007;54: 539-544.
73. Ruebner R, Keren R, Coffin S, Chu J, Horn D, Zaoutis TE. Complications of central venous catheters used for the treatment of acute hematogenous osteomyelitis. *Pediatrics.* 2006;117:1210-1215.
74. Le Saux N, Howard A, Barrowman N, Gaboury I, Sampson M, Moher D. Shorter courses of parenteral antibiotic therapy do not appear to influence response rates for children with acute hematogenous osteomyelitis: a systematic review. *BMC Infect Dis.* 2002;2:16.
75. Kaplan SL. Treatment of community-associated methicillin-resistant *Staphylococcus aureus* infections. *Pediatr Infect Dis J.* 2005;24:457-458.
76. Jantausch BA, Deville J, Adler S, et al. Linezolid for the treatment of children with bacteremia or nosocomial pneumonia caused by resistant Gram-positive bacterial pathogens. *Pediatr Infect Dis J.* 2003;22:S164-S171.
77. Kaplan SL, Afghani B, Lopez P, et al. Linezolid for the treatment of methicillin-resistant *Staphylococcus aureus* infections in children. *Pediatr Infect Dis J.* 2003;22: S178-S185.
78. Yogev R, Patterson LE, Kaplan SL, et al. Linezolid for the treatment of complicated skin and skin structure infections in children. *Pediatr Infect Dis J.* 2003;22: S172-S177.
79. Rao N, Ziran BH, Hall RA, Santa ER. Successful treatment of chronic bone and joint infections with oral linezolid. *Clin Orthop Relat Res.* 2004;427:67-71.
80. Falagas ME, Siempos II, Papagelopoulos PJ, Vardakas KZ. Linezolid for the treatment of adults with bone and joint infections. *Int J Antimicrob Agents.* 2007;29: 233-239.
81. Marty FM, Yeh WW, Wennersten CB, et al. Emergence of a clinical daptomycin-resistant *staphylococcus aureus* isolate during treatment of methicillin-resistant *staphylococcus aureus* bacteremia and osteomyelitis. *J Clin Microbiol.* 2006;44:595-597.
82. Vikram HR, Havill NL, Koeth LM, Boyce JM. Clinical progression of methicillin-resistant *Staphylococcus aureus* vertebral osteomyelitis associated with reduced susceptibility to daptomycin. *J Clin Microbiol.* 2005;43: 5384-5387.
83. Jupiter JB, Ehrlich MG, Novelline RA, Leeds HC, Keim D. The association of septic thromobophlebitis with subperiosteal abscesses in children. *J Pediatr.* 1982; 101:690-695.
84. Gorenstein A, Gross E, Houri S, Gewirts G, Katz S. The pivotal role of deep vein thrombophlebitis in the development of acute disseminated staphylococcal disease in children. *Pediatrics.* 2000;106:e87.
85. Wong AL, Sakamoto KM, Johnson EE. Differentiating osteomyelitis from bone infarction in sickle cell disease. *Pediatr Emerg Care.* 2001;17:60-63.
86. Umans H, Haramati N, Flusser G. The diagnostic role of gadolinium enhanced MRI in distinguishing between acute medully bone infarct and osteomyelitis. *J Magn Reson Imaging.* 2000;18:255-262.
87. Skaggs DL, Kim SK, Greene NW, Harris D, Miller JH. Differentiation between bone infarction and acute osteomyelitis in children with sickle-cell disease with use of sequential radionuclide bone-marrow and bone scans. *J Bone Joint Surg Am.* 2001;83:1810-1813.
88. Memon IA, Jacobs NM, Yeh TR, Lilien LD. Group B streptococcal osteomyelitis and septic arthritis: its occurrence in infants less than 2 months old. *Am J Dis Child.* 1979;133:921-923.
89. Williamson JB, Galasko CS, Robinson MJ. Outcome after acute osteomyelitis in preterm infants. *Arch Dis Child.* 1990;65:1060-1062.
90. Abril Martin JC, Aguilar Rodriguez L, Albinana Cilveti J. Flatfoot and calcaneal deformity secondary to osteomyelitis after neonatal heel puncture. *J Pediatr Orthop Part B.* 1999;8:122-124.
91. Lilien LD, Harris VJ, Ramamurthy RS. Neonatal osteomyelitis of the calcaneus: complication of heel puncture. *J Pediatr.* 1976;88:478-480.
92. Harris MC, Pereira GR, Myers MD, et al. Candidal arthritis in infants previously treated for systemic candidiasis during the newborn period: report of three cases. *Pediatr Emerg Care.* 2000;16:249-251.
93. Korakaki E, Aligizakis A, Manoura A, et al. Methicillin-resistant *Staphylococcus aureus* osteomyelitis and septic arthritis in neonates: diagnosis and management. *Jpn J Infect Dis.* 2007;60:129-131.
94. Eggink BH, Rowen JL. Primary osteomyelitis and suppurative arthritis caused by coagulase-negative staphylococci in a preterm neonate. *Pediatr Infect Dis J.* 2003;22:572-573.
95. Edwards MS, Baker CJ, Granberry WM, Barrett FF. Pelvic osteomyelitis in children. *Pediatrics.* 1978;61:62-67.
96. Mustafa MM, Saez-LLorens X, McCracken GH, Nelson JD. Acute hematogenous pelvic osteomyelitis in infants and children. *Pediatr Infect Dis J.* 1990;9:416-421.
97. Fernandez M, Carrol CL, Baker CJ. Discitis and vertebral osteomyelitis in children: an 18-year review. *Pediatrics.* 2000;105:1299-1304.
98. Correa AG, Edwards MS, Baker CJ. Vertebral osteomyelitis in children. *Pediatr Infect Dis J.* 1993;12:228-233.
99. Cushing AH. Diskitis in children. *Clin Infect Dis.* 1993;17:1-6.
100. Brown R, Hussain M, McHugh K, Novelli M, Jones D. Discitis in young children. *J Bone Joint Surg Br.* 2001;83-B:106-111.
101. Beals RK, Bryant RE. The treatment of chronic open osteomyelitis of the tibia in adults. *Clin Orthop Relat Res.* 2005;433:212-217.
102. Zalavras CG, Patzakis MJ, Holtom P. Local antibiotic therapy in the treatment of open fractures and osteomyelitis. *Clin Orthop Relat Res.* 2004;427:86-93.
103. Benson LS, Edwards SL, Schiff AP, Williams CS, Visotsky JL. Dog and cat bites to the hand: treatment and cost assessment. *J Hand Surg.* 2006;31:468-473.
104. Auh JS, Binns HJ, Katz BZ. Retropsective assessment of subactue and chronic osteomyelitis in children and young adults. *Clin Pediatr.* 2004;43:549-555.
105. Prasad KC, Prasad SC, Mouli N, Agarwal S. Osteomyelitis of the head and neck. *Acta Otolaryngol.* 2007;127: 194-205.
106. Mackowiak PA, Jones SR, Smith JW. Diagnostic value of sinus-tract cultures in chronic osteomyelitis. *JAMA.* 1978;239:2272-2275.

107. Zuluaga AF, Galvis W, Jaimes F, Vesga O. Lack of microbiological concordance between bone and non-bone specimens in chronic osteomyelitis: an observational study. *BMC Infect Dis.* 2002;2:1-7.
108. Eidelman M, Bialik V, Miller Y, Kassis I. Plantar puncture wounds in children: analysis of 80 hospitalized patients and late sequelae. *Isr Med Assoc J.* 2003;5:268-271.
109. Brand RA, Black H. *Pseudomonas* osteomyelitis following puncture wounds in children. *J Bone Joint Surg Am.* 1974;56-A:1637-1642.
110. Jacobs RF, Adelman L, Sack CM, Wilson CB. Management of *Pseudomonas* osteochondritis complicating puncture wounds of the foot. *Pediatrics.* 1982;69: 432-435.
111. Miller EH, Semian DW. Gram-negative osteomyelitis following puncture wounds of the foot. *J Bone Joint Surg Am.* 1975;57-A:535-537.
112. Vermeulen MJ, Rutten GJ, Verhagen I, Peeters MF, van Dijken PJ. Transient paresis associated with cat-scratch disease: case report and literature review of vertebral osteomyelitis caused by *Bartonella henselae. Pediatr Infect Dis J.* 2001;25:1177-1181.
113. de Kort JG, Robben SG, Schrander JJ, van Rhijn LW. Multifocal osteomyelitis in a child: a rare manifestation of cat scratch disease: a case report and systematic review of the literature. *J Pediatr Orthop B.* 2006;15: 285-288.
114. Gottesman G, Vanunu D, Maayan MC, et al. Childhood Brucellosis in Israel. *Pediatr Infect Dis J.* 1996;15:610-615.
115. Nourse C, Allworth A, Jones A, et al. Three cases of Q fever osteomyelitis in children and a review of the literature. *Clin Infect Dis.* 2004;39:e61.
116. Pasic S, Abinun M, Pistignjat B, et al. Aspergillus osteomyelitis in chronic granulomatous disease: treatment with recombinant gamma-interferon and itraconazole. *Pediatr Infect Dis J.* 1996;15:833-834.
117. Dotis J, Roilides E. Osteomyelitis due to *Aspergillus* spp. in patients with chronic granulomatous disease: comparison of Aspergillus nidulans and Aspergillus fumigatus. *Int J Infect Dis.* 2004;8:103-110.
118. Flynn PM, Magill HL, Jenkins JJ, Pearson T, Crist WM, Hughes WT. *Aspergillus* osteomyelitis in a child treated for acute lymphoblastic leukemia. *Pediatr Infect Dis J.* 1990;9:733-736.
119. Murphy SN, Parnell N. Fluconazole treatment of cryptococcal rib osteomyelitis in an HIV-negative man. A case report and review of the literature. *J Infect.* 2005;51: e309-e311.
120. Liu PY. Cryptococcal osteomyelitis: case report and review. *Diagn Microbiol Infect Dis.* 1998;30:33-35.
121. Hendrickx L, Van Wijngaerden E, Samson I, Peetermans WE. Candidal vertebral osteomyelitis: report of 6 patients, and a review. *Clin Infect Dis.* 2001;32:527-533.
122. Oppenheimer M, Embil JM, Black B, et al. Blastomycosis of bones and joints. *South Med J.* 2007;100:570-578.
123. Morris SK, Brophy J, Richardson SE, et al. Blastomycosis in Ontario, 1994-2003. *Emerg Infect Dis.* 2006;12: 274-279.
124. Holley K, Muldoon M, Tasker S. *Coccidioides immitis* osteomyelitis: a case series review. *Orthopedics.* 2002;25: 827-831.
125. Palmgren BA, Buhr BR. Histoplasmosis of the tibia. *Orthopedics.* 2005;28:67-68.
126. Rasool MN. Osseous manifestations of tuberculosis in children. *J Pediatr Orthop.* 2001;21:749-755.
127. Parsons B, Strauss E. Surgical management of chronic osteomyelitis. *Am J Surg.* 2004;188:57S-66S.
128. Yeargan SAI, Nakasone CK, Shaieb MD, Montgomery WP, Reinker KA. Treatment of chronic osteomyelitis in children resistant to previous therapy. *J Pediatr Orthop.* 2004;24:109-122.
129. Shih H-N, Shih LY, Wong Y-C. Diagnosis and treatment of subacute osteomyelitis. *J Trauma.* 2005;58:83-87.
130. Reinehr T, BuMichel E, Andler W. Chronic osteomyelitis in childhood: is surgery always indicated? *Infection.* 2000;28:282-286.
131. Zuluaga AF, Galvis W, Saldarriaga JG, Agudelo M, Salazar BE, Vesga O. Etiologic diagnosis of chronic osteomyelitis: a prospective study. *Arch Intern Med.* 2006;166:95-100.
132. Ross ER, Cole WG. Treatment of subacute osteomyelitis in childhood. *J Bone Joint Surg Br.* 1985;67:443-448.
133. Rhomberg M, Frischhut B, Ninkovic M, Schwabegger AH, Ninkovic M. A single-stage operation in the treatment of chronic osteomyelitis of the lower extremity including reconstruction with free vascularized iliac bone graft and free-tissue transfer. *Plast Reconstr Surg.* 2003;11:2353-2361.
134. Steinlechner CWB, Mkandawire NC. Non-vascrularised fibular transfer in the management of defects of long bones after sequestrectomy in children. *J Bone Joint Surg Br.* 2005;87-B:1259-1263.
135. Ezra E, Cohen N, Segev E, et al. Primary subacute epiphyseal osteomyelitis: role of conservative treatment. *J Pediatr Orthop.* 2002;22:333-337.
136. Schultz C, Holterhus PM, Seidel A, et al. Chronic recurrent multifocal osteomyelitis in children. *Pediatr Infect Dis J.* 1999;18:1008-1013.
137. King SM, Laxer RM, Manson D, Gold R. Chronic recurrent multifocal osteomyelitis: a noninfectious inflammatory process. *Pediatr Infect Dis J.* 1987;6:907-911.
138. Eyrich GKH, Harder C, Sailer HF, Langengegger T, Bruder E, Michel BA. Primary chronic osteomyelitis associated with synovitis, acne, pustulosis, hyperostosis and osteitis (SAPHO syndrome). *J Oral Pathol Med.* 1999;28:456-464.
139. Omidi CJ, Siegfried EC. Chronic recurrent multifocal osteomyelitis preceding pyodermal gangrenosum and occult ulcerative colitis in a pediatric patient. *Pediatr Dermatol.* 1998;15:435-438.
140. Gallagher KT, Roberts RL, MacFarlane JA, Stiehm R. Treatment of chronic recurrent multifocal osteomyelitis with interferon gamma. *J Pediatr.* 1997;131:470-472.
141. Huber AM, Lam P-Y, Duffy CM, et al. Chronic recurrent multifocal osteomyelitis: clinical outcomes after more than 5 years of follow-up. *J Pediatr.* 2002;141:198-203.

CHAPTER 48

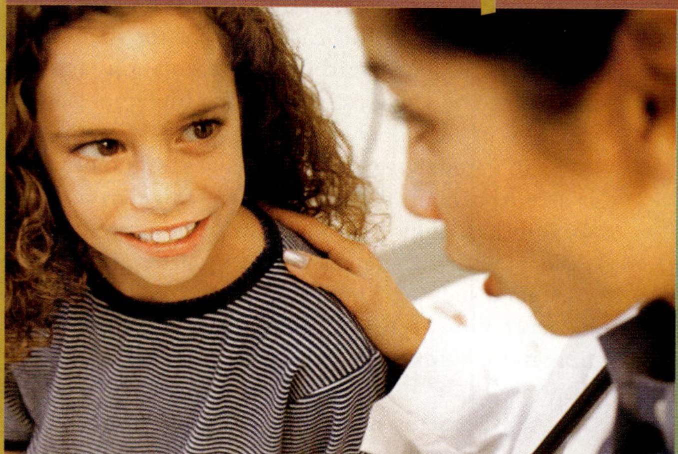

Septic Arthritis

Pablo Yagupsky

DEFINITION AND EPIDEMIOLOGY

Septic, pyogenic, and suppurative arthritis are the names given to the inflammation of the joint space caused by the presence of bacteria or fungi. Septic arthritis is more common in childhood than in any other period of human life and more than half of cases are diagnosed in individuals younger than 20 years of age. Since septic arthritis usually has a hematogenous origin, the age distribution of pediatric patients with joint infection is markedly skewed, reflecting the increased attack rate of bacteremia in early childhood. In a large series of 725 pediatric patients with joint infections compiled by Trujillo and Nelson, 52% of the children were younger than 2 years, 25% were aged 2–5 years, 15% were 6–10 years old, and the remaining 6% were aged 11–15 years.[1] Since a significant fraction of suspected cases of septic arthritis remains bacteriologically unconfirmed, the true incidence of the disease is uncertain. The estimate annual incidence of the disease in the general population ranges between 2 and 10 cases per 100,000.[2] Several pediatric subpopulations are at increased risk for septic arthritis, as summarized in Table 48–1.

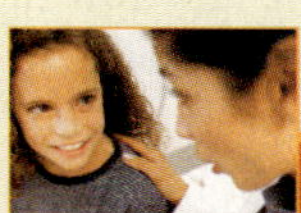

Table 48–1.

Conditions Associated with Increased Risk for Pediatric Septic Arthritis

Immunodeficiencies
Unvaccinated children
Rheumatoid arthritis
Crystal-induced arthritis
Sexually active adolescents
Intravenous drug abusers
Prematurity
Sensory neuropathies

PATHOGENESIS

The highly vascular synovial tissue lacks a limiting basement membrane, enabling easy access of circulating bacteria to the joint space during an episode of bacteremia. Once organisms have penetrated into the joint, the low fluid shear conditions facilitate microbial adherence. Occasionally, septic arthritis results by direct inoculation of bacteria in the joint by penetrating trauma, bites, intra-articular injections (particularly corticosteroids) or a surgical procedure. In neonates and young infants, bacteria may migrate from an adjacent focus of osteomyelitis into the joint traversing through capillaries that cross the metaphyseal growth plate. This capillary network recedes between 6 and 9 months of age and in the older child only the metaphyses of the hip, shoulder, and ankle bones remain intracapsular.[3]

A variety of bacterial adhesins have been implicated in anchoring organisms to the synovial layer, which explains the virulence and tropism exhibited by bacteria such as *Staphylococcus aureus*, *Streptococcus agalactiae* (group B), *Nesisseria gonorrhoeae*, and *Borrelia burgdorferi*. These adherence-promoting molecules, termed microbial surface components recognizing adhesive matrix molecules, have been best studied in *S. aureus* and include, among others, fibrinogen-, fibronectin-, and elastin-binding proteins, a collagen receptor, and an adhesin with wide specificity. Mutations in the genes encoding for these proteins markedly reduce or abolish the capability of the organism to cause septic arthritis in animal models.[3]

Trauma may facilitate the entrance of circulating bacteria into the joint space caused by increased local vascularization, whereas high concentration of a diversity of protein fibers in the synovial fluid after surgery may promote bacterial adherence to the tissue. The important role played by antecedent trauma is well exemplified by the propensity of *S. agalactiae* to invade the shoulder in newborns delivered in cervical presentation, and the occurrence of septic arthritis of the hip among those delivered in breech presentation.

In a minority of cases the host's immune system is able to contain the infection and this may account for transient arthralgias and arthritis observed in some patients with bacteremia caused by pathogens of low virulence such as *Kingella kingae*.[4,5] In most cases, however, the infection progresses and organisms multiply in the joint space to elicit an acute inflammatory response.

Both bacterial virulence factors and the host immune response appear to contribute to the progressive destruction of joint architecture in patients with septic arthritis. Following adherence, organisms such as staphylococci may be internalized into osteoblasts through membrane pseudopod formation or induction of endocytosis. Internalized bacteria may induce apoptosis or avoid the immune system defenses by surviving and multiplying inside the cell. As organisms multiply in the joint, a sequence of proliferation of the synovial lining cells, mononuclear-cell infiltration, granulation tissue, and abscess formation occurs.[3] Eventually, cartilage and bone destruction ensue as a result of release of leukocyte proteases, inflammatory cytokines (especially interleukin (IL)-1, IL6, and tumor necrosis factor-α), and bacterial toxins, as well as tissue ischemia and necrosis induced by increased intra-articular pressure.[3] Over time, cartilage degradation causes narrowing of the joint space and further erosive damage, leaving long-term orthopedic disabilities.

ETIOLOGY

In the preantibiotic era, *S. aureus*, β-hemolytic streptococci and *Streptococcus pneumoniae* were the most common organisms identified in pediatric patients with septic arthritis.[6] After the introduction of effective antimicrobial therapy, the incidence of streptococci declined and *S. aureus* remained the predominant etiology of skeletal system infections. In the 1960s, implementation of routine seeding of synovial fluid aspirates onto chocolate-agar plates, resulted in the recognition of *Haemophilus influenzae* type b as the most common cause of suppurative arthritis in young children and emphasized the crucial role played by the adequate culture techniques in the diagnosis of the disease. However, use of multiple solid media, for culturing synovial fluid aspirates obtained from children with presumptive joint infections yield the causative organism in only two-thirds of cases. Obviously, an incorrect diagnosis or previous antibiotic therapy may be responsible for a fraction of "culture-negative" septic arthritis cases. Yet, the possibility remains that some of these patients have a joint infection caused by fastidious organisms that are not detected by routine laboratory techniques.

In the late 1980s, inoculation of joint exudates into pediatric aerobic BACTEC™ blood culture vials (Becton Dickinson, Cockeysville, MD) resulted in the detection of *K. kingae*, a gram-negative commensal bacterium of the pharyngeal flora, as the most common pathogen of septic arthritis in young children, causing 48% of cases with a culture-proven etiology.[7] Attempts to isolate the organism from joint or bone exudates on routine solid media failed in most cases, although subculture of positive blood culture vials onto blood-agar or chocolate-agar plates recovered *K. kingae* without difficulties, demonstrating that routine solid media are able to support its nutritional requirements. It is postulated that pus exerts an inhibitory effect upon *K. kingae* and dilution of exudates in a large broth volume decreases the concentration of detrimental factors, improving recovery of the organism.

In recent years, use of conventional and real-time polymerase chain reaction (PCR) technology and DNA sequencing has improved detection of difficult-to-culture organisms, enabling recognition of bacteria in patients already treated with antibiotics, and reducing the time-to-detection of the pathogen. Pioneer use of these novel approaches has confirmed that *K. kingae* is the most common etiology of septic arthritis in children below the age of 3 years and shortened the time required to detect and identify the causative organism from a few days to less than 24 hours.[8–10] In a recent study by Chometon et al. that included 131 children with presumptive septic arthritis, a bacterial pathogen was identified by culture in 59 (45%) specimens, of which 25 grew *S. aureus* and 17 (29%) grew *K. kingae*.[11] The combination of culture, conventional PCR followed by sequencing of the amplicon, and real-time PCR with *K. kingae*-specific probes increased the overall bacterial identification to 61% and the fraction of specimens in which *K. kingae* was detected to 30%.[11] It is to be expected that further development and accumulative experience with nucleic acid amplification methods will substantially reduce the frustrating proportion of cases of "culture-negative septic arthritis" and contribute to a better management of these patients.

Generally, septic arthritis in children is caused by the intra-articular invasion of a single bacterial species. Isolation of multiple organisms should raise the suspicion of immunodeficiency, drug abuse, or penetrating trauma with direct inoculation of bacteria into the joint space.

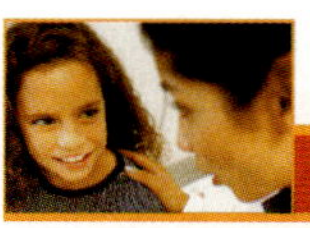

Table 48–2.

Etiology of Septic Arthritis by Age Group

Age	Organism
0–2 m	*S. aureus*
	S. agalactiae
	Enterobacteriaceae
	candida species*
	Coagulase-negative staphylococci*
<2 y	*K. kingae*
	H. influenzae type b[†]
	S. aureus
	S. pneumoniae
	S. pyogenes
<5 y	*S. aureus*
	S. pyogenes
	K. kingae
5–15 y	*S. aureus*
	S. pyogenes
>15 y	*S. aureus*
	S. pyogenes
	N. gonorrhoeae[‡]

**In premature babies with indwelling vascular catheters.*
[†]Among unvaccinated and incompletely vaccinated children.
[‡]In sexually-active adolescents.

The etiologic agents of septic arthritis show a clear age-related distribution (Table 48–2). *S. aureus* is the most common cause of joint infections in neonates and children older than 2–3 years. In recent years, methicillin-resistant strains of *S. aureus* (MRSA) are being detected in the community among patients lacking the established risk factors for nosocomial MRSA infections.[12] In some areas, an increase in the incidence and severity of skeletal system infections is being noted coinciding with the emergence of these strains, whereas the rate of infection caused by methicillin-susceptible *S. aureus* and other organisms remain stable.[13] Patients infected with community associated MRSA (CA-MRSA) organisms are usually healthy children and adolescents frequently involved in contact sports. Infecting strains harbor a unique staphylococcal chromosome cassette termed SCC*mec* type IV (and less commonly SCC*mec* typeV) that carries fewer antibiotic resistant determinants compared to MRSA isolates of nosocomial origin. Infections with CA-MRSA usually involve skin, soft tissues, the lung, and the skeletal system and are characterized by remarkable tissue destruction. More than 90% of CA-MRSA isolates possess the Panton-Valentine leucocidin, which is rarely detected in methicillin-susceptible organisms. It is unclear yet whether this toxin is the major virulence factor of CA-MRSA organisms or is merely a biological maker for some other and still unidentified bacterial component.[14]

S. agalactiae and gram-negative enteric bacilli are seen almost exclusively in the neonatal period. *S. pneumoniae* is most common between the ages of 6 months and 2 years, reflecting the increased incidence of bacteremia and invasive diseases caused by encapsulated bacteria in young children with physiological immaturity of the T-cell independent immunity.[15,16] *Streptococcus pyogenes* is isolated 10–20% of children with septic arthritis regardless of age and is especially common in patients with concomitant skin infections and varicella.[17]

H. influenzae type b was the most common cause of invasive disease in children younger than 2 years prior to the advent of the conjugated vaccine, accounting for almost one-half of the cases. The disease has become rare in countries where immunization coverage is high.[18] Children with *H. influenzae* arthritis frequently present with other suppurative foci of infection such as meningitis (in 30% of patients), osteomyelitis (in 22%), cellulitis (in 30%), pneumonia (in 4%), and otitis media (in 35%).[19]

More than 90% of all children with *K. kingae* arthritis are 6–30 months of age.[20] Antecedent or concomitant stomatitis—including that caused by primary herpetic infection—or signs of an upper respiratory tract infection are common, suggesting that invasion of the bloodstream by organisms carried in the pharynx is facilitated by mucosal breaching.

Pseudomonas aeruginosa is a rare cause of septic arthritis in the general population but it may cause infection in neonates and drug abusing adolescents.[21]

N. gonorrhoeae becomes common in sexually-active adolescents and its isolation in young children is a marker of sexual abuse. Gonococci may also invade the joint space in the course of a disseminated disease in neonates born to infected mothers.[22] Although the incidence of arthritis in invasive meningococcal disease is as high as 14%, true invasion of the joint space by *Neisseria meningitidis* is uncommon.[23] In most cases, articular involvement in patients with meningococcemia develops several days after initiation of antibiotic therapy and the synovial fluid is usually sterile. Immunocomplexes have been detected in some of these patients, suggesting a reactive nature. Recurrent disease, a prolonged course, isolation of uncommon *N. meningitidis* serogroups, and family clustering of cases should raise the possibility of complement or properdin deficiencies.[24]

Invasion of the joint space by *Salmonella enterica* has been rarely reported, usually affecting infants and young children frequently suffering from sickle cell anemia and other hemoglobinopathies.[25] In the developed world, as the result of effective public health measures, human brucellosis has been practically eradicated. In children with arthritis, residents, of endemic countries (Latin America, the Middle East, the Mediterranean basin, Eastern Europe, Asia, and Africa), and travelers returning from these regions, the possibility of brucellar arthritis (and especially that caused by *Brucella melitensis*) should be entertained.[26]

Lyme disease should be included in the differential diagnosis of children exposed to ticks in areas where the infection is prevalent who present with joint inflammation. Septic arthritis caused by *Mycoplasma* and *Ureaplasma* species is almost exclusively detected in patients with X-linked agammaglobulinemia, common variable immunodeficiency, or organ transplantation.[27]

Tuberculous septic arthritis is usually monoarticular and generally affects the hips or knees. Invasion of the joint space occurs when *Mycobacterium tuberculosis* bacilli cross the epiphyseal plate from a contiguous tuberculous bone lesion or more rarely by the direct hematogenous seeding of the organism into the synovium.[28] The lack of proteolytic enzymes preserves the joint space in early disease, but cold abscesses and draining sinus tracts may occur in long-standing, neglected disease.

Hematogenous septic arthritis caused by anaerobic organisms is exceptionally seen in children and is usually caused by a single bacterial species, generally a gram-negative bacillus. Whenever a penetrating wound or bite is the mechanism of infection, multiple organisms including both aerobes and anaerobes, may be isolated from the joint fluid culture.[29]

Rat-bite fever is a rare zoonosis caused by two members of rodents' oral flora *Streptobacillus moniliformis*, mostly in Western countries and Australia, and by *Spirilum minus* in Asia.[30] The site of inoculation of the disease usually heals before a systemic disease, characterized by fever and rash, develops. Arthritis involving multiple joints is commonly seen in rat-bite disease caused by *S. moniliformis* but it is rare in spirilar infection. Culture of the synovial fluid exudates is frequently negative, suggesting that, in some cases, involvement of the joint may represent a reactive arthritis.

CLINICAL PRESENTATION

Pediatric septic arthritis affects a single joint in 95% of cases. Involvement of multiple articulations is noted in half of the cases caused by gonococci, and in 7% of those caused by *S. aureus* or *H. influenzae* type b,[1] and is especially common among patients with rheumatoid arthritis.[31] Septic arthritis usually affects the large weight-bearing joints of the lower extremities. In a large series of 781 septic joints diagnosed in 725 patients in two medical centers in Dallas, the knee was affected in 40% of the cases, followed by the hip in 225, the elbow in 14%, the ankle in 13%, the shoulder in 5%, and the wrist in 4%. The sacroiliac, interphalangeal, metacarpal, metatarsal, acromio- and sternoclavicular joints represented less than 1% each. Involvement of the small joints of the hand and feet are overrepresented in *K. kingae* infections, and the sacroiliac joints are frequently affected in brucellosis. *Pseudomonas aeruginosa* often causes sternoclavicular joint infection in intravenous drug abusers and is a rare complication of subclavian vein catheterization. Infection of the sternoclavicular joint is frequently associated with adjacent osteomyelitis and may extend posteriorly into the mediastinum.

Most children with septic arthritis present with fever and inflammatory changes over the affected joint. Newborns, as well as young patients infected with low-grade virulence pathogens such as brucellae or *K. kingae*, may be afebrile at the time of diagnosis, requiring an increased awareness of the possibility of a joint infection.[32] Irritability, pain, abnormal (antalgic) posture, restricted range of motion or refusal to move the affected extremity ("pseudoparalysis"), and limping are frequent complaints. Arthritis of the hip is frequently difficult to localize and patients may present with pain referred to the knee or anterior thigh.[1] An infected hip is often held flexed, externally rotated, and abducted to relieve intracapsular pressure. Associated osteomyelitis should be suspected if symptoms have been present for several days and the child now has acute worsening of pain suggesting extension of the infection from bone to joint. Although, in most pediatric cases, the source of infection remains occult, associated extra-articular symptoms and signs may provide a clue to the likely bacterial etiology as shown in Table 48–3. Obviously patients should be also carefully evaluated for clinical findings that may suggest diagnoses other than infection, such as rheumatic disorders or metabolic diseases.

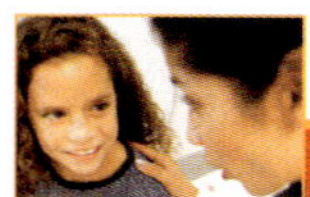

Table 48–3.

Associated Clinical Presentations in Children with Septic Arthritis Suggestive of a Specific Bacterial Etiology

Associated Condition	Possible Etiology
Pyoderma	*S. aureus*, *S. pyogenes*
Erythematous rash	*B. burgdorferi*
Endocarditis	*S. aureus*, *K. kingae*
Pneumonia	*S. pneumoniae*, *H. influenzae* type b
Meningitis	*S. pneumoniae*, *H. influenzae* type b, *N. meningitidis*
Stomatitis	*K. kingae*
Hepatosplenomegaly	*Brucella* species
Urethritis	*N. gonorrhoeae*
Multiple skeletal system involvement	*S. aureus*, *H. influenzae* type b, *Brucella* species

The presenting symptoms of Lyme arthritis and gonococcal arthritis differ from typical septic arthritis. Lyme arthritis is a late manifestation of *B. burgdorferi* infection. In one-fourth of children, clinical features consistent with Lyme disease such as erythema migrans or cranial nerve palsy precede the arthritis. Approximately 90% of cases involved the knee.[33] The affected joint is warm and swollen but only mildly tender. Signs and symptoms of systemic illness are uncommon in older children although younger children may have fever at arthritis onset.[34] Gonococcal arthritis is often preceded by disseminated gonococcal infection. This syndrome consists of fever, chills, tenosynovitis, polyarthralgias or polyarthritis, and dermatitis. The rash characteristically includes hemorrhagic papules and pustules located on the extensor surfaces of the extremities and over the affected joint. Most patients, as mentioned earlier, have asymptomatic genital, anal, or pharyngeal gonococcal infections. Some patients present without the preceding arthritis-dermatitis, making the condition difficult to distinguish from typical bacterial septic arthritis.

LABORATORY EVALUATION

The initial laboratory and radiologic evaluation of a patient with suspected infectious arthritis is summarized in Table 48–4.

Synovial Fluid

The diagnosis of bacterial arthritis in children requires a high index of clinical suspicion. Immediate synovial fluid aspiration followed by microbiological, biochemical, and cytological studies are mandatory.[35] If synovial fluid cannot be obtained by needle aspiration at the bedside, the joint should be aspirated with imaging guidance, particularly for joints that are not easily accessible such as the hip, shoulder, or sacroiliac joints.[36] Any purulent joint effusion in children should be considered infected until proven otherwise. Although acute rheumatic fever, Reiter's disease, and rheumatoid arthritis can cause a markedly inflammatory synovial fluid, the highest leukocyte counts are seen in the joint fluid of patients with septic arthritis. In children with septic arthritis, there are typically 50,000–200,000 cells per mm^3 in the synovial fluid; more than 90% are polymorphonuclear leukocytes (Table 48–5). A synovial fluid white blood cell (WBC) count higher than 50,000 leukocytes per mm^3 has been frequently proposed as a cutoff to differentiate between septic arthritis and of noninfectious joint exudates, yet lower counts may be seen in infections caused by gram-negative organisms such as *N. gonorrhoeae*, *K. kingae*, and brucellae, and early in the course of bacterial arthritis of any etiology.[35]

A low synovial fluid glucose concentration (<30–40 mg/dL) suggests infection but the sensitivity of this criterion is only 50%. Low glucose levels can also occur in patients with rheumatoid arthritis. Measurements of protein and lactate content in the synovial fluid aspirate are neither sensitive nor specificity for bacterial arthritis.[37] The only definitive proof of an infectious etiology of the joint inflammation is the demonstration of bacteria in the Gram stain or the recovery of an irrefutable pathogen in the culture. A Gram stain should be prepared from a centrifuged

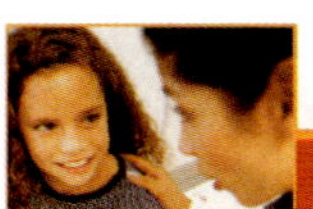

Table 48–4.

Summary of Initial Radiologic and Laboratory Evaluation of a Patient with Suspected Infectious Arthritis

- Joint radiograph to detect fracture
  - For hip, include anterior-posterior view with leg extended and slight internal rotation and frog-leg view
- Sonography to detect joint effusion and guide diagnostic aspiration
- Blood
  - Blood culture (yields organism in approximately 50% of cases)
  - CRP (elevated at presentation in 95% of patients with septic arthritis)
  - Erythrocyte sedimentation rate (elevated at presentation in approximately 90% of patients with septic arthritis)
  - Other testing as guided by clinical picture (e.g., serologic studies for *B. burgdorferi*)
- Synovial fluid (in order of priority)
  - Gram stain
  - Culture by inoculation into blood culture bottle
  - Culture by inoculation of solid media
  - WBC count
  - Glucose
  - Other testing as guided by clinical situation (e.g., PCR assays for *B. burgdorferi* or *Neisseria gonorrhoeae*)
- Consider gadolinium-enhanced magnetic resonance imaging of joint or technetium phosphate bone scintigraphy when concomitant osteomyelitis is suspected

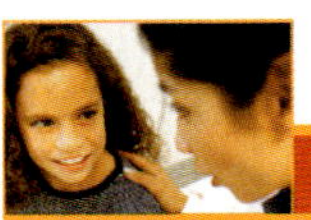

Table 48–5.

Typical Synovial Fluid WBC Counts in Normal Children and in Those with Arthritis

Diagnosis	WBC Count (per mm^3)
Normal	< 150
Bacterial arthritis	> 50,000
Gonococcal arthritis	> 50,000
Lyme arthritis	30,000–50,000
Tuberculous arthritis	10,000–20,000
Reactive arthritis	< 15,000
Juvenile rheumatoid arthritis	< 50,000

specimen (when the fluid volume is sufficient) and carefully examined. Gram's stain smears are positive in 75% of patients with staphylococcal arthritis but in less than half of those infected with gram-negative bacteria,[35,38] probably because of a lower bacterial load and the difficulties in recognizing the presence of organisms against the pink-stained fibrin background. The fluid should be inoculated bedside or promptly transported to the microbiology laboratory, seeded onto appropriate media (including a chocolate-agar plate for the isolation of *H. influenzae*), and incubated in a CO_2-enriched atmosphere.

Inoculation of a pediatric blood-culture vial, and preferably one containing antibiotic-binding resins such as the BACTEC™ 9240 Peds Plus bottle[39] or the BacT/Alert PedibacT vial (Organon Teknika Corporation, Durham, NC),)[40] is also recommended because this method significantly improves the recovery of fastidious organisms and the recovery of organisms in patients already receiving antimicrobial therapy. Anaerobic cultures are not routinely indicated in children in the absence of specific risk factors such as penetrating wounds, human and animal bites, or a sensory neuropathy. Aspiration of an amount of fluid insufficient for a comprehensive laboratory testing is a common event in young children or when a small joint is drained. In this case, performance of a Gram stain and inoculation of a blood-culture vial are probably the best diagnostic options.

Blood

Blood cultures should be drawn in all patients with suspected suppurative arthritis, not only because the accessibility of the specimen compared with drawing a joint exudate specimen, but also because the etiologic agent may be recovered from the bloodstream in up to 50% of cases, even when cultures of the synovial fluid are sterile.[35] Genital cultures should be obtained in sexually active adolescents presenting with arthritis and signs compatible with a disseminated gonococcal infection.

Acute-phase reactants such as WBC counts, erythrocyte sedimentation rate and C-reactive protein (CRP) levels are usually elevated in children with septic arthritis. A normal WBC count may be seen in neonates with infected joints. Children with septic arthritis who have a normal CRP at presentation, usually have an elevated value 8–12 hours later. Sequential measurement of CRP levels may be used to follow the disease response to therapy; the CRP is more sensitive than the ESR for this purpose. A favorable clinical course is characterized by an average normalization of CRP values (<20 mg/L) within 10 days, whereas increasing levels may represent therapeutic failure and help in the early recognition of complications.[41]

Other Studies

Lyme arthritis is suggested by serologic evidence of Lyme disease confirmed by Western blotting in a patient with documented arthritis. By the time symptoms of arthritis develop, virtually all patients have a positive serum IgG test. Since arthritis develops late in the course of infection, IgM response may no longer be present. *B. burgdorferi* DNA can be detected by PCR in the synovial tissue or joint fluid of most patients. In one study of patients with Lyme arthritis, *B. burgdorferi* PCR testing of synovial fluid was positive in 70 (96%) of 73 patients with Lyme arthritis who had received no antibiotics or short-course antibiotic therapy.[42] In contrast, the test was not positive in any of the 69 control patients diagnosed with other forms of arthritis (e.g., rheumatoid arthritis, degenerative joint disease, osteoarthritis).[42]

Although only 25–50% of patients with gonococcal arthritis have positive joint fluid cultures, PCR-based assays are extremely sensitive in detecting gonococcal DNA from synovial fluid. Cultures from mucosal surfaces (cervix, urethra, rectum, vagina, or throat) are often positive for *N. gonorrhoeae* when inoculated onto Thayer-Martin agar and incubated in an enriched CO_2 environment within 15 minutes of specimen collection. *N. gonorrhoeae* may also be detected by ligase chain reaction on first-voided urine specimens and urethral and cervicovaginal swab samples.

IMAGING STUDIES

Imaging studies are not diagnostic for septic arthritis but are helpful in supporting a clinical suspicion of the disease, detecting concomitant osteomyelitis, and excluding other conditions. The initial radiographic examination is usually normal or may reveal subtle changes such as soft tissue swelling, widening of the joint space, and osteolytic changes suggesting contiguous osteomyelitis.

When a suppurative infection of the hip is suspected, roentgenograms should be obtained in both, the "frog-leg position," as well as with the legs extended at the knees and slightly internally rotated. Displacement of the femoral head laterally and upward and of the obturador internis muscle medially by a distended joint capsule would support the diagnosis.[1] Radionuclide imaging may be useful to localize a deep infection in the hip, vertebrae, or the sacroiliac joints. Technetium phosphate joint scintigraphy is positive in any synovitis, whereas sequential gallium imaging, although not specific, may differentiate infection from other causes of joint inflammation.[43] Sonography may detect accumulation of intra-articular fluid, and bone scans may be used to localize the joint affected when in doubt. Although magnetic resonance imaging has a high resolution for skeletal system pathology, its use as a routine diagnostic test for pediatric septic arthritis is not currently recommended.

SPECIAL SITUATIONS

Septic Arthritis in the HIV-Positive Patient

Despite the profound immunosuppressive effect of the human immunodeficiency virus it remains unclear whether HIV-infected individuals have a true excess of skeletal system infections because of the confounding factors of intravenous drug abuse and frequent hospitalizations. *Staphylococcus aureus* is the most common cause of joint infection among AIDS patients and salmonellae appear to be over-represented in this population. In patients with advanced disease, and particularly in those with a CD4 count <200/mm^3, pneumococci, and opportunistic mycobacteria, *Nocardia asteroides*, *Candida* species and other yeasts, as well as a variety of fungi have also been reported.[44]

Culture-Negative Septic Arthritis

Although the accepted proportion of cases of suspected joint infections with negative cultures averages 33%,[1] percentages ranging between 16%[45] and 60%[46] have been reported. These discrepancies may be ascribable to differences in recruitment, inclusion and exclusion criteria, and performance of culture methods.[47] The epidemiological profile and clinical presentation of children with failed cultures is frequently similar to that of those in whom a pathogen is recovered, although a trend toward lower body temperature and CRP values on admission, a milder clinical course, and better prognosis have been reported in two patients' series.[48,49] Whether these observations represent infection with fastidious pathogens of lower virulence is unknown. Because of the potential serious consequences of delayed or inadequate antimicrobial therapy, patients with suspected septic arthritis and a negative culture should be administered a full course treatment with a broad-spectrum antibiotic. It is to be expected that in the future, improved microbiological culture methods and use of nucleic acid amplification essays will reduce or eliminate these cases altogether.

Neonatal Septic Arthritis

Invasion of the joint space in neonates may occur during a bacteremic episode, as a result of dissemination of the infection from a contiguous focus of osteomyelitis or, more rarely, by direct inoculation of skin organisms during a femoral venipuncture.[50] The source of the preceding bacteremic episode may be the nosocomial transmission of virulent *S. aureus* organisms, the newborn's normal skin flora, as in coagulase-negative staphylococcal or *Candida* species infections in premature babies with indwelling intravenous catheters, or acquisition of maternal flora in newborns delivered through a birth canal colonized with *Enterobacteriaceae*, *S. agalactiae* or *N. gonorrhoeae*.[1,51] Limited use of an extremity or pseudoparalysis resembling Erb's palsy, inflammatory signs over the affected joint, and multiple joint involvement may be found. A complete sepsis workout, including the performance of a lumbar puncture, is indicated.

Prosthetic Joint Infections

Infections of implanted joint prostheses are rare, and occur in 1–2% of knee arthroplasties, in 0.3–1.3% of hip replacements, and in less than 1% of shoulder arthroplasties.[52] The risk for infection is increased after revision procedures and in patients with rheumatoid arthritis. Microbial colonization of the implant may occur at the time of surgery, as a result of spreading from a contiguous wound infection, or from hematogenous seeding. Acute symptoms and signs suggestive of infection may develop in the early post operative period or infection may present as a smoldering painful process with prosthesis loosening several months or years after surgery. Virulent organisms such as *S. aureus* are recovered in only 20–25% of cases, whereas low-grade pathogens such as coagulase-negative staphylococci, non hemolytic streptococci or *Enterococcus* species, and anaerobes are isolated in more than half of the cases. Polymicrobial infections are detected in 12–19% of patients. The sensitivity of clinical examination, laboratory, radiographic or nuclear scans is insufficient to diagnose infection in a prosthetic joint, and ultimately, only identification of the etiology in the Gram stain and culture of the synovial fluid aspirate and/or histopathologic evaluation of the periprosthetic tissue confirm the clinical suspicion. The implications of septic arthritis in a prosthetic joint in terms of need for reoperation, potential loss of the prosthesis, and economic burden are substantial. Treatment of infected joint prostheses is challenging, requiring multiple surgical procedures and prolonged antimicrobial therapy and a close collaboration between orthopedic surgeons and infectious diseases specialists.[52]

TREATMENT

Antibiotic Therapy

For the reason that the potential risk for long-term orthopedic sequelae caused by the rapid joint destruction, septic arthritis should be considered a true pediatric emergency requiring a high index of clinical suspicion, early joint drainage, and prompt administration of adequate antimicrobial therapy. The initial antibiotics therapy should be administered through the parenteral route. The penetration of most antibiotics into inflamed joint effusions is sufficient providing that an adequate serum level is achieved. Therefore, antibiotics do not need to be injected intra-articularly; furthermore, this is contraindicated because of the possibility of inducing chemical synovitis.[35]

The choice of the initial antibiotic therapy should be guided by the results of the Gram stain examination of the fluid, age of the patient, clinical picture, presence of specific risk factors (such as immunodeficiency), potential exposures to organisms such as *B. burgdorferi* or brucellae, and the local prevalence of antibiotic resistance in organisms such as *S. aureus*. Once the pathogen is identified and antibiotic susceptibility is determined, antibiotic therapy should be adjusted accordingly. If no pathogen is isolated but the patient is responding adequately, therapy should be continued with the drug chosen originally. If no improvement is noted the possibility of an uncommon infectious etiology or a non infectious process should be entertained and a more extensive clinical and laboratory evaluation, including reaspiration and, eventually, a synovial biopsy should be considered.[1]

In the newborn, an antistaphylococcal penicillin, such as oxacillin or nafcillin (150–200 mg/kg per 24 hours divided q6h), in combination with a third generation cephalosporin, such as cefotaxime (150–200 mg/kg per 24 hours divided q8h), provide adequate empiric antimicrobial coverage (pending culture and antibiotic susceptibility results). In premature babies with long-term indwelling intravenous catheters, vancomycin (10–15 mg/kg per 24 hours divided in 1–3 doses, according to weight and age) instead of the penicillinase-resistant penicillins is recommended to cover nosocomial coagulase-negative staphylococci.

In preschool age children up to 5 years of age, options include cefuroxime (200–300 mg/kg per 24 hours divided q8h), cefotaxime, or ceftriaxone because each adequately covers gram-positive pathogens such as methicillin-susceptible *S. aureus*, β-hemolytic streptococci, pneumococci, as well as gram-negative organisms such as *H. influenzae* type b, *K. kingae*, *N. meningitidis*, and most of the *Enterobacteriaceae*. In children older than 5 years of age, gram-positive bacteria constitute the vast majority of isolates. Anti staphylococcal antibiotics alone would provide adequate coverage pending culture results, unless *N. gonorrhoeae* is suspected, in which case, addition of ceftriaxone is recommended. In areas where CA-MRSA organisms are prevalent, vancomycin (40–60 mg/kg per 24 hours divided q6h) or clindamycin (30–40 mg/kg per 24 hours divided tid-qid) should be administered, although resistance to the latter has been detected in a few isolates.[12] Experience with the use of linezolid for CA-MRSA is limited but the drug appears to be effective for the treatment of suppurative arthritis.[53] The use of quinopristin/dalfopristin and daptomycin as alternative drugs for skeletal infections caused by CA-MRSA has not been adequately evaluated in children, and emergence of resistance to the latter drug in the course of therapy for osteomyelitis has been reported.[54]

Immunocompromized hosts should be given broad-spectrum antibiotics to cover a large variety of common as well as rarer opportunistic organisms. Combinations of vancomycin with ceftazidime (150–200 mg/kg per 24 hours divided q4–6h) or combinations of piperacillin-clavulanate (300–400 mg/kg per 24 hours divided q6–8h) or ticarcillin-clavulanate (200–300 mg/kg per 24 hours divided q4–6h) with an aminoglycoside are currently recommended.[1] When joint infections are caused by direct penetrating wounds or bites, anti anaerobic antibiotic coverage with clindamycin should be added. *S. aureus* arthritis and infections caused by *Enterobacteriaceae* require 4 weeks of therapy, whereas arthritis caused by other organisms may be adequately treated for a total 2 weeks.

Children with Lyme arthritis may receive oral medications such as amoxicillin, doxycycline (if older than 8 years of age), or cefuroxime initially. If symptoms fail to improve substantially and the diagnosis is certain, ceftriaxone may be used. In children aged 8 years or older, brucellar arthritis is best treated with a combination of oral doxycycline (2–4 mg/kg per 24 hours, up to a maximum of 200 mg/d, divided q12h), and rifampin (15–20 mg/kg/day, maximum 600–900 mg/d, in 1 or 2 divided doses) for 6 weeks. In children younger than 8 years, oral trimethoprim-sulfamethoxazole (10 mg/kg per 24 hours of trimethoprim hours, maximum 480 mg/d, divided q12h and sulfamethoxazole, 50 mg/kg/d, maximum 2.4 g/d) should be used instead of doxycycline.[55]

Once the patient's condition has improved and surgical procedures are no longer necessary (usually within 1 week), the initial parenteral antimicrobial therapy may be shifted to oral drugs for infections involving the knee, ankle, and other small joints. The synovial fluid antibiotic concentrations after oral administration routinely exceed the serum concentrations by 60% or more.[56] Prerequisites for oral therapy include control of infection and inflammation and compliance with planned therapy and monitoring. For the oral regimen of β-lactam antibiotics, a dosage 2–3 times higher than that used for more benign infections is needed.[1] In the past, it was recommended to assess the adequacy of the antibiotic dosage and absorption of the drug in patients with osteomyelitis and septic arthritis treated with sequential parenteral-oral antibiotic therapy. The peak bactericidal activity at the steady state (after the third dose of oral antibiotics) was measured in the serum and finding of a level of 1:8 or greater was considered adequate.[1] A recent study has suggested that determining antibiotic levels may be unnecessary and patients with staphylococcal osteomyelitis may be safety managed with judicious clinical evaluation and serial CRP determinations.[57] Further experience with this simplified treatment approach and with its use in children with septic arthritis or infections caused by other organisms is required before it can be universally recommended.

The appropriate duration of antimicrobial therapy for septic arthritis is not clear but should be individualized based on the organism isolated and the clinical and laboratory response. Minimum criteria for discontinuing antibiotic therapy include resolution of signs and symptoms of infection and normalization of the CRP level. The CRP peaks on the second day of therapy and is normal within 7–9 days. In contrast, the ESR rises slowly over several days, peaks in the first week, and then normalizes slowly during the next 3–4 weeks. Since the CRP increases and decreases much more quickly than ESR, measuring the CRP may be more useful in determining response to therapy. CRP values that remain high or increase again during therapy require careful investigation. Waiting for normalization of the ESR may be an overly conservative therapeutic end point. Most infections require 2 weeks of therapy but septic arthritis caused by *S. aureus* or gram negative organisms require at least 3 weeks of therapy. Children with associated osteomyelitis should be treated for 4 weeks since a shorter duration of therapy may be inadequate for the treatment of osteomyelitis.

Lyme arthritis is treated with a 4-week course of oral amoxicillin or doxycycline, depending on age. Fewer than 10% of children fail an oral regimen but children with incomplete response to oral antibiotic therapy require intravenous ceftriaxone or penicillin for 14–21 days. Surgical irrigation of the joint is not usually required. Up to 50% of children with Lyme arthritis will have a recurrent episode of arthritis within 6 months of initial treatment.[33] Recurrences can be treated with nonsteroidal anti-inflammatory agents. The frequency and duration of recurrences, which occur more commonly in females and in older children,[34] diminish over time. Patients who receive intra-articular steroids prior to antibiotic treatment for Lyme arthritis appear to have a longer time to resolution of the arthritis.[34] Repeating Lyme serologic tests during recurrences does not alter management. Chronic arthritis rarely develops in children with Lyme arthritis.

Gonococcal arthritis should be treated with intravenous ceftriaxone or other broad-spectrum cephalosporins. Skin lesions may continue to develop during the first two days of therapy. Treatment may be switched to oral fluoroquinolones or, if penicillin-susceptible organisms are isolated, amoxicillin to complete 7–10 days of total therapy. Surgical irrigation of the joint is not routinely required. Sexually active adolescents should be evaluated for other sexually transmitted diseases, including *C. trachomatis*. Prepubertal children require evaluation for sexual abuse.

Anti-Inflammatory Therapy

Results of a recent double-blind placebo-controlled study conducted among 123 children with joint infections in Costa Rica have shown that adding intravenous dexamethasone (0.6 mg/kg per 24 hours divided q8h) for 4 days to appropriate antibiotic and surgical therapy significantly reduced the duration of symptoms and residual dysfunction compared to placebo, supporting the role played by the host's immune response in the degradation of the joint cartilage.[58] These promising results need to be confirmed before the administration of corticosteroids can be routinely recommended in patients with septic arthritis.

Surgical Treatment

Because of the deleterious effect of infected synovial fluid on the cartilage layer, removal of the accumulated exudate is recommended. A seminal study conducted by Nelson and Koontz[59] in 1966 concluded that needle aspirations (single or multiple, as clinically required) were preferable over open drainage as the initial management of infected joints, and these results have been later confirmed by others. The hip

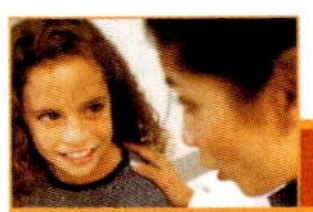

Table 48–6.

Indications for Open Surgical Drainage of a Septic Joint

Arthritis of the hip or shoulder
Presence of large amounts of fibrin, debris or loculation within the joint space
Rapid reaccumulation of fluid despite repeat aspirations
Presence of a foreign body
Arthritis not responding to medical treatment within 3 days
Adjacent osteomyelitis
Arthritis in a patient with rheumatoid arthritis
Arthritis of the sternoclavicular joint

and shoulder are the exceptions to this rule because increased intracapsular pressure of undrained fluid may compromise the vascular supply, resulting in necrosis of the femoral or humeral heads. It has been recently suggested that repeated ultrasound-guided aspirations and irrigation may spare the need for surgical drainage,[60] but this conservative approach should be confirmed by additional experience. The indications for surgery in the management of pediatric septic arthritis are summarized in Table 48–6.

PROGNOSIS

Long-term follow-up is required to assess the functional results of septic arthritis in children. A variety of functional sequelae such as limping, decrease range of motion, instability or chronic dislocation of the joint and abnormal bone growth have been reported in 10–25% of children with septic arthritis. Risk factors for a poor orthopedic outcome are listed in Table 48–7.[37,61]

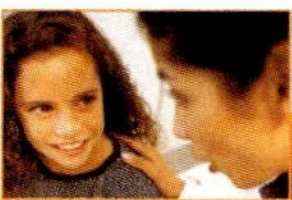

Table 48–7.

Factors Associated with Poor Prognosis in Children with Septic Arthritis

Infection in the first 6 mo of life
Involvement of the hip or shoulder
Adjacent osteomyelitis
Delay in the diagnosis of more than 4 d
Infection with *S. aureus* or gram-negative enteric organisms
Persistent positive culture after 1 w of appropriate antimicrobial therapy
Infection in a prosthetic joint

REFERENCES

1. Trujillo M, Nelson JD. Suppurative and reactive arthritis in children. *Semin Pediatr Infect Dis.* 1997;8(4):242-249.
2. Ike RW. Bacterial arthritis. *Curr Opin Rheumatol.* 1998;10(4):330-334.
3. Shirtliff ME, Mader JT. Acute septic arthritis. *Clin Microbiol Rev.* 2002;15(4):527-544.
4. Yagupsky P, Press J. Unsuspected *Kingella kingae* infections in afebrile children with mild skeletal symptoms: the importance of blood cultures. *Eur J Pediatr.* 2004;163(9):563-564.
5. Lebel E, Rudensky B, Karasik M, Itzchaki M, Schlesinger Y. *Kingella kingae* infections in children. *J Pediatr Orthop B.* 2006;15(4):289-292.
6. Welkon CJ, Long SS, Fisher MC, Alburger PD. Pyogenic arthritis in infants and children: a review of 95 cases. *Pediatr Infect Dis.* 1986;5(6):669-676.
7. Yagupsky P, Dagan R, Howard CW, Einhorn M, Kassis I, Simu A. High prevalence of *Kingella kingae* in joint fluid from children with septic arthritis revealed by the BACTEC blood culture system. *J Clin Microbiol.* 1992;30(5):1278-1281.
8. Moumile K, Merckx J, Glorion C, Berche P, Ferroni A. Osteoarticular infections caused by *Kingella kingae* in children: contribution of polymerase chain reaction to the microbiologic diagnosis. *Pediatr Infect Dis J.* 2003;22(9):837-839.
9. Rosey AL, Abachin E, Quesnes G, et al. Development of a braod-range 16S rDNA real-time PCR for the diagnosis of septic arthritis in children. *J Microbiol Methods.* 2007;68:88-93.
10. Verdier I, Gayet-Ageron A, Ploton C, et al. Contribution of a broad range polymerase chain reaction to the diagnosis of osteoarticular infections caused by *Kingella kingae*: description of twenty-four recent pediatric diagnoses. *Pediatr Infect Dis J.* 2005;24(8):692-696.
11. Chometon S, Benito Y, Boisset S, et al. Specific real-time PCR places *Kingella kingae* as the most common cause of osteoarticular infections in young children. *Pediatr Infect Dis J.* 2007;26:377-381.
12. Martinez-Aguilar G, Avalos-Mishaan A, Hulten K, Hammerman W, Mason EO, Jr., Kaplan SL. Community-acquired, methicillin-resistant and methicillin-susceptible *Staphylococcus aureus* musculoskeletal infections in children. *Pediatr Infect Dis J.* 2004;23(8):701-706.
13. Arnold SR, Elias D, Buckingham SC, et al. Changing patterns of acute hematogenous osteomyelitis and septic arthritis: emergence of community-associated methicillin-resistant *Staphylococcus aureus. J Pediatr Orthop.* 2006;26(6):703-708.
14. Voyich JM, Otto M, Mathema B, et al. Is Panton-Valentine leukocidin the major virulence determinant in community-associated methicillin-resistant *Staphylococcus aureus* disease? *J Infect Dis.* 2006;194(12):1761-1770.
15. Jacobs NM. Pneumococcal osteomyelitis and arthritis in children. A hospital series and literature review. *Am J Dis Child.* 1991;145(1):70-74.
16. Ross JJ, Saltzman CL, Carling P, Shapiro DS. Pneumococcal septic arthritis: review of 190 cases. *Clin Infect Dis.* 2003;36(3):319-327.

17. Tyrrell GJ, Lovgren M, Kress B, Grimsrud K. Varicella-associated invasive group a streptococcal disease in Alberta, Canada—2000-2002. *Clin Infect Dis.* 2005;40(7):1055-1057.
18. Howard AW, Viskontas D, Sabbagh C. Reduction in osteomyelitis and septic arthritis related to *Haemophilus influenzae* type B vaccination. *J Pediatr Orthop.* 1999;19(6):705-709.
19. Rotbart HA, Glode MP. *Haemophilus influenzae* type b septic arthritis in children: report of 23 cases. *Pediatrics.* 1985;75(2):254-259.
20. Yagupsky P. *Kingella kingae*: from medical rarity to an emerging paediatric pathogen. *Lancet Infect Dis.* 2004;4(6):358-367.
21. Brancos MA, Peris P, Miro JM, et al. Septic arthritis in heroin addicts. *Semin Arthritis Rheum.* 1991;21(2):81-87.
22. Rice PA. Gonococcal arthritis (disseminated gonococcal infection). *Infect Dis Clin North Am.* 2005;19(4):853-861.
23. Schaad UB. Arthritis in disease due to *Neisseria meningitidis. Rev Infect Dis.* 1980;2(6):880-888.
24. Mathew S, Overturf GD. Complement and properidin deficiencies in meningococcal disease. *Pediatr Infect Dis J.* 2006;25(3):255-256.
25. Syrogiannopoulos GA, McCracken GH, Jr., Nelson JD. Osteoarticular infections in children with sickle cell disease. *Pediatrics.* 1986;78(6):1090-1096.
26. Benjamin B, Annobil SH, Khan MR. Osteoarticular complications of childhood brucellosis: a study of 57 cases in Saudi Arabia. *J Pediatr Orthop.* 1992;12(6):801-805.
27. Franz A, Webster AD, Furr PM, Taylor-Robinson D. Mycoplasmal arthritis in patients with primary immunoglobulin deficiency: clinical features and outcome in 18 patients. *Br J Rheumatol.* 1997;36(6):661-668.
28. Teo HE, Peh WC. Skeletal tuberculosis in children. *Pediatr Radiol.* 2004;34(11):853-860.
29. Brook I. Joint and bone infections due to anaerobic bacteria in children. *Pediatr Rehabil.* 2002;5(1):11-19.
30. Dendle C, Woolley IJ, Korman TM. Rat-bite fever septic arthritis: illustrative case and literature review. *Eur J Clin Microbiol Infect Dis.* 2006;25(12):791-797.
31. Christodoulou C, Gordon P, Coakley G. Polyarticular septic arthritis. *BMJ.* 2006;333(7578):1107-1108.
32. Yagupsky P, Bar-Ziv Y, Howard CB, Dagan R. Epidemiology, etiology, and clinical features of septic arthritis in children younger than 24 months. *Arch Pediatr Adolesc Med.* 1995;149(5):537-540.
33. Gerber MA, Zemel LS, Shapiro ED. Lyme arthritis in children: clinical epidemiology and long-term outcomes. *Pediatrics.* 1998;102(4, pt. 1):905-908.
34. Bentas W, Karch H, Huppertz HI. Lyme arthritis in children and adolescents: outcome 12 months after initiation of antibiotic therapy. *J Rheumatol.* 2000;27(8):2025-2030.
35. Goldenberg DL, Reed JI. Bacterial arthritis. *N Engl J Med.* 1985;312(12):764-771.
36. Goldenberg DL. Septic arthritis. *Lancet.* 1998;351(9097):197-202.
37. Smith JW, Chalupa P, Shabaz Hasan M. Infectious arthritis: clinical features, laboratory findings and treatment. *Clin Microbiol Infect.* 2006;12(4):309-314.
38. Press J, Peled N, Buskila D, Yagupsky P. Leukocyte count in the synovial fluid of children with culture-proven brucellar arthritis. *Clin Rheumatol.* 2002;21(3):191-193.
39. Hughes JG, Vetter EA, Patel R, et al. Culture with BACTEC Peds Plus/F bottle compared with conventional methods for detection of bacteria in synovial fluid. *J Clin Microbiol.* 2001;39(12):4468-4471.
40. Bourbeau P, Riley J, Heiter BJ, Master R, Young C, Pierson C. Use of the BacT/Alert blood culture system for culture of sterile body fluids other than blood. *J Clin Microbiol.* 1998;36(11):3273-3277.
41. Kallio MJ, Unkila-Kallio L, Aalto K, Peltola H. Serum C-reactive protein, erythrocyte sedimentation rate and white blood cell count in septic arthritis of children. *Pediatr Infect Dis J.* 1997;16(4):411-413.
42. Nocton JJ, Dressler F, Rutledge BJ, Rys PN, Persing DH, Steere AC. Detection of *Borrelia burgdorferi* DNA by polymerase chain reaction in synovial fluid from patients with Lyme arthritis. *N Engl J Med.* 1994;330(4):229-234.
43. Namey TC, Halla JT. Radiographic and nucleographic techniques. *Clin Rheum Dis.* 1978;4:95-132.
44. Zalavras CG, Dellamaggiora R, Patzakis MJ, Bava E, Holtom PD. Septic arthritis in patients with human immunodeficiency virus. *Clin Orthop Relat Res.* 2006;451:46-49.
45. Speiser JC, Moore TL, Osborn TG, Weiss TD, Zuckner J. Changing trends in pediatric septic arthritis. *Semin Arthritis Rheum.* 1985;15(2):132-138.
46. Peltola H, Vahvanen V. Acute purulent arthritis in children. *Scand J Infect Dis.* 1983;15(1):75-80.
47. Dubost JJ. Septic arthritis with no organism: a dilemma. *Joint Bone Spine.* 2006;73(4):341-343.
48. Chang WS, Chiu NC, Chi H, Li WC, Huang FY. Comparison of the characteristics of culture-negative versus culture-positive septic arthritis in children. *J Microbiol Immunol Infect.* 2005;38(3):189-193.
49. Lyon RM, Evanich JD. Culture-negative septic arthritis in children. *J Pediatr Orthop.* 1999;19(5):655-659.
50. Asnes RS, Arendar GM. Septic arthritis of the hip: a complication of femoral venipuncture. *Pediatrics.* 1966;38(5):837-841.
51. Memon IA, Jacobs NM, Yeh TF, Lilien LD. Group B streptococcal osteomyelitis and septic arthritis. Its occurrence in infants less than 2 months old. *Am J Dis Child.* 1979;133(9):921-923.
52. Sia IG, Berbari EF, Karchmer AW. Prosthetic joint infections. *Infect Dis Clin North Am.* 2005;19(4):885-914.
53. De Bels D, Garcia-Filoso A, Jeanmaire M, Preseau T, Miendje Deyi VY, Devriendt J. Successful treatment with linezolid of septic shock secondary to methicillin-resistant *Staphylococcus aureus* arthritis. *J Antimicro b Chemother.* 2005;55(5):812-813.
54. Marty FM, Yeh WW, Wennersten CB, et al. Emergence of a clinical daptomycin-resistant *Staphylococcus aureus* isolate during treatment of methicillin-resistant *Staphylococcus aureus* bacteremia and osteomyelitis. *J Clin Microbiol* 2006;44(2):595-597.
55. AAP. Brucellosis. In: Pickering LK, Baker CJ, Long SS, McMillan JA, eds. *Red Book: 2006 Report of the Committee on Infectious Diseases.* 27th ed. Elk Grove, CA: American Academy of Pediatrics, 2006:235-237.
56. Nelson JD, Howard JB, Shelton S. Oral antibiotic therapy for skeletal infections of children. I. Antibiotic concentrations in suppurative synovial fluid. *J Pediatr.* 1978;92(1):131-134.

57. Peltola H, Unkila-Kallio L, Kallio MJ. Simplified treatment of acute staphylococcal osteomyelitis of childhood. The Finnish Study Group. *Pediatrics.* 1997;99(6):846-850.
58. Odio CM, Ramirez T, Arias G, et al. Double blind, randomized, placebo-controlled study of dexamethasone therapy for hematogenous septic arthritis in children. *Pediatr Infect Dis J.* 2003;22(10):883-888.
59. Nelson JD, Koontz WC. Septic arthritis in infants and children: a review of 117 cases. *Pediatrics.* 1966;38(6):966-971.
60. Givon U, Liberman B, Schindler A, Blankstein A, Ganel A. Treatment of septic arthritis of the hip joint by repeated ultrasound-guided aspirations. *J Pediatr Orthop.* 2004;24(3):266-270.
61. Howard JB, Highgenboten CL, Nelson JD. Residual effects of septic arthritis in infancy and childhood. *JAMA.* 1976;236(8):932-935.

CHAPTER 49

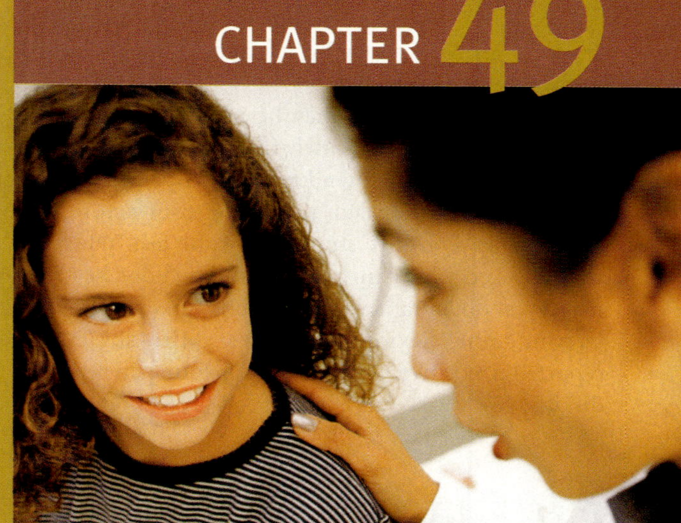

Diskitis

Gokce Mik, David A. Spiegel, and John M. Flynn

DEFINITION AND EPIDEMIOLOGY

Diskitis is an uncommon inflammatory condition affecting the intervertebral disc and adjacent vertebral end plates. The available evidence implicates a low-grade bacterial infection rather than a noninfectious inflammatory process, as was previously thought. Most cases are diagnosed in children younger than 4 years, in the age range between 7 months and 16 years,[1–8] and males are more frequently affected (male to female ratio is 1.7:1).[6–8] Diskitis involves the lumbar spine most commonly, although any area of the spine may be involved. As the findings on history and physical examination are often nonspecific, a high index of suspicion is required to make the diagnosis.

PATHOGENESIS

While several theories have been proposed including infection, noninfectious inflammation,[9,10] and trauma,[11] the weight of evidence implicates a bacterial infection involving the disc and vertebral end plate.[1,6,9,12–14] This theory is supported by cultures of intervertebral material and blood.[1,6,8–10,14] Diskitis likely represents one end of the spectrum of infection involving the anterior elements of the spine, the manifestations of which depend upon differences between the microcirculation in infants and children versus adults. Vascular channels between the vertebral body and the disc are present in infants and children, providing a portal for hematogeneous seeding of the disc. These channels are not present in adolescence and adulthood, which explains the preponderance of vertebral osteomyelitis rather than diskitis in these older age groups. While diskitis may resolve spontaneously in a subset of patients treated only by symptomatic measures, the disease process may progress and require operative debridement.[12,15,16] Ring et al. found recurrent symptoms and/or a prolonged course in 18% of patients with diskitis treated with intravenous antibiotics versus 67% who received no antibiotics.[12]

CLINICAL PRESENTATION

The clinical findings associated with diskitis differ infants and toddlers, compared with older children (Table 49–1). The presentation in infants/toddlers is usually nonspecific, often resulting in a delay in diagnosis. Occasionally, parents may report a recent infectious illness (e.g., upper respiratory tract infection) or a mild trauma. Symptoms in the infant and toddler include general irritability, crying at night, and the refusal to walk. When severe, symptoms may result in the refusal to stand or sit with a preference for bed rest.[1,3,6,13] Older children with diskitis often experience well-localized back pain, which may radiate to the hip region or legs. Gait disturbance is a common finding in this age

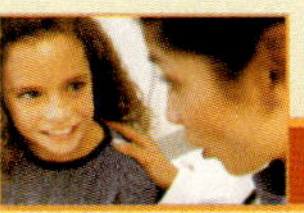

Table 49–1.

Common Signs and Symptoms of Diskitis in Infants, Toddles, and School Age Children

Infants/Toddlers	School Age Children
General irritability	Focal back pain*
Persistent crying at night	Abdominal pain
Refusal to walk	Limp
Positive coin test or Gower's sign	

**Can radiate to hips and legs.*

group,[5,7,9] and pain may be referred to the abdominal region.

Low-grade fevers may be present, but patients usually do not appear acutely ill. Physical examination can demonstrate local tenderness with palpation, paravertebral muscle spasm, hamstring contracture, and occasionally a positive straight-leg raise test. When the child is asked to pick up an object off the floor, he or she may squat down rather than bending forward, avoiding painful spinal flexion (coin test).[3] Mirovsky et al.[17] reported a positive Gower's sign in four patients with diskitis.

DIFFERENTIAL DIAGNOSIS

The differential diagnosis includes infectious, inflammatory, neoplastic, and developmental conditions (Table 49–2). Other bacterial pathogens include brucella and salmonella, often in the context of underlying sickle cell disease); granulomatous infections such as tuberculosis may present in a similar fashion. Fungal infections such as *Cryptococcus neoformans* are rare but should be considered, especially in the immunocompromised host. Neoplastic diseases such as eosinophilic granuloma, leukemia, and lymphoma must be considered. Inflammatory conditions such as juvenile idiopathic arthritis may present with symptoms similar to diskitis. Scheuermann disease, also known as juvenile kyphosis) is a deformity in the thoracic or thoracolumbar spine. Scheuermann disease can cause back pain in adolescents, and the presence of vertebral wedging (of five or more degrees with involvement of three or more consecutive vertebrae) and Schmorl's nodes (herniations of the nucleus pulposus) will establish the diagnosis though Schmorl's nodes may also be seen in Wilson disease, sickle cell disease, and spinal stenosis. In addition, symptoms may be referred from other locations such as the abdomen or the hip/pelvis. Septic arthritis of the sacroiliac joint may mimic diskitis, as may intra-abdominal causes such as appendicitis and pyelonephritis.

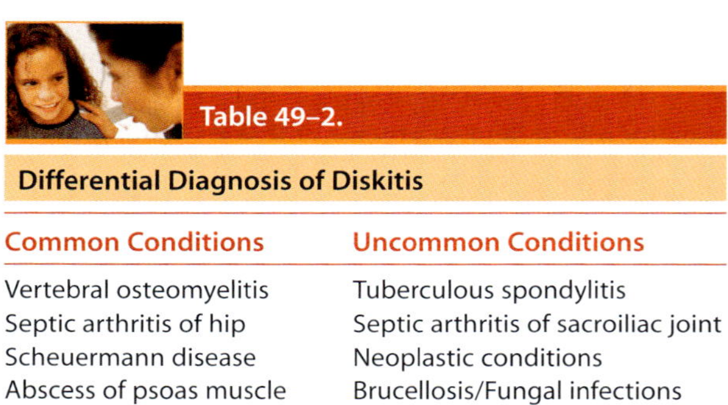

Table 49–2.

Differential Diagnosis of Diskitis

Common Conditions	Uncommon Conditions
Vertebral osteomyelitis	Tuberculous spondylitis
Septic arthritis of hip	Septic arthritis of sacroiliac joint
Scheuermann disease	Neoplastic conditions
Abscess of psoas muscle	Brucellosis/Fungal infections

DIAGNOSIS

Laboratory Studies

Laboratory examination should include complete blood cell count, erythrocyte sedimentation rate (ESR), C-reactive protein (CRP) level and blood cultures. While the WBC may be normal, the ESR is elevated in nearly all patients with diskitis. The CRP can be elevated in the early phase of infection and it is valuable to follow in observing the response to therapy. While blood cultures are negative in the majority of patients, a positive culture is more likely, when symptoms have been present for less than 6 weeks.[6] Wenger et al.[15] reported positive results in only 41% of blood cultures. Similarly, positive cultures are infrequent following open biopsy or aspiration of the disc space. Garron et al.[14] reported positive cultures in 61% following aspiration of the disc space. Factors which may decrease the likelihood of obtaining a positive culture include insufficient sampling, previous antibiotic treatment or inadequate specimen collection and culture techniques.[3,12,18,19] The most common organism isolated is *Staphylococcus aureus.*[1,6,9,12,14,20] The second most common pathogen is *Kingella Kingae,*[1,14,21] which has recently been recognized as a common organism in osteoarticular infections in young children.[22]

Radiologic Imaging

Plain radiographs are normal during the early phase of the disease, and intervertebral disc space narrowing occurs 2–4 weeks after the onset of symptoms (Figure 49–1). Additional findings may include a loss of lumbar lordosis, bony demineralization with localized erosion at the vertebral margins, and loss of vertebral height. In the recovery phase, usually after 2–3 months, sclerosis from remineralization may be observed at the margins of the adjacent vertebral bodies (Figure 49–1). While vertebral height may be restored during growth, disk space narrowing typically persists, and in some cases the adjacent vertebrae may become fused[1,9,23] or enlarged (vertebra magna).[1,10,23] Involvement of more than one disc space is rare, and the posterior elements are spared.[1] Abscess formation may be observed, but rarely requires additional measures for treatment.

A technetium bone scan may demonstrate a focal increase in uptake prior to the appearance of abnormalities on plain radiographs, and the diagnostic accuracy ranges from 72% to 100%.[3,5,6,8,9,24] Magnetic resonance imaging provides the most detailed information, including the extent of the inflammatory process, the condition of disc space and surrounding soft tissue (Figure 49–2),[25] and may potentially reduce the time to diagnosis.[3] While computed tomography provides the best bony detail,

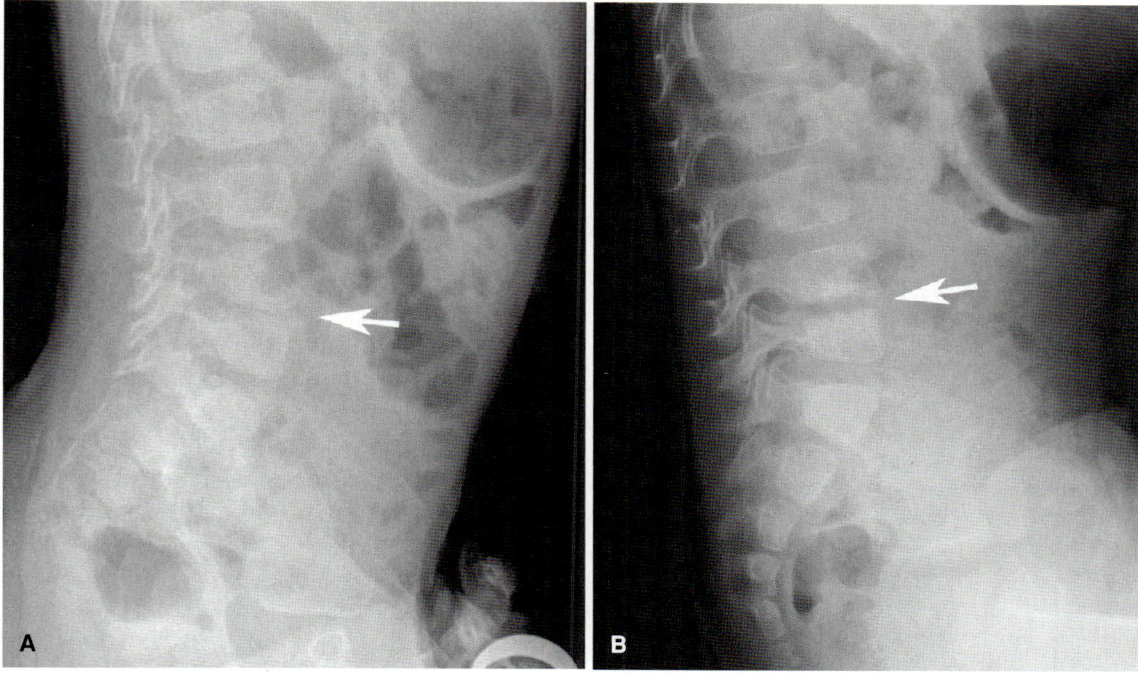

FIGURE 49–1 ■ A 16-month-old boy presented with 3-weeks history of refusal to walk. **(A)** Disc space narrowing is noted between L4-L5 (3 weeks after onset of symptoms); **(B)** Six months after presentation with erosion and sclerosis at the margins of the adjacent vertebral bodies.

and may also identify endplate irregularities/erosions and abscesses, this modality is typically utilized to guide a disc space aspiration or biopsy in selected cases. Diagnostic tests are summarized in Table 49–3.

TREATMENT

Once a diagnosis is established, the treatment is aimed at both alleviating discomfort and eradicating the disease. Symptomatic treatment measures include activity restriction (bed rest is the traditional standard) and bracing (more common today). A thoraco-lumbosacral orthosis is worn when the patient is upright for a period of at least 4–6 weeks. While many cases of diskitis resolve spontaneously (symptomatic treatment only), most authors recommend empiric antibiotic treatment based upon evidence implicating a bacterial cause for diskitis.[1,5,7,8] Empiric intravenous antibiotics (effective against staphylococci) are typically started once blood cultures have been obtained, and patients are usually converted to an oral agent depending on both the clinical response and a sequential assessment of inflammatory markers (CRP, ESR). The specific

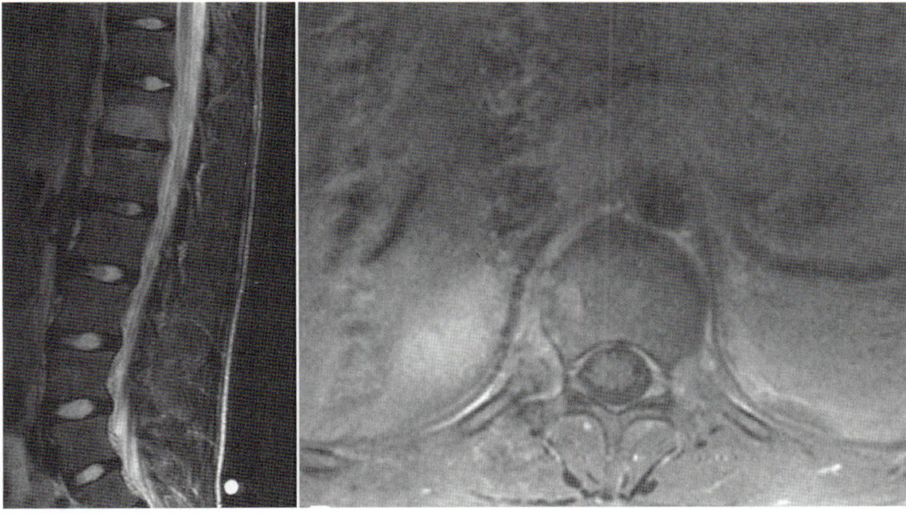

FIGURE 49–2 ■ A 16-year-old boy presented with back pain and abnormal gait. Two weeks after onset of symptoms MRI scan narrowing at the T12-L1 disc space. Hyperintense bone marrow signal abnormality is also demonstrated within the T12 and L1 vertebrae with paravertebral soft tissue enhancement and enlargement of the soft tissue.

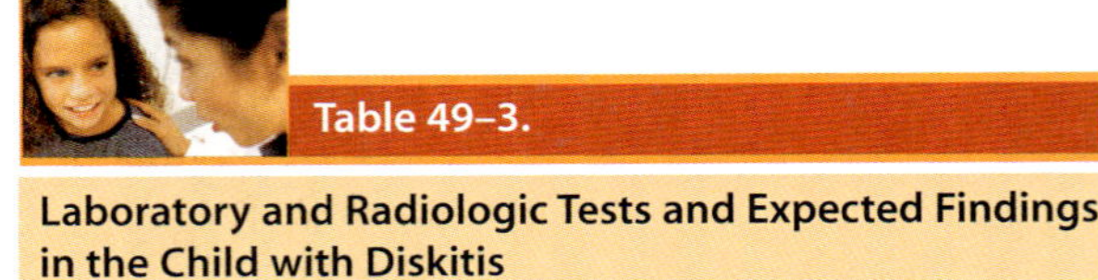

Table 49–3.

Laboratory and Radiologic Tests and Expected Findings in the Child with Diskitis

Test	Expected Findings in Diskitis
Peripheral white blood cell count	Normal or slightly elevated. Left shift and/or mild leukocytosis
ESR	Always elevated. Can be used to monitor response to antibiotics
CRP	Usually elevated earlier than ESR. Can be used to monitor response to antibiotics
Blood culture	Rarely positive. Higher yield after 6 weeks
Plain radiographs of spine	Nondiagnostic during the early phase. Disc space narrowing 2–4 weeks after onset
Tc 99 m Bone scan	Increased uptake in the first week
Computed tomography scan of spine	May demonstrate bony changes and abscess Guides disc space aspiration/biopsy
Magnetic resonance imaging of spine	Best sensitivity in detecting diskitis Excellent demonstration of disk and surrounding soft tissues

antibiotic is modified based upon culture results; the duration of therapy is typically 4–6 weeks. A computed tomography guided needle aspiration of the disc space (or open biopsy) is indicated when there has been a failure to respond to empiric antibiotic therapy. Recommended antibiotics are listed in Table 49–4.[12]

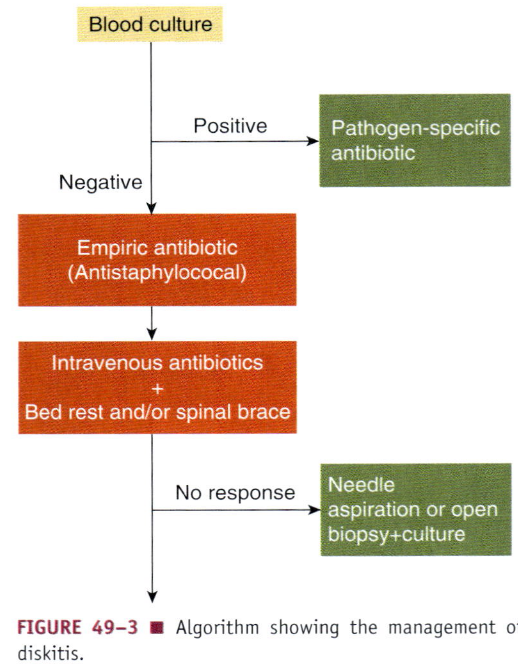

FIGURE 49–3 ■ Algorithm showing the management of diskitis.

Spontaneous interbody fusion may occur even in treated patients, but does not appear to affect the outcome.[1,9,19,23] Surgery is rarely indicated in the treatment of diskitis. An open biopsy should be considered in patients who have not responded to empiric therapy, or when another diagnosis is suspected. Decompression and/or debridement may be indicated in the extremely rare case in which there are neurologic findings on presentation, or neurologic symptoms develop during the course of treatment. An algorithm showing the management of diskitis is summarized in Figure 49–3.

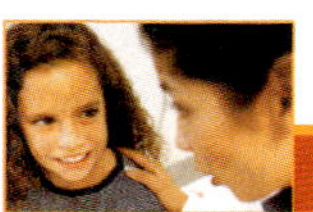

Table 49–4.

Empiric and Definitive Antibiotic Therapy in Children with Discitis

Antibiotic Route	Antibiotic	Indications
Parenteral treatment	Clindamycin	Empiric therapy; effective against many community-acquired MRSA isolates
	Vancomycin	Empiric therapy in ill-appearing child; effective against virtually all community-acquired MRSA isolates
	Cefazolin	Reserve for isolates with documented susceptibility; optimal for proven MSSA isolates
	Nafcillin/Oxacillin	Reserve for isolates with documented susceptibility; optimal for proven MSSA isolates
Oral treatment	Clindamycin*	Empiric therapy; effective against many community-acquired MRSA isolates
	Trimethoprim-Sulfamethoxazole	Empiric therapy; effective against many community-acquired MRSA isolates but poor coverage against group A beta-hemolytic streptococci
	Cephalexin*	Reserve for isolates with documented susceptibility; optimal for proven MSSA isolates
	Dicloxacillin	Reserve for isolates with documented susceptibility; optimal for proven MSSA isolates

Suggested dosing: Clindamycin, 40 mg/kg/day; cephalexin, 100–150 mg/kg/day.
MRSA, methicillin-resistant Staphylococcus aureus; MSSA, methicillin-susceptible S. aureus.

REFERENCES

1. Spiegel PG, Kengla KW, Isaacson AS, Wilson JC Jr. Intervertebral disc-space inflammation in children. *J Bone Joint Surg Am.* 1972;54:284-296.
2. Ventura N, Gonzalez E, Terricabras L, Salvador A, Cabrera M. Intervertebral diskitis in children: a review of 12 cases. *Int Orthop.* 1996;20:32-34.
3. Brown R, Hussain M, McHugh K, Novelli V, Jones D. Diskitis in young children. *J Bone Joint Surg Br.* 2001;83:106-111.
4. Fernandez M, Carrol CL, Baker CJ. Diskitis and vertebral osteomyelitis in children: an 18-year review. *Pediatrics.* 2000;105:1299-1304.
5. Fischer GW, Popich GA, Sullivan DE, Mayfield G, Mazat BA, Patterson PH. Diskitis: a prospective diagnostic analysis. *Pediatrics.* 1978;62:543-548.
6. Wenger DR, Bobechko WP, Gilday DL. The spectrum of intervertebral disc-space infection in children. *J Bone Joint Surg Am.* 1978;60:100-108.
7. Ryoppy S, Jaaskelainen J, Rapola J, Alberty A. Nonspecific diskitis in children. A nonmicrobial disease? *Clin Orthop Relat Res.* 1993;297:95-99.
8. Crawford AH, Kucharzyk DW, Ruda R, Smitherman HC Jr. Diskitis in children. *Clin Orthop Relat Res.* 1991;226:70-79.
9. Scoles PV, Quinn TP. Intervertebral diskitis in children and adolescents. *Clin Orthop Relat Res.* 1982;162:31-36.
10. Smith RF, Taylor TK. Inflammatory lesions of intervertebral discs in children. *J Bone Joint Surg Am.* 1967;49:1508-1520.
11. Doyle JR. Narrowing of the intervertebral-disc space in children. Presumably an infectious lesion of the disc. *J Bone Joint Surg Am.* 1960;42-A:1191-1200.
12. Ring D, Johnston CE II, Wenger DR. Pyogenic infectious spondylitis in children: the convergence of diskitis and vertebral osteomyelitis. *J Pediatr Orthop.* 1995;15:652-660.
13. Karabouta Z, Bisbinas I, Davidson A, Goldsworthy LL. Diskitis in toddlers: a case series and review. *Acta Paediatr.* 2005;94:1516-1518.
14. Garron E, Viehweger E, Launay F, Guillaume JM, Jouve JL, Bollini G. Nontuberculous spondylodiscitis in children. *J Pediatr Orthop.* 2002;22:321-328.
15. Ring D, Wenger DR. Magnetic resonance-imaging scans in diskitis. Sequential studies in a child who needed operative drainage: a case report. *J Bone Joint Surg Am.* 1994;76:596-601.
16. Holliday PO, III, Davis CH Jr., Shaffner LS. Intervertebral disc space infection in a child presenting as a psoas abscess: case report. *Neurosurgery.* 1980;7:395-397.
17. Mirovsky Y, Copeliovich L, Halperin N. Gowers' sign in children with diskitis of the lumbar spine. *J Pediatr Orthop B.* 2005;14:68-70.
18. Sapico FL, Montgomerie JZ. Vertebral osteomyelitis. *Infect Dis Clin North Am.* 1990;4:539-550.
19. Kayser R, Mahlfeld K, Greulich M, Grasshoff H. Spondylodiscitis in childhood: results of a long-term study. *Spine.* 2005;30:318-323.
20. Kemp HB, Jackson JW, Jeremiah JD, Hall AJ. Pyogenic infections occurring primarily in intervertebral discs. *J Bone Joint Surg Br.* 1973;55:698-714.
21. Amir J, Shockelford PG. *Kingella kingae* intervertebral disk infection. *J Clin Microbiol.* 1991;29:1083-1086.
22. Lundy DW, Kehl DK. Increasing prevalence of *Kingella kingae* in osteoarticular infections in young children. *J Pediatr Orthop.* 1998;18:262-267.
23. Jansen BR, Hart W, Schreuder O. Diskitis in childhood. 12-35-year follow-up of 35 patients. *Acta Orthop Scand.* 1993;64:33-36.
24. Nolla-Sole JM, Mateo-Soria L, Rozadilla-Sacanell A, et al. Role of technetium-99m diphosphonate and gallium-67 citrate bone scanning in the early diagnosis of infectious spondylodiscitis. A comparative study. *Ann Rheum Dis.* 1992;51:665-667.
25. Gabriel KR, Crawford AH. Magnetic resonance imaging in a child who had clinical signs of diskitis. Report of a case. *J Bone Joint Surg Am.* 1988;70:938-941.

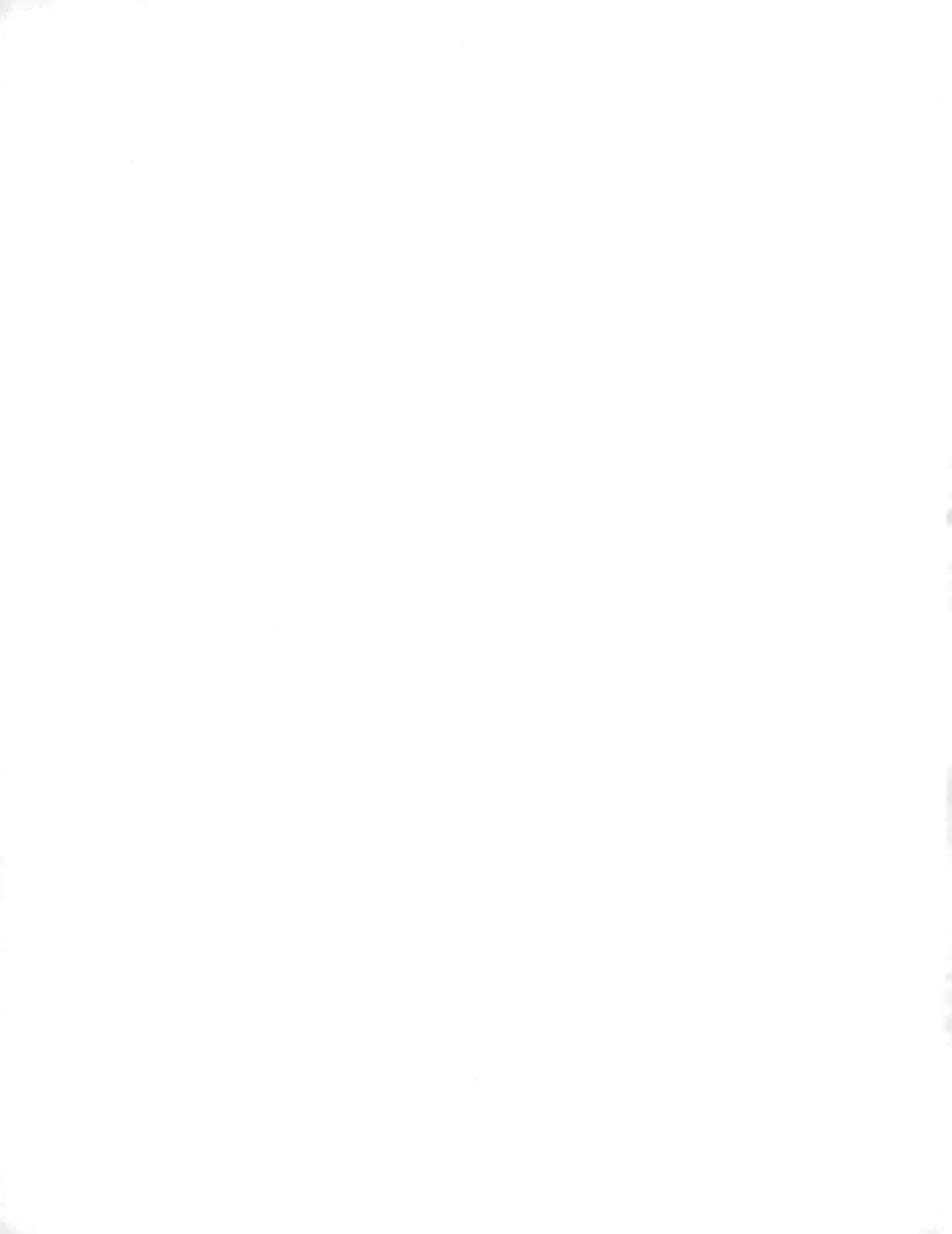

SECTION 13

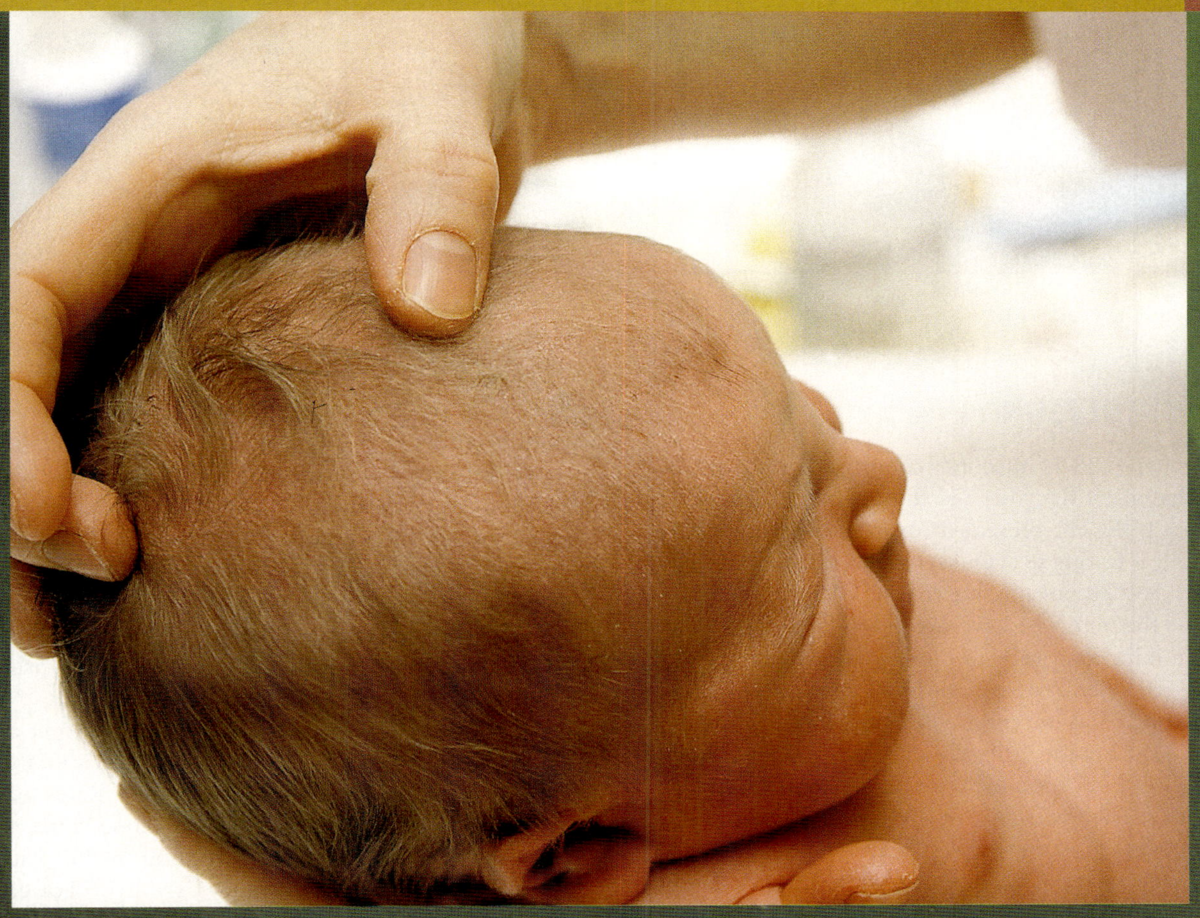

Perinatal and Neonatal Infections

CHAPTER 50

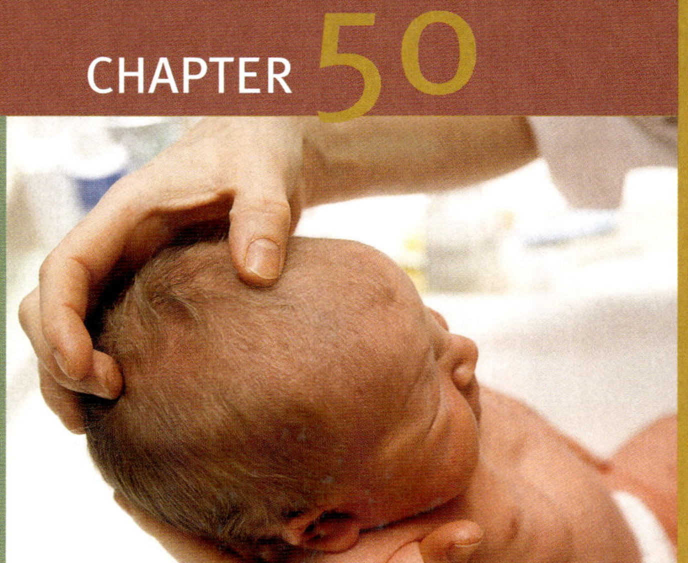

Congenital TORCH Infections

Yeisid F. Gozzo and Patrick G. Gallagher

INTRODUCTION

Congenital TORCH infections comprise a group of diseases that affect the fetus and the newborn. Classically, the term TORCH represented Toxoplasmosis, other, traditionally referring to syphilis, rubella, cytomegalovirus (CMV), and herpes simplex virus (HSV). Recent additions to the acronym have expanded its repertoire to include infections such as human immunodeficiency virus (HIV), enterovirus, parvovirus, and varicella. These congenital infections share many clinical manifestations. Consequently, the differential diagnosis of one TORCH infection includes the remaining TORCH infections. The prevalence of the TORCH infections is variable. Infection due to rubella and toxoplasmosis is rarely seen in the United States, while CMV is common, representing a significant public health concern. Table 50–1 lists the classically defined TORCH infections and their common manifestations weighted according to their prevalence among infected neonates. The following chapter will discuss the epidemiology, pathogenesis, clinical manifestations, diagnostic approaches, and management strategies for affected infants.

CYTOMEGALOVIRUS

Definitions and Epidemiology

Cytomegalovirus, a ubiquitous pathogen, is the most common cause of congenital viral infections. It is a double-stranded, species-specific DNA virus of the herpes family.[1,2] Infection in the immunoincompetent, vulnerable fetus can have devastating effects. Congenital CMV infection is a leading cause of sensorineural hearing loss (SNHL) and neurodevelopmental disturbances resulting from central nervous system involvement.[3]

The incidence of primary CMV infection in pregnancies is estimated to range from 0.15% to 4%, with vertical transmission rates as high as 40%.[2,4] Over 27,000 women per year in the United States experience a primary CMV infection during pregnancy. Primary infection in pregnancy is not evenly distributed across racial, ethnic, and socioeconomic groups. Young women of Mexican American descent and non-Hispanic blacks are disproportionately at higher risk of acquiring primary infection in pregnancy.[5]

In a study of 1018 blood donors screened over a 2-month period, Munro et al. demonstrated that CMV seroprevalence rises with increasing age. Rates of seropositivity increased from 35% in blood donors younger than 20 years old to 73% by the age of 50.[4] The seroconversion rate in pregnancy is ~2%.[6] Lower seropositivity rates in women of childbearing age pose a potential risk to their offspring. A review of multiple studies that screened infants and fetuses for CMV revealed that the maternofetal transmission rate was 32% in primary maternal infection compared to 1.4% in recurrent infection.[7]

Pathogenesis

Infants may acquire CMV infection through transplacental transmission prior to birth, during vaginal delivery through an infected birth canal, or through the administration of infected breast milk or blood products in the postpartum period. Maternal CMV infections pose the greatest threat to the fetus when they are acquired during early gestation. Postnatal infection occurs more frequently than transplacental infection and usually results in benign disease. While most infants who acquire the infection through contaminated breast milk or CMV-contaminated blood products remain

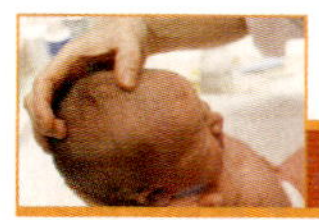

Table 50–1.

Frequency of Clinical Findings in Infants with Congenital Infections

	Congenital Infection				
Clinical Findings	**Rubella**	**Toxoplasma**	**CMV**	**Syphilis**	**HSV**
Intrauterine growth retardation	[+++]	±	++	++	±
Reticuloendothelial system					
Jaundice	+	++	[+++]	+++	+
Hepatitis	±	+	+++	+++	+
Hepatosplenomegaly	+++	++	[+++]	[+++]	+
Anemia	+	+++	++	+++	−
Thrombocytopenia	++	±	[+++]	++	+
Disseminated intravascular coagulation	−	−	±	−	++
Adenopathy	++	++	−	++	−
Dermal erythropoiesis	[+]	−	+	−	−
Skin rash	−	+	−	[++]	[+++]
Bone abnormalities	++	−	±	[++]	−
Eye					
Cataracts	[++]	±	±	±	−
Retinopathy	++	[+++]	[+]	±	[+++]
Microphthalmia	+	±	±	−	±
Central nervous system					
Microcephaly	+	+	[++]	−	±
Meningoencephalitis	++	+++	+++	++	[+++]
Brain calcification	±	[++]	[++]	−	+
Hydrocephalus	−	[++]	±	±	++
Hearing defect	+++	+	[+++]	+	−
Pneumonitis	++	+	±	+	±
Cardiovascular					
Myocarditis	+	±	±	±	−
Congenital defect	[+++]	−	−	−	−

± rare; +, 5% to 20%; ++, 20% to 50%; +++, more than 50%; □, prominent feature of particular infection; CMV, cytomegalovirus; HSV, herpes simplex virus.
Reprinted with permission from Sanchez PJ, Siegel JD. Cytomegalovirus. In: McMillan JA, Feigin RD, DeAngelis C, Jones MD, eds. Oski's Pediatrics: Principles and Practice, 4th ed. Philadelphia: Lippincott Williams and Wilkins; 2006;512.

asymptomatic, premature infants compose a unique population at higher risk for symptomatic infection. Approximately one-fourth of preterm infants develop symptoms when transfused with CMV-positive blood.[1,2,8]

The incidence of congenital CMV disease among all live-born infants has been estimated as high as 1% and this may be an underestimation. The impact on child health is significant. A recent review of 117,986 infants screened for congenital CMV reported that 12.7% of infected children manifested symptoms in the immediate newborn period and 40–58% of these infants developed long-term sequelae. In addition, 13.5% of the initially asymptomatic group also developed long-term sequelae.[1,9,10] These data indicate that congenital CMV represents a substantial burden to public health.

Consequently, prevention of CMV infection in women of childbearing age is an important step in reducing this societal burden and decreasing the numbers of affected children. Vaccines, hyperimmunoglobulin, and ganciclovir have been evaluated for their potential to reduce the risk of maternal–fetal transmission. Currently, no effective vaccine is available and the efficacy of ganciclovir has not been clearly defined in randomized controlled trials.[12] One study suggested that administration of oral valacyclovir to women carrying fetuses with symptomatic CMV infection led to therapeutic drug levels in both amniotic fluid and fetal sera and a reduction in viral load in fetal blood. Larger randomized studies are required to determine the efficacy of this therapy for congenital CMV infection.[11]

Few studies have evaluated the effect of passive immunization with CMV-specific immunoglobulin on the rate of fetal infection. One study suggested that the use of CMV-specific hyperimmunoglobulin prevented fetal infection in mothers with primary CMV infection in pregnancy.[6] No randomized controlled trials have been conducted and further investigation is required.

Clinical Presentation

Common complications associated with primary CMV infection in pregnancy include spontaneous abortion, premature delivery, intrauterine growth restriction, and hydrops fetalis. Placental dysfunction brought about by inflammation is thought to contribute to these complications,[12] as well as to complications during labor and delivery.[13]

Most (85–90%) infants with congenital CMV infection manifest no signs or symptoms of disease at the time of delivery. However, late sequelae such as developmental delay, learning disability, or SNHL occur in 8–15%.[1,14] Among symptomatic newborns, 80–90% have severe neurologic manifestations[2,14,15] and overall mortality is 20–30%.[13,14]

The virus infects many organs with a predilection for the reticuloendothelial and central nervous systems.[2] Among symptomatic newborns, the most common presenting symptoms include hepatosplenomegaly, petechiae, intrauterine growth restriction, and microcephaly.[1,15] Table 50–2 summarizes common clinical and laboratory findings in a series of 106 infants with symptomatic congenital CMV infection. Dermal erythropoiesis, commonly referred to as "blueberry muffin rash," may be seen in infants with CMV (Figure 50–1), although it is more classically identified with congenital rubella syndrome.

While many of the initial manifestations of congenital CMV infection (Table 50–2) resolve over time, central nervous system sequelae are permanent.[8] Anatomic abnormalities associated with congenital CMV infection include periventricular and intracranial calcifications (Figure 50–2), microcephaly, ventriculomegaly, and migration defects. Other findings include hypotonia, seizures, chorioretinitis, and SNHL.[1,2,12,15]

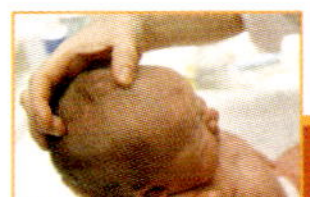

Table 50–2.

Clinical and Laboratory Findings in Infants with Symptomatic Congenital CMV Infection in the Newborn Period

Abnormalities	Abnormal/Total Examined
Prematurity*	36/106 (34)†
Small for gestational age‡	53/106 (50)
Reticuloendothelial	
Petechiae	80/106 (76)
Jaundice	69/103 (67)
Hepatosplenomegaly	63/105 (60)
Purpura	14/105 (13)
Neurologic	
One or more of the following	72/106 (68)
Microcephaly§	54/102 (53)
Lethargy/hypotonia	28/104 (27)
Poor suck	20/103 (19)
Seizures	7/105 (7)
Elevated ALT (>80 units/L)	46/58 (83)†
Thrombocytopenia	
$<100 \times 10^3/mm^3$	62/81 (77)
$<50 \times 10^3/mm^3$	43/81 (53)
Conjugated hyperbilirubinemia	
Direct serum bilirubin >2 mg/dL	55/68 (81)
Direct serum bilirubin >4 mg/dL	47/68 (69)
Hemolysis	37/72 (51)
Increased CSF protein (>120 mg/dL)¶	24/52 (46)

*Gestational age less than 38 weeks.
†Numbers in parentheses, percent.
‡Weight less than 10th percentile for gestational age.
§Head circumference less than 10th percentile based on Colorado Intrauterine Growth Charts for premature newborns.
¶Determination in the first week of life.
Reprinted with permission from Boppana SB, Fass RF, Britt WJ et al. Symptomatic congenital cytomegalovirus infection: Neonatal morbidity and mortality. Pediatr Infect Dis J 1992;11:93–99.

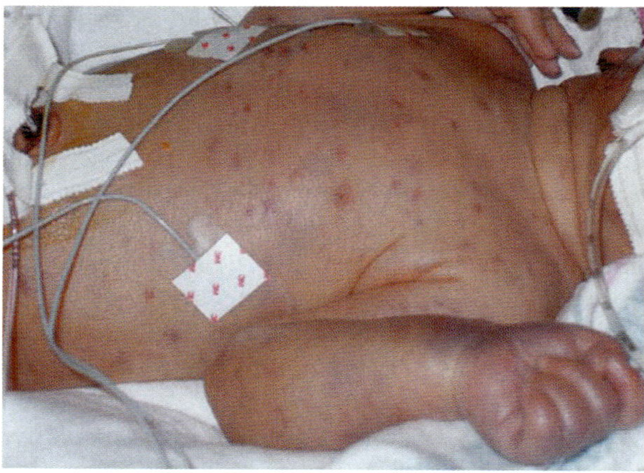

FIGURE 50–1 ■ "Blueberry muffin" rash in an infant with congenital CMV. (Dermal erythropoiesis, seen in association with congenital CMV infection, is commonly called the "blueberry muffin rash" for its classic violaceous appearance. Lesions are diffuse and appear petechial or purpuric.)

Congenital CMV infection is the most common cause of SNHL in children.[2,8] Often progressive, SNHL may be detected at birth, or in infancy and childhood.[15] Table 50–3 represents the cumulative incidence of hearing loss in a cohort of 388 children diagnosed with congenital CMV infection. Rates of SNHL rose steadily from 5.2% at birth to 8.4% by 12 months, reaching 15.4% by 6 years of age.[16] The adequacy of current hearing screening programs performed in the immediate neonatal period has been called into question because of the high numbers of initially asymptomatic infants with congenital CMV infection at risk for late onset SNHL.[16]

Diagnosis

Congenital CMV infection should be suspected in cases of primary maternal CMV infection during or

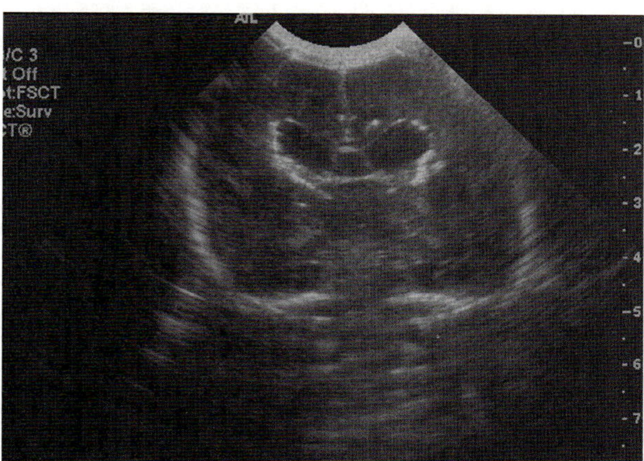

FIGURE 50–2 ■ Periventricular calcifications in congenital CMV infection. (Inflammation in the watershed region of the subependymal germinal matrix results in cystic changes and postinflammatory calcifications. These findings are distributed in the periventricular gray matter and may hinder normal migration resulting in cortical hypoplasia.)

just before pregnancy, maternal exposure to the virus during gestation, or where fetal findings on prenatal ultrasonography are attributable to CMV infection. The most common ultrasound findings suggestive of fetal CMV infection include hyperechogenic bowel, ascites, cardiomegaly, and oligohydramnios. Other common findings include ventriculomegaly, intracranial calcifications, microcephaly, intrauterine growth restriction (IUGR), hydrops, hepatic echodensities, and increased placental thickness.[17,18]

The diagnosis of congenital CMV infection must be made in the first 2–3 weeks of life; otherwise findings may reflect postnatally acquired infection (Table 50–4). The gold standard diagnostic technique is culture of the virus from samples of urine or saliva. While culture methods can take up to 2 weeks, rapid centrifugation-enhanced culture techniques combined with antibody studies can be completed in ~24 hours. Polymerase chain reaction (PCR) techniques for detection of CMV in urine, saliva, leukocytes, or other tissues are also being used more commonly to diagnose congenital CMV infection.[2,8] The limited sensitivity and specificity of CMV-specific IgM antibody assays call into question their utility in diagnosing congenital CMV infection, and its use as a diagnostic method is currently not recommended.[8,17]

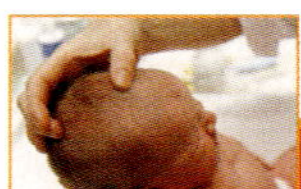

Table 50–3.

Cumulative Incidence of SNHL in 388 Children with Congenital CMV Infection

Age of Child	Cumulative Incidence of All SNHL (%)*†	Cumulative Incidence of SNHL (%)*‡
<1 month	5.2	3.9
3 months	6.5	5.3
12 months	8.4	6.8
24 months	9.9	7.2
36 months	10.8	7.6
48 months	11.3	7.6
60 months	12.4	7.6
72 months	15.4	8.3

**Estimates are based on Kaplan–Meier methods.*
†Includes any hearing loss >20 dB thresholds.
‡Includes only hearing loss ≥30 dB thresholds at 500–4000 Hz.
Reprinted with permission from Fowler KB, Dahle AJ, Boppana SB, et al. Newborn hearing screening: Will children with hearing loss caused by congenital cytomegalovirus infection be missed? J Pediatr 1999;135:60–64.

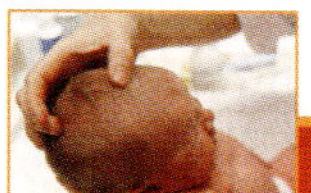

Table 50–4.

Evaluation of the Infant with a Suspected TORCH Infection

Cerebrospinal fluid
- CSF cell count, protein, glucose (enterovirus, rubella, syphilis)
- CSF PCR (enterovirus, HSV)
- CSF VDRL (syphilis)

Blood
- IgG (specify *Toxoplasma* or rubella; if positive, send IgM)
- RPR (syphilis)
- Hepatitis B surface antigen
- PCR (enteroviruses, HIV)

Skin lesions
- Dark-field examination (syphilis)
- Direct fluorescent antibody (HSV, varicella)
- PCR (HSV, varicella)
- Tzanck smear (HSV)*
- Culture (HSV)*

Urine
- PCR (CMV, enteroviruses)
- Culture (CMV)

Mucosa
- Conjunctiva culture (HSV)
- Mouth or nasopharynx culture (HSV, enterovirus)†
- Rectum culture (enterovirus, HSV)†

Other studies
- Audiologic evaluation (CMV, rubella, toxoplasmosis)
- Head CT (CMV, toxoplasmosis)
- Ophthalmologic examination (toxoplasmosis, rubella, CMV, HSV, varicella, syphilis)
- Radiograph of long bones (rubella, syphilis)

**Tzanck smear rarely used. PCR and direct fluorescent antibody testing more common. Culture may not be necessary if PCR is performed.*
†Enteroviral cultures rarely performed given the high sensitivity of enteroviral PCR for detection of enterovirus in blood, urine, and stool specimens.
CMV, cytomegalovirus; CSF, cerebrospinal fluid; CT, computed tomography; HSV, herpes simplex virus; PCR, polymerase chain reaction; RPR, rapid plasma reagin; VDRL, Venereal Disease Research Laboratory.

Once a diagnosis of congenital CMV is made, a thorough evaluation is required to assess for multisystem involvement. A complete blood cell count to detect thrombocytopenia and anemia, and liver enzymes and bilirubin levels to detect hepatitis and liver dysfunction are recommended. If respiratory symptoms are present, a chest radiograph searching for interstitial pneumonitis should be obtained. A fundoscopic examination to detect chorioretinitis and otologic evaluation to detect hearing loss should be performed.[2]

At a minimum, screening cranial ultrasonography to detect central nervous system abnormalities should be obtained. In one study, 57 newborns with congenital CMV infection were screened with cranial ultrasound and then followed with audiologic and neurodevelopmental evaluations. Neonates with signs and symptoms of congenital infection at birth had findings on cranial ultrasonography more often than asymptomatic newborns. At follow-up, all symptomatic infants with an abnormal ultrasound in the immediate neonatal period developed at least one long-term severe complication of the disease.[19]

Management/Treatment

The treatment of congenital CMV is largely supportive. Small studies have sought to describe the pharmacokinetics and safety of various oral and intravenous anti-CMV therapeutic agents in this population.[20,21] The use of ganciclovir has not yet been proven efficacious in the treatment of congenital CMV infection in randomized, blinded controlled studies. Only one study has reported any significant benefit associated with the use of ganciclovir. In 2003, Kimberlin et al. identified a cohort of congenitally infected newborns with central nervous system (CNS) abnormalities. Infants were evaluated at baseline with repeated assessments at 6 months and 1 year or later. Investigators reported that 84% of treated infants versus 59% of controls demonstrated unchanged or improved hearing. None of the treated infants versus 41% of the nontreated infants had worsened hearing loss at 6 months. Among infants assessed at 1 year or later, 21% of treated infants and 68% of untreated infants developed further hearing loss. This small study suggests that ganciclovir may reduce the progression of SNHL. Neutropenia was the most common adverse effect with 63% of treated infants developing neutropenia necessitating either a dose reduction or halt in therapy.[22] Preliminary results of further follow-up of this trial suggested that ganciclovir use may be related to improved neurodevlopmental outcome. Further investigation is required to determine the strength of this association.[23]

Serial physical examinations and follow-up hearing tests every 3 months in the first year are recommended. After the first year of life, follow-up may be modified as indicated by the presence and degree of hearing loss.[2]

NEONATAL HSV INFECTION

Definitions and Epidemiology

Neonatal infection with HSV, a double-stranded DNA virus, may be associated with severe morbidity and mortality. The majority of infections in the neonate, ~70%, are due to infection with HSV-2, the virus commonly associated with genital herpes. The remaining 30% are due to infections with HSV-1, the virus commonly associated with cold sores. HSV infections are described as primary, recurrent, and nonprimary first episodes. Primary infection occurs in an individual without prior history of the disease. Recurrent infections occur in individuals with prior history of HSV infection. A nonprimary first episode is an HSV infection in a person with history of another type of HSV infection.[2,24]

Approximately one in 3000–20,000 live births is complicated by neonatal HSV infection and disease. The infection can be acquired *in utero*, through an infected birth canal, or postnatally through contact with an infected person, for example, oral lesion(s), herpetic whitlow, etc. The majority of neonatal infections (85–95%) are acquired during labor and delivery.[2,24,25]

Pathogenesis

Several risk factors have been associated with maternal–fetal transmission of HSV with the most significant risk factor being maternal primary infection close to the time of labor and birth. Other risk factors include rupture of membranes greater than 4 hours, prematurity, and fetal instrumentation, for example, use of scalp electrodes.[2,26]

The risk of maternal–fetal transmission can be influenced by maternal serologic status and the type of maternal HSV disease.[27] The risk of perinatal HSV is 44% when the mother has a primary genital HSV infection at the time of delivery compared with 1.3% when the mother has recurrent genital lesions. Nonhispanic white women are more likely to be seronegative and their infants are at greatest risk for neonatal herpes infection.[28]

Rates of neonatal disease in infants born vaginally to women with primary HSV infection range from 33% to 50%. This high rate of infection is attributed to several factors including higher viral loads in women with primary HSV disease and decreased maternal anti-HSV antibodies. Many primary HSV infections result in vague symptomatology. As a result, more than 75% of infants with HSV infection are born to women who had no clinical history or manifestations of HSV during their pregnancy. Rates of neonatal disease in recurrent maternal infection are less than 5%.[2,24]

Clinical Presentation

The onset of neonatal disease varies from birth to 3 weeks of age, usually between days 11 and 17. The infection can manifest in one of three forms, classified as disseminated disease, localized CNS disease, or skin-eye-mouth (SEM) disease. Each type occurs with equal frequency and there can be substantial overlap between classifications.[2]

In disseminated disease, manifestations most often occur between 10 and 12 days of life, but symptoms may appear as early as the first day of life. The most common presentation is a sepsis-like syndrome with prominent liver and lung involvement. Signs and symptoms may include respiratory distress, seizures, petechiae, disseminated intravascular coagulation, hepatosplenomegaly, and vesicles. However, more than 20% of affected newborns have no vesicular skin lesions. Mortality results from respiratory failure, severe hepatic dysfunction, and/or coagulopathy.[2,24,25]

Localized CNS disease usually presents during the second to third week of life. Signs and symptoms include lethargy, bulging fontanel, irritability, temperature instability, seizures, and vesicles. Mortality is secondary to acute neurologic dysfunction secondary to the massive brain destruction caused by HSV.[2,24,25]

SEM disease most frequently presents in the first 2 weeks of life. Manifestations are limited to the skin and mucous membranes, particularly at sites of trauma. Common findings include lesions on the skin (85%), in the oropharynx, and ophthalmic manifestations including conjunctivitis and keratitis.[2,25]

Morbidity and mortality rates remain high despite appropriate treatment in infants with disseminated and CNS disease. In disseminated disease, the risk of mortality is 30% with less than 20% of survivors suffering long-term neurologic complications. In CNS disease, the risk of mortality is 5%, with greater than 60% of survivors suffering long-term neurologic sequelae including microcephaly, spastic cerebral palsy, epilepsy, blindness, and developmental delay.[2,24,25] Morbidity and mortality associated with SEM disease are low, both accounting for 1–2% of treated infants.[25]

Preterm infants are a particularly vulnerable population to HSV infection. Disseminated and CNS diseases predominate and mortality is high. These observations have been attributed to immunologic immaturity and lack of maternally derived antibodies.[26]

Differential Diagnosis

The variable manifestations of neonatal HSV infection overlap with many other newborn diseases leading to a broad differential diagnosis. Other potential infectious causes include bacteria (e.g., group B streptococci, *Staphylococcus aureus*, Listeria monocytogenes, enteric gram-negative rods, and *Treponema pallidum*) and other viruses (e.g., varicella zoster virus, enteroviruses, CMV, toxoplasmosis, and Rubella). Noninfectious causes of severe illness include surfactant deficiency, respiratory distress syndrome, intraventricular hemorrhage, and necrotizing enterocolitis. Other causes of skin rashes that may resemble the lesions of HSV include erythema toxicum, neonatal melanosis, acrodermatitis, incontinentia pigmenti, and histiocytosis.[25]

Diagnosis

The gold standard for the diagnosis of neonatal HSV infection is the identification of the virus in the culture of urine, stool, blood, cerebrospinal fluid (CSF), and lesions of the skin and mucous membranes. Of sites routinely cultured, skin and eye/conjunctival cultures yield HSV in 90% of infants with neonatal infection.[29] Rapid viral detection assays such as direct fluorescent antibody (DFA) or enzyme immunoassay (EIA) are specific but slightly less sensitive than culture.[2,24,25,29]

PCR to detect HSV DNA in CSF is the gold standard for HSV meningoencephalitis; the test, when properly performed, has nearly 100% sensitivity and more than 90% specificity. False-negative results may occur when the test is performed early in the course of illness. If the clinical findings suggest HSV but the CSF HSV PCR test is negative, the test should be repeated several days later.[25] PCR testing of vesicular swabs and mucosal surfaces is more sensitive than DFA testing. A positive HSV PCR test from peripheral blood also confirms the diagnosis of HSV, however the sensitivity of this approach is uncertain.

Other studies to consider in the evaluation of a newborn with suspected HSV disease include complete blood count, coagulation studies, and liver function testing. CSF findings, typically 50–100 WBC/mm^3 with a lymphocyte predominance, elevated protein, and low glucose, are nonspecific. In infants with respiratory symptomatology, chest radiographs demonstrate a central pattern of involvement that evolves peripherally to involve the entire lung within 1–3 days.[2] Computerized tomography or magnetic resonance imaging of the brain may reveal focal or diffuse necrosis in cases of CNS disease.

Management

Timely recognition of HSV disease in the newborn represents a unique challenge because a high index of suspicion is required and delay in initiating antiviral therapy may lead to devastating sequelae.

The management of the symptomatic infant with a positive maternal history of HSV infection or active lesions at the time of delivery is straightforward. These infants should be evaluated with surface swabs for HSV detection by PCR, DFA, or culture from the rectum, mouth, nasopharynx, and conjunctivae. Cultures from blood, urine, stool, and CSF should be obtained and CSF sent for HSV PCR. Treatment with intravenous acyclovir 60 mg/kg/d divided three times per day should be initiated. Duration of therapy is 14 days for infants with SEM disease and 21 days for those with disseminated or CNS disease.[24] Patients with a positive CSF PCR require repeat CSF examination at the end of therapy to document a negative PCR. If the test remains positive, some experts recommend continuing acyclovir until the CSF PCR is negative; while a positive CSF HSV PCR test at the end of therapy portends a worse prognosis, it is not clear whether treating for a longer period of time necessarily improves outcomes.[24]

Controversy exists in the evaluation and treatment of the asymptomatic newborn exposed to maternal HSV infection. Multiple factors such as the mode of delivery, presence of active maternal lesions, and the type of maternal disease affect the risk of transmission and should be considered in risk assessment and management decisions. Figure 50–3 outlines current recommendations for the evaluation and treatment of newborns with suspected disease or potential exposure to HSV.[2,24,30]

Neonates with HSV disease and those whose mothers had active lesions at the time of delivery should be placed in contact precautions. Contact precautions may not be necessary if a cesarean section was performed while membranes were intact or ruptured for less than 4 hours. Infants whose mothers have a history of recurrent genital herpes without active lesions at time of delivery do not require special isolation.[2,24]

Disease relapse in infants with SEM and CNS disease have been described. Management of these infants is controversial and infectious disease consultation is suggested. Infants with three or more recurrences of cutaneous vesicles within the first 6 months of life have a substantially worse neurologic outcome and the use of suppressive oral acyclovir therapy reduces the frequency of recurrences. However, the impact of suppressive therapy on long-term neurologic outcome is not clear and studies are ongoing.[24,25,31] However, infants with frequent recurrent skin lesions in the first 6 months are at increased risk for CNS disease.[2] Cutaneous recurrences can negatively impact infants and their families, interfering with family activities and ability to access childcare.[25]

Follow-up to monitor for disease recurrence, especially for infants with SEM disease, or development of long-term sequelae, especially for infants with CNS disease, is required.[25]

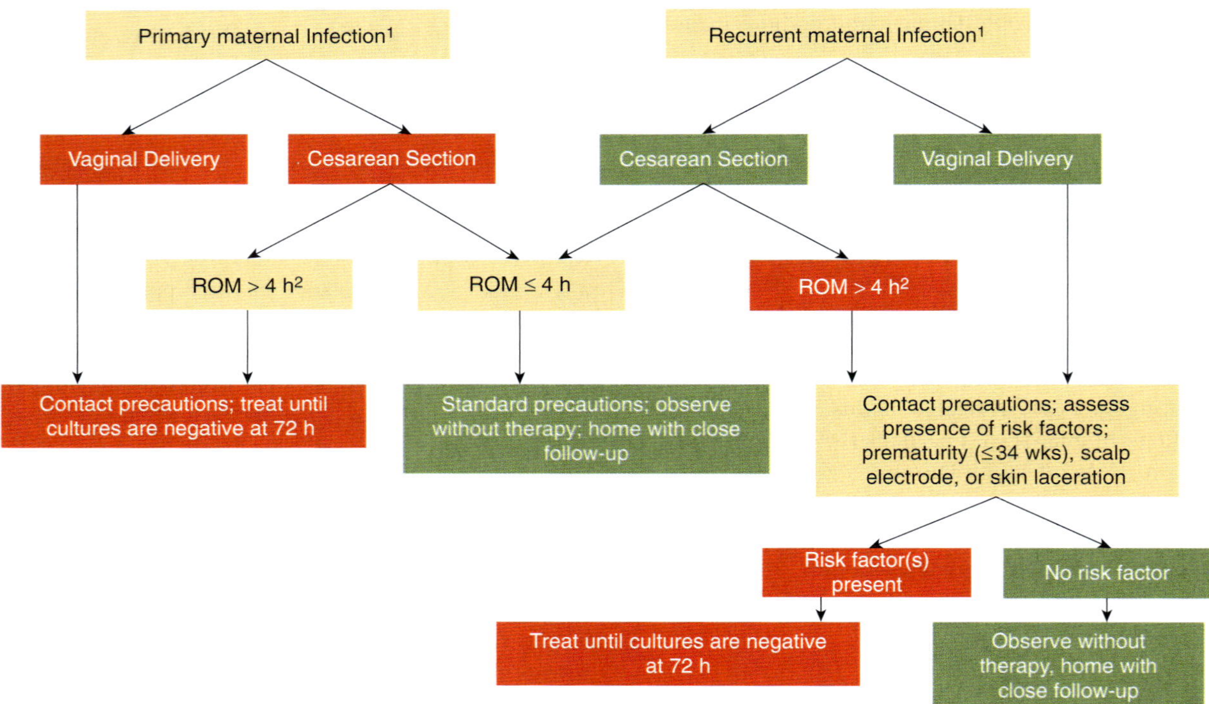

FIGURE 50–3 ■ Management of the asymptomatic newborn potentially exposed to herpes simplex virus at delivery. (HSV, herpes simplex virus; ROM, rupture of membranes; CSF, cerebral spinal fluid; PCR, polymerase chain reaction. (1) Culture conjunctiva, nasopharynx or throat, rectum, cerebrospinal fluid (CSF), and vesicle (if present). (2) Some experts would observe infant carefully and not treat unless cultures are positive for HSV or clinical signs of infection are present.)

SYPHILIS

Definitions and Epidemiology

Syphilis is one of the "great pretenders" because the disease may manifest with a broad range of signs and symptoms that mimic many other diseases. It has been a serious public health concern for centuries. The infection causes disease in both adults and children and, when acquired during pregnancy, poses a serious threat to the fetus.

Syphilis is caused by *T. pallidum*, a motile spirochete and one of four treponomemal pathogens that cause human disease. A significant peak in the incidence of acquired and congenital syphilis occurred in the late 1980s and early 1990s, with a dramatic decrease in the rates of both types of disease in the last decade (Figure 50–4). The incidence of disease varies by race and region with the highest rates of infection found in African Americans and Latinos living in urban areas of the southern and northeast United States.[2,32–34]

Pathogenesis

Outside the newborn period, syphilis is primarily transmitted through sexual contact with an infected individual. Involvement with multiple sexual partners, poverty, illicit drug use, and coinfection with HIV are the risk factors most consistently associated with disease acquisition.[34,35]

In congenital syphilis, the disease is transmitted from mother to infant via transplacental passage or through contact with infectious lesions at the time of delivery. The infection can be transmitted at any stage although risk of transmission varies with the stage of disease in the mother. Pregnant women with untreated primary or secondary syphilis have a 60–90% transmission rate compared to a 10–30% transmission rate in latent disease.[2,32] Lack of, or inadequate, prenatal care is a major contributor to vertical transmission rates of infection from mother to infant and the disease is almost completely preventable when detected and treated during pregnancy.[34,35]

Clinical Presentation

Thirty to forty percent of women with untreated syphilis in early pregnancy suffer complications such as spontaneous abortion, stillbirth, or preterm delivery. Other complications include placentomegaly, hydrops fetalis, and perinatal death.[2,34] Up to one-third of surviving infants with congenital syphilis are symptomatic at birth. Manifestations of congenital syphilis are divided into early and late findings.[34] Early signs and symptoms occur in the first 2 years of life, mainly presenting in the first 3–8 weeks. Early symptoms, attributable to active infection and inflammation, include low birth weight, failure to thrive, lymphadenopathy, hydrocephalus, edema, fever, or a maculopapular rash that later desquamates. Respiratory and gastrointestinal manifestations include respiratory distress, bloody rhinitis called "snuffles," hepatosplenomegaly, hepatitis,

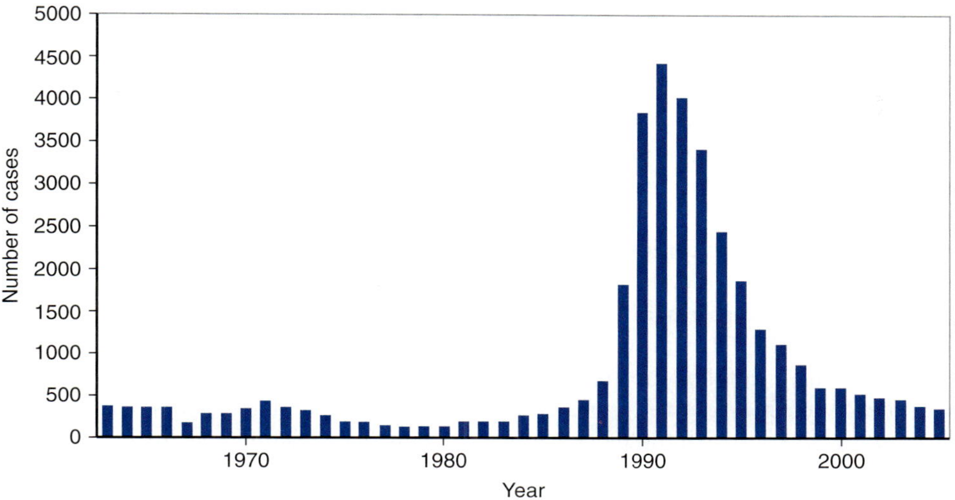

FIGURE 50–4 ■ Number of cases of congenital syphilis per year in infants younger than 1 year of age reported to the CDC from 1963 to 2005. (*Reprinted with permission from the Centers for Disease Control and Prevention, Division of STD Prevention, STD Surveillance Report 2005. http://www.cdc.gov/std/stats/toc2005.htm Bethesda, MD 2005.*) (The case definition for congenital syphilis was changed in 1988. As of 1995, cases of congenital syphilis younger than 1 year of age were obtained using case reporting form CDC 73.126. For the period 1995 through 2005, yearly case counts in this figure correspond to confirmed diagnoses of congenital syphilis among infants known to be younger than 1 year of age.)

and jaundice. Hematologic findings include Coombs-negative hemolytic anemia and thrombocytopenia. Bony lesions, frequently seen in untreated infants, are often symmetric and occur at multiple sites. They include osteochondritis of joints, periostitis, and cortical demineralization of long bones. Painful lesions give rise to "pseudoparalysis of Parrot," a condition where an infant refuses to move an affected extremity.[2,32–34]

Late manifestations, those appearing after the age of 2 years, occur in ~40% of untreated infants. These findings are typically the result of tissue scarring due to initial infection. These findings include frontal bossing, destruction of the nasal cartilage (saddle nose deformity), anterior bowing of shins (or saber shins), multicuspid first molars (mulberry molars), peg-shaped upper incisors (Hutchinson teeth), linear scars from the corners of the mouth (rhaghades), seizures, interstitial keratitis, and eighth nerve deafness.[2,32,34]

Neurosyphilis may be either an early or late manifestation of congenital infection. It is often asymptomatic and may present in an acute or chronic manner. Acutely, the disease may manifest as meningitis with signs of increased intracranial pressure and abnormal CSF findings.[32,34] Neurosyphilis may also present in a chronic manner with evidence of progressive and evolving disease, characterized by cranial nerve abnormalities, loss of developmental milestones, seizures, hydrocephalus, and strokes.[34]

Diagnosis

A variety of tests are available for the diagnosis of syphilis. A direct diagnosis can be made if spirochetes are visualized with special stains, by DFA, or by dark-field microscopy in specimens of placenta, cord, amniotic fluid, or infectious lesions. While direct visualization of the organism provides a clear and definitive diagnosis, it is not always practical or possible. Serologic diagnosis is possible using available treponemal-specific and nontreponemal-specific testing.[32–34]

Nontreponemal tests are screening tests that include the Venereal Disease Research Laboratory (VDRL) slide test, the rapid plasma reagin (RPR) test, the automated reagin test (ART). They provide quantitative results that can be used to follow treatment efficacy and disease status. Adequate treatment is indicated by a fourfold decrease in antibody titer, usually seen by 6 months, while reinfection or failure of antibiotic therapy is detected by a fourfold increase. Negative serologic status is expected after adequate treatment within 1–2 years. Nontreponemal tests have a high rate of false-positive results attributable to other infections or medical conditions such as varicella, Epstein–Barr virus, systemic lupus erythematosus, and other collagen vascular disease, or tuberculosis. A reactive nontreponemal test must be confirmed by a treponemal-specific test.[32,34]

Occasionally, a surplus of antibody in blood samples inhibits antibody–antigen complexes, resulting in false-negative reactions. This reaction, termed the prozone phenomenon, is a rare occurrence that can be overcome by dilution of the serum sample. Dilution should be performed when suspicion of infection is high, the infant or fetus has signs suggestive of congenital infection yet maternal serology is negative.[32,33]

Confirmatory treponemal-specific tests, which detect antibodies to surface proteins, include the fluorescent treponemal antibody absorption test (FTA-ABS) and the microhemagglutination for *T. pallidum* (MHA-TP). Once these tests become positive, they remain so for life and cannot be used to evaluate treatment or disease status. False positives occur in the face of infections caused by other spirochetes such as Yaws (caused by *Treponema pertenue*, a subspecies of *T. pallidum*), Pinta (caused by *Treponema carateum*), and Lyme disease (caused by *Borrelia burgdorferi*).[32,33]

Prenatal diagnosis and treatment of syphilis significantly reduces the risk of vertical transmission. With the recent resurgence of syphilis, particularly in communities with limited resources, careful and tenacious follow-up of pregnant women with the disease and efficient identification of infected newborns is critical in combating this preventable childhood infection.[36] Accordingly, the Centers for Disease Control (CDC) and American Association of Pediatrics (AAP) recommend comprehensive screening for the infection in pregnant women. Nontreponemal testing should be routinely obtained during early prenatal care at the beginning of pregnancy. For women in high-risk categories, testing should be repeated at the beginning of the third trimester as well as at the time of delivery. Maternal serology should be known prior to the discharge of all infants. A reactive VDRL or RPR should be confirmed with a treponemal-specific test. If syphilis is diagnosed in pregnancy, repeat serologies are required at the end of treatment to document response to therapy and to evaluate for possible reinfection.[32,33]

The diagnosis of congenital syphilis is classified as confirmed, presumptive, or possible based on both maternal and infant factors. The classification aids clinicians in evaluation and treatment decisions. Box 50–1 represents clinical and surveillance definitions adapted from the recommendations of the Committee on Infectious Disease, American Academy of Pediatrics.[32–34]

Any newborn whose mother has a positive serology should have a thorough physical examination and blood sent for the same serologic test as its mother to facilitate comparison of titers. Table 50–5 serves as a guide for the interpretation of serologic tests obtained in

Box 50-1. Clinical Definitions of Congenital Syphilis.

Definite	*T. pallidum* identified by dark-field microscopy, direct fluorescent antibody, or other specific stains in specimens from infant lesions, placenta, umbilical cord, amniotic fluid, or autopsy material
Probable	Infant is born to a mother who has • Untreated syphilis OR • No documentation of treatment OR • Received treatment with an antibiotic other than penicillin OR • Received penicillin treatment <30 days before delivery; OR An infant or child has a reactive treponemal test for syphilis AND • Any evidence of congenital syphilis on clinical exam OR • Any evidence of congenital syphilis on long bone radiograph OR • Reactive cerebrospinal fluid (CSF) VDRL OR • Elevated CSF white blood cell count or protein concentration (without other cause) OR • Quantitative nontreponemal serologic titer ≥fourfold higher than a maternal titer drawn near the time of birth OR • Reactive treponemal antibody test beyond age 15 months
Possible	Infant is asymptomatic AND • Treponemal or nontreponemal tests are reactive in the absence of evidence of clinical disease OR • Maternal treatment for syphilis during pregnancy but without the expected posttreatment fall in nontreponemal titers OR • Maternal treatment for syphilis before pregnancy but with insufficient serologic follow-up to assess treatment response or potential reinfection. Infants meeting all of the following criteria are unlikely to have infection but are considered by some experts to have possible congenital syphilis • The mother was treated >1 month before delivery AND • The mother has a documented fourfold or greater decline in nontreponemal antibody titers for early syphilis or remained stable for late syphilis AND • The mother has no evidence of reinfection or relapse

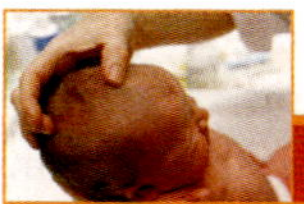

Table 50–5.

Guide for Interpretation of Syphilis Serologic Test Results of Mothers and Their Infants

Nontreponemal Test Result (e.g., VDRL, RPR, ART)		Treponemal Test Result (e.g., TP-PA, FTA-ABS)		
Mother	Infant	Mother	Infant	Interpretation*
−	−	−	−	No syphilis or incubating syphilis in the mother or infant or prozone phenomenon
+	+	−	−	No syphilis in mother or infant (false-positive result of nontreponemal test with passive transfer to infant)
+	+ or −	+	+	Maternal syphilis with possible infant infection; mother treated for syphilis during pregnancy; or mother with latent syphilis and possible infant infection[†]
+	+	+	+	Recent or previous syphilis in the mother, possible infant infection
−	−	+	+	Mother successfully treated for syphilis before or early in pregnancy; or mother with Lyme disease (i.e., false-positive serologic test result); infant syphilis unlikely

**Table presents a guide and not a definitive interpretation of serologic test results for syphilis in mothers and their newborn infants. Maternal history is the most important aspect for interpretation of test results. Factors that should be considered include timing of maternal infection, nature and timing of maternal treatment, quantitative maternal and infant titers, and serial determination of nontreponemal test titers in both mother and infant.*

[†] Mothers with latent syphilis may have nonreactive nontreponemal test results.

Reprinted with permission from Committee on Infectious Diseases American Academy of Pediatrics: Syphilis. In: Pickering LK, Baker CJ, Long SS, McMillan JA, eds. Redbook: 2006 Report of the Committee on Infectious Diseases, 27th ed.. Elk Grove Village, IL: American Academy of Pediatrics; 2006;636.

women with suspected disease and their infants. The combination of nontreponemal- and treponemal-specific tests and the comparison between maternal and infant results allows for risk assessment of disease. Infants merit a complete investigation if their titers are fourfold greater than their mothers, if they manifest disease, or if their mothers' titers have risen fourfold.[32] Due to the potentially devastating effects of untreated syphilis, evaluation of newborns is also warranted when maternal serologies are reactive and questions exist regarding the adequacy of maternal treatment.[32] Infants with suspected disease by any of the above criteria should be evaluated for stigmata of disease by physical examination, radiologic evaluation, and laboratory testing.[2,32]

Management/Treatment

Infants with congenital disease require treatment to avoid the long-term and serious sequelae of untreated congenital syphilis such as deafness, blindness, mental retardation, and facial deformities. Congenital syphilis is treated with aqueous crystalline penicillin (PCN) G 50,000 units/kg every 12 hours for first week of life and then every 8 hours for a total of 10 days or Procaine PCN G 50,000 units/kg/d administered intramuscularly for 10 days. If more than 1 day of therapy is missed, the entire treatment course must be repeated.[2,32–34]

Adequate follow-up for infants initially evaluated and treated is essential in the assessment of late manifestations of disease. After completion of treatment, current recommendations suggest follow-up clinical examination at 1, 2, 4, 6, and 12 months of age. Serologic testing is recommended at 2, 4, 6, and 12 months after completion of therapy or until the results are nonreactive or the titers have fallen fourfold. Titers should be undetectable by 6 months. Persistent or rising titers between 6 and 12 months of age are an indication for further evaluation including CSF sampling and retreatment with PCN G for 10–14 days.[2,32]

Infants with clinical or laboratory findings consistent with neurosyphilis require repeat CSF evaluations every 6 months until the CSF examination is normal. Patients whose 6-month CSF samples demonstrate positive VDRL reactivity or persistent leukocytosis at 2 years require retreatment.[2,32]

TOXOPLASMOSIS

Definitions and Epidemiology

Toxoplasmosis is a parasitic infection that is typically asymptomatic, but may cause significant disease in the fetus and the immunocompromised host. Toxoplasmosis is typically acquired through exposure to oocysts in contaminated soil, feline litter boxes, or through the ingestion of oocysts in undercooked meat.[2,37] Primary maternal infection poses a significant risk to the developing fetus. Both the rate of infection and the severity of disease vary with the gestational age at time of initial maternal infection. Maternal–fetal transmission rates are 15% in the first trimester, 30% in the second trimester, and up to 60% in the third trimester. Infants infected in the first trimester typically suffer devastating sequelae while the bulk of infants infected in the third trimester are asymptomatic at birth. However, if these asymptomatic infants are not treated, up to 85% will develop late sequelae. The severity of maternal disease has no significant impact on the transmissibility of the infection or resulting severity of fetal disease.[37]

Estimated rates of seroprevalence vary by country and region. In the National Health and Examination Survey (NHANES), the seroprevalence of individuals in the United States between the ages of 12 and 49 is estimated at 16%.[37] Up to one-third of pregnant women and nonpregnant women of childbearing age have Toxoplasma antibodies.[38] Once an individual has seroconverted, anti-Toxoplasma antibodies persist for life. As a result, the rates of seroprevalence increase with age. In the United States, the incidence of congenital toxoplasmosis infection is estimated at 1:1000–10,000 live births.[39]

Pathogenesis

Cats are the definitive hosts for the *Toxoplasma gondii* parasite. Felines shed oocysts in stool. Humans acquire infection by direct ingestion of oocysts from contaminated sources (e.g., soil, cat litter, garden vegetables) or from the ingestion of tissue cysts present in undercooked tissues from infected animals. Fetal infection typically occurs following acute maternal infection in pregnancy though it can also occur following reactivation of latent infection in immunocompromised women. After ingestion, oocysts give rise to bradyzoites or sporozoites that spread, replicate, and invade maternal tissues. The parasite becomes widely dispersed and may invade the placenta and infect the susceptible fetus.[2,37]

Clinical Presentation

Congenital toxoplasmosis infection can lead to stillbirth, premature delivery, or intrauterine growth restriction. Live born infants may (1) have manifestations of infection at birth (10–30% of all infants with congenital toxoplasmosis), (2) be asymptomatic at birth but develop manifestations in the first few months of life (70–90% of all infants with congenital toxoplasmosis), (3) develop symptoms in late infancy or childhood, typically in undiagnosed cases, or (4) the disease may remain subclinical.[2,37] Infants who are asymptomatic at birth may later develop serious sequelae such as learning difficulties or visual problems.[39]

Chorioretinitis is a complication in up to 85% of asymptomatic, untreated newborns. It is difficult to ascertain whether these infants are truly asymptomatic at birth or whether early manifestations are undiagnosed.[2,37] In one prospective, longitudinal observational study of chorioretinitis due to congenital toxoplasmosis, a subgroup of 108 infants out of an initial 132 treated with standard therapy were followed for the emergence of new eye lesions. Of these infants, 31% developed one new lesion, 14% developed new central lesions, and 25% were found to have previously undetected peripheral lesions. The development of previously undetected lesions occurred after the age of 10 years in 41% of cases, highlighting the importance of long-term follow up.[40]

In 10–30% of infants symptomatic at birth, the effects of infection may be extensive. The classic triad includes obstructive hydrocephalus, diffuse intracranial calcifications, and chorioretinits. Some infants may manifest general signs such as fever, jaundice, lymphadenopathy, hepatosplenomegaly, or maculopapular rash. Neurologic manifestations include microcephaly, seizures, diffuse intracranial calcifications, and increased CSF protein. The most common manifestation of neonatal disease is chorioretinitis. Other ophthalmologic findings include cataracts, microophthalmia, optic atrophy, glaucoma, or leukocoria.[2,38,39] Table 50–6 lists the signs and symptoms described by Couvreur et al. in 210 infants with confirmed congenital toxoplasmosis infection.

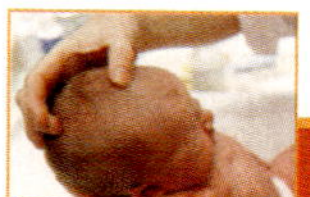

Table 50–6.

Prospective Study of Infants Born to Women Who Acquired Toxoplasma Infection During Pregnancy: Signs and Symptoms in 210 Infants with Proven Congenital Infection

Finding	Frequency
Prematurity	
Birth weight <2500 g	+
Birth weight 2500–3000 g	++
Dysmaturity (intrauterine growth retardation)	++
Postmaturity (n=108)	++
Icterus (n=201)	++
Hepatosplenomegaly	+
Thrombocytopenic purpura	+
Abnormal blood count (anemia, eosinophilia) (n=102)	+
Microcephaly	++
Hydrocephalus	+
Hypotonia	++
Convulsions	+
Psychomotor retardation	++
Intracranial calcifications on radiography	+++
Abnormal ultrasound examination (n=49)	++
Abnormal computed tomography scan of brain (n=13)	++++
Abnormal electroencephalographic result (n=191)	++
Abnormal cerebrospinal fluid (n=163)	+++
Microphthalmia	+
Strabismus	++
Chorioretinitis	
Unilateral	+++
Bilateral	++

Data from Couvreur J, Desmonts G, Tournier G, et al. A homogenous series of 210 cases of congenital toxoplasmosis in 0 to 11 month-old infants detected prospectively. Ann Pediatr 1984 (Paris) 31:815–9.
++++ ≥50%; +++ = 11% to 50%; ++ = 6% to 10%; + = ≤10%

Diagnosis

The majority of toxoplasma infections in adults result in asymptomatic infection or nonspecific manifestations of a flu-like illness.[2,37] Subsequently, clinical presentation cannot be relied upon to make a diagnosis of maternal infection, since up to 90% of cases are asymptomatic. A high index of suspicion is required for the diagnosis of infection during pregnancy.[39] Abnormalities detected on routine ultrasound such as hydrocephalus, intracranial or intrahepatic calcifications, hepatosplenomegaly, or ascites should raise suspicion of toxoplasmosis and prompt further investigation.[2,37]

The aim of prenatal diagnosis is to identify acute maternal infection and determine the timing of the infection in pregnancy. Available serologic studies include serum Toxoplasma IgG, IgM, IgA, IgE, and IgG avidity testing. Antibody levels are helpful in distinguishing acute from remote infection.[37,39,41] If maternal infection is highly suspected, fetal diagnosis should be pursued through the examination of amniotic fluid via the PCR or isolation of *T. gondii* via murine or tissue culture inoculation. The sensitivity and specificity of PCR on amniotic fluid is 64% and 100%, respectively. Monthly ultrasounds should be obtained to monitor the fetus for evolving hydrocephalus.[2,37,39]

The evaluation of infants born to women with suspected congenital toxoplasmosis should include paired maternal and infant serology, PCR of neonatal peripheral white blood cells and/or CSF, and, when available, placental and amniotic fluid samples. The diagnosis of congenital infection is made by demonstrating (1) neonatal toxoplasma-specific IgM or IgA; (2) persistently positive IgG or rising titers when compared to maternal titers; (3) detection of *T. gondii* DNA by PCR; (4) isolation of *T. gondii* from placenta, blood, or CSF.[39]

Since maternally derived IgM or IgA may result in false-positive results, titers should be repeated 10 days after initial positive results.[2,39] In one study, the specificity of serologic testing of neonatal blood (99%) was better than cord blood (92–96%) and the sensitivity of IgA antibody was better than IgM. Antibody assays were less sensitive in infants whose mothers acquired the infection in early pregnancy.[41] This led the authors to conclude that infants at greatest risk for teratogenic effects are less likely to be identified with standard serologic testing. Inclusion of placental evaluation has been found to increase the sensitivity of diagnosis of congenital infection.[42]

Infants with suspected congenital toxoplasmosis should be evaluated with a complete blood cell count, platelet count, liver function tests, CSF analyses, cranial imaging, ophthalmologic examination, and hearing screening.[2,39,43]

Treatment/Management

The efficacy of treatment of acute primary infection in pregnancy has been inconclusive.[37,39,43] All infants with congenital toxoplasmosis, whether symptomatic or not, should undergo treatment. Current therapy includes pyrethamine, sulfadiazine, and folinic acid for 1 year.[2] This regimen has potential adverse effects such as renal toxicity and risk to the glucose-6-phosphate dehydrogenase-deficient infant. Optimal doses and duration of therapy have not been conclusively defined. Consultation with an infectious disease specialist is recommended when considering treatment.[37,39]

Close followup of congenitally infected infants is critical as common complications include progressive visual loss, seizures, and cerebral palsy.[2] Serial pediatric, neurodevelopmental, and ophthalmologic assessments should be performed.[43] The development of potential adverse drug effects should be monitored.

RUBELLA

Definitions and Epidemiology

Rubella is a rare, mild, or asymptomatic infection caused by an enveloped RNA togavirus. Maternal rubella during pregnancy can result in fetal infection and ultimately the potentially devastating congenital rubella syndrome (CRS).

Rubella epidemics occurred every 6–9 years in the United States prior to introduction of the vaccination program in 1969.[44] These epidemics were followed by an increase in the numbers of infants with CRS. After adoption of routine vaccination, rates of CRS have significantly decreased. In 2005, cases of rubella decreased to record lows. Between 2001 and 2004, 9 to 23 cases of rubella infection per year were reported to the Centers for Disease Control and Prevention (CDCP). During this period, only four cases of CRS were reported, with three of the four cases occurring in the infants of mothers who were foreign born.[44–46] Figure 50–5 illustrates the decrease in rates of both rubella and CRS in the postvaccine era. Despite routine vaccination programs and an overall decrease in the number of cases of rubella, susceptibility to the virus has been reported in as many as 10% of individuals born in the United States.[44,45] Other potential reservoirs for the virus are unimmunized and inadequately immunized individuals.

A primary maternal infection during pregnancy carries the greatest risk for vertical transmission to the fetus. The risk of transmission varies inversely with the gestational age at time of infection. A maternal infection in the first trimester carries an 80% risk of transmission compared to 10–20% risk in the second and 25–50% risk in the third trimester.[2] The severity of disease is also inversely related to the timing of infection and a reliable predictor of outcome.[44,47] Fetal viremia in the first four months of pregnancy causes deleterious cellular alterations responsible for the typical manifestations associated with CRS.[48]

Pathogenesis

Rubella is transmitted hematogenously from infected mother to fetus and through contact with the infectious secretions outside of the neonatal period. Postnatal infection in susceptible hosts results in mild, vague manifestations that are rarely attributed to rubella. The duration of infectivity spans from days before rash is seen to weeks after the rash has resolved. Subsequently, the virus cycles among the reservoir of susceptible hosts, remaining an infrequent but present public health hazard.[2,44,47]

Clinical Presentation

When acquired in pregnancy, rubella may infect the placenta, resulting in spontaneous abortion, stillbirth, and intrauterine growth restriction. Fetal infection may lead to CRS. Fifty to seventy percent of the infected infants are asymptomatic at birth. However, symptomatic infants manifest the teratogenic effects of CRS with multiple organ system involvement, particularly infection of the central nervous system, heart, skin, eyes, bones, and the auditory system. Table 50–1 outlines common findings in children with congenital rubella syndrome. Common cardiac abnormalities include patent ductus arteriosus, peripheral pulmonary artery stenosis, and pulmonary vascular stenosis. Hematologic abnormalities include thrombocytopenia, hemolysis, anemia, and dermal erythropoiesis (i.e., blueberry muffin rash). Genitourinary malformations such as testicular or renal agenesis, polycystic kidneys, and renal artery

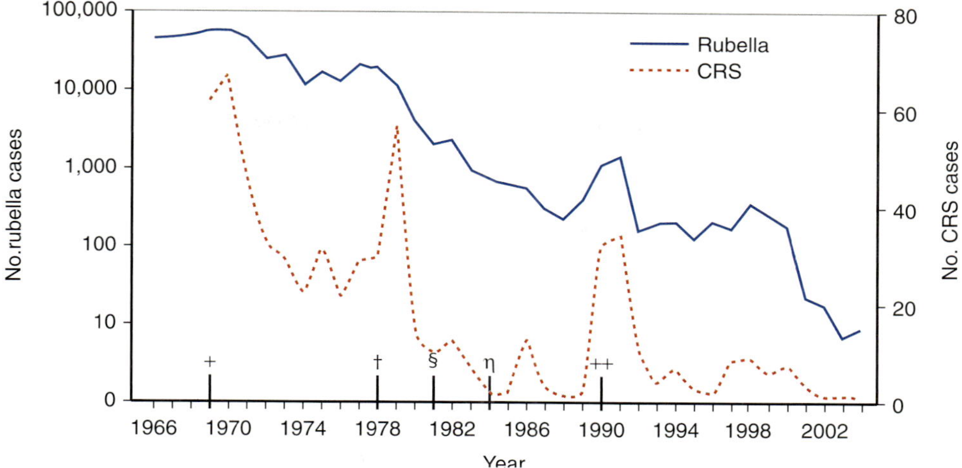

FIGURE 50–5 ■ Number of reported cases of rubella and congenital rubella syndrome (CRS), by year, and chronology of rubella vaccination recommendations by the Advisory Committee on Immunization Practices—United States, 1966–2004. *Reprinted with permission from the Centers for Disease Control and Prevention: Achievements in Public Health: Elimination of Rubella and congenital Rubella syndrome United States, 1969–2004. MMWR Weekly 2005; 54(11); 279–82. http://www.cdc.gov/mmwr/preview/mmwrhtml/ mm5411a5. htm#fig* (Number (No.) of rubella cases along the *y*-axis on the left margin/number of congenital rubella syndrome (CRS) cases along the *y*-axis on the right margin and the year along the *x*-axis from years 1966 to 2002. Cases of Rubella are represented by a solid line while cases of congenital Rubella are indicated by a dashed line. †, *1969—First official recommendations are published for the use of rubella vaccine. Vaccination is recommended for children aged 1 year to puberty.* †, *1978—Recommendations for vaccination are expanded to include adolescents and certain adults, particularly females. Vaccination is recommended for adolescent or adult females and males in populations in colleges, certain places of employment (e.g., hospitals), and military bases.* §, *1981—Recommendations place increased emphasis on vaccination of susceptible persons in training and educational settings (e.g., universities or colleges) and military settings, and vaccination of workers in health care settings.* ¶, *1984—Recommendations are published for the vaccination of workers in day care centers, schools, colleges, companies, government offices, and industrial sites. Providers are encouraged to conduct prenatal testing and postpartum vaccination of susceptible women. Recommendations for vaccination are expanded to include susceptible persons who travel abroad.* ††, *1990—Recommendations include implementation of a new two-dose schedule for measles–mumps–rubella vaccine.*)

stenosis may also occur. Mortality rates range from 10% to 15%.[2,44]

Diagnosis

Rubella is diagnosed by detection of anti-Rubella IgM or increasing anti-Rubella IgG titer over many months. Virus can be cultured from various sources including the nasopharynx, blood, urine, and CSF, especially in infants with CRS.[2,44] PCR-based strategies may detect rubella RNA or DNA. After 1 year of age, it becomes difficult to diagnose congenital infection.

The evaluation of an infant with suspected or known CRS includes a complete blood count to evaluate for neutropenia, thrombocytopenia and anemia, liver enzymes and bilirubin levels to detect hepatitis and liver dysfunction, and analysis of protein and cell count in CSF suggestive of central nervous system infection are recommended. Screening neuroimaging via cranial ultrasonography or computerized tomography of the head to detect central nervous system abnormalities should be performed. Comprehensive ophthalmic examination, audiologic evaluation, and radiographs of the long bones are also recommended.[2]

Treatment/Management

There is no specific therapy for rubella infection, with management consisting of supportive measures. Limited studies evaluating the efficacy of antiviral agents and immunoglobulin have been inconclusive.[47]

Attempts at controlling the spread of disease have consisted mainly of vaccination and isolation of infected persons.[44,47] Routine vaccination against rubella is standard practice and most individuals have received the vaccine through childhood immunization programs. The live-attenuated vaccine should not be given to pregnant women. However, in the case of vaccination during or within 28 days of becoming pregnant, the risk of symptomatic infection to the infant is very small and termination of pregnancy is not indicated.[44]

Infants with CRS, who may shed virus for greater than 1 year, represent another potential source of infection. It has been recommended that infants with confirmed or suspected CRS be placed in contact isolation during the first year of life or until two nasopharyngeal and urine cultures are negative after the age of 3 months.[44] Infants with congenital cataracts due to CRS may shed virus for years and, if hospitalized for cataract surgery, should be placed under contact precautions.[44] Neurodevelopmental, ophthalmologic, and audiologic follow-up are recommended for infants with CRS.

REFERENCES

1. Committee on Infectious Diseases American Academy of Pediatrics: Cytomegalovirus infection. In: Pickering LK, Baker CJ, Long SS, McMillan JA, eds. *Red Book: 2006 Report of the Committee on Infectious Diseases.* 27th ed. Elk Grove Village, IL, American Academy of Pediatrics; 2006:273-277.
2. Bizzarro MJ, Gallagher PG. Congenital/perinatal infections. In: Shah SS, ed. Blueprints Pediatric Infectious Diseases. Massachusetts: Blackwell Publishing; 2005: 125-134.
3. Malm G, Engman ML. Congenital cytomegalovirus infections. *Semin Fetal Neonatal Med.* 2007;12:154-159.
4. Munro SC, Hall B, Whybin LR, et al. Diagnosis of and screening for cytomegalovirus infection in pregnant women. *J Clin Microbiol.* 2005;43:4713-4718.
5. Colugnati FAB, Staras SAS, Dollard SC, et al. Incidence of cytomegalovirus infection among the general population and pregnant women in the United States. *BMC Infect Dis.* 2007;7:71.
6. Nigro G, Adler SP, La Torre R, et al. Passive immunization during pregnancy for congenital cytomegalovirus infection. *N Engl J Med.* 2005;353:1350-1362.
7. Kenneson A, Cannon MJ. Review and meta-analysis of the epidemiology of congenital cytomegalovirus (CMV) infection. *Rev Med Virol.* 2007;17:253-276.
8. Arav-Boger R, Pass RF. Diagnosis and management of cytomegalovirus infection in the newborn. *Pediatr Ann.* 2002;31:719-725.
9. Dollard SC, Grosse SD, Ross DS. New estimates of the prevalence of neurological and sensory sequelae and mortality associated with congenital cytomegalovirus infection. *Rev Med Virol.* 2007;17:355-363.
10. Stagno, S. Cytomegalovirus. In: Remington JS, Klein JO, eds. Infectious Diseases of the Fetus and Newborn Infant. 5th ed. Philadelphia: WB Saunders; 2001:389-424.
11. Jacquemard F, Yamamoto M, Costa JM et al. Maternal administration of valaciclovir in symptomatic intrauterine cytomegalovirus infection. *BJOG.* 2007;114: 1113-1121.
12. Adler SP, Nigro G, Pereira L. Recent advances in the prevention and treatment of congenital cytomegalovirus infections. *Semin Perinatol.* 2007;31:10-18.
13. Kaneko M, Sameshima H, Ikenoue T, Minematsu T. A two-step strategy for detecting intrauterine cytomegalovirus infection with clinical manifestations in the mother, fetus, and newborn. *Jpn J Infect Dis.* 2006;59:363-366.
14. Lanari M, Lazzarotto T, Venturi V, et al. Neonatal cytomegalovirus blood load and risk of sequelae in symptomatic and asymptomatic congenitally infected newborns. *Pediatrics.* 2006;117:76-83.
15. Kylat RI, Kelly EN, Ford-Jones EL. Clinical findings and adverse outcome in neonates with symptomatic congenital cytomegalovirus (SCCMV) infection. *Eur J Pediatr.* 2006;165:773-778.
16. Fowler KB, Dahle AJ, Boppana SB, et al. Newborn hearing screening: will children with hearing loss caused by congenital cytomegalovirus infection be missed? *J Pediatr.* 1999;135:60-64.
17. Revello MG, Gerna G. Diagnosis and management of human cytomegalovirus infection in the mother, fetus, and newborn infant. *Clin Microbiol Rev.* 2002;15:680-715.
18. Abdel-Fattah SA, Bhat A, Illanes S, et al. TORCH test for fetal medicine indications: only CMV is necessary in the United Kingdom. *Prenat Diagn.* 2005;25:1028-1031.
19. Ancora G, Lanari M, Lazzarotto T, et al. Cranial ultrasound scanning and prediction of outcome in newborns with congenital cytomegalovirus infection. *J Pediatr.* 2007;150:157-161.
20. Acosta EP, Brundage RC, King JR, et al. Ganciclovir population pharmacokinetics in neonates following intravenous administration of ganciclovir and oral administration of a liquid valganciclovir formulation. *Clin Pharmacol Ther.* 2007;81:867-872.
21. Galli L, Novelli A, Chiappini E, Gervaso P, et al. Valganciclovir for congenital CMV infection: a pilot study on plasma concentration in newborns and infants. *Pediatr Infect Dis J.* 2007;26:451-453.
22. Kimberlin DW, Lin CY, Sanchez PJ, et al. Effect of ganciclovir therapy on hearing in symptomatic congenital cytomegalovirus disease involving the central nervous system: a randomized, controlled trial. *J Pediatr.* 2003;143:16-25.
23. Oliver S, Cloud G, Sanchez P, et al. Effect of ganciclovir (GCV) therapy on neurodevelopmental outcomes in symptomatic congenital cytomegalovirus (CMV) infections involving the central nervous system (CNS): a randomized, controlled study. E-PAS2006;59:2540.2.
24. Committee on Infectious Diseases American Academy of Pediatrics: Herpes simplex. In: Pickering LK, Baker CJ, Long SS, McMillan JA, eds. *Red Book: 2006 Report of the Committee on Infectious Diseases.* 27th ed. Elk Grove Village, IL, American Academy of Pediatrics, 2006; 361-371.
25. Kimberlin DW. Herpes simplex virus infections of the newborn. *Semin Perinatol.* 2007;31:19-25.
26. O'Riordan DP, Golden C, Aucott SW. Herpes simplex virus infections in preterm infants. *Pediatrics.* 2006;118: e1612-e1620.
27. Brown ZA, Wald A, Morrow RA, et al. Effect of serologic status and cesarean delivery on transmission rates of herpes simplex virus from mother to infant. *JAMA.* 2003;289:203-209.
28. Xu F, Markowitz LE, Gottlieb SL, et al. Seroprevalence of herpes simplex virus types 1 and 2 in pregnant women in the United States. *Am J Obstet Gynecol.* 2007;196: 43.e1-e6.
29. Kimberlin DW. Neonatal herpes simplex infection. *Clin Microbiol Rev.* 2004;17:1-13.
30. Sanchez PJ, Siegel JD. Herpes simplex virus. In: McMillan JA, Feigin RD, DeAngelis C, Jones MD, eds. *Oski's Pediatrics: Principles and Practice.* 4th ed. Philadelphia: Lippincott Williams, and Wilkins; 2006:516-520.

31. Kimberlin DW, Lin CY, Jacobs RF, et al. Safety and efficacy of high-dose intravenous acyclovir in the management of neonatal herpes simplex virus infections. *Pediatrics.* 2001;108:230-238.
32. Committee on Infectious Diseases American Academy of Pediatrics: Syphilis. In: Pickering LK, Baker CJ, Long SS, McMillan JA, eds. *Red Book: 2006 Report of the Committee on Infectious Diseases.* 27th ed. Elk Grove Village, IL: American Academy of Pediatrics; 2006: 631-644.
33. Stoll, BJ. Congenital syphilis: Evaluation and management of neonates born to mothers with reactive serologic tests for syphilis. *Pediatr Infect Dis J.* 1994;13:845-853.
34. Woods, CR. Syphilis in children: Congenital and acquired. *Semin Pediatr Infect Dis.* 2005;16:245-257.
35. Gust DA, Levine WC, St. Louis ME, et al. Mortality associated with congenital syphilis in the United States, 1992-1998. *Pediatrics.* 2002;109:e79.
36. Chakraborty R, Luck S. Managing congenital syphilis again? The more things change. *Curr Opin Infect Dis.* 2007;20:247-252.
37. Montoya JG, Rosso F. Diagnosis and management of toxoplasmosis. *Clin Perinatol.* 2005;32:705-726.
38. Remington JS, McLeod R, Thulliez P, et al. Toxoplasmosis. In: Remington JS, Klein JO, eds. *Infectious Diseases of the Fetus and Newborn Infant.* 5th ed. Philadelphia: WB Saunders; 2001:205-346.
39. Committee on Infectious Diseases American Academy of Pediatrics: *Toxoplasma gondii* infections. In: Pickering LK, Baker CJ, Long SS, McMillan JA, eds. *Red Book: 2006 Report of the Committee on Infectious Diseases.* 27th ed. Elk Grove Village, IL, American Academy of Pediatrics; 2006:666-671.
40. Phan L, Kasza K, Jalbrzikowski J, et al. Longitudinal study of new eye lesions in treated congenital toxoplasmosis. *Ophthalmology.* 2008;115:553-559.
41. Naessens A, Jenum PA, Pollak A, et al. Diagnosis of congenital toxoplasmosis in the neonatal period: a multicenter evaluation. *J Pediatr.* 1999;135:714-719.
42. Fricker-Hidalgo H, Brenier-Pinchart MP, Schaal JP et al. Value of *Toxoplasma gondii* detection in one hundred thirty-three placentas for the diagnosis of congenital toxoplasmosis. *Pediatr Infect Dis J.* 2007;26:845-846.
43. Guerina NG, Hsu HW, Meissner HC, et al. for New England Regional Toxoplasma Working Group. Neonatal serologic screening and early treatment for congenital *Toxoplasma gondii* infection. *N Engl J Med.* 1994;330: 1858-1863.
44. Committee on Infectious Diseases American Academy of Pediatrics: Rubella. In: Pickering LK, Baker CJ, Long SS, McMillan JA, eds. *Red Book: 2006 Report of the Committee on Infectious Diseases.* 27th ed. Elk Grove Village, IL: American Academy of Pediatrics; 2006:574-579.
45. Centers for Disease Control and Prevention (CDC). Achievements in public health: elimination of rubella and congenital rubella syndrome – United States, 1969–2004, *MMWR.* 2005;54(11):279-282.
46. Meissner HC, Reef SE, Cochi S. Elimination of Rubella from the United States: a milestone on the road to global elimination. *Pediatrics.* 2006;117:933-935.
47. Cooper LZ, Alford CA: Rubella. In: Remington JS, Klein JO, eds. *Infectious Diseases of the Fetus and Newborn Infant.* Philadelphia: WB Saunders; 2001:347-388.
48. Robinson JL, Lee BE, Preiksaitis JK. Prevention of congenital Rubella syndrome—What makes sense in 2006? *Epidemiol Rev.* 2006;28:81-87.

CHAPTER 51

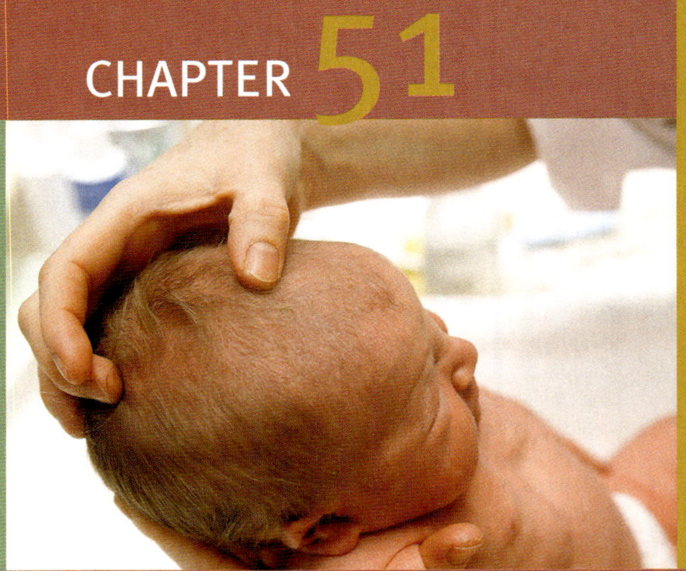

Neonatal Fever

Jeffrey R. Avner

DEFINITIONS AND EPIDEMIOLOGY

Fever in a young infant is often the only clinical sign of an underlying serious infection. This is particularly true for infants younger than 2–3 months, since they lack many of the clinical signs typically used by clinicians to judge general appearance. Although most well-appearing febrile infants in this age group have a benign; self-limited illness, as many as 10% have serious bacterial illness, including 3% with bacteremia and bacterial meningitis.[1–9] Thus, fever is an important symptom for identifying infants who need immediate evaluation and treatment.

The definition of what constitutes fever in this age is debatable. Normal body temperature varies with a variety of factors including age, sex, and time of day. There may be as much as a 0.5°C difference between the physiologic nadir in the early morning and the peak in the early evening. Older infants appear to have slightly higher basal body temperature compared to infants younger than 1 month.[10] However, despite this individual variation, several studies have shown that rectal temperatures more than 38.0°C are greater than two standard deviations above the mean for age.[2,3,10] It is important to emphasize that rectal temperature is the standard method for fever determination at this age. Other temperature-taking methods such as axillary or forehead measurements are unreliable and should not be used. Often, the parent will report a subjective fever because the infant "felt warm" or had "fever to touch." In these cases, if the infant was afebrile when examined by the clinician, there was no increase in serious bacterial illness.[11] However, if the infant had a documented fever at home by rectal thermometry, the infant remains at risk for serious bacterial illness regardless of the presence or absence of fever when the infant presents to the clinician.[11] One important caveat is the possibility of environmental factors as a cause of elevated body temperature in the infant, which often happens in the summer especially if the infant is bundled in warm clothing.

The most common organisms associated with fever in young infants are shown in Table 51–1. In infants younger than 4 weeks, infection is usually caused by organisms acquired perinatally—group B *Streptococcus* (GBS), gram-negative bacilli (*Escherichia coli*, *Klebsiella*), *Listeria monocytogenes*, and herpes simplex virus (HSV). By 6 weeks of age, the etiology shifts to community-acquired organisms—*Streptococcus pneumoniae* and less commonly *Neisseria meningitidis* and *Haemophilus influenzae* type B. During the winter months, common viral causes are influenza type A or type B and respiratory syncytial virus (RSV).

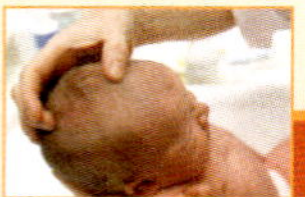

Table 51–1.

Common Bacterial Pathogens in Cases of Bacteremia & Bacterial Meningitis

Common:
- *E. coli*
- GBS
- *Staphylococcus aureus*
- *Streptococcus pneumoniae*
- Salmonella

Less Common:
- *Enterococcous faecalis*
- *Enterobacter cloacae*
- Group A *Streptococcus*
- *Klebsiella pneumoniae*
- *L. monocytogenes*

PATHOGENESIS

Infants younger than 2 months of age have lower measurable parameters of the immune response (e.g., antibody titers and proliferative responses) compared to older children and adults.[12–15] This results in an immature immune system that not only increases the infant's risk for infection but also limits the ability of the infant to contain the infection. In addition to these host factors, many organisms exhibit a varied assortment of colonization and survival factors that increases their virulence in this age group. These virulence factors contribute to disease pathogenesis by a variety of possible methods including direct tissue injury, phagocytic resistance, inhibition of neutrophil recruitment, impairment of antibody function and activation of sepsis syndrome.[14] Furthermore, the reduced ability to contain the organism may lead to the presence of only nonspecific symptoms (e.g., fever, poor feeding) early in the disease process; only when the disease progresses do the classic symptoms of sepsis or meningitis become apparent.

The mechanism of infection in the first few weeks of life is related to perinatal exposure. Infection may begin either in utero as the organism ascends through the placenta to infect the fetus or during delivery through direct contact or aspiration of infected vaginal fluid. GBS is the most common bacterial etiology causing serious illness. Approximately 20–30% of mothers are colonized with GBS and 50–70% of infants born to these mothers are also colonized.[14,16] In the first few days of life, GBS infection typically causes pneumonitis; however, outside of the newborn period, late-onset GBS may present with gradual symptoms related to bacteremia and is associated with a high incidence of meningitis.[16]

CLINICAL PRESENTATION

The history of an infant who presents with fever is directed toward identifying risk factors for serious infection. Since management strategies are dependant on the infant's prior history of being healthy, any factor that places the infant at high risk for serious infection should be identified (Table 51–2).[4,6] The duration of the febrile illness and the presence of other systemic symptoms (vomiting, diarrhea) may help in determining the underlying diagnosis.

Assessment of the infant's clinical appearance is an essential part of the physical examination. However, very young infants have not yet developed many of the social gestures, such as a social smile, that clinicians often rely on as a first step in determining whether the infant looks well or ill. Nevertheless, the presence of certain clinical signs form a reliable basis for identifying an ill or toxic infant based on global clinical assessment (Table 51–3).[3,4,17] Unfortunately, acute clinical observation scales that could identify older infants and toddlers at low risk for bacterial disease are not reliable in infants younger than 2 months.[3–5,17,18] As a result, even well-appearing febrile infants may have serious bacterial illness. In fact, up to 66% of infants with serious bacterial infection look well on initial examination.[3,4,18] Therefore, clinical observation alone does not allow the clinician to differentiate those infants who require laboratory evaluation from those with minor illness.

Further physical examination may identify an area of focal bacterial infection (Table 51–4).

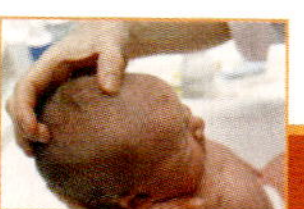

Table 51–2.

High-Risk Historical Factors for Serious Illness

Preterm gestation (less than 37 wk)
Perinatal antibiotics
Previous rehospitalization
Chronic or underlying illness
Hospitalized after birth longer than the mother
Treatment for unexplained hyperbilirubinemia
History of HSV lesions in mother in third trimester

DIFFERENTIAL DIAGNOSIS

The most common cause of fever in infants is viral illness. There are a host of viral pathogens that may be involved, and their incidence usually depends on seasonal epidemiology. In the winter months, influenza A, influenza B, and RSV predominate. The symptoms of

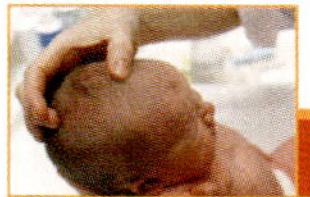

Table 51–3.

Clinical Signs of an Ill Infant

Lethargy
Weak or constant crying or moaning
Poor or absent eye contact
Pale or mottled extremities
Acrocyanosis
Signs of dehydration including prolonged capillary refill (greater than 2 s)
Abnormal respiratory pattern or tachypnea
Seizure
Rash (petechial, vesicular, macular, mucosal)
Tachypnea or apnea
Bulging fontanelle
Poor feeding
Altered sleep pattern

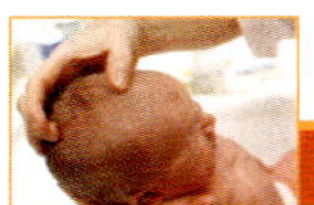

Table 51–4.

Common Sources of Focal and Nonfocal Bacterial Infections

Focal Bacterial Infection
Cellulitis
Mastitis
Omphalitis
Otitis media
Pneumonia
Osteomyelitis
Septic arthritis
Nonfocal Bacterial Infection
Urinary tract infection
Bacteremia/sepsis
Meningitis
Gastroenteritis

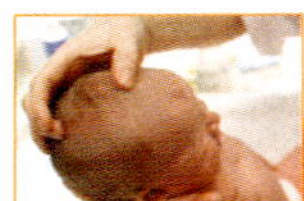

Table 51–5.

Risk Factors for possible Neonatal HSV Infection in Febrile Infants

History of HSV lesions in mother in third trimester
Skin lesions suspicious for HSV on the infant
Ill appearance
Seizure associated with acute illness
Abnormal liver function tests (more than 100 for SGOT/SGPT)
CSF pleocytosis in the absence of bacterial etiology
Fetal scalp electrode placement during delivery

influenza are often nonspecific and, in addition to fever, include upper respiratory tract symptoms, nasal discharge and tachypnea. However, especially with influenza A, the infant may appear acutely ill with symptoms that mimic bacterial sepsis. As many as 40% of febrile infants younger than 3 months during a flu season have documented influenza.[19] RSV has been identified in 22% of febrile infants who present during the winter season.[20] Typically, the infant with RSV has signs of upper and lower respiratory tract disease; however, fever may be the only presenting sign. In the summer and fall months, enteroviral infection is common and may cause aseptic meningitis.

Although HSV is a far less likely cause of fever in infants, there is high morbidity and mortality associated with this disease. The vast majority of neonatal HSV presents within the first 4 weeks of life (9% within 24 h and 30% at 1–5 days of age) and approximately 10% present with fever and no source of infection.[21,22] Neonatal HSV presents in three different clinical patterns: (1) disease localized to the skin, eye, and mouth, (2) encephalitis with or without skin involvement, and (3) disseminated infection with systemic organ system involvement. While the presence of vesicles on the skin or mucous membranes raises suspicion for HSV infection, it is important to note that a significant minority (approximately one-third) of cases of central nervous system or disseminated HSV disease do not present with accompanying skin lesions.[22] Risk factors for possible neonatal HSV infection in febrile infants are listed in Table 51–5.

Bacterial infection represents almost 10% of causes of fever in the infant.[1–4,7,23,24] Urinary tract infection accounts for approximately half of bacterial causes. More concerning is the presence of bacteremia and bacterial meningitis which are seen in 2.5% and 0.5%, respectively, of all infants with fever.[1–4,7] The incidence of bacteremia is highest in the first one month of life (1.5–4.5%) and declines in the second month of life (1–2%).[7,25]

Of the focal bacterial infections in this age group, otitis media is the most common diagnosis. Traditionally, otitis media was thought to be associated with bacterial sepsis and meningitis in less than 2-month-old infants, as a result of the infant's inability to contain a focal infection. Gram-negative enteric bacteria were reported to be responsible for a large proportion of cases; however, recent studies have shown that most cases of acute otitis media in infants younger than 2 months are caused by pathogens similar to those causing acute otitis media in older children—*S. pneumoniae* and *H. influenzae*.[26] Furthermore, some studies show that the presence of otitis media does not predict a higher risk for serious bacterial illness in well-appearing febrile infants older than 1 month.[26,27]

DIAGNOSIS

Since the clinical impression of the febrile infant is unreliable and the morbidity associated with a serious illness potentially high, various laboratory studies are needed to help determine the underlying cause of the fever. To be sure, cultures of the blood, urine, cerebrospinal fluid (CSF) and stool (if diarrhea is present) will identify serious bacterial illness. However, culture results may take days to become positive. Therefore, a series of screening tests may help identify an infant as being at high or low risk for bacterial infection.

As discussed earlier, fever is often the only sign of a urinary tract infection in infants younger than 2 months. The presence of other minor sources of infection, such as otitis media and bronchiolitis, does not exclude the presence of a urinary tract infection. Therefore, laboratory investigation for a urinary tract infection is necessary. Since the urine dipstick is unreliable in this age group, most studies use a urinalysis with a white blood cell (WBC) <10/hpf as a negative predictor. However, even the standard urinalysis and Gram stain has a sensitivity of only approximately 50%.[28,29] If available, an enhanced urinalysis, using a hemocytometer cell count and Gram stain on uncentifuged urine, has superior negative predictive value and sensitivity.[29] Of note, urine specimens should be obtained by urethral catheterization or suprapubic aspiration; bagged urine specimens have a high rate of contamination and therefore should not be used in this age group.

The peripheral WBC count by itself is a poor predictor of serious bacterial illness. However, a WBC cutoff (usually greater than 15,000/mm^3) and either absolute band count (greater than 1500/mm^3) or immature to total segmental leukocyte ratio (greater than 0.2) are often used as part of a set of predictors for serious bacterial illness.[4–6] If the infant has an abrupt onset of fever and diarrhea, a stool Gram stain and culture should be obtained. The presence of blood or WBCs on stool smear may accompany bacterial gastroenteritis. However, *Salmonella*, in particular, may not be accompanied by bloody diarrhea in this age group.[4] Febrile infants with symptoms of lower respiratory tract infection should have a chest radiograph as part of their evaluation.

The decision to perform a lumbar puncture to obtain CSF specimens for culture, cell count, chemistry and Gram stain remains somewhat variable. Most advocate a lumbar puncture for febrile infants younger than 1 month, because their risk of bacteremia and bacterial meningitis is higher, and they lack most signs typically needed for the determination of a global clinical impression of illness. The routine use of a lumbar puncture in infants 1–2 months old is debatable. Regardless of the eventual risk assessment and management strategy used, if the infant does not appear well or has other high-risk criteria, CSF studies should be obtained.

Depending on the season, rapid viral testing for RSV or influenza may prove useful in limiting the evaluation for accompanying bacterial infection. For infants with suspected HSV infection, liver function tests (for disseminated infection) or CSF HSV polymerase chain reaction (for central nervous system infection) are needed. In addition, vesicles should be unroofed and the contents sent for HSV detection by culture, direct fluorescent antibody, or polymerase chain reaction. Mucosal cultures (conjunctiva, throat, and rectum) are positive in the majority of neonates with HSV infection, even in the absence of vesicles.

MANAGEMENT

Risk Assessment

The cornerstone of management is the determination of the infant's risk of having serious illness. If the infant appears ill, then the risk is obviously high. However, since well-appearing febrile infants also have a significant risk of serious bacterial illness, clinical impression alone cannot decide management. Similarly, individual predictors of height of fever and peripheral blood WBC count are unreliable. Thus, investigators sought to combine clinical impression with history, physical examination, and a variety of laboratory tests to develop a set of criteria that could separate those febrile infants at risk for serious bacterial infection from those who may be safely managed as outpatients. The most common strategies for managing febrile infants are shown in Table 51–6.[2,4–6,30] There are notable differences among the studies including the age of infants studied, peripheral WBC cut-off, and use of empiric antibiotics. Most strategies do not include infants younger than 1 month, because of their higher risk of serious bacterial illness and their limited clinical clues on observation. Thus, for infants younger than 1 month, a complete blood count, urinalysis, CSF cell count, protein and glucose as well as cultures of the blood, urine and CSF are part of a standard evaluation; these infants should be admitted to an inpatient service for observation and given empiric parenteral antibiotics pending negative culture results. For infants older than 1 month who appear well, the clinician may defer the lumbar puncture if the other laboratory parameters fall in the low-risk range and follow-up can be assured. Recently, the Pediatric Research in Office Settings network has challenged this dogma.[7] In their study of the management of febrile infants younger than 3 months by practitioners in the office setting, 64% were managed as outpatients and 24% had no laboratory tests performed.[7] Compared to accepted guidelines for management of these infants, the Pediatric Research in Office Settings clinicians detected as many cases of bacteremia and bacterial meningitis while performing fewer tests and hospitalizing fewer infants. However, this management approach required close and reliable follow-up often only obtainable in the office setting. Furthermore, the results may not be generalizable to other populations of febrile infants. Nevertheless, the variety of existing management schemes highlights the importance of individual decision modifiers such as practice setting, experience of practitioner, ease and reliability of follow-up and patient demographics.

Treatment

For febrile infants who appear ill or meet other high-risk criteria, initial empiric antibiotic therapy should begin with a third-generation cephalosporin such as cefotaxime. Ampicillin should be added for infants younger than 1 month, to cover for Listeria. Vancomycin should be added for infants with CSF pleocytosis given the small

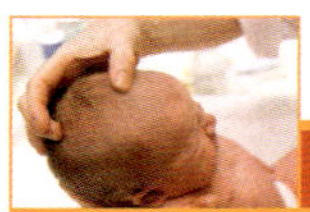

Table 51–6.

Common Strategies for the Management of Febrile Infants

Factor	Rochester Criteria	Philadelphia Criteria	Boston Criteria	Milwaukee Criteria
Age	<60 d	29–56 d	28–89 d	30–60 d
Temperature	>38.0°C	>38.2°C	>38.0°C	
History	Term infant No perinatal antibiotics No underlying disease Not hospitalized longer than the mother	Not specified	No immunizations within preceding 48 h No antimicrobial within 48 h Not dehydrated	
Physical examination	Well-appearing Unremarkable examination	Well-appearing No ear, soft tissue, or bone infection	Well-appearing No ear, soft tissue, or bone infection	Well-appearing No ear, soft tissue, or bone infection
Laboratory parameters	WBC >5000 and <15,000/mm^3 Absolute band count <1500/mm UA <10 WBC/hpf <5 WBC/hpf stool smear with diarrhea	WBC <15,000/mm^3 Band-neutrophil ratio <0.2 UA <10 WBC/hpf Urine Gram stain negative CSF <8 WBC/mm^3 CSF Gram stain negative Chest radiograph: no infiltrate Stool: no blood, few or no WBCs on smear	CSF <10/mm^3 UA <10 WBC/hpf Chest radiograph: no infiltrate WBC <20,000/mm	CSF total WBC <10/μL CBC total WBC <15,000/μL Urinalysis WBC <10/hpf, negative for bacteriuria/leukocyte esterase/nitrite No pulmonary infiltrate on chest radiograph if performed
Fail low-risk criteria	Hospitalize + empiric antibacterial agent(s)	Hospitalize + empiric antibacterial agent(s)	Hospitalize + empiric antibacterial agent(s)	Hospitalize + empiric antibacterial agent(s)
Meet low-risk criteria	Home No antibacterial therapy Follow-up required	Home No antibacterial therapy Follow-up required	Home Empiric antibacterial therapy Follow-up required	Reliable caretaker follow-up required Empiric antibacterial therapy
Reported statistics	Sensitivity 92% (83–97%) Specificity 50% (47–53%) Positive predictive value 12.3% (10–16%) NPV 98.9% (97–100%)	Sensitivity 98% (92–100%) Specificity 42% (38–46%) Positive predictive value 14% (11–175) NPV 99.7% (98–100%)	Sensitivity—not available Specificity 94.6% Positive predictive value—not available NPV—not available	

Adapted from Meltzer A, Powell K, Avner JR. Fever in children. Consensus in Pediatrics. 2005;1(7):1–19.

but real risk of pneumococcal meningitis. Well-appearing febrile infants 1–2 months old who are considered low risk, have no focal signs on physical examination, are not chronically ill and have close follow-up, may be managed as outpatients. The use of empiric antibiotics as part of outpatient management is controversial; one may choose close follow-up alone or treat with parenteral ceftriaxone once daily until cultures are negative.

Acyclovir (dosed at 60 mg/kg/day) should be started empirically in full-term infants, i.e., younger than 4 weeks, and in preterm infants, i.e, younger than 8 weeks, if any risk factors for HSV infection are present

(Table 51–5). Although febrile infants 4–8 weeks old with RSV infection, documented by rapid testing, are at significantly lower risk of serious bacterial illness than RSV negative infants, the rate of serious bacterial illness, especially urinary tract infection, remains significant.[20] Therefore, these infants should still meet low risk criteria. In febrile infants younger than 4 weeks, the risk of serious bacterial infection is substantial and not altered by the presence of RSV infection.[20] These infants should have a sepsis work-up including a lumbar puncture and be admitted to the hospital. The use of rapid influenza testing has led to less laboratory testing, hospital admission and antibiotic use for febrile infants younger than 3 months.[19] However, at this time, there is insufficient data on the risk of serious bacterial infection in febrile infants younger than 3 months with influenza to modify existing management strategies.

One approach to the management of febrile infants is shown in the algorithm (Figure 51–1). However, care should be taken when applying any algorithm

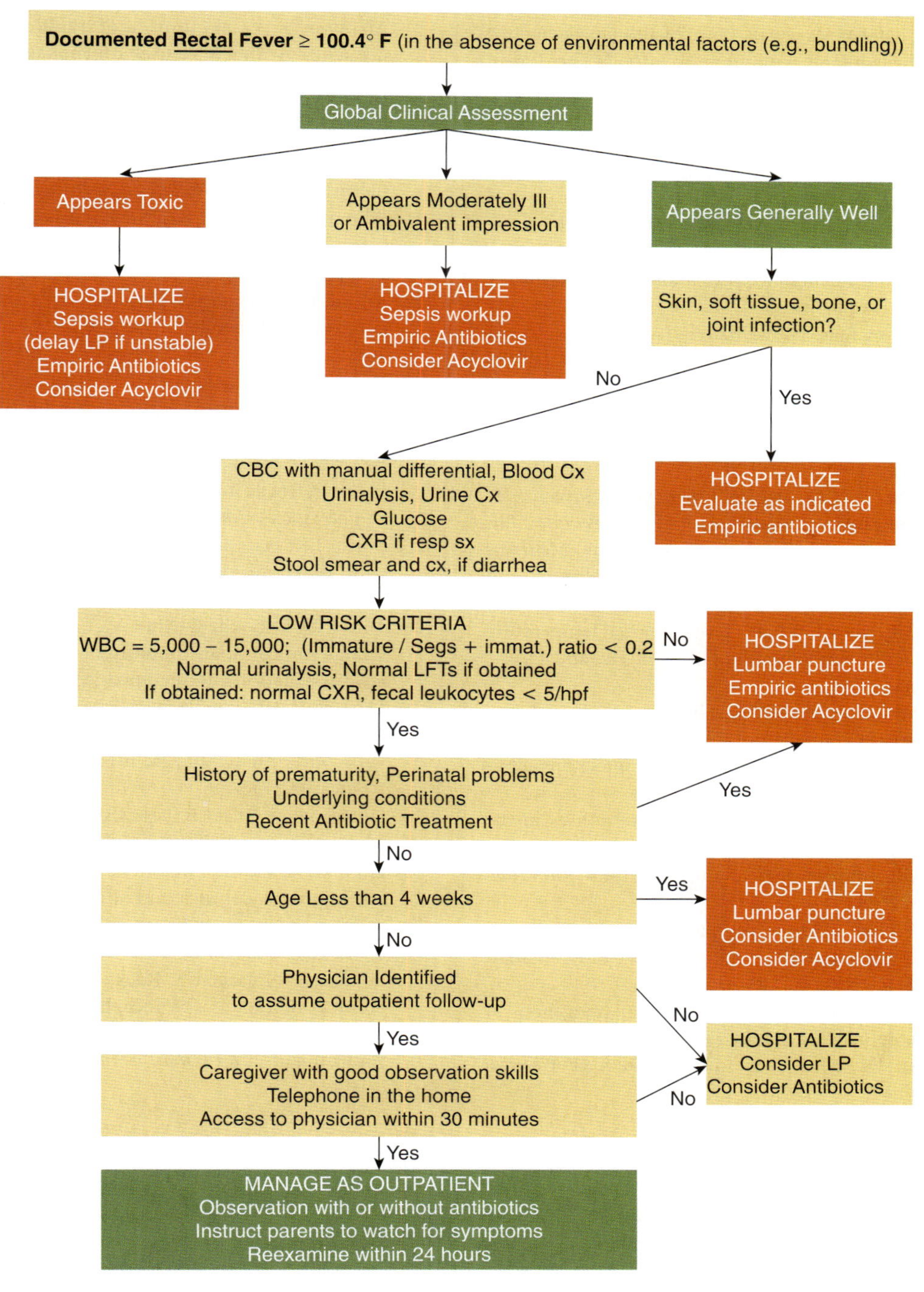

FIGURE 51–1 ■ Algorithm for the management of febrile infants.

since individual clinical decision making as well as periodic review of the literature is essential to providing the most appropriate, up-to-date management.

REFERENCES

1. Avner JR, Baker MD. Management of fever in infants and children. *Emerg Med Clin North Am.* 2002;20(1): 49-67.
2. Meltzer A, Powell K, Avner JR. Fever in children. *Consensus in Pediatrics.* 2005;1(7):1-19.
3. Baker MD, Avner JR. Fever in infants less than 2 months old. *Clin Pediatr Emerg Med.* 2000;1(2):102-108.
4. Baker MD, Bell LM, Avner JR. Outpatient management of low-risk febrile infants without antibiotics. *N Engl J Med.* 1993;329:1437-1441.
5. Baskin MN, O'Rourke EJ, Fleisher GR. Outpatient treatment of febrile infants 28 to 89 days of age with intramuscular administration of ceftriaxone. *J Pediatr.* 1992; 120:22-27.
6. Jaskiewicz JA, McCarthy CA, Richardson AC, et al. Febrile infants at low risk for serious bacterial infection—an appraisal of the Rochester Criteria and implications for management. *Pediatrics.* 1994;94:390-396.
7. Pantell RH, Newman TB, Bernzweig J, et al. Management and outcomes of care of fever in early infancy. (PROS STUDY) *JAMA.* 2004;291(10):1203-1212.
8. Slater M, Krug SE. Evaluation of the infant with fever without source: an evidence based approach. *Emerg Med Clin North Am.* 1999;17:97-126.
9. Avner JR, Sharieff GQ. Medical Emergencies. In: Fuchs S, Gausche-Hill M, Yamamoto L ed. *Advanced Pediatric Life Support (APLS): The Pediatric Emergency Medicine Resource.* 4th ed. American Academy of Pediatrics and American College of Emergency Physicians; 2004.
10. Herzog LW, Coyne LJ. What is fever? Normal temperature in infants less than 3 months old. *Clin Pediatr (Phila).* 1993;32(3):142-146.
11. Bonadio WA, Hegenbarth M, Zachariason M. Correlating reported fever in young infants with subsequent temperature patterns and rate of serious bacterial infections. *Pediatr Infect Dis J.* 1990;9:158-160.
12. Zola H. The development of antibody responses in the infant. *Immunol Cell Biol.* 1977;75:587-590.
13. Mackay CR. Immunological memory. *Adv Immunol.* 1993;53:217-265.
14. Doran KS, Nizet V. Molecular pathogenesis of neonatal group B streptococcal infection: no longer in its infancy. *Mol Microbiol.* 2004;54(1):23-31.
15. Nizet V, Ferrieri P, Rubens CE. Molecular pathogenesis of group B streptococcal disease in newborns. In: Stevens DL, Kaplan EL, eds. *Streptococcal Infections: Clinical Aspects, Microbiology, and Molecular Pathogenesis.* New York: Oxford University Press; 2000:180-221.
16. Baker CJ, Edwards MS. Group B streptococcal infections. In: Remington JS, Klien JO, eds. *Infectious Diseases of the Fetus and Newborn Infant.* Philadelphia, PA: WB Saunders; 2001:1091-1156.
17. McCarthy PL, Sharpe MR, Spiesel SZ, et al. Observation scales to identify serious illness in febrile children. *Pediatrics.*1982;70:802-809.
18. Baker MD, Avner JR, Bell LM. Failure of infant observation scales in detecting serious illness in febrile 4–8 week old infants. *Pediatrics.* 1990;85:1040-1043.
19. Benito-Fernandez J, Vazquez-Ronco M, Morteruel-Aizkuren E, et al. Impact of rapid viral testing for influenza A and B viruses on management of febrile infants without signs of focal infection. *Pediatr Infect Dis J.* 2006;25:1153-1157.
20. Levine DA, Platt SL, Dayan PS, et al. Risk of serious bacterial infection in young febrile infants with respiratory syncytial virus infections. *Pediatrics.* 2004;113:1728-1734.
21. Filippine MM, Katz BZ. Neonatal herpes simplex virus infection presenting with fever alone. *J Hum Virol.* 2001;4(4):223-225.
22. Kimberlin D. Herpes simplex virus, meningitis and encephalitis in neonates. *Herpes.* 2004;11(suppl 2): 65A-76A.
23. Baker MD, Bell LM, Avner JR. The efficacy of routine outpatient management without antibiotics of fever in selected infants. *Pediatrics.* 1999;103:660-665.
24. Baker MD, Bell LM. Unpredictability of serious bacterial illness in febrile infants from birth to 1 month of age. *Arch Pediatr Adolesc Med.* 1999;153:508-511.
25. Bonsu BK, Harper MB. Identifying febrile young infants with bacteremia: is the peripheral white blood cell count and accurate screen? *Ann Emerg Med.* 2003;42:216-225.
26. Turner D, Leibovitz E, Aran A, et al. Acute otitis media in infants younger than 2 months of age: microbiology, clinical presentation and therapeutic approach. *Pediatr Infect Dis J.* 2002;21(7):669-674.
27. Avner JR, Crain EF, Baker MD. Are well-appearing infants with otitis media at risk for serious bacterial illness? *AJDC.* 1992;146:446.
28. Hoberman A, Wald E. Urinary tract infections in young febrile children. *Pediatr Infect Dis J.* 1997;16:11-17.
29. Herr SM, Wald ER, Pitetti RD, Choi SS. Enhanced urinalysis improves identification of febrile infants ages 60 days and younger at low risk for serious bacterial illness. *Pediatrics.* 2001;108:866-871.
30. Bonadio WA, Hagen E, Rucka J, Shallow K, Stommel P, Smith D. Efficacy of a protocol to distinguish risk of serious bacterial infection in the outpatient evaluation of febrile young infants. *Clin Pediatr (Phila).* 1993;32:401-404.

SECTION 14

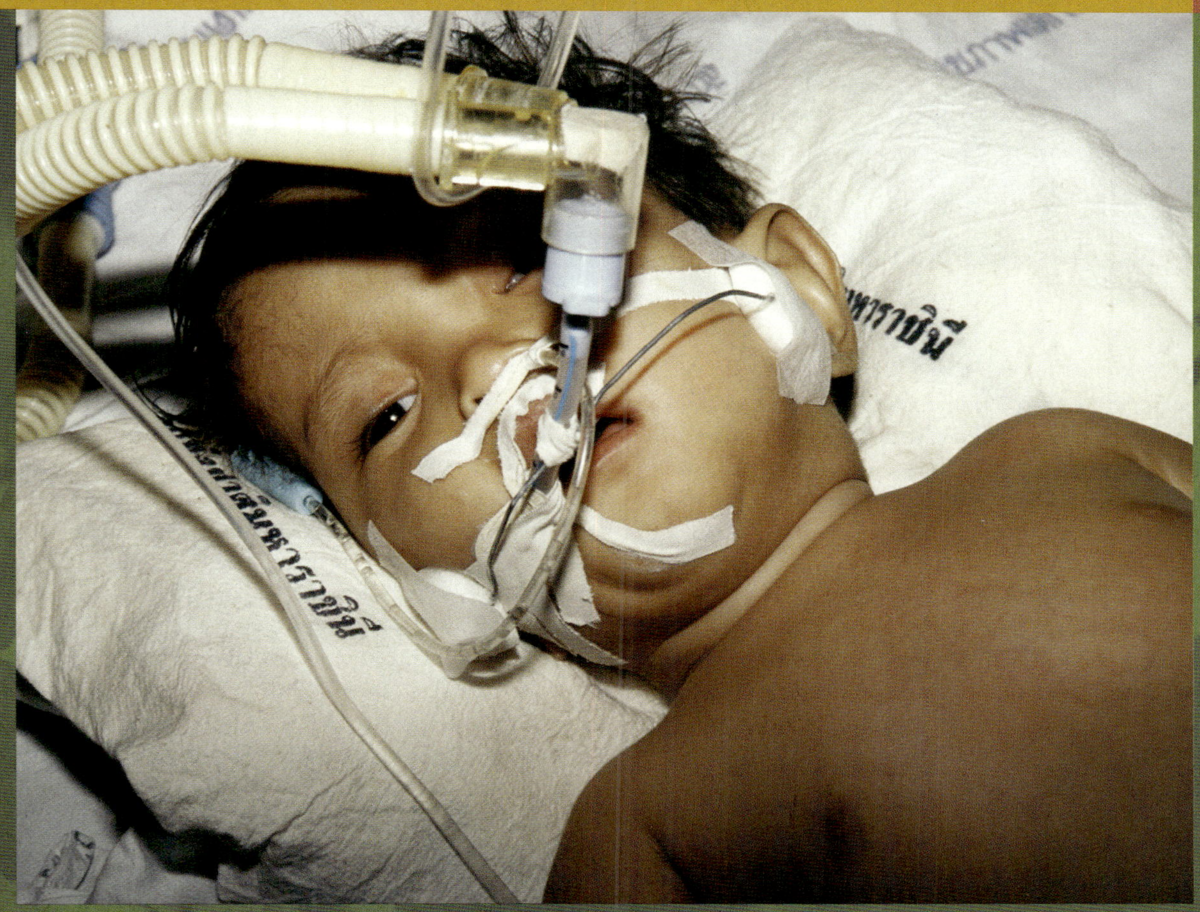

HIV Exposure and Infection

CHAPTER 52

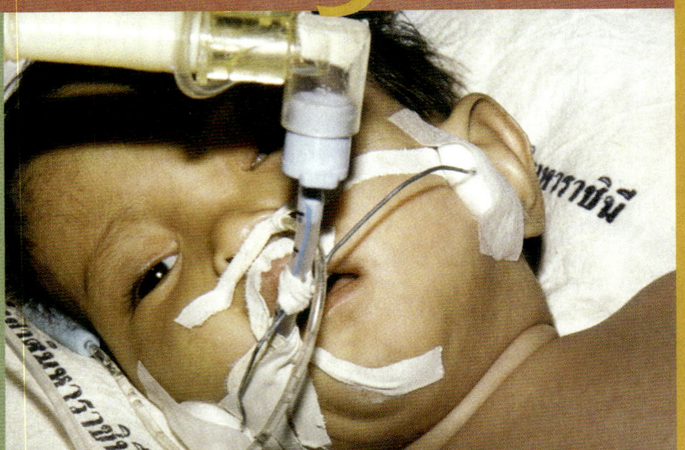

HIV-Exposed Neonate and HIV At-Risk Child

Sarah M. Wood, Richard M. Rutstein, and Andrew P. Steenhoff

Worldwide, more than 2 million children younger than 15 years are infected with HIV, with perinatal transmission the source of most of these infections.[1,2] In the developed world, where prenatal testing and safe and effective antiretroviral prophylaxis are widely available, perinatally-acquired HIV has become almost entirely preventable. With early testing and treatment of HIV-infected mothers and their newborns the risk of perinatal HIV transmission can be reduced to less than 2%.[3] The pediatric provider plays an essential role in disease reduction. By early identification of HIV-exposed infants, timely virologic testing and provision of postpartum HIV and opportunistic infection prophylaxis, pediatric care providers can intervene to dramatically reduce the risk of infection for the neonate.

DEFINITION AND EPIDEMIOLOGY

Perinatal transmission of HIV denotes infections that are acquired during the intrauterine, intrapartum and postpartum periods. In the United States, the peak years of perinatal HIV transmission occurred in the early 1990s, with 1650 new infections diagnosed in 1991 alone.[4] In recent years there has been a dramatic reduction in new HIV infections, with a 95% reduction in the incidence of perinatally acquired HIV from 1992 to 2004 in the United States.[4] In 2002, an estimated 144–236 new perinatal HIV infections were diagnosed in the United States.[4] These cases represent those women who either refused or were not offered prenatal HIV testing, had suboptimal antiretroviral adherence during pregnancy, presented at term without prenatal care, or experienced rare unexplained treatment failures.

The reduction in new infections in the developed world is a direct consequence of perinatal antiretroviral regimens. In 1994, the Pediatric AIDS Clinical Trials Group released the results of their landmark 076 study, examining the effect of a three-part regimen containing the nucleoside reverse transcriptase inhibitor (NRTI) zidovudine (ZDV). The active treatment arm consisted of maternal oral ZDV therapy beginning at 14–34 weeks gestation, intravenous ZDV in labor, and infant oral ZDV for 6 weeks. The HIV infection rate in the ZDV-treated group was 8% at 18 months versus 26% in placebo group—a remarkable 68% reduction in HIV transmission.[5] Based on the study findings, in 1994 the Centers for Disease Control and Prevention and U.S. Public Health Service issued recommendations for the routine use of the three-part ZDV regimen for all pregnant HIV-infected women.[6]

In July 1995, the U.S. Public Health Service issued recommendations for universal prenatal HIV counseling and consensual testing.[7] In 2006, the Centers for Disease Control and Prevention revised its HIV testing recommendations to increase early detection of HIV in pregnancy. The new guidelines focus on implementing HIV screening as a routine part of prenatal care, rather than as an optional test. As such, they recommend "opt-out" testing, whereby all women should receive the test as part of their care unless they specifically decline. The Centers for Disease Control and Prevention also recommends a second screening in the third trimester for women with known risk factors or those in high prevalence areas (as defined by an incidence of at least one HIV infection per thousand pregnant women).[8] Early diagnosis of pregnant women is critical for timely implementation of the recommended antiretroviral prophylaxis regimen to the mother and infant dyad.

PATHOGENESIS

In the absence of peripartum antiretroviral prophylaxis, rates of HIV transmission range from 14% to 35% in the developed world.[4,9] In the developing world, where prolonged breast-feeding is the norm and maternal HIV infection is often poorly controlled, transmission rates range from 25% to 48%.[10] With an optimized regimen of prenatal care and maternal highly active antiretroviral therapy (HAART) as well as intrapartum and postnatal ZDV prophylaxis, perinatal transmission rates are reduced to as low as 1%.[3]

Understanding the timing of perinatal HIV infection is a key step toward meaningful implementation of the perinatal prophylaxis recommendations. While it was initially believed that the majority of perinatal HIV infections occurred in utero, most transmission in fact occurs during the intrapartum period with in utero transmission accounting for less than 10% of all perinatal HIV infections.[11] Postpartum infection is largely caused by breast-feeding. A meta-analysis of prospective cohort studies estimated the risk of transmission of HIV-1 through breast-feeding as 16%.[12] The risk increases with longer duration of breast-feeding, high maternal viral load, the presence of mastitis and mixed formula and breastmilk feeding.[13]

The three-part antiretroviral regimen for prevention of mother- to -child transmission (PMTCT), based on the Pediatric AIDS Clinical Trials Group 076 ZDV-centered regimen, is constructed to prevent HIV transmission at all possible time-points.[3,6]

While alternate PMTCT regimens have been studied, the ZDV-based regimen is considered the gold-standard treatment. However, maternal monotherapy with ZDV is now believed to be suboptimal, and maternal ZDV-based HAART is warranted for all pregnant HIV-infected women in regions where combination antiretroviral therapy is available.[3,14] HAART is defined as a combination regimen of at least three drugs, from two different classes of anti-HIV agents. If an alternative prophylactic regimen must be considered, providers should consult the U.S. Public Health Service Task Force perinatal treatment guidelines, available at www.aidsinfo.nih.gov/Guidelines to obtain the most up-to-date information on perinatal prophylaxis and PMTCT regimens.[3]

Maternal antiretroviral therapy inhibits in utero infection, while intravenous ZDV in labor acts as preexposure prophylaxis against intrapartum infection.[3] As intrapartum and postpartum ZDV add additional mechanisms of protection against transmission, all HIV-infected women should receive intravenous ZDV in labor, even if they have received HAART during pregnancy. If only intrapartum and oral infant ZDV are given, transmission rates still decrease from 27% to 10%.[15] In resource-poor settings where access to prenatal care and antiretrovirals is limited, a simplified regimen consisting of a single intrapartum dose of the non-nucleoside reverse transcriptase inhibitor (NNRTI) nevirapine (NVP) followed by a single infant dose at 48–72 hours of life may be used. This regimen has been shown to reduce HIV transmission in a breast-fed population to 16% at 18 months of age compared to a 26% transmission rate in patients receiving an abbreviated regimen of oral intrapartum and neonatal ZDV[16,17] However, recent data indicate that this intervention may induce maternal and infant NVP resistance and decrease later virologic response to NNRTI-based therapy.[18] The mode of delivery also has a significant impact on the risk of transmission in the setting of poorly controlled maternal HIV infection. A meta-analysis of prospective cohort studies examining the impact of cesarean section found a 50% reduction in HIV transmission associated with cesarean delivery, independent of antiretroviral therapy.[19] Current guidelines recommend planned cesarean delivery at 38 weeks for HIV-1-infected women with viral loads greater than 1000 copies/mL near term.[20]

In the postnatal period, infant ZDV functions as postexposure prophylaxis. In the absence of prenatal or intrapartum prophylaxis, infant ZDV should still be implemented as soon as possible after birth. The initiation of infant ZDV only as postexposure prophylaxis has reduced infection rates from 27% to 9% if initiated in the first 2 days of life.[15] Starting ZDV prophylaxis after 48 hours has not been shown to reduce HIV transmission.[3]

In regions of the world where clean water and infant formula are widely available, the risk of postnatal transmission is further reduced by avoidance of breast-feeding. However, in resource-poor settings where excess infant morbidity and mortality have been associated with the use of infant formula, particularly where access to potable water is limited and formula use is hampered by cost and social stigma, HIV-infected women should continue breast-feeding.[21,22] Mixed formula and breastfeeding has been associated with an increased risk of HIV infection, and should be avoided. In resource-poor settings, HIV-infected women have been advised to exclusively breast-feed for the first 4–6 months of life, followed by rapid weaning.[13] However, recent data suggest that early weaning does not lower the risk of infection, and may increase mortality.[23] While HIV-infected women in developing nations should continue to exclusively breast-feed, the optimal time for weaning is yet to be determined.

CLINICAL PRESENTATION

There are no signs and symptoms that reliably indicate neonatal HIV infection. As such, any initial assessment of an infant with potential HIV exposure includes a thorough history detailing the prenatal course and intrapartum events. The role of the pediatric provider in the immediate postpartum period is not only to implement testing and infant prophylaxis, but also to assess the risk of infant infection. Maternal factors including high maternal plasma viral RNA level (viral load) at delivery, advanced HIV disease and the absence of HAART during pregnancy are associated with an increased risk of transmission.[9] In addition, intrapartum factors including vaginal delivery, rupture of membranes for greater than 8 hours, and preterm delivery also increase the risk. Evidence suggests that cigarette smoking, chorioamnionitis, other active sexually transmitted infections and invasive intrapartum procedures such as fetal scalp monitoring and episiotomy may also increase HIV transmission.[11]

An important role of the pediatrician is to assess the HIV status of all patients, regardless of age, race or socioeconomic status. Patients for whom maternal HIV serostatus is not known, as well as infants and children in substitute care, should undergo routine HIV testing. There are a number of clinical presentations and medical conditions, described in Table 52–1, which should raise provider suspicion of HIV infection and warrant testing. If suspicion of HIV is high in such cases, prophylaxis against *Pneumocystis jiroveci* pneumonia (PCP) should be implemented, pending receipt of test results.

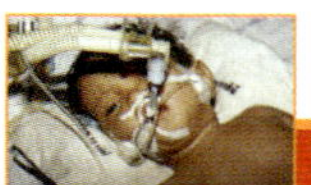

Table 52–1.

Clinical Guidelines for HIV Testing in Neonates, Children, and Adolescents

Indications for neonatal testing	Maternal HIV infection Unknown maternal HIV serostatus
Indications for child/adolescent testing	Substitute/foster care Sexual abuse Older children of women with recently diagnosed HIV infection (at any age) Unexplained clinical symptoms including: Failure to thrive Lymphadenopathy Loss of developmental milestones Hepatomegaly/splenomegaly Frequent, severe, or unusual infections Chronic or recurrent parotitis Chronic diarrhea Hepatitis without other etiology Severe overwhelming pneumonia unresponsive to usual antibiotics Recurrent episodes of bacteremia or presumed bacterial pneumonia High-risk sexual behavior in adolescents

DIFFERENTIAL DIAGNOSIS

While HIV may be the parent and provider's primary concern, pediatricians must be cognizant of the possibility of other perinatal infections which exhibit a high comorbidity with HIV, such as hepatitis B and C, syphilis, toxoplasmosis, cytomegalovirus, herpes simplex virus and tuberculosis.[24] As these conditions have a significant impact on the health of the neonate, maternal health screening and neonatal examination must also focus on these conditions.

Primary immunodeficiency diseases, particularly T-lymphocyte defects or combined B- and T-lymphocyte defects, may mimic the clinical presentation of children with the acquired immunodeficiency syndrome. Important T-lymphocyte defects include 22q deletion (DiGeorge Syndrome) and lymphocyte activation defects. Children with combined B- and T-lymphocyte defects, such as severe combined immunodeficiency syndrome, may present with PCP and other opportunistic infections commonly seen in HIV-infected children.

DIAGNOSIS

The diagnostic and treatment algorithm for the HIV-exposed infant is detailed in Figure 52–1. The most important first step for prevention of perinatal HIV infection is timely prenatal screening of all pregnant women. Knowledge of maternal serostatus allows for rapid implementation of perinatal prophylaxis and postpartum testing for the neonate. In cases where there has been no prenatal care or maternal HIV testing, maternal serostatus may be unknown at the onset of labor. In these scenarios, intrapartum HIV testing with maternal consent via expedited enzyme immunoassay (EIA) or rapid-testing kit may allow for expedient administration of intravenous ZDV prior to delivery.[25,26] Several rapid-testing kits are currently licensed for use in the United States.[25] The Mother-Infant Rapid Intervention at Delivery trial of HIV rapid testing in labor found the test to be 100% sensitive and 99.9% specific, with results available within 65 minutes.[26] Positive rapid tests must be confirmed with a separate HIV EIA or western blot assay.[25] However, empiric intrapartum ZDV and oral infant ZDV should be implemented immediately following an initial positive EIA, and should not be delayed while confirmatory results are pending.

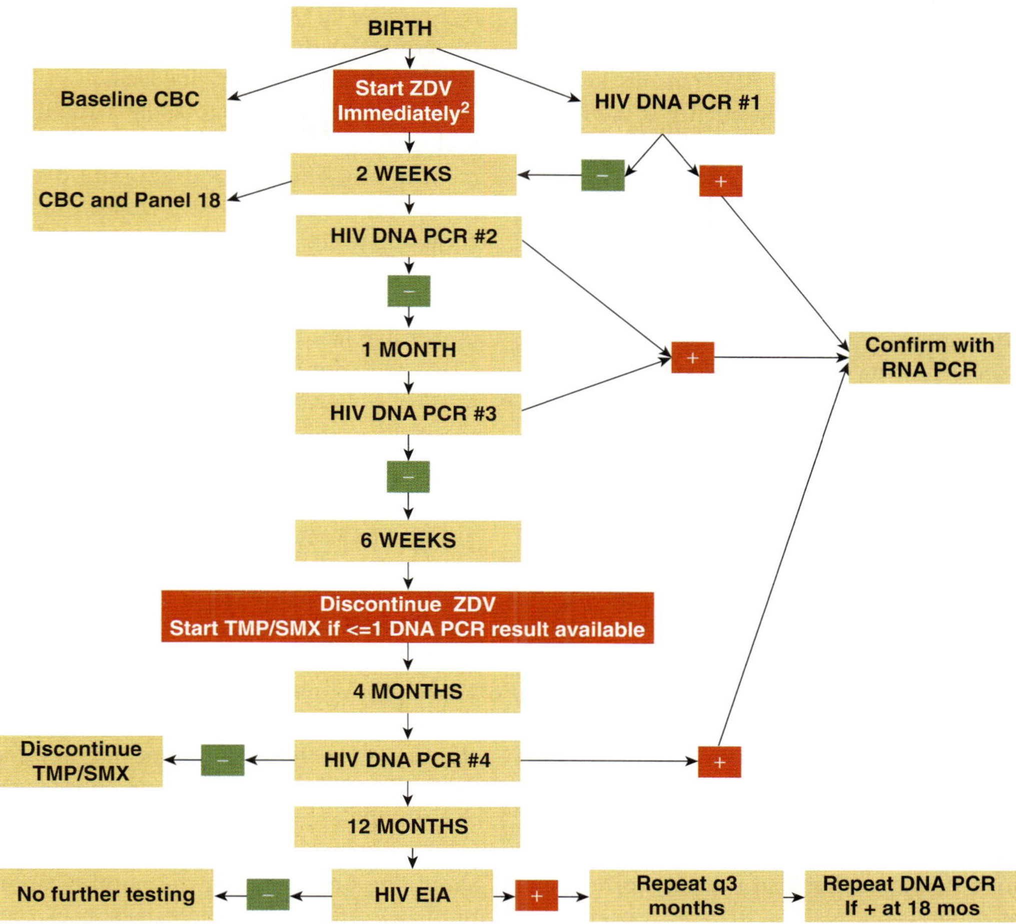

FIGURE 52–1 ■ Algorithm for testing and prophylaxis of the HIV-exposed neonate.
[1]If maternal HIV status is unknown, mother and/or infant should receive a rapid HIV test. If the test is positive, the above algorithm should be followed.
[2]For delayed diagnosis, ZDV may be started as late as 48 hr after birth. Read JS. Diagnosis of HIV-1 infection in children younger than 18 months in the United States. *Pediatrics* 2007; 120(6):e1547-62.

In cases where maternal serostatus has not been confirmed prior to delivery, the pediatrician's role is to determine the neonate's HIV-exposure status as soon as possible with expedited HIV EIA or rapid testing of the infant.[27] Owing to the placental transfer of maternal IgG in the third trimester, virtually all HIV-exposed infants will have a positive EIA at birth. A positive HIV EIA before 18 months of age indicates HIV-exposure, but cannot diagnose infection. As with maternal testing, any positive EIA or rapid test results must be confirmed by a supplemental EIA and western blot.[24] With confirmation of exposure, it is essential to initiate infant antiretroviral prophylaxis as soon as possible. If EIA results are unavailable during this period, the pediatrician should consider initiating ZDV pending test results when the pretest probability of infection is high. Procedures for obtaining documented maternal consent for infant HIV testing vary by state, and physicians should be familiar with the consent laws of their region. For infants and children in substitute care, state child welfare agencies may be able to provide consent depending on state and local law. In circumstances where the suspicion of HIV is high and parental consent has been refused, a court order may be necessary to perform HIV testing.

Virologic specific tests such as the HIV DNA polymerase chain reaction (PCR) assay or HIV culture are needed to definitively diagnose HIV infection in the neonate. The revised testing schedule recommends an initial virologic test drawn at 2–3 weeks of life, followed by a second test at 1–2 months, and a final virologic test between 4–5 months of life.[14] State guidelines may vary with respect to the specific timing of infant HIV testing, and pediatric providers should be familiar with regional practices. Many sites draw a first virologic test at day one or two of life. Testing at 48 hours of life allows for early implementation of optimal therapy should the test indicate infection.[27] A positive virologic test at or before 48 hours indicates in utero infection, whereas a negative virologic test in the first week of life followed by a subsequent positive test after 2 weeks suggests intrapartum infection.[14] While early neonatal testing is essential, up to 60% of HIV-infected infants will have negative test results at 48 hours of life. While a positive test strongly indicates infection, a negative test in this early period does not exclude the possibility of HIV transmission.[14]

The standard virologic test in infancy is the HIV DNA PCR assay.[28] This qualitative test gives a "yes, HIV was detected" or "no, HIV was not detected" answer. It indicates either the presence or absence of HIV DNA in peripheral blood mononuclear cells, but does not quantify the number of detectable copies. Sensitivity of the test is 40% within the first 2 weeks of life, but increases to 93% by 14 days. By 1 month of life, the test is 96% sensitive and 99% specific in identifying HIV.[14] Cord blood should not be used in postpartum testing, as it may contain maternal blood cells resulting in a false positive assay.[24] The sensitivity of the currently available HIV-1 DNA PCR assays are reduced for non-B subtypes of HIV. While the B subtype of HIV is predominant in the United States, there is extensive global variation in HIV subtypes and clades. In cases where maternal infection with a non-B subtype is known or suspected, the infant should be tested for HIV with a branched-chain DNA (bDNA) test of HIV culture as well as the standard DNA PCR.[29]

Quantitative HIV RNA PCR assay, the test typically used to evaluate viral load in confirmed HIV infection, has a sensitivity comparable to the DNA test, but a higher false positive rate. Although minor, this decrease in specificity limits its utility as the primary test for HIV-exposed infants.[30] However, infant viral load is highly correlated with disease progression, making RNA PCR assay an excellent confirmatory test for a positive DNA PCR assay. Finally, HIV-1 peripheral blood cell culture is considered the gold standard for the detection of HIV infection. Its sensitivity is equal to that of the HIV DNA PCR and it is 100% specific. However, its use is often limited by its significant expense, limited availability and long (up to 28 days) turn-around time for results.[24] In facilities where HIV culture is available, it may be used in tandem with the DNA PCR assay at 1 month to assess infection. All positive virologic tests must be confirmed by a second test on a separate sample. Infection is defined by at least two positive virologic tests drawn at different times.

HIV infection can be excluded with some confidence in a non–breast-fed; 5-month-old infant who has had at least two negative virologic tests provided these tests occurred at least 1 month and 4 months after birth.[14] In infants who are presumed to be uninfected by virologic testing, serologic testing by HIV EIA should be performed at 1 year to confirm the disappearance of maternal anti-HIV IgG. If the EIA remains positive, the test should be repeated between 15 and 18 months.[14,24] While in rare cases, HIV-uninfected children may retain maternal antibodies after 18 months, it is generally accepted that a confirmed positive EIA after ≥18 months of age indicates HIV infection. Virologic testing should be repeated in this instance.[14,24] For children older than 2 years, initial testing may be done using the HIV EIA. Infection is confirmed by 2 positive HIV antibody tests (each with confirmatory western blots), drawn on different days. HIV RNA PCR should follow to quantify viral load.

In resource poor areas, the feasibility of repeated testing is often limited. Numerous ongoing trials aim to identify cost-effective and accurate diagnostic algorithms. HIV EIA testing at 6 weeks, which is relatively cheap and widely available, may be used to identify HIV-exposed infants. EIA samples may be saved as dried blood spots on filter paper, and sent to the nearest comprehensive laboratory facility for PCR confirmation. $CD4^+$ cell count at 1 and 3 months may be used as another surrogate marker for infection, although the specificity of this method is poor.

TREATMENT

The HIV-exposed neonate should be assessed in the immediate postpartum period, and then followed in the outpatient setting at 1 week, 1 month, and 2, 4, 6, 9, 12 months. Virologic testing should be performed at the 1- and 4-month visits, and serologic testing should commence at 12 months. All routine immunizations should be given to HIV-exposed infants, with the exception of the recently approved rotavirus vaccine.[24] As this vaccine is not yet approved in HIV-infected children, it should be omitted from the immunization schedule until HIV infection has been reliably excluded. If HIV infection is confirmed, immunization guidelines for HIV infected children should be followed.

Treatment of the HIV-exposed neonate begins with implementation of ZDV therapy in the immediate postpartum period. In cases where risk of infection is high, that is, failure to implement prenatal or intrapartum prophylaxis or known maternal nonadherence to HAART, clinicians may consider adding a second antiretroviral to the infant regimen. The antiretrovirals of choice in these scenarios are those for which infant dosing is well established—the NRTI lamivudine 2′,3′-dideoxy-3′-thiacytidine (3TC) and/or the NNRTI NVP. However, evidence to support this treatment approach is limited, and such complicated cases should be managed in consultation with a specialist in pediatric HIV. Antiretroviral dosing for preterm and full-term infants is detailed in Table 52–2.

After discharge from the hospital, the infant and primary caregiver should be seen for a full outpatient assessment at 1 week of life. Comprehensive management of the HIV-exposed neonate includes a thorough review of maternal health information in order to garner information about the perinatal course and assess the risk of infant infection with HIV and other related pathogens. Counseling should be provided to the primary caregivers regarding the duration of therapy, testing schedule, and the importance of avoiding

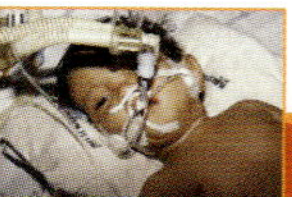

Table 52–2.

Neonatal Antiretroviral Dosing

Medication	Preterm Dosing (< 36 weeks EGA)	Full-Term Dosing
ZDV*	1.5 mg/kg IV or 2 mg/kg po q12h ■ ↑ to q8h at 2 wks of age, if ≥ 30 weeks EGA at birth ■ ↑ at 4 weeks of age if < 30 wks EGA at birth	2 mg/kg po q6h or 1.5 mg/kg IV q6h
Epivir (3TC)	Consult an HIV specialist	2 mg/kg bid
NVP	Consult an HIV specialist	Through age 2 mo: 5 mg/kg or 120 mg/m^2 once daily for the first 14 d, followed by 200 mg/m^2 bid for 14 d, followed by 200 mg/m^2 bid

**Preferred regimen.*

EGA, estimated gestational age; IV, intravenous; po, by mouth; q12h, every 12 hours; ↑, "increase the dose"; bid, twice a day.

breast-feeding to prevent late postnatal transmission. As the mother may be recently diagnosed, referral to support services and HIV treatment is an essential aspect of family-oriented care. In addition, all siblings of the infant should undergo HIV testing, following the testing schema detailed above, if their serostatus is unknown, regardless of their age.[24] One of the primary roles of the pediatrician is to monitor infant ZDV therapy during the 6-week prophylactic regimen. Antiretroviral adherence and adverse effects should be assessed at each encounter. The most common adverse effect associated with neonatal ZDV treatment is a mild, macrocytic anemia that generally resolves after 2 months.[28,31] Neutrophil, lymphocyte and platelet counts may also decrease.[31] A complete blood count with differential should be performed at birth, 2 weeks, and 4 months to monitor any changes in hematologic parameters.[24]

The potential toxicity of ZDV has been a topic of some debate. As an inhibitor of DNA polymerase gamma, ZDV is known to act as a human mitochondrial toxin. Large cohorts of ZDV-treated HIV-exposed infants in the United States have failed to find any cases of mitochondrial toxicity.[32] However, 12 cases of confirmed, and 14 cases of possible, mitochondrial toxicity have been reported within a French cohort of ZDV-treated infants. Neurologic signs of mitochondrial toxicity included encephalopathy, seizures, and developmental delay. The overall incidence of mitochondrial toxicity in this cohort was 0.26%, with findings occurring more commonly in infants treated with a combination of ZDV and the NRTI lamivudine (3TC).[33] Because of this potential risk, ZDV and/or 3TC-treated infants should receive a thorough neurologic examination at all routine visits. While maternal prenatal ZDV treatment has not been associated with an increased risk of congenital anomalies,[34] less information is available about the risks of in utero exposure to the various other antiretroviral components of HAART. Efavirenz is a known teratogen, and infants exposed to this NNRTI are at risk for congenital anomalies. All infants with in utero exposure to HAART should be assessed for congenital anomalies at birth, 6 months, and yearly thereafter.[3,24] Any instances of suspected adverse effects or congenital anomalies related to antiretroviral exposure should be reported the Antiretroviral Pregnancy Registry.[35] Ongoing trials examining long-term outcomes of uninfected ZDV-treated and HAART-exposed infants are underway in the hopes of resolving these questions.

At 6 weeks of age ZDV prophylaxis should be discontinued provided the infant has had two negative DNA PCRs, with one drawn at 2 weeks of life, and the second after 4 weeks of life. In such cases, HIV infection is presumptively excluded and prophylaxis against *Pneumocystis jiroveci* (formerly Pneumocystis carinii) pneumonia (PCP) does not need to be initiated. In the era prior to routine prophylaxis, PCP was the most common opportunistic infection in HIV-infected children. Disease incidence peaks at 3–6 months of age and tends toward an acute and severe course. Unlike many other opportunistic infections, PCP may occur at relatively high CD4$^+$ cell counts.[28] As it is difficult both to ascertain which HIV-infected infants are at risk for PCP and to confirm HIV-infection during the period of peak incidence, trimethoprim/sulfamethoxazole (TMP/SMX) prophylaxis is recommended for HIV-exposed infants of indeterminate status and all HIV-infected infants starting at 4–6 weeks of age regardless of their CD4$^+$ cell count.[36] TMP/SMX prophylaxis should generally be delayed until 6 weeks to avoid both the additive hematologic marrow suppression effects of combined ZDV and TMP/SMX prophylaxis, and the concern for neonatal hyperbilirubinemia associated with early administration of sulfa antibiotics. Prophylaxis with TMP/SMX is continued until a second negative virologic test is available at 4 months of age. If virologic test results are unavailable or if the infant is found to be HIV-infected, TMP/SMX prophylaxis should be continued until a minimum of 1 year of age. The incidence of PCP decreases dramatically after

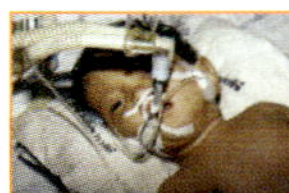

Table 52–3.

Dosing for PCP Prophylaxis for HIV-Exposed Newborns Older Than 4 Weeks

Medication	Dosing	Adverse Effects
TMP/SMX*	TMP 150 mg/m^2 with SMX 750 mg/m^2 twice daily for 3 days weekly (e.g., every Monday, Wednesday, Friday).	■ Common: Rash, anemia, GI upset. ■ Rare and severe: Stevens-Johnson syndrome, toxic epidermal necrolysis, aplastic anemia, agranulocytosis, hepatic necrosis. ■ Use with caution in patients with G6PD deficiency.
Dapsone	2 mg/kg (not to exceed 100 mg) po once daily.	■ Common: Rash, anemia, GI upset. ■ Rare and severe: See TMP/SMX. ■ Use with caution in patients with G6PD deficiency, methemoglobin reductase deficiency or hemoglobin M.
Atovaquone		■ Common: Rash, GI upset, anemia.
1–3 mo of age	30 mg/kg po once daily.	■ Rare and severe: Neonatal gasping syndrome.
3–6 mo of age	45 mg/kg po once daily.	■ Solution contains benzyl alcohol; may cause allergic reactions in susceptible infants.
Pentamidine	4 mg/kg IV every 2–4 wk. Aerosolized pentamidine is not recommended until age ≥ 5 ys	■ Common: Rash, anemia, nausea. ■ Rare and severe: Hypotension, arrhythmias, nephrotoxicity. ■ Adjust dose in renal impairment.

**Preferred regimen.*
PO, by mouth; IV, intravenous; G6PD, glucose-6-phosphate-dehydrogenase; GI, gastrointestinal.

the first year of life, and only those HIV-infected children with a past history of PCP or CD4$^+$ cell counts suggesting severe immunosuppression should remain on prophylaxis past 1 year of age. In the case of sulfa allergy, oral atovaquone or dapsone therapy may be used. Monthly intravenous pentamidine is another option for PCP prophylaxis, however, the cumbersome route of delivery makes it a less feasible option for HIV-exposed children and their families. Dosing schedules for TMP/SMX and alternative regimens are detailed in Table 52–3.

Comprehensive care of the HIV-infected mother and the HIV-exposed infant have dramatically lowered the rate of new perinatal HIV infections. Virtually, all perinatal HIV infections in the developed world are now preventable through antiretroviral prophylaxis. Great strides are still to be made in sub-Saharan Africa and other HIV-endemic regions of the world where over 1500 new pediatric infections occur everyday.[2] Globally, the increased availability of PMTCT programs, combined with educational interventions to produce sustainable changes in risk behavior, will be key to improving the outcomes of all children with perinatal HIV exposure.

PEARLS

1. All infants should undergo rapid HIV testing if maternal HIV serostatus is unknown.
2. ZDV should be initiated as soon as possible and not later than 48 hours for all infants with known perinatal HIV exposure.
3. Virologic testing of the HIV-exposed neonate by DNA PCR should be performed at birth, 1 and 4 months of age, and serologic testing by HIV EIA should commence at 12 months.
4. A positive HIV EIA before 18 months of age confirms HIV exposure, not infection, and virologic testing such as DNA or RNA PCR is needed to confirm infection.
5. A positive HIV EIA after 18 months of age suggests infection and requires immediate confirmation with a second HIV EIA and western blot.

REFERENCES

1. UNICEF, UNAIDS, WHO. *Children and AIDS: A Stocktaking Report*. New York: UNICEF, January 2007, 16. http://www.unicef.org/publications/index_38048.html
2. De Baets AJ, Bulterys M, Abrams EJ, Kankassa C, Pazvakavambwa IE. Care and treatment of HIV-infected children in Africa: issues and challenges at the district hospital level. *Pediatr Infect Dis J*. 2007;26(2):163-173.
3. Recommendations for use of Antiretroviral Drugs in Pregnant HIV-1 Infected Women for Maternal Health and Interventions to Reduce Perinatal HIV-1 Transmission in the United States. Rockville, MD: U.S. Public Health Service Task Force November 17, 2005.
4. Achievements in public health. Reduction in perinatal transmission of HIV infection–United States, 1985–2005. *MMWR*. 2006;55(21):592-597.
5. Connor EM, Sperling RS, Gelber R, et al. Reduction of maternal-infant transmission of human immunodeficiency

virus type 1 with zidovudine treatment. Pediatric AIDS Clinical Trials Group Protocol 076 Study Group. *N Engl J Med.* 1994;331(18):1173-1180.

6. Recommendations of the U.S. Public Health Service Task Force on the use of zidovudine to reduce perinatal transmission of human immunodeficiency virus. *MMWR Recomm Rep.* 1994;43(RR–11):1-20.
7. Centers for Disease Control and Prevention. U.S. Public Health Service recommendations for human immunodeficiency virus counseling and voluntary testing for pregnant women. *MMWR.* 1995;44(No. RR–7):1-15.
8. Branson BM, Handsfield HH, Lampe MA, et al. Revised recommendations for HIV testing of adults, adolescents, and pregnant women in health-care settings. *MMWR Recomm Rep.* 2006;55(RR-14):1-17; quiz CE1-4.
9. Mofenson LM. Mother-child HIV-1 transmission: timing and determinants. *Obstet Gynecol Clin North Am.* 1997; 24(4):759-784.
10. De Cock KM, Fowler MG, Mercier E, et al. Prevention of mother-to-child HIV transmission in resource-poor countries: translating research into policy and practice. *JAMA.* 2000;283(9):1175-1182.
11. Bulterys M, Nolan ML, Jamieson D, Dominguez K, Fowler MG. Advances in the prevention of mother-to-child HIV-1 transmission: current issues, future challenges. *AIDScience.* 2002;2(4). http://aidscience.org/Articles/aidscience017.htm. Accessed August 18, 2008.
12. John GC RB, Naduati RW, Mbori-Ngacha D, Kreiss JK. Timing of breast milk HIV-1 transmission: a meta analysis. *East Afr Med J.* 2001;78(2):75-79.
13. Read JS. Human milk, breastfeeding, and transmission of human immunodeficiency virus type 1 in the United States. American Academy of Pediatrics Committee on Pediatric AIDS. *Pediatrics.* 2003;112(5):1196-1205.
14. Working Group of Antiretroviral Therapy and Medical Management of HIV-Infected Children. Guidelines for the use of Antiretroviral Agents in Pediatric HIV Infection. July 29, 2008, 1-134.
15. Wade NA, Birkhead GS, Warren BL, et al. Abbreviated regimens of zidovudine prophylaxis and perinatal transmission of the human immunodeficiency virus. *N Engl J Med.* 1998;339(20):1409-1414.
16. Guay LA, Musoke P, Fleming T, et al. Intrapartum and neonatal single-dose nevirapine compared with zidovudine for prevention of mother-to-child transmission of HIV-1 in Kampala, Uganda: HIVNET 012 randomised trial. *Lancet.* 1999;354(9181):795-802.
17. Jackson JB, Musoke P, Fleming T, et al. Intrapartum and neonatal single-dose nevirapine compared with zidovudine for prevention of mother-to-child transmission of HIV-1 in Kampala, Uganda: 18-Month follow-up of the HIVNET 012 randomised trial. *Lancet.* 2003;362(9387): 859-868.
18. Lockman S, Shapiro RL, Smeaton LM, et al. Response to antiretroviral therapy after a single, peripartum dose of nevirapine. *N Engl J Med.* 2007;356(2):135-147.
19. The mode of delivery and the risk of vertical transmission of human immunodeficiency virus type 1—a meta-analysis of 15 prospective cohort studies. The International Perinatal HIV Group. *N Engl J Med.* 1999;340(13): 977-987.
20. ACOG committee opinion scheduled Cesarean delivery and the prevention of vertical transmission of HIV infection. Number 234, May 2000 (replaces number 219, August 1999). *Int J Gynaecol Obstet.* 2001;73(3):279-281.
21. Ali FM HM, Pugh RN. The associations between feeding modes and diarrhoea among urban children in a newly developed country. *Public Health.* 1997;111:239-243.
22. Nicoll A, Killewo JZ, Mgone C. HIV and infant feeding practices: epidemiological implications for sub-Saharan African countries. *AIDS.* 1990;4(7):661-665.
23. Kuhn L, Aldrovandi GM, Sinkala M, Kankasa C, Semrau K, Mwiya M, et al. Effects of early, abrupt weaning on HIV-free survival of children in Zambia. *N Engl J Med* 2008;359(2): 130-141.
24. King SM. Evaluation and treatment of the human immunodeficiency virus-1–exposed infant. *Pediatrics.* 2004;114(2):497-505.
25. Rapid HIV test distribution–United States, 2003–2005. *MMWR.* 2006;55(24):673-676.
26. Bulterys M, Jamieson DJ, O'Sullivan MJ, et al. Rapid HIV-1 testing during labor: a multicenter study. *JAMA.* 2004;292(2):219-223.
27. Committee on Pediatric AIDS, American Academy of Pediatrics. Identification and care of HIV-exposed and HIV-infected infants, children, and adolescents in foster care. *Pediatrics.* 2000;106(1, pt 1):149-153.
28. Mofenson LM. Committee on Pediatric AIDS, American Academy of Pediatrics. Technical report: perinatal human immunodeficiency virus testing and prevention of transmission. *Pediatrics.* 2000;106(6):E88.
29. Zaman MM, Recco RA, Haag R. Infection with non-B subtype HIV type 1 complicates management of established infection in adult patients and diagnosis of infection in newborn infants. *Clin Infect Dis.* 2002;34(3):417-418.
30. Nesheim S, Palumbo P, Sullivan K, et al. Quantitative RNA testing for diagnosis of HIV-infected infants. *J Acquir Immune Defic Syndr.* 2003;32(2):192-195.
31. Pacheco SE, McIntosh K, Lu M, et al. Effect of perinatal antiretroviral drug exposure on hematologic values in HIV-uninfected children: an analysis of the women and infants transmission study. *J Infect Dis.* 2006;194(8): 1089-1097.
32. Dominguez K, Bertolli J, Fowler M, et al. Lack of definitive severe mitochondrial signs and symptoms among deceased HIV-uninfected and HIV-indeterminate children ≤ 5 years of age, pediatric spectrum of HIV disease project (PSD), USA. *Ann N Y Acad Sci.* 2000;918:236-246.
33. Barret B, Tardieu M, Rustin P, et al. Persistent mitochondrial dysfunction in HIV-1-exposed but uninfected infants: clinical screening in a large prospective cohort. *AIDS.* 2003;17(12):1769-1785.
34. Culnane M, Fowler M, Lee SS, et al. Lack of long-term effects of in utero exposure to zidovudine among uninfected children born to HIV-infected women. Pediatric AIDS clinical trials group protocol 219/076 teams. *JAMA.* 1999;281(2):151-157.
35. Antiretroiral Pregnancy Registry. http://www.apregistry.com/. Accessed August 18, 2008.
36. 1995 revised guidelines for prophylaxis against Pneumocystis carinii pneumonia for children infected with or perinatally exposed to human immunodeficiency virus. National Pediatric and Family HIV Resource Center and National Center for Infectious Diseases, Centers for Disease Control and Prevention. *MMWR Recomm Rep.* 1995;44(RR-4):1-11.

CHAPTER 53

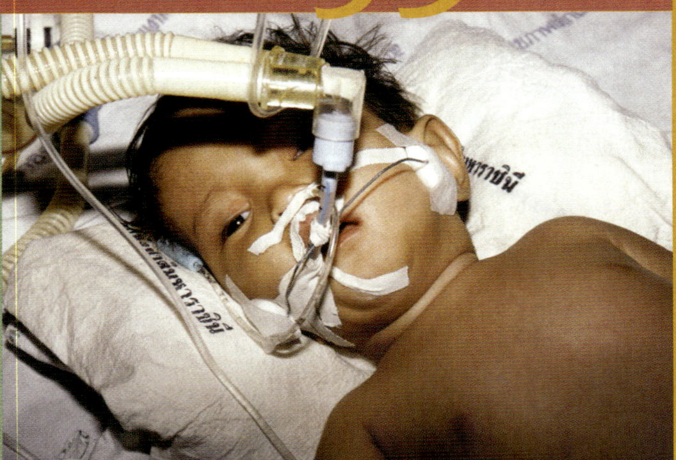

Care of the HIV-Infected Child

Andrew P. Steenhoff, Wolfgang Rennert, and Richard M. Rutstein

DEFINITION AND EPIDEMIOLOGY

In June 1981, the first cases in the United States of what was later called acquired immunodeficiency syndrome (AIDS) were reported.[1] In the decades since, the human immunodeficiency virus (HIV) epidemic in the United States has resulted in more than 900,000 individuals diagnosed with AIDS, as reported to the Centers for Disease Control by the end of 2004.[2] In general population, the number of new AIDS cases reported annually increased rapidly in the 1980s and peaked in 1992 with an estimated 78,000 cases diagnosed. In 1998, the epidemic stabilized and since then approximately 40,000 AIDS cases have been diagnosed annually.

Among children younger than 13 years, the proportion of all AIDS cases decreased from 1.4% (7668 cases) in 1981–1995 to 0.2% (341 cases) in 2001–2004.[3] The number of children reported with newly diagnosed AIDS dropped to 48 in 2004, primarily because of the identification of HIV-infected pregnant women and the effectiveness of antiretroviral prophylaxis in reducing mother-to-child transmission of HIV.[2,4] The successes achieved in controlling perinatal infection have not been mirrored in other at-risk pediatric groups. The 2005 Youth Risk Behavior Survey reported that 47% of high school students engaged in sexual intercourse at least once and 37% of sexually active students had not used a condom during their most recent act of sexual intercourse.[5] More than half of all HIV-infected adolescents are estimated to be unaware of their infection.[6] In a survey of 18–24-year-old men who have sex with men (MSM), 14% were found to be HIV-infected and 79% of these HIV-infected MSM were unaware of their infection.[7] This is an area where the pediatric practitioner can make a difference—among adolescents who were tested for HIV, 58% cited their provider's recommendation as their reason for testing.[8]

These national achievements are, however, overshadowed by the global picture of the AIDS epidemic. Despite increased access to effective treatment and prevention programs, both the number of people living with HIV and the number of deaths due to AIDS continue to grow. In each day of 2006, new HIV infections occurred in 1450 children and 10,400 adults while 1000 children and 7000 adults died as a result of AIDS.[9] The social fabric of nations is being altered by HIV, a virus that has resulted in 12 million AIDS orphans in Africa alone.

This chapter will focus on the care of the HIV-infected child in the United States. See Chapter 52 for an approach to the HIV-exposed child, Chapter 54 for a more detailed discussion of infections in HIV-infected children, and Chapter 55 for a discussion on postexposure prophylaxis.

The diagnosis of HIV infection depends on the laboratory detection of human immunodeficiency virus, or antibody directed against the virus, in a body fluid. This is performed either directly by virologic testing or indirectly by demonstrating the antibody to the virus. The diagnosis of AIDS combines clinical skills with laboratory diagnostics and is based on the detection of one or more AIDS-defining diagnoses in an individual who is HIV-infected (Table 53–1).

In 2006, it is estimated that there were 11,000 children younger than 15 years in North America who were living with HIV. In the same time period, there were less than 100 AIDS-related pediatric deaths. Despite these encouraging figures, prevention of mother-to-child transmission (PMTC) is an area that requires additional attention—estimates suggest that

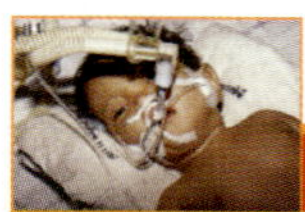

Table 53–1.

1993 Revised Case Definition of AIDS-Defining Conditions for Adolescents 13 Years of Age and Older.[36,37]

AIDS-Defining Condition
Candidiasis of bronchi, trachea or lungs
Candidiasis of the esophagus
Cervical cancer, invasive
Coccidioidomycosis, disseminated or extrapulmonary
Cryptococcosis, extrapulmonary
Cryptosporidiosis, chronic intestinal (>1 mo duration)
Cytomegalovirus disease (other than liver, spleen, or nodes)
Cytomegalovirus retinitis (with loss of vision)
Encephalopathy, HIV-related
Herpes simplex: chronic ulcers (>1 mo duration) or bronchitis, pneumonitis or esophagitis
Histoplasmosis, disseminated or extrapulmonary
Isosporiasis, chronic intestinal (>1 mo duration)
Kaposi sarcoma
Lymphoma, Burkitt (or equivalent term)
Lymphoma, immunoblastic (or equivalent term)
Lymphoma, primary or brain
Mycobacterium avium complex or *Mycobacterium kansasii*, disseminated or extrapulmonary
Mycobacterium tuberculosis, any site, pulmonary or extra pulmonary
Mycobacterium, other species or unidentified species, disseminated or extrapulmonary
Pneumocystis jiroveci pneumonia (PCP)
Pneumonia, recurrent
Progressive multifocal leukoencephalopathy
Salmonella septicemia, recurrent
Toxoplasmosis of the brain
Wasting syndrome attributable to HIV
$CD4^+$ T-lymphocyte count <200/μL or $CD4^+$ percentage <15%

AIDS, acquired immunodeficiency syndrome; HIV, human immunodeficiency virus.

100–200 North American children were infected with HIV in 2006 alone. The pediatrician has an important role to play when screening all newborns for HIV—initially by history and then by targeted testing of those whose mothers have not been tested for HIV during pregnancy or by retesting in those whose mothers have engaged in high-risk activity since their initial HIV test which usually occurs early in pregnancy. HIV-infected infants are still slipping through the net in the United States—the reasons for this include not offering the mother HIV testing, maternal refusal of HIV testing, or lack of maternal prenatal care. In addition, a single negative HIV test in early pregnancy will miss those women who seroconvert later in that pregnancy. The latter situation has resulted in the CDC guidelines recommending repeat HIV testing in the 36th week of gestation in all pregnant women where the population HIV seroprevalence is >1/1000.[10]

PATHOGENESIS

HIV is an RNA virus of the retrovirus family. HIV replicates via DNA intermediaries using the viral enzyme reverse transcriptase, a replication pathway that differs from the usual flow of genetic material in which cells use DNA to form RNA intermediaries. The retrovirus family is classified into seven different groups or genera. HIV is one of the primate lentiviruses, a group which includes HIV-1, HIV-2, and simian immunodeficiency virus (SIV). Primate lentiviruses infect T-lymphocytes thereby having the potential to cause severe immunodeficiency. See Chapter 54 for a more detailed discussion of the pathogenesis of immunodeficiency caused by HIV.

HIV is a zoonosis that resulted from a primate-to-human cross-species transmission. Chimpanzees are the host for SIV_{cpz}. The chimpanzee subspecies *Pan troglodytes troglodytes* is the origin of HIV-1. Transmission is estimated to have occurred between 1920 and 1930 in western equatorial Africa. Sooty mangabey monkeys are the host for SIV_{smm}. HIV-2 is closely related to SIV_{smm} and transmission is estimated to have occurred in the 1940s also in western Africa. The mode of cross species transmission in both types of HIV is thought to be exposure of humans to infected primate blood during hunting. Phylogenetic studies using molecular clock analyses have revealed that HIV-1 and HIV-2 have each arisen several times: in the case of HIV-1, the three groups (M, N, and O) are the result of independent cross-species transmission events.[11]

A hallmark of HIV is the broad genomic diversity of viruses within an individual and between infected individuals. This diversity of genetic material results from the high replication rate of the virus coupled with a high mutation rate and the occurrence of recombinations. In an infected person, about 10 billion viral particles are produced each day. The high mutation rate is the product of an "error-prone" viral reverse transcriptase, which lacks the ability to proofread DNA. Recombination may occur when a cell is coinfected by two different but related viruses; when these parent virions replicate, one RNA strand from each provirus can be encapsulated into a single new virion. The reverse transcriptase of this new "heterozygous" virion may move back and forth between the two RNA templates thus synthesizing a recombinant DNA sequence, which is a hybrid of the two parent HIV virions. The process of recombination may result in dramatic evolution of the virus and has proved to be a major obstacle to the development of a broadly effective HIV vaccine.

HIV-1 has three groups—O, M, and N. Ninety-five percent of global infections are caused by Group M subtypes A, B, C, or D or circulating recombinant forms (CRF), most commonly CRF_AE or CRF_AG. The greatest variation of HIV subtypes occurs in Cameroon

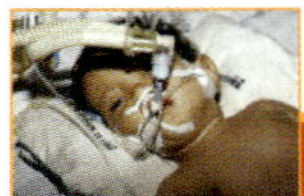

Table 53–2.

Pediatric HIV Classification for Children Younger Than 13 Years of Age.[37,38]

	Clinical Classifications*				Immunologic Categories†					
					<12 mo		1–5 y		6–12 y	
Immunologic Definitions	N: No Signs or Symptoms	A: Mild Signs and Symptoms	B: Moderate Signs and Symptoms	C: Severe Signs and Symptoms	No./μL	%	No./μL	%	No./μL	%
1: No evidence of suppression	N1	A1	B1	C1	≥1500	≥25	≥1000	≥25	≥500	≥25
2: Moderate suppression	N2	A2	B2	C2	750-1499	15-24	500-999	15-24	200-499	15-24
3: Severe suppression	N3	A3	B3	C3	<750	<15	<500	<15	<200	<15

*See Table 53–3 for which diseases fall into clinical categories N-C; the severity of each HIV-infected child's immunosuppression is categorized by one of the symbols represented in the pale gray area.
†Age-specific CD4+ T-lymphocyte count and percentage of total lymphocytes.

in west Africa. HIV-1 subtypes differ from each other by about 10% of their nucleotide sequences coding for the enzymes reverse transcriptase and protease. The clinical significance of HIV-1 subtypes is an active area of research—group O is resistant to a class of antiretrovirals, the nonnucleoside reverse transcriptase inhibitors (NNRTIs) and group N susceptibility has yet to be studied in detail. Subtype C has greater genetic variability than subtype B and this may result in different clinical outcomes including greater transmission potential.

HIV-2 is found predominantly in western Africa and the countries that were former Portuguese colonies such as Mozambique, Angola, and Brazil. With an increasing number of west Africans relocating to the United States, it is important that pediatricians are aware of some of the features of HIV-2. Compared to HIV-1, HIV-2 is less easily transmitted. Coinfection with HIV-1 may occur but initial infection with HIV-2 confers a significant reduction of 50–70% in the subsequent risk of acquiring HIV-1. Commercially available assays detect both HIV-1 and HIV-2 antigen but do not discriminate between the two types. However, there is no commercially available assay to detect HIV-2 plasma viral load. Clinically, HIV-2 presents with a similar spectrum of illnesses to HIV-1 but demonstrates a slower rate of progression to AIDS, a lower viral load, a lower rate of viral diversity, and a slower CD4 decline. Similar to HIV-1 group O, HIV-2 is also resistant to the NNRTI class of antiretrovirals.

The majority of cases of pediatric HIV infection in the United States are acquired perinatally or by sexual contact during adolescence. Less commonly HIV may be acquired through breastfeeding, sexual abuse, contaminated blood transfusion, or by exposure to premasticated food.[12] Risk factors for perinatal acquisition of HIV include maternal, delivery, and neonatal factors. Maternal factors include acute HIV infection during pregnancy, advanced HIV disease with low CD4 count, and poor prenatal care including poor or nonadherence to antiretroviral therapy (ART). Delivery by vaginal route, rupture of membranes for more than 4 hours, use of a fetal scalp electrode, and episiotomy all increase the risk of viral transmission. Neonatal factors include prematurity (gestational age less than 36 weeks) due to immaturity of the immune system and poor compliance with postnatal zidovudine prophylaxis (see Chapter 52).

Adolescence is a time of experimentation and limit testing where unsafe sexual practices place many young men and women at risk for HIV infection. Additional risk factors include multiple sexual partners, traumatic sex, genital ulcer disease, such as syphilis, herpes simplex or chancroid, and anal sex. The most efficient transmission of HIV occurs during the phase of acute infection—a 26-fold increase relative to the rate in chronic infection. Appropriate use of highly active antiretroviral therapy (HAART) resulting in an undetectable viral load substantially reduces the risk of transmission in HIV-discordant couples although condom use is still advocated to decrease the risk even further. Male circumcision has been conclusively shown to decrease the risk of transmission from female to male and may also decrease the risk from male to female.[13]

The safety of the blood supply in North America relies on numerous steps including donor interview, selection, and serologic screening.[14] Although all blood donations are tested for HIV-1 and HIV-2, a small residual risk of infections remains from donations collected during the "window period," the period immediately following acute infection when a donor is highly infectious but screening tests are negative. Beginning in 1999, nucleic acid amplification (NAA) testing of blood and plasma donations was introduced in the United States. Estimates suggest that NAA testing on pooled units has decreased the preantibody seroconversion "window period" from 22 days to 13–15 days for HIV.[14] The rigorous approach to optimizing the safety of the US blood supply has decreased the risk of acquiring HIV-1 or HIV-2 from a single unit of blood to an estimate of one in 2 million.

The pathogenesis of HIV is affected by the pathogenicity of the infecting virus itself as well as the immune system of the host. For example, three main variants of HIV-1 can be distinguished based on their ability to use the naturally occurring membrane receptors, CCR5 and CXCR4, during viral entry. Both of these receptors occur on T cells and are involved in immune system interactions. The three HIV-1 variants are those that selectively use CCR5 (called R5 variant), those that use CXCR4 (the X4 variant), and those that use either coreceptor (R5X4). R5 variants are most commonly responsible for transmission of HIV from one person to another and are also the predominant type of HIV during the long asymptomatic phase experienced by most adults. Genetically determined features of the host's immune system also play a role in pathogenesis. HIV infection is extremely rare, for example, in persons who are homozygous for a 32 base pair deletion within the CCR5 gene. In those who are heterozygous, HIV infection shows a more attenuated course.

Viral reservoirs represent an important aspect of HIV pathogenesis and a stumbling block to the eradication of HIV in individuals who are adherent to their HAART regimen. These reservoirs are resting CD4 cells and macrophages that can harbor proviral DNA. The long lifespan of these cells provides HIV with a long-lived latent reservoir of up to 30 years. Other hidden reservoirs or sanctuary sites for HIV include the central nervous system (CNS), the genitourinary system, and the gastrointestinal tract. Not only do these reservoirs help to prevent the eradication of HIV but they also archive drug-resistant virions for the lifetime of the patient. This explains the importance of considering all previous resistance tests when planning a change in antiretroviral regimen for a child.

CLINICAL PRESENTATION

HIV infection may present with an array of symptoms and signs. A history focused on risk factors for, and symptoms of, HIV is the first step toward evaluating the risk of infection. Pertinent risk factors include maternal HIV status, body fluid exposure such as intravenous drug use, sexual abuse, intercourse, and transfusion of blood products. Symptoms of HIV include a history of AIDS-defining conditions (Table 53–1), an unexplained chronic cough or any of the conditions listed in Table 53–3.

A developmental assessment should exclude features of HIV encephalopathy such as delay, regression, or

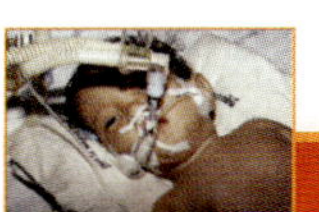

Table 53–3.

Clinical Categories for Children Younger Than 13 Years of Age with HIV Infection.[37,38]

Category	Clinical Conditions
N: Not symptomatic	No signs or symptoms considered to be the result of HIV infection or have only 1 of the conditions listed in Category A.
A: Mildly symptomatic	Children with two or more of the conditions listed but none of the conditions listed in categories B and C.
	■ Lymphadenopathy (≥0.5 cm at more than two sites; bilateral at one site)
	■ Hepatomegaly
	■ Splenomegaly
	■ Dermatitis
	■ Parotitis
	Recurrent or persistent upper respiratory tract infection, sinusitis or otitis media
B: Moderately symptomatic	Children who have symptomatic conditions other than those listed for category A or C that are attributed to HIV infection.
	■ Anemia (hemoglobin <8g/dL), neutropenia (white cell count <1000/μL) and/or thrombocytopenia (platelet count $<100 \times 10^3/\mu L$) persisting for ≥30 d
	■ Bacterial meningitis, pneumonia or sepsis (single episode)
	■ Candidiasis, oropharyngeal (thrush) persisting for >2 mo in children >6 mo of age
	■ Cardiomyopathy
	■ Cytomegalovirus infection with onset before 1 mo of age
	■ Diarrhea, recurrent or chronic

(continued)

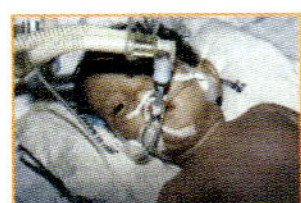

Table 53–3. (continued)

Clinical Categories for Children Younger Than 13 Years of Age with HIV Infection.[37,38]

Category	Clinical Conditions
	■ Hepatitis ■ Herpes simplex virus (HSV) stomatitis that is recurrent (less than two episodes in 1 year) ■ HSV bronchitis, pneumonitis or esophagitis with onset before 1 mo of age ■ Herpes zoster (shingles) involving at least two distinct episodes or more than one dermatome ■ Leiomyosarcoma ■ Lymphoid interstitial pneumonia (LIP) or pulmonary lymphoid hyperplasia complex ■ Nephropathy ■ Nocardiosis ■ Persistent fever (lasting >1 mo) ■ Toxoplasmosis with onset before 1 mo of age ■ Varicella, disseminated (complicated chickenpox)
C: Severely symptomatic	Serious bacterial infections, multiple or recurrent (less than two culture-confirmed infections in a 2-y period) of: Septicemia, pneumonia, meningitis, bone or joint infection, abscess of an internal organ or body cavity (excluding otitis media, superficial skin or mucosal abscesses, and indwelling catheter-related infections). ■ Candidiasis, esophageal or pulmonary (bronchi, trachea, lungs) ■ Coccioidomycosis, disseminated (at site other than or in addition to lungs or cervical or hilar lymph nodes) ■ Cryptococcosis, extrapulmonary ■ Cryptosporidiosis or isosporiasis with diarrhea persisting >1 mo ■ Cytomegalovirus disease with onset of symptoms after 1 mo of age (at a site other than liver, spleen or lymph nodes) ■ Encephalopathy (at least 1 of the following progressive findings present for >2 mo in the absence of a concurrent illness other than HIV infection that could explain the findings): (1) Failure to attain or loss of developmental milestones or loss of intellectual ability, verified by standard developmental tests; (2) impaired brain growth or acquired microcephaly demonstrated by head circumference measurements or brain atrophy seen by CT or MRI; (3) acquired symmetric motor deficit manifested by 2 or more of: paresis, pathologic reflexes, ataxia or gait disturbance. ■ HSV mucocutaneous ulcer that persists for >1 mo or HSV bronchitis, pneumonitis or esophagitis for any duration in a child >1 mo of age ■ Histoplasmosis, disseminated (at a site other than or in addition to lungs or cervical or hilar lymph nodes) ■ Kaposi sarcoma ■ Lymphoma, primary in the brain ■ Lymphoma, small, noncleaved cell (Burkitt), immunoblastic or large-cell lymphoma of B-cell or unknown immunologic phenotype. ■ *Mycobacterium tuberculosis*, disseminated or extrapulmonary ■ *Mycobacterium*, other species or unidentified species, disseminated (at a site other than or in addition to lungs, skin or cervical or hilar lymph nodes) ■ *Pneumocytis jiroveci* pneumonia (PCP) ■ Progressive multifocal leukoencephalopathy ■ *Salmonella* (nontyphoid) septicemia, recurrent ■ Toxoplasmosis of the brain with onset after 1 mo of age Wasting syndrome in the absence of a concurrent illness other than HIV infection that could explain the following findings: (1) Persistent weight loss >10% of baseline; (2) downward crossing of at least two of the following percentile lines on the weight-for-age chart (e.g., 95th, 75th, 50th, 25th, 5th) in a child >1 y of age; OR (3) <5th percentile on weight-for-height chart on two consecutive measurements >30 d apart; PLUS chronic diarrhea (at least two loose stools/d for >30 d) OR documented fever (for >30 d, intermittent or constant).

d, days; mo, month; y, year; CT, computed tomography; MRI, magnetic resonance imaging.

stasis in developmental milestones. In the absence of antiretroviral therapy, HIV encephalopathy is progressive and three subtypes are recognized: subacute progressive, plateau, and static. The most severe symptoms are seen in children with subacute progressive encephalopathy who develop one or more of the following findings over weeks to months: loss of milestones, particularly motor or expressive language, cognitive deterioration, and apathy.[15] Those with more advanced CNS diseases may present with seizures, choreoathetoid movements, and cerebellar signs.[16] The plateau form of encephalopathy may present with any of these features but has a more indolent course. Typically there is no loss of existing skills; rather, the rate of acquisition of new skills is slowed. Static encephalopathy by contrast presents with nonprogressive neuromotor and cognitive impairments. These children continue to develop but at a slower rate than their uninfected peers. Intelligence quotient (IQ) testing reveals an IQ below the norm but this does not deteriorate over time.

An organ system-based approach to the physical examination facilitates an astute clinical assessment of the risk of HIV infection. Growth parameters may reveal failure to thrive (Figure 53–1) or stunting, particularly where the infection has followed a more indolent course. Acquired microcephaly in the setting of developmental delay (especially with loss of previously acquired skills) and pyramidal tract neuromuscular deficits, such as brisk deep tendon reflexes, completes the classic triad of HIV encephalopathy.[15] Less severely affected children with HIV encephalopathy demonstrate brisk reflexes and hypertonicity that are confined to the legs. In severe case, all limbs are affected. Rarely, either hypotonicity or opisthotonus is the presenting sign of HIV encephalopathy. Neuroimaging of children with HIV encephalopathy classically reveals brain atrophy and bilateral calcifications of the basal ganglia and frontal white matter.[17,18]

The retinas need to be carefully examined for signs of opportunistic infectious retinitis such as cytomegalovirus (CMV) although evidence suggests that only children with CD4 counts less than 20/μL are at high risk for CMV retinitis.[19]

HIV-infected children may present with a number of signs localized to the respiratory tract. Upper respiratory clues include recurrent suppurative otitis media, recurrent or severe sinusitis, and episodes of epistaxis resulting from HIV-induced thrombocytopenia. The most common pulmonary conditions in HIV-infected children are *Pneumocytis jiroveci* pneumonia (PCP), lymphocytic interstitial pneumonitis (LIP), tuberculosis, and recurrent bacterial infections including bacterial pneumonia. Pulmonary infections in the HIV-infected child are discussed in Chapter 54.

LIP is an example of a condition seen in HIV-infected children that is rare in HIV-infected adults.[20] In the era before effective antiretrovirals, LIP was diagnosed in 30–40% of children in the first decade of life.[21] History may reveal a 2–4-year-old child with gradual progression of a nonproductive cough with decreasing exercise tolerance and the insidious onset of hypoxia. Presentation to hospital is often precipitated by an intercurrent viral infection with worsening of pulmonary symptoms. Clinical signs of LIP may include clubbing of the fingers, parotidomegaly (Figure 53–2), hepatosplenomegaly, and a diffuse reticulonodular pattern on chest radiography (Figure 53–3). Radiologically, the infiltrate may be difficult to differentiate from miliary tuberculosis, with a reticulonodular pattern present in all lobes, including the periphery. Pathologically, LIP is characterized by diffuse infiltration of the small airways and bronchi by lymphocytes and plasma cells. The cause of LIP is poorly defined. It is postulated that LIP is caused by an exaggeration of the host's pulmonary immune response to local infection, most commonly Epstein–Barr virus (EBV). In the era of antiretrovirals and following

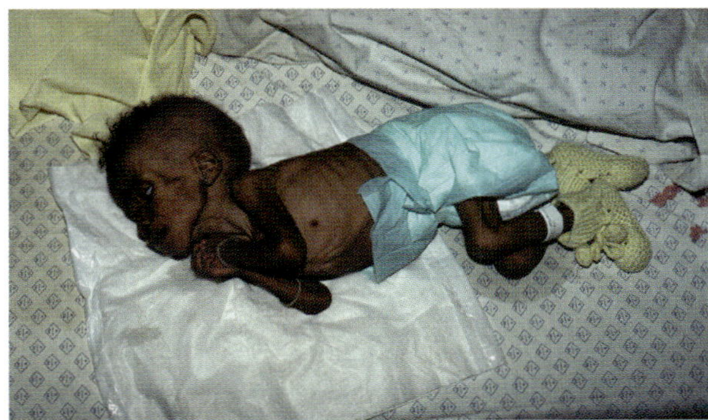

FIGURE 53–1 ■ Slim's disease. HIV may present as failure to thrive with severe wasting.

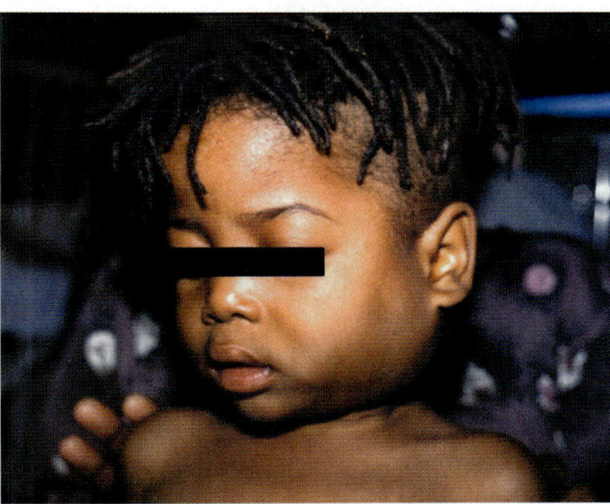

FIGURE 53–2 ■ Parotidomegaly may be a presenting sign of HIV, particularly in the child who also has lymphocytic interstitial pneumonitis.

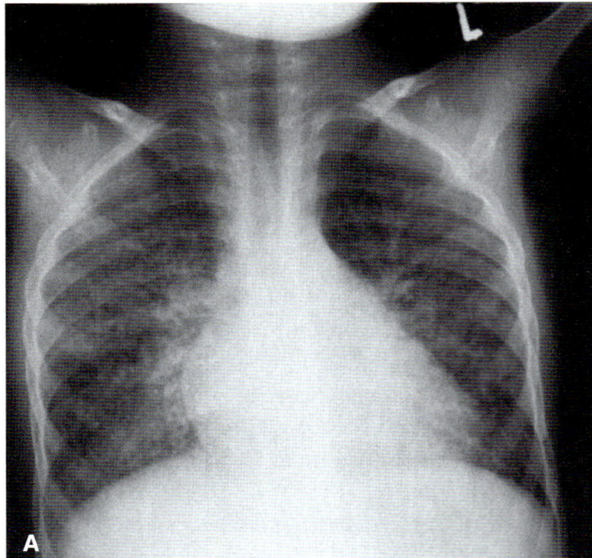

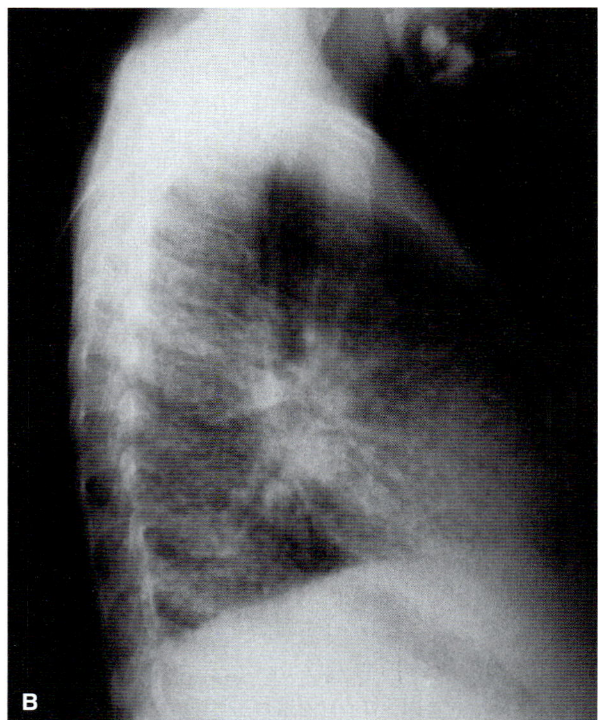

FIGURE 53–3 ■ (A) Lymphocytic interstitial pneumonitis (frontal view). A chest X-ray demonstrating a diffuse interstitial infiltrate in an HIV-infected child who may have clubbing of the fingers, is highly suggestive of this diagnosis. **(B)** Lymphocytic interstitial pneumonitis (lateral view).

reconstitution of the host's immune system, this condition has all but disappeared.

The cardiovascular system may be affected primarily by HIV, such as HIV-cardiomyopathy, or secondarily, such as the development of cor pulmonale following recurrent bouts of pneumonia or LIP, or hyperlipidemia as a consequence of antiretrovirals. In the pre-HAART era, subclinical cardiac abnormalities in HIV-infected children were common, persistent, and often progressive.[22] Cardiac manifestations such as dilated cardiomyopathy and inappropriate left ventricular (LV) hypertrophy have been shown to limit survival in children not on HAART and depressed LV function correlates with the degree of baseline immune dysfunction. In HIV-infected children with cardiac involvement, carnitine, selenium, and multivitamin supplementation should be considered, especially in those with wasting or diarrhea syndromes.[23] Monthly intravenous immunoglobulin (IVIG) infusions have been demonstrated to preserve LV parameters in HIV-infected children including ventricular recovery in some children with recalcitrant HIV-related cardiomyopathy. HAART, particularly the protease inhibitors (PI), maybe associated with the development of dyslipidemia and the metabolic syndrome necessitating monitoring of lipid profiles in all children on PI therapy. The pericardium may also be affected in HIV-infected children. Small asymptomatic effusions in end-stage children with AIDS are often nonspecific in nature, and maybe caused by the proinflammatory milieu found in advanced AIDS. In contrast, large or symptomatic effusions are often associated with infection or malignancy, and warrant thorough investigation and etiology-specific treatment.[23]

HIV nephropathy is characterized by progressive proteinuria, at times a nephrotic syndrome, late stage azotemia, normal blood pressure, and enlarged, hyperechoic kidneys with eventual progression to end-stage renal disease (ESRD) in the absence of HAART.[24] The clinical course of HIV nephropathy in children is less fulminant than adults. Renal biopsy results are variable but the most common findings are those of focal segmental glomerulosclerosis.[25] Advances in management including HAART and angiotensin antagonists to control proteinuria have decreased the incidence of renal failure. In addition, HAART may itself lead to renal damage. Of the antiretrovirals, the nucleotide reverse transcriptase inhibitor, tenofovir, has been most frequently associated with impaired renal function. Indinavir, a PI, may induce renal stones particularly when it is boosted with ritonavir and in patients who are not adequately hydrated.

The cutaneous findings in HIV-infected children are numerous and generally relate to integumentary manifestations of the host's immune dysfunction. These vary from recalcitrant eczema to severe forms of cutaneous infections such as scabies, zoster, or herpes. Drug reactions, such as Stevens Johnson syndrome (Figure 53–4), may be precipitated by trimethoprim-sulfamethoxazole or other agents such as nevirapine or abacavir. Kaposi's sarcoma was a cutaneous malignancy of elderly males in the pre-HIV era but in now an AIDS-defining condition. It is less frequently seen in pediatrics but a careful examination of the skin and palate is important to help rule out this condition (Figure 53–5).

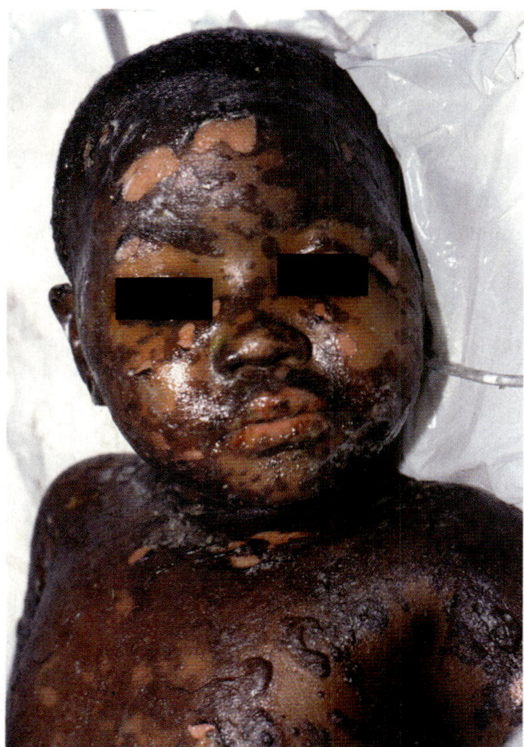

FIGURE 53–4 ■ Stevens-Johnson syndrome associated with trimethoprim-sulfamethoxazole (TMP-SMX) use. TMP-SMX is generally a very safe drug but this side effect necessitates choosing another agent which is active against PCP.

The gastrointestinal tract may be affected at any point from the mouth to the anus with most presentations being a manifestation of impaired immunity. In the mouth, oral thrush and dental caries are the most common features. Esophageal candidiasis may present with dysphagia, odynophagia or failure to thrive. Herpes simplex and CMV can also cause a painful esophagitis. Chronic diarrhea was a frequent presentation in the pre-HAART era; refer to Chapter 54 for a list of potential opportunistic pathogens. Many HIV-infected children will have clinically signs localized to the reticuloendothelial system such as diffuse lymphadenopathy or hepatosplenomegaly.

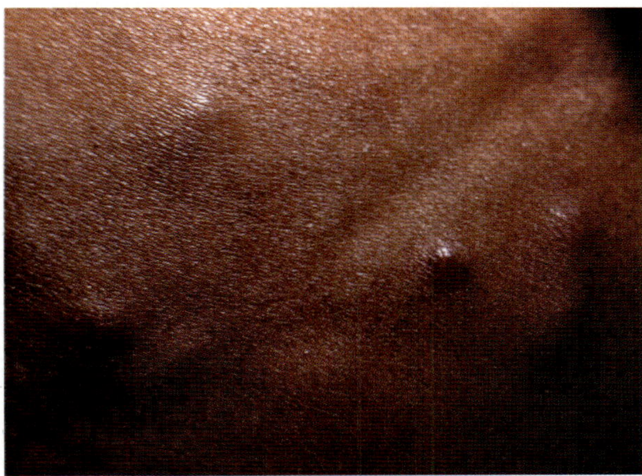

FIGURE 53–5 ■ Kaposi's sarcoma seen in the skin of an HIV-infected child. Certain malignancies including Kaposi's sarcoma and lymphoma are more common in children with HIV.

Musculoskeletal findings are not usually a characteristic feature of HIV-infected children. When they do occur, they are usually the result of an opportunistic infection of a muscle, bone, or joint.

Hematologically, in the late stage of HIV infection, anemia, leukopenia, and lymphopenia may result from HIV itself, or from opportunistic infections, such as disseminated MAC infection. In contrast, idiopathic thrombycytopenic purpura (ITP), secondary to HIV, may be seen earlier in the course of the illness. Up to 10% of children and adults may present with thrombocytopenia.

DIFFERENTIAL DIAGNOSIS

Children infected with HIV may present with a broad range of signs and symptoms. The complete differential diagnosis includes consideration of the different causes of immune deficiency as well as the varying presentations of opportunistic infections. The differential diagnosis is also affected by the age of a child—a 3-month-old who presents with failure to thrive secondary to recurrent urinary tract infections may show many clinical features suggestive of HIV whereas an adolescent presenting with features suggesting acute EBV infection may in fact have acute HIV seroconversion illness. Noninfectious conditions such as malignancies or autoimmune diseases may also mimic the clinical picture of HIV.

DIAGNOSIS

The tests used to diagnose HIV infection and their relative merits are summarized in Table 53–4. The broad principles to remember when testing a child for HIV are the following:

1. Maternal anti-HIV IgG antibody may persist for as long as 18 months necessitating viral specific testing in children under 18 months of age.
2. It is currently not possible to reliably diagnose HIV in children under the age of 2 weeks:
   a. The sensitivity of a single HIV DNA PCR test performed at $<$48 hours of age is less than 40%, but increases to over 90% by 2–4 weeks of age.
   b. By 28 days of age, HIV DNA PCR has a 96% sensitivity and 99% specificity.
3. A single positive HIV test should always be confirmed with a second test to minimize the chance of a false-positive result.

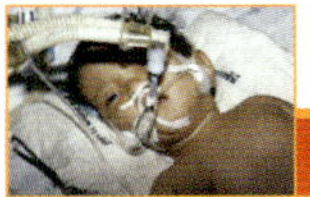

Table 53–4.

Laboratory Diagnosis of HIV Infection.[37]

Test Type	Test	Comment
Virologic	HIV DNA PCR on peripheral blood mononuclear cells	Preferred test to diagnose HIV infection in infants and children ≤18 months of age. Highly sensitive and specific by 2 weeks of age. Easily available.
	HIV culture	Gold standard BUT expensive, not easily available and requires 4 weeks for result.
	HIV RNA PCR	Not used to diagnose HIV infection due to both false positive and negative results in this setting; rather is used to quantify the concentration of HIV in the blood.
Antibody	HIV ELISA	Preferred test to diagnose HIV infection in children >18 months of age. Highly sensitive, needs confirmatory western blot. Easily available. Rapid version allows faster result but is more expensive.
	HIV Western Blot	Confirmatory test after positive HIV ELISA. High specificity, easily available.
Antigen	HIV p24 Ag	Not recommended: less sensitive than DNA PCR, false positive results in first month of life.
	ICD p24 Ag	Not recommended: negative test does not rule out infection.

HIV, human immunodeficiency virus; PCR, polymerase chain reaction; ELISA, enzyme linked immunosorbent assay; Ag, antigen; ICD, immune complex dissociated.

4. HIV DNA PCR is used to diagnose HIV whereas the HIV RNA PCR assay is used to quantify HIV plasma viral RNA (the viral load) in a child who is already known to be HIV-infected.
5. HIV culture is regarded as the gold standard but is not widely available.

The high sensitivity and specificity of currently available DNA PCR tests is reassuring when testing a child with possible subtype B HIV infection. However, false-negative results have been reported in infants infected with nonsubtype B HIV.[26,27] Currently available HIV RNA PCR assays have improved sensitivity to detect non-subtype B infection but even these assays may miss some non-B HIV subtypes.[28,29] The cautious clinician will therefore take a careful history to establish which children are at high risk of non-B subtype infection—those whose parents are from Africa or Southeast Asia—and these children should not only be tested by HIV DNA PCR but also have repeat testing using one of the newer RNA assays. Occasionally nonsubtype B infection will continue to be suspected in children who test negative on both DNA and RNA testing. These children should be followed by an HIV expert, be monitored clinically, and have HIV serologic testing at 18 months of age.

MANAGEMENT

Following the introduction in 1996 of effective antiretroviral medications in the form of HAART, HIV has been changed from a progressive illness with certain mortality to a chronic disease more similar to asthma or diabetes. This dramatic change in the outlook of children infected with HIV depends on early diagnosis, appropriate management, and excellent adherence to HAART regimens. Significant advances have been made in all of these areas but challenges remain, particularly in ensuring an early diagnosis and optimizing adherence.

Management of the HIV-infected child may be conveniently divided into two areas—HIV-specific management and general pediatric care. Key aspects of HIV specific management include regular follow-up visits with a clinician and team experienced in caring for HIV-infected children and monitoring of salient laboratory tests. Children who are stable on HAART are seen every 3 months by a multidisciplinary team including a pediatrician, social worker, nurse, and nutritionist. Annual neurodevelopmental testing is also suggested to screen for subtle signs of HIV encephalopathy. A psychologist is also a key member of the team given that many HIV-infected children benefit from regular counseling sessions. If the psychosocial aspect of care is neglected, it is likely that the child will be nonadherent both to clinic visits and to the rigorous medication regimen.

At the three-monthly visit, a careful history, physical examination, review of the previous laboratory tests, and selected follow-up laboratory tests are done. The history reviews current medications including possible side effects and a careful discussion of adherence. Where available, adherence by history should be correlated with pharmacy refill data as the earlier nonadherence is detected, the less likely resistance to the current HAART regimen is to develop. A brief developmental screen, particularly in children under the age of 2 years, will reveal the need for more detailed testing. A general physical examination focuses on appropriate growth and features of HIV as discussed in the clinical presentation section. Laboratory monitoring of HIV-infected children is somewhat center-specific but most practitioners would do a minimum of the following:

- Every 3 months: CBC, CD4 count and percentage, RNA PCR quantitative viral load, electrolytes, and liver transaminases
- Every 6 months: full liver function tests, lipid screening, urine analysis

Additional testing may be warranted depending on the findings on history and examination. Age group specific laboratory testing may also be indicated such as screening for sexually transmitted diseases and Papanicolaou smears in adolescents.

The need for prophylactic antibiotics should be reviewed at each visit. Trimethoprim sulfamethoxazole is used to prevent PCP and a weekly macrolide is used to prevent *Mycobacterium avium* complex (MAC) infection. See Chapter 54 for a more detailed discussion of prophylaxis including indications of when to start prophylactic antibiotics.

The diagnosis of HIV, unlike many other illnesses, may still result in stigmatization in many communities in the United States. When considering the best way to communicate with an HIV-infected child about his/her illness, a thoughtful approach to HIV disclosure is particularly important. As with all chronic illnesses of childhood, the pediatrician needs to adhere to the following tenets:

1. Communicate with the child in a developmentally appropriate way.
2. Always tell the truth:
   a. There is no merit in telling a child that she takes her HIV medications to treat her cough as when the cough resolves, there is a good chance that her adherence will suffer as a result.
3. Maintain a positive relationship with both the child and family.
4. Understand the family's dynamics and social situation.

The timing and technique of disclosing a child's HIV status varies from clinic to clinic. Disclosing the diagnosis of HIV to a child is a controversial and emotionally charged issue among both the health care team and parents and caregivers of these children.[30] There is emerging evidence that complete disclosure by caregivers to their children coupled with strong parental relationships predict good adherence.[31] Less clear is the effect and timing of disclosure in families where the parental relationship is poor. The benefits of disclosure include that the child can participate more actively in their health care, improvement in the child–caregiver relationship, the veil of secrecy has been lifted allowing for more open support and a result dispelling of any false reasons for the child taking medicine such as, "I have cancer and no one has told me." The risks of disclosure include inadvertent disclosure of the "family's secret" by the child, stigma, breakdown of the child–parent relationship particularly if disclosure occurs in late or mid-adolescence, and a lack of support in the home. Many practitioners advocate a staged approach to disclosure where the child is gradually introduced to some of the broad concepts of HIV. The actual time of full disclosure is usually a negotiated one between the caregivers and the health team and takes into account the developmental level of the child.

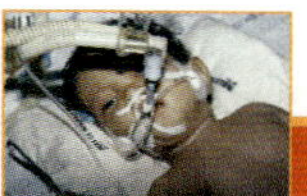

Table 53–5.

Recommendations for Routine Immunization of HIV-Infected Children in the United States.[37]

Vaccines	Known Asymptomatic HIV Infection	Symptomatic HIV Infection
Hepatitis B	Yes	Yes
DTaP	Yes	Yes
IPV	Yes	Yes
MMR	Yes	Consider*
Hib	Yes	Yes
Pneumococcal	Yes†	Yes†
Influenza	Yes	Yes
Varicella	Consider	Consider‡
Meningococcal	Yes	Yes
BCG	No	No
Hepatitis A	Yes	Yes
Rotavirus	No data	No data

**The measles vaccine is withheld if the CD4 percentage is <15%.*
†The heptavalent conjugate pneumococcal vaccine (Prevnar) is given using the usual pediatric schedule, but pneumovax (pneumococcal polysaccharide 23-valent vaccine) is given at age 2 and age 5–7 y.
‡The varicella vaccine is withheld if the CD4 percentage is <15%.

In many urban settings, general pediatric care is provided by the HIV clinic but in more rural areas this is frequently the responsibility of the general pediatrician. Table 53–5 describes the recommendations for immunization in an HIV-infected child. In addition to standard pediatric practice, the annual visit should pay particular attention to adherence, development, psychosocial wellbeing, and medication side effects. A proactive approach to healthy eating habits is another important area as the PIs are associated with changes in the blood lipid profile and a predilection to the metabolic syndrome.

TREATMENT

Recommendations for the initiation of HAART are more aggressive in children than adults as HIV disease progresses more rapidly in children. The decision to

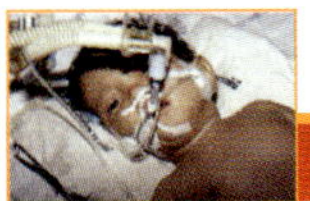

Table 53–6.

Six Classes of Antiretroviral Classes.

Three Established Classes			Three New Classes		
NRTI/NtRTIs	**NNRTIs**	**PIs**	**Fusion Inhibitors**	**Integrase Inhibitors**	**Chemokine Receptor Inhibitors**
AZT/ZDV (Zidovudine)	EFV (Efavirenz)	DRV (Darunavir)	ENF (Enfuvirtide)	Raltegravir	MRV (Maraviroc)
3TC (Lamivudine)	NVP (Nevirapine)	LPV/r (lopinavir/ritonavir)			
d4T (Stavudine)	DLV (Delavirdine)	NFV (Nelfinavir)			
ddI (Didanosine)	ETV (Etravirine)	SQV (Saquinavir)			
ABC (Abacavir)		RTV (Ritonavir)			
TDF (Tenofovir)		IDV (Indinavir)			
FTC (Emtricitabine)		APV (Amprenavir)			
ddC (Zalcitabine)		ATV (Atazanavir)			
		FPV (Fosamprenavir)			
		TPV (Tipranavir)			

NRTI, nucleoside reverse transcriptase inhibitors; NtRTIs, nucleotide reverse transcriptase inhibitors; NNRTIs, nonnucleoside reverse transcriptase inhibitors; PIs, protease inhibitors.
Consult the latest guidelines at www.aidsinfo.nih.gov/Guidelines to determine which of the above are currently approved for pediatric use.

initiate or withhold HAART should be made in conjunction with an HIV specialist and after consulting the latest HIV guidelines available at www.aidsinfo.nih.gov/Guidelines. The general trend is to recommend the initiation of HAART in all HIV-infected children under the age of 12 months. Reasons include that the youngest children are at greatest risk for rapid disease progression including HIV encephalopathy and life-threatening opportunistic infections. After the age of 12 months, clinical, immunologic, and social parameters are used to decide when to initiate therapy.

The six classes of antiretrovirals are shown in Table 53–6. HAART is defined as the initiation of at least three antiretrovirals, usually from at least two different classes. Occasionally a regimen of three NRTIs is used but this is unusual. Triple therapy is important to minimize the development of resistant virus. This was well illustrated when in the early days of antiretroviral development zidovudine monotherapy was used—patients initially showed a clinical and immunologic response but the response usually waned within 6 months due to viral resistance to zidovudine.

The goals of HAART include the following:

- Restoring and preserving immune function
- Rapid and sustained maximal suppression of viral replication as measured by an undetectable viral load
- Minimizing drug side effects and maximizing adherence
- Normal growth and development
- Improved quality of life
- Minimizing HIV-related morbidity and mortality

The first time a patient commences HAART is generally their best chance of achieving a favorable response. This is not to say that second or third line regimens do not work; rather it speaks to nonmedication factors that play a vital role in adherence to a lifelong medication. Hence, the decision to start HAART is a process and commitment which includes family, child, and the health team. The goal is to aim for 100% adherence and studies have shown that anything less than 95% adherence is associated with the development of resistant viral mutants. Adherence is optimized by selecting one person in the home who will supervise the medication regimen and take full responsibility for the child's therapy. Other important factors include the palatability of medications and the frequency of the regimen. The former may be addressed by consultation with an experienced HIV nurse who will advise giving medications with certain foods. Failing this, a gastrostomy tube may be required. Medication regimens are now more patient friendly with daily or twice daily regimens being the rule. This represents a dramatic improvement from the initial antiretroviral regimens, which required much more frequent dosing and a larger daily pill count.

After initiation of HAART, the viral load decreases in two phases. Initially in the first 6–10 weeks after commencing HAART, there is a rapid decrease secondary to inhibition of viral replication in activated CD4 cells. The second phase occurs over the subsequent 24 weeks and is characterized by a slower decrease due to inhibition of viral replication in resting CD4 cells and macrophages. The rate and magnitude of CD4 response vary from one child to another. In children with a sluggish increase in CD4 cells following HAART initiation, most HIV specialists would watch and wait as long as the viral load remains undetectable and the child is improving

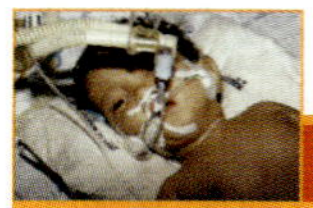

Table 53–7.

Antiretroviral Class-Related Adverse Drug Effects.

Adverse Effect	Drug Class	Key Points	Diagnosis
Anemia/neutropenia	NRTIs	Particularly common with zidovudine	Examination and macrocytic anemia
Peripheral neuropathy and/or pancreatitis	NRTIs	Particularly common with didanosine or stavudine.	History, examination and pancreatic enzymes
Hepatotoxicity	All ARVs	NNRTIs > NRTIs/NtRTIs > PIs Increased risk in those with preexisting hepatitis	History, examination and LFTs
Lipodystrophy	NRTIs, NNRTIs, PIs	Two types occur – fat accumulation and fat loss (lipoatrophy). Higher risk of progressing to the metabolic syndrome	History, examination, waist-hip ratios, skin fold measurement, DEXA, CT or MRI
Hyperlipidemia	NNRTIs, PIs, d4T	Hypertriglyceridemia may present with pancreatitis	Fasting lipid profile at least once/year
Insulin resistance	PIs	Common in patients with lipoatrophy and those with HCV co-infection	History, examination, fasting blood sugar every 3–6 months in patients on PIs
Injection site reactions	FIs	Fewer injection reactions are seen with the new needle-free gas powered injection system	History, examination

ARV, antiretroviral; NRTI, nucleoside reverse transcriptase inhibitors; NtRTIs, nucleotide reverse transcriptase inhibitors; NNRTIs, nonnucleoside reverse transcriptase inhibitors; PIs, protease inhibitors; FIs, fusion inhibitors; HCV, hepatitis C virus; LFTs, liver function tests; DEXA, dual energy X-ray absorptiometry; CT, computer tomography; MRI, magnetic resonance imaging.

clinically. For treatment naïve children, the expectation is that the viral load should decrease by at least 1 log by 12 weeks of therapy, and be undetectable by 24 weeks of therapy, or soon thereafter.

All antiretrovirals are associated with some side effects. The common class-specific ones are summarized in Table 53–7. For a more complete list of drug side effects, consult the latest pediatric HIV treatment guidelines at www.aidsinfo.nih.gov/Guidelines. It is vital that the treating pediatrician is aware of both the common and uncommon side effects of these drugs as well as the various drug–drug interactions. The skills of a clinical pharmacist are often required with the latter as dose adjustments may be required. Initiating and maintaining HAART in an HIV-infected individual is always best done in close consultation with an HIV-treatment specialist.

COURSE AND PROGNOSIS

The outlook for HIV-infected children has been dramatically altered for the better since the introduction of HAART. HIV-infected children now have the opportunity to grow and develop normally and to live healthy and productive lives. The caveat to this is that they are adherent to their medications. Without >95% adherence, the residual virus will develop resistance to one or more of the medications, resulting in a subsequent increase in viral load and finally a fall in CD4 count and percentage.

Clinically the key is to provide ongoing counseling and support around adherence. The master clinician will endeavor to discover a drop-off in adherence before laboratory markers alert him/her that this has occurred. The technique of using pharmacy refill data to check a patient's adherence record is a valuable aid in this regard.[32]

Although the acute threat of immune suppression caused by rampant HIV infection is now avoidable due to effective HAART, the long-term prognosis for HIV-infected children is still being studied. HIV-infected children are now surviving into adulthood and having families of their own. However, the long-term effects of HIV and HAART on longevity remain to be seen. There are conflicting data regarding cardiovascular risk and HAART; some studies have shown an increased risk, while others have shown no greater risk than the general population.[33,34]

The search for a cure for HIV is ongoing. Thus far viral eradication has proved elusive due to the immense mutational potential of the virus and ability to seek sanctuary in a number of sites including dormant CD4 cells. These resting CD4 cells and macrophages can harbor replication-competent virus for the duration of their lifespan of up to 30 years. Potential interventions to eradicate these latent reservoirs include attempts to induce the latent virions to replicate, hence making them susceptible to HAART.

Future directions in pediatric HIV include careful monitoring of long-term outcomes, optimizing adherence, minimizing new infections particularly in adolescents, and the roll out of antiretrovirals to the developing world. The prospect of an HIV vaccine, either therapeutic or preventative, is still some way off. [35]

PEARLS

- There remains no cure for HIV although the virus can be controlled with HAART.
- A minimum of 95% adherence is required in order to prevent the development of viral resistance to HAART.
- All HIV-infected children under the age of a year should be commenced on HAART.

REFERENCES

1. Pneumocystis pneumonia—Los Angeles. *MMWR.* 1981; 30(21):250-252.
2. CDC. HIV/AIDS surveillance report 2004. 2004 [cited April 1, 2007]; Available from:http://www.cdc.gov/hiv/topics/surveillance/resources/reports/2004report/default.htm.
3. Epidemiology of HIV/AIDS—United States, 1981-2005. *MMWR.* 2006;55(21):589-592.
4. Lindegren ML, Byers RH, Jr., Thomas P, et al. Trends in perinatal transmission of HIV/AIDS in the United States. *JAMA.* 1999;282(6):531-538.
5. Eaton DK, Kann L, Kinchen S, et al. Youth risk behavior surveillance—United States, 2005. *MMWR Surveill Summ.* 2006;55(5):1-108.
6. Rotheram-Borus MJ, Futterman D. Promoting early detection of human immunodeficiency virus infection among adolescents. *Arch Pediatr Adolesc Med.* 2000; 154(5):435-439.
7. Centers for Disease Control and Prevention. HIV prevalence, unrecognized infection, and HIV testing among men who have sex with men—five U.S. cities, June 2004–April 2005. *MMWR.* 2005;54(24):597-601.
8. Murphy DA, Mitchell R, Vermund SH, Futterman D. Factors associated with HIV testing among HIV-positive and HIV-negative high-risk adolescents: The REACH Study. *Reaching for Excellence in Adolescent Care and Health. Pediatrics.* 2002;110(3):e36.
9. UNAIDS. Global summary of the AIDS epidemic December 2006. 2006 [cited April 3, 2007]; Available from: http://data.unaids.org/pub/EpiReport/2006/02-Global_Summary_2006_EpiUpdate_eng.pdf
10. Public Health Service Task Force: Recommendations for the Use of Antiretroviral Drugs in Pregnant HIV-Infected Women for Maternal Health and Interventions to Reduce Perinatal HIV Transmission in the United States In: NIH/CDC, ed.; November 2, 2007.
11. Sharp PM, Bailes E, Chaudhuri RR, Rodenburg CM, Santiago MO, Hahn BH. The origins of acquired immune deficiency syndrome viruses: where and when? *Philos Trans Royal Soc Lond.* 2001;356(1410):867-876.
12. Gaur AH DK, Kalish M, Rivera-Hernandez D, Donohoe M, Mitchell C. Practice of offering a child pre-masticated food: an unrecognized possible risk factor for HIV Transmission. Boston: CROI 2008; 2008.
13. Abdool Karim Q. Prevention of HIV by male circumcision. *BMJ.* 2007;335(7609):4-5.
14. AAP. *Red Book Report of the Committee on Infectious Diseases.* 27th ed. Elk Grove, IL: American Academy of Pediatrics; 2006.
15. Belman AL. HIV-1-associated CNS disease in infants and children. Research publications. *Assoc Res Nervous Mental Dis.* 1994;72:289-310.
16. Mitchell CD. HIV-1 encephalopathy among perinatally infected children: neuropathogenesis and response to highly active antiretroviral therapy. *Mental Retard Dev Disab Res Rev.* 2006;12(3):216-222.
17. Belman AL, Diamond G, Dickson D, et al. Pediatric acquired immunodeficiency syndrome. Neurologic syndromes. American J Dis Child (1960) 1988;142(1):29-35.
18. Scarmato V, Frank Y, Rozenstein A, et al. Central brain atrophy in childhood AIDS encephalopathy. *AIDS.* 1996;10(11):1227-1231.
19. Du LT, Coats DK, Kline MW, et al. Incidence of presumed cytomegalovirus retinitis in HIV-infected pediatric patients. *J Aapos.* 1999;3(4):245-249.
20. Pitt J. Lymphocytic interstitial pneumonia. *Ped Clin North Am.* 1991;38(1):89-95.
21. Scott GB. HIV infection in children: clinical features and management. *J Acq Immune Defic Synd.* 1991;4(2):109-115.
22. Lipshultz SE, Easley KA, Orav EJ, et al. Left ventricular structure and function in children infected with human immunodeficiency virus: the prospective P2C2 HIV Multicenter Study. Pediatric Pulmonary and Cardiac Complications of Vertically Transmitted HIV Infection (P2C2 HIV) Study Group. *Circulation.* 1998;97(13):1246-1256.
23. Harmon WG, Dadlani GH, Fisher SD, Lipshultz SE. Myocardial and pericardial disease in HIV. *Curr Treat Options Cardiovasc Med.* 2002;4(6):497-509.
24. Strauss J, Zilleruelo G, Abitbol C, Montane B, Pardo V. Human immunodeficiency virus nephropathy. *Pediatr Nephrol.* 1993;7(2):220-225.
25. Abitbol CL, Friedman LB, Zilleruelo G. Renal manifestations of sexually transmitted diseases: sexually transmitted diseases and the kidney. *Adolesc Med Clin.* 2005; 16(1):45-65.
26. Haas J, Geiss M, Bohler T. False-negative polymerase chain reaction-based diagnosis of human immunodeficiency virus (HIV) type 1 in children infected with HIV strains of African origin. *J Infect Dis.* 1996;174(1):244-245.
27. Kline NE, Schwarzwald H, Kline MW. False negative DNA polymerase chain reaction in an infant with subtype C human immunodeficiency virus 1 infection. *Ped Infect Dis J.* 2002;21(9):885-886.
28. Swanson P, de Mendoza C, Joshi Y, et al. Impact of human immunodeficiency virus type 1 (HIV-1) genetic diversity on performance of four commercial viral load assays: LCx HIV RNA Quantitative, AMPLICOR HIV-1 MONITOR v1.5, VERSANT HIV-1 RNA 3.0, and NucliSens HIV-1 QT. *J Clin Microbiol.* 2005;43(8):3860-3868.
29. Geelen S, Lange J, Borleffs J, Wolfs T, Weersink A, Schuurman R. Failure to detect a non-B HIV-1 subtype by the HIV-1 Amplicor Monitor test, version 1.5: a case of unexpected vertical transmission. *AIDS.* 2003;17(5):781-782.

30. Wiener L, Mellins CA, Marhefka S, Battles HB. Disclosure of an HIV diagnosis to children: history, current research, and future directions. *J Dev Behav Pediatr.* 2007;28(2):155-166.
31. Bikaako-Kajura W, Luyirika E, Purcell DW, et al. Disclosure of HIV status and adherence to daily drug regimens among HIV-infected children in Uganda. *AIDS Behav.* 2006;10(4 suppl):S85-S93.
32. Gross R, Yip B, Lo Re V, 3rd, et al. A simple, dynamic measure of antiretroviral therapy adherence predicts failure to maintain HIV-1 suppression. *J Infect Dis.* 2006; 194(8):1108-1114.
33. Jones CY. Metabolic syndrome in HIV-infected patients: no different than the general population? *Clin Infect Dis.* 2007;44(5):735-738.
34. Friis-Moller N, Reiss P, Sabin CA, et al. Class of antiretroviral drugs and the risk of myocardial infarction. *N Engl J Med.* 2007;356(17):1723-1735.
35. Berkley SF, Koff WC. Scientific and policy challenges to development of an AIDS vaccine. *Lancet.* 2007;370(9581): 94-101.
36. 1993 revised classification system for HIV infection and expanded surveillance case definition for AIDS among adolescents and adults. *MMWR Recomm Rep.* 1992; 41(RR-17):1-19.
37. American Academy of Pediatrics. Human immunodeficiency virus infection. In: Pickering LK, Baker CJ, Long SS, McMillan JA, eds. *Red Book: 2006 Report of the Committee on Infectious Diseases.* 27th ed. Elk Grove, IL: American Academy of Pediatrics. 2006:378-401.
38. CDC. 1994 revised guidelines for the performance of CD4+ T-cell determinations in persons with human immunodeficiency virus (HIV) infections. Centers for Disease Control and Prevention. *MMWR Recomm Rep.* 1994;43(RR-3):1-21.

CHAPTER 54

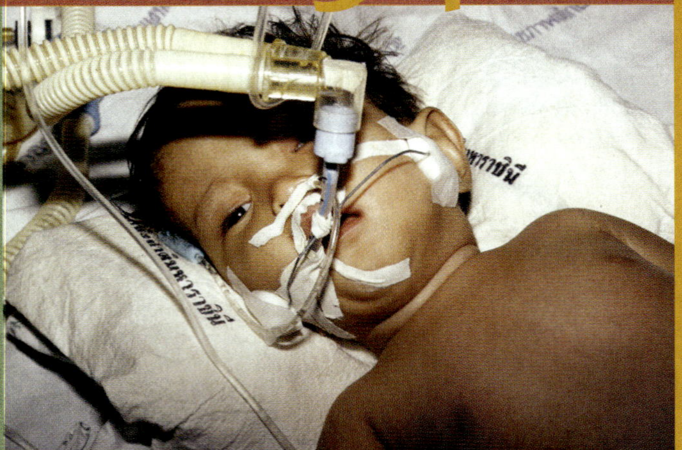

Infections in HIV-Infected Children

Andrew P. Steenhoff, Wolfgang Rennert, and Richard M. Rutstein

DEFINITION AND EPIDEMIOLOGY

Infection with the human immunodeficiency virus (HIV) induces a secondary immune deficiency, rendering the host susceptible to infection. The immunosuppressive combination of HIV infection in the setting of the immature pediatric immune system represents an ideal medium for opportunistic pathogens to thrive and the challenge rests with the pediatrician to diagnose, treat, and prevent these infections.

Infections in HIV-infected children occur in two broad groups: opportunistic infections (OI) and nonopportunistic infections. OI are defined by the Centers for Disease Control and Prevention (CDC) disease classification of pediatric HIV infection (see Table 53–1 in Chapter 53).[1,2] Nonopportunistic infections represent all other known pathogens. The description of an infection as an OI is helpful in defining an AIDS-related illness (ARI), but does not mean that the nonopportunistic infections are any less common or severe.

In the United States, earlier detection of HIV infection through screening of pregnant women as well as the widespread use of highly active antiretroviral therapy (HAART) and pneumocystis prophylaxis have dramatically decreased the rates of AIDS-related OI in children. These advances have converted pediatric HIV in most children from an acute life-threatening condition to a chronic illness. Despite these advances, OI continue to occur in this population.

The epidemiology of infections in the HIV-infected child in the United States has dramatically altered after the introduction of HARRT in 1996 and its subsequent widespread use. In the pre-HAART era, the five most common OI, which all occurred at an event rate of greater than 1 per 100 patient-years, were serious bacterial infection, herpes zoster, disseminated *Mycobacterium avium* complex (MAC), *Pneumocystis jiroveci* pneumonia (PCP, formerly called *Pneumocystis carinii* pneumonia), and mucosal candidiasis (Table 54–1).[3] Other less common opportunistic conditions included cytomegalovirus (CMV) disease particularly retinitis, tuberculosis, invasive fungal disease other than mucosal candidiasis, toxoplasmosis, and progressive multifocal leukoencephalopathy. In the HAART era, opportunistic illnesses occur mainly in two settings: as the presenting sign of a child in whom the diagnosis of HIV was previously unknown and in known HIV-infected children with a persistently low $CD4^+$ T-lymphocyte percentage.[4] Following the introduction of HAART, the four most common OI, all of which occur at a lower event rate than the pre-HAART era, are now bacterial pneumonia, herpes zoster, oral candidiasis, and dermatophyte infections (Table 54–1).[5]

This chapter will focus on the care of infections in the HIV-infected child in the United States. See Chapter 55 for an approach to the HIV-exposed child and Chapter 53 for a more general approach to managing the HIV-infected child.

PATHOGENESIS

The immunodeficiency caused by HIV-infection is due to a progressive decline in both number and function of T-lymphocytes.[6] Effective antiretroviral therapy has addressed one of these shortcomings—immune reconstitution is associated with a rise in T-lymphocytes, often into the normal range for age. However, a critical question is whether this new T-cell population is fully functional or not.[7] Recent work in a group of HIV-infected children following HAART demonstrated poor cellular immune responses, which may indicate persistent functional immune deficits in these children despite a normal $CD4^+$ T-lymphocyte count.[7]

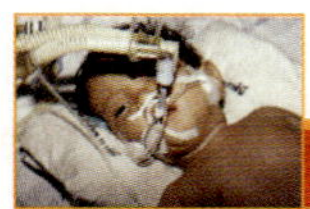

Table 54–1.

Overall Incidence Rates of Most Common First-time Infections in HIV-infected Children Before and After the Introduction of HAART[3,5]

	Pre-HAART	HAART Era
Opportunistic infection category	Incidence rate of events/ 100 person-years (95% CI)	Incidence rate of events/ 100 person-years (95% CI)
Serious bacterial infection	15.1 (14.2–16.1)	Unknown
Pneumonia	11.1 (10.3–12.0)	2.15 (1.79–2.56)
Bacteremia	3.3 (2.9–3.8)	0.35 (0.22–0.51)
Herpes Zoster	2.9 (2.6–3.3)	1.11 (0.88–1.39)
Disseminated *Mycobacterium avium* complex	1.8 (1.5–2.1)	0.14 (0.07–0.25)
Pneumocystis jiroveci pneumonia	1.3 (1.1–1.6)	0.09 (0.04–0.19)
Candidiasis of mucous membranes	1.3 (1.0–1.5)	0.93 (0.70–1.22)
Invasive fungal infections	0.1 (0.05–0.2)	0.08 (0.03–0.17)
Dermatophyte infections	Unknown	0.88 (0.67–1.14)

In the absence of HAART, infection with HIV leads to chronic immune activation and the progressive functional impairment and loss of $CD4^+$ cells.[8–11] HIV infection also causes $CD8^+$ T-cell depletion in up to 50% of patients.[12–14] The resultant T-cell dysregulation leads to immunodeficiency and AIDS, but the mechanisms leading to T-cell depletion remain controversial.[15] Evidence exists for a number of mechanisms including impaired thymic production, direct lysis of $CD4^+$ cells, and apoptosis of uninfected bystander T cells. Impaired thymic production of naïve T cells over time reduces the size of the T-cell pool.[16,17] Direct lysis of infected $CD4^+$ cells also contributes to T-cell depletion.[18] However, most of the apoptotic T cells in the peripheral blood and lymph nodes of HIV-infected patients are uninfected.[13,19–23] Apoptosis of uninfected bystander T cells is caused by activation-induced cell death of mature T cells following chronic immune activation in addition to HIV-mediated mechanisms.[11,24,25] HIV-1 induces apoptosis in uninfected T cells by several mechanisms including cytotoxic effects of HIV-1 proteins and envelope glycoproteins (Env), which have been implicated as the major cause of bystander cell death in T cells and other cell types.[26–34] Nonreplicating virions induce a proapoptotic signal in uninfected $CD4^+$ T cells through a CXCR4- or CXCR5-mediated pathway that does not require CD4 signaling or membrane fusion.[31,35] In addition, soluble, virion, or cell-associated HIV-1 envelope glycoproteins can prime uninfected T cells for activation-induced apoptosis.[28,30]

The slope of the $CD4^+$ cell decline depends on the viral load. In one adult study the median rate of decline in the absence of therapy was 4%/year for each $\log_{10}$HIV RNA c/mL.[36] The slope of $CD4^+$ cell decline increases in late-stage disease. The catastrophic decline in numbers of $CD4^+$ and $CD8^+$ T-lymphocytes is usually reversed by an appropriate HAART regimen.

In the United States, the goal is to offer prenatal HIV testing for all pregnant women. In reality, however, not all women are screened for HIV and as a result, there are still children who acquire HIV perinatally and are diagnosed only when they present with symptomatic HIV infection. In these children, the pathogenesis of their symptoms is usually because of a progressive decline in both number and function of T-lymphocytes. When the CD4 percentage falls below 25%, their risk for infection is increased and when it falls below 15%, they are at substantial risk for opportunistic pathogens.

The exact pathogenesis of the immune reconstitution syndrome is still being elucidated. In an HIV-infected individual who has received several weeks of HAART, the cell-mediated immune response is restored, which may result in an inflammatory reaction to hitherto dormant pathogens, such as MAC antigens, and lead to local symptoms. Manifestations of the immune reconstitution syndrome are varied and depend on the causative pathogen and on the vigor of the host's immune response. Symptoms vary from painful lymphadenopathy 1–12 weeks after initiating HAART, as is seen in some cases of MAC-induced immune reconstitution, to severe symptoms requiring hospitalization in others.[37,38] The clinician needs to be vigilant for symptoms and signs of this syndrome when commencing HAART in children who have a low CD4 count.

CLINICAL PRESENTATION

The clinical diagnosis of an opportunistic infection in an HIV-infected child depends on a high index of suspicion as signs and symptoms are frequently more nuance than in the immunocompetent child. The clinical features of the most important OI in HIV-infected children are summarized in Table 54–2.

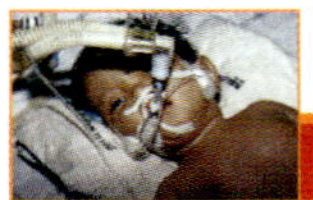

Table 54–2.

Epidemiology and Clinical Features of Selected Opportunistic Infections in HIV-Infected Children

Pathogen	Epidemiology	Clinical Presentation
Candida infections	■ Oral thrush and diaper dermatitis occur in 50–85% of HIV-infected children ■ *C. albicans* is the most common cause ■ *Candida esophagitis* may be seen in children not responding to HAART ■ Disseminated candidiasis is infrequent in HIV+ children	■ Oral thrush may present with angular cheilitis-red, fissured lesions in the corners of the mouth ■ Odynophagia, dysphagia, or retrosternal pain may be the presentation of esophageal candidiasis ■ Oropharyngeal candidiasis may be absent in children on HAART who have esophageal candidiasis ■ Barium swallow in esophageal candidiasis reveals classic cobblestoning appearance
Coccidiodomycosis	■ Caused by *Coccidioides immitis*, which is endemic in southwestern US, northern Mexico, and Central and South America ■ In utero and perinatal transmission occur	■ Common symptoms include fever and dyspnea as well as weight loss, lymphadenopathy, headache, and chest pain ■ Pulmonary disease may present with bilateral diffuse reticulonodular infiltrates, persistent nodules, or thin-walled cavities ■ Features of disseminated disease are rash including but not limited to erythema nodosum, arthralgias, bone, joint, or CNS disease
Cryptococcosis	■ Less frequent infection in HIV-infected children (1%) than in HIV+ adults ■ Most frequent in children aged 6–18 years and with CD4%<15%	■ Initially, meningitis is most frequent presentation-indolent course of fever, headache, and altered mental status ■ Disseminated cryptococcosis may involve the skin and has a varied presentation including umbilicated papules indistinguishable from molluscum contagiosum ■ Pulmonary disease may be clinically subtle—recurrent fever with pulmonary nodules, dry cough, intrathoracic lymphadenopathy, or pulmonary infiltrates (focal or diffuse)
Cryptosporidiosis	■ Highly infectious parasite transmitted by ingested oocytes ■ Predilection for the jejunum and terminal ileum	■ Severe profuse, nonbloody, persistent, watery diarrhea with abdominal cramps ■ Can be chronic in immunocompromised children and complicated by malnutrition ■ Migration into the biliary system may cause acalculous cholecystitis and sclerosing cholangitis ■ Pulmonary or disseminated infection occurs rarely
CMV	■ The commonest perinatal infection in the United States (incidence of 0.2–2.2% of live-born infants)—this rate is probably even higher is infants with perinatal HIV exposure ■ Rate of congenital infection is 30–40% in mothers with primary CMV infection during pregnancy ■ The rate of congenital CMV is lower (0.15–1.0%) after recurrent maternal CMV during pregnancy caused by reactivation or by infection with a different strain of CMV	■ Only 10% of infants with in utero infection are symptomatic at birth ■ Features of newborns with symptomatic CMV disease include small for gestational age, microcephaly, intracranial calcifications, impaired hearing, purpura/petechiae, jaundice, chorioretinitis, and hepatosplenomegaly ■ Long-term sequelae of congenital infection are seen in 90% of those with symptomatic infection at birth-hearing loss, mental retardation, chorioretinitis, optic atrophy, seizures, or learning disabilities

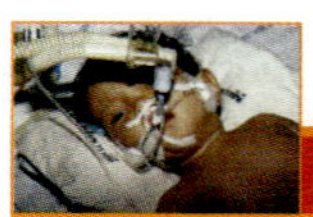

Table 54–2. (continued)

Epidemiology and Clinical Features of Selected Opportunistic Infections in HIV-Infected Children

Pathogen	Epidemiology	Clinical Presentation
	■ 50–80% of US women of childbearing age are seropositive for CMV ■ 90% of HIV-infected pregnant women are co-infected with CMV ■ HIV-infected children are at higher risk of acquiring CMV infection, particularly in first 4 years of life ■ Overall, a third of HIV-infected children shed CMV (up to 60% in those with AIDS) ■ CMV causes 8–10% of pediatric AIDS-defining illness with CMV retinitis accounting for 25% of these	■ Of the 90% of infants with in utero infection who are asymptomatic at birth, 10–15% develop long-term sequelae such as hearing loss ■ In HIV-infected children, CMV co-infection doubles the rate of progression of HIV disease ■ CMV retinitis: frequently asymptomatic in young HIV-infected children; may be discovered on screening eye examination; older children present with floaters, loss of peripheral, or reduced central vision ■ Extraocular disease may involve lungs (interstitial pneumonia with nonproductive cough), GI tract, sinuses, or CNS (20% have normal CSF) ■ GI manifestations include colitis (most commonly), oral or esophageal ulcers, hepatitis, ascending cholangitis, or gastritis ■ CNS manifestations include myelitis, subacute encephalopathy, and polyradiculopathy
Herpes simplex virus	■ Risk for neonatal HSV is greatest (30–50%) with primary maternal HSV infection ■ Maternal reactivation of HSV is associated with a lower risk (0%–5%) of neonatal infection ■ 75% of neonatal infection in the United States are caused by HSV type 2 ■ HIV-infected women more commonly shed HSV from the vulva and cervix than HIV uninfected women ■ The risk for maternal genital HSV reactivation and shedding increases with decreasing CD4 count ■ In 6% of pediatric AIDS cases, recurrent or persistent HSV infection is the AIDS-indicator condition	■ Neonatal HSV may present as disseminated multiorgan disease (25%), localized CNS disease (35%) or diseases localized to the skin, eyes, and mouth (40%) ■ Orolabial HSV is the most common presentation outside of the neonatal period and may be severe in HIV-infected children ■ Rarely, primary orolabial HSV disseminates with visceral and generalized skin involvement ■ Other sites of HSV in severely immunocompromised children include esophagus, CNS, genitalia or dissemination to the liver, adrenals, kidney, spleen, lung, and brain ■ HSV proctitis may be seen in sexually active children or adolescents
Histoplasmosis	■ Incidence is 0.4% in United States HIV-infected children but is higher in HIV-infected children in Latin America (2.7–3.8%) ■ No evidence for congenital disease	■ Disseminated disease most frequently presents with prolonged fever ■ Other symptoms include malaise, nonproductive cough and weight loss ■ Interstitial pneumonitis is rare in children but a primary pulmonary focus may lead to dissemination in HIV+ children ■ Signs of dissemination include hepatosplenomegaly (89% of infants), skin lesions, anemia, thrombocytopenia, elevated transaminases ■ Disseminated histoplasmosis is fatal if not treated

(continued)

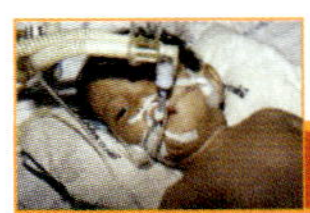

Table 54–2. (continued)

Epidemiology and Clinical Features of Selected Opportunistic Infections in HIV-Infected Children

Pathogen	Epidemiology	Clinical Presentation
Human papillomavirus	■ Transmission occurs by close person-to-person contact e.g., sexual intercourse or passage through an infected birth canal ■ HPV DNA detection rates may be as high as 95% in nonpregnant HIV+ women ■ Predominant risk factors for HPV in adolescents are number of lifetime and recent sexual partners ■ Persistent HPV infection, particularly with types 16, 18, 31, or 33 is associated with a high risk of developing carcinoma	■ Wart lesions occur most frequently on the cutaneous and mucosal squamous epithelium of hands, feet, face, and genitalia ■ Other sites include skin and mucus membranes of the anus, nose, conjunctiva, gastrointestinal, and respiratory systems ■ Warts may be smooth and flat or pedunculated ■ HPV immunization should still be given to those with HPV lesions—this is because the vaccine may protect them from acquiring HPV infection with a second or third serotype
MAC	■ Acquired through inhalation, inoculation or ingestion ■ Respiratory and GI colonization may act as portal for dissemination ■ Frequency of pediatric disseminated MAC increases with age and falling CD4%, particularly with CD4%<50%	■ Disseminated MAC: recurrent fever, weight loss, night sweats, fatigue, abdominal pain, anemia, leucopenia, thrombocytopenia, occasionally elevated alkaline phosphatase ■ Less commonly: pulmonary MAC or cutaneous disease, including lymphadenitis
Mycobacterium tuberculosis	■ Incidence of TB may be as much as 100-fold higher in HIV-infected vs uninfected children in the United States ■ Infection usually represents primary TB rather than reactivation disease ■ Identify and treat the source patient-usually an adult in the child's home	■ Congenital TB has nonspecific signs: poor feeding, failure to thrive, enlarged liver/spleen, fever, occasionally progressive pneumonia, meningitis ■ Pediatric pulmonary TB often presents in a nonspecific way: weight loss, fever, pulmonary infiltrate with hilar adenopathy ■ Common extrapulmonary sites include lymph nodes, military (via hematogenous), CNS, bone, pericardium, pleura, and peritoneum
Pneumocystis jiroveci pneumonia	■ Highest incidence in first year of life, peak age is 3–6 months ■ CD4 counts are not a good indicator of risk for PCP in infants <1 year old	■ Tachypnea, dyspnea, and cough ■ Fever in some ■ Bibasilar rales and hypoxia ■ Extrapulmonary disease is rare ■ Coinfection with CMV is a poor prognostic feature
Serious and recurrent bacterial infections	■ *S. pneumoniae* is the most prominent invasive pathogen in HIV-infected children ■ Pseudomonas and Salmonella species are the most common causes of gram-negative bacteremia ■ *S. aureus* is the most commonly isolated pathogen in catheter-related infections	■ Acute presentation with fever is most common ■ Leukocytosis may be absent in severely immunocompromised children ■ Recurrence of a previous infection is more likely
Syphilis	■ Can be transmitted from mother to child at any stage of pregnancy ■ Rate of congenital syphilis may be 50 times greater among infants of HIV+ women in the United States ■ Of HIV+ adolescents, 9% girls and 6% boys have syphilis	■ Sixty percent of infants with congenital syphilis are asymptomatic ■ Early features of congenital syphilis hepatosplenomegaly, peeling rash on palms and soles, jaundice, bloody nasal discharge, pseudoparalysis, bone marrow suppression

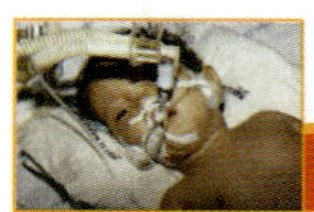

Table 54–2. (continued)

Epidemiology and Clinical Features of Selected Opportunistic Infections in HIV-Infected Children

Pathogen	Epidemiology	Clinical Presentation
		■ Late features of congenital syphilis: abnormalities of CNS, bone, teeth, eyes, and skin
Toxoplasmosis	■ Major mode of transmission is congenital ■ Infection of the fetus in early gestation results in more severe disease ■ Older children acquire disease through eating poorly cooked meat containing parasitic cysts or by ingesting sporulated oocysts in soil, food or water	■ Majority of newborns are asymptomatic ■ When symptoms occur, they are localized to the neurologic system (calcifications, hydrocephalus, retinitis, seizures, microcephaly) or a generalized disease (rash, hepatosplenomegaly, bone marrow suppression, jaundice, lymphadenopathy) ■ Reactivated chronic toxoplasmosis may present as pneumonitis, hepatitis, and cardiomyopathy/myocarditis.
Varicella zoster virus	■ Mortality and morbidity is higher in HIV+ immunocompromised children than HIV- children ■ Congenital VZV: it is unknown whether this occurs more frequently in the newborns of HIV+ women ■ Zoster is unusual among HIV+ children who had primary VZV when their CD4% was normal ■ Zoster is common (rate of up to 70%) among HIV+ children who had primary VZV when their CD4% was <15% ■ This high rate of zoster is decreased when these children are exposed to HAART and VZV immunization	■ Congenital infection is characterized by skin scarring, limb hypoplasia, microcephaly, cortical atrophy, seizures, mental retardation, ocular damage (chorioretinitis, microopthalmia, cataracts), renal anomalies, swallowing dysfunction, and aspiration pneumonia ■ Primary VZV classically presents with fever and a generalized pruritic vesicular rash ■ Persistent lesions may be atypical and lack a vesicular component ■ Chronic VZV (appearance of new lesions for >1 month after primary or recurrent VZV infection) is associated with low CD4% ■ Viral isolates may become acyclovir resistant during prolonged therapy ■ Typically, zoster presents with a frequently painful vesicular eruption in a dermatomal distribution but atypical forms occur in this population ■ VZV retinitis: a rare complication in HIV+ children, which may be confused with CMV retinitis ■ Rarely may present as a progressive encephalitis

HIV, human immunodeficiency virus; AIDS, acquired immune deficiency syndrome; CMV, cytomegalovirus; GI, gastrointestinal tract; CNS, central nervous system; CSF, cerebrospinal fluid; HPV, human papilloma virus; HSV, herpes simplex virus; VZV, varicella zoster virus.
Adapted from CDC. Treating opportunistic infections among HIV-exposed and infected children: recommendations from CDC, the National Institutes of Health, and the Infectious Diseases Society of America. Morb Mortal Wkly Rep 2004;2004;53(No. RR-14).

Bacterial Pneumonia

Bacterial pneumonia may present with classic symptoms of fever, cough, and labored breathing, but more subtle signs such as a change in exercise tolerance may be the only presenting feature. Symptoms are frequently more indolent when the cause of pneumonia is an opportunistic pathogen, such as *Pneumocystis jiroveci* or *Mycobacterium tuberculosis.* With the latter, systemic symptoms such as weight loss, night sweats, and intermittent fever may be prominent. Clinical examination may reveal lobar or diffuse pulmonary involvement depending on the pathogen. In PCP, the lungs are often remarkably clear to auscultation. The finding of a tachypneic child with oxygen saturation lower than expected for the clinical picture is highly suggestive of

PCP. Sinusitis may complicate a preceding viral upper respiratory tract infection and requires a high index of suspicion, particularly in patients who are nonverbal.

Varicella

Chickenpox caused by varicella zoster virus (Figure 54–1) may be seen in HIV-infected children and presents with fever and skin lesions at multiple stages of development. It may be complicated by pneumonia or secondary bacterial infection of the skin. After primary infection, the virus becomes latent in the dorsal root ganglia and may reactivate to cause herpes zoster (Figure 54–2). Zoster occurs 7–20 times more frequently in HIV-infected children than in their HIV-uninfected peers.[39] The incidence of zoster has declined since 2000, likely representing the combined effects of varicella zoster immunization and immune reconstitution secondary to HAART.[40] Children who are on HAART at the time of their primary varicella infection have been shown to be at lower risk of subsequently developing zoster than those who develop primary varicella off HAART. In HIV-infected children, zoster occurs in a dermatomal distribution and may be single or multidermatomal.[40] In the early phases of zoster, patients may present with a sharp or burning dermatomal pain in the absence of skin lesions. Careful follow-up will reveal the diagnosis when the characteristic rash appears a day or two later.

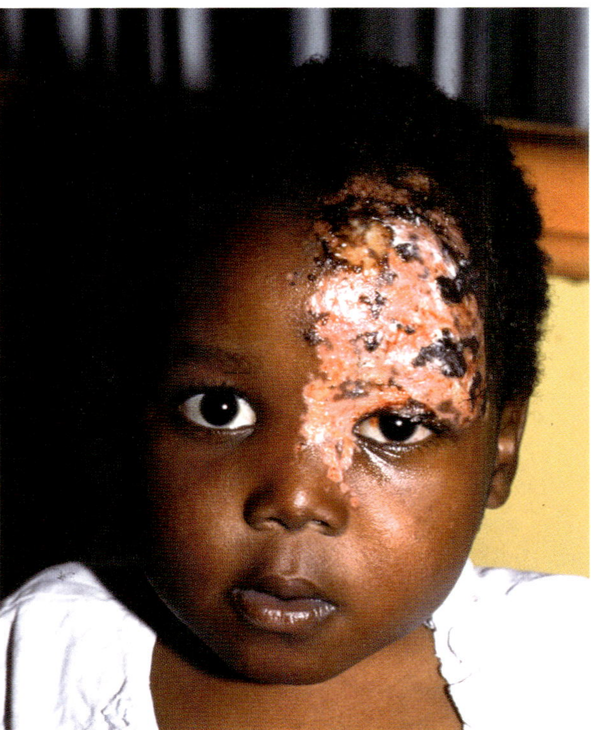

FIGURE 54–2 ■ Herpes zoster in an HIV-infected boy. Zoster is the second most common opportunistic infection in the HAART era.

Mucosal and Cutaneous Fungal Infections

Oropharyngeal candidiasis (Figure 54–3) is a frequent finding in many children in the first few months of life. However, thrush that is particularly unresponsive to therapy, is recurrent, occurs in a child older than a year of age, and is not preceded by a course of antibiotics or inhaled steroids should prompt the clinician to consider the diagnosis of a coexistent immunodeficiency, such as HIV.

A detailed skin examination of an HIV-infected child may reveal cutaneous dermatophyte infections (Figure 54–4), widespread molluscum contagiosum,

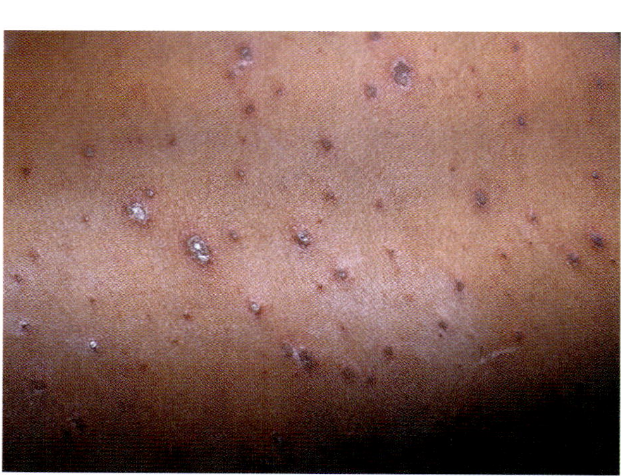

FIGURE 54–1 ■ An episode of chicken pox in HIV-infected children may be complicated by secondary infection with group A *Streptococcus*, causing hemorrhagic varicella.

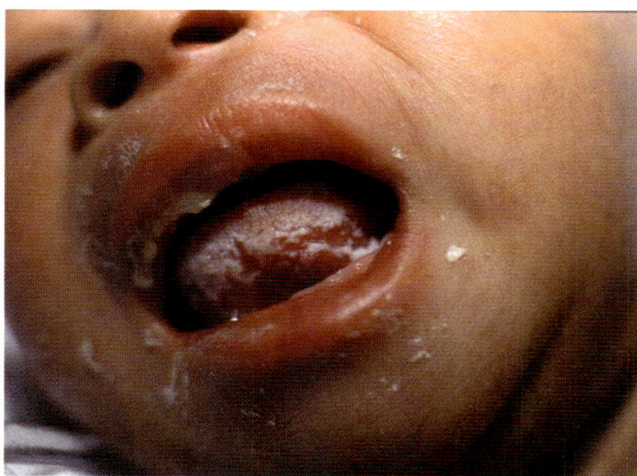

FIGURE 54–3 ■ Severe oral thrush or thrush occurring in a child older than a year raise the suspicion for an immunodeficiency such as HIV infection.

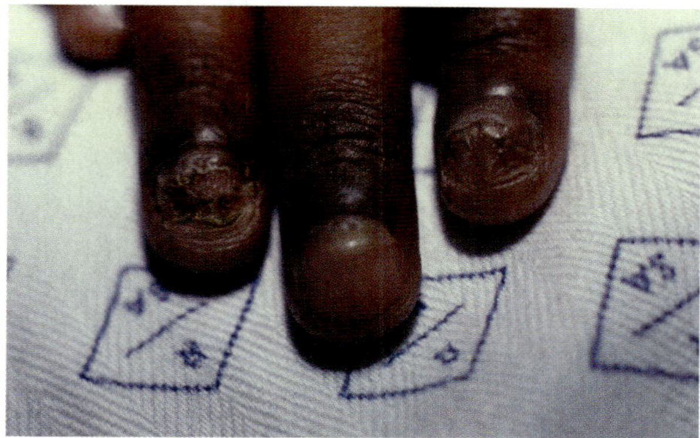

FIGURE 54–4 ■ Cutaneous fungal infections such as onychomycosis are one of the commonest opportunistic infections in HIV-infected children in the HAART era.

severe scabies (Figure 54–5), or pronounced genital warts caused by human papilloma virus (Figure 54–6). Any of these signs may also be found in a child who has been a long-term nonprogressor. This small group of children who acquire HIV perinatally are relatively asymptomatic as they coexist with HIV for up to a decade or more while their CD4 count slowly declines. Eventually they present with features of AIDS, which may include cutaneous findings.

Central Nervous System Infections

Central nervous system infections such as cryptococcal meningitis may have an indolent course. Subtle symptoms reported by parents include behavior changes, headaches, and a gradual decline in school achievement. If the diagnosis is not made during this phase, symptoms progress to reflect the underlying meningitis or space-occupying lesion. CMV or toxoplasmosis may present with changes in visual acuity. These visual changes may be reported by older HIV-infected children but annual ophthalmology screening visits are advocated for children who are not able to give a reliable visual history and have a low CD4 count. On Fundoscopic examination, CMV retinitis is characterized by white and yellow retinal infiltrates often associated with retinal hemorrhages.

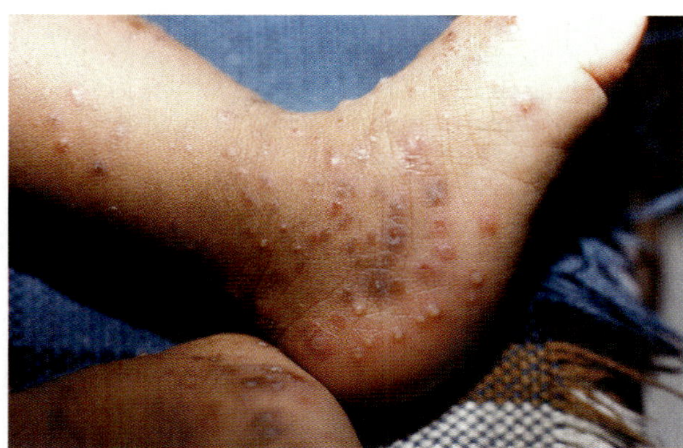

FIGURE 54–5 ■ Severe scabies may be seen in HIV-infected children. Lesions occur more frequently on the peripheries, including hands and feet.

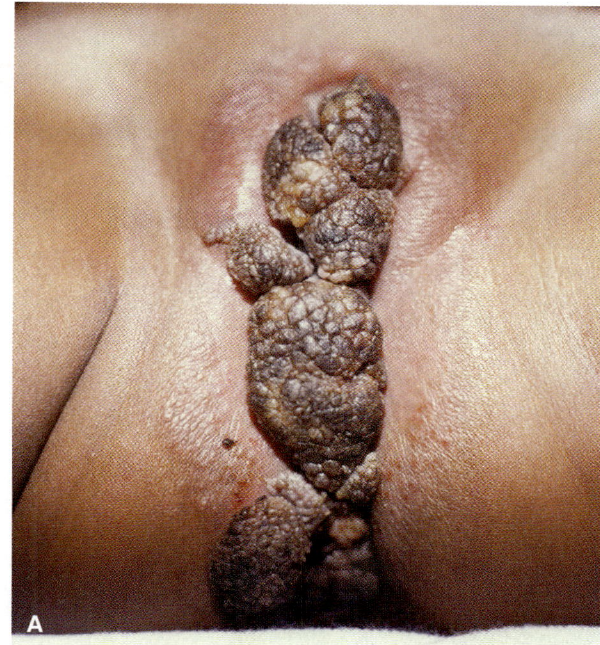

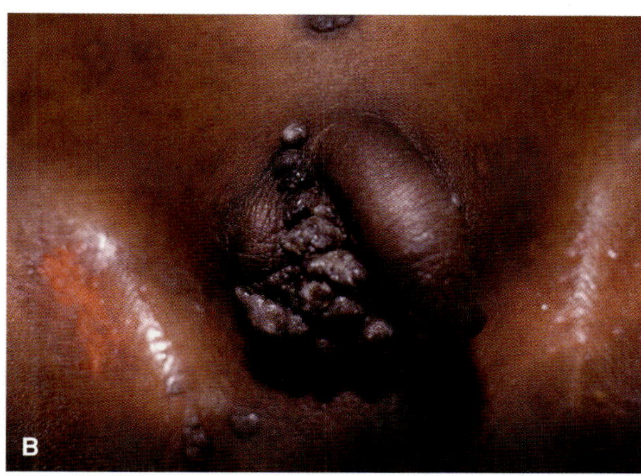

FIGURE 54–6 ■ **(A)** Condyloma acuminata in the genital area of an HIV-infected girl. This condition, caused by human papilloma virus, may respond to a combination of HAART and topical therapy. **(B)** Condyloma acuminata in the genital area of an HIV-infected boy.

DIFFERENTIAL DIAGNOSIS

The discipline of carefully constructing and reviewing one's differential diagnosis is a valuable one when caring for an HIV-infected child with a possible OI. We recommend constructing a differential diagnosis based on the presenting symptoms and signs (Table 54–3).

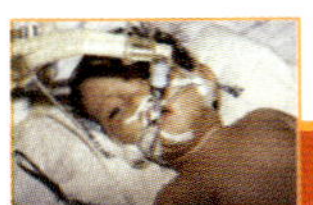

Table 54–3.

Clinical Approach to the Differential Diagnosis of an HIV-infected Child with a Suspected Opportunistic Infection.

Symptoms and Signs	Differential Diagnosis of Clinical Syndrome	Differential Diagnosis of Etiology Includes*
Tachypnea hypoxia, and fever	Community-acquired pneumonia	Bacterial
		Streptococcus pneumoniae
		Staphylococcus aureus
		Mycoplasma pneumoniae
		Group A *streptococcus*
		Viral
		Influenza A or B
		Respiratory syncytial virus
		Parainfluenza virus 1, 2, or 3
		Adenovirus
		Metapneumovirus
	Opportunistic organisms	*Pneumocystis jiroveci*
		Mycobacterium tuberculosis
	Cardiac failure	HIV cardiomyopathy
	Gastroenteritis, dehydration, and acidosis	See diarrhea for possible causes
Failure to thrive, intermittent fever	Infection	TB
		MAC
		Recurrent urinary tract infection
	Malignancy	HIV-associated lymphoma
	HIV nephropathy	HIV-associated
Visual problems	Infectious	CMV
		Toxoplasmosis
	Noninfectious	Hydrocephalus
CNS symptoms or signs such as Photophobia Meningism Behavior changes	Bacterial meningitis	*Streptococcus pneumoniae*
		Neisseria meningitidis
		Listeria monocytogenes
	Viral meningitis	CMV
		Enterovirus
		Herpes simplex virus
	Fungal meningitis	*Cryptococcal meningitis*
	Progressive multifocal leukoencephalopathy	JC virus
	HIV encephalopathy	
	Brain abscess	Anaerobes
		Nocardia spp.
	CNS malignancy	Lymphoma
Skin rashes	Vesicular rash	Chicken pox (primary infection)
		Herpes zoster (dermatomal)
		Herpes simplex
		Smallpox
	Pustular or nodular	Scabies
		Insect bites
		Kaposi's sarcoma
		Erythema nodosum
	Eczema	Eczema
	Scalded skin	Scalded skin syndrome
		e.g., Staphylococcus aureus
		Group A streptococcus
		Steven's Johnson syndrome
Diarrhea	Infectious enteritis	Viral
		Rotavirus
		Adenovirus
		Norwalk
		CMV
		Herpes simplex virus
		Bacterial
		Salmonella spp.

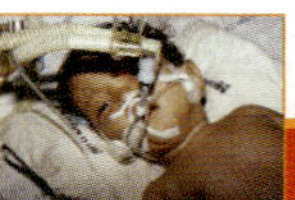

Table 54–3. (continued)

Clinical Approach to the Differential Diagnosis of an HIV-infected Child with a Suspected Opportunistic Infection.

Symptoms and Signs	Differential Diagnosis of Clinical Syndrome	Differential Diagnosis of Etiology Includes*
Diarrhea (continued)		*Shigella* spp.
		E. coli
		Clostridium difficile
		Campylobacter jejuni
		MAC
		TB
		Parasitic
		Giardia lamblia
		Entamoeba histolytica
		Cryptosporidium
		Isospora belli
		Strongyloides stercoralis
	Noninfectious enteritis	Gastrointestinal lymphoma

**Differential diagnosis includes infections and some noninfectious causes.*
HIV, human immunodeficiency virus; TB, tuberculosis; MAC, mycobacterium tuberculosis; CMV, cytomegalovirus.

Careful observation of the clinical course and underlying pathologic mechanisms may also provide the key to making a microbiologic diagnosis.

DIAGNOSIS

The accurate microbiologic diagnosis of infection in HIV-infected children ensures targeted and effective therapy in a population who are prone to infection with a plethora of organisms. Using a carefully crafted list of differential diagnoses, the clinician should prioritize testing for those infections that are most likely in each clinical setting. While a microbiologic diagnosis is the ultimate goal this should be obtained with due thought to any possible morbidity from the diagnostic procedure itself.

Rapid diagnostic tests such as pharyngeal streptococcal antigen, stool rotavirus antigen, or nasopharyngeal viral antigen screening are frequently revealing in children with the appropriate clinical syndrome. For example, the diagnosis of varicella zoster infection, which can be challenging in an immunocompromised host, has been revolutionized by newer molecular diagnostic techniques. Where available, polymerase chain reaction (PCR) testing has become the gold standard. Rapid antigen testing is less sensitive, but is useful in an emergency department setting given its faster turnaround time. Culture of the virus is sometimes available and reference laboratories use this technique to assess whether the infecting strain was vaccine or wild type varicella virus. The Tzanck smear, whereby cells from a fresh blister are smeared on a slide and stained to look for characteristic herpes-related changes, is no longer recommended because of its relatively poor sensitivity and specificity.[41]

A blood culture to screen for bacteremia should be performed in a febrile HIV-infected child when the source of fever is not readily apparent. When infection with MAC is suspected (Figure 54–7), multiple blood cultures sent in using isolator tubes might be required to detect the organism.[38] The microbiology laboratory will then place the blood directly onto mycobacterial broth media, such as Lowenstein-Jensen medium, or they will concentrate the blood and place it in mycobacterial broth media. Standard blood cultures may detect

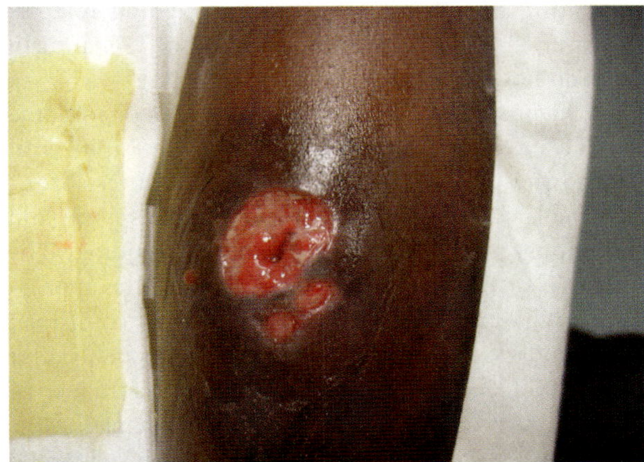

FIGURE 54–7 ■ Cutaneous MAC infection on the posterior calf in an adolescent boy. This is presented as a manifestation of the immune reconstitution syndrome within 3 months of commencing HAART.

rapid-growing mycobacteria but will not detect MAC leading to the potentially false assumption that the patient is not infected by this organism. A negative acid-fast stain performed on a blood culture specimen should be interpreted with caution—the majority of these stains are negative even in patients whose blood cultures subsequently culture MAC.

Patients with subtle features suggesting meningitis, such as a chronic headache or behavioral changes, should have a lumbar puncture to assess the cell count, chemistry, and culture of the cerebrospinal fluid (CSF). The early diagnosis of meningitis in an immune-compromised child is difficult, given the propensity for underwhelming symptoms and signs. A high index of suspicion and a low threshold to rule out meningitis with a spinal tap will enhance the clinician's chances of making this challenging diagnosis. If there is clinical suspicion for an intracranial space occupying lesion or hydrocephalus such as is sometimes seen in cryptococcal meningitis, this should be evaluated by head imaging.

In an HIV-infected child who has a low CD4 count, cryptococcal infection should be suspected, particularly if the child is in the age range of 6–12 years. Blood and CSF should be sent for cryptococcal antigen testing. Antigen is detected in CSF or serum specimens from more than 90% of patients with cryptococcal meningitis. Where antigen detection is not available, cryptococcus may also be visualized by examining India ink-stained samples of CSF. Occasionally, CSF cryptococcal antigen detection may be negative in patients with culture-proven meningitis. Three possible reasons for this include infection with a nonencapsulated strain of cryptococcus, low antigen titers, or very high antigen titers, which give a false negative result—the prozone phenomenon.[42,43] The latter reverts to positive when the antigen test is repeated after diluting the sample of CSF. Cryptococcal antigen titers in CSF can be helpful in evaluating response to therapy or ongoing relapse. However, changes in serum, rather than CSF, antigen titers do not correlate with clinical response.[44]

Identifying the microbiologic cause of pneumonia in HIV-infected children is challenging. Rapid viral diagnostics, blood cultures, sputum cultures, bronchoalveolar lavage specimens, pleural fluid aspirate, and lung biopsy may all be used to diagnose the etiology. The diagnosis of PCP is suggested by a ground glass appearance on chest radiography but is usually only confirmed after identifying the organism from bronchoalveolar lavage fluid. Serum lactate dehydrogenase is frequently elevated in children with PCP but is not specific for this condition.[44] *Mycobacterium tuberculosis* may be isolated from early morning gastric aspirates and, because of the variable yield of this technique, at least three samples are usually sent for both Ziehl-Neelsen staining and mycobacterial culture.

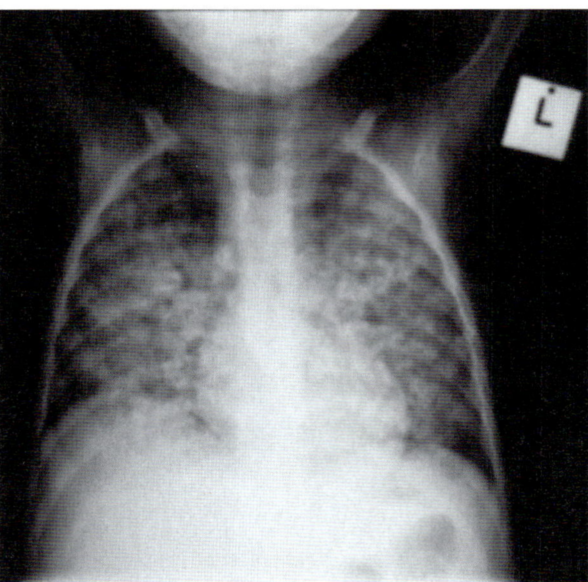

FIGURE 54–8 ■ Bronchogenic tuberculosis in an HIV-infected child. Note the diffuse nodular airspace opacities which represent bronchogenic spread of tuberculosis from a site of primary infection.

Imaging of the affected organ system frequently clinches the diagnosis. The chest radiograph is particularly helpful in cases of pneumonia and pulmonary tuberculosis (Figures 54–8 and 54–9). Computed tomography of the head may reveal sinusitis, hydrocephalus or an intracranial abscess. Magnetic resonance imaging is often required to diagnose the early features of progressive multifocal leukoencephalopathy. In this setting,

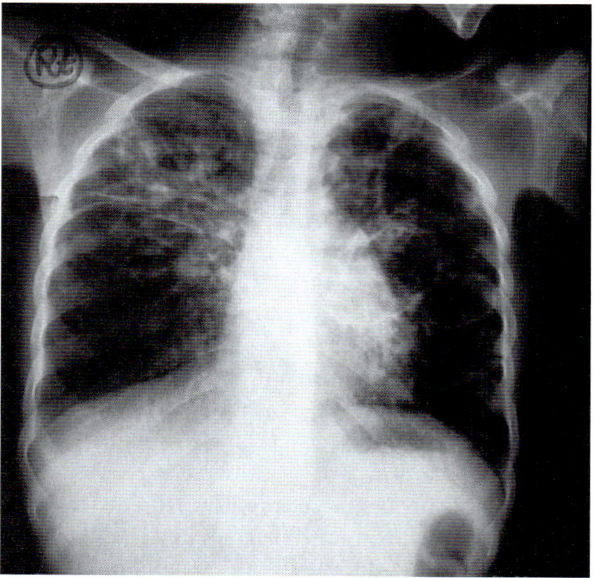

FIGURE 54–9 ■ Cavitary disease secondary to tuberculosis. This is rare in children but may be seen in children with advanced HIV disease.

CSF should be tested for JC virus by PCR. In a child who has had untreated HIV for some time, the electrocardiogram may reveal evidence of left ventricular hypertrophy caused by HIV-associated cardiomyopathy. In more severe cases, the echocardiogram demonstrates cardiac dysfunction.

MANAGEMENT

The management of infections in HIV-infected children is focused primarily on preventing infection using a three-tiered approach. The primary goal is immune reconstitution using HAART. The HIV-infected child is further protected by inducing active immunity to common childhood pathogens by vaccination. In patients without documented immune response to vaccines or where vaccination may not have occurred, passive immunization is practiced, following exposure to certain pathogens such as varicella zoster virus. The third tier is the use of antibiotic prophylaxis.

HIV clinicians use the CDC guidelines to decide when to initiate antibiotic prophylaxis and the reader is referred to this source for pathogen-specific recommendations.[45] Table 54–4 summarizes key elements of the CDC treatment and prophylaxis guidelines and Table 54–5 tabulates selected adverse reactions of antimicrobials commonly used to manage infections in HIV-infected children. The decision to commence prophylaxis depends on the child's age, $CD4^+$ T-lymphocyte percentage and count. For example, PCP prophylaxis with an agent such as trimethoprim-sulfamethoxazole is recommended for all HIV-infected children younger than the age of a year regardless of their $CD4^+$ T-lymphocyte percentage and count, as even those children with counts in the normal range carry a higher risk of acquiring PCP. For MAC, the risk of infection increases as the child's $CD4^+$ T-lymphocyte percentage and count fall—the prophylaxis guidelines reflect this.

Despite recent improvements in microbiologic diagnostic capabilities, including the introduction of PCR-based molecular technology, the clinician may still be faced with the challenge of caring for an HIV-infected child with an acute fever of unknown origin. Figure 54–10 describes an approach to such a patient.

TREATMENT

Treatment of infections in HIV-infected children is targeted at the causative organism. In the acute setting where the cause is not yet known, broad-spectrum antibacterial coverage may be necessary for a 24–48-hour period. Local antibiograms should be consulted when choosing empiric antimicrobial therapy. Empiric coverage may also include fungal, mycobacterial, or viral agents depending on the clinical syndrome. A valuable resource is the CDC recommendations on treating OI among HIV-infected children.[44] When PCP is suspected, it is important to begin therapy as soon as possible as this may prove lifesaving in a condition that still carries a high mortality. The clinician does not need to wait until a bronchoalveolar lavage has been performed to confirm the diagnosis, as this will remain positive for PCP for at least 48 hours after therapy has commenced.

The duration of therapy depends on the underlying condition. For tuberculosis or MAC therapy lasts for at least 6–9 months and frequently longer. Treatment of these conditions should be done in consultation with a pediatric infectious diseases expert with expertise in pediatric HIV infection. For tuberculosis, principles for treating the HIV-infected child are the same as for the HIV-uninfected child except that ceratin modifications may be required given drug interactions with HAART. For initial therapy, before culture and sensitivity data are known, a four-drug regimen is recommended to allow for the possibility of a resistant organism. For MAC, initial empiric therapy should include at least two drugs, a macrolide (clarithromycin or azithromycin are frequently used) and ethambutol. Rifabutin is frequently added as a third drug, particularly in children with disseminated disease or more severe symptoms. For uncomplicated bacterial pneumonia, a 5–7 day course of antibiotics is sufficient. PCP is usually treated for 21 days and is followed by commencing prophylaxis (see Chapter 52 for prophylaxis recommendations and dosing). Trimethoprim-sulfamethoxazole at a high dose of 15–20 mg/kg/day is the recommended treatment for PCP. A short course of corticosteroids in moderate to severe cases of PCP should be started within 72 hours of diagnosis and has been associated with decreased mortality, less need for ventilation and reduced respiratory failure.[46–48]

COURSE AND PROGNOSIS

The course and prognosis of infection in HIV-infected children is determined by three main factors—the host, the organism, and the treatment. Key host factors include age and immune status. Younger children are generally more likely to experience a stormy course and a higher mortality particularly from PCP. By contrast, immune reconstitution syndrome seems to be less common in younger children who perhaps have not had the same degree of exposure to the causative pathogens such as *Mycobacterium tuberculosis* or MAC. The child's immune status, as measured by $CD4^+$ T-lymphocyte percentage and count, impacts their ability to clear the organism and those with lower counts are more likely to fare more poorly.

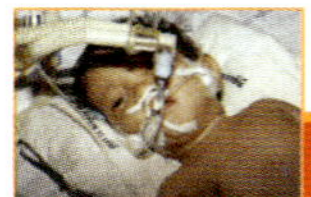

Table 54–4.

Treatment and Prophylaxis of Infections in HIV-Infected Children[44,45*]

Pathogen	Treatment	Indication for Prophylaxis	Prophylaxis
Candida infections	*Oropharyngeal* Topical therapy e.g., nystatin If failure—Fluconazole 3–6 mg/kg daily PO for 7–14 days *Esophageal* Fluconazole 6 mg/kg/day on day 1, then 3–6 mg/kg daily PO for 14–21 days If failure—Voriconazole *Invasive*: Amphotericin B 0.5–1.5 mg/kg daily IV-but may change to fluconazole depending on which species of candida	Frequent or severe recurrences of candida infections	Consider fluconazole 3–6 mg/kg daily PO
Coccidiodomycosis	All therapies are followed by chronic suppressive therapy[†] *Diffuse pulmonary or disseminated nonmeningitic disease*: Amphotericin B 0.5–1-mg/kg IV daily until clinical improvement (minimum of several weeks) *Meningeal infection*: Fluconazole 5–6 mg/kg IV or PO twice daily (max 800 mg/day)	No primary prophylaxis recommended-only suppressive therapy once diagnosed and treated for this infection	Fluconazole 6-mg/kg PO daily *Alternative*: Itraconazole 2–5 mg/kg PO every 12–48 hrs
Cryptococcus neoformans	All therapies are followed by chronic suppressive therapy[†] *Isolated pulmonary disease*: Mild-fluconazole 3–6-mg/kg PO daily Severe-amphotericin B 0.7–1.5 mg/kg IV daily (usually with an initial 2 weeks of flucytosine) until stable, then fluconazole suppression *Meningeal and extrameningeal disseminated disease*: Two week induction followed by suppressive therapy – Amphotericin B 0.7–1.5-mg/kg IV daily **PLUS** flucytosine 25-mg/kg PO four times daily (monitor levels)	Prophylaxis not usually recommended in HIV-infected children	N/A
Cryptosporidiosis	HAART *Alternative* Nitazoxanide 100-mg PO twice daily (age 1–3 yr) and 200 mg PO twice daily (age 4–11 yr)	None apart from HAART	HAART
Cytomegalovirus	*Symptomatic congenital infection*: Consult infectious diseases Consider ganciclovir 6-mg/kg IV every 12 hrs for 6 weeks *Disseminated disease and retinitis*: Ganciclovir 5–7.5-mg/kg IV every 12 hrs for 2–3 weeks, then 5 mg/kg per day for 5–7 days/week for chronic suppression *Alternative*: Foscarnet 60 mg/kg IV every 8 hrs for 2–3 weeks, then 90–120 mg/kg daily for chronic suppression	Prophylaxis not usually recommended in HIV-infected children	In unusual circumstances, may consider ganciclovir 30-mg/kg PO three times daily
Herpes simplex virus	*Neonatal CNS or disseminated disease*: Acyclovir 20 mg/kg IV three times daily for 21 days *Alternative for acyclovir-resistant HSV*: Foscarnet 40 mg/kg IV in three divided doses or 60 mg/kg in two divided doses	Frequent or severe recurrences	Acyclovir 80-mg/kg PO in 3–4 divided doses *Alternative if >12 years*: Valacyclovir 500 mg twice daily

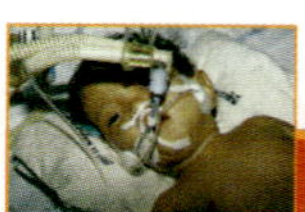

Table 54–4. (continued)

Treatment and Prophylaxis of Infections in HIV-Infected Children[44,45*]

Pathogen	Treatment	Indication for Prophylaxis	Prophylaxis
	Neonatal skin, eye, or mouth disease: Acyclovir 20 mg/kg IV three times daily for 14 days *CNS or disseminated disease in children outside neonatal period*: Acyclovir 10 mg/kg IV three times daily for 21 days *Alternative for acyclovir-resistant HSV*: Foscarnet 120 mg/kg IV in two to three divided doses *Moderate-to-severe gingivostomatitis*: Acyclovir 5–10 mg/kg IV three times daily for 7–14 days *For genital HSV (adolescents)*: Valacyclovir 1 g PO twice daily for 7–10 days		
Histoplasmosis	Both treatment regimens are followed by chronic suppressive therapy *Disseminated disease or Immunocompromised host*: Amphotericin B 1 mg/kg for 4–6 weeks (12–16 weeks for meningitis), followed by itraconazole 2–5 mg/kg (max 200 mg/dose) PO twice daily for 3–6 months *Mild disseminated disease*: Itraconazole 4–10 mg/kg (max 600 mg/day) IV or PO twice daily for 3 days, followed by 2–5 mg/kg (max 200 mg/dose) PO twice daily for 12–16 weeks	Severe immuno-suppression in endemic geographic area	Itraconazole 2–5-mg/kg PO every 12–24 hrs[†]
Human papillomavirus	Individual lesions can be removed by electrodessication or cryotherapy—this can be repeated every 1–2 weeks ≤4 times *Alternative topical therapies*: Podofilox solution/gel 0.5% applied topically twice daily for 3 consecutive days/week for ≤4 weeks Imiquimod cream 5% topically at night and washed off in the morning for 3 consecutive days/week for up to 16 weeks Trichloroacetic acid topically weekly for ≤3–6 weeks Podophyllin resin applied topically and washed off several hrs later, repeated weekly for 3–6 weeks	N/A	N/A
MAC	*Minimum of two drugs* Clarithromycin 7.5–15-mg/kg PO twice daily (max 500 mg twice daily) **OR** azithromycin 10–12 mg/kg PO daily (max 500 mg daily) plus ethambutol 15–25 mg/kg PO daily (max 1 g) *Add* rifabutin in disseminated or more severe disease	Age ≥6 yr if CD4 count <50/μL; age 2–6 yr if CD4 count <75/μL; age1–2 yr CD4 count <500/μL; age <1 yr if CD4 count <750/μL	Clarithromycin 7.5–15 mg/kg PO twice daily (max 500 mg twice daily) **OR** Azithromycin 20-mg/kg PO weekly (max 1200 mg weekly)
Mycobacterium tuberculosis	Same regimens as for HIV-uninfected child *For TB meningitis add* Prednisone 1–2 mg/kg/day for 6–8 weeks	TST ≥5 mm or contact with any person with active TB	Isoniazid 10–15 mg/kg/day daily for 9 months (max 300 mg) Alternative if INH-resistant: Rifampin 10–20 mk/kg PO for 4–6 months

(continued)

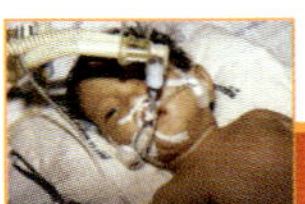

Table 54–4. (continued)

Treatment and Prophylaxis of Infections in HIV-Infected Children[44,45*]

Pathogen	Treatment	Indication for Prophylaxis	Prophylaxis
Pneumocystis jiroveci pneumonia	*First choice*: TMP-SMX 15–20 mg/kg of trimethoprim per day in four divided doses and Corticosteroids e.g., prednisone 1 mg/kg/day twice daily for days 1–5, 0.5 mg/kg/day for days 6–10 and 0.5 mg/kg/day for days 11–21. *Alternative*: Pentamidine 4 mg/kg/day IV	If <12 months and HIV-infected or indeterminate; or if ≥1 yr, HIV infected and CD4%<15	*First choice*: TMP-SMX 150/750 mg/m²/day in 2 divided doses PO three times weekly on consecutive days *Alternatives*: Pentamidine aerosolized, dapsone PO
Serious and recurrent bacterial infections	Antibiotics targeting likely organism/s while considering local antimicrobial susceptibility patterns	>2 severe infections in a 1-year period	TMP-SMX 150/750 mg/m²/day in 2 divided doses PO daily *Alternative* IVIG 400 mg/kg every 2–4 weeks
Syphilis	*Congenital*: Aqueous crystalline penicillin G 50,000–75,000 units/kg given twice daily for 7 days, then thrice daily for the next 3 days If diagnosed after 1 month of age, then dose at 200,000–300,000 units/kg IV every 6 hrs for 10 days *Acquired*: Early stage-benzathine penicillin 50,000 units/kg (max: 2.4 million units) IM for one dose Late latent-same medication but give once weekly for 3 weeks Neurosyphilis-aqueous penicillin G 200,000–300,000 units/kg IV every 6 hrs (max: 18–24 million units/day) for 10–14 days	N/A	N/A
Toxoplasmosis	*Congenital*: Pyrimethamine (load with 2 mg/kg/day for 2 days, then 1 mg/kg/day for 2–6 months, then 1 mg/kg 3/week to complete 12 months total) and Sulfadiazine (50 mg/kg/dose twice daily) *Alternative* to sulfadiazine is clindamycin	Previous infection with toxoplasmosis IgG antibody to Toxoplasma and CD4%<15%	TMP-SMX 150/750 mg/m²/day in two divided doses PO daily *Alternative* Dapsone, pyrimethamine and leucovorin **OR** atovaquone *If prior toxoplasmic encephalitis* Sulfadiazine 85–120 mg/kg/day in 2–4 divided doses PO daily plus pyrimethamine 1-mg/kg PO daily plus leucovorin 5-mg PO every 3 days
Varicella zoster virus	*Chickenpox*: Moderate or severe immune suppression, high fever, or necrotic lesions:	Substantial exposure to VZV with no history of	Varicella zoster immune globulin 1.25 mL/10 kg

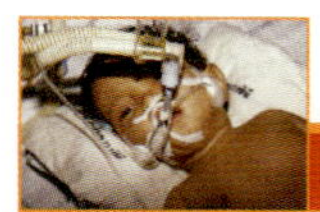

Table 54–4. (continued)

Treatment and Prophylaxis of Infections in HIV-Infected Children[44,45*]

Pathogen	Treatment	Indication for Prophylaxis	Prophylaxis
	Acyclovir 10 mg/kg IV three times daily for 7 days or until no new lesions have appeared for 48 hrs Mild immune suppression and mild disease: Acyclovir 20 mg/kg PO (max 800 mg/dose) four times daily for 7 days or until no new lesions have appeared for 48 hrs *Zoster*: Children with severe immune suppression, trigeminal nerve involvement or extensive multidermatomal zoster: Acyclovir 10 mg/kg IV three times daily for 7–10 days Children with mild immune suppression and mild disease: Acyclovir 20 mg/kg PO (max 800 mg/dose) four times daily for 7–10 days Alternative for patients not responding to acyclovir: Foscarnet 40–60 mg/kg IV three times daily for 7–10 days	chickenpox or shingles	(max 5 vials) intramuscularly, given within 48 to max of 96 hrs of exposure If not available, consider regular immune globulin

**Clinicians should consult the latest CDC guidelines to inform clinical care.*
†Safety of stopping secondary prophylaxis in children receiving HAART and with immune reconstitution has not been extensively studied.
TMP-SMX, trimethoprim-sulfamethoxazole; IV, intravenous; PO, by mouth; IM, intramuscular; GI, gastro-intestinal; VA, visual acuity; IVIG, intravenous immune globulin; N/A, not applicable.

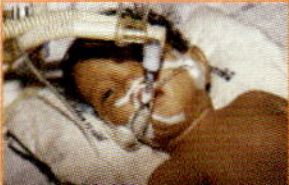

Table 54–5.

Selected Adverse Reactions of Antimicrobials, Antivirals, and Antifungals Recommended in Table 54–4

Medication Class	Medication	Adverse Reaction*
Antibiotics	TMP-SMX	Rash, bone marrow suppression, GI, interstitial nephritis
	Clarithromycin	GI upset, drug interactions
	Azithromycin	GI upset, ototoxicity, less drug interactions
	Ethambutol	Optic neuritis-monitor VA and color discrimination
	Rifabutin	↑cytochrome P3A activity → HAART drug interactions
	Penicillin	Pain at injection site, rash, hemolytic anemia, interstitial nephritis, hypersensitivity, anaphylaxis, Jarisch-Herxheimer reaction
Antivirals	Acyclovir	Renal, phlebitis, nausea, vomiting, rash, neutropenia in neonates
	Valacyclovir	Renal, thrombotic microangiopathy
	Ganciclovir	Myelosuppression, renal toxicity, CNS, GI, hepatitis, thrombophlebitis
	Foscarnet	Renal, electrolyte imbalances, elevated transaminases, CNS
	Podophyllin resin	Systemic absorption → nausea, vomiting or CNS effects
Antifungals	Amphotericin B	Infusion side effects, nephrotoxicity
	Fluconazole	GI, hepatitis, rash, alopecia
	Flucytosine	Bone marrow suppression, liver, GI, kidney, skin
	Itraconazole	GI, skin rash, elevated transaminases, thrombocytopenia, leucopenia
Antiparasitics	Pentamidine	Renal toxicity, arrhythmias, electrolyte abnormalities
	Nitazoxanide	GI upset, headache, yellow sclera
	Pyrimethamine	Rash including photosensitivity, nausea. Hematologic toxicity-supplement with leucovorin to minimize this
	Sulfadiazine	Rash including photosensitivity, fever, leucopenia, hepatitis, GI, crystalluria

**Medication adverse reactions refer to those seen more commonly.*
TMP-SMX, trimethoprim-sulfamethoxazole; GI, gastro-intestinal.

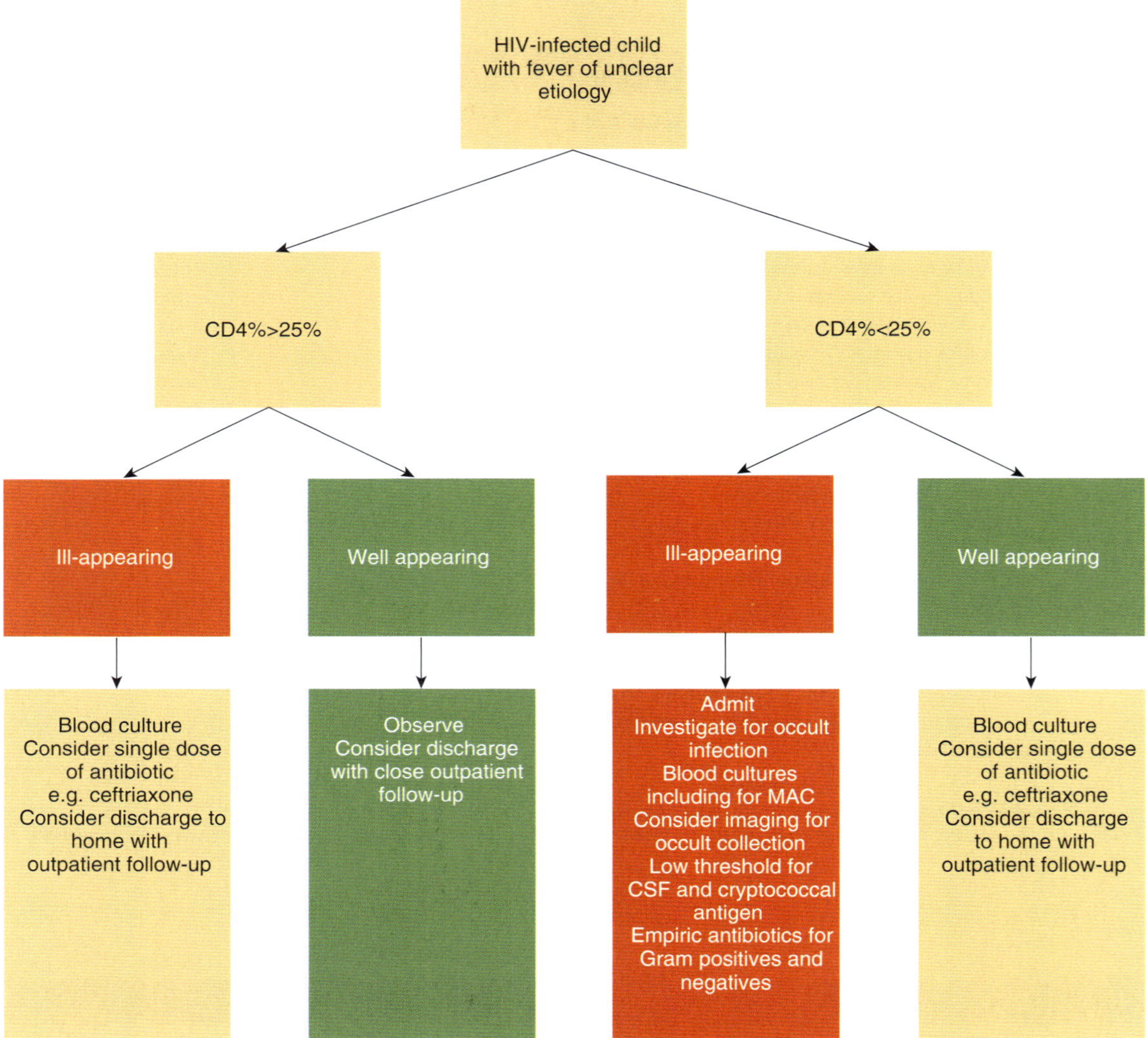

FIGURE 54–10 ■ Approach to the HIV-infected child with a fever of unknown cause. (*Note*: Given the complexity of management, this figure represents a broad guideline. Specific management often requires consultation with a pediatric HIV expert.)

Virulence and disease burden of the offending organism both play an important role in diseases course and prognosis. Invasive bacterial disease caused by pneumococcus or secondary group A streptococcal infection following chicken pox can both be rapidly fatal. More indolent infections, such as those caused by MAC or dermatophytes, generally follow a less fulminant course.

Prompt commencement of appropriate antimicrobial therapy impacts disease course and prognosis. Early consideration of drug interactions will ensure appropriate dosing. Once the patient is nearing discharge, attention to issues that may affect adherence will be time well spent.

PEARLS

1. The four most prevalent infections in the post-HAART era are bacterial pneumonia, herpes zoster, dermatophyte infections, and oral candidiasis.
2. In children with a $CD4^+$ T-lymphocyte count<100 cells/mL, PCP and MAC infection can be prevented in the majority of cases by using appropriate antimicrobial prophylaxis.
3. In the initial stages, signs and symptoms of cryptococcal meningitis are subtle requiring a high index of suspicion to make the diagnosis.
4. A high lactate dehydrogenase level is not specific for PCP—start treatment and organize a Bronchial Alveolar Lavage (BAL) to confirm the diagnosis.
5. For the latest guidelines on treating or preventing infections in HIV-infected children, visit http://aidsinfo.nih.gov/Guidelines and click on the appropriate, updated guideline.

REFERENCES

1. CDC. 1993 revised classification system for HIV infection and expanded surveillance case definition for AIDS among adolescents and adults. *MMWR Recomm Rep.* 1993;41(RR-17):1-19.
2. CDC. 1994 revised guidelines for the performance of CD4+ T-cell determinations in persons with human immunodeficiency virus (HIV) infections. Centers for Disease Control and Prevention. *MMWR Recomm Rep.* 1994;43(RR-3):1-21.
3. Dankner WM, Lindsey JC, Levin MJ. Correlates of opportunistic infections in children infected with the human immunodeficiency virus managed before highly active antiretroviral therapy. *Pediatr Infect Dis J.* 2001;20(1): 40-48.
4. Ylitalo N, Brogly S, Hughes MD, et al. Risk factors for opportunistic illnesses in children with human immunodeficiency virus in the era of highly active antiretroviral therapy. *Arch Pediatr Adolesc Med.* 2006;160(8): 778-787.
5. Gona P, Van Dyke RB, Williams PL, et al. Incidence of opportunistic and other infections in HIV-infected children in the HAART era. *JAMA.* 2006;296(3):292-300.
6. Borkowsky W, Steele CJ, Grubman S, Moore T, La Russa P, Krasinski K. Antibody responses to bacterial toxoids in children infected with human immunodeficiency virus. *J Pediatr.* 1987;110(4):563-566.
7. Ching N, Deville JG, Nielsen KA, et al. Cellular and humoral immune responses to a tetanus toxoid booster in perinatally HIV-1-infected children and adolescents receiving highly active antiretroviral therapy (HAART). *Eur J Pediatr.* 2007;166(1):51-56.
8. Clerici M, Stocks NI, Zajac RA, et al. Detection of three distinct patterns of T helper cell dysfunction in asymptomatic, human immunodeficiency virus-seropositive patients. Independence of CD4+ cell numbers and clinical staging. *J Clin Invest.* 1989;84(6):1892-1899.
9. Grossman Z, Meier-Schellersheim M, Sousa AE, Victorino RM, Paul WE. CD4+ T-cell depletion in HIV infection: are we closer to understanding the cause? *Nat Med.* 2002;8(4):319-323.
10. Hazenberg MD, Hamann D, Schuitemaker H, Miedema F. T cell depletion in HIV-1 infection: how CD4+ T cells go out of stock. *Nat Immunol.* 2000;1(4):285-289.
11. McCune JM. The dynamics of CD4+ T-cell depletion in HIV disease. *Nature.* 2001;410(6831):974-979.
12. Margolick JB, Munoz A, Donnenberg AD, et al. Failure of T-cell homeostasis preceding AIDS in HIV-1 infection. The Multicenter AIDS Cohort Study. *Nat Med.* 1995;1(7): 674-680.
13. Meyaard L, Otto SA, Jonker RR, Mijnster MJ, Keet RP, Miedema F. Programmed death of T cells in HIV-1 infection. *Science.* 1992;257(5067):217-219.
14. Roederer M, Dubs JG, Anderson MT, Raju PA, Herzenberg LA, Herzenberg LA. CD8 naive T cell counts decrease progressively in HIV-infected adults. *J Clin Invest.* 1995; 95(5): 2061-2066.
15. Holm GH, Gabuzda D. Distinct mechanisms of CD4+ and CD8+ T-cell activation and bystander apoptosis induced by human immunodeficiency virus type 1 virions. *J Virol.* 2005;79(10):6299-6311.
16. Douek DC, McFarland RD, Keiser PH, et al. Changes in thymic function with age and during the treatment of HIV infection. *Nature.* 1998;396(6712):690-695.
17. McKeating JA, McKnight A, Moore JP. Differential loss of envelope glycoprotein gp120 from virions of human immunodeficiency virus type 1 isolates: effects on infectivity and neutralization. *J Virol.* 1991;65(2):852-860.
18. Cao J, Park IW, Cooper A, Sodroski J. Molecular determinants of acute single-cell lysis by human immunodeficiency virus type 1. *J Virol.* 1996;70(3):1340-1354.
19. Badley AD, Dockrell DH, Algeciras A, et al. In vivo analysis of Fas/FasL interactions in HIV-infected patients. *J Clin Invest.* 1998;102(1):79-87.
20. Carbonari M, Cibati M, Pesce AM, et al. Frequency of provirus-bearing CD4+ cells in HIV type 1 infection correlates with extent of in vitro apoptosis of CD8+ but not of CD4+ cells. *AIDS Res Hum Retroviruses.* 1995;11(7): 789-794.
21. Finkel TH, Tudor-Williams G, Banda NK, et al. Apoptosis occurs predominantly in bystander cells and not in productively infected cells of HIV- and SIV-infected lymph nodes. *Nat Med.* 1995;1(2):129-134.
22. Katsikis PD, Wunderlich ES, Smith CA, Herzenberg LA, Herzenberg LA. Fas antigen stimulation induces marked apoptosis of T lymphocytes in human immunodeficiency virus-infected individuals. *J Exp Med.* 1995;181(6): 2029-2036.
23. Muro-Cacho CA, Pantaleo G, Fauci AS. Analysis of apoptosis in lymph nodes of HIV-infected persons. Intensity of apoptosis correlates with the general state of activation of the lymphoid tissue and not with stage of disease or viral burden. *J Immunol.* 1995;154(10):5555-5566.
24. Gougeon ML. Apoptosis as an HIV strategy to escape immune attack. *Nat Rev.* 2003;3(5):392-404.
25. Mohri H, Perelson AS, Tung K, et al. Increased turnover of T lymphocytes in HIV-1 infection and its reduction by antiretroviral therapy. *J Exp Med.* 2001;194(9):1277-1287.
26. Geleziunas R, Xu W, Takeda K, Ichijo H, Greene WC. HIV-1 Nef inhibits ASK1-dependent death signalling providing a potential mechanism for protecting the infected host cell. *Nature.* 2001;410(6830):834-838.
27. Stewart SA, Poon B, Song JY, Chen IS. Human immunodeficiency virus type 1 vpr induces apoptosis through caspase activation. *J Virol.* 2000;74(7):3105-3111.
28. Westendorp MO, Frank R, Ochsenbauer C, et al. Sensitization of T cells to CD95-mediated apoptosis by HIV-1 Tat and gp120. *Nature.* 1995;375(6531):497-500.
29. Herbein G, Van Lint C, Lovett JL, Verdin E. Distinct mechanisms trigger apoptosis in human immunodeficiency virus type 1-infected and in uninfected bystander T lymphocytes. *J Virol.* 1998;72(1):660-670.
30. Herbein G, Mahlknecht U, Batliwalla F, et al. Apoptosis of CD8+ T cells is mediated by macrophages through interaction of HIV gp120 with chemokine receptor CXCR4. *Nature.* 1998;395(6698):189-194.
31. Holm GH, Zhang C, Gorry PR, et al. Apoptosis of bystander T cells induced by human immunodeficiency virus type 1 with increased envelope/receptor affinity and coreceptor binding site exposure. *J Virol.* 2004;78(9): 4541-4551.
32. Jekle A, Keppler OT, De Clercq E, Schols D, Weinstein M, Goldsmith MA. In vivo evolution of human

immunodeficiency virus type 1 toward increased pathogenicity through CXCR4-mediated killing of uninfected CD4 T cells. *J Virol.* 2003;77(10):5846-5854.

33. Ohagen A, Ghosh S, He J, et al. Apoptosis induced by infection of primary brain cultures with diverse human immunodeficiency virus type 1 isolates: evidence for a role of the envelope. *J Virol.* 1999;73(2):897-906.
34. Vlahakis SR, Algeciras-Schimnich A, Bou G, et al. Chemokine-receptor activation by env determines the mechanism of death in HIV-infected and uninfected T lymphocytes. *J Clin Invest.* 2001;107(2):207-215.
35. Esser MT, Bess JW, Jr., Suryanarayana K, et al. Partial activation and induction of apoptosis in CD4(+) and CD8(+) T lymphocytes by conformationally authentic noninfectious human immunodeficiency virus type 1. *J Virol.* 2001;75(3):1152-1164.
36. Gottlieb GS, Sow PS, Hawes SE, et al. Equal plasma viral loads predict a similar rate of CD4+ T cell decline in human immunodeficiency virus (HIV) type 1- and HIV-2-infected individuals from Senegal, West Africa. *J Infect Dis.* 2002;185(7):905-914.
37. Race EM, Adelson-Mitty J, Kriegel GR, et al. Focal mycobacterial lymphadenitis following initiation of protease-inhibitor therapy in patients with advanced HIV-1 disease. *Lancet.* 1998;351(9098):252-255.
38. Steenhoff AP, Wood SM, Shah SS, Rutstein RM. Cutaneous Mycobacterium avium complex infection as a manifestation of the immune reconstitution syndrome in a human immunodeficiency virus-infected child. *Pediatr Infect Dis J.* 2007;26(8):755-757.
39. Vafai A, Berger M. Zoster in patients infected with HIV: a review. *Am J Med Sci.* 2001;321(6):372-380.
40. Wood SM, Shah SS, Steenhoff AP, Rutstein RM. Primary Varicella and Herpes Zoster Among HIV-Infected Children from 1989-2006. *Pediatrics.* 2008;121:e150-e156.
41. Perkins D, Chong H, Irvine B, Domagalski J. Genital co-infection with herpes simplex viruses type 1 and 2: Comparison of real-time PCR assay and traditional viral isolation methods. *J Cell Mol Med.* 2007;11(3):581-584.
42. Chuck SL, Sande MA. Infections with Cryptococcus neoformans in the acquired immunodeficiency syndrome. *N Engl JMed.* 1989;321(12):794-799.
43. Currie BP, Freundlich LF, Soto MA, Casadevall A. False-negative cerebrospinal fluid cryptococcal latex agglutination tests for patients with culture-positive cryptococcal meningitis. *J Clin Microbiol.* 1993;31(9):2519-2522.
44. CDC. Treating opportunistic infections among HIV-exposed and infected children: recommendations from CDC, theNational Institutes of Health, and the Infectious Diseases Society of America. *Morb Mortal Wkly Rep* 2004. 2004;53(No. RR-14).
45. CDC. Guidelines for preventing opportunistic infections among HIV-infected persons-2002 recommendations of the U.S. Public Health Service and the Infectious Diseases Society of America. *Morb Mortal Wkly Rep* 2002. 2002; 51(No. RR-8).
46. Sleasman JW, Hemenway C, Klein AS, Barrett DJ. Corticosteroids improve survival of children with AIDS and Pneumocystis carinii pneumonia. *Am J Dis Child* (1960). 1993;147(1):30-34.
47. Bye MR, Cairns-Bazarian AM, Ewig JM. Markedly reduced mortality associated with corticosteroid therapy of Pneumocystis carinii pneumonia in children with acquired immunodeficiency syndrome. *Arch Pediatr Adolesc Med.* 1994;148(6):638-641.
48. McLaughlin GE, Virdee SS, Schleien CL, Holzman BH, Scott GB. Effect of corticosteroids on survival of children with acquired immunodeficiency syndrome and Pneumocystis carinii-related respiratory failure. *J Pediatr.* 1995;126(5, pt 1):821-824.

CHAPTER 55

Preventing HIV Infection: Postexposure Prophylaxis

Richard M. Rutstein and Andrew Steenhoff

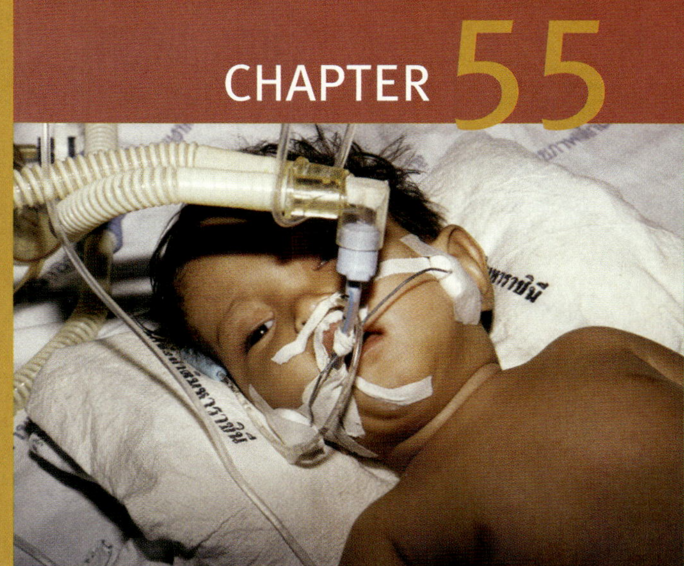

DEFINITIONS AND EPIDEMIOLOGY

Until an effective HIV vaccine is in widespread use, taming the HIV epidemic will require the prevention of exposure to the virus. Activities such as on-site rapid HIV testing with early treatment of infected persons, universal precaution training, safer sex education, and needle exchange programs all are important aspects of an effective preventative strategy. However, in cases where exposure has already occurred, it is possible to decrease the risk of transmission of HIV infection through the use of postexposure prophylaxis (PEP).

The best-documented success of HIV PEP has been through the prevention of maternal to child transmission. In the National Institutes of Health, U.S. Department of Health and Human Services funded Pediatric AIDS Clinical Trials Group 076 trial, a three-arm intervention with zidovudine (prenatal, intrapartum, and postpartum) decreased the risk of neonatal HIV infection from 21% to 8%.[1] Subsequent studies indicated that a significant part of the decrease in the transmission risk was based on the receipt of postnatal medication. In situations where mothers did not receive any prenatal antiretroviral therapy, the provision of antiretroviral medication to the HIV-exposed newborns within 48 hours of life decreased the risk of transmission by up to 50%.[2]

HIV-related PEP is now used routinely in hospitals following occupational exposure and in emergency departments following accidental or unprotected exposure to body fluids—termed nonoccupational exposure. It is important for all health care providers to be aware of current PEP recommendations, and to know how to rapidly access such information and/or consultation. This chapter will discuss HIV PEP as it relates to occupational and nonoccupational exposure to HIV.

OCCUPATIONAL PEP

Through June 2000, the Centers for Disease Control of the U.S. Department of Health and Human Services reported 56 cases of HIV infection in health care workers (HCWs) documented to follow occupational exposure, with an additional 138 possible cases.[3] The risk of occupational exposure to potentially infectious body fluid is highest among surgical staff, followed by nonsurgical nurses (especially those in the Emergency Department), phlebotomists, and resident physicians. General surgeons report an average of 4 intraoperative percutaneous injuries per year.[4] Among pediatric residents, 13–70% report at least one needle stick exposure per year.[5,6]

The risk of transmission of HIV from a single percutaneous injury from a contaminated needle is approximately 1 in 300 (0.3%) (Table 55–1).[7] An increased risk of transmission has been associated with exposures to patients with late stage HIV infection/AIDS, hollow bore needles, a deep puncture wound, and blood observed in the involved needle.[8,9] The risk of transmission of HIV from nonpercutaneous exposures is much less. For exposure to bloody fluid across mucus membranes, the risk is estimated to be less than 1/1000 (0.1%), and even less when the exposure is across intact skin.

The interest in using antiretroviral agents in an attempt to abort HIV infection following exposure arose from animal studies. In these studies, there was some evidence of protection through the administration of

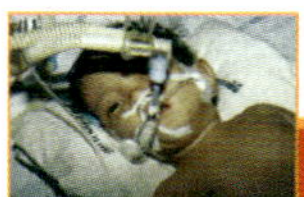

Table 55–1.

Estimated Risk of Transmission of HIV Based on Exposure

Exposure	Risk (%)	Per 1000 Encounters
Transfusion of HIV+blood	90	900
Needle sharing	0.6	6
Receptive anal sex	0.5	5
Needle stick, occupational	0.3	3
Receptive vaginal sex	0.1	1
Insertive anal sex	0.07	0.7
Insertive vaginal sex	0.05	0.5
Receptive oral sex	0.01	0.1

For maternal–child transmission, the risk is 13–25%, excluding breast-feeding. The risk of breast-feeding 14–29% based on time of maternal infection, and length of breast-feeding: 0.7% per month up to age 5 months, 0.6% 6–11 months and 0.3% per month thereafter (therefore, at time of greatest risk, 7/1000 per month, or 2/1000 per day breast-feeding, or approximately 0.5–0.3/1000 each episode of feeding)[1,25–29]

Adapted from MMWR 2005;54(No. RR-2):1-20.[20]

zidovudine if given immediately after exposure to retroviral infections.[10,11]

The Centers for Disease Control of the U.S. Department of Health and Human Services performed a retrospective case-control study of HCWs with occupational exposure to known HIV-infected blood. Many of the HCWs had received zidovudine for PEP. The results showed an 81% decrease in the risk of transmission if the employee received zidovudine.[9] With these results, and the proven success of zidovudine and other agents in maternal to child transmission prevention trials, the use of PEP for high-risk occupational exposures has become the standard of care.

When evaluating an employee with an exposure to blood or other potentially infectious body fluid, the immediate task is an assessment of the risk involved with the exposure (Table 55–1). The exposure must be categorized as to its potential for transmission of HIV. As noted, deep injury from visibly contaminated blood carries the highest risk of transmission of HIV. In contrast, mucus membrane exposure to nonbloody body fluids carries a much lower risk, and exposure across intact skin does not carry a risk of HIV-infection.

Of equal importance is whether or not the source patient is known to be HIV-infected. If the patient's serostatus is unknown, efforts should be made to immediately obtain HIV testing, consistent with existing local policies on testing and consent. The use of HIV rapid assays for testing of the source patient can result in cost savings (through decreased medications dispensed to exposed HCWs) and alleviating emotional stress, as it allows for immediate discontinuation of PEP should the source patient test negative. For exposures where the patient's status is unknown, and testing is not possible, an assessment must be made of the potential HIV risk status of the source patient, based on local HIV seroprevalence.

NONOCCUPATIONAL PEP (nPEP)

Epidemiology

In urban emergency departments, the most common scenario for consideration of nPEP involves a patient presenting for evaluation following a high-risk sexual encounter, consensual or not. Again, the first issue is to assess the degree of risk, based on exposure characteristics (Table 55–1). In instances where one partner is known to be HIV infected, the risk of anal intercourse is higher than for vaginal intercourse. Receptive anal intercourse with an HIV-infected partner carries an estimated risk of HIV transmission of 0.3–0.5%. Vaginal intercourse carries a risk estimated at one-tenth that of anal sex (0.03–0.09%), with receptive partners more at risk than the insertive partner. Oral sex is associated with a minimal, but not zero, risk of transmission. Intercourse during menses, and traumatic intercourse, as in cases of sexual assault, carry an increased risk of transmission.

For the pediatrician, the consideration of nPEP is generally in relation to exposures from common childhood behaviors, such as biting between children, or puncture wounds from discarded needles found on playgrounds. Although in certain conditions viable virus can be recovered from 8% of syringes and needles up to 21 days later, the risk is quite low. To date there have been no cases of documented transmission of HIV from puncture wounds from discarded needles.

There are several cases of purported transmission of HIV through biting or other in-home exposures, but there are no well-documented cases of HIV transmission between children through biting. HIV is rarely isolated from the saliva, and there are inhibitory molecules in saliva that reduce infectivity, therefore the risk of transmitting HIV through biting is believed to be extremely low. The few cases of in-household nonsexual transmission of HIV have involved direct exposure to infected blood.

In a pediatric hospital setting, inadvertent exposure to breast milk may occur as well, through the inadvertent offering of stored breast milk to the wrong infant. A meta-analysis of prospective cohort studies estimated the risk of transmission of HIV-1 through breast-feeding in infancy as 16%.[12] The risk increases with longer duration of breast-feeding, high maternal viral load, the presence of mastitis and mixed formula and breast-feeding.[13] However, the risk from a single feeding of infected breast milk is quite low, estimated to be 1–4/100,000. In addition, in the United States most women are HIV-tested during pregnancy and, if HIV-infected, strongly instructed to avoid breast-feeding. The likelihood, therefore, that a breast-feeding woman is HIV-infected, and that a one time exposure to her milk will transmit HIV, is minimal.

In the Emergency Department, or the Pediatric office, the first step in assessing the need for nPEP is in evaluating the significance of the exposure, as the risk of transmission of HIV varies greatly based on the type of exposure (Table 55–1). The risk is highest following transfusion of HIV-infected blood, where up to 90% of recipients will convert to HIV positive status. Other common exposures carry a risk of infection ranging from 13% to 25%, for perinatal exposure in the absence of breast-feeding, to 0.01% (for receptive oral sexual encounters).

TREATMENT OF A SIGNIFICANT EXPOSURE

PEP is recommended for exposures with a significant risk of HIV transmission and should be started as soon as possible after the exposure (Tables 55–2 and 55–3). It must be stressed, however, that for occupational as well as nPEP this must be done in consultation with experts after a detailed analysis of the characteristics of each individual case. In occupational settings, procedures should be in place to allow for administration of the first dose within hours of exposure. If the mode of exposure is significant, initiation of PEP should not be delayed while the source patient is tested. From animal and case review studies, treatment started 48–72 hours after exposure is much less likely to be effective. If HIV testing of the source patient does occur postexposure, ideally by rapid assay methods, PEP therapy can be discontinued if the results are negative.

Employees should have a baseline HIV antibody drawn, along with hepatitis B surface antibody (to confirm immune status) and hepatitis C antibody (Figure 55–1). Treatment should not be delayed while waiting to obtain or receive the results of baseline blood tests.

Current guidelines recommend a two or three-drug regimen given for 4 weeks. There is no evidence that a three-drug regimen for PEP is more efficacious than a two-drug regimen. However, based on results from HIV-infected adult and pediatric treatment trials, three-drug regimens result in more rapid and prolonged suppression of viral replication than two-drug regimens. Theoretically, three-drug regimens might offer an increased chance of efficacy. The difficulty is that adherence to three-drug regimens is much more difficult than to two-drug regimens, related to the increased toxicity associated with the most common third agents employed. All antiretroviral agents have side effects, and

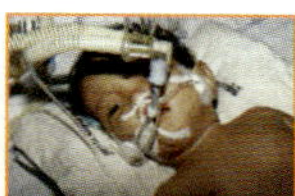

Table 55–2.

Assessment of Risk*

Risk of HIV Infection in Source Patient	
Highest Risk:	Known to be HIV infected Late stage illness, high viral load
Intermediate Risk:	Unknown HIV status, but known risk factors (e.g., discarded needle found in area of high injecting drug use)
Low Risk:	Unknown HIV status, no known risk factors
Significance of Exposure	
Highest Risk:	Percutaneous needle injury, concentrated viral sample (e.g., laboratory injury from HIV+ patient blood specimen Percutaneous needle injury, hollow bore) Receptive anal intercourse Sharing injecting drug equipment
Intermediate Risk:	Injury from suture or lancet Other forms of intercourse Exposure to infected blood across nonintact skin, mucus membranes
Low Risk:	Oral sex One time exposure to breast milk Wounds from discarded needles on playground
No Known Risk:	Bites, without blood/significant trauma Exposure to nonblood containing body fluids such as urine, stool, tears, saliva Exposure to blood across intact skin Kissing, sharing utensils

**PEP is recommended for high-risk exposures, from known HIV positive, or at-risk, source. PEP should be considered for all other exposures on a case by case basis.*

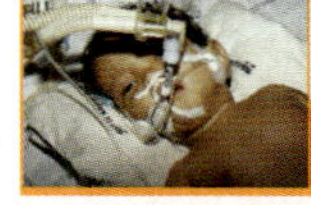

Table 55–3.

Drugs Frequently Used for PEP

NRTI	NNRTI	PI
Zidovudine (AZT, ZDV)	Efavirenz	Lopinavir/ritonavir
Lamivudine (3TC)		Nelfinavir
Tenofovir*		Atazanavir*
Emtriva (FTC)		
Stavudine (d4T)		
Didanosine (ddI)		

**Drugs without pediatric formulation and/or no dosing information available*
NRTI, nucleoside analog reverse transcriptase inhibitors; NNRTI, nonnucleoside analog reverse transcriptase inhibitor; PI, protease inhibitors.

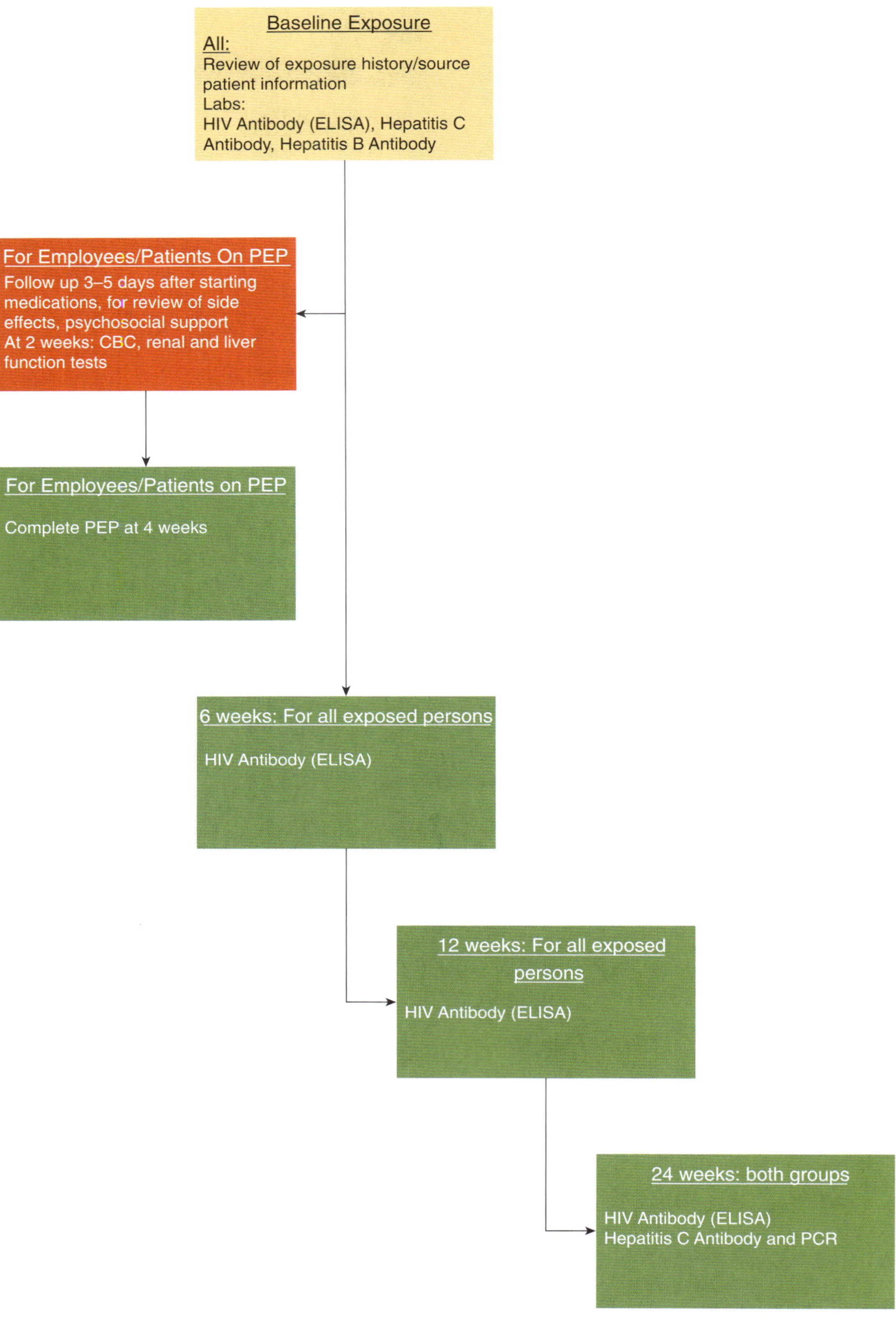

FIGURE 55-1 ■ Testing and follow-up for significant exposures. (PEP, postexposure prophylaxis; HIV, human immunodeficiency virus; ELISA, enzyme linked immunosorbent assay; PCR, polymerase chain reaction.)

there is a high rate of discontinuation associated with three-drug regimens, particularly those containing a protease inhibitor (PI). This dilemma, the potential for more pronounced side effects, has to be balanced with the potentially increased efficacy, and should be discussed with both the patient and parents.[14,15]

The choice of antiretroviral agents for PEP must be individualized, and is best done in consultation with an HIV treatment specialist. Emergency departments and hospital employee health offices must be able to dispense a starter supply of medications, based on usual prescribing patterns, but then the treatment regimen should be reviewed as soon as possible with treatment experts.

The selection of the PEP regimen is more complicated when the source patient or partner is known to be HIV-infected, and on treatment. Ideally, when selecting a treatment regimen for PEP, the source patient will be naïve to at least two of the agents used to treat the exposed person.

Most treatment experts recommend a minimum of two nucleoside reverse transcriptase (NRTI) agents, most commonly zidovudine and lamivudine, each given twice daily. For older children and adolescents, the two drugs come in a coformulated tablet (Combivir). For the younger-aged child, they are available in suspension form with a reasonably palatable taste. Alternative NRTI agents include stavudine and didanosine (although not given together, as a result of overlapping toxicities). Abacavir is not recommended for PEP because of its high rate of early hypersensitivity reactions.

Tenofovir is widely used for adults, and in animal studies had a high rate of success in experimental PEP trials.[16] However, tenofovir is not yet approved for those younger than 18 years, and is only available in tablet form. For those older than 18 years, the combination of a once daily tablet coformulation of tenofovir and emtriva is one of the preferred regimens.

Prescribing physicians must balance the risk of transmission versus risk of side effects from therapy. At times enhanced potency of three-drug regimens is offset by the increased risk of side effects leading to patients discontinuing therapy prematurely. Some authors feel that the optimal strategy to modify the risk of transmission is to recommend a two-drug regimen for improved compliance and follow-up.

When constructing a three-drug regimen, the U.S. Public Health Service recommends adding a PI. Among the PIs, lopinavir/ritonavir is the preferred agent. However, its' use is associated with significant gastrointestinal side effects. In addition, the pediatric liquid formulation is significantly unpalatable. Nelfinavir is a PI available as both a powder and tablet. In very young infants and children, however, it requires 3-times-a-day dosing. Atazanavir is a newly released PI, taken once daily, with minimal gastrointestinal side effects (with the exception of asymptomatic elevations of total bilirubin levels). Although available only in capsule formulation at this time, it is expected a powder formulation will be available by 2009.

One alternative to a PI-based three-drug regimen would be using the nonnucleoside reverse transcriptase inhibitor (NNRTI), efavirenz. Efavirenz has an easy dosing schedule, one tablet, once daily. For infants and children, the small capsules can be sprinkled on food. However, in primate drug trails, efavirenz was associated with a high rate of birth defects, so it should not be used in women of childbearing potential. Nevirapine, the other widely used NNRTI, has been associated with severe hepatic toxicity, including several cases of liver failure, when included in PEP regimens.

In recent years, many practitioners have used a three-drug nucleoside and nucleotide regimen, generally zidovudine, lamivudine and tenofovir. In 2001, the New York State Department of Health AIDS Institute issued new guidelines that listed this combination as the preferred regimen for PEP. The rationale for this approach included the efficacy noted in primate studies, the ease of administration and low incidence of side effects, compared to NRTI–PI or NRTI–NNRTI combinations. Despite the expectation that this would be a relatively well-tolerated regimen, one center reported that for the initial 65 patients prescribed the zidovudine/lamuvidine/tenofovir combination for nPEP or oPEP, 66% complained of nausea, and 25% of emesis.[17] In contrast, a study from Australia found a better 28-day completion rate for nPEP (85%) using a tenofovir, stavudine and lamuvidine regimen, with a 23% incidence of nausea.[18]

FOLLOW-UP

PEP always follows stressful events, whether related to occupational or nonoccupational exposures. Follow-up measures should include provision or referral for psychological support services. Sexually active adolescents and adults must be cautioned about the potential for transmission of newly acquired HIV through sexual contact. Because of the teratogenic potential of PEP regimens, women of childbearing potential should use reliable birth control contraception during treatment.

Once PEP is prescribed, patients should be carefully monitored for side effects (Figure 55–1). More than 50% of those on PEP report side effects, with gastrointestinal symptoms and general fatigue the most common. Among HCWs prescribed oPEP, more than 20% fail to complete the 28-day regimen, most commonly from medication side effects.

During the 28-day PEP regimen, ideally the patient's blood counts and chemistries should be monitored at baseline, 2 weeks and 4 weeks.

Box 55–1. Online Resources

1. The Centers for Disease Control Guidelines can be accessed at www.cdc.gov/hiv/resources/guidelines/index.htm
2. HIV Guidelines, New York State Department of Health AIDS Institute can be accessed at www.hivguidelines.org/
3. The U.S. Department of Health and Human Services (HHS) issues guidelines documents for the medical management of HIV infection and issues surrounding HIV infection can be accessed at www.aidsinfo.nih.gov/guidelines/

Testing for HIV infection should be by antibody, and not by direct viral methods such as HIV DNA or RNA assays. The DNA and RNA assays have false positive rates of 1–2%, which generally exceeds the risk of infection in the exposed patient. Antibody testing should be performed at 6 weeks, 12 weeks, and 24 weeks postexposure. Although recent data from one study group suggests that virtually all infected patients will seroconvert to antibody positive status by 12 weeks following exposure,[19] the present guidelines recommend testing at least through 24 weeks postexposure.[20]

It is important to realize that there have been failures of PEP both for occupational and nonoccupational exposure.[21] Through 2005, there have been at least six cases of transmission of HIV among HCWs despite PEP. When following patients post exposure, providers must be attuned to symptoms of acute retroviral syndrome. Although nonspecific, symptoms noted in 70% or more of patients with the acute retroviral syndrome include fever, adenopathy, pharyngitis and rash.[22] Should these occur, urgent consultation with an HIV treatment specialist is necessary for evaluation and management.

Among adolescents and adults receiving nPEP for sexual assault there is a very high rate of failure to complete the prescribed 28-day therapy. Of the 97 patients referred from two emergency departments in Boston for follow-up, only 37 (38%) made at least one follow-up visit, and only 16% finished 28 days of PEP. Almost half of the patients reported an adverse event from the medication.[23] In a study form Vancouver, 71 of 258 sexual assault victims were prescribed nPEP regimens, but only eight patients completed a 4-week course of therapy and follow-up visits.[24] The reasons for poor compliance with prescribed regimens and scheduled follow-up visits were multifactorial, but illustrate the difficulties in implementing successful nPEP programs.

Emergency departments and hospital employee health divisions must have established policies to provide immediate assessment, support, and treatment to employees and patients with potentially significant exposures to HIV. The treatment of HIV is a rapidly evolving area, even in this third decade of the epidemic. Providers must remain current with new treatment guidelines, and be able to access up-to-date changes. Online references are invaluable, as treatment options are always expanding (Box 55–1).[20]

REFERENCES

1. Connor EM, Sperling RS, Gelber R, et al. Reduction of maternal-infant transmission of human immunodeficiency virus type 1 with zidovudine treatment. Pediatric AIDS Clinical Trials Group Protocol 076 Study Group. *N Engl J Med.* 1994;331(18):1173-1180.
2. Wade NA, Birkhead GS, Warren BL, et al. Abbreviated regimens of zidovudine prophylaxis and perinatal transmission of the human immunodeficiency virus. *N Engl J Med.* 1998;339(20):1409-1414.
3. Updated U.S. Public Health Service Guidelines for the management of occupational exposures to HBV, HCV, and HIV and recommendations for postexposure prophylaxis. *MMWR Recomm Rep.* 2001;50(RR-11):1-52.
4. Leentvaar-Kuijpers A, Dekker MM, Coutinho RA, et al. Needlestick injuries, surgeons, and HIV risks. *Lancet.* 1990;335(8688):546-547.
5. Melzer SM, Vermund SH, Shelov SP. Needle injuries among pediatric housestaff physicians in New York city. *Pediatrics.* 1989;84(2):211-214.
6. Pettit LL, Gee SQ, Begue RE. Epidemiology of sharp object injuries in a children's hospital. *Pediatr Infect Dis J.* 1997;16(11):1019-1023.
7. Henderson DK, Fahey BJ, Willy ME, et al. Risk for occupational transmission of human immunodeficiency virus type 1 (HIV-1) associated with clinical exposures. A prospective evaluation. *Ann Intern Med.* 1990;113(10):740-746.
8. Case-control study of HIV seroconversion in health-care workers after percutaneous exposure to HIV-infected blood–France, United Kingdom, and United States, January 1988-August 1994. *MMWR Morb Mortal Wkly Rep.* 1995;44(50):929-933.
9. Cardo DM, Culver DH, Ciesielski CA, et al. A case-control study of HIV seroconversion in health care workers after percutaneous exposure. Centers for Disease Control and Prevention Needlestick Surveillance Group. *N Engl J Med.* 1997;337(21):1485-1490.
10. Ruprecht RM, O'Brien LG, Rosson LD, Nusinoff-Lehrman S. Suppression of mouse viraemia and retroviral disease by 3'-azido-3'-deoxythymidine. *Nature.* 1986;323(6087):467-469.
11. Tavares L, Roneker C, Johnston K, et al. 3'-Azido-3'-deoxythymidine in feline leukemia virus-infected cats: a model for therapy and prophylaxis of AIDS. *Cancer Res.* 1987;47(12):3190-3194.
12. John GC, Richardson BA, Naduati RW, Mbori-Ngacha D, Kreiss JK, Timing of breast milk HIV-1 transmission: a meta analysis. *East Afr Med J.* 2001;78(2):75-79.
13. Read JS. Human milk, breastfeeding, and transmission of human immunodeficiency virus type 1 in the United States. American Academy of Pediatrics Committee on Pediatric AIDS. *Pediatrics.* 2003;112(5):1196-1205.
14. Bassett IV, Freedberg KA, Walensky RP. Two drugs or three? Balancing efficacy, toxicity, and resistance in postexposure

prophylaxis for occupational exposure to HIV. *Clin Infect Dis.* 2004;39(3):395-401.

15. Panlilio AL, Cardo DM, Grohskopf LA, et al. Updated U.S. Public Health Service guidelines for the management of occupational exposures to HIV and recommendations for postexposure prophylaxis. *MMWR Recomm Rep.* 2005; 54(RR–9):1-17.
16. Otten RA, Smith DK, Adams DR, et al. Efficacy of postexposure prophylaxis after intravaginal exposure of pig-tailed macaques to a human-derived retrovirus (human immunodeficiency virus type 2). *J Virol.* 2000;74(20): 9771-9775.
17. Luque A, Hulse S, Wang D, et al. Assessment of adverse events associated with antiretroviral regimens for postexposure prophylaxis for occupational and nonoccupational exposures to prevent transmission of human immunodeficiency virus. *Infect Control Hosp Epidemiol.* 2007;28(6): 695-701.
18. Winston A, McAllister J, Amin J, Cooper DA, Carr A. The use of a triple nucleoside-nucleotide regimen for nonoccupational HIV post exposure prophylaxis. *HIV Med.* 2005;6:191-197.
19. Lindback S, et al. Diagnosis of primary HIV-1 infection and duration of follow-up after HIV exposure. Karolinska institute primary HIV infection study group. *AIDS.* 2000; 14(15):2333-2339.
20. Centers for Disease Control and Prevention. Antiretroviral postexposure prophylaxis after sexual, injection-drug use, or other nonoccupational exposure to HIV in the United States: recommendations from the U.S. Department of Health and Human Services. *MMWR Recomm Rep.* 2005;54(RR–2):1-20.
21. Roland ME, Neilands TB, Krone MR, et al. Seroconversion following nonoccupational postexposure prophylaxis against HIV. *Clin Infect Dis.* 2005;41(10):1507-1513.
22. Hecht FM, Busch MP, Rawal B, et al. Use of laboratory tests and clinical symptoms for identification of primary HIV infection. *AIDS.* 2002;16:1119-1129.
23. Olshen E, Hsu K, Woods ER, et al. Use of human immunodeficiency virus postexposure prophylaxis in adolescent sexual assault victims. *Arch Pediatr Adolesc Med.* 2006;160(7):674-680.
24. Wiebe ER, Comay SE, McGregor M, Ducceschi S. Offering HIV prophylaxis to people who have been sexually assaulted: 16 months' experience in a sexual assault service. *CMAJ.* 2000;162(5):641-645.
25. Miotti PG, Taha TE, Kumwenda NI, et al. HIV transmission through breastfeeding: a study in malawi. *JAMA.* 1999;282(8):744-749.
26. Coutsoudis A, Dabis F, Fawzi W, et al. Late postnatal transmission of HIV-1 in breast-fed children: an individual patient data meta-analysis. *J Infect Dis.* 2004;189(12): 2154-2166.
27. Gray RH, Wawer MJ, Brookmeyer R, et al. Probability of HIV-1 transmission per coital act in monogamous, heterosexual, HIV-1-discordant couples in Rakai, Uganda. *Lancet.* 2001;357(9263):1149-1153.
28. Dunn D, Newell ML, Ades AE, Peckham CS. Risk of human immunodeficiency virus type 1 transmission through breastfeeding. *Lancet.* 1992;340:585-588.
29. Van de Perre P. Postnatal transmission of human immunodeficiency virus type 1: the breast-feeding dilemma. *Am J Obstet Gynecol.* 1995;173:483-487.

SECTION 15

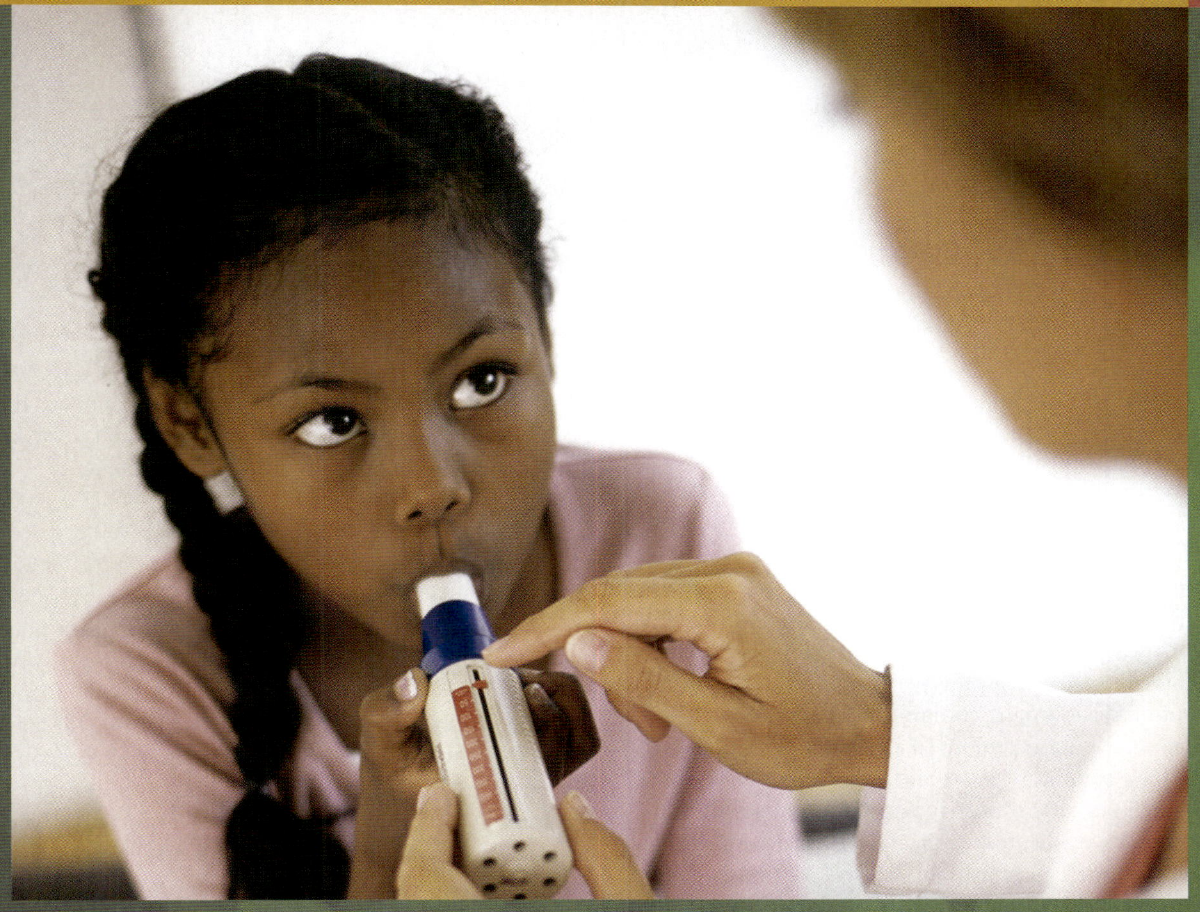

Infections Complicating Chronic Diseases

CHAPTER 56

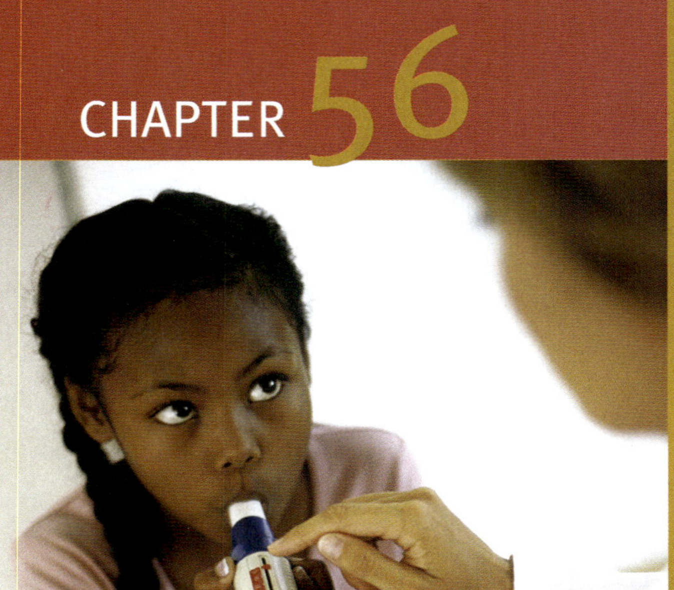

Infections in Children with Tracheostomy

Jay Berry, Shannon Manzi, and Laura Hammitt

INTRODUCTION

Tracheotomy is one of the most common surgical airway procedures performed in children. Approximately 5000 children undergo tracheotomy each year.[1] In the past, tracheotomy was predominately performed in older children with acute upper airway compromise secondary to infection such as epiglottitis and croup.[2] Currently, these acute upper airway infections represent less than 5% of tracheotomy performed in children.[1,3] Tracheotomy is now more commonly being performed in children who require prolonged mechanical ventilation or who have significant anatomic rather than infectious causes of upper airway obstruction. The changes in the indications for tracheotomy reflect the extended survival of children born prematurely as well as those with chronic underlying illnesses such as neuromuscular disease and congenital anomalies.[2–4] These underlying illnesses influence the etiology of tracheotomy-related infections encountered in children. This chapter focuses on the childhood tracheotomy-related infections of stoma cellulitis, tracheitis, and bacterial pneumonia.

TRACHEOSTOMY STOMA CELLULITIS

Definition and Epidemiology

Tracheostomy stoma cellulitis is a bacterial infection of the epidermis lining of the tracheostomy opening. It is a dangerous infection that, if untreated, can spread contiguously through the tracheostomy site into the trachea or into the deep tissues of the neck and mediastinum. In the past, stoma infections occurred approximately in one-third of patients undergoing surgical tracheotomy placement.[5] In more recent studies the rates of stoma infection have been significantly lower, ranging from 0% to 3%.[6,7]

Pathogenesis

There is limited information on the pathogens responsible for tracheostomy stoma cellulitis. It appears that the bacteria colonizing the granulation tissue surrounding the tracheostomy cause most cases of stoma cellulitis. The epithelial granulation tissue lining the tracheostomy site is colonized with bacteria by direct contact with the bacterial flora of the surrounding skin. Polymicrobial colonization has been reported in the majority of tracheostomy granulation tissue specimens, with a mixture of gram-positive, gram-negative, and anaerobic bacteria. Approximately 6 bacteria are detected in each granulation tissue specimen sent for culture.[8,9] The bacteria most frequently recovered from granulation tissue culture include alpha-hemolytic streptococci, *Staphylococcus aureus*, *Peptostreptococcus* species, *Bacteroides* species, *Fusobacterium* species, and *Pseudomonas aeruginosa*.[9,10] Most isolates produced beta-lactamase, including all isolates of *S. aureus* and *Bacteroides* species.[9]

The tracheostomy tube itself may also become colonized as it provides a portal of entry from the outside directly into the normally sterile trachea. Tracheostomy tubes are typically composed of plastic, with differing degrees of flexibility depending on the specific type of material (i.e., silicone or polyvinyl chloride). Bacteria with a polysaccharide shell can bond to the surface of a tracheostomy tube lumen, forming organized matrices of bacterial colonies. The colonies are often referred to as biofilm.[11] The longer that a tracheostomy tube is used, the more likely that it will develop biofilm.

The bacteria that most frequently colonize the tracheostomy tube include *S. aureus* and *P. aeruginosa.*[12] Exposure to these pathogens likely occurs in the hospital. Most children undergo tracheotomy in an intensive care setting. Pretracheotomy intubation times may exceed more than 1 month[4,13,14] while overall hospital lengths of stay associated with tracheotomy placement may exceed 50 days.[1] This significant nosocomial exposure provides ample opportunity for colonization with flora endemic to the intensive care unit setting.

Although many of the bacterial species that colonize granulation tissue and tracheostomy tubes are considered normal skin flora and are typically nonpathogenic, others can cause clinically significant infection. The most common bacterial pathogens believe to be responsible for tracheostomy stoma cellulitis include group A β-hemolytic streptococci, *S. aureus,* and *P. aeruginosa* in addition to various anaerobic bacteria. Additionally, *candida* species may also be responsible for tracheostomy stoma cellulitis

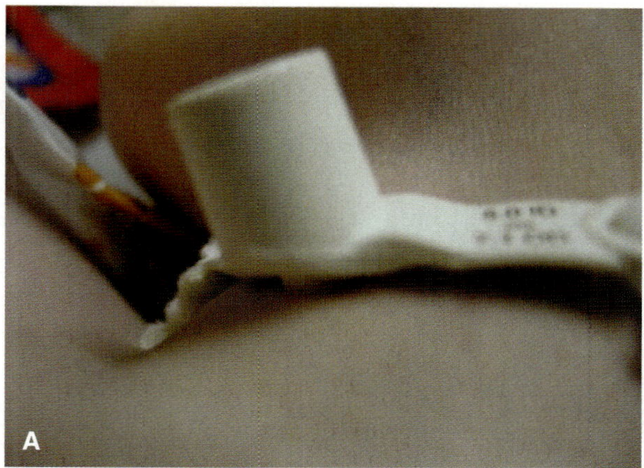

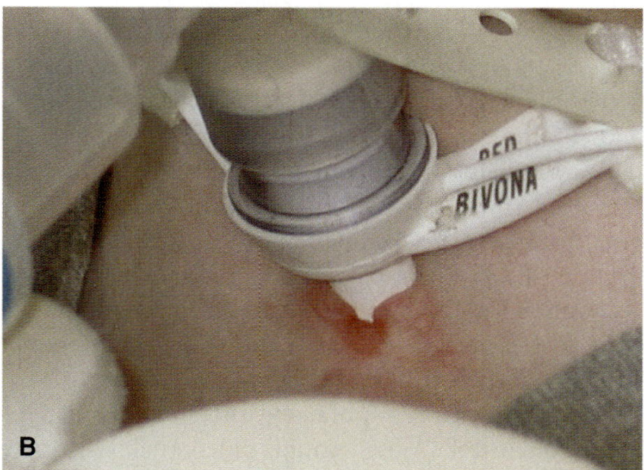

FIGURE 56–1 ■ **(A)** Healthy stoma with no visible granulation tissue; **(B)** Healthy stoma with noninfected granulation tissue.

Clinical Presentation

On history, parents of children with tracheotomy who have stoma cellulitis will commonly report a change in color of the granulation tissue of the tracheostomy stoma from pink to red. This redness may spread circumferentially throughout the skin surrounding the tracheostomy. Foul-smelling, yellow/green drainage and bleeding at the site have also been reported. The infection may be accompanied by a history of fever, malaise, overall discomfort, and localized pain.

On physical examination, children may be febrile, tachycardic, and ill-appearing. Frank erythema, edema, and/or induration of the skin surrounding the tracheostomy site may be observed. Bleeding may be present. The skin may also feel warm to the touch. Purulent exudate may be visualized emerging from the stoma tissue. Supraclavicular and cervical lymphadenopathy may be palpable. Confluent papular erythema with erythematous satellite papules may be present with candidal tracheostomy cellulitis.

Differential Diagnosis

Noninfected, healthy granulation tissue or fibrous scar tissue is commonly mistaken for cellulitis. Most children with tracheotomy will likely develop pink granulation stoma epithelium to some degree (Figure 56–1). Characteristics that distinguish health stoma granulation tissue from stoma cellulitis are shown in Table 56–1. Stoma cellulitis is unlikely in the presence of exudate without other clinical features of infection.

Superficial stoma cellulitis should also be differentiated from the extremely rare but life-threatening deep tissue infections such as cervical necrotizing fasciitis and mediastinitis.[15] In these deep tissue infections, the erythema may progress rapidly; the patient is often ill-appearing with systemic signs of toxicity.[16] In cases with cervical necrotizing fasciitis, the skin may appear gray, green, or purple. Subcutaneous emphysema may also be observed.[16] Mediastinitis is difficult to recognize early; however, significant respiratory distress or even respiratory failure will likely be present.[17] Patients who have undergone tracheotomy in relation to cardiac surgery are at increased risk for deep-tissue infection.[18]

Diagnosis

Tracheostomy stoma cellulitis is a clinical diagnosis. Laboratory and radiographic diagnostic tests are not

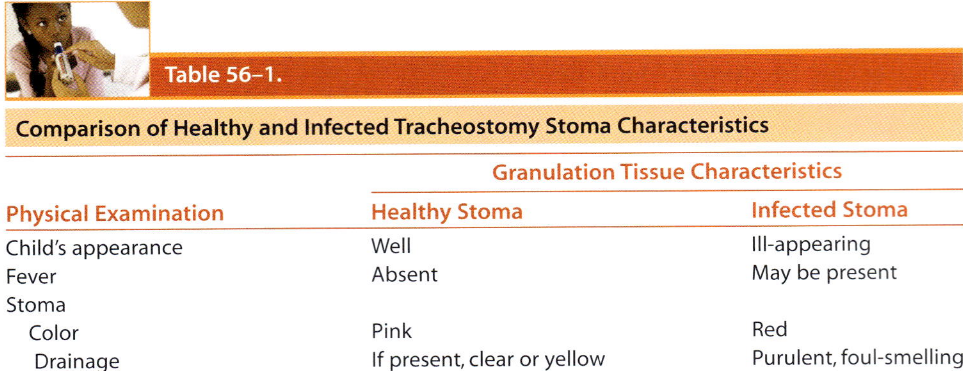

Table 56–1.

Comparison of Healthy and Infected Tracheostomy Stoma Characteristics

	Granulation Tissue Characteristics	
Physical Examination	**Healthy Stoma**	**Infected Stoma**
Child's appearance	Well	Ill-appearing
Fever	Absent	May be present
Stoma		
Color	Pink	Red
Drainage	If present, clear or yellow	Purulent, foul-smelling
Bleeding	Rare	Common

helpful in making the diagnosis but may help guide empiric antibiotic therapy and facilitate early detection of complications such as deep-tissue infection. Gram stain and culture from the tracheotomy stoma tissue or exudates may help identify potential causative pathogens. However, since polymicrobial colonization of healthy granulation tissue is common, the presence of bacteria in a culture alone does not necessarily indicate cellulitis. We recommend that Gram stain and culture be obtained prior to treatment as a guide to antibiotic therapy, rather than as a diagnostic indicator of stoma cellulitis.

The diagnostic role of blood inflammatory markers (white blood cell [WBC] count, differential, C-reactive protein, etc.) has not been evaluated in children with tracheostomy stoma bacterial infections. WBC counts less than 15,400 cells/mm^3 have a negative predictive value of 99% excluding necrotizing fasciitis in adult patients with stoma cellulitis.[19] Chest radiography or magnetic resonance imaging provide evidence of deep-tissue infection such as subcutaneous emphysema (on radiograph or magnetic resonance imaging) and fascia inflammation or abscess formation (on magnetic resonance imaging).

Treatment

Evidence-based guidelines for the treatment of tracheostomy stoma cellulitis do not currently exist. Clinical trials of antibiotic therapy for this infection have not been performed. However, since polymicrobial infections are common, initial antibiotic therapy should be broad-spectrum. Therapy should also be directed toward the most common pathogens (Table 56–2).

Intravenous antibiotics are recommended for the ill-appearing patients and those with significant or rapidly progressing cellulitis. Close follow-up is recommended, especially given the possible direct route of bacterial spread into the trachea and into the deep tissues of the neck and chest if the infection progresses. For this reason, hospitalization is strongly encouraged for the initial portion of therapy for ill-appearing patients with stoma cellulitis. Intravenous options for single initial therapy may include ampicillin-sulbactam or, if *Pseudomonas* species are strongly suspected, piperacillin-tazobactam or imipenem. Children with severe penicillin allergy may receive imipenem alone or a combination of

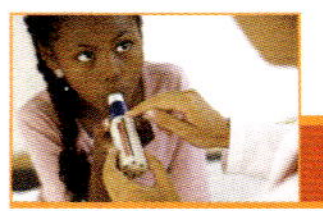

Table 56–2.

Suggested Antibiotics for the Treatment of Tracheostomy Stoma Cellulitis

	Penicillin Allergy			
	Absent		Present	
Route	**Single Therapy**	**Combination Therapy**	**Single Therapy**	**Combination Therapy**
Intravenous				
MRSA absent	Ampicillin-sulbactam or pipercillin-tazobactam	Plus a third-generation cephalosporin	Clindamycin	Clindamycin plus an aminoglycoside
MRSA	Vancomycin	Plus a third-generation cephalosporin or clindamycin	Vancomycin	Vancomycin plus a third-generation cephalosporin or clindamycin
Enteral	Amoxicillin-clavulanate		Clindamycin or Trimethoprim-sulfamethoxazole	

clindamycin and an aminoglycoside (i.e., tobramycin, amikacin, or gentamicin).[20] Additional broad-spectrum coverage may be provided with the addition of either ciprofloxacin or cephalosporins with activity against *P. aeruginosa*, such as ceftazidime or cefepime. The stoma culture antibiotic susceptibilities may be used to adjust or narrow antibiotic therapy. Vancomycin may be required if methicillin-resistant *S. aureus* (MRSA) is suspected.[21]

Transition from intravenously to enterally administered antibiotics is reasonable for patients who have initial treatment as indicated by decreased stoma site erythema, exudate, and induration. Reasons for failure in treatment response may include resistant organisms and extension of infection into the trachea or soft tissues. Surgical debridement may be warranted for deep-tissue infections.[18]

Initial enteral antibiotic therapy may be appropriate for the nontoxic appearing patient with mild cellulitis, assuming that antibiotic absorption is not compromised by conditions such as diarrhea or short gut syndrome. In previous studies, bacteria present in granulation tissue at the tracheostomy site have been susceptible to amoxicillin-clavulanate or ciprofloxacin, suggesting that these antibiotics may be options for enteral therapy.[8] The American Academy of Pediatrics does not endorse the use of fluoroquinolones for skin or soft-tissue infections in children younger than 18 years, unless there is no other available alternative therapy.[22] Other enteral choices include clindamycin or trimethoprim-sulfamethoxazole.[21] If candidal cellulitis is suspected, therapy with a topical antifungal medication (e.g., nystatin) may be appropriate.

Most clinical trials of skin infections in children have used 10 days of antibiotic therapy.[21] Current data suggests that 10–14 days of antibiotic therapy should be considered for children with tracheostomy stoma cellulitis. It is important to dispose or thoroughly clean home tracheostomy equipment at risk for bacterial contamination when a child experiences a stoma infection. This equipment may include trach ties, suction catheters, suction tubing, humidification nose, oxygenation and ventilation tubing.[23] Consultation with an otolaryngologist and intensivist should be undertaken in situations where a tracheostomy tube must be replaced secondary to stoma cellulitis.

BACTERIAL TRACHEITIS IN CHILDREN WITH TRACHEOTOMY

Definition and Epidemiology

Bacterial tracheitis is a serious infection of the tracheal epithelium. The prevalence rate in children with tracheostomy has not been reported, although it is believed to be very rare. Bacterial tracheitis is associated with significant morbidity. Respiratory failure requiring intubation and mechanical ventilation is commonly reported.[24] Mortality rates have been reported as high as 18–40%.[25]

Pathogenesis

Children with tracheostomy are at risk for bacterial infection in the trachea as a result of direct airway exposure to exogenous pathogens, colonized bacteria on the tracheostomy tube, and tracheal injury. Over time, the presence of the tracheostomy tube within the trachea may result in epithelial ulceration and denudation, which may predispose the trachea to infection.[26] Some children with tracheostomy may have a history of gastroesophageal reflux disease that, with chronic tracheal aspiration, may result in tracheal injury as a predicate to tracheitis.[27] *S. aureus*, group A *Streptococcus*, and *Haemophilus influenzae* have been reported as the leading bacterial causes of tracheitis in children, with *S. aureus* isolated in the majority of cases.[24,27] Although gram-negative organisms are rarely isolated in tracheitis, *P. aeruginosa* should be considered given the high rates of tracheostomy colonization with this organism.[12]

Clinical Presentation

On history, children with bacterial tracheitis have a 2–4 day prodrome of upper respiratory tract infection symptoms, including rhinorrhea, low-grade fever, cough, and sore throat. The hoarseness and "barky" cough frequently encountered in otherwise healthy children with tracheitis may be more difficult to recognize in children with tracheostomy.

Typically, the child with tracheitis will rapidly develop signs of respiratory distress following this prodrome. Increased work of breathing, airway compromise, higher fever, and toxic appearance are commonly observed.[27] Parents may also report changes in the quantity and quality of tracheal secretions. With bacterial tracheitis, the amount of secretions may increase dramatically and change from thin and clear to thick and yellow or green in color.

On physical examination, the child with bacterial tracheitis may appear ill. Biphasic (inspiratory and expiratory) stridor may be audible over the tracheostomy if the infection is severely compromising the airway. Tracheostomy suctioning may reveal continuous, thick, purulent secretions. Auscultation of the lower airways may reveal gurgling sounds transmitted from the upper airways. If pneumonia is absent, the lower airways may be clear, without focal findings. Signs of respiratory distress, including tachypnea and retractions, are common.

Differential Diagnosis

The most common condition confused with bacterial tracheitis in children with tracheostomy is viral laryngotracheobronchitis (croup). Differentiating croup from *early* bacterial tracheitis in children with tracheostomy can be challenging. Typically, children with bacterial tracheitis have progressive respiratory distress despite the use of racemic epinephrine and corticosteroids. Pneumonia should also be considered in the differential diagnosis, as up to 25% of children with bacterial tracheitis may have concurrent pneumonia.[28]

Diagnosis

If bacterial tracheitis is suspected in the child with tracheostomy, maintaining patency of the upper airway requires immediate medical attention. Delaying attention to the airway secondary to obtaining diagnostic tests could place the child in immediate danger of respiratory collapse.

The diagnosis of bacterial tracheitis is usually made by direct visualization with laryngoscopy or tracheoscopy.[29] Direct visual examination of the trachea can help distinguish trachieitis from croup and epiglottitis. A normal-appearing epiglottis and larynx with visual evidence of tracheal inflammation, the presence of purulent tracheal secretions, and a sloughing tracheal pseudomembrane is diagnostic for tracheitis.[27,30]

A Gram stain of tracheal secretions to evaluate for the presence of polymorphonuclear leukocytes and bacteria may be a helpful initial screen. This Gram stain should be compared with the child's previous tracheal aspirate results. If the previous aspirate revealed gram-negative rods and few white cells, but now demonstrates gram-positive organisms and sheets of white blood cells, the index of suspicion must be significantly higher for a tracheitis, especially if there is no evidence of pneumonia.[27] Bacterial culture of the tracheal secretions and a blood culture are recommended with suspected tracheitis in children with tracheostomy. These cultures may be used to determine bacterial sensitivities and guide antibiotic therapy.

Radiographs of the upper airway may be performed in stable children without signs of impending respiratory collapse. An anterior–posterior neck film may demonstrate a "steeple sign" that is also commonly seen in children with croup. A lateral neck film may demonstrate a tracheal air column that appears diffusely hazy, with multiple luminal soft tissue irregularities. These irregularities may be indicative of pseudomembrane detachment.[29]

Treatment

Children with tracheostomy and suspected bacterial tracheitis should be considered to have a critical airway. At least half of all children with bacterial tracheitis require endotracheal intubation although some clinicians recommend routine intubation for airway protection.[31,32] Prompt airway stabilization with transfer to an intensive care unit with a team of experienced nurses, respiratory therapists, and practitioners skilled in advanced airway management in children should be considered.

Once the airway is stabilized, antibiotic therapy should be initiated. Empiric broad-spectrum antibiotic administration provides coverage for *S. aureus*, *Streptococcus* spp., and *H. influenzae*. Parental antibiotics are strongly recommended. Vancomycin may be appropriate for initial therapy if MRSA is suspected.[27] Combination therapy with a third-generation cephalosporin, such as cefotaxime, and/or clindamycin may also be considered. If MRSA is not suspected, therapy may be narrowed from vancomycin to a penicillinase-resistant penicillin pending bacterial sensitivities. Ten to fourteen days of intravenous antibiotics is recommended given the high morbidity and mortality associated with bacterial tracheitis.

Tracheoscopy may be therapeutic for bacterial tracheitis in children with tracheostomy. Frequently, a thick inflammatory exudate with sloughed mucosa that obstructs the lumen of the trachea and main bronchi can be visualized. This thick material may be removed with suction and foreign body forceps if necessary.[29]

BACTERIAL PNEUMONIA IN CHILDREN WITH TRACHEOTOMY

Definition and Epidemiology

Pneumonia is defined as an infection of the lower airways. In children with tracheostomy, there is a high prevalence of pneumonia. Eighty-eight percent of patients with tracheotomy will develop a lower airway infection within one year of tracheotomy placement. Children with tracheotomy have an average of 2.8 episodes of pneumonia annually.[33]

Pathogenesis

Children with tracheotomy are at increased risk for developing both community- and hospital-acquired pneumonia caused by impaired respiratory immunity, enhanced exposure to pathogens during routine tracheotomy care, bacterial colonization of the lower airways, and impaired cough reflex which compounds the difficulties with bacterial clearance from the airway.

The lower airways of healthy children are sterile. Healthy lungs have integral defense mechanisms designed to maintain sterility. These mechanisms, often referred to as the "mucociliary escalator," include mucus secretion, upward beating cilia and secretory immunologlobulin A.[12] In children with tracheotomy, this defense mechanism is impaired. The tracheotomy itself provides direct exposure of these pathogens to the lower airway, bypassing the humidification and warming from the nose and oropharynx. This decreased humidification and warming impairs tracheal cilliary activity, resulting in thicker secretions and decreased mucous clearance.[34] For those children with tracheotomy who have coexisting neurologic-impairment, a weakened or absent cough reflex further prevents the expulsion of respiratory secretions and infectious pathogens.

Impaired respiratory immunity is largely responsible for bacterial colonization of the airways of children with tracheotomy. Colonization refers to the presence of bacteria in the lower airways without evidence of infection. Up to 95% of children with tracheotomy are colonized with bacterial pathogens in their lower airways.[33] *S. aureus* and *P. aeruginosa* have been reported as the most common exogenous bacteria responsible for colonization.[12,35] Over time, colonized bacteria in the lower airways may replicate, infecting the lower airways.[35]

Routine tracheostomy care provides a portal for exogenous pathogens to enter the lower airways of children. Daily respiratory care maintenance for a child with a tracheostomy requires suctioning and tube tie changes. Routine suctioning is necessary to ensure a patent airway. This involves the placement of a suction catheter through the tracheostomy into the trachea to remove mucus and other debris. Improper cleaning of the suction catheter or poor hand hygiene of the caregiver may lead to direct contamination of the trachea with exogenous pathogens.

Clinical Presentation

Caregivers of children with a tracheotomy-related pneumonia will often report an increase in the quantity of secretions suctioned. Secretions that become thicker and change color from clear to yellow, brown, or green may be associated with pneumonia. Overall, caregivers often report that the child sounds "more junky." Children with tracheotomy who require oxygen may demonstrate desaturations and increased oxygen requirement. Constitutional signs of fever, malaise, and increased somnolence may be present. Caregivers may also report signs of respiratory distress, including tachypnea and retractions.

On physical examination, children with tracheotomy who have pneumonia may be ill-appearing, febrile, and tachycardic. Lung auscultation may reveal crackles, rhonchi, or decreased breath sounds over the affected area. Additionally, percussion of the affected lung field(s) may reveal muffled tones. It is important to auscultate the child immediately following suctioning or a solid cough. Upper airway mucous plugging can be mistaken for lower airway rhonchi. Tachypnea and retractions may be noted in children who are experiencing respiratory distress.

Differential Diagnosis

The most common condition confused with bacterial pneumonia in children with tracheotomy is an upper respiratory infection in a child with "noninfectious" bacterial colonization of the lower airways. Almost all children with tracheotomy will eventually become colonized with bacteria such as *S. aureus* and *P. aeruginosa.* These bacteria may be present in the child's lower airway without inducing an inflammatory response or pneumonia. When these bacteria are isolated in a patient without fever, cough, sputum changes, lung auscultation findings, or respiratory distress, the child likely does not have pneumonia. The distinction between bacterial colonization and pneumonia becomes less clear when children exhibit one or two of the above symptoms, such as sputum change and cough. These symptoms are not specific for pneumonia. They can be associated with a self-limiting upper respiratory infection.

Viral pneumonia and aspiration pneumonia should also be considered in the differential diagnosis of pneumonia in a child with trachesotomy and respiratory distress. Viral pneumonia, such as influenza or RSV infection, will be more likely to occur during seasonal peaks of incidence in the late fall and winter. Aspiration pneumonia may be associated with a temporal history of a choking, gagging, or vomiting event 1–2 days prior to the development of respiratory symptoms.

Diagnosis

Features that may help distinguish bacterial pneumonia from bacterial colonization are summarized in Table 56–3. The use of sputum culture or tracheal aspirate to diagnose bacterial pneumonia in children with tracheotomy is complicated because of the difficulty of differentiating bacterial colonization of the trachea from bacterial infection of the lower airways. The presence of a high bacterial load and leukocytes are also not specific for lower-airway infection.[23] Bacteria isolated from the trachea may not correlate with bacteria found in the lower airways. Previous studies support the use of bronchoalveolar lavage (BAL) or quantitative deep endotracheal aspirate (QDEA) for diagnosing ventilator-assisted pneumonia in adult patients.[36,37] Clinical studies using these techniques to diagnose ventilator-associated pneumonia in children are in progress. It is unlikely that sputum or tracheal aspirate will assist greatly in the diagnosis of pneumonia in children with

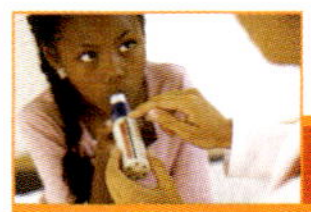

Table 56–3.

Comparison of Bacterial Colonization and Bacterial Pneumonia in Children with Tracheostomy

Features of Comparison	Bacterial Colonization without Infection	Bacterial Pneumonia
History		
Appearance	Well	Ill-appearing
Temperature	Afebrile	Fever may be present
Cough	May be present	Increased from baseline
Respiratory Distress	Absent	May be present
Secretions		
Quantity	Minimal	Moderate to large
Color	Clear, yellow	Yellow, green, brown
Tracheal Aspirate		
Bacteria presence	May be present	May be present
Bacteria quantity	Low or high	Low or high
White cells	May be present	May be present
Chest Radiograph		
Infiltrate	Absent	May be present
Atelectasis	May be present	May be present

tracheostomy. However, these specimens may be useful to determine antibiotic sensitivities of the bacteria present in the airway and direct antibiotic therapy.

Chest radiograph is the gold-standard for diagnosing pneumonia, if the pneumonia is visible on chest radiograph. A substantial number of children suspected of pneumonia will not have radiographic evidence of an infiltrate on initial chest X-ray.[38] Comparing prior chest radiographs to the current film is extremely important in assessing pneumonia in children with tracheostomy. Children with neurologic impairment who have a tracheostomy may exhibit chronic lung findings on radiographs, including chronic atelectasis at the lung bases. These markings may be confused with a pneumonia infiltrate (Figure 56–2).

The utility of laboratory diagnostic tests to assist in the diagnosis of bacterial pneumonia is variable. Evaluation of these tests to diagnose pneumonia in children with tracheotomy has not been performed. Increased rates of pneumonia have been reported in children with fever and WBC counts greater than 15,000 cells/mm^3.[39,40] High procalcitonin ($\geq$2 ng/mL) and C-reactive protein ($\geq$65 mg/L) have exhibited 90% or greater sensitivity in diagnosing bacterial compared with viral lower-respiratory infection in children.[41]

The combination of symptoms, laboratory and radiographic findings has been the most useful in diagnosing pneumonia in adult, ventilated patients. A new radiographic infiltrate with at least two of the following: fever, leukocytosis, or purulent sputum has been shown to increase the likelihood of pneumonia.[42] The absence

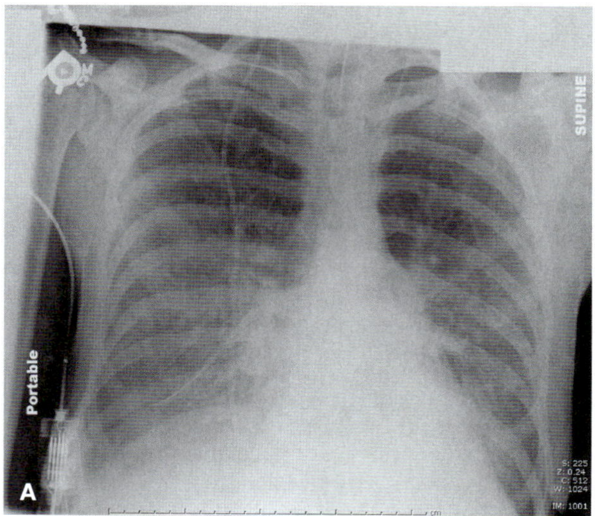

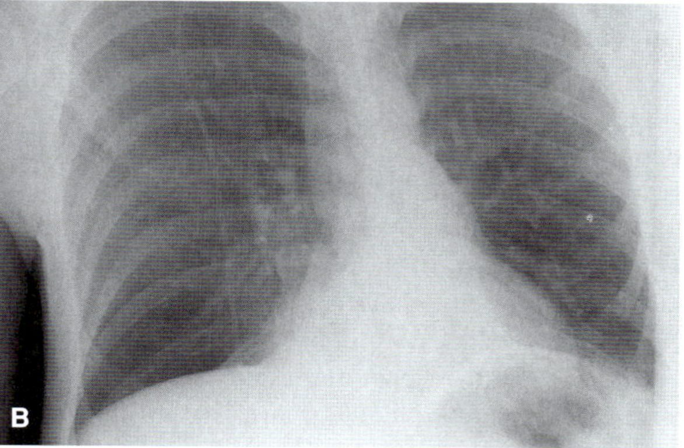

FIGURE 56–2 ■ **(A)** Bilateral pneumonia in a child with tracheostomy; **(B)** Chronic atelectasis in the same child with tracheostomy.

of a new infiltrate on a plain chest radiograph and fewer than 50% neutrophils on cell count analysis lowered the likelihood of pneumonia.[42]

Blood culture has not proved useful in the diagnosis or initial treatment of pneumonia in hospitalized adult patients.[43] Following the introduction of *H. influenzae* type B vaccine, rates of bacteremia in healthy children with pneumonia have been reported as less than 2%.[44] Rates of bacteremia associated with pneumonia in children with tracheostomy have not been described. The rates may be higher in children with tracheostomy, given their impaired respiratory immunity. Until further data is available, we recommend that blood culture be performed in children with tracheostomy and suspected pneumonia.

Treatment

Evidence-based guidelines for the treatment of pneumonia in children with tracheotomy do not exist. The recommendations described below are based on studies of patients with ventilator-assisted pneumonia or chronic bacterial colonization. The antibiotic options discussed are intended for the treatment of bacterial pneumonia without effusion or empyema.

Early broad-spectrum antibiotic administration has been associated with decreased morbidity and mortality in adult patients with ventilator-assisted pneumonia.[45] Initial intravenous antibiotic therapy for tracheostomy-related pneumonia should be based on the recent bacterial colonization pattern of the patient (Table 56–4). Pipercillin-tazobactam, ticarcillin-clavulanate,[46] or ceftazidime may be necessary for children previously-colonized with antibiotic-susceptible *P. aeruginosa*. Therapy with multiple antibiotics is often necessary. Clindamycin may be added for children colonized with methicillin-sensitive *S. aureus* or if aspiration pneumonia is suspected.[47] Vancomycin may be recommended as antibiotic therapy for MRSA pneumonia depending on individual institutional guidelines.[48] For children not colonized with *P. aeruginosa* or *S. aureus*, a third-generation cephalosporin is suggested for coverage of *S. pneumoniae*, group A β-hemolytic *Streptococcus*, and typeable or nontypeable *H. influenzae*.[49,50]

Narrowing the spectrum of therapy, once final sputum, tracheal or blood culture results are available, is recommended if the child has clinically responded to initial therapy. Once the child's respiratory status has returned close to baseline, a transition to enteral antibiotics is suggested. Options for enteral therapy include amoxicillin-clavulanate, clindamycin, or cefdinir.[51,52] Fluoroquinolones have been endorsed for the exacerbation of pulmonary disease in patients with cystic fibrosis who have colonization with *P. aeruginosa*, when no alternative therapies are available, and the child can be treated in an ambulatory setting.[22] Fluoroquinolones may be an option for enteral therapy in the ambulatory setting for children with tracheostomy who are colonized with *P. aeruginosa*, when no other alternative is available. Consultation with a pulmonary specialist is recommended under these circumstances.

Previous studies evaluating duration of therapy suggest that at least 14 days of therapy for patients with *P. aeruginosa* pneumonia is necessary to avoid recurrence.[53]

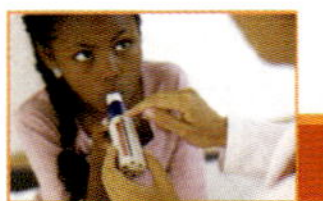

Table 56–4.

Suggested Antibiotics for the Treatment of Bacterial Pneumonia in Children with Tracheostomy

	Penicillin Allergy			
	Absent		Present	
Route	Single Therapy	Combination Therapy	Single Therapy	Combination Therapy
Intravenous				
P. aeruginosa colonization	Pipercillin-tazobactam or ticarcillin-clavulanate	Plus a third-generation cephalosporin (ceftazidime)	Third-generation cephalosporin (ceftazidime)	Plus an aminoglycoside
MRSA colonization	Vancomycin	Plus a third-generation cephalosporin or clindamycin	Vancomycin	Plus a third-generation cephalosporin or clindamycin
No colonization History	Third-generation cephalosporin (ceftriaxone)		Third-generation cephalosporin (ceftriaxone)	
Enteral	Amoxicillin-clavulanate		Clindamycin or Trimethoprim-sulfamethoxazole	

For other pathogens, 10–14 days of therapy may be generally appropriate. Children with tracheostomy and pneumonia who are ill-appearing, dehydrated, in respiratory distress, or in need of enhanced oxygenation or ventilatory support should be cared for initially in a hospital setting. Children who respond to initial therapy may be eligible for treatment completion as an outpatient.

REFERENCES

1. Lewis CW, Carron JD, Perkins JA, Sie KC, Feudtner C. Tracheotomy in pediatric patients: a national perspective. *Arch Otolaryngol Head Neck Surg.* 2003;129(5):523-529.
2. Arcand P, Granger J. Pediatric tracheostomies: changing trends. *J Otolaryngol.* 1988;17(2):121-124.
3. Kremer B, Botos-Kremer AI, Eckel HE, Schlondorff G. Indications, complications, and surgical techniques for pediatric tracheostomies—an update. *J Pediatr Surg.* 2002;37(11):1556-1562.
4. Tantinikorn W, Alper CM, Bluestone CD, Casselbrant ML. Outcome in pediatric tracheotomy. *Am J Otolaryngol.* 2003;24(3):131-137.
5. Stauffer JL, Olson DE, Petty TL. Complications and consequences of endotracheal intubation and tracheotomy. A prospective study of 150 critically ill adult patients. *Am J Med.* 1981;70(1):65-76.
6. Mohammedi I, Vedrinne JM, Ceruse P, Duperret S, Allaouchiche B, Motin J. Major cellulitis following percutaneous tracheostomy. *Intensive Care Med.* 1997;23(4):443-444.
7. Mittendorf EA, McHenry CR, Smith CM, Yowler CJ, Peerless JR. Early and late outcome of bedside percutaneous tracheostomy in the intensive care unit. *Am Surg.* 2002;68(4):342-346.
8. Brown MT, Montgomery WW. Microbiology of tracheal granulation tissue associated with silicone airway prostheses. *Ann Otol Rhinol Laryngol.* 1996;105(8):624-627.
9. Brook I. Microbiological studies of tracheostomy site wounds. *Eur J Respir Dis.* 1987;71(5):380-383.
10. Brook I. Role of anaerobic bacteria in infections following tracheostomy, intubation, or the use of ventilatory tubes in children. *Ann Otol Rhinol. Laryngol.* 2004;113(10):830-834.
11. Jarrett WA, Ribes J, Manaligod JM. Biofilm formation on tracheostomy tubes. *Ear Nose Throat J.* 2002;81(9):659-661.
12. Morar P, Singh V, Jones AS, Hughes J, van Saene R. Impact of tracheotomy on colonization and infection of lower airways in children requiring long-term ventilation: a prospective observational cohort study. *Chest.* 1998;113(1):77-85.
13. Puhakka HJ, Kero P, Valli P, Iisalo E. Tracheostomy in pediatric patients. *Acta Paediatr.* 1992;81(3):231-234.
14. Da Silva PS, Waisberg J, Paulo CS, Colugnati F, Martins LC. Outcome of patients requiring tracheostomy in a pediatric intensive care unit. *Pediatr Int.* 2005;47(5):554-559.
15. Wang RC, Perlman PW, Parnes SM. Near-fatal complications of tracheotomy infections and their prevention. *Head Neck.* 1989;11(6):528-533.
16. Berlucchi M, Galtelli C, Nassif N, Bondioni MP, Nicolai P. Cervical necrotizing fasciitis with mediastinitis: a rare occurrence in the pediatric age. *Am J Otolaryngol.* 2007;28(1):18-21.
17. Cai XY, Zhang WJ, Zhang ZY, Yang C, Zhou LN, Chen ZM. Cervical infection with descending mediastinitis: a review of six cases. *Int J Oral Maxillofac Surg.* 2006;35(11):1021-1025.
18. Force SD, Miller DL, Petersen R, et al. Incidence of deep sternal wound infections after tracheostomy in cardiac surgery patients. *Ann Thorac Surg.* 2005;80(2):618-621.
19. Anaya DA, Dellinger EP. Necrotizing soft-tissue infection: diagnosis and management. *Clin Infect Dis.* 2007; 44(5):705-710.
20. Vayalumkal JV, Jadavji T. Children hospitalized with skin and soft tissue infections: a guide to antibacterial selection and treatment. *Paediatr Drugs.* 2006;8(2):99-111.
21. Ladhani S, Garbash M. Staphylococcal skin infections in children: rational drug therapy recommendations. *Paediatr Drugs.* 2005;7(2):77-102.
22. American Academy of Pediatrics. The use of systemic fluoroquinolones. *Pediatrics.* 2006;118(3):1287-1292.
23. Sherman JM, Davis S, Albamonte-Petrick S, et al. Care of the child with a chronic tracheostomy. This official statement of the american thoracic society was adopted by the ATS board of directors, July 1999. *Am J Respir Crit Care Med.* 2000;161(1):297-308.
24. Hopkins A, Lahiri T, Salerno R, Heath B. Changing epidemiology of life-threatening upper airway infections: the reemergence of bacterial tracheitis. *Pediatrics.* 2006;118(4):1418-1421.
25. Seigler RS. Bacterial tracheitis: recognition and treatment. *J S C Med Assoc.* 1993;89(2):83-87.
26. Friedberg SA, Griffith TE, Hass GM. Histologic changes in the trachea following tracheostomy. *Ann Otol Rhinol Laryngol.* 1965;74(3):785-798.
27. Graf J, Stein F. Tracheitis in pediatric patients. *Semin Pediatr Infect Dis.* 2006;17(1):11-13.
28. Marcos Alonso S, Molini Menchon N, Rodriguez Nunez A, Martinon Torres F, Martinon Sanchez JM. Bacterial tracheitis: an infectious cause of upper airway obstruction to be considered in children. *An Pediatr (Barc).* 2005;63(2):164-168.
29. Stroud RH, Friedman NR. An update on inflammatory disorders of the pediatric airway: Epiglottitis, croup, and tracheitis. *Am J Otolaryngol.* 2001;22(4):268-275.
30. Bernstein T, Brilli R, Jacobs B. Is bacterial tracheitis changing? A 14-month experience in a pediatric intensive care unit. *Clin Infect Dis.* 1998;27(3):458-462.
31. Salamone FN, Bobbitt DB, Myer CM, Rutter MJ, Greinwald JH Jr. Bacterial tracheitis reexamined: is there a less severe manifestation? *Otolaryngol Head Neck Surg.* 2004;131(6):871-876.
32. Chan PW, Goh A, Lum L. Severe upper airway obstruction in the tropics requiring intensive care. *Pediatr Int.* 2001;43(1):53-57.
33. Brook I. Bacterial colonization, tracheobronchitis, and pneumonia following tracheostomy and long-term intubation in pediatric patients. *Chest.* 1979;76(4):420-424.
34. Toews GB, Hansen EJ, Strieter RM. Pulmonary host defenses and oropharyngeal pathogens. *Am J Med.* 1990;88(5A):20S-24S.

35. Rao AR, Splaingard MS, Gershan WM, Havens PL, Thill A, Barbieri JT. Detection of *Pseudomonas aeruginosa* type III antibodies in children with tracheostomies. *Pediatr Pulmonol.* 2005;39(5):402-407.
36. Mondi MM, Chang MC, Bowton DL, Kilgo PD, Meredith JW, Miller PR. Prospective comparison of bronchoalveolar lavage and quantitative deep tracheal aspirate in the diagnosis of ventilator associated pneumonia. *J Trauma.* 2005;59(4):891-895.
37. Canadian Critical Care Trials Group. A randomized trial of diagnostic techniques for ventilator-associated pneumonia. *N Engl J Med.* 2006;355(25):2619-2630.
38. Wilkins TR, Wilkins RL. Clinical and radiographic evidence of pneumonia. *Radiol Technol.* 2005;77(2):106-110.
39. Bachur R, Perry H, Harper MB. Occult pneumonias: empiric chest radiographs in febrile children with leukocytosis. *Ann Emerg Med.* 1999;33(2):166-173.
40. Murphy CG, van de Pol AC, Harper MB, Bachur RG. Clinical predictors of occult pneumonia in the febrile child. *Acad Emerg Med.* 2007;14(3):243-249.
41. Prat C, Dominguez J, Rodrigo C, et al. Procalcitonin, C-reactive protein and leukocyte count in children with lower respiratory tract infection. *Pediatr Infect Dis J.* 2003;22(11):963-968.
42. Klompas M. Does this patient have ventilator-associated pneumonia? *JAMA.* 2007;297(14):1583-1593.
43. Ramanujam P, Rathlev NK. Blood cultures do not change management in hospitalized patients with community-acquired pneumonia. *Acad Emerg Med.* 2006;13(7):740-745.
44. Shah SS, Alpern ER, Zwerling L, McGowan KL, Bell LM. Risk of bacteremia in young children with pneumonia treated as outpatients. *Arch Pediatr Adolesc Med.* 2003; 157(4):389-392.
45. Davis KA. Ventilator-associated pneumonia: a review. *J Intensive Care Med.* 2006;21(4):211-226.
46. Kristjansson K, Cox F, Taylor L. Ticarcillin/clavulanic acid combination. Treatment of bacterial infections in hospitalized children. *Clin Pediatr (Phila).* 1989;28(11): 521-524.
47. Martinez-Aguilar G, Hammerman WA, Mason EO Jr., Kaplan SL. Clindamycin treatment of invasive infections caused by community-acquired, methicillin-resistant and methicillin-susceptible *Staphylococcus aureus* in children. *Pediatr Infect Dis J.* 2003;22(7):593-598.
48. Maclayton DO, Hall RG, II. Pharmacologic treatment options for nosocomial pneumonia involving methicillin-resistant *Staphylococcus aureus. Ann Pharmacother.* 2007; 41(2):235-244.
49. Whitney CG, Farley MM, Hadler J, et al. Increasing prevalence of multidrug-resistant streptococcus pneumoniae in the united states. *N Engl J Med.* 2000;343(26): 1917-1924.
50. Yu VL, Chiou CC, Feldman C, et al. An international prospective study of pneumococcal bacteremia: correlation with in vitro resistance, antibiotics administered, and clinical outcome. *Clin Infect Dis.* 2003;37(2):230-237.
51. Perry CM, Scott LJ. Cefdinir: a review of its use in the management of mild-to-moderate bacterial infections. *Drugs.* 2004;64(13):1433-1464.
52. McCracken GH Jr. Diagnosis and management of pneumonia in children. *Pediatr Infect Dis J.* 2000;19(9): 924-928.
53. Chastre J, Wolff M, Fagon JY, et al. Comparison of 8 vs 15 days of antibiotic therapy for ventilator-associated pneumonia in adults: a randomized trial. *JAMA.* 2003; 290(19):2588-2598.

CHAPTER 57

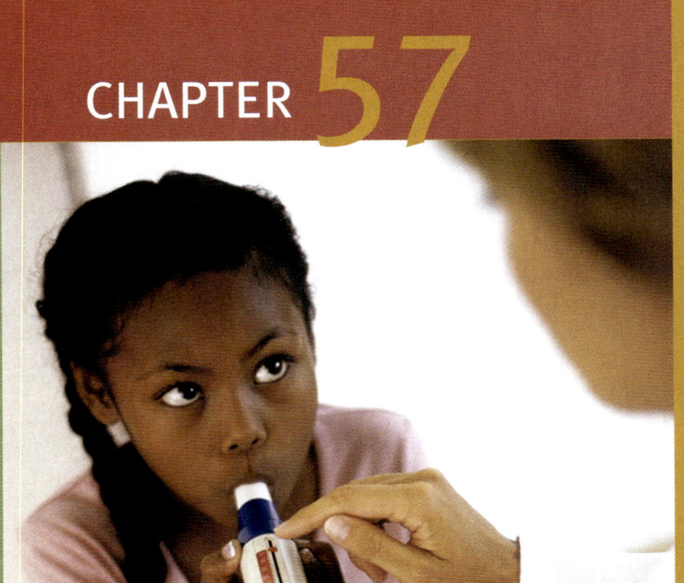

Infections in Asplenic Children

Catherine Yen and Adam J. Ratner

DEFINITIONS AND EPIDEMIOLOGY

Long thought of as an unessential organ that could be removed without adverse effects, the spleen and its significance in defense against infections were not well recognized until 1952, when King and Shumacker published a seminal paper describing an association between splenectomy and subsequent susceptibility to overwhelming infection.[1] Since then, severe infection in asplenic individuals has become a well-known entity, termed postsplenectomy sepsis or overwhelming postsplenectomy sepsis. This chapter will provide an overview of the basic functions of the spleen and the infectious complications associated with asplenia.

Causes of Asplenia

A child may be asplenic for anatomic or functional reasons. Anatomic reasons include: (1) congenital asplenia, which can be isolated, or part of Ivemark syndrome, which is associated with cardiovascular defects and heterotaxy and (2) splenectomy. Splenectomy may be performed for various reasons. In children, the most common reasons are trauma-associated splenic rupture, malignancy, hypersplenism, and splenomegaly associated with persistent anemia and/or thrombocytopenia.[2] Functional asplenia results from having an anatomically intact but poorly working spleen. There are various conditions that can cause functional asplenia, including sickle cell disease (Table 57–1). Some of the mechanisms leading to functional asplenia include infarction, infiltration, and impaired phagocyte function.[2–4]

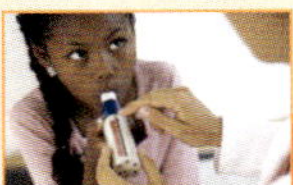

Table 57–1.

Causes of Asplenia

Congenital asplenia
Splenectomy
- Trauma
- Malignancy
- Splenomegaly
- Hypersplenism

Functional asplenia
- *Hematologic*—sickle cell disease, thalassemia
- *Autoimmune*—biliary cirrhosis, chronic active hepatitis, Graves disease, Hashimoto's thyroiditis, rheumatoid arthritis, Sjogren's syndrome, systemic lupus erythematosis, polyarteritis nodosa
- *Gastrointestinal*—celiac disease, Crohn's disease, ulcerative colitis, dermatitis herpetiformis, intestinal lymphangiectasias, Whipple's disease
- *Infiltrative*—amyloidosis, sarcoidosis, storage diseases (Gaucher, Niemann Pick)
- *Therapy-induced*—radiation therapy, corticosteroid therapy, intravenous IgG (transient)
- *Other*—bone marrow transplant (chronic graft versus host disease)

Epidemiology

Rates of overwhelming infection in asplenic children vary, depending on age and underlying reason for asplenia. Past studies have found that younger age, underlying illnesses including hemoglobinopathies, and splenectomy within the prior 3 years are associated with increased risk.[2,5,6] However, it is important to note that there is a lifelong risk for overwhelming infection.

PATHOGENESIS

Anatomy

The spleen is comprised of a fibrous capsule, a trabecular framework of fibers and smooth muscle, cell-rich red and white pulp interspersed among this framework, and a blood supply arising from the splenic artery[2,7,8]:

- *Fibrous capsule*: The splenic capsule is highly elastic, containing smooth muscle that allows for the distension and splenomegaly seen in many pathologic states.
- *White pulp*: White pulp contains aggregates of lymphoid follicles (B-lymphocytes) found in the periarterial sheaths of the medium-sized splenic arteries. These follicles can form germinal centers with antigenic stimulation. At the edge of each follicle is a region called the marginal zone, where antigen trapping and processing occur.
- *Red pulp*: Red pulp is composed of venous sinusoids and splenic cords with reticular cells, macrophages, neutrophils, and elements of circulating blood. Blood flows through the red pulp via open circulation or closed circulation. Approximately 90% of the spleen's blood supply travels through open circulation via the venous sinusoids, a slower route allowing for filtration of the blood.
- *Blood supply*: The splenic artery divides into many branches prior to entering the hilum of the spleen as the trabecular artery. This arterial network is surrounded by periarterial sheaths and continues to divide, eventually ending as arterioles in the red pulp.

Normal Functions of the Spleen

Immune response

The main immune functions of the spleen include antigen processing, antibody production, and phagocytosis.[2,4,8] Antigens are trapped and processed in the marginal zone, which contains T-lymphocytes and macrophages. From there, the antigen moves into the germinal center of the lymphoid follicle where B-lymphocytes are activated and become memory B cells and plasma cells. The plasma cells then travel to the red pulp and release antibody into the blood. Although liver macrophages are very efficient at clearing opsonized blood-borne bacteria, splenic macrophages are better at responding to bacteria with little or no opsonic coating, such as the encapsulated organisms.[3,8] In addition to the immune functions mentioned above, the spleen is capable of making the alternate complement component properdin and other opsonins, such as tuftsin.

Hematopoiesis

The spleen plays an active role in hematopoiesis in the second and third trimesters of fetal development. Although not a normal site for hematopoiesis after birth, it can become active in certain disease states in which extramedullary hematopoiesis occurs. Examples include the thalassemias, myelofibrosis, and certain tumors such as hemangiomas, hepatoblastomas, and leiomyomas.[8]

Filtration

Apart from its responsibility to remove microorganisms and immune complexes from the circulation, the spleen also plays a role in the removal or repair of damaged erythrocytes.[4,8] Deformed cells are removed by macrophages, a process known as culling, and cells containing particulate material, such as Howell-Jolly bodies, Heinz bodies, or vesicles, undergo a process known as pitting. Pitting occurs when macrophages remove the particulate material and the erythrocyte subsequently returns to the normal circulation.

Storage

Platelets, granulocytes, and factor VIII are stored in the spleen. Normally, up to 30–40% of the body's platelets are stored in the spleen. This percentage can increase greatly in pathologic states, resulting in severe thrombocytopenia. Additionally, the spleen can hold up to 45% of the body's erythrocyte mass in pathologic states such as splenic sequestration associated with sickle cell disease.[2]

Why Infections Occur with Asplenia

In the child with asplenia or functional asplenia, there is impaired antigen recognition, impaired production of antibodies (namely antigen specific IgM), altered T cell function, and altered phagocytic activity with impaired removal of particles unable to be compensated by liver and lung macrophages.[8–10] This leads to an increased risk of infection, especially with encapsulated microorganisms.

CLINICAL PRESENTATION

History and Physical Examination

Symptoms are usually nonspecific. A child may present with a short prodrome of fever, chills, and other complaints such as malaise, myalgias, sore throat, headache, nausea, vomiting, diarrhea, and/or abdominal pain. He or she initially may appear nontoxic, but then rapidly progress to a more classical septic picture, with respiratory distress, cardiovascular instability, disseminated intravascular coagulation, purpura fulminans, hypoglycemia, or coma within hours of presentation.[2,3,11–15] In many cases, there is no identifiable focus of infection. When a defined infectious focus is found, meningitis and pneumonia are common.[1,13]

DIFFERENTIAL DIAGNOSIS

Sepsis should always be suspected, worked up, and empirically treated when faced with a febrile or ill-appearing child with a history of asplenia. While many other etiologies may explain the child's constellation of symptoms, it is important to address this potentially fatal cause first. Many organisms may cause infections in asplenic children; however, certain ones occur more frequently and should be kept in mind:

Most Common Organisms Associated with Infections in Asplenic Children

- *Streptococcus pneumoniae:* The most commonly identified organism, accounting for 50–90% of septic episodes.[16,17] However, the incidence of invasive pneumococcal disease may be decreasing. A recent study by Halasa et al. noted a marked decrease in the incidence of invasive pneumococcal disease among children with sickle cell disease after the introduction of routine immunization with the pneumococcal conjugate vaccine.[18]
- *Haemophilus influenzae* type b: The second most common organism, although invasive disease is rare now with the use of the Hib vaccine.
- *Neisseria meningitidis*: The third most common organism. It can be associated with fulminant sepsis.

Other Organisms

- *Capnocytophaga canimorsus*: A gram-negative rod that is usually acquired following close contact with dog or cat saliva.
- *Babesia* species: Asplenic individuals are a greater risk for morbidity and mortality secondary to babesiosis.
- *Plasmodium* species: Malarial parasite clearance is delayed in asplenic individuals.[19]
- *Escherichia coli*
- *Klebsiella* species
- *Staphylococci*
- Other *Streptococci* (i.e., *Streptococcus suis*, *Streptococcus bovis*)
- *Salmonella* species
- *Bordetella holmesii*: A rare gram-negative rod associated with bacteremia, endocarditis, and respiratory illness in humans, it has been isolated from asplenic individuals in the past.[14,20]

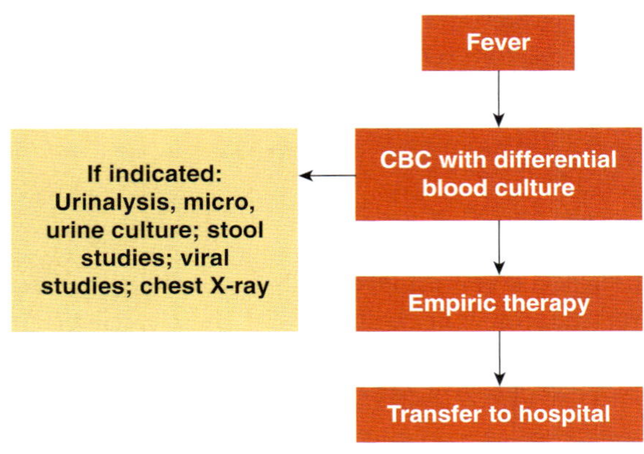

FIGURE 57–1 ■ Algorithm for evaluation of fever in the asplenic child.

DIAGNOSIS

General Evaluation

When faced with a febrile, asplenic child in the outpatient setting, a preliminary workup may be initiated if the situation permits (Figure 57–1). Following a thorough history and physical, preliminary diagnostic testing should include a complete blood count with differential (look for organisms on the peripheral smear) and a blood culture. Other tests to consider are urinalysis with microscopy, urine culture, cerebrospinal fluid studies and culture, stool studies such as bacterial culture, assay for *Clostridium difficile* toxin if the child has been on prophylactic antibiotics, and assays for adenovirus and rotavirus, viral studies to help determine the etiology of the child's fever should a bacterial etiology be ruled out, and chest radiograph, if indicated based on age, symptoms, and physical examination findings. Ideally, bloodwork should be drawn prior to the administration of antibiotics. *However, the diagnostic workup should never delay empiric therapy.*

TREATMENT

Empiric Therapy (Tables 57–2 and 57–3)

In general, empiric therapy should be targeted toward the most common organisms associated with asplenia. In the outpatient setting, an empiric dose of antibiotics should be given prior to transferring the child to an emergency department or inpatient facility. If the child is in a location far from any medical provider or medical center, primary caretakers should be instructed to give the child a dose of oral antibiotics immediately. Efforts should be made to ensure that families always keep the antibiotic on hand.

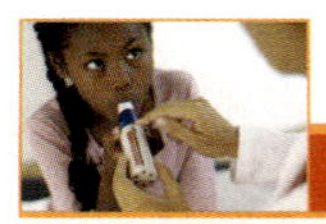

Table 57–2.

Suggested Therapeutic Options for Asplenic Children in the Outpatient Setting Prior to Transfer to Hospital

Antibiotic	Pediatric Dose	Adult Dose
Ceftriaxone	100 mg/kg IM or IV × 1 dose	1–2 g IM or IV × 1 dose
Amoxicillin/clavulanic acid	40 mg/kg PO × 1 dose	875 mg PO × 1 dose
Trimethoprim/sulfamethoxazole (TMP/SMX) if penicillin allergic	5 mg TMP/kg PO × 1 dose	1 double strength tab PO × 1 dose

Targeted Therapy

Once an organism is identified, more targeted therapy can be initiated. Therapeutic decisions should be based on the child's clinical status, organism identification, and antibiotic susceptibility pattern.

PREVENTION

Chemoprophylaxis

Chemoprophylaxis against pneumococcal infections is recommended for most children with asplenia, such as those with congenital asplenia, sickle cell disease, splenectomy secondary to hemolytic anemias, malignancies, liver transplants, and during the first year following splenectomy for any reason.[21,22] Chemoprophylaxis is also recommended for children younger than 5 years of age with asplenia for any reason. In the United States, the duration of chemoprophylaxis may vary with the underlying reason for being asplenic. Chemoprophylaxis is recommended during the first year following splenectomy at any age. For other children, the recommendation for continuing chemoprophylaxis until the age of five is based on past experience with sickle cell disease in which the risk for development of pneumococcal bacteremia or meningitis may be lower in school-aged children.[23]

Prophylactic regimens may include the following:

- Penicillin VK 125 mg PO bid for children < 5 years
- Penicillin VK 250 mg PO bid for children ≥ 5 years
- Amoxicillin 20 mg/kg/day
- Trimethoprim/sulfamethoxazole (TMP/SMX) 5 mg TMP/kg PO daily for those with penicillin allergies (based on dosing for *Pneumocystis jiroveci* prophylaxis). Higher rates of pneumococcal resistance with TMP/SMX have been reported.[24]

Primary caretakers and patients should be informed that chemoprophylaxis does not guarantee complete protection against infection. Regarding dental procedures, there are no current recommendations regarding prophylaxis for those no longer on daily chemoprophylaxis without cardiac conditions.[25,26]

Vaccinations

Vaccines are not contraindicated. Children should be vaccinated according to the schedule recommended by the Advisory Committee on Immunization Practices, the American Academy of Pediatrics, and the American Academy of Family Physicians with appropriate modifications for children with asplenia as emphasized below. An updated schedule may be found on the following Web site provided by the Centers for Disease Control and

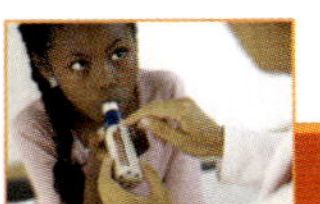

Table 57–3.

Suggested Empiric Therapy for Asplenic Children in the Inpatient Setting

Antibiotic	Pediatric Dose	Adult Dose
Ceftriaxone or	100 mg/kg/d IV divided every 12–24 h	2 g IV every 12–24 h (give every 12 h if meningitis suspected)
Cefotaxime*,†	200–300 mg/kg/d IV divided every 6 h	2 g IV every 6–8 h
PLUS Vancomycin* if meningitis suspected	60 mg/kg/d IV divided every 6 h	30–45 mg/kg/day divided every 8–12 h **or** 500–750 mg every 6 h; maximum dose 2–3 g/d

**Dose should be adjusted with renal impairment.*
†Dose should be adjusted with severe liver disease.

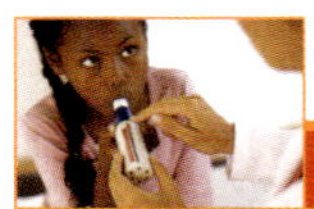

Table 57–4.

Indicated Vaccines for Asplenic Children

Vaccine	Recommended Schedule	Revaccination
Pneumococcal conjugate vaccine PCV7 (Prevnar)	*2–6 mo of age*: 3 doses, 6–8 wk apart, 1 dose at 12–15 months *7–11 mo*: 2 doses, 6–8 wk apart, 1 dose at 12–15 mo *12–23 mo*: 2 doses, 6–8 wk apart *≥ 24 mo*: 1 dose	See Table 58–5
H. influenzae type b conjugate vaccines HibTITER, ActHIB	*2–6 mo of age*: 3 doses, 8 wk apart, 1 dose at 12–15 mo *7–11 mo*: 2 doses, 8 wk apart, 1 dose at 12–15 mo, at least 8 wk after prior dose *12–14 mo*: 2 doses, 8 wk apart *15–59 mo*: 1 dose	Not currently recommended
H. influenzae type b conjugate vaccine PedvaxHIB	*2–6 mo of age*: 2 doses, 8 wk apart, 1 dose at 12–15 mo *7–11 mo*: 2 doses, 8 wk apart, 1 dose at 12–15 mo, at least 8 wk after prior dose *12–14 mo*: 2 doses, 8 wk apart *15–59 mo*: 1 dose	Not currently recommended
DTaP-Hib combination vaccine TriHIBit	Not to be used for primary series. May be given for the fourth dose of the DTaP and Hib series	Not currently recommended
Hepatitis B-Hib combination vaccine Comvax	Three doses at 2, 4, and 12–15 mo of age	Not currently recommended
MPSV (Menomune)	One dose at 2–10 y of age	Consider: 1 dose 2–3 y after 1st dose, if given at age < 4 y; else 1 dose 3–5 y after 1st dose, if not old enough for MCV
MCV (Menactra)	One dose at 11–55 y of age if no prior MPSV given—MPSV may be given, if MCV not available	Not currently recommended

Prevention: http://www.cdc.gov/vaccines/recs/schedules. Recommended vaccines for asplenic children include the following (see Tables 57–4 to 57–5)[22,27–29]:

- *Pneumococcal conjugate and/or polysaccharide vaccine.* In addition to receiving their primary and booster series, asplenic children should be revaccinated as recommended in Table 57–5 since they continue to remain at a greater risk for overwhelming pneumococcal sepsis.
- *H. influenzae* type b *vaccine.* Severe infection with *H. influenzae* type b, seen frequently prior to the advent of the vaccine, is now rare, although still possible.
- *Meningococcal polysaccharide or conjugate vaccine.* Asplenic children as young as 2 years of age should be given the meningococcal polysaccharide vaccine (MPSV), as opposed to the meningococcal conjugate vaccine (MCV), which should be given at 11–12 years of age. Revaccination should be considered given the continued risk for meningococcal disease.[29] Of note, although it is not approved currently for use in younger children, the recommendations regarding use of MCV may change in the future.
- *Influenza vaccine.* Although not specifically indicated for asplenia, it is a recommended vaccine which may be important for those with asplenia as influenza can be associated with bacterial coinfection, especially with *Staphylococcus aureus*, *S. pneumoniae*, and *N. meningitidis.*

Education

Primary caretaker and patient education are crucial in helping to prevent severe infections. Studies have indicated that many patients and their caretakers are not well informed about the risk for infection and the

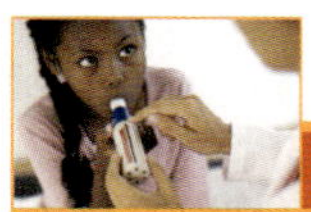

Table 57–5.

Recommendations for Pneumococcal Vaccination for Children at High Risk

Age	Previous Doses	Recommended Schedule
≤23 mo	None	Primary series (see Table 57–4)
24–59 mo	4 doses of PCV7*	1 dose of PPV23 at 24 mo 1 dose of PPV23 3–5 y after 1st dose of PPV23
24–59 mo	1–3 doses of PCV7	1 dose of PCV7 1 dose of PPV23 6–8 wk later 1 dose of PPV23 3–5 y after 1st dose of PPV23
24–59 mo	1 dose of PPV23	2 doses of PCV7, 6–8 wk apart (should be given at least 6–8 wk following PPV23 dose) 1 dose of PPV23 3–5 y after 1st dose of PPV23
24–59 mo	None	2 doses of PCV7, 6–8 wk apart 1 dose of PPV23 6–8 wk after last dose of PCV7 1 dose of PPV23 3–5 y after 1st dose of PPV23

Adapted from American Academy of Pediatrics. Committee on infectious diseases. Policy statement: Recommendations for the prevention of pneumococcal infections, including the use of pneumococcal conjugate vaccine (Prevnar), pneumococcal polysaccharide vaccine, and antibiotic prophylaxis. Pediatrics 2000;106(2 Pt. 1):362–366.
PCV7, pneumococcal conjugate vaccine (Prevnar); PPV23, pneumococcal polysaccharide vaccine (Pneumovax).

importance of chemoprophylaxis, vaccination, and/or empiric therapy.[30–32] In addition, those who are not well informed may be less likely to seek medical care in a timely fashion. The risk of severe infection with asplenia and the need for the preventive measures mentioned previously should be discussed repeatedly.[11,33] Emphasis should be placed on the need to seek medical attention at the start of any illness as the progression to fulminant sepsis can be rapid. Medical care should also be sought with any animal or human bites.[34] All health care professionals should be made aware of the child's diagnosis. The use of medical alert bracelets, portable immunization records, or portable cards outlining steps for what to do in the case of illness have also been suggested.[16,35,36]

PEARLS

Individuals with asplenia are at risk for overwhelming infections. Asplenic children are at greater risk for overwhelming sepsis than their adult counterparts. Preventive measures and timely medical care are crucial in averting serious morbidity and mortality. Main points to keep in mind when caring for an asplenic child are the following:

- Chemoprophylaxis: An important measure in preventing invasive pneumococcal disease in children with asplenia, although breakthrough infection can still occur, especially with penicillin-resistant strains.
- Education: Emphasis on the risk for infection and the need to seek early medical attention should occur on routine basis.
- Diagnosis and treatment: Never let the diagnostic workup delay empiric therapy.

REFERENCES

1. King H, Shumacker HB Jr. Splenic studies. I. Susceptibility to infection after splenectomy performed in infancy. *Ann Surg.* 1952;136(2):239-242.
2. Chesney PJ. Asplenia. In: Patrick CC, ed. *Clinical Management of Infections in Immunocompromised Infants and Children.* Philadelphia: Lippincott Williams & Wilkens; 2001:307-326.
3. Lutwick LI. Infections in Asplenic Patients. In: Mandell GI, Bennett JE, Dolin R, eds. *Mandell, Douglas, and Bennett's Principles and Practice of Infectious Diseases.* 6th ed. Philadelphia: Elsevier/Churchill Livingstone; 2005:3524-3530.
4. Sumaraju V, Smith LG, Smith SM. Infectious complications in asplenic hosts. *Infect Dis Clin North Am.* 2001; 15(2):551-565.
5. Bisharat N, Omari H, Lavi I, Raz R. Risk of infection and death among post-splenectomy patients. *J Infect.* 2001; 43(3):182-186.
6. Kyaw MH, Holmes EM, Toolis F, et al. Evaluation of severe infection and survival after splenectomy. *Am J Med.* 2006;119(3):276.e1-276.e7
7. Kumar V, Abbas AK, Fausto N, Robbins SL, Cotran RS. *Robbins and Cotran Pathologic Basis of Disease.* 7th ed. Philadelphia: Elsevier Saunders; 2005.
8. Shurin SB. The spleen and its disorders. In: Hoffman R, ed. *Hematology: Basic Principles and Practice.* 4th ed. Philadelphia: Churchill Livingstone; 2005: 901-908.
9. Ejstrud P, Kristensen B, Hansen JB, Madsen KM, Schonheyder HC, Sorensen HT. Risk and patterns of bacteraemia after splenectomy: A population-based study. *Scand J Infect Dis.* 2000;32(5):521-525.

10. Wang JK, Hsieh KH. Immunologic study of the asplenia syndrome. *Pediatr Infect Dis J.* 1991;10(11):819-822.
11. Hansen K, Singer DB. Asplenic-hyposplenic overwhelming sepsis: postsplenectomy sepsis revisited. *Pediatr Dev Pathol.* 2001;4(2):105-121.
12. Kanthan R, Moyana T, Nyssen J. Asplenia as a cause of sudden unexpected death in childhood. *Am J Forensic Med Pathol.* 1999;20(1):57-59.
13. Schutze GE, Mason EO Jr., Barson WJ, et al. Invasive pneumococcal infections in children with asplenia. *Pediatr Infect Dis J.* 2002;21(4):278-282.
14. Shepard CW, Daneshvar MI, Kaiser RM, et al. Bordetella holmesii bacteremia: a newly recognized clinical entity among asplenic patients. *Clin Infect Dis.* 2004;38(6): 799-804.
15. Ward KM, Celebi JT, Gmyrek R, Grossman ME. Acute infectious purpura fulminans associated with asplenism or hyposplenism. *J Am Acad Dermatol.* 2002;47(4):493-496.
16. Brigden ML, Pattullo AL. Prevention and management of overwhelming postsplenectomy infection–an update. *Crit Care Med.* 1999;27(4):836-842.
17. Waldman JD, Rosenthal A, Smith AL, Shurin S, Nadas AS. Sepsis and congenital asplenia. *J Pediatr.* 1977;90(4): 555-559.
18. Halasa NB, Shankar SM, Talbot TR, et al. Incidence of invasive pneumococcal disease among individuals with sickle cell disease before and after the introduction of the pneumococcal conjugate vaccine. *Clin Infect Dis.* 2007;44(11):1428-1433.
19. Chotivanich K, Udomsangpetch R, McGready R, et al. Central role of the spleen in malaria parasite clearance. *J Infect Dis.* 2002;185(10):1538-1541.
20. Lindquist SW, Weber DJ, Mangum ME, Hollis DG, Jordan J. Bordetella holmesii sepsis in an asplenic adolescent. *Pediatr Infect Dis J.* 1995;14(9):813-815.
21. Riddington C, Owusu-Ofori S. Prophylactic antibiotics for preventing pneumococcal infection in children with sickle cell disease. *Cochrane Database Syst Rev.* 2002(3): CD003427.
22. American Academy of Pediatrics. Immunization in Special Clinical Circumstances. In: Pickering LK, Baker CJ, Long SS, McMillan JA, eds. *Red Book: 2006 Report of the Committee on Infectious Diseases.* 27th ed. Elk Grove Village: American Academy of Pediatrics; 2006:83-85.
23. Falletta JM, Woods GM, Verter JI, et al. Discontinuing penicillin prophylaxis in children with sickle cell anemia. Prophylactic Penicillin Study II. *J Pediatr.* 1995;127(5): 685-690.
24. Price VE, Dutta S, Blanchette VS, et al. The prevention and treatment of bacterial infections in children with asplenia or hyposplenia: practice considerations at the hospital for sick children, Toronto. *Pediatric Blood Cancer.* 2006;46(5): 597-603.
25. Wilson W, Taubert KA, Gewitz M, et al. Prevention of Infective Endocarditis. Guidelines from the American Heart Association. A Guideline from the American Heart Association Rheumatic Fever, Endocarditis, and Kawasaki Disease Committee, Council on Cardiovascular Disease in the Young, and the Council on Clinical Cardiology, Council on Cardiovascular Surgery and Anesthesia, and the Quality of Care and Outcomes Research Interdisciplinary Working Group. *Circulation.* 2007; 116: 1736-1754.
26. De Rossi SS, Glick M. Dental considerations in asplenic patients. *J Am Dent Assoc.* 1996;127(9):1359-1363.
27. Centers for Disease Control and Prevention. *Epidemiology and Prevention of Vaccine Preventable Diseases.* Atkinson W, Hamborsky J, McIntyre L, Wolfe S, eds. 10th ed. Washington DC: Public Health Foundation; 2007:115-128, 257-282, A-19.
28. American Academy of Pediatrics. Committee on infectious diseases. Policy statement: recommendations for the prevention of pneumococcal infections, including the use of pneumococcal conjugate vaccine (Prevnar), pneumococcal polysaccharide vaccine, and antibiotic prophylaxis. *Pediatrics.* 2000;106(2, pt. 1):362-366.
29. Centers for Disease Control and Prevention. Prevention and control of meningococcal disease: Recommendations of the advisory committe on immunization practices. *Morb Mortal Wkly Rep.* 2005;54(RR–7).
30. Corbett SM, Rebuck JA, Rogers FB, et al. Time lapse and comorbidities influence patient knowledge and pursuit of medical care after traumatic splenectomy. *J Trauma.* 2007; 62(2):397-403.
31. de Montalembert M, Lenoir G. Antibiotic prevention of pneumococcal infections in asplenic hosts: admission of insufficiency. *Ann Hematol.* 2004;83(1):18-21.
32. Waghorn DJ. Overwhelming infection in asplenic patients: current best practice preventive measures are not being followed. *J Clin Pathol.* 2001;54(3):214-218.
33. Castagnola E, Fioredda F. Prevention of life-threatening infections due to encapsulated bacteria in children with hyposplenia or asplenia: a brief review of current recommendations for practical purposes. *Eur J Haematol.* 2003; 71(5):319-326.
34. Davidson RN, Wall RA. Prevention and management of infections in patients without a spleen. *Clin Microbiol Infect.* 2001;7(12):657-660.
35. Davies JM, Barnes R, Milligan D. Update of guidelines for the prevention and treatment of infection in patients with an absent or dysfunctional spleen. *Clin Med.* 2002;2(5): 440-443.
36. Melles DC, de Marie S. Prevention of infections in hyposplenic and asplenic patients: an update. *Neth J Med.* 2004;62(2):45-52.

CHAPTER 58

Infections in Atopic Dermatitis

Jessica K. Hart and Kara N. Shah

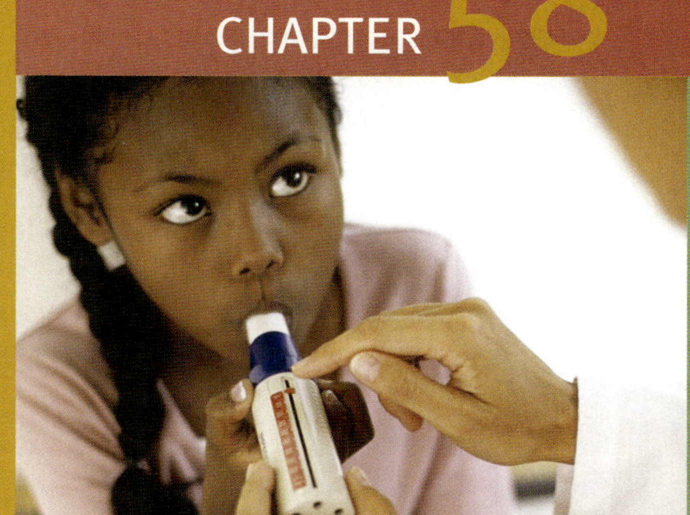

OVERVIEW OF ATOPIC DERMATITIS

Epidemiology and Pathogenesis

Atopic dermatitis (AD) is a common inflammatory skin disorder that affects 10–20% of children younger than 14 years of age.[1,2] The prevalence of AD has increased two- to threefold in the past three decades in industrialized countries and it remains the most common dermatitis of childhood. The pathogenesis of AD is not completely understood and is likely multifactorial, involving complex interactions between environmental triggers, defects in skin barrier function, and systemic and local immunologic responses.[3] AD is often the initial presentation of atopic disease in children, and according to the theory of the "atopic march," poorly controlled AD is believed to contribute to the development of asthma and allergic rhinitis in older children in 50–80% of affected patients.[2,3]

Clinical Presentation and Diagnosis

The diagnosis of AD is made on clinical evaluation. The majority of cases arise within the first 2 years of life.[4] The key features of AD as defined by Hanifin and Rajka in 1980 and modified in 2001 include a chronic and relapsing course, typical morphology and distribution of cutaneous findings, and pruritus.[5,6] Pruritus is a universal finding in AD and can be severe, leading to sleep disturbances and irritability. Pruritus also leads to scratching, which causes secondary skin changes such as lichenification (thickening and hyperpigmentation of skin with accentuation of skin lines), excoriations, skin breakdown, and infection.

The cutaneous manifestations of AD may be classified as acute or chronic. In an acute exacerbation of AD, erythematous papules and patches associated with scaling, excoriations, and serous exudates are seen (Figure 58–1). Chronic AD is characterized by hyperpigmented, lichenified plaques and nodules that result from chronic rubbing and scratching (Figure 58–2). Acute and chronic changes may coexist in the same patient. Most AD patients also have dry lackluster skin (xerosis), and a significant number also have ichthyosis vulgaris, a genetic skin disorder that results from mutations in the gene for filaggrin.[7–9] Filaggrin is a key component of the cornified cell envelope, which forms the epidermal skin barrier. Disruption of the epidermal barrier is thought to increase epicutaneous exposure to potential environmental allergens, which can contribute to the development of atopic disease.

The presentation of AD varies with the patient's age. In infants, AD typically presents acutely with erythematous scaling or crusted patches that involve the

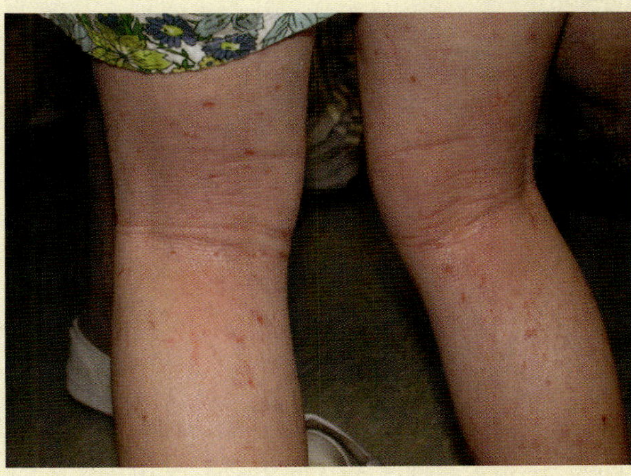

FIGURE 58–1 ■ Acute presentation of AD with erythema and scaling.

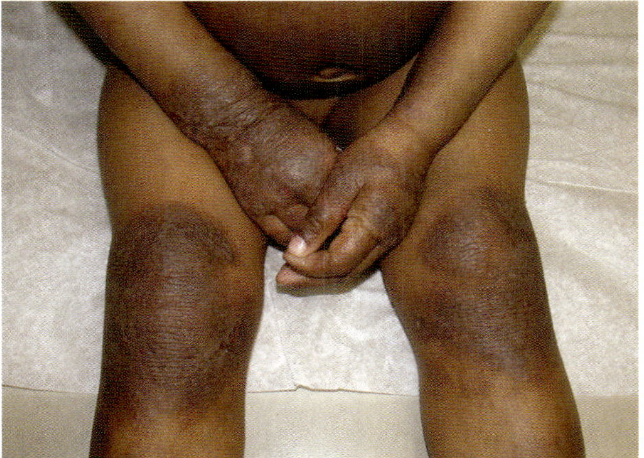

FIGURE 58–2 ■ Chronic AD with the development of hyperpigmentation and lichenification.

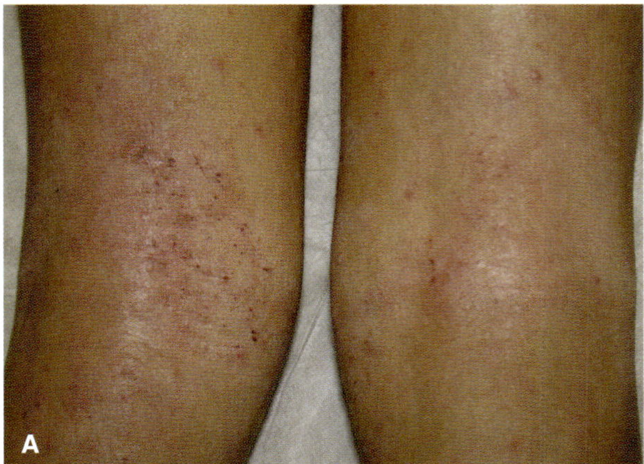

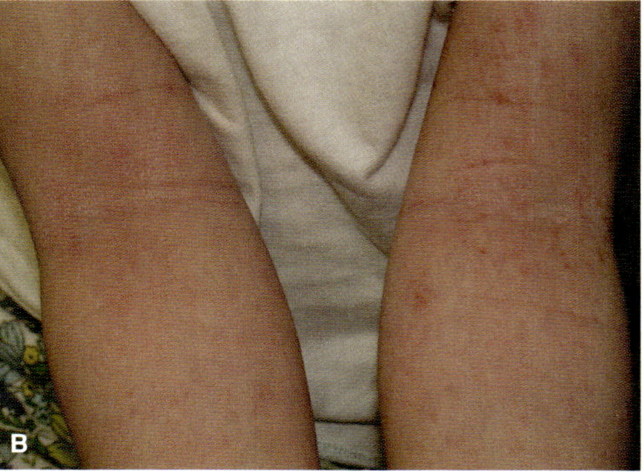

FIGURE 58–4 ■ Typical appearance of AD in childhood and adolescence with involvement of the flexure surfaces of the extremities. **(A)** Popliteal fossae; **(B)** Antecubital fossa.

face, especially the cheeks, the scalp, and the extensor surfaces of the extremities; the diaper area, periocular areas, and perinasal areas are usually spared (Figure 58–3). In childhood and adolescence, AD typically involves the feet, the hands, and flexural areas such as the antecubital fossae, popliteal fossae, and neck (Figure 58–4). Both acute and chronic cutaneous manifestations can be seen. Other cutaneous manifestations associated with AD include periorbital hyperpigmentation, Dennie–Morgan folds (prominent folds of skin under the lower eyelid), hyperlinearity of the palms and soles, pityriasis alba, and follicular prominence, especially on the trunk.

There are a number of exposures that may aggravate AD in susceptible children, including foods, skin irritants such as wool clothing and sweating, and environmental allergens such as dog dander and dustmites. Substantial clinical improvement may occur when patients are removed from environments that contain allergens or irritants to which they react.[2] If food or environmental allergen sensitivity is suspected, patients should be evaluated with prick skin testing under the supervision of a pediatric allergist. The majority of children with AD, however, do not have clearly identifiable allergens as a component of their disease. In many patients, disease flares are also reported in association with concurrent upper respiratory infection or a change of season. Extremes of temperature and low humidity both commonly exacerbate AD.

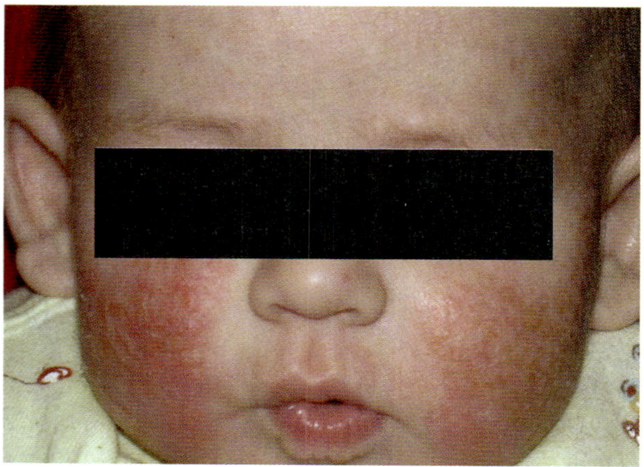

FIGURE 58–3 ■ Infantile AD with striking involvement of the cheeks and chin and perinasal and periocular sparing.

Treatment Regimens

The treatment of AD requires a systematic, multifaceted approach that incorporates skin hydration, topical anti-inflammatory agents, identification and elimination of exacerbating factors, and, if necessary, systemic therapy. Patients and their families should be counseled about the chronic nature of AD and the need for continued adherence to proper skin care. In children with cutaneous infection associated with a flare of their AD, appropriate management of the underlying AD is a key component of the treatment regimen.

Atopic skin care

Patients with AD have decreased skin barrier function, which is exacerbated during cold, dry weather, and with overbathing. Skin hydration and the frequent use of topical emollients to repair the impaired skin barrier function is a key part of management. Reasonable recommendations for atopic skin care include:

- Infrequent bathing (1–3 times per week) with lukewarm water for no more than 5–10 minutes.
- Use of mild nonsoap cleansers, such as Dove™ soap or Cetaphil™ liquid cleanser.
- Application of an emollient immediately following bathing (pat skin with towel to remove excess water and apply emollient while skin is still damp, ideally within 2–3 minutes). Ointment formulations such as Aquaphor™ or Vaseline™ are preferred.
- Keeping child's fingernails filed short to avoid injury to the skin from scratching.
- Severely affected skin can be optimally hydrated by the wet wrap technique. Immediately after bathing, topical corticosteroids and/or emollients are applied, followed by occlusion with damp pajamas or gauze wraps, followed by dry pajamas or clothing.
- Occasional soaks in tar (Cutar™) baths or with colloidal oatmeal (Aveeno™) can be used to treat pruritus.

Topical corticosteroids

Topical corticosteroids have been the mainstay of anti-inflammatory treatment of AD for many years. They are effective in the control of both acute and chronic skin inflammation. Topical corticosteroids are grouped into seven potency categories (Table 58–1), with group 1 containing the most potent agents and group 7 containing the least potent agents. A general principle in treating AD with topical corticosteroids is to use the least potent agent required and to limit the frequency of application. Topical glucocortocoids are available as lotions, foams, ointments, solutions, creams, and gels. In general, lotions and foams are avoided when treating AD, as these preparations often contain alcohol and can be irritating. Ointments (water-in-oil emulsions) are generally preferred over creams (oil-in-water emulsions), as ointments provide better skin hydration. In general, ointment preparations of a given corticosteroid are also more potent than cream formulations of the same corticosteroid, and the same steroid in a different vehicle can differ in potency by one or two classes. Some areas of the body dictate the type of vehicle needed. For example, the scalp is best treated with a solution. In addition, some patients do not tolerate ointments because of their greasy consistency, especially in hot, humid weather.

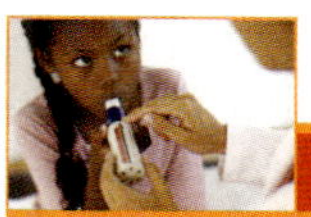

Table 58–1.

Topical Corticosteroid Potencies

Topical Corticosteroid Potencies
Class I (super potent)
Clobetasol (Temovate) 0.05% ointment, cream, gel, solution
Clobetasol (Olux) 0.05% foam
Clobetasol (Clobex) 0.05% shampoo, spray
Halobetasol (Ultravate) 0.05% ointment, cream
Betamethasone diproprionate augmented (Diprolene) 0.05% ointment, gel
Fluocinonide (Vanos) 0.1% cream
Class 2 (potent)
Fluocinonide (Lidex) 0.05% ointment, cream, gel
Desoximetasone (Topicort) 0.25% ointment, cream
Desoximetasone (Topicort) 0.05% gel
Betamethasone diproprionate (Diprosone) 0.05% ointment
Betamethasone diproprionate augmented (Diprolene) 0.05% cream, lotion
Class 3 (potent)
Fluticasone (Cutivate) 0.005% ointment
Betamethasone diproprionate (Diprosone) 0.05% cream
Betamethasone valerate (Valisone) 0.1% ointment
Fluocinonide (Lidex) 0.05% cream
Mometasone (Elocon) 0.1% ointment
Triamcinolone (Kenalog) 0.1% ointment
Class 4 (mid-potent)
Hydrocortisone valerate (Westcort) 0.2% ointment
Mometasone (Elocon) 0.1% cream
Prednicarbate (Dermatop) 0.1% ointment
Triamcinolone (Kenalog) 0.1% cream
Fluocinolone (Synalar) 0.025% ointment
Desoximetasone (Topicort LP) 0.05% cream
Betamethasone (Luxiq) 0.12% foam
Clocortolone (Cloderm) 0.1% cream
Class 5 (mid-potent)
Hydrocortisone valerate (Westcort) 0.2% cream
Betamethasone valerate (Valisone) 0.1% cream
Hydrocortisone butyrate (Locoid) 0.1% cream, ointment, solution
Betamethasone (Diprosone) 0.05% lotion
Triamcinolone (Kenalog) 0.1% lotion
Fluticasone (Cutivate) 0.05% cream
Fluocinolone (Synalar) 0.025% cream
Prednicarbate (Dermatop) 0.1% cream
Class 6 (mild)
Alclometasone (Aclovate) 0.05% ointment, cream
Desonide (Desowen) 0.05% cream
Betamethasone valerate (Valisone) 0.1% lotion
Fluocinolone (Synalar) 0.01% solution
Desonide (Verdeso) 0.05% foam
Desonide (Desonate) 0.05% hydrogel
Fluocinolone (Dermasmoothe FS) 0.01% scalp oil
Class 7 (mild)
Hydrocortisone 2.5% ointment, cream
Hydrocortisone 1% ointment, cream

The majority of infants with AD respond well to low potency corticosteroids (class 6–7), but others will require short treatment courses of a more potent corticosteroid. Olderchildren and adolescents, especially those with more severe disease, may require intermittent use of a medium potency corticosteroid (class 4–5). Short 1–2-week courses of higher potency topical corticosteroids (class 2–3) may be required in some patients with acute flares and to treat moderate-to-severe chronic AD. Group 1 topical corticosteroids are generally best avoided in children younger than 12 years. Topical corticosteroids should be used no more than twice daily, as more frequent application has not been shown to increase efficacy, only to result in more adverse sequelae.

Compared with adults, children (especially infants) are at higher risk for the local and systemic side effects of topical corticosteroids (Table 58–2). Use of higher potency topical corticosteroids (class 1–4) should be avoided in intertriginous areas such as the groin and axillae and on the face, as the risk of systemic absorption and cutaneous atrophy is high in these areas. Use of any topical corticosteroid under occlusion (e.g., a diaper or dressing) also increases systemic absorption and the risk of local side effects. Chronic use of topical corticosteroids may result in cutaneous atrophy at the sites of application, with thinning and dyspigmentation of the skin. Permanent striae may occur (Figure 58–5). In addition, chronic application of topical corticosteroids over large areas of inflamed skin may result in systemic absorption and hypothalamic-pituitary-adrenal axis suppression. Adverse effects are related to the potency of the topical corticosteroid, the site of application, the percentage of body surface area covered, and the duration of use.

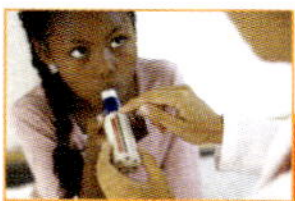

Table 58–2.

Local and Systemic Adverse Effects of Topical Corticosteroids

Local

- Atrophy
- Striae
- Telangiectasias
- Perioral dermatitis
- Acneiform rash
- Allergic contact dermatitis

Systemic

- Growth suppression
- Hypothalamic-pituitary-adrenal axis suppression
- Immunosuppression
- Cushing syndrome

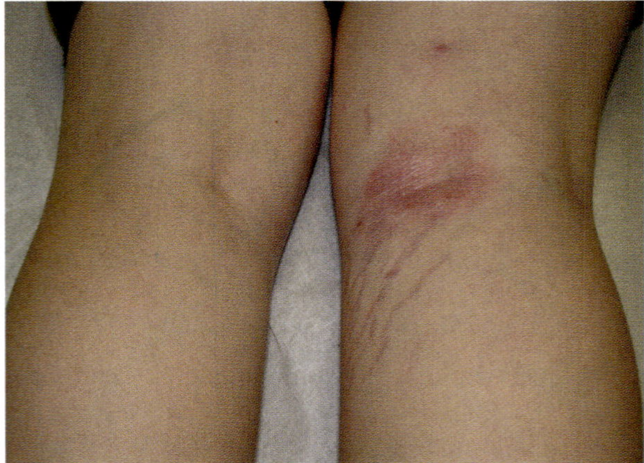

FIGURE 58–5 ■ Topical corticosteroid-induced striae.

Topical immunomodulators

The topical calcineurin inhibitors tacrolimus (available as 0.03% and 0.1% ointments) and pimecrolimus 1% cream appear to be effective for the treatment of AD, and unlike topical corticosteroids, do not have the potential to cause skin atrophy or hypothalamic-pituitary-adrenal axis suppression. For this reason, they are particularly useful on the face and in intertriginous areas. They are also useful in the treatment of chronic AD as corticosteroid-sparing agents. Topical tacrolimus and pimecrolimus are applied twice daily. Adverse effects include local irritation or stinging, pruritus, and rash, which generally resolve with continued use.[1] Although both topical preparations are approved by the U.S. Food and Drug Administration (FDA) for the treatment of AD in children older than 2 years, there are concerns regarding the possibility of an increased risk of both skin malignancies and lymphoma, which have been demonstrated in animal-model studies.[10–12] Although in controlled human trials in adults and children use of the topical calcineurin inhibitors appears to be safe, in 2006, the FDA placed a "black box" warning on the prescribing information for these medications.[13–16] While further study is underway, the FDA has made the following recommendations:

- Use these agents only as second-line therapy in patients unresponsive to or intolerant of other treatments.
- Avoid the use of these agents in children younger than 2 years of age; clinical studies have found higher rates of upper respiratory infections, fever, otitis media and diarrhea in children younger than 2 years of age who were treated with pimecrolimus.
- Use these agents only for short periods of time and use the minimum amount necessary to control symptoms, avoid continuous use.
- Avoid the use of these agents in patients with compromised immune systems.

Antihistamines

Antihistamines are widely used as a therapeutic adjunct in patients with AD to treat associated pruritus. The evidence supporting their use is relatively weak since no large, randomized, placebo-controlled trials with definitive conclusions have been performed.[17] Nevertheless, the sedating oral antihistamines appear to be most effective (e.g., diphenhydramine and hydroxyzine). However, these agents can affect a child's ability to learn and play as a result of their sedating effects, and are often best utilized at bedtime to faciliate sleep. Higher than normal doses may be necessary because of the development of tachyphylaxis. In our clinical experience, the use of nonsedating preparations such as fexofenadine or loratidine is less helpful in mitigating the pruritus associated with AD. The use of topical antihistamines is discouraged, as there is no evidence that they are effective in ameliorating the pruritus associated with AD, and overuse may lead to significant systemic absorption and potential side effects.

Systemic therapy

If patients with severe disease fail appropriate topical treatment, systemic therapy is warranted. Some patients may benefit from phototherapy with either psoralen-UVA, broadband UVB, or narrow-band UVB treatments.[18,19] Ultraviolet light has immunodulatory effects on the skin-immune system and reduces cutaneous inflammation. Treatment is usually initiated 2–3 times weekly and the frequency decreased as clinical improvement is seen. Rarely, systemic immunosuppressive therapy may be required. Such therapy should generally be prescribed by a specialist because of the potential for adverse effects and requirements for routine monitoring. The most widely used oral immunosuppressive agent is cyclosporine, although the use of other agents such as mycophenlate mofetil have been reported to be efficacious in children in several published case reports and small case series.[20–23]

INFECTIOUS COMPLICATIONS OF AD

Patients with AD, especially those with disseminated or severe disease, tend to develop the following infections with higher frequency than children without AD: impetigo, bacterial folliculitis, viral warts, herpes simplex virus infections (eczema herpeticum), and molluscum contagiosum.[24] A number of factors may favor higher rates of these bacterial and viral infections in children with AD. Xerosis, pruritus, and subsequent scratching help to inoculate, maintain, and disseminate infection. Recent studies suggest that primary and/or secondary defects in the innate immune system in patients with AD are important contributing factors to the development of cutaneous infections in these patients.[25] In particular, patients with AD appear to exhibit a deficiency in the secretion of antimicrobial peptides (beta-defensins and cathelicidins) that contributes to the high incidence of cutaneous bacterial and viral infections.[26] There is also emerging evidence to suggest that Staphylococcal superantigens play a role in promoting a Th2-mediated cutaneous inflammatory response and in promoting IgE production.[27] At present, there is no clear evidence that the use of topical corticosteroids or topical immunomodulators increases the risk of cutaneous infection in children with AD.

Bacterial Superinfections

Secondary bacterial infection of atopic eczema is a common complication, with *Staphylococcus aureus* being the most common etiology, followed by *Streptococcus pyogenes*. Of patients with AD, more than 90% are colonized with *S. aureus*.[28] In contrast, *S. aureus* can be found on the skin of only 5–30% of normal individuals. *S. aureus* is isolated from clinically affected and unaffected skin, and both acute and chronic AD lesions may be colonized.[29] Recent studies suggest that the skin of patients with AD has increased avidity for binding to *S. aureus* and is deficient in its ability to generate antimicrobial peptides needed to eradicate infectious agents.[30] Impaired skin integrity, increased *S. aureus* adherence, and abnormal innate immune responses all predispose patients to more invasive cutaneous infections (e.g., cellulitis, furuncles, abscesses).[31] Recurrence of bacterial infection, usually with *S. aureus,* is common, occurring in up to 40% of children with AD.[24]

Clinical presentation

Clinical signs of impetiginization, such as weeping and crusting, fissuring, or small superficial pustules are very common signs indicating that skin colonization with *S. aureus* may have occurred (Figure 58–6).[32] Extensive crusting, folliculitis, or impetigo, or the development of pyoderma, are indicators of bacterial skin infection that requires antibiotic therapy. Regional lymphadenopathy is common in such patients. Patients with extensive skin involvement may develop an exfoliative dermatitis as a result of superinfection with toxin-producing *S. aureus.* This is associated with generalized redness, scaling, weeping, crusting, systemic toxicity, lymphadenopathy, and fever. In contrast to impetiginization with *S. aureus,* infection with *S. pyogenes* often presents with either well-demarcated erythematous, eroded patches favoring intertriginous areas such as the popliteal and antecubital fossae, or with impetigo.

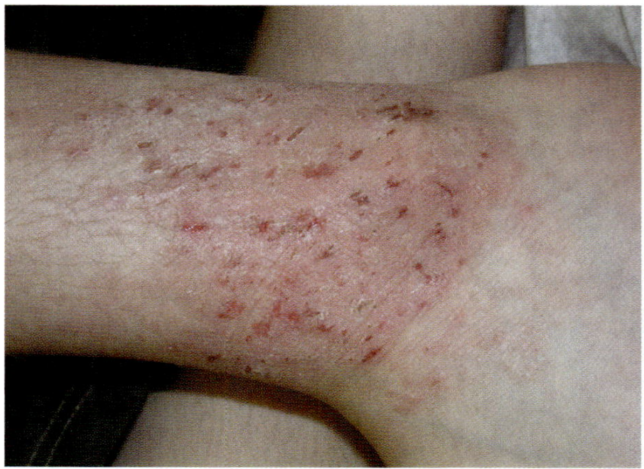

FIGURE 58–6 ■ Impetiginized AD.

Diagnosis

The diagnosis of a bacterial superinfection can usually be made based upon the appearance of the skin. Given the increasing prevalence of antibiotic-resistant strains of *S. aureus*, the identification of the organism from superficial skin lesions or bullae by Gram stain and culture is recommended prior to the initiation of systemic antibiotics.

Treatment

Standard treatment for bacterial infection with *S. aureus* often involves topical and/or oral administration of antibacterial agents; however, resistance to standard antibacterial regimens is an increasing problem, and mupirocin-resistant and methicillin-resistant *S. aureus* are present worldwide. While the use of a topical antibiotic such as mupirocin or bacitracin may be adequate for mild, localized disease, systemic antibiotic therapy may be necessary to treat AD when more widespread bacterial infection with *S. aureus* or *S. pyogenes* is present or in the presence of systemic symptoms such as fever or pain. Semisynthetic penicillins or first- or second-generation cephalosporins given for 7–10 days are usually effective. Rarely, longer treatment courses of up to 14 days may be required. Erythromycin-resistant organisms are fairly common, making macrolides less useful alternatives. The presence of an atypical skin infection in patients with AD, particularly those unresponsive to conventional penicillinase-resistant penicillins and cephalosporins, should alert the clinician to the possibility of methicillin-resistant *S. aureus* as the underlying etiology, and intervention should be directed accordingly. Methicillin-resistant strains may be treated with clindamycin, trimethoprim-sulfamehoxazole, or a tetracycline, although antibiotic resistance to these agents also occurs. Infections with *S. pyogenes* are best treated with penicillin or amoxicillin.

Unfortunately, recolonization of the skin after a course of antistaphylococcal therapy occurs rapidly. Maintenance antibiotic therapy, however, should be avoided, because it may result in colonization by antibiotic-resistant organisms. The use of topical regimens to control skin colonization with *S. aureus* may be more helpful. Although antibacterial skin cleansers are effective in reducing bacterial skin flora, they can cause significant skin irritation. Additionally, studies of antiseptics have shown conflicting evidence in the treatment of AD.[33,34] A recent double-blind, placebo-controlled study found that daily bathing with an antimicrobial soap containing 1.5% triclocarban resulted in reductions in *S. aureus* colonization and significantly greater clinical improvement than with the placebo soap.[33] Other agents that may be used intermittently (1–2 times per week) to reduce colonization with *S. aureus* include chlorhexidine topical cleanser (Hibiclens®), benzoyl peroxide 5% wash, and 0.25% sodium hypochlorite soaks (1 capful of Clorox® bleach per gallon of water). Topical mupirocin applied three times daily to the nares, fingertips, and perianal area for 5 contiguous days per month may also be effective in reducing colonization rates.

Although significant reduction of bacterial colonization in the skin of AD patients by oral antibiotics has been demonstrated, there is little evidence for clinical improvement in the severity of the dermatitis.[35] Several studies have demonstrated that the combination of appropriate topical corticosteroids with a topical antibiotic is significantly more effective at reducing skin inflammation caused by AD than using the topical corticosteroid or topical antibiotic alone.[30,31,36] However, there is no conclusive clinical evidence suggesting that patients with AD may benefit from specific antibiotic treatment in the absence of clinical signs of infection.[37]

As a result of the increased risk of bacterial resistance that may occur with frequent use of antibiotics, it is important to combine antimicrobial therapy with effective skin care since it is well established that the impaired skin barrier in patients with poorly-controlled AD predisposes to *S. aureus* colonization and infection. Use of topical emollients and an appropriate skin care regimen as detailed above to restore skin barrier function, combined with use of effective anti-inflammatory therapy, is the most efficacious way to reduce the frequency of cutaneous superinfection.[30]

Viral Superinfections

Children with AD are also predisposed to the development of viral skin infections. Infection with the human papillomavirus (HPV), herpes simplex virus (HSV), varicella-zoster virus (VZV) and molluscum contagiosum virus is common in children with AD. Extensive infection with these viruses may develop in children with poorly controlled AD caused by the impaired skin barrier. Eczema vaccinatum is a potentially fatal complication of inadvertent exposure to the vaccinia virus in a patient with AD. Close contact with a patient with AD is a contraindication to receiving the smallpox vaccine.

Eczema herpeticum

Eczema herpeticum is an acute cutaneous HSV infection in a patient with AD. Children of all ages and ethnic groups may be affected by eczema herpeticum, with the highest incidence occurring in children 2–3 years of age.[38] A history of a close relative with recurrent HSV labialis is common. Patients with AD may also develop widespread varicella during a primary infection with the varicella zoster virus.

Clinical presentation Eczema herpeticum usually presents as an acute deterioration of the child's AD. Monomorphous punched-out erosions are the most common lesions seen but papules, vesicles, pustules, and crusts may also be seen (Figure 58–7). Although lesions initially develop as vesicles, rupture of the vesicles commonly occurs as a result of scratching, leaving punched-out erosions in the skin. Oozing may occur from raw areas. Lesions may be discrete or confluent and tend to occur in crops. Associated clinical symptoms include fever, itching, malaise, vomiting, anorexia, diarrhea, and lymphadenopathy.[38] At the height of the vesicular phase, widespread dissemination of virus may occur and lead to systemic involvement.[38]

Diagnosis The diagnosis of HSV infection can be made by a variety of techniques including viral culture, direct immunofluorescence, polymerase chain reaction (PCR), or a Tzanck preparation. Proper technique in obtaining a specimen for analysis is crucial. An intact vesicle should be gently "unroofed" with a sterile blade. The base of the vesicle should be rubbed vigorously with a sterile cotton swab and placed in viral culture medium. If no intact vesicles are available for sampling, an erosion or crusted lesion may be used; however, any exudates or crust should be removed prior to sampling. While viral culture has remained the standard diagnostic method for isolating HSV, real-time HSV PCR assays have emerged as a more sensitive method to confirm HSV infection. The Tzanck smear, which relies on the demonstration of multinucleated giant cells in infected tissue, is now of predominantly historical interest, although it can be performed at the bedside by specialists who are trained in processing and interpreting the specimen. Differentiating between HSV-1 and HSV-2 infection is rarely indicated. Although much less common, evaluation for VZV infection should also be considered in any patient with suspected eczema herpeticum. PCR, direct immunofluorescence, and viral culture are all available diagnostic tests.

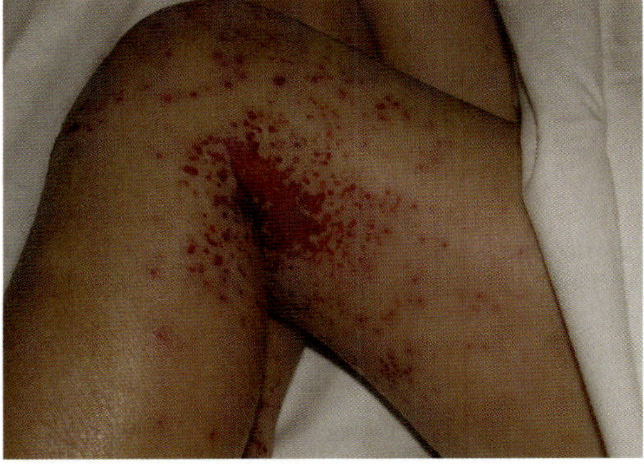

FIGURE 58–7 ■ Eczema herpeticum. Note the characteristic monomorphous, punched-out erosions.

Treatment Early recognition of infection and initiation of appropriate treatment is important as the virus may disseminate rapidly, especially in immunocompromised patients. Infants and children who appear ill may require intravenous acyclovir. Children who do not have systemic symptoms and have localized involvement usually respond well to oral acyclovir. Adolescents may be treated with valacyclovir. Topical or systemic antibiotic therapy may be required if secondary bacterial infection develops. The use of tap water soaks twice daily may help to remove any adherent crusts. Topical steroid therapy is often discontinued in the acute phase of eczema herpeticum because of the concern that concomitant use of topical steroids may perpetuate the spread of the infection, although there is no clear evidence to support this conjecture. In our practice, use of topical steroids on involved areas is held for 24–48 hours after initiation of antiviral therapy and until further development of new lesions has ceased.

Complications Following peripheral inoculation, HSV undergoes retrograde axonal transport and establish chronic latent infections in sensory neurons of the trigeminal and dorsal root ganglia. Intermittent reactivation of HSV leads to peripheral shedding of infectious virus particles, which under favorable conditions cause inflammation and lesion formation on cutaneous and mucosal surfaces. Shedding of HSV in and around the eyes occurs frequently.[39] Conjunctivitis and keratoconjunctivitis may occur as manifestations of either a primary or a recurrent infection. The conjunctiva may appear congested and swollen, but there is usually little, if any, purulent discharge. Corneal lesions may be superficial, in the form of a dendritic ulcer, or deep, as a disciform keratitis. Dendritic keratitis is unique to HSV eye involvement. The diagnosis is suggested by the presence of herpetic vesicles on the lids; it is established by the isolation of the virus. Topical corticosteroid use will worsen HSV ocular disease. Recurrent herpetic corneal infection may result in scarring of the cornea and vision impairment. Any patient with periocular involvement should be evaluated by an ophthalmologist for evidence of keratitis.

Secondary bacterial infection of the skin may also be present, usually caused by *S. aureus* and group A β-hemolytic *Streptococcus*, which may be a potential focus for the development of septicemia. Evaluation with surface cultures for bacteria and initiation of appropriate antibiotic therapy is recommended in all cases of eczema herpeticum.

Molluscum contagiosum

Molluscum contagiosum is a common pediatric skin infection caused by the molluscum contagiosum virus, a large double-stranded virus that is the most common poxvirus infecting humans.[40] Infection in otherwise healthy children is self-limiting. The infection can spread rapidly and produce hundreds of lesions in children with AD.

Clinical presentation The lesions of molluscum contagiosum are discrete, pearly, skin-colored, dome-shaped, smooth papules varying in size from 1 to 5 mm (Figure 58–8). Typically, they have a central umbilication from which a plug of keratinaceous material can be expressed. Papules can occur anywhere on the body, but there is predilection for the face, eyelids, neck, axillae, and thighs.

Diagnosis The diagnosis of molluscum contagiosum is generally a clinical one. A magnifying lens and illumination aids in the visualization of the pathognomonic central umbilication. If the diagnosis is uncertain, a Tzank preparation can be performed on a scraping of a lesion, which will demonstrate numerous discrete ovoid intracytoplasmic inclusion bodies, called molluscum bodies.

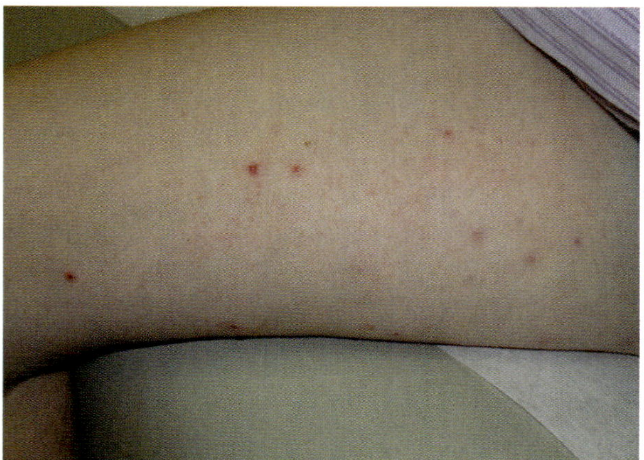

FIGURE 58–8 ■ Molluscum contagiosum with molluscum dermatitis in AD.

Treatment The average infection lasts 9–15 months, although lesions can persist for years. Affected persons should be advised to avoid sharing baths and towels until the infection has cleared. The use of swimming pools while infected should also be discouraged as water is thought to facilitate transmission of the virus. Active nonintervention has been the most common therapy; however, in patients with AD, therapy may indicated. Optimization of the treatment of the underlying AD is critical in minimizing the dissemination of the infection. Use of a rapid mechanical or localized treatment such as curettage or cryotherapy is preferable to use of a topical agent such as a topical retinoid or cantharidin, which may cause significant skin irritation and worsening of underlying AD.

Cryotherapy, or topical application of liquid nitrogen or another cryogen, is very effective and, in many instances, is the treatment of choice. Each lesion should be frozen with liquid nitrogen on a cotton-tipped swab for 5–10 seconds; this should be repeated at 2–4 week intervals as needed. There is a small risk of postinflammatory hyperpigmentation and hypopigmentation after cryotherapy.

Curettage has the advantage of providing tissue specimens to confirm the diagnosis. The major disadvantages are that there is a small risk of scarring with the procedure, and the procedure is messy (because of local bleeding) and uncomfortable. In children, curettage must be accompanied by the use of a local anesthetic. Application of topical anesthetic (e.g., lidocaine/prilocaine cream) 15–30 minutes prior to the procedure has been shown to significantly reduce any associated pain.[41] Manual extraction with the use of a comedo extractor may also be efficacious but is associated with pain and bleeding.

Particularly in younger children in whom liquid nitrogen therapy and curettage are not well tolerated, cantharidin 0.9% can be applied to each lesion without occlusion; this agent causes the development of an epidermal blister with sloughing of infected skin. There is no pain during the actual application of the drug. Furthermore, there is a greater than 90% efficacy rate with limited local discoloration or scarring. There is also a high satisfaction rate (95%) among parent of children treated with cantharidin. The substance is generally washed off in 2–6 hours with little discomfort afterward, although the occasional side effects of blistering and pain may be disturbing, especially if this medication is injudiciously applied or left on too long. For this reason, application on the face or genital area is not recommended.

Tylenol may be used adjunctively at home to reduce any pain associated with vesiculation. On average, 2 treatment sessions are required to clear most patients.[42] Due to the risk of systemic absorption and toxicity, application should generally be limited to no more than 20 lesions per session. In addition, cantharidin should never be dispensed to the family for home use. Applications should always be performed in the office.

Other topical therapies include the off-label use of topical retinoids and topical imiquimod. Imiquimod 5% cream is a topical immunomodulator that is approved by the FDA for the treatment of genital warts in adults. It is of questionable efficacy in the treatment of molluscum infections in healthy children, with clearance rates of approximately 40% reported in several small clinical trials; local irritation is the most common side effect.[43–47] New FDA labeling changes for imiquimod 5% cream states that two large clinical trials failed to demonstrate efficacy for the treatment of molluscum. Although there are no clinical studies addressing the use of topical retinoids to treat molluscum in children, use of a topical retinoid such as tretinoin 0.025% cream or tretinoin 0.1% gel may also be efficacious, although significant irritation can develop during treatment.[48] With both topical retinoids and imiquimod, treatment of a few selected lesions may enhance the ability of the child's immune system to eliminate additional lesions. Use of these agents in patients with poorly-controlled AD is discouraged because of the risk of an exacerbation of the underlying AD should significant irritation develop.

Complications Particularly common in patients with AD is the development of an eczematous dermatitis around individual lesions or groups of lesions, also known as "molluscum dermatitis," which should be treated with topical corticosteroids and antihistamines. The presence of molluscum dermatitis increases the risk of autoinoculation and spreading of the virus.[42] The issue of superinfection is a controversial one, as bacterial superinfection of molluscum contagiosum is uncommon with the exception of children with AD and those who scratch or manipulate the lesions. In cases where bacterial superinfection is suspected, use of a topical antibiotic such as mupirocin is usually sufficient unless widespread involvement develops, in which case use of an oral anti-Staphylococcal antibiotic such as a cephalexin is warranted.

Cutaneous warts

HPV infects epithelial tissues of skin and mucous membranes. The most common clinical manifestation of these viruses is warts (verrucae). There are more than 150 distinct HPV subtypes; some tend to infect specific body sites and produce characteristic lesions at those sites. Warts commonly occur in children and young adults, especially in infants and toddlers. AD predisposes patients with warts for either more extensive or recalcitrant involvement.

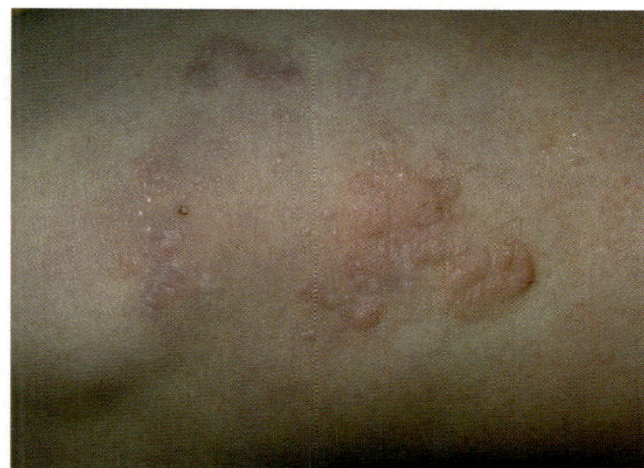

FIGURE 58–9 ■ Extensive verruca vulgaris on the knee of a patient with AD.

Clinical presentation Warts typically present as single or grouped flesh-colored, scaly, keratotic papules from 1–10 mm in diameter (Figure 58–9). They are most commonly located on the hands and knees but may be found on any skin area. Several general types of warts can be distinguished clinically. The common wart (*verruca vulgaris*) appears as a solitary papule with an irregular, rough surface. *Filiform* warts appear as spiny projections with a narrow stalk; these are usually smaller and are found on the face, with a predilection for the nares and periorbital area. *Flat* warts, as the name suggests, appear as flat, smooth, flesh- colored papules, usually 1–5 mm in diameter. They are most commonly located on the face, hands, and shins. *Plantar* warts present as rough papules on the weight-bearing areas on the feet and may also occur on the palms. Unlike most warts, which are usually asymptomatic, plantar warts are often very painful when they occur on weight-bearing surfaces. *Periungual* warts occur around the cuticles of fingers and toes. Plantar and periungual warts are often recalcitrant to therapy. Venereal warts (*condylomata acuminata*) are multiple discrete or confluent papules with a rough surface that appear on the genital mucosa or skin. Common warts also appear on genital or perigenital skin, particularly in toddlers.[49]

Diagnosis The diagnosis of warts is based upon clinical appearance. Useful clinical signs include the presence of multiple small black dots (thrombosed capillaries) within the lesion that may be more readily visualized if the lesion is pared down with a sharp blade; the disruption of normal dermatoglyphics on the palms and soles also indicates the presence of warts. Rarely, a shave biopsy is indicated to confirm the diagnosis.

Treatment The type and aggressiveness of therapy for verrucae will depend upon the type of wart, its location, the degree of symptoms, and the patient's cooperation and immune status. Most warts will resolve spontaneously within several months to years, and therefore active nonintervention is a viable option for many children. The presence of recalcitrant warts, those that are actively spreading through autoinoculation, or the presence of a significant number of warts or warts in cosmetically sensitive areas such as the face and that cause emotional distress to the child warrant treatment.

It is important to remember when treating verrucae that the virus is microscopic and, although the skin may look normal after treatment, there often is virus still present in the remaining tissue. Unless that tissue also is removed, a few months later the warts will recur. Thus, most topical treatments are more effective if the wart is pared down with a sharp blade or pumice stone after a brief soak in warm water before the application of any topical agents. This strategy helps to remove excess stratum corneum and allows for better penetration of the medication into the lower layers of the epidermis.[48]

Current therapies for HPV are not specific for the virus; all work by tissue destruction, with the goal of destroying the virus-containing epidermis and preserving as much uninvolved tissue as possible. The most commonly employed treatments involve destroying the affected tissue by freezing, burning, curetting, or applying topical acids. The least painful methods should be used initially, especially in young children. More destructive therapies should be reserved for areas where scarring is not a consideration or for recalcitrant lesions.

Heat. Warts exposed to heat—either through immersion in hot water or application of exothermic patches—appear to clear more quickly when compared with controls. This is a benign, well-tolerated modality that may be used adjunctively with other therapies.[48]

Occlusion. The simple method of occlusion of warts with duct tape or waterproof medical tape, either alone or in combination with other treatment modalities, is a relatively pain-free method that can be useful in younger children. The mechanism for its utility remains unknown, although some hypothesize that occlusion slows the abnormal keratinization within the wart or may induce a local irritant contact dermatitis. In addition, removal of the tape often aids in the debridement of the affected area.

Snip excision. Snip excision is useful for the removal of filiform warts. The area is anesthetized with subcutaneous lidocaine 1%, then the wart is removed with curved scissors. Hemostasis can be achieved with electrocautery or aluminum chloride.

Salicylic acid. Salicylic acid functions as a keratolytic. It is generally well tolerated and is among the best-studied modalities for the treatment of warts, with several placebo-controlled trials available to validate its effectiveness.[50–52] Seventeen percent salicylic acid solutions are readily available as an over the counter remedy for common warts, while 40% salicylic acid plasters are available for the treatment of plantar warts. Salicylic acid formulations can also be combined with occlusion for home use following an office-based treatment such as cryotherapy or cantharidin. Advantages of this treatment modality are that it is available over the counter and is inexpensive. The main disadvantage is that clinical resolution may require several months of treatment.

Cantharidin. Cantharidin 1% preparations that are combined with 8% podophyllin and 30% salicylic acid are available for the treatment of warts. Despite its widespread use, no controlled trials evaluating its use in the treatment of warts have been performed. Because of its toxicity when ingested, in-office application is recommended. Occlusive tape is generally applied to the treated area. The lipophilic medication is then washed off by the parent or caregiver at home after 1–4 hours using soap and water. It may be particularly useful for patients with multiple lesions and in young children because application is painless in the office. However, pain may occur 2–24 hours after application, and repeat applications may be required every 2–4 weeks until clear. Side effects include significant blistering, although scarring is unlikely unless subsequent superinfection has occurred. As with treatment for molluscum, cantharidin products are not recommended on the face or genital areas as a result of the potential for excessive blistering.[48]

Cryotherapy. Liquid nitrogen therapy is useful in older children and adults but is painful for younger children. Up to 75% of warts eventually resolve with liquid nitrogen therapy, although plantar warts may be somewhat more resistant. In general, liquid nitrogen is applied so that there is a freeze ball of the lesion and 1–2 mm of surrounding normal tissue, usually 10–20 seconds for common, plantar, or palmar warts, and 5–10 seconds or less for flat warts. Treatment intervals every 2–3 weeks produce a cure rate of between 70% and 80%, while intervals greater than 4 weeks have a significantly lower cure rate of 40%.[48,53] Liquid nitrogen must be used cautiously on the digits, especially where nerves are located, to prevent severe pain and possible neuropathy, and to avoid over-treatment in the periungual region, which can result in permanent nail dystrophy.

Side effects include pain, blistering, and, rarely, scarring. Hypopigmentation may occur in the treated area; thus, dark skinned patients should be treated cautiously with cryotherapy. The use of a topical anesthetic such as lidocaine/prilocaine cream may be helpful for those with large lesions and in younger children.

Pulsed dye laser. Pulsed dye laser therapy can selectively target hemoglobin contained in blood vessels within the wart, leading to cauterization of blood vessels. The result is a necrotic wart that eventually sloughs off.[54] Studies examining the effectiveness of pulsed dye laser therapy after an average of two or three treatments have reported overall cure rates of 48–93% for warts located at various sites.[55,56] Advantages of pulsed dye laser therapy include minimal pain, little risk of scarring, and ease and speed of use. Disadvantages include the expense and the need to refer patients to a specialist.

Imiquimod. Imiquimod is a topical immunomodulator that is believed to act by local cytokine induction. Although more commonly used for anogenital warts, imiquimod 5% cream (Aldara) can be used to treat nongenital warts as well. Various imiquimod regimens have been used and none has been extensively studied. One small study in children has documented moderate efficacy in the treatment of recalcitrant warts in children.[57] Imiquimod is nonscarring and it is painless to apply. Local irritation is common and can be significant, and there are rare reports of systemic side effects including flu-like symptoms. Imiquimod may be useful in the treatment of periungual and subungual warts, which are often recalcitrant to standard therapy. Imiquimod is expensive compared with many other therapies for warts.

Topical retinoids The purported mechanism of action of topical retinoids such as tretinoin in the treatment of warts is the induction of a local inflammatory response, although there are no good studies documenting its efficacy. It is applied once or twice a day, with a goal of inducing mild irritation. Several months of treatment are often required. Benefits of this therapy include the ability to easily treat multiple lesions, including smaller lesions. It can also be safely used to treat warts on the face or on other sensitive areas. Local irritation, secondary eczematization, and photo-sensitivity may be seen but are usually well tolerated.[48]

5-Fluorouracil. 5-Fluorouracil is an antimetabolite that inhibits DNA synthesis and topical 5% 5-fluorouracil (Efudex 5% cream) is FDA-approved for the treatment of actinic keratoses, a precursor to squamous cell carcinoma, and superficial basal cell carcinomas. It has been reported to be efficacious in the treatment of warts, in a small number of clinical studies.[58–60] Its use is limited by the potential for significant local irritation. The cream is applied to affected areas twice daily for 3–5 weeks. Sun protection is essential because the drug is photosensitizing.

Cimetidine. Cimetidine, an H_2-receptor antagonist, has been used to treat recalcitrant warts based upon the theory that H_2-receptor antagonists stimulate cell-mediated immunity and have been reported to enhance the resolution of warts in immunocompetent children.[61–64] This is usually used in conjunction with another treatment modality and should be reserved for treatment-resistant warts. Side effects include impaired metabolism of drugs that use the cytochrome P450 enzyme system with risk of systemic toxicity, renal impairment, and sedation.

Alternative therapies. More aggressive therapies reported for recalcitrant warts include the use of intralesional bleomycin, intralesional interferon-alpha, intralesional immunotherapy with candida antigen and topical or intravenous cidofovir, which is a potent but prohibitively expensive antiviral drug. These therapies are reserved for patients who have failed multiple standard therapies or who are immunosuppressed.

Fungal Superinfections

Fungi may play an important role as aggravating factors in AD.[65,66] Colonization of the skin with *Malassezia* species is more prevalent in AD patients compared to healthy individuals and a substantial proportion of AD patients have positive prick tests, positive intradermal reactions and positive scarification patch tests to *Malassezia* antigens.[67–69] An anti-*Malassezia*-specific immunoglobulin E antibody is produced in patients with AD who have disrupted skin barrier function, while healthy subjects do not produce the immunoglobulin E antibody.[70] Although generally considered to be nonpathogenic, *Malassezia* yeasts can, under appropriate circumstances, cause skin diseases such as pityriasis versicolor and folliculitis, and have also been associated with seborrheic dermatitis. Because these yeasts are also frequently isolated from healthy control subjects, it has been hypothesized that they act as allergens in patients who are susceptible, rather than as infectious agents, leading to skin inflammation that may exacerbate the underlying dermatitis.[71,72] The use of antifungal agents in selected patients has been shown to improve the symptoms of AD.[68,73] Patients with AD also develop chronic dermatophyte infections more easily, which are often more severe and more difficult to eradicate.[65]

Optimal treatment dosages and duration remain to be determined. Comparative placebo-controlled, double-blind clinical studies are warranted to determine the place of antimycotic therapy in the management of AD.[66]

REFERENCES

1. Losek JD. Atopic dermatitis and treatment with topical immunomodulators. *Pediatr Emerg Care.* 2004;20(12): 852-854; quiz 5-7.
2. Correale CE, Walker C, Murphy L, Craig TJ. Atopic dermatitis: a review of diagnosis and treatment. *Am Fam Physician.* 1999;60(4):1191-1198, 1209-1210.
3. Leung DY, Boguniewicz M, Howell MD, Nomura I, Hamid QA. New insights into atopic dermatitis. *J Clin Invest.* 2004;113(5):651-657.
4. Abramovits W. Atopic dermatitis. *J Am Acad Dermatol.* 2005;53(1 suppl 1):S86-S93.
5. Hanifin J. Defining AD and assessing its impact: eeking simplified, inclusive, and internationally applicable criteria. Paper presented at: the International Symposium on Atopic Dermatitis, National Eczema Association for Science and Education; September 6–9, 2001; Portland, OR.
6. Hanifin JM, Rajka G. Diagnostic features of atopic dermatitis. *Acta Derm Venereol (Stockh).* 1980;92(Suppl): 44-47.
7. Barker JN, Palmer CN, Zhao Y, et al. Null mutations in the filaggrin gene (FLG) determine major susceptibility to early-onset atopic dermatitis that persists into adulthood. *J Invest Dermatol.* 2007;127(3):564-567.
8. Palmer CN, Irvine AD, Terron-Kwiatkowski A, et al. Common loss-of-function variants of the epidermal barrier protein filaggrin are a major predisposing factor for atopic dermatitis. *Nat Genet.* 2006;38(4):441-446.
9. Sandilands A, O'Regan GM, Liao H, et al. Prevalent and rare mutations in the gene encoding filaggrin cause ichthyosis vulgaris and predispose individuals to atopic dermatitis. *J Invest Dermatol.* 2006;126(8):1770-1775.
10. Paul C, Cork M, Rossi AB, Papp KA, Barbier N, de Prost Y. Safety and tolerability of 1% pimecrolimus cream among infants: experience with 1133 patients treated for up to 2 years. *Pediatrics.* 2006;117(1):e118-e128.
11. Ashcroft DM, Dimmock P, Garside R, Stein K, Williams HC. Efficacy and tolerability of topical pimecrolimus and tacrolimus in the treatment of atopic dermatitis: meta-analysis of randomised controlled trials. *BMJ.* 2005; 330(7490):516.
12. Topical tacrolimus for treatment of atopic dermatitis. *Med Lett Drugs Ther.* 2001;43(1102):33-34.
13. Aoyama H, Tabata N, Tanaka M, Uesugi Y, Tagami H. Successful treatment of resistant facial lesions of atopic dermatitis with 0.1% FK506 ointment. *Br J Dermatol.* 1995;133(3):494-496.
14. Reitamo S, Rustin M, Ruzicka T, et al. Efficacy and safety of tacrolimus ointment compared with that of hydrocortisone butyrate ointment in adult patients with atopic dermatitis. *J Allergy Clin Immunol.* 2002;109(3): 547-555.
15. Reitamo S, Wollenberg A, Schopf E, et al. Safety and efficacy of 1 year of tacrolimus ointment monotherapy in adults with atopic dermatitis. The European Tacrolimus Ointment Study Group. *Arch Dermatol.* 2000;136(8): 999-1006.
16. Boguniewicz M, Fiedler VC, Raimer S, Lawrence ID, Leung DY, Hanifin JM. A randomized, vehicle-controlled trial of tacrolimus ointment for treatment of atopic dermatitis in children. Pediatric Tacrolimus Study Group. *J Allergy Clin Immunol.* 1998;102(4, pt 1): 637-644.
17. Nuovo J, Ellsworth AJ, Larson EB. Treatment of atopic dermatitis with antihistamines: lessons from a single-patient, randomized clinical trial. *J Am Board Fam Pract.* 1992;5(2):137-141.
18. Clayton TH, Clark SM, Turner D, Goulden V. The treatment of severe atopic dermatitis in childhood with narrowband ultraviolet B phototherapy. *Clin Exp Dermatol.* 2007;32(1):28-33.
19. Jury CS, McHenry P, Burden AD, Lever R, Bilsland D. Narrowband ultraviolet B (UVB) phototherapy in children. *Clin Exp Dermatol.* 2006;31(2):196-199.
20. Berth-Jones J, Finlay AY, Zaki I, et al. Cyclosporine in severe childhood atopic dermatitis: a multicenter study. *J Am Acad Dermatol.* 1996;34(6):1016-1021.
21. Harper JI, Berth-Jones J, Camp RD, et al. Cyclosporin for atopic dermatitis in children. *Dermatology (Basel).* 2001; 203(1):3-6.
22. Heller M, Shin HT, Orlow SJ, Schaffer JV. Mycophenolate mofetil for severe childhood atopic dermatitis: experience in 14 patients. Br J Dermatol. 2007;157(1):127-132.
23. Zaki I, Emerson R, Allen BR. Treatment of severe atopic dermatitis in childhood with cyclosporin. *Br J Dermatol.* 1996;135 (Suppl 48):21-24.
24. Ruiz-Maldonado R, Parish LC, Beare JM. *Textbook of Pediatric dermatology.* Philadelphia, PA: Grune & Stratton; 1989.
25. McGirt LY, Beck LA. Innate immune defects in atopic dermatitis. *J Allergy Clin Immunol.* 2006;118(1):202-208.
26. Ong PY, Ohtake T, Brandt C, et al. Endogenous antimicrobial peptides and skin infections in atopic dermatitis. *N Engl J Med.* 2002;347(15):1151-1160.
27. Cardona ID, Cho SH, Leung DY. Role of bacterial superantigens in atopic dermatitis: implications for future therapeutic strategies. *Am J Clin Dermatol.* 2006;7(5):273-279.
28. Behrman RE KR, Arvin AM, Nelson WE. *Nelson Textbook of Pediatrics.* 17th ed. Philadelphia, PA: Saunders; 2004.
29. Breuer K, S HA, Kapp A, Werfel T. Staphylococcus aureus: Colonizing features and influence of an antibacterial treatment in adults with atopic dermatitis. *Br J Dermatol.* 2002;147(1):55-61.
30. Leung DY. Infection in atopic dermatitis. *Curr Opin Pediatr.* 2003;15(4):399-404.
31. Gong JQ, Lin L, Lin T, et al. Skin colonization by Staphylococcus aureus in patients with eczema and atopic dermatitis and relevant combined topical therapy: a double-blind multicentre randomized controlled trial. *Br J Dermatol.* 2006;155(4):680-687.
32. Lubbe J. Secondary infections in patients with atopic dermatitis. *Am J Clin Dermatol.* 2003;4(9):641-654.
33. Breneman DL, Hanifin JM, Berge CA, Keswick BH, Neumann PB. The effect of antibacterial soap with 1.5% triclocarban on Staphylococcus aureus in patients with atopic dermatitis. *Cutis.* 2000;66(4):296-300.

34. Stalder JF, Fleury M, Sourisse M, et al. Comparative effects of two topical antiseptics (chlorhexidine vs KMn04) on bacterial skin flora in atopic dermatitis. *Acta Derm Venereol Suppl.* Stockh. 1992;176:132-134.
35. Hanifin JM, Cooper KD, Ho VC, et al. Guidelines of care for atopic dermatitis, developed in accordance with the American Academy of Dermatology (AAD)(American Academy of Dermatology Association "Administrative Regulations for Evidence-Based Clinical Practice Guidelines". *J Am Acad Dermatol.* 2004;50(3):391-404.
36. Lever R, Hadley K, Downey D, Mackie R. Staphylococcal colonization in atopic dermatitis and the effect of topical mupirocin therapy. *Br J Dermatol.* 1988;119(2): 189-198.
37. Darsow U, Lubbe J, Taieb A, et al. Position paper on diagnosis and treatment of atopic dermatitis. *J Eur Acad Dermatol Venereol.* 2005;19(3):286-295.
38. Harper JI, Oranje AP, Prose N. *Textbook of Pediatric Dermatology. London.* UK: Blackwell Publishing Professional; 2000.
39. Prabriputaloong T, Margolis TP, Lietman TM, Wong IG, Mather R, Gritz DC. Atopic disease and herpes simplex eye disease: a population-based case-control study. *Am J Ophthalmol.* 2006;142(5):745-749.
40. Braue A, Ross G, Varigos G, Kelly H. Epidemiology and impact of childhood molluscum contagiosum: a case series and critical review of the literature. *Pediatr Dermatol.* 2005;22(4):287-294.
41. de Waard-van der Spek FB, Oranje AP, Lillieborg S, Hop WC, Stolz E. Treatment of molluscum contagiosum using a lidocaine/prilocaine cream (EMLA) for analgesia. *J Am Acad Dermatol.* 1990;23(4, pt 1):685-688.
42. Brown J, Janniger CK, Schwartz RA, Silverberg NB. Childhood molluscum contagiosum. *Int J Dermatol.* 2006; 45(2): 93-99.
43. Skinner RB, Jr. Treatment of molluscum contagiosum with imiquimod 5% cream. *J Am Acad Dermatol.* 2002;47(4 suppl):S221-S224.
44. Bayerl C, Feller G, Goerdt S. Experience in treating molluscum contagiosum in children with imiquimod 5% cream. *Br J Dermatol.* 2003;149(suppl 66):25-29.
45. Theos AU, Cummins R, Silverberg NB, Paller AS. Effectiveness of imiquimod cream 5% for treating childhood molluscum contagiosum in a double-blind, randomized pilot trial. *Cutis.* 2004;74(2):134-138, 141-142.
46. Arican O. Topical treatment of molluscum contagiosum with imiquimod 5% cream in Turkish children. *Pediatr Int.* 2006;48(4):403-405.
47. Hanna D, Hatami A, Powell J, et al. A prospective randomized trial comparing the efficacy and adverse effects of four recognized treatments of molluscum contagiosum in children. *Pediatr Dermatol.* 2006;23(6): 574-579.
48. Smolinski KN, Yan AC. How and when to treat molluscum contagiosum and warts in children. *Pediatr Ann.* 2005;34(3):211-221.
49. Weston WL, Lane AT, Morelli JG. *Color Textbook of Pediatric Dermatology.* 3rd ed. St. Louis: Mosby; 2002.
50. Parish LC, Monroe E, Rex IH, Jr. Treatment of common warts with high-potency (26%) salicylic acid. *Clin Ther.* 1988;10(4):462-466.
51. Steele K, Irwin WG. Liquid nitrogen and salicylic/lactic acid paint in the treatment of cutaneous warts in general practice. *J R Coll Gen Pract.* 1988;38(311):256-258.
52. Steele K, Shirodaria P, O'Hare M, et al. Monochloroacetic acid and 60% salicylic acid as a treatment for simple plantar warts: effectiveness and mode of action. *Br J Dermatol.* 1988;118(4):537-543.
53. Bacelieri R, Johnson SM. Cutaneous warts: an evidence-based approach to therapy. *Am Fam Physician.* 2005; 72(4):647-652.
54. Hruza GJ. Laser treatment of epidermal and dermal lesions. *Dermatol Clin.* 2002;20(1):147-164.
55. Goldman MP. FRE. *Cutaneous Laser Surgery: The Art and Science of Selective Photothermolysis.* 2nd ed. St. Louis: Mosby; 1999.
56. Borovoy MA, Borovoy M, Elson LM, Sage M. Flashlamp pulsed dye laser (585 nm). Treatment of resistant verrucae. *J Am Podiatr Med Assoc.* 1996;86(11):547-550.
57. Grussendorf-Conen EI, Jacobs S. Efficacy of imiquimod 5% cream in the treatment of recalcitrant warts in children. *Pediatr Dermatol.* 2002;19(3):263-266.
58. Lee S, Kim JG, Chun SI. Treatment of verruca plana with 5% 5-fluorouracil ointment. *Dermatologica.* 1980;160(6): 383-389.
59. Hursthouse MW. A controlled trial on the use of topical 5-fluorouracil on viral warts. *Br J Dermatol.* 1975;92(1): 93-96.
60. Goncalves JC. 5-Fluorouracil in the treatment of common warts of the hands. A double-blind study. *Br J Dermatol.* 1975;92(1):89-91.
61. Orlow SJ, Paller A. Cimetidine therapy for multiple viral warts in children. *J Am Acad Dermatol.* 1993;28(5, pt 1): 794-796.
62. Fischer G, Rogers M. Cimetidine therapy for warts in children. *J Am Acad Dermatol.* 1997;37(2, pt 1):289-290.
63. Bauman C, Francis JS, Vanderhooft S, Sybert VP. Cimetidine therapy for multiple viral warts in children. *J Am Acad Dermatol.* 1996;35(2, pt 1):271-272.
64. Choi YS, Hann SK, Park YK. The effect of cimetidine on verruca plana juvenilis: clinical trials in six patients. *J Dermatol.* 1993;20(8):497-500.
65. Faergemann J. Atopic dermatitis and fungi. *Clin Microbiol Rev.* 2002;15(4):545-563.
66. Nikkels AF, Pierard GE. Framing the future of antifungals in atopic dermatitis. *Dermatol (Basel).* 2003;206(4): 398-400.
67. Waersted A, Hjorth N. Pityrosporum orbiculare–a pathogenic factor in atopic dermatitis of the face, scalp and neck? *Acta Derm Venereol Suppl (Stockh).* 1985;114:146-148.
68. Back O, Scheynius A, Johansson SG. Ketoconazole in atopic dermatitis: Therapeutic response is correlated with decrease in serum IgE. *Arch Dermatol Res.* 1995;287(5): 448-451.
69. Kolmer HL, Taketomi EA, Hazen KC, Hughs E, Wilson BB, Platts-Mills TA. Effect of combined antibacterial and antifungal treatment in severe atopic dermatitis. *J Allergy Clin Immunol.* 1996;98(3):702-707.
70. Sugita T, Tajima M, Tsubuku H, Tsuboi R, Nishikawa A. A new calcineurin inhibitor, pimecrolimus, inhibits the growth of Malassezia spp. *Antimicrob Agents Chemother.* 2006;50(8):2897-2898.

71. Gupta AK, Batra R, Bluhm R, Boekhout T, Dawson TL, Jr. Skin diseases associated with Malassezia species. *J Am Acad Dermatol.* 2004;51(5):785-798.
72. Aspres N, Anderson C. Malassezia yeasts in the pathogenesis of atopic dermatitis. *Australas J Dermatol.* 2004;45(4): 199-205; quiz 6-7.
73. Lintu P, Savolainen J, Kortekangas-Savolainen O, Kalimo K. Systemic ketoconazole is an effective treatment of atopic dermatitis with IgE-mediated hypersensitivity to yeasts. *Allergy.* 2001;56(6):512-517.

SECTION 16

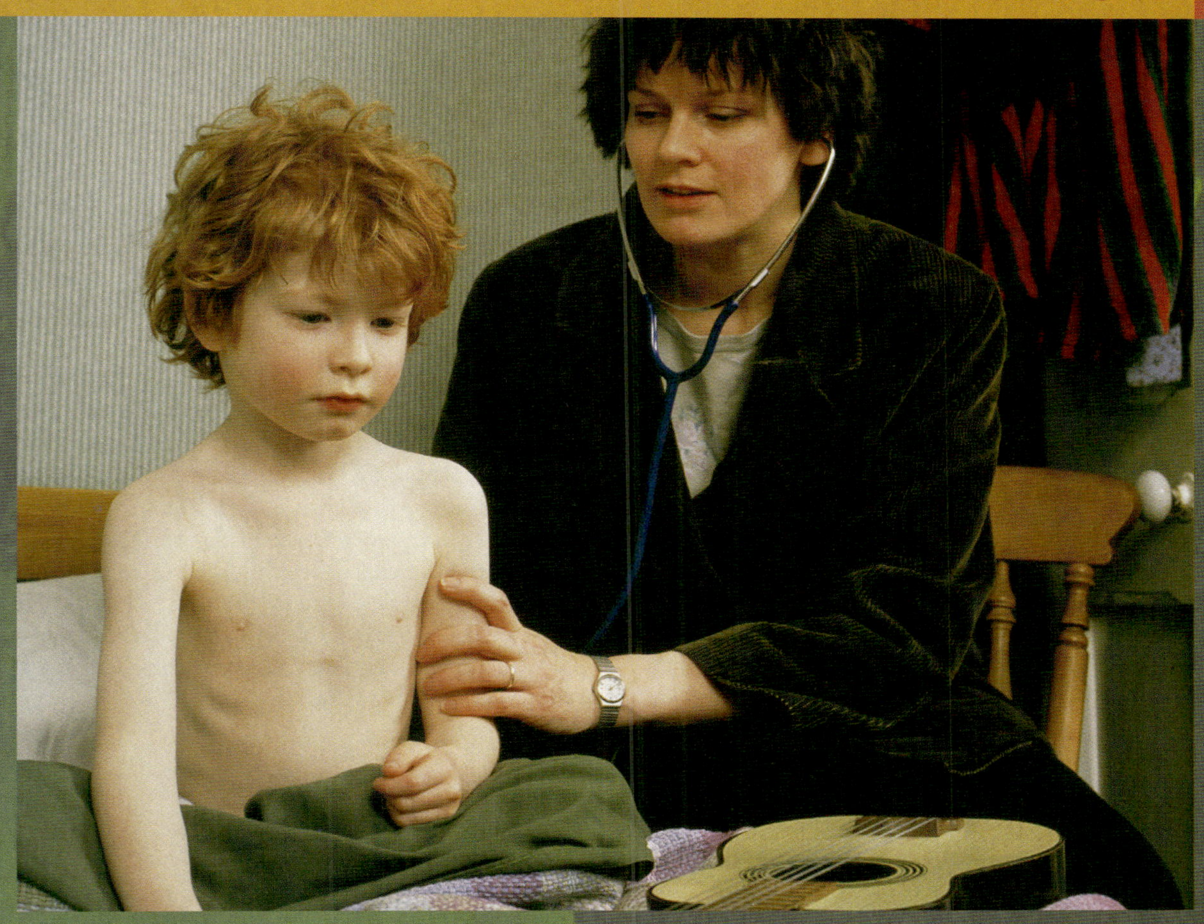

Congenital Immunodeficiency Syndromes

CHAPTER 59

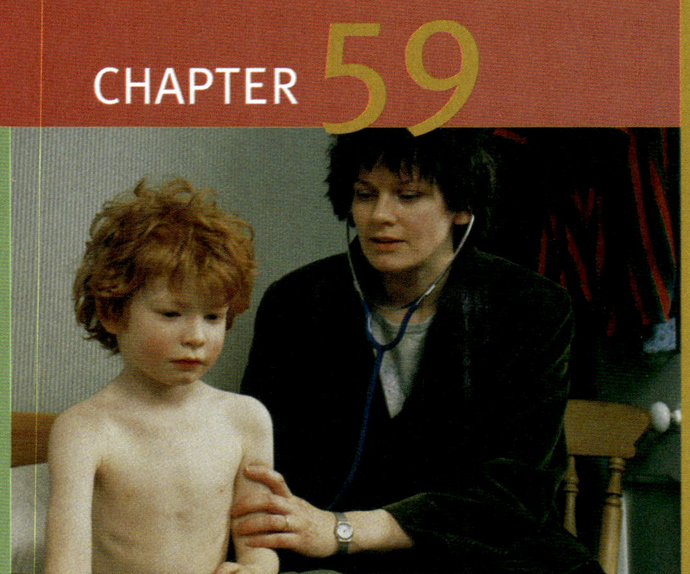

Evaluation of the Child with Suspected Immune Deficiency

Timothy R. La Pine and Harry R. Hill

DEFINITIONS AND EPIDEMIOLOGY

Primary immune deficiencies represent a class of disorders in which there is an intrinsic defect in the immune system. In contrast, acquired or secondary immune deficiency states occur as a consequence of external agents such as infection or chemotherapy. Over 150 distinct primary immune deficiency syndromes have been recognized. The true prevalence of primary immune deficiencies is not known as routine screening for these defects is not performed at birth or at any time during life. One well-conducted telephone survey of 10,000 households found that the population rate for the diagnosis of primary immune deficiency was 0.0863%, which translates into approximately 250,000 persons (95% confidence interval: 151,769 to 361,408) with primary immune deficiency in the United States.[46]

The diagnosis of a primary immune deficiency in a child is one of the more challenging diagnoses in medicine. It requires both an understanding of immune function and development and a clinical understanding of age-related infections and relevant genetic risks and environmental exposures. Children with primary immunodeficiency diseases most commonly present with recurrent infections. When evaluating a child with recurrent infections, it is important to remember the normal pattern of infections for different ages and situations. For example, a normal child living at home may have 6 to 12 infections per year if living only at home, and up to 18 infections per year when cared for at a day care center. Children with primary immunodeficiencies commonly have a positive family history. A thorough physical examination may reveal subtle scaring from previous infections, eczema, lymphadenopathy, or prior surgery.

A history suggestive of childhood immunodeficiency usually contains one or more "red flags" (Table 59–1). Situations that warrant consideration of a primary immune deficiency include frequent chronic infections without any other explanation. Always consider immunodeficiency in children with recurrent infections and associated failure to thrive. Likewise, any severe or unusual infection, in particular, infections with opportunistic organisms warrants consideration of an immunodeficiency state.

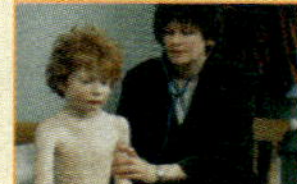

Table 59–1.

Patient History Suggestive of Immunodeficiency

- Patients with increased frequency of infections compared with patients of similar age and exposure risk:
  - ≥8 episodes of otitis media in 1 year
  - ≥2 episodes of serious sinusitis in 1 year
  - ≥2 episodes of pneumonia in 1 year.
- Patients whose infections with common, often nonpathogenic or usually inconsequential pathogens, are more severe than would be normally expected.
- Patients whose infections are of prolonged duration and require prolonged antimicrobial therapy with often incomplete clearing between episodes or requiring surgical intervention (e.g., recurrent deep skin or organ abscesses).
- Patients with multiple, complicated infections often involving different organ systems.
- Patients who have infections with unusual or opportunistic organisms.
- Patients with autoimmunity and poor wound healing.
- Persistent or recurrent mucosal candidiasis after 1 year of age.
- Failure to thrive.

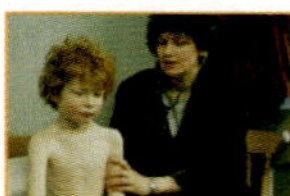

Table 59–2.

Distribution of Primary Immune Deficiencies by Category

Category	Percent (%)
B-cell defects	50
Combined B- and T-cell defects	25
Phagocyte defects	15
T-cell defects	7
Complement system defects	3

PATHOGENESIS

The components of the immune response are exceedingly complex and require the close cooperation and orchestration of a variety of cellular elements. For clinical utility, however, the functional categories of immunodeficiency can be categorized as follows: (1) Defects in the T-lymphocyte system (including T cells and lymphokines); (2) defects in the B-lymphocyte system (including B cells and immunoglobulins); (3) defects in the phagocyte system (including neutrophils and macrophages), and (4) defects in the complement system. Combined B- and T-cell defects also occur. Among these functional categories of immunodeficiency, about 75% are either B-cell or combined B- and T-cell defects (Table 59–2). Severe combined immunodeficiencies (typically combined B- and T-cell defects), phagocytic and complement deficiencies tend to manifest in the neonatal period. B-lymphocyte system defects tend to manifest after 4 to 6 months of life, when the maternally passed antibodies have decreased.[1,3–5]

Each of these functional categories of the immune response provides protection against specific classes of microorganisms. Deficiencies in a particular function of the immune response can lead to infections with certain types of infectious pathogens. Gram-negative bacteria, for example, are recognized by neutrophils. Neutrophils are able to recognize outer membrane molecules on the cell wall of gram-negative bacteria. Encapsulated bacteria have a polysaccharide coat, which hides their cell walls. The immune system responds to these pathogens by generating antibodies to the polysaccharide coat. The antibody–pathogen complex then activates the complement system, leading to further opsonization and subsequent killing by phagocytes. Intracellular pathogens such as viruses and mycobacteria require T-lymphocyte responses for their elimination. When evaluating a patient, frequent infections and suspected immunodeficiency the type of infecting organism and the type of infection can suggest which functional category of the immune response is defective (Table 59–3).[5–7]

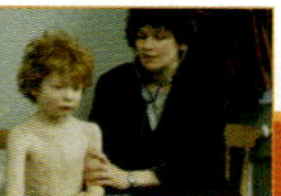

Table 59–3.

Immunodeficiencies and their Commonly Associated Infections and Pathogens

T-lymphocyte defects	Severe respiratory viral infections
	Herpes/varicella infections
	Pneumocystis jiroveci pneumonia
	Cryptococcus
	Candidiasis
	Aspergillosis
	Salmonellosis
	Mycobacteria
	Cytomegalovirus infections
B-lymphocyte defects	Sepsis/meningitis
	Recurrent otitis media
	Recurrent sinopulmonary infections
	Streptococcus pneumoniae
	Hemophilus influenzae
	Pseudomonas aeruginosa
	Persistent viral infections
	Gastroenteritis—*Giardia lamblia,* rotavirus, *Cryptosporidium parvum*
	Chronic enteroviral infections
Phagocytic disorders	Skin and cutaneous abscesses
	Gram-negative bacilli
	Staphylococcus aureus
	Escherichia coli
	Burkholderia
	Aspergillus
Complement disorders	*Neisseria meningitidis*
	Streptococcus pneumoniae
	Haemophilus influenzae

CLINICAL PRESENTATION

Clinical presentation of immune deficiencies varies by category (Table 59–4). Clinical presentations of specific common primary immune deficiencies are discussed further in the Special Considerations section of this chapter.

DIFFERENTIAL DIAGNOSIS

Acquired immune deficiency states should always be considered in the differential diagnosis of primary immune deficiencies. Specific acquired causes include drug therapies (e.g., corticosteroids, cytotoxic drugs, chemotherapies; the antiepileptic medications carbamazepine and valproate can cause hypogammaglobulinemia), nutritional or vitamin deficiencies (e.g., zinc), alcoholism, diabetes, cachexia, myelophthistic disorders, various hematologic and nonhematologic malignancies, and acquired immunodeficiency syndrome (AIDS).[1–5] Nonimmunologic causes such as structural or anatomic defects should always be considered when evaluating a child with recurrent infections. It is important

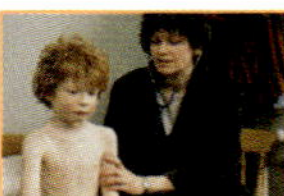

Table 59–4.

Common Clinical Manifestations by Category of Immunodeficiency

T-lymphocyte system defects	Chronic oral candidiasis or mucocutaneous candidiasis presenting early in infancy and persisting after 6 months of age with resistance to therapy Systemic illness after vaccinations with live virus or *Mycobacterium* bacille Calmette-Guérin vaccine Graft-versus-host disease after blood transfusions Persistently low absolute lymphocyte counts Hypocalcemia/tetany with thymic aplasis/hypoplasic and DiGeorge facies Intracellular infections (caused by viruses, fungi, protozoa, and some bacteria).
B-lymphocyte system defects	Recurrent sinopulmonary and/or gastrointestinal infections Recurrent bacterial pneumonias, meningitis, or severe sepsis without lymphadenopathy Enteroviral or other viral infections Absent or incomplete responses to certain vaccinations Nodular lymphoid hyperplasia and malignancies Autoimmunity
Phagocytic system defects	Recurrent cutaneous bacterial abscesses, cellulitis, and mucocutaneous candidiasis Frequent pneumonias, sinusitis, and draining otitis media Delayed separation of the umbilical cord Osteomyelitis Periodontitis and lymphadenitis Granulomatous lesions
Complement system defects	Recurrent encapsulated bacteria infections Immune complex diseases Recurrent sepsis with *Neisseria* species

to query the family for possible environmental or drug exposures. Structural defects such as eczema, burns, urinary tract obstruction, and asplenia can predispose a child to an increased number of infections. Recurrent infections in the same location should raise suspicion of an anatomic defect or foreign body (e.g., right middle lobe pneumonia and an inhaled peanut).

DIAGNOSIS

Laboratory tests used to screen for and confirm and define suspected immunodeficiency syndromes are listed in Table 59–5 and Table 59–6, respectively.

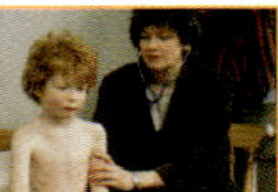

Table 59–5.

Laboratory Testing to Screen for Immunodeficiency

T-lymphocyte deficiency	■ Total lymphocyte count ■ Delayed hypersensitivity skin tests (diphtheria, tetanus, candida, PPD, mumps) for T-cell function ■ Tests for HIV antibodies if suspected ■ Lymphocyte antigen and mitogen stimulation
B-lymphocyte deficiency	■ Serum IgM, IgG, IgA levels ■ IgG antibody response to protein (diphtheria, tetanus, influenzae) and polysaccharide (*S. pneumoniae*) antigens ■ Isohemagglutinin titers for IgM antibody response ■ Serum IgG subclass levels ■ Urinalysis (protein loss)
Phagocytic system defects	■ Complete blood count with absolute neutrophil count ■ Dihydrorhodamine stimulation for respiratory burst activity (defect in CGD) ■ Serum IgE levels for HIE (Job) syndrome
Complement deficiency	■ Total hemolytic complement activity ■ Alternative pathway hemolytic activity ■ Serum C2, C3, C4, C5, and Factor B levels

T-Lymphocyte Defects

Defects in the T-lymphocyte system generally present shortly after birth as severe infections and failure to thrive. They may also present as recurrent viral infections, systemic illness, or both after vaccination with live viruses. A complete blood count and differential, quantitation of T-cell and T-cell subsets (CD4 and CD8), skin testing, and mitogen/antigen proliferation assays are useful aides in the diagnosis of T-lymphocyte defects.

B-Lymphocyte Defects

Defects in the B-lymphocyte system are generally characterized by recurrent sinopulmonary and gastrointestinal infections presenting after the first 4 to 6 months of life. A complete blood count with differential, quantitation of B cells, quantitation of serum immunoglobulins (Table 59–7) with specific IgG subclasses, and IgG challenge testing, which determines the ability of the patient to mount an IgG response, are useful aids in the diagnosis of B-lymphocyte defects. IgG challenge testing includes vaccination with the following substances, followed by serum titer measurements (diphtheria and tetanus vaccination predominantly for IgG1; pneumococcal vaccination with the adult 23-valent polysaccharide

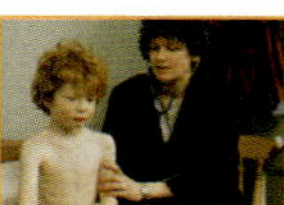

Table 59–6.

Laboratory Testing to Confirm and Define a Primary Immune Deficiency

T-lymphocyte deficiency	■ Enumerate total T cell and T-cell subsets (i.e., CD3, CD4, CD8) ■ Measure T-cell proliferation with mitogens, antigens, and allogeneic cells (MLR) along with cytokine production ■ Enzyme assays for ADA or PNP deficiency ■ Molecular assays to detect mutations
B-lymphocyte deficiency	■ B-cell enumeration (total B cells, CD19, CD20) and surface IgM, IgG, IGA, IgD bearing B cells ■ In vitro Ig biosynthesis ■ Molecular assays for specific mutations
Phagocytic system defects	■ Leukocyte adhesive glycoprotein analysis (CD11a/CD18, CD11b/CD18, CD11c/CD18, and sialyl Lewis-X) ■ Adherence and aggregation ■ Chemotaxis and random motility ■ Phagocytosis and killing of bacteria ■ Assays for respiratory burst activity (dihydrorhodamine stimulation, chemiluminescence, oxygen radical production) ■ Enzyme assay (MPO, G6PD) for phagocyte enzyme defects ■ Cytochrome B or cytosolic protein measurements for CGD ■ Molecular assays for specific mutations
Complement deficiency	■ Specific component determinations ■ Molecular assays for specific mutations

vaccine to evaluate the response IgG2; and influenza vaccination to evaluate IgG3 production can be utilized). Do not, however, give live virus vaccines to patients suspected of having immunodeficiency as serious illness may ensue.

Phagocytic System Defects

Defects in the phagocytic system are characterized by perianal or periodontal abscesses; recurrent soft tissue abscesses, with or without a history of delayed separation of the umbilical cord (greater than one month). A complete blood count with differential, dihydrorhodamine oxidation assays, quantitation of the beta-2 integrins CD11/18 by flow cytometry and myeloperoxidase assays are useful aids in the diagnosis of phagocytic defects.

Complement System Defects

Complement system defects are characterized by recurrent infections with encapsulated bacteria (deficiencies of C3 and C5) and *Neisseria* species (deficiencies of C5-8 and properdin). Collagen vascular diseases are associated with deficiencies of C1, C2, and C4. Total hemolytic complement activity and specific complement component assays are useful diagnostic aids. It is important to note that complement levels in neonates are half that of adults and complement levels may be reduced in patients with rheumatoid arthritis, nephritis, and immune complex diseases.[3,5,8–15]

SPECIAL CONSIDERATIONS: FUNCTIONAL CATEGORIES OF IMMUNODEFICIENCY

T-Lymphocyte System

Thymus-dependent T cells are derived from pluripotent hematopoietic stem cells in developing bone marrow stores. By the eighth gestational week, immature T cells infiltrate the thymus where they differentiate and mature and present specific outer membrane glycoproteins before migrating to their target lymphoid tissues. The main function of the T-lymphocytic systems is in

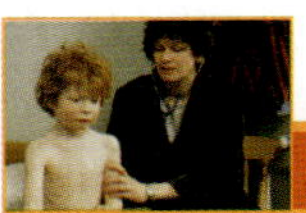

Table 59–7.

Interpretation of Serum Immunoglobulin Levels

IgG	IgM	IgA	Suggested Diagnosis
Normal	Normal	Decreased	IgA deficiency
Decreased	Normal	Normal	IgG deficiency (check specific subclasses) Evaluate for protein-losing enteropathy or nephrotic syndrome
Decreased	Decreased	Decreased	Bruton's agammaglobulinemia (males)
Decreased	Increased or normal	Decreased	Hypogammaglobulinemia with normal to increased IgM
Decreased	Low-normal	Low-normal	Common variable immune deficiency

host defense against intracellular pathogens (viruses, fungi, protozoa, and intracellular bacteria such as mycobacterial and *Listeria* species).[16]

The T-lymphocyte system is also involved in delayed hypersensitivity reactions, tumor surveillance, and graft-versus-host disease. The T-lymphocyte system orchestrates pathogen annihilation through antigen-dependent cellular interactions. Deficiency of T-cell-mediated immunity can result from defects in (1) the maturation, differentiation, and activation T-cell precursors, (2) the thymus and the thymic microenvironment, (3) the T cell itself, and (4) the production of regulatory cytokines or their receptors. Defects in T-cell immunity are usually associated with variable degrees of B-cell deficiency because most of the maturation, differentiation, and activation processes of B-cells require T-cell help. The patient with abnormal cell-mediated immunity usually has an increased incidence of infections with intracellular pathogens and a predisposition for malignancy.[10,16,17]

Selected T-lymphocyte system disorders

The most severe forms of immunodeficiency are the syndromes of severe combined immunodeficiency (SCID). Diseases in this category include a spectrum of at least five X-linked and autosomal recessive genetic defects characterized by the inability to mount normal cell-mediated and humoral immunity. SCID diseases lead to severe and often fatal infections with failure to thrive that usually present shortly after birth. Infections include persistent oral candidiasis, diarrhea, and pneumonia (usually interstitial, often caused by *Pneumocystis jiroveci*). Seventy-five percent of the patients with SCID are male. A prenatal diagnosis of SCID may be made in some cases by fetal blood sampling at 20 weeks' gestation through enumeration of lymphocyte subsets and functional studies.[18,19] SCID variants include the following:

X-linked SCID X-linked SCID is the most common SCID variant and the diagnosis can be confirmed by the identification of the mutation for the IL-2 receptor gamma chain on the X chromosome. This defect will produce T-cell maturational arrest, as this receptor is the mediator of T-cell growth by several cytokines. B-cell development is affected as well. Maternal carriers can be identified by the pattern of X-chromosome inactivation in T cells. Bone marrow transplantation and more recently retroviral mediated gene therapy have been used successfully in treating these patients.[10,16,17,19]

Purine metabolic pathway abnormalities Adenosine deaminase deficiency accounts for about 20% of all SCID cases and 50% of the patients with autosomal recessive SCID have an associated adenosine deaminase (ADA) deficiency. The gene for ADA deficiency has been mapped to chromosome 20q-13. Absence of this enzyme leads to the accumulation of toxic metabolites including adenosine and deoxyadenosine triphosphate, which is capable of killing T-cells. This results in reduced numbers of T- and B-cells. In addition to the classic symptoms of SCID, this disease is characterized by the presence of skeletal abnormalities, particularly abnormalities of the ribs and scapula. The diagnosis is made by measuring ADA levels in hemolyzed red blood cells. Heterozygotes are symptom-free but have half the normal enzyme concentration. Prenatal diagnosis is possible by measuring ADA levels in cultured amniotic cells during the second trimester. Bone marrow transplantation or enzyme replacement using bovine ADA have been used with some success in the management of this disease. Promising recent attempts in treatment of patients with ADA deficiency has been the use of autologous lymphocytes corrected in vitro with retroviral-vector-inserted normal human ADA DNA, especially after myeloablative therapy to give an advantage to the corrected cells.[10,11,16,17]

Purine–nucleoside phosphorylase deficiency

Purine–nucleoside phosphorylase deficiency is an autosomal recessive disorder characterized by a deficiency in the enzyme purine–nucleoside phosphorylase, leading to the accumulation of deoxyguanosine triphosphate, which destroys dividing T cells. B-cell function is often spared and the defect has been localized to chromosome 14q13.12. Patients can have anemia and usually have recurrent viral, bacterial, and fungal infections. Two-thirds of the patients have evidence of neurologic disorders ranging from mild developmental delay or muscle spasticity to severe mental retardation. The diagnosis is made by measuring purine–nucleoside phosphorylase in hemolysed erythrocytes. Heterozygous individuals have half the normal level of this enzyme. Serum uric acid levels are low in these patients because of the absence of this enzyme and a normal uric acid level may help rule out this disease. Prenatal diagnosis is made possible by assaying purine–nucleoside phosphorylase levels cultured in amniotic cells during the second trimester. Bone marrow transplant is the only successful therapy at present. However, enzyme replacement therapy and animal models of vitro viral gene transfer are currently being investigated as promising future therapies.[10,11,16,17]

Ataxia telangiectasia

Ataxia telangiectasia is a multisystem disease characterized by progressive cerebellar ataxia, oculocutaneous telangiectasia, chronic sinopulmonary disease, and a high incidence of malignancy. This autosomal recessive disorder has been identified as a single gene disease encoded to chromosome 11q22.23. This gene encodes a protein that is involved signal transduction, recombination, and cell cycle control important in T-cell and B-cell rearrangement and the ability to repair damaged DNA. The defect observed in DNA repair in these patients after X-ray irradiation results in a high incidence of chromosomal translocation, specifically in chromosome 7, 14, and the X chromosome. Progressive ataxia due to Purkinje cell degeneration becomes apparent when the child begins to walk by 2 years of age. Telangiectasia develops between 2 and 8 years of age on the bulbar conjunctiva and exposed flexor surfaces of the arms. Approximately, 70% have a selective IgA deficiency and more than one-half of these patients have an associated IgG-2 subclass deficiency. Approximately 80% of these patients have depressed or absent IgE levels. The most notable T-cell abnormalities are leukopenia and a decrease in helper T-cell/suppressor T-cell ratios. Serum alpha-fetoprotein levels are persistently elevated in these patients, which may aid in the diagnosis. Therapy for these patients consists of intravenous immunoglobulin therapy to reduce the incidence of recurrent infections in patients with IgG-2 subclass deficiency. Gene therapy for ataxia telangiectasia is currently under investigation.[10,11,16,20]

Wiskott Aldrich syndrome

Wiskott Aldrich syndrome is an X-linked recessive disease characterized by recurrent pyogenic infections within the first years of life. The decreased production of antipolysaccharide antibody in these patients can lead to overwhelming pneumococcal disease or other encapsulated bacterial infections. These patients also have an associated thrombocytopenia characterized by small-sized and poorly functioning platelets predisposing to bleeding and bruising. Eczema is characteristically found in most patients. The Wiskott Aldrich syndrome gene has been mapped to the short arm of the X chromosome. Patients with Wiskott Aldrich syndrome have low serum levels of IgM. IgA and IgE concentrations are high and the IgG level is normal, elevated, or only slightly depressed. These patients are unable to produce antibody in response to polysaccharide antigens. Both T cell numbers and function progressively decrease in this disorder and a profound leukopenia becomes apparent at approximately 6 years of age. Prenatal diagnosis can be facilitated by fetal blood sampling for the analysis of thrombocyte numbers and size. First trimester diagnosis of Wiskott Aldrich syndrome is possible by DNA markers and analysis of an unbalanced pattern of X chromosome inactivation. Early bone marrow transplantation may correct the immunologic defects and platelet disorders observed in these patients.[10,11,16,17,21]

DiGeorge syndrome

DiGeorge syndrome mainly affects the structures derived from third, fourth, and fifth pharyngeal pouches. This is due to a failure of a population of neural crest cells to migrate and interact with endodermally derived cells of the branchial pouches and arches. This syndrome can present as neonatal tetany associated with hypocalcemia caused by hypoparathyroidism. Malformation of the cardiac outflow tract is seen in many DiGeorge patients (e.g., interrupted aortic arch, truncus arteriosus, tetralogy of Fallot). Abnormal facial features include low-set ears with or without malformation, hyperpelorism, short philtrum, micrognathia, and a fish-mouth. The thymus of the infants may be absent, hypoplastic, or atopic, and the parathyroid glands may be absent or reduced in number. T-cell immunity in patients with DiGeorge syndrome is variable and ranges from diminished T-cell numbers with low function to complete absence of T-cell immunity. Some patients with DiGeorge syndrome have normal B-cell immunity as measured by normal levels of immunoglobulin and normal antibody response after immunization. DiGeorge syndrome has been isolated to monosomy of chromosome 22q11. Prenatal diagnosis of DiGeorge syndrome can be performed by fluorescence in situ hybridization (FISH) of fetal tissue. Treatment of patients with DiGeorge syndrome has included the implantation of fetal thymic tissue, fetal thymic epithelium, or fetal thymus in a diffusion chamber and has met with limited success. Full restoration of immune function has not been realized in these patients. Bone marrow transplantation, which provides donor postthymic T cells to reconstitute the patient's immunity, has been used successfully to treat patients with DiGeorge syndrome and severe T-cell immunodeficiency.[10,11,16,22,23]

The B-Lymphocyte System

The humoral or adaptive immune system starts with B stem cells in the bone marrow derived from hematopoietic stem cells. These stem cells produce cytoplasmic IgM heavy chains and become pre-B cells. The pre-B cells continue to differentiate to become mature surface IgM-bearing B cells, which seed peripheral lymphoid tissue. Upon stimulation, IgM-bearing B cells undergo class switching to IgG-, IgA-, or IgE-bearing B cells. These B cells can then differentiate to immunoglobulin-secreting plasma cells with the help of T cells and T-cell-derived lymphokines. Some of the B cells further differentiate into small memory B cells, which are responsible for the secondary immune response. The major function of B cells and plasma cells is to produce antibodies to protein and carbohydrate antigens on microorganisms, toxins, or other antigenetic substances potentially harmful to the host. These antibodies can be classified into nine different immunoglobulin isotypes (IgM, IgD, IgG1, IgG2, IgG3, IgG4, IgA1, IgA2, and IgE).

IgM antibodies are made first and are the most efficient in activating the classical complement system to facilitate the opsonization and ingestion of microorganisms. IgG antibodies are the only maternal antibodies that are transplacentally passed to the developing fetus. These antibodies are responsible for much of the newborn infant's defense against invading microorganisms and toxic substances. IgA antibodies are selectively transported across mucus membranes by a secretory moiety and the attachment of microorganisms or absorption of harmful antigens through mucus membranes. IgE antibodies are mainly responsible for allergic reactions and parasite defense. Any defect in the maturation and differentiation of B cells, from the hematopoietic stem cells to plasma cells and their secretory immunoglobulins, or T cells and their lymphokines may produce B-cell immunodeficiency syndromes.[10,11,16,24]

The clinical presentation of antibody deficiencies results from a decreased defense against the extracellular phases of bacterial and viral infections. Patients with B-cell deficiencies usually have recurrent pyogenic infections without lymphadenopathy or tonsillar enlargement. Sinopulmonary infections are most commonly seen (90–100%) then gastrointestinal infections (usually chronic diarrhea 50–60%). Systemic infections usually involve encapsulated bacteria and blunted or absent responses to certain vaccinations can be seen. Patients with B-cell deficiencies are predisposed to autoimmunity and lymphoreticular malignancies as well (25%).[10,11,24–26]

Selected B-lymphocyte system disorders

B-lymphocyte disorders are characterized by decreased humoral immunity with variable to absent antibody isotype production. Select B-lymphocyte disorders are described below.

Bruton's agammaglobulinemia Bruton's agammaglobulinemia is an X-linked recessive disease that affects only males. The underlying defect is the arrested development of B-cell precursors due to the absence of Bruton's tyrosine kinase. This defect is characterized by recurrent pyogenic infections starting in early infancy after transplacental maternal antibody has disappeared. Affected individuals may not be symptomatic before 6 months of age because of maternal transplacentally acquired IgG antibodies. The absence is of immunoglobulins of all classes, panhypogammaglobulinemia, absence of circulating immunoglobulins bearing mature B cells and functional serum antibody, and the absence of plasma cells in lymphoid tissue are hallmarks of Bruton's agammaglobulinemia. T lymphocytes are present in normal numbers and function. Approximately half of the patients have a family history of an affected male sibling or maternal male relative who is affected. Infections are usually caused by encapsulated bacterial organs, including *Streptococci*, *Meningococci*, and *Hemophilis influenza*. Sinopulmonary infections predominant but gastrointestinal infections particularly with Giardia are common. Patients with this syndrome have an unusual susceptibility to persistent echo or Coxsackie virus infection, including lethal meningoencephalitis as well as vaccine-associated polio myelitis. Female carriers do not exhibit antibody deficiency and can be detected by analyzing the unbalanced pattern of X chromosome inactivation in peripheral blood monocytes. Prenatal diagnosis can be made by sex determination of the fetus or direct sampling of fetal blood and finding the absence of mature immunoglobulin-bearing B cells. Therapy consists of monthly intravenous immunoglobulin administration and close surveillance for infection associated with prompt aggressive therapy of infections.[10,11,24,26,27]

Hypogammaglobulinemia with normal to increased IgM concentrations Patients with this immune deficiency have increased IgM concentration, recurrent pyogenic infections, autoimmune disease, and lymphoproliferative disease, especially IgM surface-bearing B-cell lymphomas of the intestinal tract. The hyper-IgM syndrome can be inherited in an X-linked or an autosomal recessive fashion. The defect results from a block in the further differentiation of the B-cell IgM isotypes, and little to no class switching occurs to IgG, IgA, or IgE isotypes. The gene for the T-cell CD40 ligand, which binds B cells and promotes class switching, is absent in 80% of the patients. This gene defect has been cloned and mapped to Xq26.3-27.1. In 20% of the cases, an autosomal recessive CD40 receptor signal transduction defect is present. The patients have normal or increased concentrations of serum IgM and, in some cases, IgD but decreased or absent IgG, IgA, and IgE. T-cell numbers and function usually appear to be normal. The interaction of CD40 with its ligand may also participate in thymic development. It may explain the susceptibility to opportunistic infections such as *P. jiroveci* pneumonia. Neutropenia is commonly associated with this disease, and about 50% of patients have hepatosplenomegaly. Prenatal diagnosis can be performed by flow cytometry looking for expression of CD40 ligand on T cells. In some patients, IgG replacement therapy results in decreased serum levels of IgM and the regression of lymphoid hyperplasia. Bone marrow transplantation has recently been tried in the treatment of children affected with immunodeficiency with hyper-IgM syndrome and results are promising. Replacement therapy with a recombinant, soluble form of the CD40 ligand or gene therapy may be developed in the future.[10,11,24,26]

IgA deficiency IgA deficiency is the most common immunodeficiency with an incidence of about one in

400 to one in 1000; these estimates are based on screening studies of blood bank donor. In IgA deficiency, there is a terminal block in B-cell differentiation into plasma cells capable of secreting IgA. The susceptibility gene is probably in the class III MCH region on chromosome 6. The T cells, B cells, and other antibody isotypes are usually normal. Many patients (about 30%) are asymptomatic and have no definite increase in infections, presumably because of the protective effects of IgG and IgM. The patients with symptoms usually have recurrent infections of the respiratory and gastrointestinal tracts, autoimmune disease, arthritis, allergy, and malignancy. Patients with IgA deficiency can develop anti-IgA antibodies, which can cause severe anaphylactic reactions when they are transfused with blood containing IgA. IgA deficiency has been defined as a serum IgA concentration of less that 5 mg/dL in severe deficiency, and more than 5 mg/dL (but less than 2 SD below the age-normal mean) in partial deficiency. In partially deficient patients, the low serum concentrations of IgA often return to normal within 2–4 years of diagnosis. Therapy with IgA is not possible in patients with IgA deficiency because (1) the half-life of IgA is short (about 7 days), (2) administered IgA is not transported to the mucosal surfaces, and (3) the presence of anti-IgA autoantibodies in 30–40% of the patients. In approximately 20% of the IgA-deficient patients who have frequent infections, there is an associated IgG2 and/or IgG4 subclass deficiency. Some of these patients, including ones with anti-IgA antibodies, can tolerate treatment with intravenously administered immune globulin, particularly, the preparations containing low levels of IgA.[10,11,24,26,28,29]

Common variable immunodeficiency Common variable immunodeficiency (CIVD), or late-onset hypogammaglobulinemia, is characterized by markedly decreased serum immunoglobulin levels, normal or nearly normal numbers of circulating immunoglobulin-bearing mature B cells, impaired antibody responses, and recurrent bacterial (usually sinopulmonary) infections. The underlying problem in common variable immunodeficiency is that B cells do not differentiate into plasma cells, resulting in a slow decline of all immunoglobulin classes. IgA levels usually decrease first. Several mechanisms can cause common variable immunodeficiency. It may be caused by a primary B-cell defect (failure to terminally glycosylate and secrete immunoglobulins), decreased IL-2 production, or abnormalities in specific T cell helper/suppressor functions. The immunologic defects are not limited to B cells but also affect macrophages and immunoregulatory T cells. Although some patients appear to have only intrinsic B-cell defects, more than half also have abnormalities of T-cell activation and deficient secretion lymphokines including IL-2, and a B-cell differentiation factor. The defects in T-cell immunity usually progress with age. Clinical manifestations include sinopulmonary infections (90–100%), chronic diarrhea (50–60%), and these patients may also have malabsorption syndromes. Autoimmune disease, hepatitis, gastric carcinoma, and lymphoreticular malignancy may occur in older patients. Nodular lymphoid hyperplasia of the intestine and a sarcoid-like syndrome associated with hepatosplenomegaly are additional features of the disease. Many patients have had first-degree relatives with IgA-deficiency. Similar to IgA deficiency, a susceptibly gene is located in the class III MCH region located on chromosome 6, and affects both males and females. Management of CVID includes immunoglobulin replacement therapy, antimicrobial and pulmonary therapy, and immunomodulatory therapies including recombinant human IL-2 conjugated with polyethylene glycol, IL-20, and cimetidine.[10,11,24,26,29]

Phagocytic System

The phagocytic system belongs to the nonspecific or innate immune system, which includes polymorphonuclear leukocytes (e.g., neutrophils, eosinophils) and mononuclear phagocytes (e.g., circulating monocyte, tissue macrophage, and fixed macrophages). Phagocytic cell development occurs within the fetal bone marrow by five months gestation. Major phagocytic functions include adherence to endothelial cells, diapedesis, chemotaxis, phagocytosis, and degranulation, leading to pathogen annihilation. Neonatal neutrophils are depressed in their ability to migrate toward and kill bacteria. The phagocytic system is responsible for defense against extracellular bacterial invasion in association with opsonins (e.g., antibodies, complement, and some acute-phase proteins). Neutrophils are one of the first lines of defense against bacterial invasion of the tissues. If there is a defect in number or function of neutrophils, the patients usually have recurrent pyogenic tissue infections (e.g., impetigo, furunculosis, abscesses, deep tissue infections, or pneumonias).[9,30–32]

Selective phagocytic system disorders

Defects in neutrophil production Neutropenia is an absolute neutrophil count less than 1500 cells/μL. Clinically significant neutropenia occurs with absolute neutrophil counts of less than 500 cells/μL. Neutropenia can be either acquired or congenital. Acquired neutropenia can be due to (1) bone marrow stem cell suppression, as in the case of pharmacologic toxicity; (2) increased neutrophil adherence to the microvasculature, as observed with complement activation, and in severe burn patients; and (3) increased neutrophil destruction, as in hypersplenism or in the cases of autoimmune or alloimmune neutropenia. Acquired neutropenia has also been associated with vitamin B12 or folate deficiency. Transient neutropenia is observed in some infants of mothers with pregnancy induced hypertension. Primary or metastatic bone marrow malignancy can present with neutropenia, and transient neutropenia can follow viral infections (Epstein–Barr virus, cytomegalovirus, parvovirus, and human immunodeficiency virus) or immunizations.[9,30–33]

Congential neutropenia consists of inherited neutrophil production defects. Always think of neutropenia as a sign of sepsis in the newborn. Kostmann syndrome or congenital agranulocytosis is one of a few of the inherited neutropenias. Neutorphil counts are reduced from birth and patients present with sepsis or septic shock. Bone marrow stores in these patients show maturational arrest of the promyelocytes and myelocytes. Kostmann syndrome is associated with an increased risk for acute myeloid leukemia. Defects in the granulocyte colony-stimulating factor (G-CSF) receptors are accountable for some, but not all, cases of Kostmann syndrome and more than 90% of these patients respond to exogenous recombinant G-CSF. In patients refractory to G-CSF, stem cell transplantation from an HLA-matched sibling has shown to be beneficial. Cyclic neutropenia is another form of congenital neutropenia and is characterized by regular fluctuations in circulating neutrophil pools, usually occurring in 21-day cycles. Treatment of cyclic neutropenia with recombinant G-CSF enhances absolute neutrophil counts but does not eliminate the cycling of cell counts. Other congenital disorders associated with a neutropenia include Shwachman–Diamond syndrome, a rare autosomal recessive disorder that usually manifests in infancy characterized by exocrine pancreatic insufficiency, rib abnormalities, short stature, bone marrow dysfunction, and associated neutropenia. These patents respond to treatment with recombinant G-CSF or bone marrow transplantation and are also predisposed to leukemic transformation. Metabolic diseases (glycogen storage disease Ib and Gaucher disease) are also associated with neutropenia in the newborn period.[9,17,30–35]

Leukocyte adhesion deficiency Three types of leukocyte adhesion deficiency (LAD) exist: LAD I is transmitted as an autosomal recessive trait and features the absence of the neutrophil CD11b/CD18 integrin complex, which prevents tight adhesion of the neutrophil to endothelial cell surfaces. LAD II is also an autosomal recessive trait, which features the absence of the neutrophil sialyl Lewis X ligand that promotes tethering (loose adhesion) to the P and E selectin ligands on endothelial cells. LAD III is a recently described defect in the regulation of integrin complex activation, which prevents tight adhesion. The underlying defect results from heterogenous mutations affecting the CD18 gene, which has been mapped to chromosome 21 at 21q22.3.[9,17,30,32,33,36]

This disorder is characterized by defective neutrophil mobilization and frequent infections in patients with poor wound healing, leukocytosis, and a history of delayed umbilical cord separation (more than 2 weeks after birth). Patients usually suffer from recurrent skin abscesses, otitis media, periodontitis, omphalitis, perirectal abscesses, sepsis, and pneumonia. The striking feature of these infections is the almost total absence of leukocytes in the lesions despite high peripheral white cell counts. The most prevalent invading microorganisms are *Staphylococcus aureus*, group A streptococci, *Proteus mirabilis, Pseudomonas aeruginosa,* and *Escherichia coli.* The diagnosis of this disease can be made by assessing the expression of CD11b/ CD18 on the patient's neutrophils by flow cytometry. Therapy consists mainly of early, aggressive antibiotic therapy for bacterial infection, long-term trimethoprim-sulfamethoxazole prophylaxis, or both and early bone marrow transplantation. In severe infection, granulocyte transfusions in addition to antibiotic therapy have been reported to have therapeutic benefit. Bone marrow transplantation has been used successfully to treat these patients; it is the definitive therapy at this time. Successful gene therapy, replacing the defective subunit (CD18) gene into the patient's myeloid precursor cells, may become available in the future. In vitro correction of CD18-deficient lymphocytes by retrovirus-mediated gene transfer has been accomplished. A transfection efficiency of 5–10% may be sufficient to change the course from fatal to moderate.[9,17,30,32,33,37,38]

Chediak–Higashi syndrome This syndrome is an autosomal recessive disorder, which involves abnormal granules and abnormal microtubule formation. Giant lysosomal granules exist in phagocytes, melanocytes, and other cells. The neutrophils of these patients have an inhibited ability to degranulate, which results in poor bacterial killing and a predisposition to infection. Defective melanosomes cause partial albinism. The defective neutrophil microtubule formation leads to decreased chemotaxis, diapedesis, and engulfment of bacteria. Chediak–Higashi syndrome is characterized by recurrent pyogenic infections, a bleeding tendency caused by a platelet storage pool deficiency, partial oculocutaneous albinism, and giant granules in the cytoplasm of many cells, particularly peripheral leukocytes. The underlying defect is likely a result of abnormal membrane fusion, leading to defects in chemotaxis, degranulation, and bactericidal activity. Symptoms generally begin in early childhood with recurrent pyoderma, subcutaneous abscesses, otitis, sinusitis, severe periodontal disease, bronchitis, and pneumonia. The most common microorganisms are *S. aureus* and hemolytic streptococci. Approximately 85% of patients have an accelerated phase characterized by widespread organ infiltration by histiocytes and atypical lymphocytes. Hepatosplenomegaly, lymphadenopathy, neurologic abnormalities, pancytopenia, and a bleeding tendency are also common. The diagnosis is made by identification of the characteristic large azurophilic cytoplasmic granules in the patient's leukocytes or microscopic examination of hair shafts for abnormal giant melanosomes. Prenatal diagnosis can be made by measuring the largest acid phosphatase-positive lysosomes in cultured amniotic fluid cells, chorionic villus cells, or fetal blood leukocytes. In addition to prophylaxis with antibiotics and prompt treatment of acute infection with antimicrobial agents, high doses of ascorbate (500 mg/day orally) and bone marrow transplantation may have benefit in some patients.[9,17,30–33]

Chronic granulomatous disease Chronic granulomatous disease (CGD) is an X-linked or autosomal disorder characterized by an absent neutrophil respiratory burst activity. The lack of O_2 uptake by granulocytes and absent superoxide production, as well as and other oxygen radicals, in response to phagocytosis leads to diminished bactericidal activity for catalase-positive microorganisms. The catalase-negative species, including pneumococci, streptococci, and *H. influenzae,* rarely cause serious infections in these patients. CGD should be suspected in any patient with a subcutaneous abscess or furunculosis associated with abscess formation in a lymph node, the liver, or the lung. The underlying defect in X-linked CGD is due to a defect in a gene (C4BB) encoded by the X chromosome for the 91 kD heavy chain of cytochromes b558. The diagnosis of CGD is based on the demonstration of an absent or greatly diminished respiratory burst by stimulated phagocytes. Available assays now include dihydrorhodamine fluorescence, nitroblue tetrazolium dye reduction, and measurement of oxygen consumption and the products of oxidative metabolism (superoxide anion and hydrogen peroxide). A documented inability of blood granulocytes to kill ingested catalyze-positive bacteria provides confirmatory evidence of CGD. The symptom-free carrier of the X-linked form of CGD can be identified by determining the respiratory burst activity of their neutrophils, which shows a population of both normal and abnormal cells. Prenatal diagnosis can be made during the second trimester by direct sampling of fetal blood followed by tests, which screen for superoxide production. Prophylaxis with trimethoprim–sulfamethoxazole may prolong infection-free intervals by preventing infections, especially with staphylococci and aspergillous. Interferon-gamma administration showed significant reduction in serious infections (70%) among CGD patients, especially when the patient was younger than 10 years. Alternative therapy includes bone marrow transplantation. Patients with CGD are potential candidates for gene therapy because the specific genetic lesions have been identified and the genes cloned.[9,17,30–33,37,39–42]

Job's syndrome The syndrome of hyperimmunoglobulin E (HIE) and recurrent infections is transmitted by autosomal dominant inheritance. It is characterized by extremely high serum IgE values (often greater than 2000 IU/mL), recurrent serious infections and chronic eczematoid dermatitis usually beginning early in infancy. The infections primarily involve the skin and sinopulmonary tract and usually present with recurrent furunculosis, cutaneous abscess formation, bronchitis, pneumonia, chronic otitis media, and sinusitis. Some of the skin abscesses are cold without classical signs and symptoms of inflammation (e.g., redness, heat and pain). The most common infecting microorganisms are *S. aureus,* and *Candida albicans,* but infections caused by *H. influenzae,* group A streptococci, gram-negative pathogens and fungi are also observed. Pneumatoceles, bronchiectasis, and bronchopleural fistula formation are seen after episodes of acute or chronic pneumonia. Chronic mucocutaneous candidiasis, primarily involving the mouth, nails, skin and vagina, is found in about half of the patients. Associated features include coarse facial features with a broad nasal base, growth retardation, osteoporosis, keratoconjunctivitis, asymmetric sterile polyarthritis, and eosinophilia. In addition to markedly elevated serum IgE concentrations, other immunologic abnormalities include elevated specific anti-*S. aureus* and Candida IgE antibodies, an intermittent defect in neutrophi chemotaxis in 80%, low anamnestic antibody response to booster immunizations and poor antibody and cell-mediated response to newly encountered antigens. The anti-*S. aureus* IgE antibodies may appear in early infancy before the development of staphylococcal infections. The underlying defect in the hyperimmunoglobulin E syndrome may be associated with a T-cell abnormality characterized by inadequate production of gamma-interferon, which normally suppresses IgE production. The genetic defect in HIE has been recently described.[43] Differentiation of the HIE syndrome from atopic dermatitis is sometimes difficult and is mainly dependent on the presence of recurrent deep abscesses and pneumonia in the hyperimmunoglobulin E syndrome.

Management of this syndrome consists of the control of the pruritic eczematoid dermatitis with emollient creams, topical steroids, and antihistamines. Prophylactic oral dicloxacillin or trimethoprim-sulfa-methoxazole for *S. aureus* or oral ketoconazole for preventing *C. albicans* infections can benefit patients. Plasmapheresis has been used for a few patients who do not respond to other more conservative therapies. Other reported experimental immunomodulatory therapies include the use of levamisole, ascorbic acid, cimetidine, and transfer factor. Gamma-interferon therapy may increase these patient's neutrophil chemotactic response and reduce symptoms.[9,17,30,44,45]

The Complement System

The complement system is composed of an interacting series of glycoproteins that, upon activation, interact in an orderly sequence to produce biologically active substances, which enhance the inflammatory reaction and may cause lysis of cells or microorganisms (Figure 59–1). The system can be activated through two major pathways: the classical pathway, which is activated by binding of IgG1, IgG2, IgG3, or IgM to antigens and the alternative pathway, which is initiated by direct attachment of activated C3 to the surface of bacteria, viruses, fungi, and virus-infected cells. Once the alternative pathway is triggered, an amplification loop is activated, which induces more C3b formation. Surface-bound C3b in conjunction with C3 convertase, C4b2a (classical pathway), or C3bBb (alternative pathway) serves as a C5 convertase, which initiates the formation of the membrane attack complex (MAC: C5b678[9]n). All of the activated components of the complement system are tightly controlled by regulatory proteins including C1 esterase inhibitor, Factor I, C4 binding protein, Factor H, decay accelerating factor, S protein, and C8-binding protein. The major effects of active complement components include anaphylotoxic (C3a, C5a), opsonic (C3b, C3bi, C4b), chemotactic (C5a), and cytolytic activity (MAC). Deficiency of early components of the classical pathway results in a high incidence of collagen vascular-like disease (C1q, C1r, C1s, C4, or C3 deficiency). Patients who lack these components often present with some combination of recurrent infections (usually pneumococcal), arthritis, skin rash, and glomerulonephritis. This is most likely a result of suboptimal removal of circulating immune complexes from the circulation.[8,17,46]

Selected complement system disorders

Deficiency of C2 This deficiency is transmitted as an autosomal recessive trait and is the most commonly reported complement deficiency. The incidence of homozygous C2 deficiency is about one in 28,000 to 40,000 whereas the heterozygous carrier rate is estimated at about 1.2% in the general population based on screening of normal blood donors. Patients usually have recurrent pneumonias, bacteremia, or meningitis caused by *S. pneumoniae, H. influenzae,* and *Neisseria*

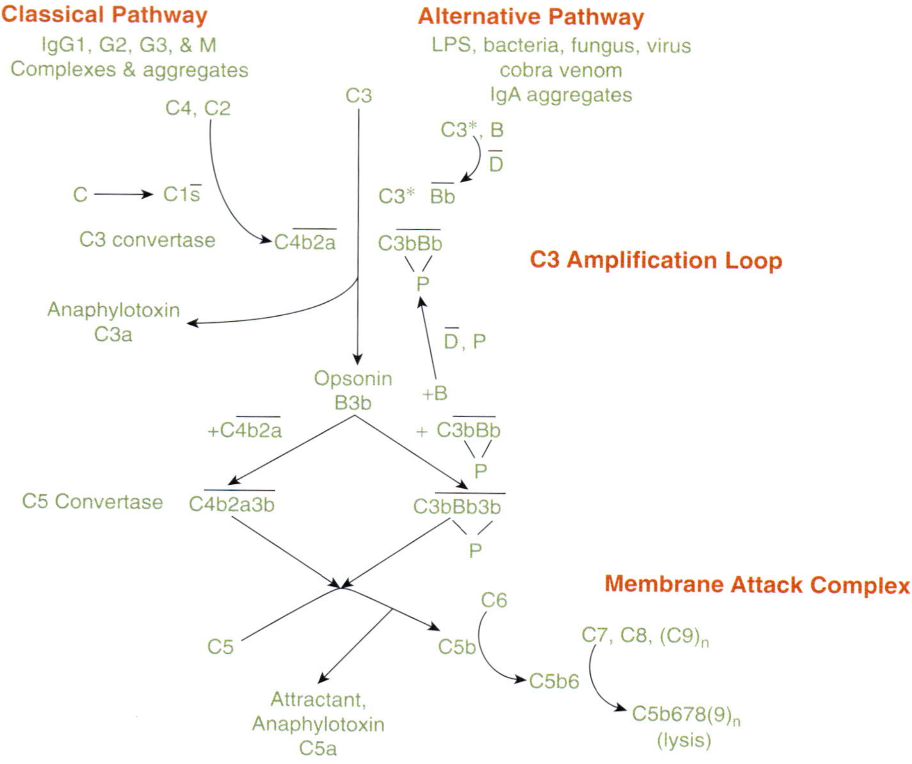

FIGURE 59–1 ■ The complement cascade.

meningitides. Autoimmune or rheumatic complications are present in about half of the patients. The lupus-like disease in C2-deficient patients is characterized by early onset, marked photosensitivity, low titers, or absent antinuclear antibody.[8,17,46]

Deficiency of C3 This deficiency is transmitted by autosomal recessive inheritance. C3 is positioned at the junction of the classical and alternative complement pathways and is important for opsonization of most encapsulated bacteria; generation of C3a, C5a, and initiation of the MAC. Patients with total C3 deficiency have severe episodes of recurrent pneumonia, sepsis, meningitis, and peritonitis. The most common pathogens isolated are *S. pneumoniae, H. influenzae, N. meningitides*, and *S. aureus*. Lupus-like illness and glomerulonephritis occur in 15–21% of the patients. Heterozygous carriers have C3 concentrations about 50% of normal but are asymptomatic.[8,17,46]

Deficiency of C1 complex and C4 These deficiencies are also transmitted by autosomal recessive inheritance. Activation of the alternative pathway through C3 may be sufficient for host defense against many pathogens, but deficient patients still tend to have pneumococcal infectious. Lupus-like illnesses (e.g. nephritis, arthritis, and facial rashes) and autoimmune disorders characterize a majority of the patients.[8,17,46]

Deficiency of C5–C9 Some individuals with deficiency of C5–C9 (the MAC) have an unusual susceptibility to recurrent *Neisseria* infections (*N. meningitides* or *Neisseria gonorrhoeae*). Deficiency of these terminal components is also transmitted by autosomal recessive inheritance. Recurrent episodes of meningococcemia, meningococcal meningitis, and disseminated gonococcal infection have occurred in about 50% of reported patients. The rate of C5–C9 deficiency in patients with disseminated *Neisseria* infections may be as high as 10–15%. In contrast to early complement component deficiencies, autoimmune diseases are only occasionally diagnosed in these patients. The management of complement deficiencies is symptomatic with antibiotic therapy as clinically indicated.[8,17,46]

REFERENCES

1. Holland SM, Gallin JI. Evaluation of the patient with suspected immunodeficiency. In: Mandell GL, Bennett JE, Dolin R, eds. *Principles and Practice of Infectious Diseases*. New York: Elsevier; 2005:149-60.
2. Bonella F, Bernstein IL, Khan DA, et al. Practice parameter for the diagnosis and management of primary immunodeficiency. *Ann Allergy Asthma Immunol.* 2005;94(5):S1-S63.
3. Kavanaugh A. Evaluation of patients with suspected immunodeficiency. *Am Fam Physician.* 1994;49:1167-1172.
4. Ballow M, O'Neil KM. Approach to the patient with recurrent infections. In: Adkinson NF, Yunginger JW, Busse WW, Bochner BS, Holgate ST, Simons FE, eds. *Middleton's Allergy Principles and Practice*. Philadelphia: Mosby; 2004:1043-1072.
5. Azar AE, Zuhair K, Ballas MD. Evaluation of the adult with suspected immunodeficiency. *Am J Med.* 2007;120: 764-768.
6. Christenson JC, Hill HR. Infections complicating congenital immunodeficiency syndromes. In: Rubin RH, Young LS, eds. *Clinical Approach to Infection in the Compromised Host.* New York: Kluwer Academic/Plenum Publishers; 2002:465-495.
7. Yang KD, Hill HR. Immune responses to infectious diseases: an evolutionary perspective. *Pediatr Infect Dis J.* 1996:15:355-336.
8. La Pine TR, Hill HR. Complement disorders. In: Osborn LM, DeWitt TG, First LR, Zenel JA, eds. *Pediatrics.* Philadelphia: Elsevier Mosby; 2005:1118-1122.
9. La Pine TR, Hill HR. Phagocytic and leukocyte abnormalities. In: Osborn LM, DeWitt TG, First LR, Zenel JA, eds. *Pediatrics.* Philadelphia: Elsevier Mosby; 2005:1123-1127.
10. La Pine TR, Hill HR. T- and B-lymphocyte disorders. In: Osborn LM, DeWitt TG, First LR, Zenel JA, eds. *Pediatrics.* Philadelphia: Elsevier Mosby; 2005:1127-1131.
11. Puck JM. Primary immunodeficiency diseases. *JAMA.* 1997;278(22):1835-1841.
12. Fleisher TA, Tomar RH. Introduction to diagnostic laboratory immunology. *JAMA.* 1997;278(22):1823-1834.
13. Fleisher TA, Oliveria JB. Functional and molecular evaluation of lymphocytes. *J Allergy Clin Immunol.* 2004;114: 227-234.
14. Shyur SD, Hill HR. Recent advances in the genetics of primary immunodeficiency syndromes. *J Pediatr.* 1996; 129: 8-24.
15. Casanova JL, Abel L. Primary immunodeficiencies: a field in its infancy. *Science.* 2007;317(5838):617-619.
16. Wilson CB, Edelmann KH. The T-lymphocyte system. In: Stiehm ER, Ochs HD, Winkelstein JA, eds. *Immunologic Disorders in Infants and Children.* Philadelphia: Elsevier Saunders; 2004:20-52.
17. Shyur SD, Hill HR. Immunodeficiency in the 1990s. *Pediatr Infect Dis J.* 1991:10:595-611.
18. Fischer A, Notarangelo LD. Combined immunodeficiencies. In: Stiehm ER, Ochs HD, Winkelstein JA, eds. *Immunologic Disorders in Infants and Children.* Philadelphia: Elsevier Saunders; 2004:447-449.
19. Puck JM. X-linked severe combined immunodeficiency. In: Ochs HD, Smith CIE, Puck JM, eds. *Primary Immunodeficiency Diseases.* New York: Oxford University Press; 1999:99-110.
20. Nowak-Wegrzyn A, Crawford TO, Winkelstein JA, et al. Immunodeficiency and infections in ataxia-telangiectasia. *J Pediatr.* 2004;144(4):505-511.
21. Sullivan KE. Genetic and clinical advances in Wiskott–Aldrich syndrome. *Curr Opin Pediatr.* 1995;7: 683-687.
22. Driscoll DA, Sullivan KE. DiGeorge syndrome: A chromosome 22q11.s deletion syndrome. In: Ochs HD, Smith CIE, Puck JM, eds. *Primary Immunodeficiency Diseases.* New York: Oxford University Press; 1999:198-208.

23. Hong R. The DiGeorge anomaly. *Immunodefic Rev.* 1991; 3(1):1-14.
24. Ochs HD, Stiehm ER, Winkelstin JA. Antibody deficiencies. In: Stiehm ER, Ochs HD, Winkelstein JA, eds. *Immunologic Disorders in Infants and Children.* Philadelphia: Elsevier Saunders; 2004:356-426.
25. Wald ER. Sinusitis in children. *Curr Concept.* 1995;128(3): 440-442.
26. Stiehm ER. The B-lymphocyte system: Clinical immunology. In: Stiehm ER, Ochs HD, Winkelstein JA, eds. *Immunologic Disorders.* Philadelphia: Elsevier Saunders; 2004: 85-108.
27. Kainulainen L, Suonpaa J, Nikoskelainnen J, et al. Bacteria and viruses in maxillary sinuses of patients with primary hypogammaglobulinemia. *Arch Otolaryngol Head Neck Surg.* 2007;133(6):597-602.
28. Cunningham-Rundels C. Selective IgA deficiency. In: Stiehm ER, Ochs HD, Winkelstein JA, eds. *Immunologic Disorders in Infants and Children.* Philadelphia: Elsevier Saunders; 2004:427-446.
29. Hammarstrom L, Voreschovsky I, Webster D. Selective IgA deficiency (SIgAD) and common variable immunodeficiency (CVID). *Clin Exp Immunol.* 2000;120:225-231.
30. Johnston RB, Babior BM. The polymorphonuclear leukocyte system. In: Stiehm ER, Ochs HD, Winkelstein JA, eds. *Immunologic Disorders in Infants and Children.* Philadelphia: Elsevier Saunders; 2004:109-128.
31. Yang KD, Hill HR. Neutrophil function disorders: pathophysiology, prevention, and therapy. *J Pediatr.* 1991; 119(30):343-354.
32. Yang KD, Quie PG, Hill HR. Phagocytic system. In: Ochs HD, Smith CIE, Puck JM, eds. *Primary Immunodeficiency Diseases.* New York: Oxford University Press; 1999:82-89.
33. Rosenzweig SD, Uzel G, Holland SM. Phagocyte disorders. In: Stiehm ER, Ochs HD, Winkelstein JA, eds. *Immunologic Disorders in Infants and Children.* Philadelphia: Elsevier Saunders; 2004: 618-651.
34. Lieschke GJ, Burgess AW. Granulocyte colony-stimulating factor and granulocyte-macrophage colony-stimulating factor. *New Engl J Med.* 1992;327(1):28-35.
35. Yang KD, Hill HR. Disorders of leukocyte function. In: Rimoin DL, Connor JM, Pyeritz RE, Korf BR, eds. *Principles and Practice of Medical Genetics.* London: Churchill Livingstone; 2007:1868-1888.
36. Pasvolsky R, Feigelson SW, Kilic SS, et al. A LAD-III syndrome is associated with defective expression of the Rap-1 activator CalDAG-GEFI in lymphocytes, neutrophils, and platelets. *J Exp Med.* 2007;204(7):1571-1582.
37. Blaese RM, Culver KW. Gene therapy for primary immunodeficiency disease. *Immunodefic Rev.* 1992:3(4): 329-349.
38. Cavazzana-Calfo, Dal-Cortivo L, Andre-Schmutz I, et al. Cell therapy for inherited diseases of the hematopoietic system. *C R Biol.* 2007;330(6–7):538-542.
39. Gonzalez LA and Hill HR. Advantages and disadvantages of antimicrobial prophylaxis in chronic granulomatous disease of childhood. *Pediatr Infect Dis J.* 1988;7(2): 83-85.
40. Ott MG, Seger R, Stein S, et al. Advances in the treatment of chronic granulomatous disease by gene therapy. *Curr Gene Ther.* 2007;7(3):155-161.
41. Mouy R, Fischer A, Vilmer E, et al. Incidence, severity, and prevention of infections in chronic granulomatous disease. *J Pediatr.* 1989;114(4):555-560.
42. Quie PG. Chronic granulomatous disease of childhood: a saga of -discovery and understanding. *Pediatr Infect Dis J.* 1993:12:395-398.
43. Minegishi Y, Saito M, Tsuchiya S, et al. Dominant-negative mutations in the DNA-binding domain ofSTAT3 cause hyper-IgE syndrome. *Nature.* 2007;448:1058-1063.
44. La Pine TR, Hill HR. Hyperimmunglobulin E syndrome. In: Rose BD, ed. *UpToDate.* Wellesley, MA: www.uptodate.com; 2007.
45. Hill HR. Modulation of host defenses with interferon-gamma in pediatrics. *J Infect Dis.* 1993;167(1):S23-S28.
46. Boyle JM, Buckley RH. Population prevalence of diagnosed primary immune deficiency diseases in the United States. *J Clin Immunol.* 2007;27:497-502.

SECTION 17

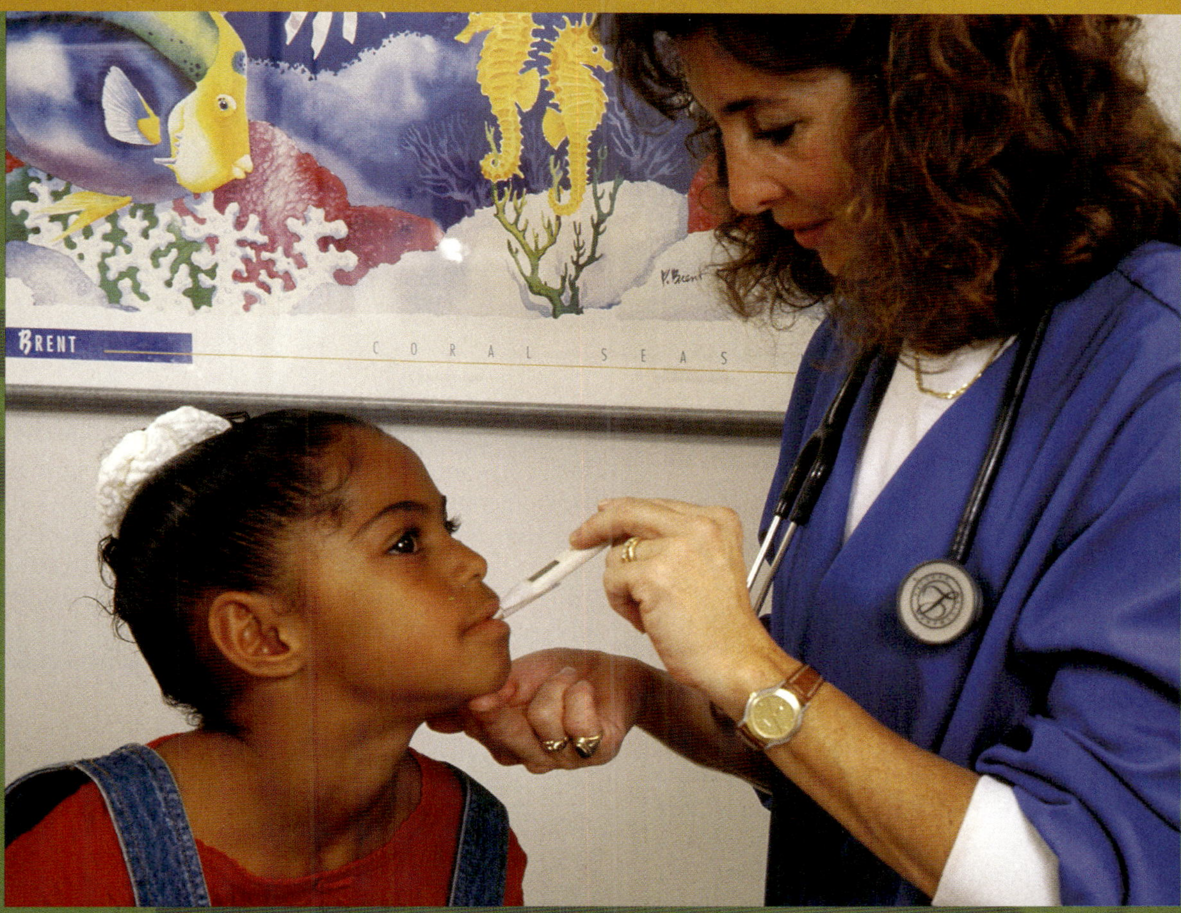

Fever Syndromes

CHAPTER 60

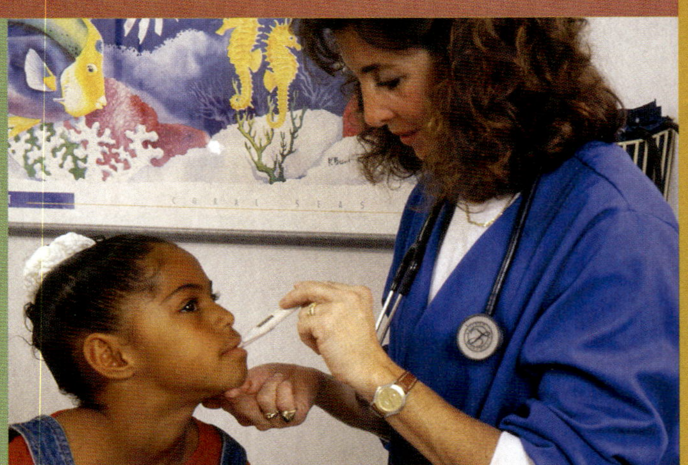

Fever of Unknown Origin

Jason G. Newland and Mary Anne Jackson

DEFINITIONS AND EPIDEMIOLOGY

Physiologic Temperature Variation

The first historical reference of fever was observed on a Sumerian pictogram in the sixth century BC with the first robust scientific study to address normal temperature variation performed by Carl Reinhold Wunderlich in the nineteenth century. Over 1 million temperature measurements were obtained on approximately 25,000 subjects establishing a normal value for the healthy human as 37°C.[1] It is now clear that "normal" temperature represents a range of values rather than a single value. Furthermore, diurnal variation in temperature exists such that the lowest body temperature occurs in the early morning (approximately 4 am) and the highest in the early evening (approximately 4 pm). Significant elevations of core body temperature can also occur from endogenous or exogenous factors. Among the exogenous factors that can influence this rate, ambient temperature and humidity are most important.

Fever Syndromes and Definition of Fever of Unknown Origin

Fever in a child is an everyday occurrence in an office-based pediatric setting and accounts for 19–30% of all physician encounters.[2] Prolonged fevers account for only a minority of these visits.

The term fever of unknown origin (FUO) was first coined in 1961 by Petersdorf and Beeson and directed the evaluation of the adult patient.[3] They introduced the concept that FUO be defined as a temperature higher than 38.3°C on several occasions and lasting longer than 3 weeks, with a diagnosis that remains uncertain after 1 week of investigation. The classic spectrum of disease they outlined included "no diagnosis," infections, inflammatory diseases, and malignancies. Deep vein thrombosis and temporal arthritis in the elderly were important considerations. Conventional bias at that time held that most adult patients presenting with FUO had serious, potentially life-threatening disease. The traditional approach for evaluation of FUO in the adult patient involved a staged evaluation culminating in tissue diagnosis.

In the first observational survey of children with FUO, Pizzo et al. in 1975 described 100 children with fever greater than 38.5°C for longer than 2 weeks and identified infections as the most commonly established diagnoses.[4] Pizzo's experience suggested that an aggressive staged approach to diagnosis was not necessary in most pediatric cases as most patients had reversible or treatable disease, usually an infection. They emphasized that most children recovered and prognosis was usually good. Diagnoses that were age-based were described and infectious diseases predominated. A small percent of those younger than 6 years had malignancy (neuroblastoma or leukemia) or rheumatoid disease (juvenile arthritis). Similarly, children older than age 6 years on occasion had an oncologic or rheumatologic diagnosis (leukemia, lymphoma, systemic lupus erythematosus). An organized approach in such cases was felt to be essential to identify those children with prolonged fever related to treatable infection or noninfectious disease to avoid morbidity and occasional mortality.

From a practical standpoint, we often use the term "prolonged fever" interchangeably with FUO. This term implies (1) fever of prolonged duration (at least 2 weeks); (2) documented temperature higher than 38.3°C (101°F) on multiple occasions and, preferably, by different care providers; and (3) uncertain cause.[5] Up to half of the patients referred for evaluation of FUO will have multiple, unrelated, self-limited viral infections, parental misinterpretation of normal temperature variation, or complete absence of fever at the time of referral.

PATHOGENESIS

The definition of fever from the International Union of Physiological Sciences Commission for Thermal Physiology defines it as "a state of elevated core temperature, which is often, but not necessarily, part of the defense responses of multicellular organisms (host) to the invasion of live (microorganisms) or inanimate matter recognized as pathogenic or alien by the host."[6] This scenario typically relates to the endogenous production of pyrogens. Both endogenous and exogenous pyrogens exist. Endogenous pyrogens are proteins produced by host cells. Examples of common endogenous pyrogens are interleukin-1, tumor necrosis factor-α, IL-6, and interferon. Exogenous pyrogens are substances produced by invading microorganisms. Many times these substances induce the production of endogenous pyrogens. Recent studies suggest that bacterial lipopolysaccharide (LPS) can directly induce fever without the use of endogenous cytokines.[6]

Once the pyrogens are present, they interact with receptors on many host cells throughout the body. They also interact with receptors in the major thermocenter, the preoptic area of the anterior hypothalamus. This interaction leads to the production of prostaglandin E2, which activates thermosensitive neurons. Some scientists believe this pathway is oversimplified and that other pathways probably exist.

DIAGNOSIS

An evaluation for fever should occur in any ill child and in more contemporary approaches, in the child where it is prolonged beyond 5–7 days. For example, it is critical that the child with Kawasaki disease be identified before the 10th day of illness as treatment with intravenous immune globulin is essential to prevent coronary artery complications.[7] Children with occult bacterial infection that is skeletal, intra-abdominal, or urinary tract in origin often do not have defining findings early in the course but the persistent course of fever coupled with observations of focal pain will lead to a diagnosis before the traditionally established definition of FUO. The ability of current technology and interventions to define these processes at an earlier time is reflected in more present-day descriptions of FUO where such diagnoses appear much less frequently. Certain epidemiologic clues may guide the evaluation (Table 60–1).

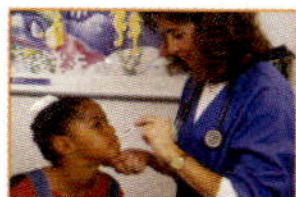

Table 60–1.

List of Pertinent Diagnostic Clues and Their Potential Diagnoses

Pertinent Diagnostic Clues	Potential Diagnoses
Foreign travel	Malaria, typhoid fever, TB
Palpebral conjunctivitis	EBV
Fever without reflex tachycardia	Typhoid fever
Consumption of unpasteurized milk	Brucellosis
Contact with kittens	Bartonellosis
Contact with birthing animals	Q fever
Contact with ticks	Tularemia, RMSF
Contact with reptiles	Salmonellosis
Contact/consumption of pond, lake, or river water	Leptospirosis
Bone pain	Leukemia, osteomyelitis
Evanescent rash	Systemic JRA

Whether fever has been present for 4 hours, 4 days, or 4 weeks, the clinician's approach to evaluation should follow five basic tenets as described below (Table 60–2).

Definition of Fever

Even though Barton Schmitt reported on the numerous parental misconceptions about fever in children more than 25 years ago, if one surveys parents and even many physicians today, an accurate definition of fever may not be consistent.[8] When Schmitt coined the term "fever phobia," he noted that many caregivers worried that high fever was associated with brain damage and death. He also noted that inappropriate dosing of antipyretics could contribute to toxicity in as many as 25% of children. The importance of accurate measurement of temperature was emphasized and an attempt was made to destigmatize fever. These are still important messages

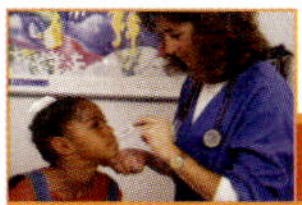

Table 60–2.

Approach to Evaluating the Child with Fever of Unknown Origin

- Use of a clear-cut definition of fever
- Confirm the duration and pattern of the fever
- Use of a carefully outlined history and meticulous physical examination
- Develop a thorough differential diagnosis
- Plan a cost-effective approach to utilization of the laboratory to confirm a diagnosis that allows for prompt initiation of appropriate therapy

today but the medical profession has not standardized their definition of fever to assist in this venture.

While much is written about the approach to the febrile infant and child, neither the Society of Pediatric Nurses nor the American Academy of Pediatrics has published position statements, which outline temperature measurement or give a definition of fever in children.[9,10] The Community Pediatrics section of the Canadian Pediatric Society published a 2007 revision of a position statement, which delineates recommendations for temperature measurement in children. Still only one line is relegated to defining fever stating a fever is present if rectal temperature is above 100.4°F (38.0°C).[11] This is consistent with publications which target the evaluation for fever in young infants.

Understanding the definition of fever, how to take the temperature and the reliability of temperature recordings from newer digital electronic products is important for the clinician. Temperatures can be measured rectally, orally, by electronic pacifier, or by ear canal. Accuracy of the measurement depends on what method the parents choose to measure temperature and most importantly, if the parents use the thermometers appropriately. Most experts agree that temperatures measured rectally are the most accurate and the standard for detecting fever in infants younger than 3 months. A rectal temperature of 38°C (100.4°F) generally is regarded as fever in the neonate 0–28 days of age. The definition of fever in the 1- to 3-month-old varies from 38°C to 38.2°C (100.4°F to 100.7°F).

Digital ear thermometers are most popular and have the advantage of measuring temperature in less than 2 seconds. Axillary temperatures can be performed but generally take longer. The thermometer is placed in a dry armpit and by holding the elbow against the chest for 4–5 minutes. It is generally regarded to be the least accurate but may be preferred in the youngest infants as it is easy to perform. However, if the axillary temperature is above 99.0°F (37.2°C), there is general agreement that it should be confirmed with another method, usually a rectal temperature in the young and an oral temperature in children older than 4–5 years of age. Digital pacifier thermometers are available but are not recommended as they do not accurately measure core body temperature.[12]

Finkelstein et al. reported a series of over 20,000 children in a single office practice and identified 5000 randomly chosen patients aged 3–36 months who presented for evaluation of fever of ≥38°C.[13] While fever was a common clinical presentation, they did not identify any patients over a 4-year period with FUO, underscoring the fact that while fever is a common symptom, FUO is a rare encounter in clinical practice. This in itself highlights the importance of having a systematic approach to evaluating fever in a child.

Confirmation of the Duration and Pattern of the Fever

There are a number of different approaches to the evaluation of fever in a pediatric patient depending on the patient's age, height, duration, and pattern of fever. Fever in the young infant (younger than 3 months), without a source for instance, may signal a serious bacterial infection.[14] The literature is full of recommendations to guide the physician's evaluation in such cases. Fever, which presents in the older infant or child where no localizing signs are present, can similarly raise concern for invasive bacterial disease though in the vast majority of cases, a viral pathogen is the etiologic culprit.

While fever patterns are not sensitive or specific in making FUO diagnoses, the pattern may aid in establishing an etiology of the fever. Patterns of fever that have been described include intermittent, remittent, hectic, and sustained.[15,16] Intermittent fevers refer to patients experiencing elevated temperature that return to normal at least one time during the day. This pattern of fever may signal a pyogenic infection such as abdominal abscesses and has been described with tuberculosis, lymphoma, and juvenile idiopathic arthritis (JIA). Hectic fevers are described as high fevers with a rapid rate of defervescence. Conditions associated with this pattern include juvenile rheumatoid arthritis and bacteremia. Patients with elevated temperatures that fluctuate but never return to normal are described as having remittent fevers. This pattern of fevers has been observed in patients with viral infection and bacterial infections such as endocarditis. Sustained fevers have little fluctuation in temperature and do not return to normal. Malaria, typhoid fever, and central nervous system (CNS) damage have been associated with this pattern. In addition, patients with typhoid fever lack the normal physiologic tachycardia seen in the presence of fever.[16] Physicians must be aware that antipyretics can cause remittent and persistent fever patterns to appear as intermittent fevers.

History and Physical Examination

A complete history and physical examination are essential to correctly diagnose all patients, but in the setting of FUO, this information can direct the evaluation and suggest an analytic algorithm for the clinician. Lohr et al. observed that among patients with FUO, the majority of diagnostic confirmations occurred through available laboratory tests, clinical course, tissue diagnosis, history, and physical examination.[17] The diagnosis was delayed due to an incomplete history and physical examination in 17% and 7% of all patients, respectively.[17] This study underscores the importance of utilizing available information and the history and physical examination.

The initial aspects of the history should focus on the fever. It is important to confirm the presence of fever (temperature >38°C) on consecutive days for 14 days. Any days the patient is afebrile would result in starting over in counting the days of fever. In many cases, patients will have days without fever. Additionally, an understanding of when the fever occurs in the day may provide important information. For example, a patient with mildly elevated temperatures in the evening without other systemic signs might represent normal diurnal variation.

After understanding the pattern of fever, clinicians must elicit symptoms that occur in conjunction with the fever. Patients lacking symptoms such as fatigue and/or malaise are potential clues for factitious fever. In addition to questioning patients and their families on common symptoms such as rhinorrhea, cough, vomiting, diarrhea, and rashes, clinicians should also be mindful of inquiring about symptoms such as oral ulcers, dental pain, night sweats, dysuria, bone pain, abdominal pain and weight gain or loss.

Further history should be focused on exposures. It is important to divide these exposures into animal contacts, ill contacts, diet, and travel. Contact with certain types of animals provides potential diagnostic clues for patients with FUO. Kittens, reptiles, and parturient farm animals, especially lambs, could indicate infection with *Bartonella henselae, Salmonella sp., and Coxiella burnetti,* respectively.[18] Other animals that should be inquired about include dogs, wild rodents, birds, and bats. Additionally, contact with insects such as ticks is important. Tick exposure might suggest tularemia or Rocky Mountain spotted fever; however, the latter is invariably diagnosed before the 7th day of illness as this disease is fatal if not recognized early in the clinical course.[19]

It is essential to inquire about ill contacts of the patient. Day care attendance is important as patients have a greater likelihood of coming in contact with ill children. Often, children with fevers who have just entered day care are experiencing recurrent viral infections. Persons at home with a history of a chronic cough and night sweats might indicate an exposure to tuberculosis (TB). Additional questions for potential TB exposures include persons at home who work in healthcare, in prisons, and have traveled or lived in a TB endemic area.[20]

The travel history is an important part of all FUO evaluations. The history should encompass the entire life of the patient. Malaria can present years after a person travels to an endemic area. Also, foreign travel might suggest the diagnosis of malaria or typhoid fever. Furthermore, living or traveling to parts of the United States with histoplasmosis, blastomycosis, and coccidiomycosis are important. The travel history should not be limited to just where they went but also what activities they participated in and the type of food consumed.

The diet history is an essential element of the FUO evaluation. Questions should focus on the consumption of raw meat, poultry, or fish as well as game meat and raw shellfish. Unpasteurized milks and cheeses as well as pica may provide clues to the diagnoses of brucellosis, toxoplasmosis, or cutaneous larva migrans.[21]

Other important historical information in an FUO evaluation includes the use of medications and the receipt of immunizations. All medications should be outlined. It is not uncommon for parents to forget to mention drugs taken daily by their child for conditions such as acne for instance. As ibuprofen and other antipyretics have been implicated as a cause for FUO, the specific drug, dosing, and duration should be described. The list of drugs that may cause fever is long and includes antimicrobials, nonsteroidal anti-inflammatory agents, anticonvulsants, antihistamines, cardiovascular agents, histamine blockers, iodides, and phenothiazides. The antibiotics that have been identified include carbapenems, cephalosporins, minocycline, nitrofurantoin, penicillins, rifampin, and sulfonamides. The most common anticonvulsants are barbiturates, carbamazepine, and phenytoin. Cardiovascular drugs include hydralazine, procainamide, and quinidine.[22,23] Receipt of immunizations are also important as they often times cause fever. In such cases, the duration of the fever is usually not more than 72 hours. While it is unusual for them to be a cause of FUO, they may contribute to fever in the setting of a concurrent illness.

School attendance and high-risk behaviors in adolescents are additional information that should be obtained in patients with FUO. Knowledge of school attendance aids the clinician in further understanding the extent of the illness. In some cases, numerous school absences could suggest a behavioral issue. For adolescents, it is essential to talk to them without their parents present and to inquire about drug and alcohol use and sexual activity. Finally, all records and laboratory data that have been obtained should be thoroughly reviewed.

A thorough physical examination is essential. Initially the examination should focus on the child's overall appearance including growth parameters and the pattern of growth. Weight loss, while nonspecific, might suggest a diagnosis of inflammatory bowel disease, cancer, or chronic disease. Attention should be paid to the lymph node examination assuring palpation occurs in the cervical, supraclavicular, axillary, epitrochlear, and inguinal areas. A careful assessment of the abdomen for hepatosplenomegaly and the joints for effusions should be performed. A thorough skin examination may also provide helpful clues in determining the diagnosis of a child with FUO. Patients with systemic JIA can present with fever and an evanescent rash.[24]

Confirming the Diagnosis: Laboratory Evaluation

Practically speaking, fever related to simple uncomplicated viral infection generally resolves in 48–72 hours. Depending on the patient's age, height of fever, and associated symptoms, when the febrile infant or child presents and no focus of infection is obvious by examination, initial laboratory testing often includes a complete blood count and urinalysis. Fever that persists for longer than 5–7 days requires a careful evaluation to avoid missing the diagnosis of Kawasaki disease. Similarly, occult bacterial infection may cause a persistent fever course. The evaluation at this point often includes inflammatory markers (sedimentation rate, C-reactive protein), liver function studies, a basic metabolic panel, and blood and urine cultures.

The rest of the laboratory evaluation of children with FUO should be directed toward the information obtained in the history and physical examination. At the same time, the clinician should utilize the results of the basic laboratory testing. Serologic studies likely to be of help include Bartonella and Epstein–Barr virus (EBV) testing. We generally advise that in the setting of FUO, HIV serologies should be obtained and a tuberculin skin test placed. Routine imaging studies should be limited to a chest radiograph, obtaining both a posterior–anterior (PA) and lateral view. In the patient with nonspecific gastrointestinal complaints, abdominal ultrasound may be helpful. Diagnoses including bartonellosis, abdominal abscess, pyelonephritis and inflammatory bowel disease may be identified by a skilled ultrasonographer. Additional imaging studies might include a bone scan evaluating for osteomyelitis and computed tomography scan of the abdomen in patients with histories suggestive of an intra-abdominal abscess. Magnetic resonance imaging (MRI) imaging of bones and joints may be helpful if a focal site of involvement is suggested by examination.

Other laboratory tests should be based on the history, physical examination, and course of illness. Based on the history, physical examination, and local geography, obtaining serologic tests for histoplasmosis, blastomycosis, tularemia, Brucella, CMV, or toxoplasmosis might be indicated. In patients with contact with reptiles, stool cultures could be useful in identifying salmonellosis. A bone marrow examination may be useful in patients where leukemia, neuroblastoma, or hemophagocytic syndrome is being considered.

The use of subspecialists can also be helpful in patients with FUO. The referral to these physicians should be based on the information collected during the initial evaluation. Infectious diseases, rheumatologist, and oncologist are the most likely subspecialist to be utilized. An ophthalmology consultation is another service that can utilized to evaluate for uveitis, which can be present in some rheumatologic disorders such as JIA.[25]

Following the initial evaluation, monitoring the fever and maintaining close follow-up is essential. A fever log that records the temperature and the symptoms experienced during the fever is helpful. In some instances, the diagnosis will become apparent while monitoring the clinical course. Therefore, follow-up is imperative and provides clinicians further opportunities to obtain additional historical facts and to potentially discover new physical examination findings. Follow-up also provides the parents and child with reassurance that you are continuing to care for and are willing to be diligent in determining a diagnosis. However, it is important to discuss with the patient and the parents that a diagnosis is not established in up to 50% of patients with FUO.[26, 27]

The use of empiric antibiotics in patients with FUO is not indicated. Treatment with antimicrobials should only be initiated when a diagnosis is established. The use of antimicrobials before a diagnosis is known could obscure and change the clinical course, potentially delaying the diagnosis and the appropriate treatment. Similarly, the use of corticosteroids should be avoided in such patients as even short courses can mask the diagnosis of oncologic and rheumatologic diseases.[28]

Differential Diagnosis: Causes of FUO in Children

A recent single center study confirms what older studies have previously noted in that viral infection is still the most common cause of FUO.[27] This review identified 131 (70%) patients in whom a diagnosis in the setting of FUO was established. Seventy (37.8%) had an infectious disease and EBV infection was the most common infection. Autoimmune disorders were diagnosed in 24 (12.9%), Kawasaki disease in 12 (6.4%), malignant diseases in 12 (6.4%), and miscellaneous conditions in 15 (8.1%) patients. In the remaining 54 (30%) patients, diagnosis was not established though most of them had self-limited disease. During the investigation, 26 (14%) patients developed serious organ dysfunction. Virus-associated hemophagocytic syndrome accounted for two deaths.

COURSE AND PROGNOSIS

The development of a differential diagnosis is essential in determining the extent of which a diagnostic evaluation will be performed. In studies describing diagnoses of patient with FUO, an infectious etiology is the most common diagnosis making up 25–52% of the cases.[4,17,26,27] In the sections below, the most common infectious clinical manifestations, infectious pathogens, and noninfectious diagnoses will be discussed.

Infectious Mononucleosis

The most common infectious clinical syndrome reported in case series of children with FUO is mononucleosis.[26, 27] Infectious mononucleosis (IM) is caused by EBV or cytomegalovirus (CMV) with EBV being most frequently identified. The transmission of EBV occurs primarily by contact with infected secretions. The incubation period is approximately 4–6 weeks.[29]

Clinically, patients initially present with malaise, headache, and fatigue that lasts 3–5 days. These prodromal symptoms are followed by fever that can be as high as 40°C and last typically for 1–2 weeks. In some cases, the fever has been observed to be present for up to 5 weeks.

The classic physical findings in cases of infectious mononucleosis are lymphadenopathy and tonsillopharyngitis. The lymphadenopathy is commonly located in the anterior and posterior cervical chain but can also be generalized throughout the body. The enlarged nodes are often times described as 2–4 cm in size, firm and mildly tender. The pharyngitis observed in IM can resemble that of group A streptococcal pharyngitis. In up to 50% of cases, of IM exudates are present on the tonsils.[30]

Additional findings that may be present in cases of IM include splenomegaly, hepatitis, and skin rashes.[30] Splenomegaly is present in 50% of cases during the second and third week of illness. Hepatomegaly is found in 10% of cases and elevated transaminases are present in up to 80% of cases. Skin rashes are seen primarily in children and adolescents with IM. The rash, found primarily on the trunk and arms, can be erythematous macular, papular, or morbilliform. Additionally in young adults with IM, a rash may appear after a patient receives ampicillin.[31]

Laboratory abnormalities include leucopenia or leukocytosis. Additionally patients with IM may have aplastic anemia or thrombocytopenia.[32,33] A potential clue for a patient having IM is greater than 10% atypical lymphocytes. Diagnostically, patients older than 4 years produce a heterophile antibody. This IgM antibody is produced during the second week of illness and can be present for up to 6 months. Monospot™ test attempts to detect this antibody and are positive in 85% of patients with IM after the first 1–2 weeks of illness.[29] More specific EBV serologies should be obtained even in children older than 4 years of age as 20% of such patients will have negative heterophile testing in the face of EBV infection.[34]

The primary therapy for patients with IM is supportive care. Only in cases of severe tonsillopharyngitis with airway obstruction should corticosteroids be used.[35] Unfortunately, IM can have a prolonged resolution phase with fatigue lasting for up to 3 months.

Urinary Tract Infections

Urinary tract infections (UTIs) are one of the more common causes of FUO in children. In two recent FUO pediatric case series, UTIs were the third most common infectious etiology comprising up to 10% of infectious diseases diagnoses.[26,27] In general, UTIs are more common in girls. During the first 6 years of life, Hellstrom et al. noted the incidence of symptomatic UTIs as being 8.4% in girls and 1.7% in boys.[36]

Clinical signs and symptoms often vary based on the age of the child. Infants may present with fever, poor feeding, vomiting, and possibly failure to thrive. In toddlers, fever and abdominal pain are common. Patients older than 5 years of age are more likely to complain of dysuria, urgency, and costovertebral angle tenderness. New onset of bedwetting in a child previously potty trained may also be a presenting symptom.

Diagnosis of a UTI is confirmed by obtaining a quantitative urine culture. Colony counts of greater than 10^5 CFU/mL organisms have been established as a definite infection in adults. Some experts have recommended that greater than 50,000 CFU/mL in children younger than 2 years is indicative of an acute infection.[37] In infants, a suprapubic tap or obtaining urine by a catheterization is ideal. Collecting urine from a bag specimen is not appropriate for diagnosis as 25% are contaminated usually with enteric flora, and sometimes with a single pathogen.[38] Bag urine may be acceptable if negative in the child who is not receiving antibiotics. In any case, where a bag urine culture is positive, it should always be confirmed with an appropriate catheterized urine specimen *before* antibiotic therapy is initiated. A midstream void from an older child is appropriate. Urinalysis can also be helpful in suggesting a diagnosing of UTIs. A positive nitrite test from a freshly voided urine is highly suggestive of a UTI. Additionally, a negative leukocyte esterase and a microscopic examination that does not observe any bacteria has a high negative predictive value.[39]

The empiric choice of therapy for children with UTI should be based on the susceptibilities found within one's own hospital. For those with known anatomic kidney defects including vesicoureteral reflux, ampicillin and gentamicin are recommended. Otherwise, parenteral ceftriaxone is appropriate for the vast majority of those who require hospitalization. Outpatient therapy with trimethoprim–sulfamethoxazole may no longer be appropriate as resistance rates have become significant in the last 5–10 years. An oral cephalosporin like cefixime can be utilized while awaiting the urine culture and susceptibilities in those with simple, uncomplicated UTIs.[40]

In the patient with complicated UTI causing FUO, CT imaging is helpful to confirm the diagnosis and to direct adjunctive therapy including drainage in case of sizeable renal abscess.[41,42] Inflammatory markers may be helpful to follow the clinical course. Parenteral therapy should be continued until clinical, microbiologic, and inflammatory marker improvement before a change to oral therapy.

Inflammatory Bowel Disease

The incidence of inflammatory bowel disease in the United States is increasing with prevalence data showing children and adolescents currently account for approximately 30% of all patients with this condition.[43] It is estimated that approximately 5% of children with inflammatory bowel disease (IBD) will present with FUO.[30] Other symptoms, which may be noted on review include anorexia, or abdominal pain; only 25% have the classic triad of abdominal pain, weight loss, and diarrhea[44]. Often the gastrointestinal complaints have not been brought to the physician's attention. Failure to grow and gain weight, however, may be noted when the growth chart is examined. That being said, recent data confirms that while 22–24% of children with Crohn's disease and 7–9% of children with ulcerative colitis were undergrown, most had a normal body mass index (BMI) and 10% of children with Crohn's disease and 20–30% of children with ulcerative colitis had a BMI at diagnosis consistent with overweight or risk for overweight.[45] A family history of inflammatory bowel disease should be elicited if IBD is suspected; one recent study suggests that 36.4% versus 17.5% of Caucasian and African-American children, respectively, will have a positive family history.[45] In 20–40% of cases, extraintestinal manifestations of IBD may be present.[46] Most commonly, these include peripheral arthritis, erythema nodosum, and pyoderma gangrenosum. Ocular manifestations may include uveitis and episcleritis. Confirming the diagnosis is usually definitive with endoscopy with biopsy.

Osteomyelitis

Most children with osteomyelitis have an acute presentation and the diagnosis is made within days to a week of symptom onset.[47] While fever, antalgic gait, and point tenderness over the metaphysis of a long bone is the common clinical presentation for osteomyelitis in a child, often times, the child does not localize pain, particularly if they are not weight bearing. Careful examination in such cases may identify the site of involvement. However, in the child with vertebral or pelvic osteomyelitis, fever and irritability are often the only clinical signs and a longer clinical prodrome is typical.[48,49] In most cases, inflammatory markers are elevated and if the child has had more than 1 week of fever, anemia may be present, raising the concern for an oncologic or rheumatologic diagnosis. It is important to note that blood cultures may not be positive in as many as 40% of patients.[50] CT (pelvis) or MRI imaging (spine) should be obtained depending on the suspected site of infection. While *Staphylococcus aureus* is usually the etiologic pathogen, unusual organisms including *Brucella*, *Bartonella*, and *Mycobacterium tuberculosis* should be considered if other epidemiologic risk factors are elicited.[51–53]

Kawasaki Disease and Polyarteritis Nodosa

Most pediatricians readily recognize the patient with fever and typical stigmata of Kawasaki disease. The clinical manifestations are well outlined and include polymorphous rash, nonexudative bulbar conjunctivitis, a single large cervical lymph node, indurative swelling of the hands and feet, and mucositis generally manifesting as red, cracked lips. Irritability refractory to any comforting maneuvers and high spiking fever for 5 or more days is typical.[54]

While Kawasaki disease most commonly occurs in children with a mean age of 2 years, it can occur in those as young as 6 weeks and even into the adolescent age group. Incomplete clinical presentations are most frequently noted in those <1 year of age but can occur in any age group. Fever without any clinical stigmata is for the most part only seen in those <6 months of age.[55]

The fever course of this inflammatory process is persistent and may last 10–14 days before fever abates. The major clinical concern then is related to the known sequelae of coronary artery involvement. Coronary arteritis with aneurysm formation occurs 10–40 days after the fever onset in 20–30% of untreated patients and can be documented by transthoracic echocardiography.[56] IVIG and aspirin treatment prevents coronary artery involvement if it is given in the first 2 weeks of symptoms.[54]

Polyarteritis nodosa (PAN) and Kawasaki disease share clinical and pathologic features, and many consider them to be the same disorder. The difference between KD and polyarteritis nodosa relates to the multiorgan involvement in the latter, particularly with involvement of mesenteric vessels.[57] Extensive coronary involvement with giant aneurysms may be present (Figure 60–1). In PAN, the febrile course is often longer and morbidity and mortality is high. Treatment of PAN often involves immunosuppressive therapy and the involvement of a pediatric rheumatologist is necessary.

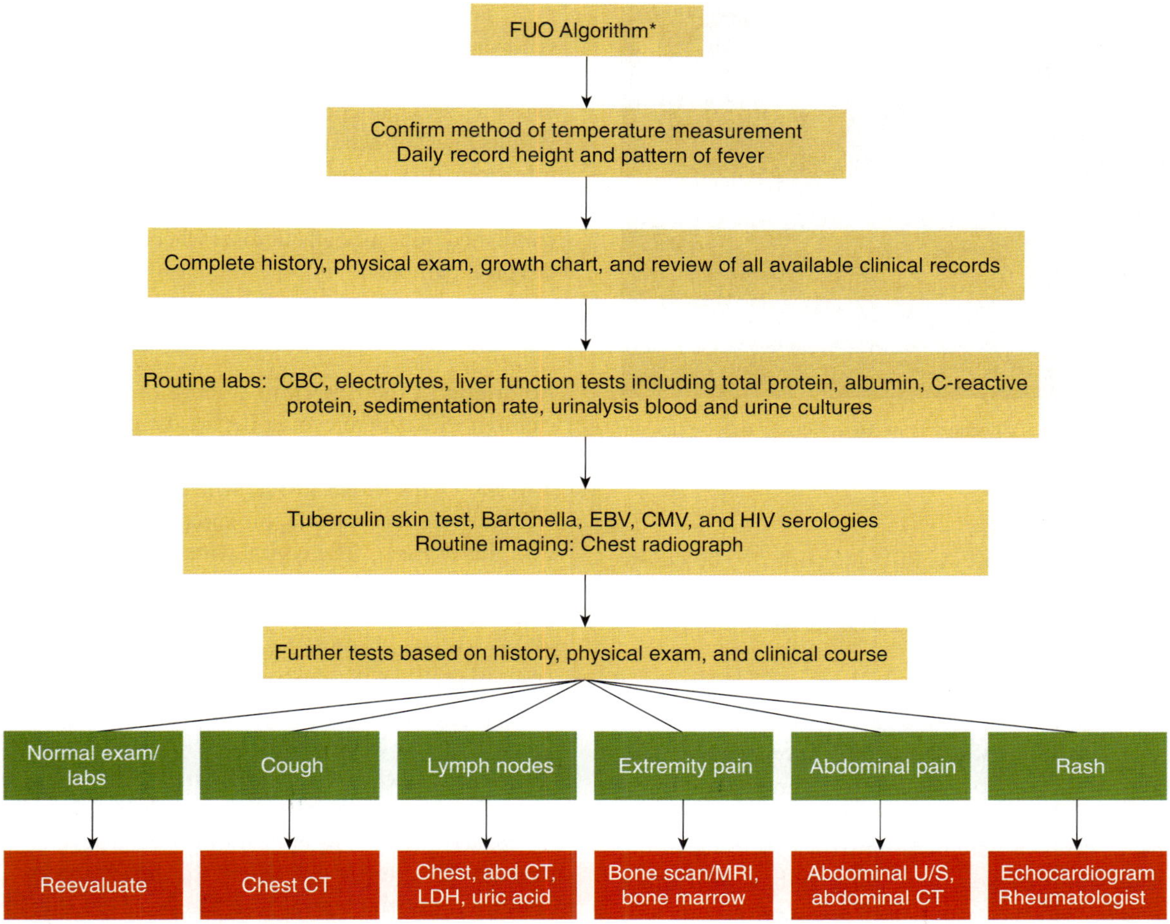

FUO Algorithm*

Confirm method of temperature measurement
Daily record height and pattern of fever

Complete history, physical exam, growth chart, and review of all available clinical records

Routine labs: CBC, electrolytes, liver function tests including total protein, albumin, C-reactive protein, sedimentation rate, urinalysis blood and urine cultures

Tuberculin skin test, Bartonella, EBV, CMV, and HIV serologies
Routine imaging: Chest radiograph

Further tests based on history, physical exam, and clinical course

Normal exam/labs	Cough	Lymph nodes	Extremity pain	Abdominal pain	Rash
Reevaluate	Chest CT	Chest, abd CT, LDH, uric acid	Bone scan/MRI, bone marrow	Abdominal U/S, abdominal CT	Echocardiogram Rheumatologist

FIGURE 60–1 ■ Algorithm for proceeding with FUO evaluation.

Hematologic/Oncologic Diagnoses: Leukemia, Hodgkin's Disease, Neuroblastoma, and Virus-Associated Hemophagocytosis

The diagnosis of malignancy should be considered carefully in the child with FUO. Most children have no other localizing findings though joint pain may be voiced and lead to consideration of the diagnosis of systemic onset JIA. It is helpful to note that while children with the JIA are uncomfortable and may have swollen joints, the joint pain elicited by examination of the child with leukemia may be severe and generally seems out of proportion to the degree of observed swelling.[58] Neuroblastoma and leukemia should be considered in the differential for FUO in the young child and leukemia and lymphoma in the child who is school aged or older. In children with Hodgkin's disease, a relapsing fever pattern may be present. In such cases, high-grade fever reaching 40–40.5°C (105–106°F) may be present with a periodicity of 7–10 days. The fever spikes abruptly and resolves abruptly but the baseline temperature does not return to normal.

In all cases where oncologic disease is suspected, LDH, uric acid, and ferritin measurement should be added to standard laboratories. CT imaging of chest and abdomen may be helpful depending on the tumor type. Bone scan and bone marrow aspirate and biopsy should be pursued in such cases after consultation with the pediatric oncologist (Figure 60–2).

A syndrome that is not common but important to understand is viral-associated hemophagocytic syndrome. Hemophagocytosis refers to the pathologic finding that includes activated macrophages, engulfing erythrocytes, leukocytes, platelets, and their precursor cells The literature refers to this phenomena as hemophagocytic lymphohistiocytosis (HLH).[59] Characterized by fever, pancytopenia, splenomegaly, the diagnosis maybe confirmed by finding hemophagocytosis in bone marrow, liver, or lymph nodes. HLH was initially thought to be a sporadic disease caused by neoplastic proliferation of histiocytes but the familial form of the disease, which is X-linked, has been associated with an aberrant

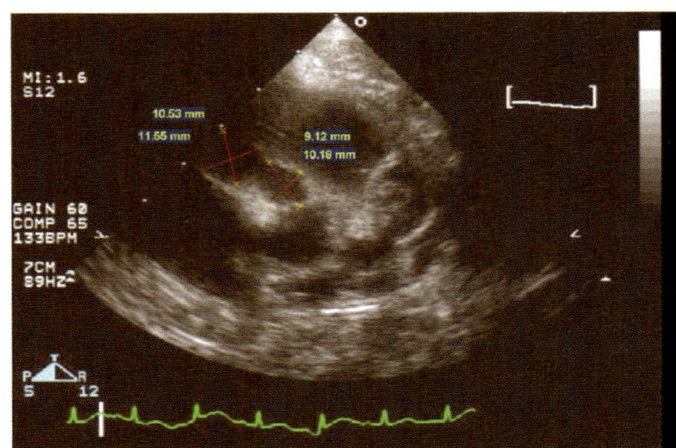

FIGURE 60–2 ■ Giant aneurysms on transthoracic echocardiogram in a 5-month-old infant with PAN.

immunologic response to EBV infection.[60] The classic laboratory findings include high triglycerides, ferritin, transaminases, and bilirubin and decreased fibrinogen.[60]

Fictitious Fever

There are two cases where fictitious fever may be considered: Parental misconception regarding definition of fever and falsification of symptoms by the patient or parent. In cases of parenteral misconception regarding the definition of fever, the child may have had other evaluations, which have provoked great concern for serious disease. In such cases, careful delineation of the manner and height of fever should be documented. If true fever is not present, no further evaluation is necessary other than parental education. This requires careful explanation as diagnoses such as leukemia or immune deficiency may have been raised. In such instances, the family must know that you have carefully reviewed all history, performed careful examination, and reviewed all laboratory testing before a conclusion has been made. A follow-up evaluation is mandatory to make sure that the child has remained well and is back to normal activities.

In 1977, the first report of a new form of child abuse was published and coined Munchausen syndrome by proxy (MSBP) after the syndrome that first had been reported by Asher in 1951.[61,62] This term is applied when an adult, usually the mother, presents a false history to the physician regarding a child who is not suffering from any of the fabricated symptoms. This history causes the physician to perform unnecessary diagnostic procedures that do not result in any specific diagnosis. MSBP has been called Polle syndrome, named after Baron von Munchausen's only child. In 2002, a new terminology, pediatric condition falsification (PCF), was suggested by the American Professional Society on the Abuse of Children (APSAC).[63]

Fever may be a presenting complaint with this syndrome and in some cases, the perpetrator has actually caused a febrile illness with clinical infection. In extreme cases, patients have injected bacteria into intravenous lines for instance to produce sepsis. Inclusion of infectious disease specialists is mandatory in any scenario where bacteria bloodstream infection has been confirmed but especially in cases where the isolate is not a typical pathogen.

Juvenile Idiopathic Arthritis

According to the American College of Rheumatology, children with systemic onset JIA are defined as those who display a daily or twice daily intermittent fever for at least 2 weeks.[24] This subset of JIA, which was formerly called Still's disease, occurs in approximately 20% of children with this disease.[24] The typical patient is under the age of 5 years and sexes are equally affected. The typical triad is fever, rash, and arthritis although the extraarticular manifestations are often more prominent. It is clear that while arthritis is a manifestation of disease, which is necessary for a definitive diagnosis, it may not be noted in the early course of the disease.

Fever is characteristically high and spiking but virtually always returns to normal during some time in the day. The child appears ill during fevers but is dramatically improved when the fever abates. The appearance of the typical rash can be diagnostic but is sometimes not even mentioned by parents and has to be sought with careful questioning. It is most prominently noted when the child is febrile and is often described by parents as more prominent when the child is bathed as heat is a well described trigger (Figure 60–3). The skin

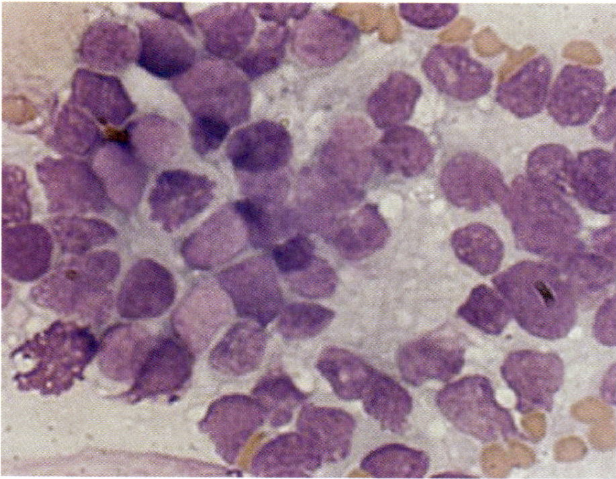

FIGURE 60–3 ■ Histologic picture of a neuroblastoma that shows many tumor cells in the enter and right separated by "neuropil," tumor cell neuritic cell process (axonal and dendrite-like). Tumor cells range in size from smaller poorly differentiated neuroblasts to larger cells with feature similar to Ganglion cells (differentiated neuroblasts). (Courtesy of David Zwick, MD.)

lesions are typically macular, salmon pink lesions, and are seen in the axillae and around the waist.[24] The so-called Koebner phenomenon may be helpful in that the rash can be provoked by stroking the skin.

It is important to note that children with systemic onset JIA may have additional findings on examination including joint pain with effusion, hepatomegaly, splenomegaly, and lymphadenopathy, which may raise the clinical suspicion for leukemia.[58] Associated laboratory findings include anemia, leuckocytosis, and thrombocytosis. Unfortunately, in this subset of JIA patients, who have the greatest visceral involvement, ANA and rheumatoid factor are generally negative. As clinical manifestations often lead to the inclusion of malignancy in the differential diagnosis, a bone marrow examination is almost always performed and is typically normal in systemic onset JIA. It is important to recognize that this disease has been found to display a wide range of severity. Many patients have a short monocyclic course with good prognosis; a prolonged chronic course with severe destructive arthritis occurs in a quarter to a third of patients.[64] Lastly, it is critical that the practitioner be aware that careful monitoring is necessary in the patient with systemic onset JIA as complications such as macrophage activation syndrome may lead to significant morbidity and occasional mortality.[65]

Bartonellosis

B. henselae is a fastidious slow growing Gram-negative bacillus and the implicated cause of cat scratch infection.[66] While the true incidence of this disease is unknown, the classical clinical presentation and epidemiology is well documented. More than 90% of children with cat-scratch disease (CSD) have a history of cat exposure, most often kittens.[67] This historical piece of information must be carefully sought, however, because the child may be exposed outside of the household. Since the presentation may be remote by up to 2 months from the time of exposure, asking the parent to identify these exposures requires them to consider other family members and friends who may have cats.

A peak of cases is generally noted in the late summer and fall.[29] A primary skin lesion may occur 1–2 weeks after the scratch but this lesion may be gone at the time of the child's presentation with classical disease, which is a subacute lymphadenitis.[67] The involved lymph node is generally adjacent to the scratch and most commonly noted in the neck (33%), axillary (27%), or inguinal (18%) regions.

Atypical or systemic CSD occur in up to 20% of patients, and FUO accounts for nearly one-fifth of such presentations.[6] In a study by Jacobs and Schutze, 146 children with FUO or prolonged fever (documented daily temperature of ≥38°C for at least 14 days without diagnostic signs or symptoms and fever for at least 14 days and no diagnosis at the time of referral for evaluation) were identified from 1990 to 1996. A diagnosis was established for just over half of the patients with the most common infectious disease diagnoses of Epstein-Barr virus infection, osteomyelitis, bartonellosis, and occult UTI. In the patients with bartonellosis, a subset of patients had occult hepatosplenic involvement.[26] Occult bone involvement caused by *B. henselae* infection has similarly been noted in the child with FUO.[51]

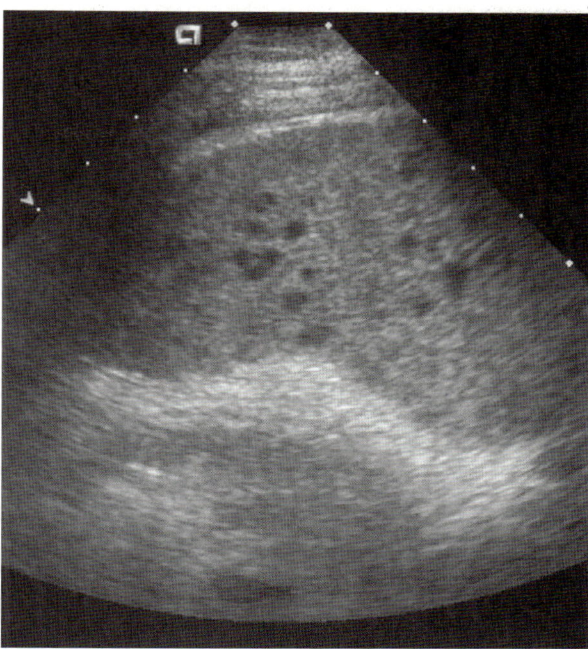

FIGURE 60–4 ■ Transverse images of the spleen show several scattered hypoechoic foci throughout both organs without mass effect. (Courtesy of Lisa Lowe, MD.)

Typically, an elevated erythrocyte sedimentation rate is noted but even in children with hepatosplenic involvement, liver transaminases tend to be normal.[67] Abdominal ultrasound or CT scan of the abdomen can confirm the typical hepatosplenic lesions (Figure 60–4). Liver biopsy, which would show necrotizing granuloma analogous to that found in the typical lymph node presentation, can be obviated by careful consideration of this diagnosis early in the child's course. Diagnosis can be confirmed serologically and virtually all such patients have a confirmatory positive titer at the time of presentation with FUO.[68]

Endocarditis

While the diagnosis of infective endocarditis (IE) in the pediatric patient is uncommon, characterizing the patient at risk is not usually difficult. The diagnosis is usually promptly considered in the child with fever and underlying congenital heart disease, particularly those

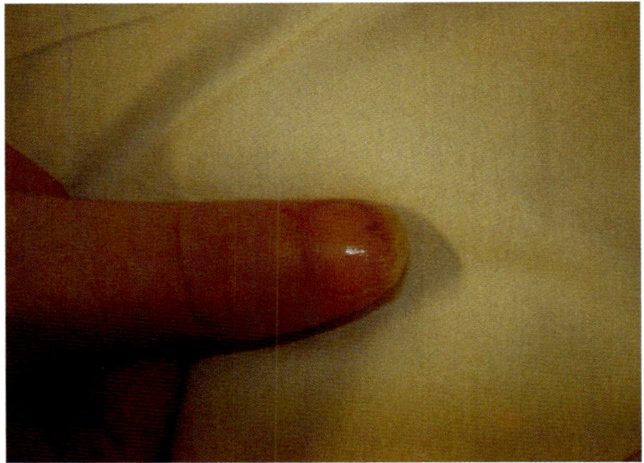

FIGURE 60–5 ■ Splinter hemorrhages in child with endocarditis.

with vascular shunts or grafts. In addition, this diagnosis is considered early in the course of children with fever and indwelling central vascular catheters, and in those who are persistently bacteremic with typically virulent pathogens. However, there is a small subset of patients where an underlying valvular lesion is not known and the clinical presentation is indolent, with prolonged low-grade fever and a variety of somatic complaints, including fatigue, weakness, arthralgias, myalgias, weight loss, rigors, and diaphoresis.[68] It is helpful for the clinician to consider that the clinical findings of IE in children relate to four underlying phenomena: bacteremia (or fungemia), valvulitis, immunologic responses, and emboli.[68] The classic change in murmur relates generally to valvulitis. The findings of petechiae, hemorrhages, Roth's spots, Janeway lesions, Osler nodes, or splenomegaly are less common in children than in adults but may be the clue to diagnosis (Figure 60–5).

The diagnosis of IE is usually promptly considered and confirmed when a child has positive blood cultures in the setting of a known underlying congenital heart defect. However, this diagnosis can be very difficult in instances where the patient has been partially treated with antibiotics or has an indolent, hard to culture pathogen (i.e., culture-negative endocarditis). This is particularly true in the approximately one-third of children who have no antecedent identification of a predisposing cardiac lesion at disease onset. The presence of low-grade clinical symptoms or atypical features may result in delayed diagnosis. The diagnosis of IE is based upon a careful history and physical examination, blood culture and laboratory results, an electrocardiogram (ECG), a chest radiograph, and an echocardiogram.[68] For those younger than 10 years, transthoracic echocardiogram is appropriate; a transesophageal study should be considered for the older pediatric patient.[69]

REFERENCES

1. Mackowiak PA, Wasserman SS, Levine MM. A critical appraisal of 98.6 degrees F, the upper limit of the normal body temperature, and other legacies of Carl Reinhold August Wunderlich. *JAMA.* 1992;268:1578-1580.
2. Wright PF, Thompson J, McKee KT, Jr., Vaughn WK, Sell SH, Karzon DT. Patterns of illness in the highly febrile young child: epidemiologic, clinical, and laboratory correlates. *Pediatrics.* 1981;67:694-700.
3. Petersdorf RG, Beeson PB. Fever of unexplained origin: report on 100 cases. *Medicine.* (Baltimore). 1961;40:1-30.
4. Pizzo PA, Lovejoy FH, Jr., Smith DH. Prolonged fever in children: review of 100 cases. *Pediatrics.* 1975;55:468-473.
5. Shah SS, Alpern ER. Prolonged fever and fever of unknown origin. In: Zaoutis LB, Chiang VW, eds. *Comprehensive Pediatric Hospital Medicine.* Philadelphia: Mosby; 2007:324-328.
6. Reynolds MG, Holman RC, Curns AT, O'Reilly M, McQuiston JH, Steiner CA. Epidemiology of cat-scratch disease hospitalizations among children in the United States. *Pediatr Infect Dis J.* 2005;24:700-704.
7. Durongpisitkul K, Gururaj VJ, Park JM, Martin CF. The prevention of coronary artery aneurysm in Kawasaki disease: a meta-analysis on the efficacy of aspirin and immunoglobulin treatment. *Pediatrics.* 1995;96:1057-1061.
8. Schmitt BD. Fever phobia: misconceptions of parents about fevers. *Am J Dis Child.* 1980;134:176-181.
9. Society of Pediatric Nurses. Society of Pediatric Nurses, 2008. http://www.pedsnurses.org. Accessed February 6, 2008.
10. American Academy of Pediatrics. American Academy of Pediatrics, 2008. http://www.aap.org. Accessed February 6, 2008.
11. Community Paediatrics Committee CPS. Temperature measurement in paediatrics. Canadian Paediatric Society. 2007.
12. Callanan D. Detecting fever in young infants: reliability of perceived, pacifier, and temporal artery temperatures in infants younger than 3 months of age. *Pediatr Emerg Care.* 2003;19:240-243.
13. Finkelstein JA, Christiansen CL, Platt R. Fever in pediatric primary care: occurrence, management, and outcomes. *Pediatrics.* 2000;105:260-266.
14. Baraff LJ, Bass JW, Fleisher GR, et al. Practice guideline for the management of infants and children 0 to 36 months of age with fever without source. Agency for Health Care Policy and Research. *Ann Emerg Med.* 1993;22:1198-1210.
15. Cunha BA. The clinical significance of fever patterns. *Infect Dis Clin North Am.* 1996;10:33-44.
16. Davis TM, Makepeace AE, Dallimore EA, Choo KE. Relative bradycardia is not a feature of enteric fever in children. *Clin Infect Dis.* 1999;28:582-586.
17. Lohr JA, Hendley JO. Prolonged fever of unknown origin: a record of experiences with 54 childhood patients. *Clin Pediatr* (Phila). 1977;16:768-773.
18. Lorin MI, Feigin RD. Fever without source and fever of unknown origin. In: Feigin RD, Cherry J, Demmler GJ, Kaplan S, eds. *Textbook of Pediatric Infectious Diseases.* Philadelphia: Saunders; 2004:825-836.
19. Kirkland KB, Wilkinson WE, Sexton DJ. Therapeutic delay and mortality in cases of Rocky Mountain spotted fever. *Clin Infect Dis.* 1995;20:1118-1121.

20. Froehlich H, Ackerson LM, Morozumi PA. The Pediatric Tuberculosis Study Group of Kaiser Permanente NC. Targeted testing of children for tuberculosis: validation of a risk assessment questionnaire. *Pediatrics.* 2001;107:e54.
21. Tenter AM, Heckeroth AR, Weiss LM. *Toxoplasma gondii*: from animals to humans. *Int J Parasitol.* 2000;30:1217-1258.
22. Lipsky BA, Hirschmann JV. Drug fever. *JAMA.* 1981;245: 851-854.
23. Johnson DH, Cunha BA. Drug Fever. *Infect Dis Clin North Am.* 1996;10:85-91.
24. Schneider R, Passo MH. Juvenile rheumatoid arthritis. *Rheum Dis Clin North Am.* 2002;28:503-530.
25. Wright T, Cron RQ. Pediatric rheumatology for the adult rheumatologist II: Uveitis in juvenile idiopathic arthritis. *J Clin Rheumatol.* 2007;13:205-210.
26. Jacobs RF, Schutze GE. Bartonella henselae as a cause of prolonged fever and fever of unknown origin in children. *Clin Infect Dis.* 1998;26:80-84.
27. Pasic S, Minic A, Djuric P, et al. Fever of unknown origin in 185 paediatric patients: a single-centre experience. *Acta Paediatr.* 2006;95:463-466.
28. Chessels JM. Pitfallis in the diagnosis of childhood leukaemia. *Br J Haematol.* 2001;114:506-511.
29. Diseases CoI. Epstein–Barr virus infections. In: Pickering LK, ed. *Red Book.* Washington, DC: American Academy of Pediatrics; 2006:286-288.
30. Leach CT, Fumaya CV. Epstein–Barr virus. In: Feigin RD, Cherry J, Demmler GJ, Kaplan S, eds. *Textbook of Pediatric Infectious Diseases.* Philadelphia: Saunders; 2004:1932-1948.
31. Kerns D, Shira JE, Go S, Summers RJ, Schwab JA, Plunket DC. Ampicillin rash in children. Relationship to penicillin allergy and infectious mononucleosis. *Am J Dis Child.* 1973;125:187-190.
32. Jenson HB. Acute complications of Epstein-Barr virus infectious mononucleosis. *Curr Opin Pediatr.* 2000;12: 263-268.
33. Lazarus KH, Baehner RL. Aplastic anemia complicating infectious mononucleosis: a case report and review of the literature. *Pediatrics.* 1981;67:907-910.
34. Sumaya CV, Ench Y. Epstein–Barr virus infectious mononucleosis in children. II. Heterophile antibody and viral-specific responses. *Pediatrics.* 1985;75:1011-1019.
35. Ganzel TM, Goldman JL, Padhya TA. Otolaryngologic clinical patterns in infectious mononucleosis. *Am J Otolaryngol.* 1996;17:397-400.
36. Hellstrom A, Hanson E, Hansson S, Hjalmas K, Jodal U. Association between urinary symptoms at 7 years old and previous urinary tract infection. *Arch Dis Child.* 1991;66: 232-234.
37. Hoberman A, Wald ER, Reynolds EA, Penchansky L, Charron M. Pyuria and bacteriuria in catheterized urine specimens obtained from young children with fever. *J Pediatr.* 1994;124:513-519.
38. Alam MT, Coulter JB, Pacheco J, et al. Comparison of urine contamination rates using three different methods of collection: clean-catch, cotton wool pad and urine bag. *Ann Trop Paediatr.* 2005;25:29-34.
39. Whiting P, Westwood M, Watt I, Cooper J, Kleijnen J. Rapid tests and urine sampling techniques for the diagnosis of urinary tract infection (UTI) in children under five years: a systematic review. *BMC Pediatr.* 2005;5:4.
40. Hoberman A, Wald ER, Hickey RW, et al. Oral versus initial intravenous therapy for urinary tract infections in young febrile children. *Pediatrics.* 1999;104:79-86.
41. Reid BS, Bender TM. Radiographic evaluation of children with urinary tract infections. *Radiol Clin North Am.* 1988; 26:393-407.
42. Wang YT, Lin KY, Chen MJ, Chiou YY. Renal abscess in children: a clinical retrospective study. *Acta Paediatr Taiwan.* 2003;44:197-201.
43. Kappelman MD, Rifas-Shiman SL, Kleinman K, et al. The prevalence and geographic distribution of Crohn's disease and ulcerative colitis in the United States. *Clin Gastroenterol Hepatol.* 2007;5:1424-1429.
44. Beattie RM, Croft NM, Fell JM, Afzal NA, Heuschkel RB. Inflammatory bowel disease. *Arch Dis Child.* 2006;91: 426-432.
45. Kugathasan S, Nebel J, Skelton JA, et al. Body mass index in children with newly diagnosed inflammatory bowel disease: observations from two multicenter North American inception cohorts. *J Pediatr.* 2007;151:523-527.
46. Su CG, Judge TA, Lichtenstein GR. Extraintestinal manifestations of inflammatory bowel disease. *Gastroenterol Clin North Am.* 2002;31:307-327.
47. Kaplan SL. Osteomyelitis in children. *Infect Dis Clin North Am.* 2005;19:787-797, vii.
48. Fernandez M, Carrol CL, Baker CJ. Discitis and vertebral osteomyelitis in children: an 18-year review. *Pediatrics.* 2000;105:1299-1304.
49. Zvulunov A, Gal N, Segev Z. Acute hematogenous osteomyelitis of the pelvis in childhood: diagnostic clues and pitfalls. *Pediatr Emerg Care.* 2003;19:29-31.
50. Goergens ED, McEvoy A, Watson M, Barrett IR. Acute osteomyelitis and septic arthritis in children. *J Paediatr Child Health.* 2005;41:59-62.
51. Hajjaji N, Hocqueloux L, Kerdraon R, Bret L. Bone infection in cat-scratch disease: a review of the literature. *J Infect.* 2007;54:417-421.
52. Colmenero JD, Ruiz-Mesa JD, Plata A, et al. Clinical findings, therapeutic approach, and outcome of brucellar vertebral osteomyelitis. *Clin Infect Dis.* 2008;46:426-433.
53. Rasool MN. Osseous manifestations of tuberculosis in children. *J Pediatr Orthop.* 2001;21:749-755.
54. Newburger JW, Takahashi M, Gerber MA, et al. Diagnosis, treatment, and long-term management of Kawasaki disease: a statement for health professionals from the Committee on Rheumatic Fever, Endocarditis and Kawasaki Disease, Council on Cardiovascular Disease in the Young, American Heart Association. *Circulation.* 2004;110:2747-2771.
55. Rosenfeld EA, Corydon KE, Shulman ST. Kawasaki disease in infants less than one year of age. *J Pediatr.* 1995; 126:524-529.
56. Kato H, Sugimura T, Akagi T, et al. Long-term consequences of Kawasaki disease. A 10- to 21-year follow-up study of 594 patients. *Circulation.* 1996;94:1379-1385.
57. Brogan PA, Davies R, Gordon I, Dillon MJ. Renal angiography in children with polyarteritis nodosa. *Pediatr Nephrol.* 2002;17:277-283.
58. Jones OY, Spencer CH, Bowyer SL, Dent PB, Gottlieb BS, Rabinovich CE. A multicenter case-control study on predictive factors distinguishing childhood leukemia from juvenile rheumatoid arthritis. *Pediatrics.* 2006;117: e840-e844.

59. Fisman DN. Hemophagocytic syndromes and infection. *Emerg Infect Dis.* 2000;6:601-608.
60. Imashuku S. Clinical features and treatment strategies of Epstein–Barr virus-associated hemophagocytic lymphohistiocytosis. *Crit Rev Oncol Hematol.* 2002;44:259-272.
61. Asher R. Munchausen's syndrome. *Lancet.* 1951;1:339-341.
62. Meadow R. Munchausen syndrome by proxy. The hinterland of child abuse. *Lancet.* 1977;2:343-345.
63. Schreier H. Munchausen by proxy defined. *Pediatrics.* 2002;110:985-988.
64. Spiegel LR, Schneider R, Lang BA, et al. Early predictors of poor functional outcome in systemic-onset juvenile rheumatoid arthritis: a multicenter cohort study. *Arthritis Rheum.* 2000;43:2402-2409.
65. Tristano AG, Casanova-Escalona L, Torres A, Rodriguez MA. Macrophage activation syndrome in a patient with systemic onset rheumatoid arthritis: rescue with intravenous immunoglobulin therapy. *J Clin Rheumatol.* 2003;9:253-258.
66. Massei F, Gori L, Macchia P, Maggiore G. The expanded spectrum of bartonellosis in children. *Infect Dis Clin North Am.* 2005;19:691-711.
67. Carithers HA. Cat-scratch disease. An overview based on a study of 1200 patients. *Am J Dis Child.* 1985;139:1124-1133.
68. Baddour LM, Wilson WR, Bayer AS, et al. Infective endocarditis. Diagnosis, antimicrobial therapy, and management of complications: a statement for healthcare professionals from the Committee on Rheumatic Fever, Endocarditis, and Kawasaki Disease, Council on Cardiovascular Disease in the Young, and the Councils on Clinical Cardiology, Stroke, and Cardiovascular Surgery and Anesthesia, American Heart Association: endorsed by the Infectious Diseases Society of America. *Circulation.* 2005;111:e394-e434.
69. Humpl T, McCrindle BW, Smallhorn JF. The relative roles of transthoracic compared with transesophageal echocardiography in children with suspected infective endocarditis. *J Am Coll Cardiol.* 2003;41:2068-2071.

CHAPTER 61

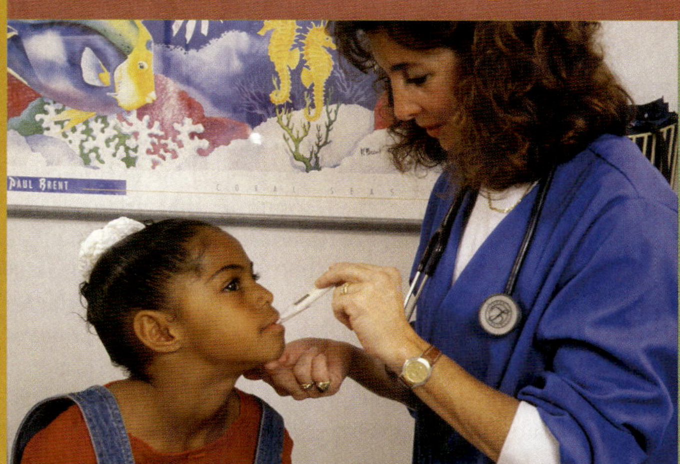

Hereditary Periodic Fever Syndromes

Evelien J. Bodar, Anna Simon, and Joost P.H. Drenth

DEFINITIONS AND EPIDEMIOLOGY

Hereditary periodic fever syndromes are defined by the presence of recurrent incapacitating episodes or fluctuating degrees of fever and inflammation in the absence of infection. Unlike autoimmune diseases, hereditary periodic fever syndromes are marked by the absence of significant levels of autoantibodies and autoreactive T-cells. As a consequence, the name autoinflammatory syndromes has been advocated as a common descriptive denominator for this group of rare disorders.[1,2] Since 1997, ten of the major syndromes have been linked to mutations in seven specific genes, facilitating the specific diagnosis of these conditions rather than relegating them to diagnoses of exclusion[3] (Table 61–1). The nomenclature of the various autoinflammatory syndromes is complicated, comprising a mix of syndromes described by various typical manifestations and syndromes characterized by identification of specific genetic defects. Most terms originated from the period preceding the discovery of the implicated genetic defects. To confound matters even more, most autoinflammatory syndromes are known by more than one name based on personal and geographical preferences.

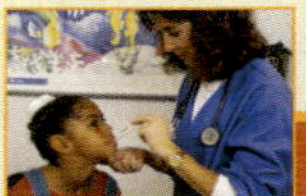

Table 61–1.

Main Periodic Fever Syndromes Overview

Mode of Inheritance	Gene	Chromosome	Mutated Protein	Group Name	Disease
Autosomal dominant	*CIAS1*	1q44	Cryopyrin/NALP3/ PYPAF1	CAPS	FCAS/FCU Muckle-Wells syndrome NOMID/CINCA
	TNFRSF1A	12p13	TNF receptor type 1	-	TRAPS
	PSTPIP1/CD2BP1	15q24	PSTPIP1	-	PAPA syndrome
	NOD2/CARD15	16q12	NOD2	-	Blau syndrome/early onset sarcoidosis
Autosomal recessive	*MEFV*	16p13	Pyrin/marenostrin	-	Familial Mediterranean Fever (FMF)
	MVK	12q24	Mevalonate kinase	Mevalonate kinase deficiencies	HIDS Mevalonic aciduria
	LPIN2	18p	Lipin 2	-	Majeed syndrome
Acquired	-		-	-	PFAPA syndrome

CINCA, Chronic infantile neurological cutaneous and articular syndrome; FCU, Familial cold urticaria; FCAS, familial cold autoinflammatory syndrome; HIDS, hyper-ID with periodic fever syndrome; NOMID, neonatal onset multisystem inflammatory diseases; PAPA, pyogenic sterile arthritis, pyoderma gangrenosum, and acne; PFAPA, Periodic fever, aphthous stomatitis, pharyngitis and cervical adenopathy; TRAPS, tumor necrosis factor receptor-associated periodic fever syndrome

For the purpose of this chapter we use the most accepted terms as retained in the literature.

Epidemiology

The incidence and prevalence of autoinflammatory syndromes vary by ethnicity and geographic location. For instance, FMF, the most common autoinflammatory syndrome, has a high prevalence among Sephardic Jews (100–400 patients per 100,000 persons) and among residents of Turkey (93 patients per 100,000 inhabitants) but a much lower prevalence among Western Europeans (2.5 patients per 100,000 inhabitants).[4,5] The prevalence of the other syndromes, while not specifically known, is estimated to be much lower than FMF. The syndrome of periodic fever, aphthous stomatitis, pharyngitis, and cervical adenopathy (PFAPA) is the most common of the remaining syndromes with more than 400 cases reported in English literature since 1989.[6] Pyogenic sterile arthritis, pyoderma gangrenosum, and acne (PAPA) and Majeed syndrome are probably the least common with five and three affected families reported, respectively.[7–9] The prevalence of other autoinflammatory syndromes is unclear, but each probably affects no more than several hundreds of patients.

Mendelian Inheritance

Most autoinflammatory syndromes show a clear Mendelian inheritance pattern. The following six display an autosomal dominant inheritance pattern: Familial cold autoinflammatory syndrome (FCAS), Muckle-Wells syndrome, neonatal onset multisystem inflammatory diseases (NOMID), tumor necrosis factor (TNF) receptor-associated periodic syndrome (TRAPS), PAPA, and Blau syndrome. There are four autosomal recessive syndromes: FMF, Majeed syndrome, and the mevalonate kinase deficiencies, which include both hyper-IgD with periodic fever syndrome (HIDS) and mevalonic aciduria. PFAPA syndrome is acquired and important to pediatricians because of its relative frequent presentation at an early age.[10,11]

PATHOGENESIS

Stimuli

It is thought that trivial stimuli cause a generalized inflammatory response in children with autoinflammatory syndromes with the immune system being either too sensitive to a stimulus or unable to stop the inflammatory response. In most cases, no obvious trigger can be identified as a cause of an attack. Immunological stimuli (vaccinations, upper respiratory tract infections), mechanical stimuli (insect bites, skin trauma, surgery, exercise), physical stimuli (cold exposure) and emotional stress have been reported to elicit an attack.

Genes and Proteins

In the last decade, the genetic defects of several autoinflammatory syndromes have been discovered. FMF was the first autoinflammatory syndrome that was elucidated at the molecular level; mutations in *MEFV* which encodes pyrin underlie FMF. TRAPS was termed as such following the discovery of *TNFRSF1A, the type 1 TNF-receptor,* as the susceptibility gene. FCAS, NOMID, and Muckle-Wells syndrome, syndrome were first seen as three different disorders but genetic research showed that they were allelic and that *CIAS1* mutations encoding cryopyrin are responsible for all three syndromes. Therefore, they are collectively termed the cryopyrin-associated periodic syndromes (CAPS). *CARD15* gene mutations are responsible for Blau syndrome but are also found in sporadic cases of Crohn's disease. HIDS and mevalonic aciduria are caused by deficiency of mevalonate kinase as a result from *MVK* mutations. In mevalonic aciduria there is a (near) complete deficiency of mevalonate kinase activity (<1%) while there is some residual activity in HIDS (5–10%). PAPA syndrome is caused by missense mutations in the *PSTPIP1* gene. Majeed syndrome is caused by mutations in *LPIN2*. The discovery of the mutated proteins for all these syndromes has led to an appreciation that most of the proteins involved, including pyrin (in FMF), cryopyrin (in CAPS), TNF receptor type 1 (in TRAPS) and PSTPIP1 (in PAPA) are members of the death domain fold superfamily and are implicated in regulation of apoptosis, NFκB activation and proinflammatory cytokine production. They are molecules intimately involved in innate immunity and play a key role in the hyperinflammatory response found in autoinflammatory syndromes (Table 61–1).[3]

CLINICAL PRESENTATION

The common denominator of the autoinflammatory syndromes is lifelong recurrent episodes of fever and other inflammatory symptoms. The acquired PFAPA syndrome is the exception to this rule because it is usually self-limiting and in most cases attacks disappear after childhood.[12] Attacks in patients with autoinflammatory syndromes generally occur at irregular intervals without obvious periodicity. Therefore the term recurrent is favorable over periodic.[13] In individual patients symptomatology during different attacks is usually similar and the course predictable when it comes to duration and the order in which the symptoms occur.[14] The recurrent nature of these diseases in children often leads to frequent absence at school and sometimes inability to finish education despite the presence of normal intellectual capacities.

Common Features

Most of these syndromes are invariably marked by episodes of high spiking fever (often >40°C) accompanied by chills and sweating. For example, in Blau syndrome and PAPA syndrome, fever is not a major symptom. One of the hallmarks, common to all autoinflammatory syndromes, is the accompanying acute phase response with elevated C-reactive protein (CRP) (often 10–30 mg/dL), erythrocyte sedimentation rate, serum amyloid A and leukocytosis (often 15–30 × 10^9/L) usually caused by neutrophilia. Parents and patients often describe a short but recognizable prodromal phase with aspecific symptoms like fatigue, irritability, headache, and malaise before the onset of fever. Recurrent inflammation can cause general symptoms such as normocytic anemia, fatigue, weight loss, or growth retardation. With the exception of PFAPA syndrome, all other syndromes are associated with a positive family history for comparable symptoms. A negative family history does not exclude an autoinflammatory syndrome since sporadic cases have been described in all hereditary autoinflammatory syndromes except PAPA and Majeed syndrome. Symptoms resolve spontaneously, and in between inflammatory attacks patients are asymptomatic although also in asymptomatic periods an acute phase response can be present. In the more severe syndromes (mevalonic aciduria, NOMID, Muckle-Wells syndrome), there is usually a fluctuating degree of inflammation without complete resolution between episodes.[2]

Distinguishing Features

Skin rash, if present, is an important clue for the diagnosis (Figure 61–1, 61–2 and 61–3). The urticarial-like rash in CAPS patients (Figure 61–3) can be distinguished from classical urticaria as histopathology demonstrates neutrophils and lymphocytes instead of mast cells. Both the migratory erythematous rash and

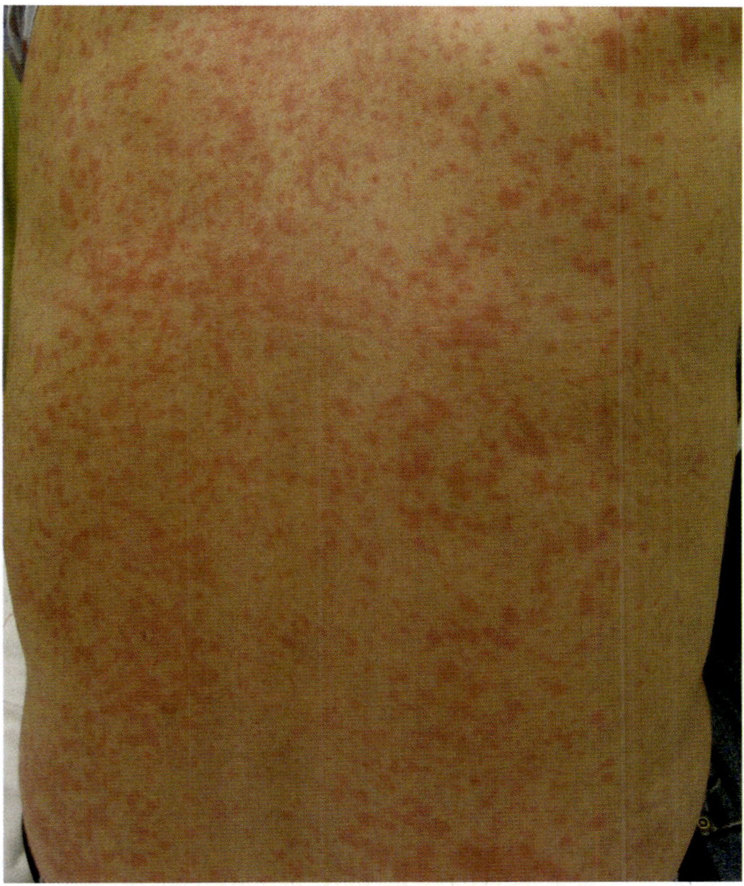

FIGURE 61–1 ■ Maculopapular rash in HIDS.

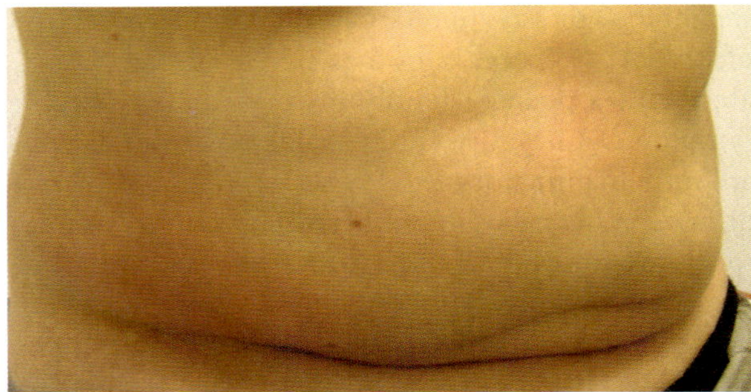

FIGURE 61–2 ■ Migratory erythematous rash in TRAPS.

erysipeloid erythema in TRAPS (Figure 61–2) and FMF, respectively, are very painful and mimic skin infections caused by *Staphylococcus aureus* and streptococci. The erysipeloid erythema is usually localized on the distal lower extremities (ankle, calf) and expands. The migratory rash is usually localized on the trunk, abdomen and proximal extremities slowly migrating from one location to the next. The maculopapular rash in Blau syndrome and mevalonate kinase deficiencies mimics varicella and other viral infections. In Blau syndrome histopathology shows noncaseating granulomas while cultures for mycobacteria remain negative.

Peritonitis in FMF, TRAPS, and occasionally HIDS can lead to intra-abdominal adhesion formation and unnecessary abdominal surgery with removal of an uninflamed appendix (appendix sana). Painful scrotal swelling in FMF and TRAPS is caused by involvement of the tunica vaginalis testis and has to be distinguished from other conditions such as testicular torsion and epididymitis. Pleuritis causes chest pain and dyspnoea. Pericardial involvement (pericarditis) is rare, but can be seen in FMF.

The lymphadenopathy in HIDS can be prominent and is tender at palpation. In PFAPA syndrome only cervical nodes are involved. Another feature both PFAPA and HIDS have in common is the painful aphthous stomatitis. Dysmorphic features, mental retardation and neurological symptoms are seen in NOMID, Muckle-Wells syndrome, and mevalonic aciduria. Perceptive deafness is an important feature of Muckle-Wells syndrome, and usually develops before adolescence. Uveitis is one of the characterizing symptoms of Blau syndrome but is also seen in mevalonic aciduria and NOMID.

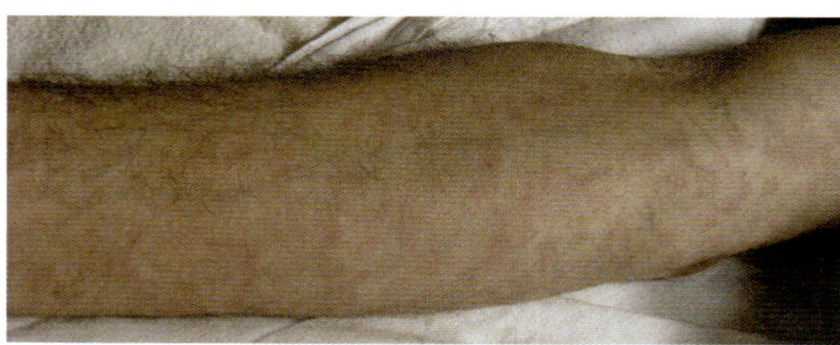

FIGURE 61–3 ■ Urticarial rash in CAPS.

An overview of distinguishing symptoms and characteristics for each syndrome can be found in Tables 61–2 to 61–3. It is important to realize that FCAS, Muckle-Wells syndrome, and NOMID are three syndromes representing a continuous phenotypic spectrum (cryopyrin-associated periodic syndromes or CAPS) and symptoms may overlap. HIDS and mevalonic aciduria also represent two ends of the same phenotypic spectrum (mevalonate kinase deficiencies).[15,16]

Complications

Reactive amyloidosis (type AA) is a serious complication sometimes leading to renal failure. The first sign usually is proteinuria and regular checks for its presence are necessary in all patients with autoinflammatory syndromes. The risk of amyloidosis is the highest for FMF and Muckle-Wells syndrome, and low in HIDS.[17,18] Reduction of the acute phase response with serum amyloid A levels $<$10 mg/L decreases the risk of amyloidosis and can halt its progression. Therefore early diagnosis and treatment of autoinflammatory syndromes is necessary. Several forms of vasculitis sometimes leading to renal impairment have occasionally been reported in TRAPS, FMF, Blau syndrome and mevalonate kinase deficiency patients (Table 61–2 to 61–3).

DIFFERENTIAL DIAGNOSIS

Inflammation and fever caused by autoinflammatory syndromes must be distinguished from other and more frequent causes of chronic and recurrent fever. Patients with prolonged recurrent fever present a diagnostic challenge for physicians especially since the chance of reaching a diagnosis is significantly smaller than in patients with continuous fever.[19] In young children, it is important to differentiate between the multiple self-limiting viral infections and other more pathological conditions. It has been estimated that the viral infections can occur up to ten times a year in the first three years of life.[14] The differential diagnosis of recurrent fever is extensive and includes among others vasculitis, rheumatological conditions, metabolic diseases, infections, and malignancies as listed in Table 61–4.[4,13,20,21] In approximately one-third of FMF patients fulfilling

Table 61–2.

Distinguishing Clinical Features of Autosomal Dominant Autoinflammatory Syndromes*

Clinical Features	FCAS	Muckle-Wells Syndrome	NOMID	TRAPS	Blau Syndrome	PAPA
Age at onset (y)	< 1	< 20	< 1	< 20	< 2, Up to 27	< 16
Duration attack (d)	< 2	1–3	Continuous, flares	> 7	Weeks–months	3–7
Specific trigger	Cold exposure	No	No	No	No	Trauma
Attack frequency	<1/d	per month-continuous	Continuous, flares	0.5/Mo	Months	0.5 per month
Ethnicity	Western European	Western European	Western European	Western European	All races	All races
Amyloidosis	Rare	Common	Rare	Yes	No	co
Development	Normal	Normal	Saddle-nose, frontal bossing, digital clubbing, mental and growth retardation	No	Campylodactyly	Normal
Skin	Urticarial rash, histological findings: lymphocytes and neutrophils	Urticarial rash, histological findings: lymphocytes and neutrophils	Urticarial rash, histological findings: lymphocytes and neutrophils	Migratory erythematous rash, periorbital edema, histological findings: mainly neutrophils	Maculopapular/nodular erythema, histological findings: noncaseating granulomas	Pyoderma gangrenosum, cystic acne, sterile abscess
Neurology	Headache	Perceptive deafness, headache, perceptive deafness	Aseptic meningitis, headache, perceptive deafness	Under debate	No	No
Lympadenopathy	No	Rare	Occasional	Rare	Granulomatous	No
Joints/muscles/ bone	Arthralgia, myalgia	Arthralgia, myalgia, lancing limb pain	Arthralgia, epiphyseal bone formation	Migratory myalgia, arthralgia, epiphyseal overgrowth	Tendonitis	Arthralgia
Lung	No	No	No	No	Pneumonitis	No
Serositis	No	Arthritis, rare: pleuritis	Erosive arthritis, rare: pleuritis	Peritonitis, pleuritis, pericarditis, (mono-) arthritis, tunica vaginalis testis	Granulomatous arthritis	Destructive pyogenic sterile arthritis
Abdominal	Nausea	Pain	Hepato-splenomegaly	Pain, constipation, diarrhea, Splenomegaly	Granulomatous hepatic and kidney involvement	No
Eye	Conjunctivitis	Conjunctivitis, optic nerve elevation, episcleritis	Papil edema, visual loss, uveitis, conjunctivitis	Conjunctivitis	Uveitis, iritis	No
Vasculitis	No	No	Rare	Henoch-Schönlein purpura, lymphocytic vasculitis	Granulomatous large vessel vasculitis	No

*Only typical features given; some may be highly variable (e.g., duration and frequency attacks).

FCAS, familial cold autoinflammatory syndrome; NOMID, neonatal onset multisystem inflammatory diseases; PAPA, pyogenic sterile arthritis, pyoderma gangrenosum, and acne; TRAPS, tumor necrosis factor receptor-associated periodic fever syndrome.

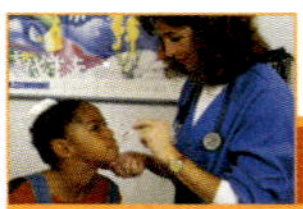

Table 61–3.

Distinguishing Clinical Features of Autosomal Recessive and Acquired Autoinflammatory Syndromes*

Clinical Features	FMF	HIDS/Mevalonic Aciduria	Majeed Syndrome	PFAPA
Age at onset (y)	< 20	< 1	< 2	< 10
Duration attack (d)	1–3	3–7	3–4	3–6
Specific trigger	No	Vaccination	No	No
Attack frequency	1–2 per mo	0.5–1 per mo	1–2 per mo	0.5–1 per mo
Ethnicity	Jewish, Armenian, Arab, Italian, Turkish	Western European	Arab	All races
Amyloidosis	Common	Rare	No	No
Development	Digital clubbing	Dysmorphic features†, mental retardation†, growth retardation†	Growth retardation, contractures	Normal
Skin	Erysipeloid erythema, histological findings: mainly neutrophils	Maculo-papular/nodular rash, histological findings: perivascular lymphocytic and polymorphonuclear infiltrates	Sweet syndrome, cutaneous pustulosis, histological findings: neutrophils	Rash
Neurology	Aseptic meningitis	Headache, cerebellar ataxia†	No	Headache, cranial neuritis, aseptic encephalitis
Lympadenopathy	Rare	Painful mainly cervical, histological findings: aspecific reactive changes	No	Cervical
Joints/muscles/ bone	Poly-arthralgia, myalgia, myopathy	arthralgia, hypotonia†, myopathy†	Osteomyelitis	Arthralgia, myalgia
Mucosa	No	Aphthous stomatitis, genital ulcera	No	Pharyngitis, aphthous stomatitis, tonsillitis
Serositis	Peritonitis, pleuritis, Pericarditis, (mono-/ oligo-) arthritis, tunica vaginalis testis	Rare: peritonitis, pleuritis, (poly-) arthritis	No	No
Abdominal	Pain, constipation, Splenomegaly	Pain, diarrhea, vomiting, splenomegaly	Hepato-splenomegaly	Pain, nausea, vomiting, diarrhea
Eye	Rare	Conjunctivitis†, uveitis†, cataract†	No	No
Blood/ bone marrow	No	High serum IgD and IgA (not in young children)	Hypochromic microcytic dyserythropoetic anemia‡	High IgD and IgA has been reported
Urine	No	High mevalonate during attacks	No	No
Vasculitis	Henoch-Schönlein purpura, polyarteritis nodosa	Skin vasculitis, Henoch-Schönlein purpura	No	No

*Only typical features given some may be highly variable (e.g., duration and frequency attacks)
†Features exclusively seen in MA.
‡Peripheral smear and bone marrow.
HIDS, hyper-ID with periodic fever syndrome; PFAPA, periodic fever, aphthous stomatitis, pharyngitis, and cervical adenopathy.

clinical criteria (Table 61–5)[22] a positive genetic diagnosis can be made. Furthermore, only in a minority of the patients (<30%) fitting the clinical phenotype of an autoinflammatory syndrome a genetic diagnosis can be made.[2,3,23] These things suggest that there are more, as yet unknown genetic defects that can lead to periodic fever and that the list of autoinflammatory disorders is probably incomplete at this moment.

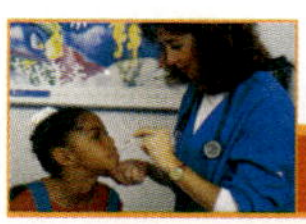

Table 61–4.

Differential Diagnosis of Chronic and Recurrent Fever in Children[4,13,20,21]

Category	Examples
Infectious	
Viral nonspecific	Multiple viral infections of different origin
Viral specific	Epstein-Barr virus, cytomegalovirus, herpes simplex virus, parvo B19
Bacterial nonspecific	Multiple bacterial infections of the same organ caused by anatomic deformities (e.g., urinary tract, airways), endocarditis, spondylodiscitis, osteomyelitis
Bacterial specific	Salmonella typhi, Yersinia, Campylobacter, cat scratch disease (Bartonella), Brucella melitensis, tuberculosis other mycobacteria, Borrelia (hermsii/parkeri), Lyme disease, Coxiella burnetii (Q-fever), tularemia, melioidosis, Whipple's disease, syphilis
Parasitic	Malaria, toxoplasmosis, babesiosis, trypanosomiasis, visceral leishmaniasis
Compromised host	HIV, cystic fibrosis, ciliary dyskinesia, common variable immunodeficiency, humoral immune deficiency, cyclic neutropenia
Noninfectious	
Neoplasia/lymphoproliferative	Neuroblastoma, atrial myxoma, leukemia, lymphoma, masto cytosis, Castleman's disease, histiocytosis (Letterer-Siwe disease)
Rheumatologic	Systemic onset juvenile rheumatoid arthritis, juvenile idiopathic arthritis, systemic lupus erythematosus, juvenile dermatomyositis, connective tissue disease, inflammatory bowel disease
Vasculitis	Kawasaki disease, Wegener granulomatosis, microscopic polyangeiitis, Churg-Straus, Takayashu, Behcet disease, polyarteritis nodosa, Henoch-Schönlein purpura
Miscellaneous	Hemophagocytic syndrome, urticaria pigmentosa, drug induced, diabetes insipidus, Fabry disease, Gaucher's disease, Mucha Haberman disease, familial dysautonomia (Riley-Day syndrome), anhidrotic dysplasia, factitious fever, Munchausen by proxy
Autoinflammatory	FMF, CAPS, Mevalonate kinase deficiencies, TRAPS, PFAPA, PAPA, Blau syndrome/early onset sarcoidosis, Majeed syndrome

CAPS, cryptoporin-associated periodic syndromes (i.e., familial cold autoinflammatory syndrome, neonatal onset multisystem inflammatory disorder, Muckle-Wells syndrome); PAPA, pyogenic sterile arthritis, pyoderma gangrenosum, and acne; PFAPA, Periodic fever, aphthous stomatitis, pharyngitis and cervical adenopathy; TRAPS, tumor necrosis factor receptor-associated periodic fever syndrome.

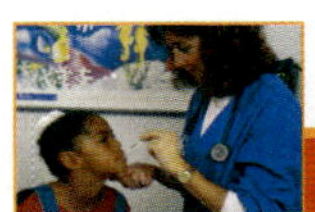

Table 61–5.

Diagnostic Criteria of FMF[22]

Major Criteria	Minor Criteria
≥ 3 attacks of ≤ 3 d duration with fever and peritonitis	Recurrent chest pain (incomplete attack)
≥ 3 attacks of ≤ 3 d duration with fever and pleuritis or pericarditis	Recurrent monoarthritis (incomplete attack)
≥ 3 attacks of ≤ 3 d duration with fever and monoarthritis	Exertional leg pain
≥ 3 attacks of ≤ 3 d duration with fever	Favorable response to colchicine
≥ 3 attacks of ≤ 3 d duration with fever	
Recurrent abdominal pain (incomplete attack)	

Requirements for clinical diagnosis of FMF are one or more major criteria or two or more minor criteria.

DIAGNOSIS

When a patient presents with a history of recurrent episodes of fever, meticulous evaluation is necessary to exclude the presence of infection and the other conditions mentioned earlier (Table 61–4).[14,24] In patients with a long history of recurrent fever episodes in the absence of symptom progression or additional complaints, malignant and infectious causes become less likely. Patients with autoinflammatory syndromes often go undiagnosed for many years after the onset of their first symptoms. The presence of an autoinflammatory syndrome is suggested by recurrent inflammatory attacks with predictable course and set of symptoms especially when family members are affected as well.

The clinician should elicit a detailed medical history with special attention for features of autoinflammatory syndromes (Tables 61–2 to 61–3), family history and previous febrile episodes (including reactions after vaccination and hospital admissions). Parents should be asked to take photographs of potentially important clues such as transient skin lesions and to keep a temperature and symptom diary. Since medical history, physical examination, and laboratory tests to evaluate the acute phase response (serum amyloid A levels, CRP, erythrocyte sedimentation rate, peripheral leukocyte count and differential) are usually unremarkable during asymptomatic periods, these tests should be repeated during a febrile episode. Hospital admission during an attack for clinical observation, cultures, and laboratory and radiological examination may be warranted. The evaluation of a child suspected of having an autoinflammatory syndrome largely depends on the presence of potential diagnostic clues, however, suggestions for initial evaluation are provided in Table 61–6.[14,20,21]

Apart from high plasma IgD and IgA (which can be normal in young children) and high urinary mevalonate during attacks in mevalonate kinase deficiency patients, there are no specific nongenetic laboratory tests to distinguish one autoinflammatory syndrome from another. Genetic confirmation is warranted if an autoinflammatory syndrome remains in the differential diagnosis after initial evaluation. Specialized clinical genetic laboratories perform these tests. The specimen can be placed in 2 × 10 mL EDTA tubes kept and shipped at room temperature. Studies have shown that the DNA quality from buccal swabs is comparable to that of isolated blood leukocytes. The yield from EDTA blood is considerably higher, reason that we prefer this as the source for DNA preparation. It is important to bear in mind that genetic testing is expensive and not covered by all insurance companies. The yield of genetic testing is low in patients without clinical features suggestive of a specific autoinflammatory syndrome. In two studies, more extensive genetic testing was performed in patients suffering recurrent fever episodes in whom no genetic diagnosis was established after 1 or 2 specific tests for the most likely syndromes based on clinical findings. This additional testing revealed the presence of a hereditary autoinflammatory syndrome in only 5% and 6.8% of patients, respectively.[23,25] Because of this low yield of random genetic analysis, it is important to focus the differential diagnosis based on several characteristics: Inheritance pattern, age of onset, duration of attacks, attack frequency, geographical region of origin, symptoms, and complications.[25]

Although the mainstay of the diagnosis is clinical evaluation by an experienced clinician, we propose an algorithm that can guide the performance of specific diagnostic testing. It is important to consider that clinical presentation can vary highly in terms of symptom constellation, attack duration and frequency within one disease entity. Especially in young children the full-blown phenotype might not have fully developed (e.g., deafness and neurological symptoms in Muckle-Wells syndrome, and CINCA or uveitis in Blau syndrome). Furthermore, a small group of patients fulfilling clinical criteria for a specific diagnosis will be

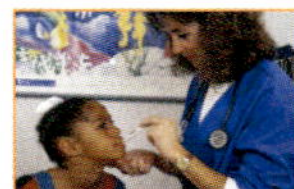

Table 61–6.

Suggested Focus of Attention During Initial Evaluation in Patients with Suspected Autoinflammatory Syndrome

Evaluation	Suggestions
History	Family members with autoinflammatory symptoms
	Previous febrile episodes, frequency, hospital admissions, triggers (vaccination)
	Symptoms during episodes (ask for specific features in Table 61–2 and 61–3)
	Duration of symptoms and order of appearance during episodes
	Duration of fever and maximum temperature
	Equal and recognizable course for each episode, prodromal phase
	Ethnicity, travel history
Physical	Development: growth chart, speech, fine motor, gross motor, vision, hearing
	General physical examination especially temperature, lymph nodes, skin rashes, joint function, hepato-splenomegaly*
	Neurological evaluation, including fundoscopy
Laboratory	Hemoglobin, leucocytes, differentiation, trombocytes, erythrocyte sedimentation rate, CRP, AST, ALT, LDH, kreatinine, creatine kinase*
	Serum immunoglobulin levels, ANA, ANCA, IgM reumafactor
	Urine analysis (proteinuria, hematuria); if HIDS suspected: mevalonate†
	Serial blood cultures (n = 3) urine culture, paired serology EBV, CMV, HIV†
Other	Chest X-ray, abdominal ultrasonography†
	Tuberculin skin test
PDC	Skin lesions consider biopsy†
	Lymphadenopathy consider excision for PA and bone marrow biopsy (including culture)†
	Hepato-splenomegaly consider liver biopsy
	Bone pain consider X-ray and radionuclide scanning (osteomyelitis)
No PDCs	Bone marrow biopsy (including culture), CT chest, abdomen†

*Both during symptomatic and asymptomatic phase.
†During attack.
PDC, potential diagnostic clue.

mutation negative. If the phenotype is typical for a specific disease a clinical diagnosis will be made although clinicians should be aware that in the future the diagnosis might have to be reconsidered. *If a clinical diagnosis cannot be confirmed by genetic testing, the terms variant HIDS, variant NOMID, and clinical FMF are used.*[26,27]

A continuously updated list of mutations responsible for autoinflammatory syndromes and the associated phenotypes can be found at the INFEVERS

Web site: http://fmf.igh.cnrs.fr/infevers/ There are associations between certain genotypes and phenotype. In mevalonate kinase deficiencies the V377I mutation is associated with higher residual mevalonate kinase enzyme activity and a less severe phenotype, therefore most HIDS patients carry at least one copy. In CAPS the association between genotype and phenotype seems less strict and the same mutations can be found in for instance FCAS, Muckle-Wells syndrome, and NOMID patients. There are also low penetrance mutations with a high prevalence in the normal population found in patients with less severe phenotypes. Examples are R92Q and P46L in *TNFRSF1A* and E148Q in *MEFV*. These mutations are no longer considered disease defining but rather disease modifying polymorphisms.[28]

TREATMENT

FMF

Continuous treatment with colchicine prevents attacks and development of amyloidosis in FMF. It can safely be used during conception, pregnancy and lactation. Failure to this therapy is usually as a result of poor compliance but in 5% of FMF patients there is a genuine lack of efficacy in terms of preventing attacks. However, these patients should still use continuous colchicine therapy to reduce the risk of amyloidosis. Small series and single case reports demonstrate beneficial responses to treatment with interferon-α, anakinra, etanercept, and infliximab combined with colchicine. However, the actual benefit is unclear as larger observational studies and randomized trials never have been performed.[29–31] Systemic corticosteroids are only warranted in FMF patients with prolonged febrile myalgia or vasculitis.[32,33]

HIDS

The first placebo-controlled crossover trial in HIDS showed that thalidomide was not effective, and toxicity remains the limiting factor.[34] A crossover trial demonstrated some benefits of simvastatin in terms of reduction of the number of days of illness in HIDS.[35] Some cautions are warranted when simvastatin treatment is started in mevalonic aciduria since two patients developed severe inflammatory attacks during simvastatin treatment.[36] Anakinra treatment seems to be more effective than etanercept treatment[37] and some patients benefit from systemic corticosteroids during attacks.

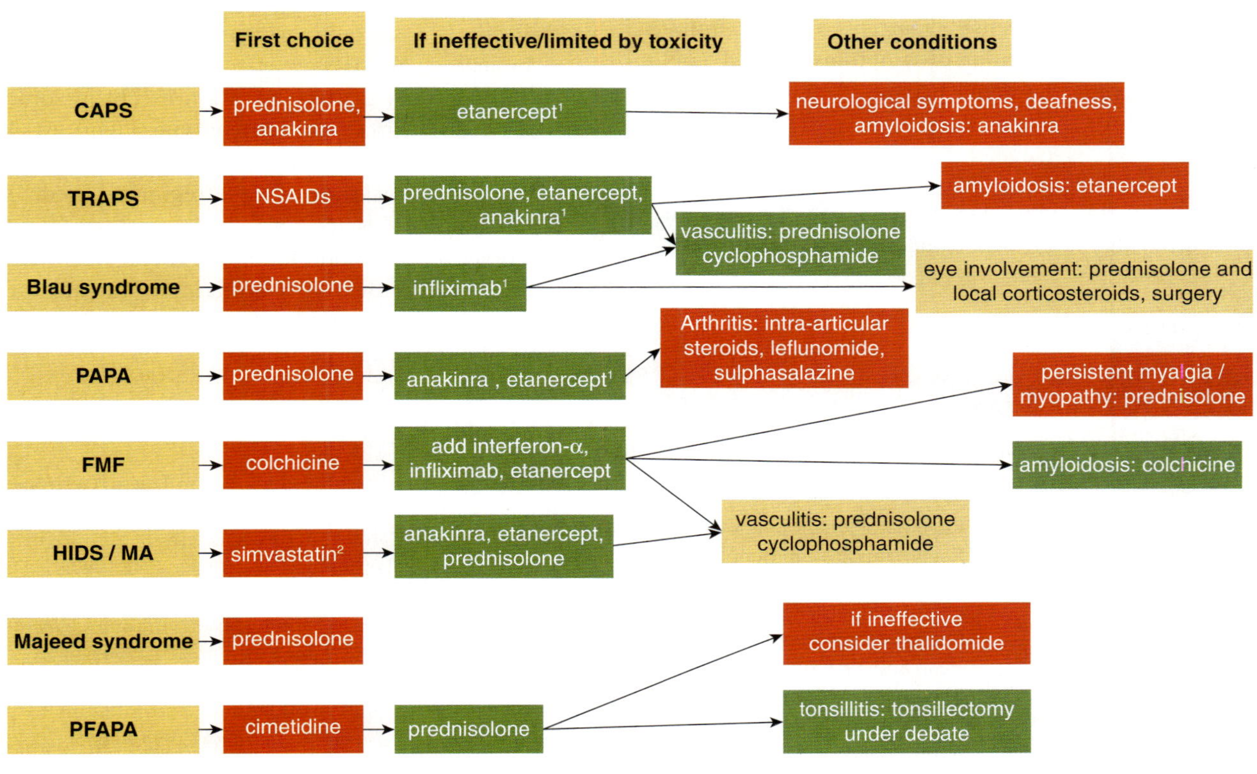

FIGURE 61–4 ■ Treatment algorithm.
[1]Evidence anecdotic.
[2]Caution warranted in MA: no formal proof of its efficacy exists.

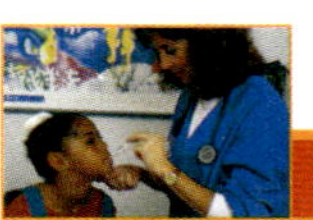

Table 61–7.

Medication and Most Frequently Used Dose

Medication	Dose Children	Dose Adults
Prednisolone	0.5–2 mg/kg/d*	30–60 mg/d*
Colchicine	1–2 mg/d	1–2 mg/d
Anakinra	1–2 mg/kg/d	100 mg/d
Etanercept	2 × 0.4 mg/kg/w	2 × 25 mg/w
Infliximab	1 × 3–5 mg/kg/mo	1 × 3–5 mg/kg/mo
Interferon-α	1–2 × 3–5 × 10^6 IU/wk	1–2 × 3–5 × 10^6 IU/wk
Simvastatin	10–20 mg/d	40–80 mg/d
Leflunomide	10–20 mg/d	10–20 mg/d
Sulphasalazine	30 mg/kg/d	1–3 g/d
Cimetidine	20–40 mg/kg/d	1–2 × 150 mg/kg/d
Thalidomide	1–6 mg/kg/d	50–200 mg/d

To be tapered to the lowest possible dose.

TRAPS

TRAPS patients generally respond well to NSAIDs and on-demand corticosteroid treatment during attacks but often escalating doses are necessary and treatment becomes chronic leading to toxicity. Some, but not all, TRAPS patients respond well to etanercept and there were reports that etanercept is effective in treating amyloidosis. There is a single report that one TRAPS patient developed amyloidosis despite effective etanercept treatment. Infliximab results in exacerbation of symptoms in TRAPS but anakinra was effective in one patient.[38,39]

PFAPA

Continuous cimetidine treatment was effective in some patients with PFAPA syndrome, but later results have not substantiated the early successes.[6] Systemic corticosteroid treatment reduced attack duration, but sometimes leads to a shorter asymptomatic period. One steroid-resistant PFAPA patient responded well to thalidomide. The role of tonsillectomy in these patients is still under discussion.[6,40]

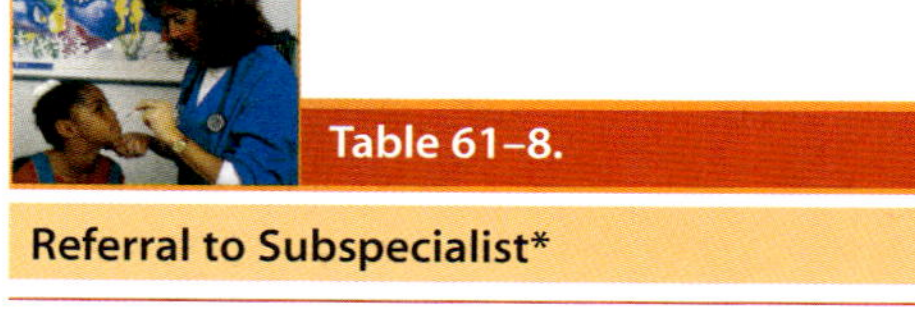

Table 61–8.

Referral to Subspecialist*

Indication	Specialist
Neurological symptoms	Rheumatologist/immunologist
Perceptive deafness	Rheumatologist/immunologist
Uveitis, iritis	Ophtalmologist
Amyloidosis	Rheumatologist/immunologist
Erosive arthritis	Rheumatologist/immunologist
Tonsillitis	Head and neck surgeon
Vasculitis	Rheumatologist/immunologist
Severe skin defects	Dermatologist
Renal function impairment	Nephrologist

**All patients should be referred to a rheumatologist or immunologist when despite maximum treatment (as allowed by toxicity) patients remain continuously symptomatic.*

CAPS

CAPS patients generally respond well to on demand corticosteroid treatment during attacks but often escalating doses are necessary and treatment becomes chronic leading to toxicity. Anakinra has shown to be remarkably effective in CAPS patients and leads to stabilization or even improvement of neurological symptoms and amyloidosis.[41–45]

Other Autoinflammatory Syndromes

PAPA patients generally respond well to on-demand corticosteroid treatment, but if limited by toxicity it was shown that anakinra (on demand) and etanercept (continuous) was also effective in PAPA syndrome. Leflunomide and sulphasalazine were able to induce remission in a PAPA patient primarily suffering from arthritis. Isolated arthritis also responds to intra-articular steroids.[7,8] There are few reports on effective treatment for Majeed and Blau syndrome, but systemic corticosteroid treatment is effective and in Blau syndrome infliximab was used effectively as steroid sparing treatment.[46–48]

In general, NSAIDs are effective for pain control but do not influence attack duration except in some TRAPS patients with a mild phenotype. Figure 61–4 shows an algorithm for treatment options and Table 61–7 gives an indication of dose regimens used. If asymptomatic periods are long, on-demand treatment is to be preferred over continuous treatment. Treatment with colchicine, simvastatin, and cimetidine are the exceptions to this rule. Table 61–8 lists the indications for referral to other subspecialists.

REFERENCES

1. McDermott MF, Aksentijevich I, Galon J, et al. Germline mutations in the extracellular domains of the 55 kDa TNF receptor, TNFR1, define a family of dominantly inherited autoinflammatory syndromes. *Cell.* 1999;97(1): 133-144.
2. Kastner DL. Hereditary periodic fever syndromes. *Hematology Am Soc Hematol Educ Program.* 2005;2005:74-81.
3. Simon A, van der Meer JW. Pathogenesis of familial periodic fever syndromes or hereditary autoinflammatory syndromes. *Am J Physiol Regul Integr Comp Physiol.* 2007; 292(1):R86-R98.
4. Hofer M, Mahlaoui N, Prieur AM. A child with a systemic febrile illness—differential diagnosis and management. *Best Pract Res Clin Rheumatol.* 2006;20(4):627-640.

5. Deltas CC, Mean R, Rossou E, et al. Familial Mediterranean fever (FMF) mutations occur frequently in the greek-cypriot population of cyprus. *Genet Test.* 2002;6(1): 15-21.
6. Pinto A, Lindemeyer RG, Sollecito TP. The PFAPA syndrome in oral medicine: differential diagnosis and treatment. *Oral Surg Oral Med Oral Pathol Oral Radiol Endod.* 2006;102(1):35-39.
7. Tallon B, Corkill M. Peculiarities of PAPA syndrome. *Rheumatology.* 2006;45(9):1140-1143.
8. Dierselhuis MP, Frenkel J, Wulffraat NM, Boelens JJ. Anakinra for flares of pyogenic arthritis in PAPA syndrome. *Rheumatology.* 2005;44(3):406-408.
9. Al-Mosawi ZS, Al-Saad KK, Ijadi-Maghsoodi R, El-Shanti HI, Ferguson PJ. A splice site mutation confirms the role of LPIN2 in majeed syndrome. *Arthritis Rheum.* 2007; 56(3):960-964.
10. Touitou I. INFEVERS: an online database for autoinflammatory mutations. http://fmf.igh.cnrs.fr/ISSAID/infevers/. Accessed August 18, 2008.
11. Touitou I, Lesage S, McDermott M, et al. Infevers: an evolving mutation database for auto-inflammatory syndromes. *Hum Mutat.* 2004;24(3):194-198.
12. Leong SC, Karkos PD, Apostolidou MT. Is there a role for the otolaryngologist in PFAPA syndrome? A systematic review. *Int J Pediatr Otorhinolaryngol.* 2006;70(11):1841-1845.
13. Majeed HA. Differential diagnosis of fever of unknown origin in children. *Curr Opin Rheumatol.* 2000;12(5): 439-444.
14. Long SS. Distinguishing among prolonged, recurrent, and periodic fever syndromes: approach of a pediatric infectious diseases subspecialist. *Pediatr Clin North Am.* 2005;52(3):811-835.
15. Simon A, Kremer HP, Wevers RA, et al. Mevalonate kinase deficiency: evidence for a phenotypic continuum. *Neurology.* 2004;62(6):994-997.
16. Arostegui JI, Aldea A, Modesto C, et al. Clinical and genetic heterogeneity among Spanish patients with recurrent autoinflammatory syndromes associated with the CIAS1/PYPAF1/NALP3 gene. *Arthritis Rheum.* 2004;50(12): 4045-4050.
17. van der Hilst JC, Simon A, Drenth JP. Hereditary periodic fever and reactive amyloidosis. *Clin Exp Med.* 2005;5(3): 87-98.
18. Samuels J, Ozen S. Familial Mediterranean fever and the other autoinflammatory syndromes: evaluation of the patient with recurrent fever. *Curr Opin Rheumatol.* 2006; 18(1):108-117.
19. Vanderschueren S, Knockaert D, Adriaenssens T, et al. From prolonged febrile illness to fever of unknown origin: the challenge continues. *Arch Intern Med.* 2003;163(9): 1033-1041.
20. Frenkel J, Kuis W. Overt and occult rheumatic diseases: the child with chronic fever. *Best Pract Res Clin Rheumatol.* 2002;16(3):443-469.
21. Bleeker-Rovers C, van der Meer JW. Fever of unknown origin. *Medicine.* 2005;33(3):33-36.
22. Livneh A, Langevitz P, Zemer D, et al. Criteria for the diagnosis of familial mediterranean fever. *Arthritis Rheum.* 1997;40(10):1879-1885.
23. Federici L, Rittore-Domingo C, Kone-Paut I, et al. A decision tree for genetic diagnosis of hereditary periodic fevers in unselected patients. *Ann Rheum Dis.* 2006; 65(11):1427-1432.
24. Drenth JP, van der Meer JW. Hereditary periodic fever. *N Engl J Med.* 2001;345(24):1748-1757.
25. Simon A, van der Meer JW, Vesely R, et al. Approach to genetic analysis in the diagnosis of hereditary autoinflammatory syndromes. *Rheumatology.* 2006;45(3):269-273.
26. Simon A. Approach to the diagnosis of hereditary autoinflammatory syndromes. *Future Rheumatology.* 2007; 2(1):5-8.
27. Aksentijevich I, Putnam D, Remmers EF, et al. The clinical continuum of cryopyrinopathies: novel CIAS1 mutations in north american patients and a new cryopyrin model. *Arthritis Rheum.* 2007;56(4):1273-1285.
28. Grateau G. Clinical and genetic aspects of the hereditary periodic fever syndromes. *Rheumatology.* 2004;43(4): 410-415.
29. Mor A, Pillinger MH, Kishimoto M, Abeles AM, Livneh A. Familial mediterranean fever successfully treated with etanercept. *J Clin Rheumatol.* 2007;13(1):38-40.
30. Calguneri M, Apras S, Ozbalkan Z, Ozturk MA. The efficacy of interferon-alpha in a patient with resistant familial mediterranean fever complicated by polyarteritis nodosa. *Intern Med.* 2004;43(7):612-614.
31. Belkhir R, Moulonguet-Doleris L, Hachulla E, Prinseau J, Baglin A, Hanslik T. Treatment of familial mediterranean fever with anakinra. *Ann Intern Med.* 2007;146(11):825-826.
32. Gdynia HJ, Sperfeld AD, Haerter G. Histologic signs of inflammatory myopathy in familial mediterranean fever. *J Clin Rheumatol.* 2006;12(5):265-266.
33. Soylu A, Kasap B, Turkmen M, Saylam GS, Kavukcu S. Febrile myalgia syndrome in familial mediterranean fever. *J Clin Rheumatol.* 2006;12(2):93-96.
34. Drenth JP, Vonk AG, Simon A, Powell R, van der Meer JW. Limited efficacy of thalidomide in the treatment of febrile attacks of the hyper-IgD and periodic fever syndrome: a randomized, double-blind, placebo-controlled trial. *J Pharmacol Exp Ther.* 2001;298(3):1221-1226.
35. Simon A, Drewe E, van der Meer JW, et al. Simvastatin treatment for inflammatory attacks of the hyperimmunoglobulinemia D and periodic fever syndrome. *Clin Pharmacol Ther.* 2004;75(5):476-483.
36. Hoffmann GF, Charpentier C, Mayatepek E, et al. Clinical and biochemical phenotype in 11 patients with mevalonic aciduria. *Pediatrics.* 1993;91(5):915-921.
37. Bodar EJ, van der Hilst JC, Drenth JP, van der Meer JW, Simon A. Effect of etanercept and anakinra on inflammatory attacks in the hyper-IgD syndrome: introducing a vaccination provocation model. *Neth J Med.* 2005;63(7): 260-264.
38. Simon A, Bodar EJ, van der Hilst JC, et al. Beneficial response to interleukin 1 receptor antagonist in traps. *Am J Med.* 2004;117(3):208-210.
39. Church LD, Churchman SM, Hawkins PN, McDermott MF. Hereditary auto-inflammatory disorders and biologics. *Springer Semin Immunopathol.* 2006;27(4):494-508.
40. Marque M, Guillot B, Bessis D. Thalidomide for treatment of PFAPA syndrome. *Oral Surg Oral Med Oral Pathol Oral Radiol Endod.* 2007;103(3):306-307.
41. Goldbach-Mansky R, Dailey NJ, Canna SW, et al. Neonatal-onset multisystem inflammatory disease responsive to

interleukin-1beta inhibition. *N Engl J Med.* 2006;355(6): 581-592.

42. Frenkel J, Rijkers GT, Mandey SH, et al. Lack of isoprenoid products raises ex vivo interleukin-1beta secretion in hyperimmunoglobulinemia D and periodic fever syndrome. *Arthritis Rheum.* 2002;46(10):2794-2803.
43. Hawkins PN, Lachmann HJ, Aganna E, McDermott MF. Spectrum of clinical features in muckle-wells syndrome and response to anakinra. *Arthritis Rheum.* 2004;50(2): 607-612.
44. Hawkins PN, Bybee A, Aganna E, McDermott MF. Response to anakinra in a de novo case of neonatal-onset multisystem inflammatory disease. *Arthritis Rheum.* 2004; 50(8):2708-2709.
45. Ramos E, Arostegui JI, Campuzano S, Rius J, Bousono C, Yague J. Positive clinical and biochemical responses to anakinra in a 3-yr-old patient with cryopyrin-associated periodic syndrome (CAPS). *Rheumatolog.* 2005;44(8): 1072-1073.
46. Milman N, Andersen CB, Hansen A, et al. Favourable effect of TNF-alpha inhibitor (infliximab) on blau syndrome in monozygotic twins with a de novo CARD15 mutation. *APMIS.* 2006;114(12):912-919.
47. Becker ML, Martin TM, Doyle TM, Rose CD. Interstitial pneumonitis in blau syndrome with documented mutation in CARD15. *Arthritis Rheum.* 2007;56(4): 1292-1294.
48. Al-Mosawi ZS, Al-Saad KK, Ijadi-Maghsoodi R, El-Shanti HI, Ferguson PJ. A splice site mutation confirms the role of LPIN2 in majeed syndrome. *Arthritis Rheum.* 2007; 56(3):960-964.

CHAPTER 62

Kawasaki Disease

Adriana H. Tremoulet and Jane C. Burns

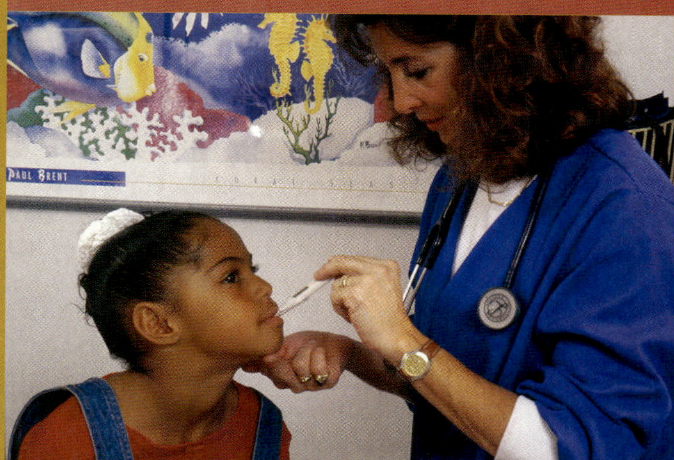

Since the original description in 1967 by Tomisaku Kawasaki of 50 children with a unique constellation of clinical signs and symptoms that did not fit any known disease, children worldwide of various racial and ethnic backgrounds have been described with Kawasaki Disease (KD).[1,2] While we have learned much about KD over the last 40 years, there is still much about this disease, including its etiology, pathogenesis, and long-term prognosis that eludes us.

KD, an acute, self-limited vasculitis, can affect children of any age. It is the most common cause of acquired heart disease in children of the developed world. KD is identified by a constellation of clinical signs and the exclusion, as appropriate, of similar appearing conditions. The case definition of KD, as outlined in the recent guidelines by the American Heart Association, is described in Table 62–1.

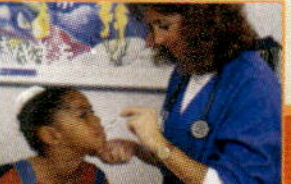

Table 62–1.

Diagnostic Clinical Criteria for KD[32]

Fever ≥ 4 days with at least four of the following:
Bilateral conjunctival injection
Mucous membrane changes: injected, fissured lips; strawberry tongue; injected pharynx
Changes of the peripheral extremities: edema or erythema of the hands and feet; periungal desquamation
Polymorphous rash
Cervical lymphadenopathy
OR
Patients with fever for ≥5 days, with <4 clinical features and echocardiographic evidence of coronary artery disease*

**Echocardiographic evidence of coronary artery disease based on the dimensions of proximal right and left anterior descending coronary arteries; Normal = Z-score ≤ 2.5 standard deviations from the mean internal diameter normalized for body surface area; Dilated = Z-score > 2.5 but < 4.0; Aneurysm = focal or diffuse dilatation of coronary artery segment with Z-score > 4.0.*

EPIDEMIOLOGY

The epidemiologic patterns of KD have been documented in multiple nationwide surveys in Japan.[3–5] During a 14-year period (1987–2000), the mean incidence of KD in Japan was 6059 cases per year.[6] The annual incidence of KD, approximately 150 per 100,000 children, younger than 5 years, is increasing steadily.

The epidemiology of KD has been less well characterized in the continental United States, where the annual incidence ranges from 9 to 45.2 cases per 100,000 children younger than 5 years.[7,8] The variation in estimates reflects the different regions and ethnic groups that have been studied. The rate of KD hospitalizations was highest in Asian/Pacific Islander children, followed by black children (39 and 19.7 cases per 100,000 children, respectively).[9] In Hawaii, where there is a large Japanese-American population, the incidence of KD in Japanese-American children is as high as 197.7 per 100,000 children younger than 5 years.[10]

GENETICS

The increased incidence in Asian/Pacific Islanders in the United States and in Japan suggests a genetic influence on KD susceptibility. In addition, researchers have described KD pedigrees with multiple affected members.[11–13] A retrospective study, evaluating 18 families found no clear pattern of inheritance, suggesting that multiple genetic polymorphisms may contribute to KD susceptibility.[14] A genome-wide linkage analysis of KD using affected sibling pairs has identified 10 regions on different chromosomes that are linked to KD susceptibility.[15]

PATHOGENESIS

While a number of infectious agents, including bacteria, viruses such as human coronavirus NL-63, and mycobacteria, have been investigated, the cause of KD remains unknown.[16,17] Seasonal peaks in winter/spring and mid-summer, as well as geographical clusters, have been noted in several countries, suggesting an infectious cause.[5,18,19] Standard microbiological methods to isolate the causative agent as well as searches for highly conserved viral and bacterial nucleic acid sequences have not revealed the etiologic agent in KD.[1,20,21] Given the similarities between KD and bacterial toxin-mediated diseases, a recent hypothesis was that bacterial superantigens could trigger the vasculitis.[22] However, further studies, including a multicenter, prospective study, did not detect a difference in the overall isolation rate of superantigen-producing bacteria between patients with KD and febrile controls.[23,24]

Activation of the immune system is a driving force in the vasculitis of KD. Levels of several proinflammatory cytokines, including tumor necrosis factor-α and interleukins 1 and 6, are elevated during the acute phase of KD.[25,26] In addition, the number of activated, circulating monocytes and macrophages increases during acute KD, and appears to be higher in patients with coronary artery lesions as compared to those without lesions.[27]

Autopsy studies have documented that $CD8^+$ T-cells, macrophages, and Immunoglobulin (Ig) A plasma cells infiltrate the wall of coronary artery aneurysms.[28,29] The IgA antibody response is oligoclonal, suggesting that the immune system is responding to a specific antigen.[30] Studies are currently underway to establish the target of these antibodies, and thus identify the etiologic agent or trigger of KD.

CLINICAL PRESENTATION

The classic definition of KD has been ≥5 days of fever and ≥4 of the 5 principal clinical features (Figure 62–1).[31] However, the recent American Heart Association Scientific Statement on KD modified this definition so that in the presence of ≥4 principal criteria, the diagnosis of KD can be made on day 4 of illness (Table 62–1).[32] In addition, patients with fever for ≥5 days, <4 principal criteria, and echocardiographic evidence of coronary artery disease also qualify as having KD.

Although none of the clinical signs of KD are pathognomonic when considered in isolation, the constellation of clinical findings makes an easily recognizable syndrome. The bilateral conjunctival injection in KD usually involves the bulbar conjunctivae, sparing the limbus (less vascular area around the iris) (Figure 62–1A). There is usually no exudate or corneal ulceration and biopsy studies have documented the absence of inflammation. Thus, the term "conjunctivitis" is a misnomer in this disease. A slit lamp examination may reveal mild anterior uveitis if performed during the first week of illness and prior to treatment.[33] The mucous membrane changes include (1) dry, cracked, fissured lips, (2) a "strawberry tongue" (identical to what is found in toxin-mediated streptococcal or staphylococcal infection), and (3) an injected pharynx without exudate (Figures 62–1B to 62–1C). The palms and soles may be diffusely erythematous, and the dorsum of the hands and feet may be edematous (Figures 62–1D to 62–1E). Between 2 and 3 weeks after the onset of fever, peeling may occur, beginning in a periungal distribution (Figure 62–1F). The rash of KD usually presents as a diffuse maculopapular rash which is accentuated in the perineal region in 50% of patients (Figures 62–1E, 62–1G, and 62–1H). Although the rash can take many forms, including urticarial or micropustular, it has never been described as bullous or vesicular. The least commonly fulfilled principal criterion is cervical lymphadenopathy. This is classically a unilateral mass measuring >1.5 cm in diameter, with or without overlying erythema. As compared to bacterial lymphadenitis, which presents as a solitary node with a hypoechogenic center on imaging studies, the lymphadenopathy of KD involves a grape-like cluster of multiple nodes.[34]

DIFFERENTIAL DIAGNOSIS

Not all the clinical features of KD may be present at a single point in time. Thus, the differential diagnosis of KD can be separated into different categories, depending on the number of criteria present (Figure 62–2). A delayed diagnosis often occurs when a child presents with fewer principal criteria, a common occurrence in the infant <6 months of age.[35,36] Errors in the diagnosis of KD can occur in the following settings: (1) the infant with sterile pyuria is thought to have pyelonephritis, (2) the infant with CSF pleocytosis and a rash is thought to have viral meningitis, (3) the older child with unilateral lymphadenopathy is thought to have bacterial lymphadenitis and the subsequent appearance of the rash is thought to be an allergic reaction to the antibiotics, and (4) the older child with rash and strawberry tongue is thought to have scarlet fever despite negative cultures for group A β-hemolytic *Streptococcus*.

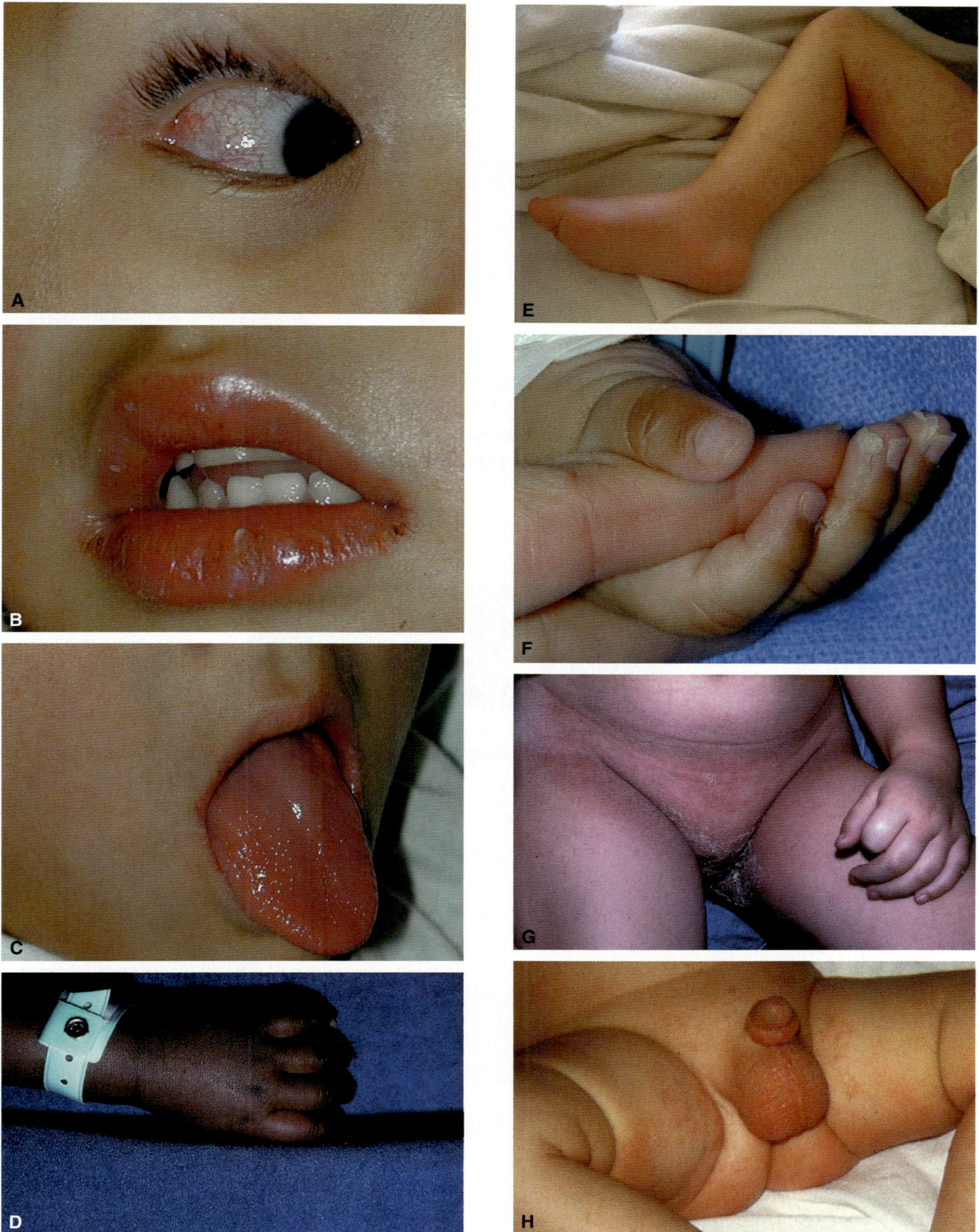

FIGURE 62–1 ■ Clinical Features of KD. **(A)** Conjunctival injection with limbal sparing and without exudate; **(B)** Dry, cracked lips; **(C)** "Strawberry tongue," an erythematous tongue with raised papillae; **(D)** Swelling of the hand's dorsum with dimpling at the base of each digit; Erythema over the proximal interphalangeal joints may be more subtle in the dark skinned patient; **(E)** Diffuse erythema of the sole of the foot that abruptly ends at the ankle; Maculopapular rash on the leg; **(F)** Peeling of the hands that starts in the periungal area can occur 2–3 weeks after the onset of fever; **(G)** Accentuation of the rash in the perineal area which can include some fine peeling; **(H)** Accentuation of the rash in the perineal area which can include inflammation of the urethral meatus.

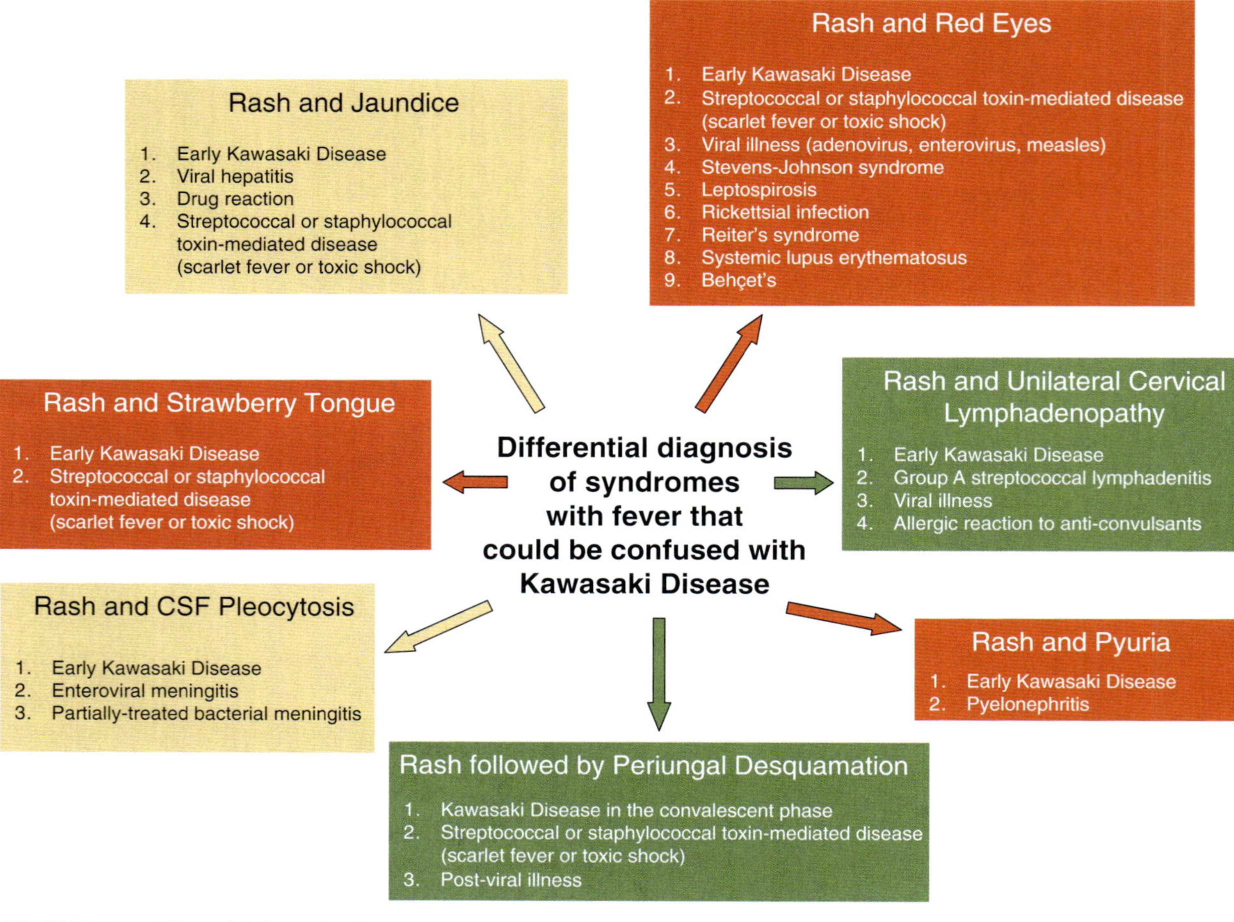

Rash and Jaundice
1. Early Kawasaki Disease
2. Viral hepatitis
3. Drug reaction
4. Streptococcal or staphylococcal toxin-mediated disease (scarlet fever or toxic shock)
Rash and Red Eyes
1. Early Kawasaki Disease
2. Streptococcal or staphylococcal toxin-mediated disease (scarlet fever or toxic shock)
3. Viral illness (adenovirus, enterovirus, measles)
4. Stevens-Johnson syndrome
5. Leptospirosis
6. Rickettsial infection
7. Reiter's syndrome
8. Systemic lupus erythematosus
9. Behçet's
Rash and Strawberry Tongue
1. Early Kawasaki Disease
2. Streptococcal or staphylococcal toxin-mediated disease (scarlet fever or toxic shock)
Differential diagnosis of syndromes with fever that could be confused with Kawasaki Disease
Rash and Unilateral Cervical Lymphadenopathy
1. Early Kawasaki Disease
2. Group A streptococcal lymphadenitis
3. Viral illness
4. Allergic reaction to anti-convulsants
Rash and CSF Pleocytosis
1. Early Kawasaki Disease
2. Enteroviral meningitis
3. Partially-treated bacterial meningitis
Rash and Pyuria
1. Early Kawasaki Disease
2. Pyelonephritis
Rash followed by Periungal Desquamation
1. Kawasaki Disease in the convalescent phase
2. Streptococcal or staphylococcal toxin-mediated disease (scarlet fever or toxic shock)
3. Post-viral illness

FIGURE 62–2 ■ Differential diagnosis of KD.
The differential diagnosis of syndromes with fever that could be confused with KD can be separated by the presence or absence of specific clinical features.

DIAGNOSIS

As there is no definitive diagnostic test for KD, a thorough history, including duration of fever as well as presence of any of the clinical signs that may have already resolved, are central to making the diagnosis. The algorithm for the diagnosis of KD includes a high index of clinical suspicion as well as laboratory testing and an echocardiogram (Figure 62–3). Laboratory studies that can be helpful in establishing the diagnosis are listed in Table 62–2. The new guidelines from the American Heart Association encourage the use of laboratory studies as an adjunct to making the diagnosis of KD. In a study comparing KD patients with febrile controls who were referred for evaluation of possible KD, the KD patients were more likely to be anemic, have a higher ESR, and have an elevated ALT (Figure 62–4).[37] Although infants younger than 6 months may present with fewer clinical signs of KD, they usually have a higher white blood cell count and higher platelet count than older children.[38]

Approximately one-third of KD patients who undergo lumbar puncture prior to intravenous immunoglobulin (IVIG) infusion will have cerebrospinal fluid pleocytosis (median, 22.5 cells/μl) with mononuclear cell predominance (median, 91.5%) and a normal glucose and protein.[39]

If there is doubt about the diagnosis of KD, consultation with an ophthalmologist during the first week of fever may be helpful to look for anterior uveitis by a slit lamp examination; this condition is present in up to 85% of children with KD. In addition, consultation with a rheumatologist or an infectious disease specialist may be necessary to identify another source of the fever.

Some patients do not fulfill the clinical criteria for the diagnosis of KD, but have had ≥5 days of fever with only 2 or 3 of the clinical signs. These children may have "incomplete KD" and are still at risk for the cardiovascular complications. Incomplete KD is more common in the infant younger than 6 months of age,

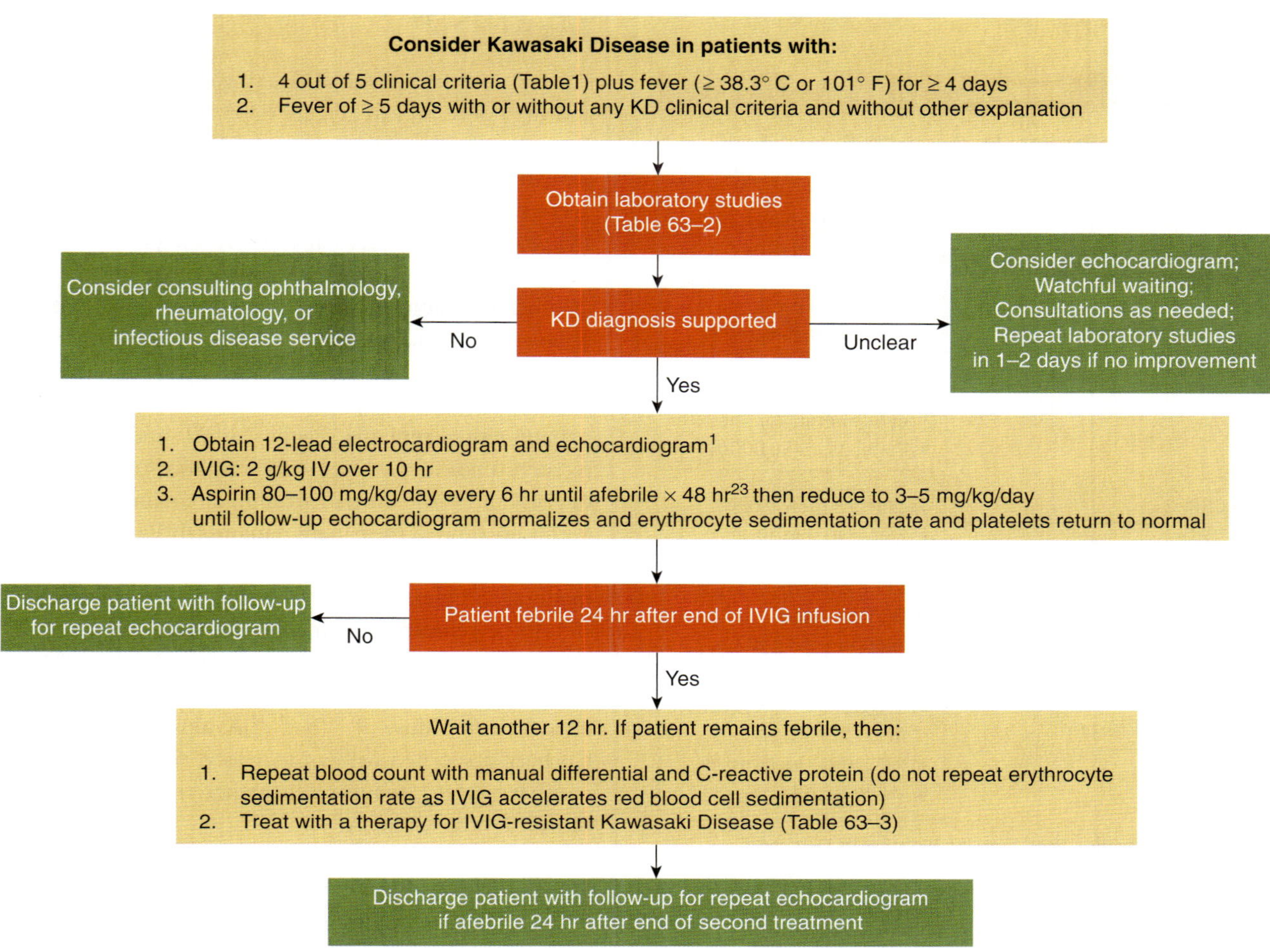
Consider Kawasaki Disease in patients with:
1. 4 out of 5 clinical criteria (Table1) plus fever (≥ 38.3° C or 101° F) for ≥ 4 days
2. Fever of ≥ 5 days with or without any KD clinical criteria and without other explanation
Obtain laboratory studies (Table 63–2)
KD diagnosis supported
No
Consider consulting ophthalmology, rheumatology, or infectious disease service
Unclear
Consider echocardiogram; Watchful waiting; Consultations as needed; Repeat laboratory studies in 1–2 days if no improvement
Yes
1. Obtain 12-lead electrocardiogram and echocardiogram¹
2. IVIG: 2 g/kg IV over 10 hr
3. Aspirin 80–100 mg/kg/day every 6 hr until afebrile × 48 hr²³ then reduce to 3–5 mg/kg/day until follow-up echocardiogram normalizes and erythrocyte sedimentation rate and platelets return to normal
Patient febrile 24 hr after end of IVIG infusion
No
Discharge patient with follow-up for repeat echocardiogram
Yes
Wait another 12 hr. If patient remains febrile, then:
1. Repeat blood count with manual differential and C-reactive protein (do not repeat erythrocyte sedimentation rate as IVIG accelerates red blood cell sedimentation)
2. Treat with a therapy for IVIG-resistant Kawasaki Disease (Table 63–3)
Discharge patient with follow-up for repeat echocardiogram if afebrile 24 hr after end of second treatment

FIGURE 62–3 ■ Algorithm for the diagnosis and treatment of a patient with suspected KD.
[1]Echocardiographic evidence of coronary artery disease based on the dimensions of proximal right and left anterior descending coronary arteries; Normal = Z-score = 2.5 standard deviations from the mean internal diameter normalized for body surface area; Dilated = *Z*-score > 2.5 but < 4.0; Aneurysm = focal or diffuse dilatation of coronary artery segment with *Z*-score > 4.0.
[2]Day 1 of illness = first day of fever.
[3]For high dose aspirin, round off dose to nearest one-half baby aspirin tablet (81 mg). IV, intravenous; kg, kilograms; mg, milligrams; g, grams.

which can delay treatment in this group that is at high risk for coronary artery abnormalities.[38,40] In such patients, laboratory studies and echocardiography can be helpful in making the diagnosis of KD. A recent study documented that patients at the extremes of the pediatric age range (patients younger than 6 months and older than 8 years) may be misdiagnosed because of lack of awareness of the occurrence of KD in these age groups.[36]

An echocardiogram with choral hydrate sedation as appropriate (80–100 mg/kg orally up to 1 g) should be obtained in all patients with confirmed or suspected KD. Measurements of the internal luminal diameter of the coronary arteries should be expressed in standard deviation units (*Z*-score) for the proximal right coronary artery and the left anterior descending coronary artery.[41] A normal *Z*-score is ≤2.5 standard deviations from the mean internal diameter normalized for body surface area. A dilated right coronary artery or left anterior descending coronary artery has a *Z*-score >2.5 but <4.0, while an aneurysm has a *Z*-score >4.0 (Figure 62–5). In a retrospective study, 15.3% of patients had coronary artery dilatation based on measurements normalized for body surface area on the initial echocardiogram.[41] Delayed diagnosis results in an increased incidence of coronary artery abnormalities.[42] In another retrospective study, patients with incomplete KD were treated significantly later (median, 10 days) and had a significantly higher occurrence of coronary artery aneurysms (37%) than those

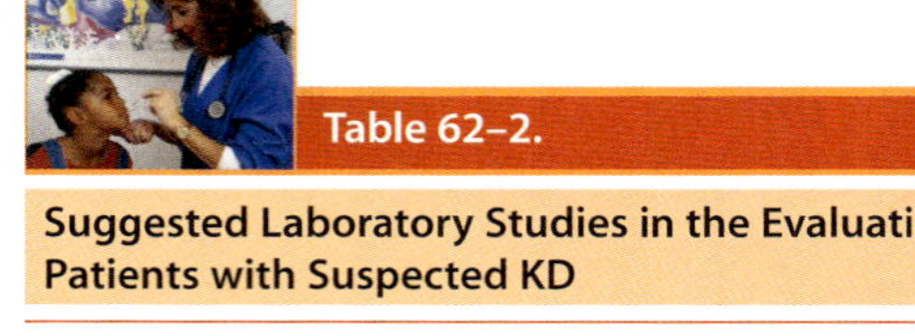

Table 62–2.

Suggested Laboratory Studies in the Evaluation of Patients with Suspected KD

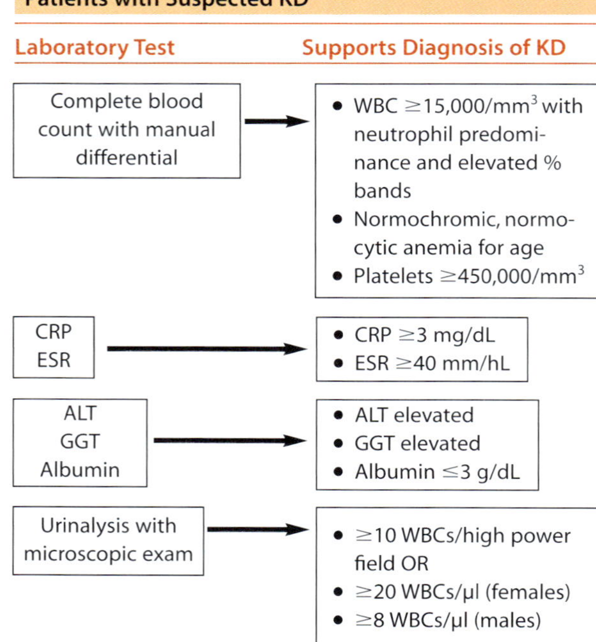

Laboratory Test	Supports Diagnosis of KD
Complete blood count with manual differential	• WBC ≥15,000/mm^3 with neutrophil predominance and elevated % bands • Normochromic, normocytic anemia for age • Platelets ≥450,000/mm^3
CRP ESR	• CRP ≥3 mg/dL • ESR ≥40 mm/hL
ALT GGT Albumin	• ALT elevated • GGT elevated • Albumin ≤3 g/dL
Urinalysis with microscopic exam	• ≥10 WBCs/high power field OR • ≥20 WBCs/µl (females) • ≥8 WBCs/µl (males)

Ancillary Studies that May be Helpful in Selected Patients with Suspected KD

1. Blood culture & lumbar puncture if patient is <6 months or presentation suggests meningitis. KD associated with increased CSF WBC count with normal CSF protein level.
2. Direct fluorescent antibody test or viral culture for adenovirus
3. Polymerase chain reaction (PCR) on plasma and/or CSF for enterovirus
4. Throat culture or rapid streptococcal antigen test
5. Streptococcal serology: anti-streptolysin O or anti-Dnase B*
6. Epstein Barr virus serology if hepatomegaly, splenomegaly, or generalized lymphadenopathy present
7. Plasma titers for bartonella henselae
8. Purified protein derivative test (PPD)†

**A single elevated titer does not exclude KD as polyclonal B cell activation is associated with KD and could result in an elevated titer. Serology should be performed by neutralization test as other methods are unreliable.*

†Children with KD are commonly anergic.

WBC, white blood cell; CRP, C-reactive protein; ESR, erythrocyte sedimentation rate; ALT, alanine aminotransferase; GGT, γ-glutamyl transferase; CSF, cerebrospinal fluid.

with complete KD, who were treated at a median of 7 days ($p < 0.001$) and had a 12% aneurysm rate ($p = 0.009$).[43] A pediatric cardiologist should be consulted for any child with significant abnormalities on the echocardiogram. A 12-lead electrocardiogram should be performed as a baseline study.

TREATMENT

The first-line therapy for KD is a single 2 g/kg dose of IVIG and high dose aspirin (Figure 62–3 and Table 62–3).[44,45] Treatment with a single dose of IVIG and high-dose aspirin results in resolution of fever and a significant decrease in the rate of coronary artery aneurysms (from 18% to 4% seven weeks after initial diagnosis) in most cases. Although corticosteroids are the treatment of choice in other vasculitides, a recent multicenter, randomized, double-blind, placebo-controlled trial by Newburger et al. failed to demonstrate any benefit of intravenous methylprednisolone in the primary treatment of KD.[46] If a patient either remains febrile for 24 hours or has a recrudescence of the fever within 24 hours of the end of the IVIG infusion, the patient should remain hospitalized for observation. If the patient remains febrile over the next 12 hours, laboratory examinations to evaluate for inflammation (complete blood counts and C-reactive protein) should be repeated and therapy for IVIG-resistant KD should be given (Table 62–3). Between 10% and 20% of children with KD have persistent or recrudescent fever after their first dose of IVIG.[47,48] As this IVIG resistance has been associated with an increased risk of developing coronary artery aneurysms, further treatment is warranted in these patients.[49]

No clinical trials have established the optimal therapy for IVIG-resistant patients. Retreatment with IVIG has been shown to be safe and is frequently used to treat IVIG-resistant patients.[50] As not all patients remain afebrile after a second dose of IVIG, several other therapies have been evaluated in such IVIG-resistant cases. Since the serum levels of the proinflammatory cytokine tumor necrosis factor-α are elevated in acute patients with KD, a retrospective case review was recently conducted to evaluate the role of infliximab, a chimeric murine/human tumor necrosis factor a-specific monoclonal antibody, in patients who fail to become afebrile after their first dose of IVIG.[51] In the published experience to date, there have been no infusion reactions or complications attributed to infliximab administration in this patient population. Corticosteroids have also been used to treat patients who remain febrile after initial IVIG therapy. A small randomized Japanese study comparing the efficacy and safety of pulse steroid therapy with a second dose of IVIG showed that patients in the steroid group had a shorter duration of fever.[52] However, there was no significant difference in the incidence of coronary artery aneurysms. Plasmapheresis has also been used in IVIG-resistant patients, presumably to remove proinflammatory cytokines.[53]

The mortality of individuals with a history of KD was evaluated in Japan by comparing the survival of more than 6500 patients to healthy age-matched

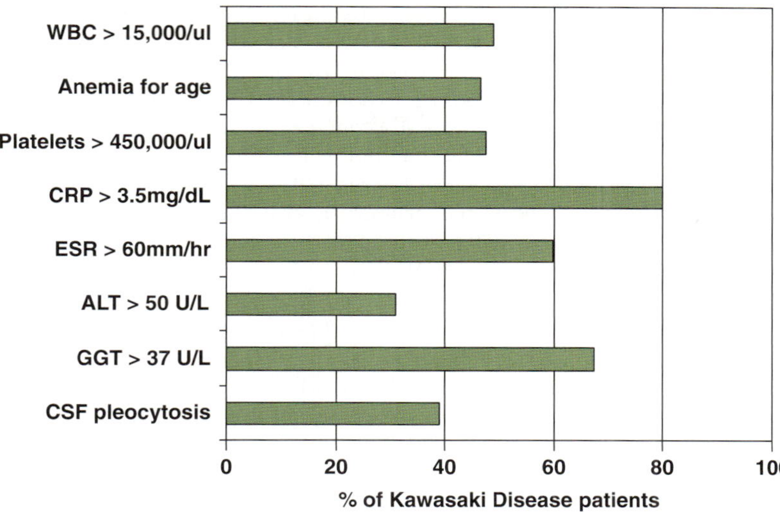

FIGURE 62–4 ■ Laboratory abnormalities in acute KD. (These data are based on studies of KD patients presenting within the first ten days after onset of fever.[37,39,55])

controls.[54] In the first 2 months after the diagnosis of KD, the ratio of the observed number of deaths in KD patients to the expected number of deaths was elevated (8.2). After the acute phase, the mortality ratio was elevated only in males with cardiac sequelae.

SUMMARY

KD is a clinical diagnosis supported by laboratory results that reflect severe inflammation. As KD can present without all of its clinical features, it is important for the clinician to keep a high index of suspicion for this disease in a child of any age who presents with fever without a source. This is especially true for the infant younger than 6 months. Only through heightened awareness of KD can we hope to reduce the rate of coronary artery sequelae in these children.

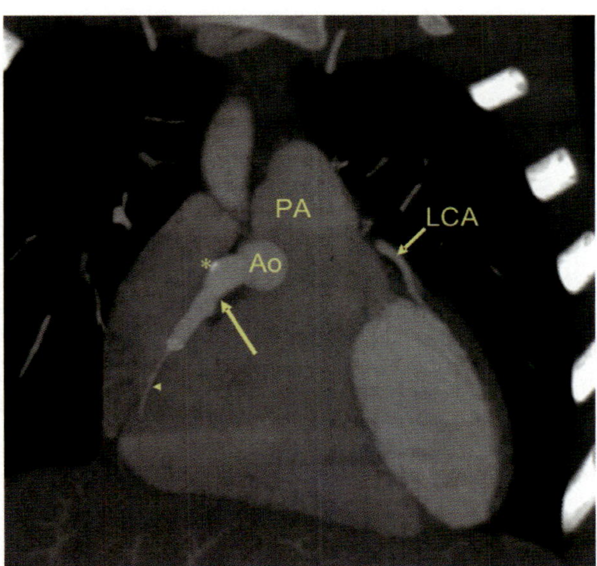

FIGURE 62–5 ■ Computerized tomography of aneurysms in a KD patient.

This is a 64-slice Computerized tomography angiogram of the coronary arteries in a 12-year-old patient, 11 years after KD. Note the dilated right coronary artery with fusiform aneurysms (arrow) in comparison to normal, nondilated coronary artery (arrow head). There is calcification noted in the proximal aneurysm (star).

[2]Ao, aorta; PA, pulmonary artery; LCA, left coronary artery.

Acknowledgments

The authors thank Dr. Jeffrey Frazer for his contribution of the computerized tomography angiogram and Dr. John Kanegaye for clinical photographs.

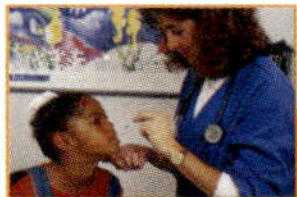

Table 62–3.

Treatment for Kawasaki disease

Initial Therapy for KD
IVIG 2 g/kg IV over 10 h
Aspirin 80–100 mg/kg/d every 6 h through illness day 14*,†
Therapy for IVIG-resistant KD
Repeat IVIG dose at 2 g/kg
If fever persists, consider one of the following therapies:
Infliximab 5 mg/kg
Repeat IVIG at 2 g/kg
Methylpredinisolone IV 30 mg/kg/d × 1–3 doses; consider oral prednisone 2 mg/kg with slow taper
Plasmapheresis

**Day 1 of illness = 1st day of fever.*

†Practices regarding the duration of aspirin vary by institution, and many centers reduce the dose of aspirin after the child has been afebrile for 48–72 h[32]

REFERENCES

1. Kawasaki T. Acute febrile mucocutaneous syndrome with lymphoid involvement with specific desquamation of the fingers and toes in children. *Arerugi.* 1967;16(3):178-222.
2. Kawasaki T. Acute febrile mucocutaneous syndrome with lymphoid involvement with specific desquamation of the fingers and toes in children: my clinical observation of fifty cases. *Pediatr Infect Dis J.* 2002;21(11):1-38.
3. Yanagawa H, Nakamura Y, Yashiro M, et al. Results of the nationwide epidemiologic survey of kawasaki disease in 1995 and 1996 in Japan. *Pediatrics.* 1998;102(6):E65.
4. Yanagawa H, Yashiro M, Nakamura Y, Kawasaki T, Kato H. Epidemiologic pictures of kawasaki disease in japan: from the nationwide incidence survey in 1991 and 1992. *Pediatrics.* 1995;95(4):475-479.
5. Yanagawa H, Nakamura Y, Yashiro M, Uehara R, Oki I, Kayaba K. Incidence of kawasaki disease in Japan: the nationwide surveys of 1999-2002. *Pediatr Int.* 2006;48(4):356-361.
6. Burns JC, Cayan DR, Tong G, et al. Seasonality and temporal clustering of kawasaki syndrome. *Epidemiology.* 2005;16(2):220-225.
7. Belay ED, Holman RC, Clarke MJ, et al. The incidence of kawasaki syndrome in west Coast health maintenance organizations. *Pediatr Infect Dis J.* 2000;19(9):828-832.
8. Kao AS, Getis A, Brodine S, Burns JC. Spatial and temporal clustering of kawasaki syndrome cases. *Pediatr Infect Dis J.* (In Press).
9. Holman RC, Curns AT, Belay ED, Steiner CA, Schonberger LB. Kawasaki syndrome hospitalizations in the united states, 1997 and 2000. *Pediatrics.* 2003;112(3, pt. 1):495-501.
10. Holman RC, Curns AT, Belay ED, et al. Kawasaki syndrome in hawaii. *Pediatr Infect Dis J.* 2005;24(5):429-433.
11. Matsubara T, Furukawa S, Ino T, Tsuji A, Park I, Yabuta K. A sibship with recurrent kawasaki disease and coronary artery lesion. *Acta Paediatr.* 1994;83(9):1002-1004.
12. Mori M, Miyamae T, Kurosawa R, Yokota S, Onoki H. Two-generation kawasaki disease: mother and daughter. *J Pediatr.* 2001;139(5):754-756.
13. Uehara R, Yashiro M, Nakamura Y, Yanagawa H. Clinical features of patients with kawasaki disease whose parents had the same disease. *Arch Pediatr Adolesc Med.* 2004;158(12):1166-1169.
14. Dergun M, Kao A, Hauger SB, Newburger JW, Burns JC. Familial occurrence of kawasaki syndrome in north america. *Arch Pediatr Adolesc Med.* 2005;159(9):876-881.
15. Onouchi Y, Tamari M, Takahashi A, et al. A genomewide linkage analysis of kawasaki disease: evidence for linkage to chromosome 12. *J Hum Genet.* 2007;52(2):179-190.
16. Shimizu C, Shike H, Baker SC, et al. Human coronavirus NL63 is not detected in the respiratory tracts of children with acute kawasaki disease. *J Infect Dis.* 2005;192(10):1767-1771.
17. Dominguez SR, Anderson MS, Glode MP, Robinson CC, Holmes KV. Blinded case-control study of the relationship between human coronavirus NL63 and kawasaki syndrome. *J Infect Dis.* 2006;194(12):1697-1701.
18. Chang RK. Hospitalizations for kawasaki disease among children in the united states, 1988-1997. *Pediatrics.* 2002;109(6):e87.
19. Huang GY, Ma XJ, Huang M, et al. Epidemiologic pictures of kawasaki disease in shanghai from 1998 through 2002. *J Epidemiol.* 2006;16(1):9-14.
20. Chua PK, Nerurkar VR, Yu Q, Woodward CL, Melish ME, Yanagihara R. Lack of association between kawasaki syndrome and infection with parvovirus B19, human herpesvirus 8, TT virus, GB virus C/hepatitis G virus or chlamydia pneumoniae. *Pediatr Infect Dis J.* 2000;19(5):477-479.
21. Rowley AH, Wolinsky SM, Relman DA, et al. Search for highly conserved viral and bacterial nucleic acid sequences corresponding to an etiologic agent of kawasaki disease. *Pediatr Res.* 1994;36(5):567-571.
22. Meissner HC, Leung DY. Superantigens, conventional antigens and the etiology of kawasaki syndrome. *Pediatr Infect Dis J.* 2000;19(2):91-94.
23. Leung DY, Meissner HC, Shulman ST, et al. Prevalence of superantigen-secreting bacteria in patients with kawasaki disease. *J Pediatr.* 2002;140(6):742-746.
24. Terai M, Miwa K, Williams T, et al. The absence of evidence of staphylococcal toxin involvement in the pathogenesis of kawasaki disease. *J Infect Dis.* 1995;172(2):558-561.
25. Furukawa S, Matsubara T, Yone K, Hirano Y, Okumura K, Yabuta K. Kawasaki disease differs from anaphylactoid purpura and measles with regard to tumour necrosis factor-alpha and interleukin 6 in serum. *Eur J Pediatr.* 1992;151(1):44-47.
26. Maury CP, Salo E, Pelkonen P. Circulating interleukin-1 beta in patients with kawasaki disease. *N Engl J Med.* 1988;319(25):1670-1671.
27. Furukawa S, Matsubara T, Yabuta K. Mononuclear cell subsets and coronary artery lesions in kawasaki disease. *Arch Dis Child.* 1992;67(6):706-708.
28. Brown TJ, Crawford SE, Cornwall ML, Garcia F, Shulman ST, Rowley AH. CD8 T lymphocytes and macrophages infiltrate coronary artery aneurysms in acute kawasaki disease. *J Infect Dis.* 2001;184(7):940-943.
29. Rowley AH, Eckerley CA, Jack HM, Shulman ST, Baker SC. IgA plasma cells in vascular tissue of patients with kawasaki syndrome. *J Immunol.* 1997;159(12):5946-5955.
30. Rowley AH, Shulman ST, Spike BT, Mask CA, Baker SC. Oligoclonal IgA response in the vascular wall in acute kawasaki disease. *J Immunol.* 2001;166(2):1334-1343.
31. Dajani AS, Taubert KA, Gerber MA, et al. Diagnosis and therapy of kawasaki disease in children. *Circulation.* 1993;87(5):1776-1780.
32. Newburger JW, Takahashi M, Gerber MA, et al. Diagnosis, treatment, and long-term management of kawasaki disease: a statement for health professionals from the committee on rheumatic fever, endocarditis and kawasaki disease, council on cardiovascular disease in the young, american heart association. *Circulation.* 2004;110(17): 2747-2771.
33. Burns JC, Joffe L, Sargent RA, Glode MP. Anterior uveitis associated with kawasaki syndrome. *Pediatr Infect. Dis* 1985;4(3):258-261.
34. Tashiro N, Matsubara T, Uchida M, Katayama K, Ichiyama T, Furukawa S. Ultrasonographic evaluation of cervical lymph nodes in kawasaki disease. *Pediatrics.* 2002;109(5):E77-77.
35. Anderson MS, Todd JK, Glode MP. Delayed diagnosis of kawasaki syndrome: an analysis of the problem. *Pediatrics.* 2005;115(4):e428-e433.

36. Pannaraj PS, Turner CL, Bastian JF, Burns JC. Failure to diagnose kawasaki disease at the extremes of the pediatric age range. *Pediatr Infect Dis J.* 2004;23(8):789-791.
37. Burns JC, Mason WH, Glode MP, et al. Clinical and epidemiologic characteristics of patients referred for evaluation of possible kawasaki disease. United states multicenter kawasaki disease study group. *J Pediatr.* 1991; 118(5):680-686.
38. Chang FY, Hwang B, Chen SJ, Lee PC, Meng CC, Lu JH. Characteristics of kawasaki disease in infants younger than six months of age. *Pediatr Infect Dis J.* 2006;25(3): 241-244.
39. Dengler LD, Capparelli EV, Bastian JF, et al. Cerebrospinal fluid profile in patients with acute kawasaki disease. *Pediatr Infect Dis J.* 1998;17(6):478-481.
40. Burns JC, Wiggins JW, Jr., Toews WH, et al. Clinical spectrum of kawasaki disease in infants younger than 6 months of age. *J Pediatr.* 1986;109(5):759-763.
41. de Zorzi A, Colan SD, Gauvreau K, Baker AL, Sundel RP, Newburger JW. Coronary artery dimensions may be misclassified as normal in kawasaki disease. *J Pediatr.* 1998;133(2):254-258.
42. Wilder M, Palinkas L, Kao A, Bastian J, Turner C, Burns J. Delayed diagnosis by physicians contributes to the development of coronary artery aneurysms in children with kawasaki syndrome. *Pediatr Infect Dis J.* 2007;26(3): 256-260.
43. Baer AZ, Rubin LG, Shapiro CA, et al. Prevalence of coronary artery lesions on the initial echocardiogram in kawasaki syndrome. *Arch Pediatr Adolesc Med.* 2006; 160(7):686-690.
44. Newburger JW, Takahashi M, Burns JC, et al. The treatment of kawasaki syndrome with intravenous gamma globulin. *N Engl J Med.* 1986;315(6):341-347.
45. Newburger JW, Takahashi M, Beiser AS, et al. A single intravenous infusion of gamma globulin as compared with four infusions in the treatment of acute kawasaki syndrome. *N Engl J Med.* 1991;324(23):1633-1639.
46. Newburger JW, Sleeper LA, McCrindle BW, et al. Randomized trial of pulsed corticosteroid therapy for primary treatment of kawasaki disease. *N Engl J Med.* 2007;356(7): 663-675.
47. Durongpisitkul K, Soongswang J, Laohaprasitiporn D, Nana A, Prachuabmoh C, Kangkagate C. Immunoglobulin failure and retreatment in kawasaki disease. *Pediatr Cardiol.* 2003;24(2):145-148.
48. Han RK, Silverman ED, Newman A, McCrindle BW. Management and outcome of persistent or recurrent fever after initial intravenous gamma globulin therapy in acute kawasaki disease. *Arch Pediatr Adolesc Med.* 2000;154(7): 694-699.
49. Burns JC, Capparelli EV, Brown JA, Newburger JW, Glode MP. Intravenous gamma-globulin treatment and retreatment in kawasaki disease. US/Canadian kawasaki syndrome study group. *Pediatr Infect Dis J.* 1998;17(12): 1144-1148.
50. Chiyonobu T, Yoshihara T, Mori K, et al. Early intravenous gamma globulin retreatment for refractory kawasaki disease. *Clin Pediatr (Phila).* 2003;42(3):269-272.
51. Burns JC, Mason WH, Hauger SB, et al. Infliximab treatment for refractory kawasaki syndrome. *J Pediatr.* 2005; 146(5):662-667.
52. Hashino K, Ishii M, Iemura M, Akagi T, Kato H. Retreatment for immune globulin-resistant kawasaki disease: a comparative study of additional immune globulin and steroid pulse therapy. *Pediatr Int.* 2001;43(3): 211-217.
53. Mori M, Imagawa T, Katakura S, et al. Efficacy of plasma exchange therapy for kawasaki disease intractable to intravenous gamma-globulin. *Mod Rheumatol.* 2004;14(1):43-47.
54. Nakamura Y, Aso E, Yashiro M, et al. Mortality among persons with a history of kawasaki disease in Japan: can paediatricians safely discontinue follow-up of children with a history of the disease but without cardiac sequelae? *Acta Paediatr.* 2005;94(4):429-434.
55. Ting EC, Capparelli EV, Billman GF, Lavine JE, Matsubara T, Burns JC. Elevated gamma-glutamyltransferase concentrations in patients with acute kawasaki disease. *Pediatr Infect Dis J.* 1998;17(5):431-432.

CHAPTER 63

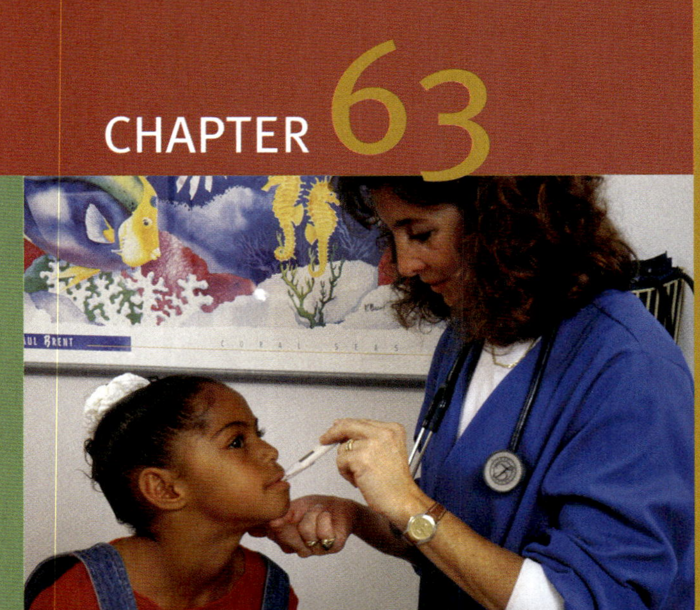

Mononucleosis Syndromes

Beth C. Marshall and William C. Koch

DEFINITION AND EPIDEMIOLOGY

Infectious mononucleosis is a clinical syndrome classically defined by the presence of fever, lymphadenopathy, pharyngitis, and fatigue. The illness was first recognized in the late 19th century and termed "glandular fever" or "Drusenfieber" by German physicians who noted its frequent occurrence in the context of family outbreaks.[1,2] In a 1920 Johns Hopkins Medical Bulletin, Sprunt and Evans described 6 previously healthy young adults with a febrile illness similar to glandular fever, and noted the presence of atypical lymphocytes in the peripheral blood smear; because of the predominance of these unusual mononuclear cells, they termed the syndrome "infectious mononucleosis."[3] Twelve years later while investigating rheumatic disease, Paul and Bunnell[4] serendipitously noted that the serum of patients with symptoms of infectious mononucleosis contained high titers of antibodies that agglutinated sheep red blood cells, thus the detection of these "heterophile antibodies" became the first laboratory marker available to diagnose the illness. The association of Epstein-Barr virus (EBV) with infectious mononucleosis followed in the late 1960s when a laboratory technician working with specimens from patients with Burkitt's lymphoma, a condition which had recently been shown to be associated with EBV, accidentally became infected and developed clinical infectious mononucleosis.[5,6]

We now know that the majority of patients with infectious mononucleosis have an acute EBV infection; the symptoms are caused by another infectious agent in up to 10% of patients. This chapter will concentrate on EBV, the major infectious cause, but other important diagnostic considerations will also be addressed.

More than 95% of adults worldwide are EBV-seropositive.[7,8] In lower socioeconomic classes and in underdeveloped countries, most children acquire the infection before the age of 5.[9] Fewer than 10% of children younger than the age of 4, develop clinically apparent symptoms of EBV infection.[10] This parallels the epidemiology of several of the other differential etiologies of infectious mononucleosis, including cytomegalovirus (CMV) and hepatitis A infections. Therefore, patients who present with symptomatic infectious mononucleosis are most often older children, adolescents, and young adults of middle to upper socioeconomic status.[11]

EBV is transmitted primarily by direct contact with oral secretions. Transmission via aerosol or fomites is uncommon given the virus' poor ability to survive outside host body fluids. The incubation period, during which the virus may be communicated but the patient is asymptomatic, is approximately 4–6 weeks.[12] Epidemics of viral spread have not been reported, suggesting fairly low transmission rates, and no seasonal predominance has been identified. Transmission by blood product transfusion has occasionally been documented. Additionally, the presence of the virus in cervical secretions suggests that sexual transmission may also occur. As is characteristic of the other members of the herpesvirus family, EBV exhibits the property of latency in the host, so that those who have been previously infected, often continue to intermittently shed virus, further contributing to the transmission of EBV. Immunosuppression in the host from any etiology will increase viral shedding in secretions.

PATHOGENESIS

After the initial infection and replication in oropharyngeal epithelial cells, EBV exhibits a predilection for B cells, which upon infection, have the potential for subsequent unlimited proliferation. Large numbers of these infected B cells circulate during the first few days of illness; these cells resemble plasma cells and produce large quantities of nonspecific antibodies, including the heterophile antibodies. The host immune response to this massive B-cell proliferation is to mount a counter suppressive T cell response, many of which are reactive and appear atypical, hence the atypical lymphocytosis seen on peripheral smear. This cellular (T cell) immune response is crucial to limiting EBV replication and EBV-induced B-cell proliferation; accordingly, the most severe disease manifestations occur in individuals with impaired cellular immunity.[13]

Both infected and reactive lymphocytes infiltrate the entire reticuloendothelial system, including the liver, spleen, and lymph nodes, which accounts for the enlargement of these organs on physical examination. Massive cytokine production and release by reactive T lymphocytes result in fever and the profound fatigue associated with acute infectious mononucleosis.[13] Additionally, the large quantities of antibodies produced by infected B cells, some of which have been shown to be autoantibodies, are believed to account for some of the other diverse manifestations of infectious mononucleosis, including hematologic abnormalities such as hemolytic anemia, thrombocytopenia, and neutropenia.[14]

CLINICAL PRESENTATION

Common Manifestations

Most young children (toddlers and preschool aged) who become infected with EBV exhibit no or few nonspecific viral symptoms. Quite often, the acute illness mimics a viral upper respiratory infection with cough, rhinitis, and mild fever. For older children and adolescents, acute EBV infection is heralded by an initial prodrome, lasting up to 1 week, that consists of nonspecific constitutional symptoms including fatigue, malaise, anorexia, and headache. These symptoms usually increase in intensity as the classic triad of fever, pharyngitis and lymphadenopathy emerges as a prominent feature in more than 50% of adolescents and adults with infectious mononucleosis. The most common symptoms associated with infectious mononucleosis are presented in Table 63–1.

Less Common Manifestations

A number of multisystem clinical signs and symptoms are manifested by a smaller number of patients. Children of all ages may complain of rhinitis, mild cough or periorbital edema, the latter of which may have resolved prior to presentation. Some patients may report diffuse vague abdominal pain, and a few may even demonstrate localized left upper quadrant pain that may occur with significant splenic enlargement. Splenomegaly can be detected on physical examination in approximately half of all patients with acute infectious mononucleosis. In such cases, the spleen is rarely palpable more than 3 cm below the left costal margin; massive splenomegaly is rare.

A few patients may present with a rash during the acute symptomatic of infectious mononucleosis. This rash is highly variable in appearance and may be maculopapular, scarlatinaform, urticarial, or erythema multiforme; it is more common in older children.[15] A minority of patients may present with symptoms of hepatitis including jaundice and right upper quadrant abdominal pain or with other gastrointestinal complaints, including anorexia and nausea. In males, unilateral orchitis may be an initial complaint suggesting acute EBV infection.

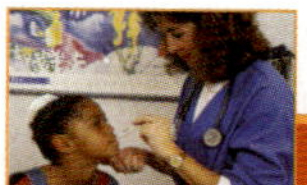

Table 63–1.

Frequency of Presenting Signs and Symptoms of Infectious Mononucleosis*

Study	Frequency (%) Maeda et al.[29]	Glade et al.[30]	Finch et al.[31]
Lymphadenopathy	100	100	94–95
Fever	98	80–95	92–100
Malaise/fatigue		90–100	
Pharyngitis	85	80–85	
Splenomegaly	75	50–60	53–82
Headache		40–70	
Cough		30–50	15–51
Periorbital edema	33	25–40	14
Hepatomegaly		15–25	30–63
Rhinitis		10–25	
Rash	3	3–6	17–34

Data compiled from References 29, 30, and 31.

Physical Examination

Almost 95% of children with acute EBV infection demonstrate nontender lymphadenopathy. The adenopathy is most often confined to the anterior and posterior cervical chains, but is occasionally generalized and involves the axillary and inguinal nodes. Inflamed tonsillopharyngeal tissue, often with an exudate and palatal petechiae resembling a streptococcal pharyngitis, is seen in infectious mononucleosis. In fact, up to 18% of children with infectious mononucleosis may demonstrate the presence of group A beta-hemolytic *Streptococcus* on rapid testing or culture, although it is unclear whether these children are actually coinfected or represent streptococcal carriers. The lack of clinical improvement within 48 hours on appropriate antibiotics should suggest infectious mononucleosis as the underlying etiology of the pharyngitis.[16] Hepatic and/or splenic enlargement is common in all patients with acute infectious mononucleosis, but is more common in children younger than 4 years of age.[15]

DIFFERENTIAL DIAGNOSES

Other disease entities may produce infectious mononucleosis-like syndromes, most of which are caused by other infections (Table 63–2). The most common of these is acute CMV infection which also may produce generalized lymphadenopathy, fever, splenomegaly and malaise in acutely infected, previously healthy hosts. Unlike with EBV, in CMV infections, pharyngitis and atypical lymphocytosis on peripheral blood smear are less prominent presenting features. Toxoplasmosis can also cause a clinical presentation quite similar to acute EBV infection, so obtaining pertinent history regarding cat exposures (e.g., litterbox contact, soil contamination) may be helpful. It is also crucial to ask about relevant risk factors on interview as acute HIV infection may be indistinguishable from infectious mononucleosis as well.

Other infectious etiologies that may present like acute infectious mononucleosis include viral hepatitis (hepatitis A especially), adenovirus, or rubella, however, history or physical or laboratory findings can often help to differentiate these entities. Patients with viral hepatitis usually demonstrate significant elevations in liver enzymes as opposed to the modest increases seen with infectious mononucleosis and the diagnosis of rubella becomes apparent once the exanthem appears. The pharyngitis of EBV infection may clinically mimic group A streptococcal pharyngitis.

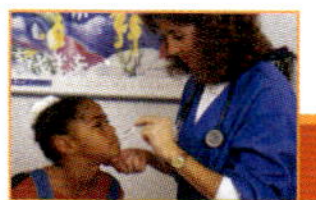

Table 63–2.

Differential Diagnosis of Infectious Mononucleosis Syndrome

Infectious
EBV
CMV
Toxoplasma gondii
Group A streptococcal pharyngitis
Human immunodeficiency virus
Adenovirus
Hepatitis A virus
Rubella virus
Influenza A and B viruses

Noninfectious
Malignancy (lymphoma, leukemia)
Drug reactions

Malignancies, particularly leukemias and lymphomas, may also mimic infectious mononucleosis when presenting as fever, malaise, fatigue, and lymphadenopathy. On occasion, patients with a drug reaction to certain medications, particularly dilantin or sulfa-containing drugs, may have fever and lymphadenopathy that mimic infectious mononucleosis.

DIAGNOSIS

Isolation of EBV is possible using specialized laboratory techniques, but given the complexity of the methods required for cell culture, these tests are primarily conducted in research laboratories and are not widely available. Studies have demonstrated that real-time polymerase chain reaction assays that quantitate EBV in the blood are quite sensitive for diagnosing acute infectious mononucleosis, particularly early in infection and in young children[17,18]; however, these tests are very expensive and often not readily available commercially. Given these restrictions, neither of these methods of laboratory diagnosis has utility in the setting of diagnosing infectious mononucleosis in otherwise healthy children.

The diagnosis of acute EBV infection relies on serologic testing that is readily available from most hospital-based and commercial laboratories. The most rapid methods detect the presence of heterophile antibodies. The heterophile antibody is a non-specific IgM (immunoglobulin M) antibody response to a variety of infectious, inflammatory, and autoimmune stimuli. The heterophile antibody test for EBV includes an intermediate step that removes most non-EBV stimulated heterophile antibody. In EBV-infected patients, it appears during the first 2 weeks after infection and may last up to 6 months. Detection of these antibodies identifies up to 85% of older children and adolescents from the second week of illness and beyond; these tests are less reliable in younger children and are often negative in EBV-infected children younger than 4 years. False-positive results have been reported in several disorders including leukemia, lymphoma, and Gaucher disease.

Specific EBV serologies are required for younger children with illness suspicious for infectious mononucleosis and for those who test negative on heterophile antibody testing but have a clinical presentation and history compatible with acute infectious mononucleosis. Unlike with many other viral infections where paired acute and convalescent specimens are needed, a single serum sample can usually confirm the diagnosis of acute EBV given the varying kinetics of the antibodies produced after primary infection.

The first antibodies made against EBV are the IgM and Immunoglobulin G (IgG) antibodies directed

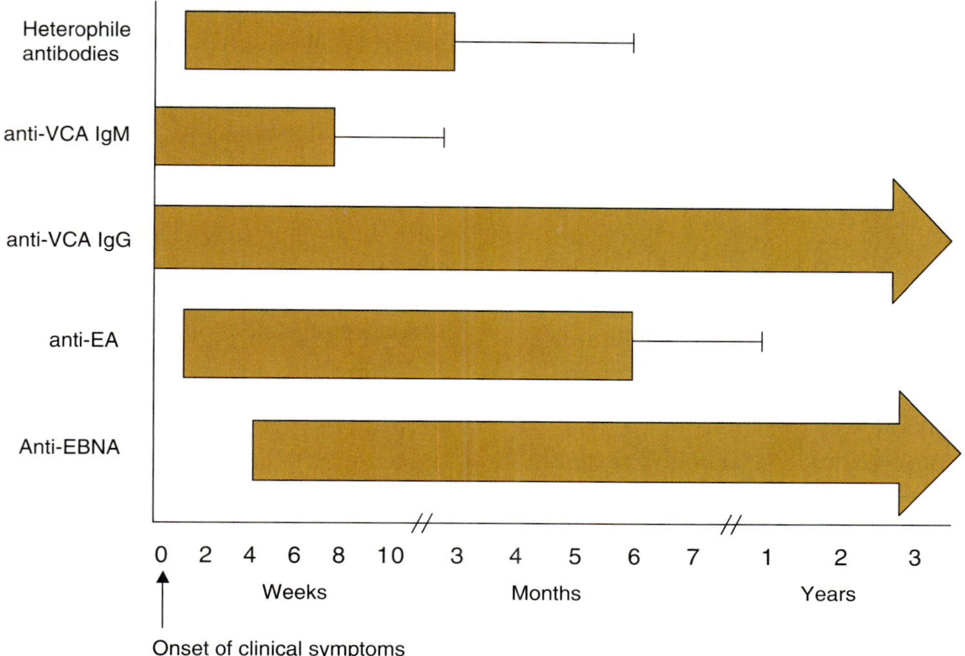

FIGURE 63-1 ■ Timing of EBV serologies.[19] (Schematic representation of the timing of Epstein-Barr antibodies starting from the onset of clinical symptoms. Bars represent timing where the majority of patients will demonstrate antibody production, while lines illustrate the outer limits of antibody detection in a lesser number of individuals. Arrows designate antibodies that persist indefinitely.)

against the viral capsid antigen of EBV (anti-VCA IgM and IgG). Anti-VCA IgM antibody occurs within 1–2 weeks after infection but usually is gone by 3 months after infection; likewise, anti-VCA IgG occurs early after infection, but persists for life.[19] Antibodies against the EBV early antigen (anti-EA) occur next, several weeks to months after infection; in most individuals, these antibodies disappear by 6–12 months, but occasionally may last for several years after infection.[20] The anti-EBNA (EBV nuclear antigen) antibody occurs several weeks to months after acute infection and also persists indefinitely (see Figure 63–1).

As with other IgM laboratory methodologies, there are numerous technical difficulties and a relatively high number of false positives as a result of rheumatoid factors in the blood, such that a positive anti-VCA IgM antibody alone is not diagnostic. The presence of anti-VCA IgM in combination with anti-VCA IgG, while in the absence of anti-EBNA, is diagnostic for acute EBV infection. The presence of anti-VCA IgG and anti-VCA EBNA is diagnostic for a past infection (see Table 63–3).

Although not diagnostic, other laboratory markers are suggestive and corroborate clinical suspicion for EBV infectious mononucleosis. Even without the clinical finding of hepatomegaly or jaundice, hepatic enzymes are often elevated, although usually only 2–3 fold. On a peripheral blood smear, lymphocytes account for more than 50% of the peripheral white blood cells and, typically, at least 10% are atypical lymphocytes. However, atypical lymphocytosis is a nonspecific finding and can be seen with other infectious etiologies of infectious mononucleosis-like illness. Other abnormal hematologic parameters may also be revealed on a complete blood count that may be attributed to a variety of immune-mediated events, including anemia, neutropenia and/or thrombocytopenia. The neutropenia is mild with absolute neutrophil counts ranging from 2000/mm^3 to 3000/mm^3, although profound neutropenia has also been reported. Most children develop a mild thrombocytopenia but the platelet count is rarely less than 100,000/mm^3. Abnormalities of prothrombin and

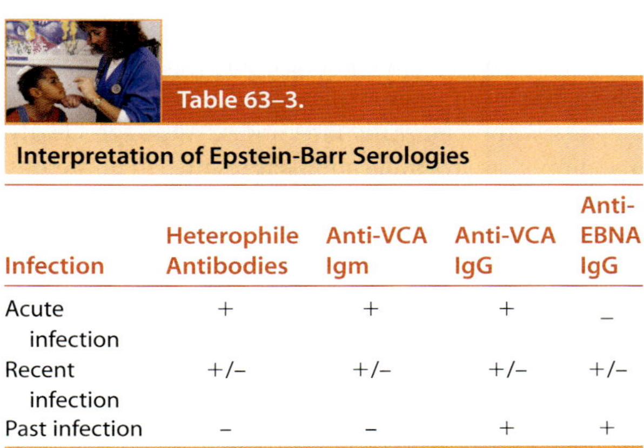

Table 63-3.

Interpretation of Epstein-Barr Serologies

Infection	Heterophile Antibodies	Anti-VCA Igm	Anti-VCA IgG	Anti-EBNA IgG
Acute infection	+	+	+	–
Recent infection	+/–	+/–	+/–	+/–
Past infection	–	–	+	+

partial thromboplastin times are uncommon and typically occur in the context of EBV-related septicemia or severe hepatitis. Hematologic abnormalities typically resolve within one month of diagnosis.

COMPLICATIONS

For most patients with a primary EBV infection, infectious mononucleosis is a self-limited disease with no sequelae. In rare instances, however, serious or life-threatening consequences may occur and should be recognized.

One serious and somewhat common complication of acute infectious mononucleosis is significant tonsillar hypertrophy resulting in airway compromise. This complication may occur at any age but younger children are more often and more severely affected. When administered early, corticosteroids may prevent severe obstruction otherwise resulting in endotracheal intubation, but occasionally the onset of airway compromise may be precipitous.

A variety of central nervous system complications may occur in a small number of patients including meningitis or encephalitis, cranial nerve palsies, transverse myelitis, Guillain-Barré syndrome or Reye syndrome. Occasionally there have been descriptions of patients with the so-called metamorphopsia or the "Alice in Wonderland Syndrome" in which there are bizarre perceptual distortions of size, shape, and spatial relationships.

Hematologic abnormalities resulting from immune-mediated mechanisms of cell destruction may vary in degree of severity. If Coombs test is positive hemolytic anemia may be seen as well as neutropenia secondary to anti-neutrophil antibodies. More than 50% of all patients will develop a mild thrombocytopenia, usually not less than 100,000/mm^3 but rarely a clinical picture of thrombotic thrombocytopenic purpura will result in platelet counts low enough to result in bleeding.

Cardiac manifestations including myocarditis or pericarditis may be life-threatening and must be recognized early for possible therapy. Rarely, EBV infection may cause pneumonia.

The most feared complication is splenic rupture, which has been estimated to occur in 0.1–0.5% of patients with acute EBV infection.[21] Although clearly uncommon, this complication has resulted in numerous deaths and careful evaluation for the presence of splenomegaly and subsequent appropriate patient counseling is critical. This complication is more often seen in males, usually within the first 3 weeks of acute illness,[22] and may be spontaneous, without history of antecedent trauma.

One important complication to note is the rare instance of death associated with EBV infection in children. This complication most often occurs when there is an uncontrolled lymphoproliferative response to EBV infection and often is associated with hemophagocytic syndrome.[23] This syndrome, also called hemophagocytic lymphohistiocytosis, occurs when activated macrophages engulf bone marrow cells (leukocytes, erythrocytes, and platelets, including their precursors); clinically these patients demonstrate fever, splenomegaly, pancytopenia, and an extremely elevated serum ferritin. This syndrome may occur sporadically, most often in association with EBV,[24] but has also been associated with a number of other viral infections (viral-associated hemophagocytic syndrome). Most significantly, this syndrome may often be seen in children with an underlying immunodeficiency of the cellular immune response called X-linked lymphoproliferative syndrome (XLP).[23] These children present with fulminant disseminated primary EBV infection and have an inadequate or deficient cellular response resulting in lack of control of viral replication. Children with XLP are usually boys who present in the first decade of life with no prior history consistent with immune deficiency. They present with an infectious mononucleosis-like illness that rapidly progresses to fulminant hepatic failure and multiple cytopenias. It is fatal in approximately two-thirds of these individuals, and survivors often go on to develop hypogammaglobulinemia and/or B-cell lymphoma.[25]

MANAGEMENT

For the most part, the management of infectious mononucleosis from acute EBV infection in a healthy patient is supportive. Rest, hydration, and analgesics for both fever and pharyngitis relief are encouraged. It is important to inform patients and their families of the often protracted nature of the recovery from infectious mononucleosis, as many patients have persistent fatigue for up to 3 or 4 months.

Of significant importance is the assessment of splenomegaly in patients with acute infectious mononucleosis; these patients and their parents must be counseled to ensure strenuous exercise and contact sports are avoided for at least 3–4 weeks after the onset of symptoms, or longer if the spleen is still palpably enlarged, to reduce the risk of splenic rupture.[22]

The use of steroids to ameliorate the duration of symptoms of EBV infectious mononucleosis has been debated, however, current recommendations are to reserve them for the most extreme and life-threatening complications of the illness. These situations may include: Marked tonsillar hypertrophy with resulting airway compromise, cardiac impairment, massive splenomegaly, hemolytic anemia or hemophagocytic syndrome. Steroids, when used for severe complications of infectious mononucleosis, are usually of short course; variable regimens have been suggested, but one commonly recommended is 1 mg/kg/day (maximum dose, 20 mg) for 7 days with subsequent tapering.[26]

Although acyclovir has in vitro activity against many herpesviruses including EBV, numerous studies have demonstrated this antiviral agent has little or no clinical benefit in the situation of uncomplicated infectious mononucleosis in a previously healthy child.[27] Likewise, unless there is a demonstrable concurrent bacterial infection, antibiotics should not be used. If antibiotic therapy is indicated, ampicillin and amoxicillin should be avoided as these agents will precipitate a significant rash in more than 80% of EBV-infected patients. This rash is usually maculopapular in nature and presents 5–9 days into therapy, but does not represent a true penicillin allergy.

COURSE AND PROGNOSIS

Most healthy children, adolescents and young adults recover within 1–2 months with no medical intervention and no resulting sequelae. Numerous attempts to associate EBV infection with other disease syndromes have been made, but none have been definitively substantiated. The best studied of these entities is Chronic Fatigue Syndrome, an illness characterized by persisting fatigue, weakness, myalgia and arthralgias, and occasionally lymphadenopathy, pharyngitis and low-grade fevers. Although studies have not supported an association with chronic fatigue syndrome, experts do recognize the entity of chronic active EBV in the rare patient with fever, hepatosplenomegaly, and fatigue persisting for a year or occasionally more after an acute infectious mononucleosis illness. These patients are distinct in that they have demonstrable organ dysfunction directly attributable to EBV by immunohistochemical staining.[28] Additionally, they have extremely high serum EBV viral loads by polymerase chain reaction, and markedly elevated anti-VCA and EA antibody titers, but never demonstrate antibody to EBNA.[29]

PEARLS

- Infectious mononucleosis is defined by the clinical triad of fever, pharyngitis and lymphadenopathy.
- The EBV is responsible for most infectious mononucleosis cases.
- Heterophile antibody tests are sensitive for the diagnosis of infectious mononucleosis in older children and adults, but EBV-specific serologic testing is necessary for children younger than 4 years.
- A common complication of infectious mononucleosis is splenomegaly with the associated risk of splenic rupture; thorough counseling regarding avoidance of contact sports for at least one month after diagnosis, or until the spleen is no longer palpable, is crucial.

REFERENCES

1. Filatov NF. Lektuse ob ostrikh infektsion Nikh Lolienznyak (Lectures on Acute Infectious Disease of Children). Moscow, U. Deitel; 1885.
2. Pfeiffer E. Drusenfieber. *Jahrb Kinderheilkd.* 1889;29: 257.
3. Sprunt TP, Evans FA. Mononucleosis leukocytosis in reaction to acute infections (infectious mononucleosis). *John Hopkins Hosp Bull.* 1920;31:409.
4. Paul JR, Bunnell WW. The presence of heterophile antibodies in infectious mononucleosis. *Am J Med Sci.* 1932; 183:90-104.
5. Epstein MS, Achong BG, Barr YM. Virus particles in cultured lymphoblasts from Burkitt's lymphoma. *Lancet.* 1964;1:702-703.
6. Henle G, Henle W, Diehl V. Relation of Burkitt's tumor-associated herpes-type virus to infectious mononucleosis. *Proc Natl Acad Sci.* 1968;59:94-101.
7. Henle G, Henle W, Clifford P, et al. Antibodies to epstein-barr virus in Burkitt's lymphoma and control groups. *J Natl Cancer Inst.* 1969:43:1147-1154.
8. Pereira MS, Blake JM, Macrae AD:EB virus antibody at different ages. *Br Med J.* 1969;4:526-527.
9. Chetham MM, Roberts KB. Infectious mononucleosos in adolescents. *Pediatr Ann.* 1991;20:206-213.
10. Auwaerter PG. Infectious mononucleosis in middle age. *JAMA.* 1999;281:454-459.
11. Sumaya CV, Henle W, Henle G, et al. Seroepidemiologic sudy of Epstein-Barr virus infections in a rural community. *J Infect Dis.* 1975;131:403-408.
12. Fleischer GR, Pasquariello PS, warren WS, et al. Intrafamilial transmission of epstein-barr virus infections. *J Pediatr.* 1981;98:16-19.
13. Strauss SE, Fleisher GR. Infectious mononucleosis epidemiology and pathogenesis. In: Schlossberg D, ed. *Clinical Topics in Infectious Disease: Infectious Mononucleosis.* 2nd ed. New York: Springer-Verlag; 1989:8-28.
14. Pearson GR. Infectious mononucleosis: The humoral response. In: Schlossberg D, ed. *Clinical Topics in Infectious Disease: Infectious Mononucleosis.* 2nd ed. New York: Springer-Verlag; 1989:89-99.
15. Sumaya CV, Ench Y. Epstein-Barr infectious mononucleosis in children I. Clinical and general laboratory findings. *Pediatrics.* 1985;75:1003-1010.
16. Rush MC, Simon MW. Occurrence of Epstein-Barr virus illness in children diagnosed with group A streptococcal pharyngitis. *Clin Pediatr.* 2003;42:417-420.
17. Bauer CC, Aberly SW, Popow-Kraupp T, Kapitan M, Hofmann H, Puchhammer-Stockl E. Serum epstein-barr virus DNA load in primary Epstein-Barr infection. *J Med Virol.* 2005;75:54-58.

18. Piterri RD, Laus S, Wadowsky RM. Clinical evaluation of a quantitative real time polymerase chain reaction assay for diagnosis of primary Epstein-Barr virus infection in children. *Pediatr Infect Dis J.* 2003;22:736-739.
19. Sumaya CV, Ench Y. Epstein-Barr virus infectious mononucleosis in children II. Heterophil antibody and viral-specific responses. *Pediatrics.* 1985;75:1011-1018.
20. Horwitz CA, Henle W, Henle G, et al. Long term serological follow-up of patients for Epstein-Barr virus after recovery from infectious mononucleosis. *J Infect Dis.* 1985;151:1150-1153.
21. Rothwell S, McAuley D. Spontaneous splenic rupture in infectious mononucleosis. *Emerg Med (Fremantle).* 2001; 13:364-366.
22. Waninger KN, Harcke HT. Determination of safe return to play for athletes recovering from infectious mononucleosis: a review of the literature. *Clin J Sport Med.* 2005; 15:410-416.
23. Mroczek EC, Weisenburger DD, Grierson HL, et al. Fatal infectious mononucleosis and virus-associated hemophagocytic syndrome. *Arch Pathol Lab Med.* 1987;111: 530-535.
24. Okano M, Gross TG. Epstein-Barr virus-associated hemophagocytic syndrome and fatal infectious mononucleosis. *Am J Hematol.* 1996;53:111-115.
25. Jensen HB. Acute complications of Epstein-Barr virus infectious mononucleosis. *Curr Opin Pediat.* 2000;12: 263-268.
26. American Academy of Pediatrics. Epstein-Barr Virus Infections (Infectious Mononucleosis). In: Pickering LK, Baker CJ, Long SS, McMillan JA, eds. *Red Book: 2006 Report of the Committee on Infectious Diseases.* 27th ed. Elk Grove Village, IL: American Academy of Pediatrics; 2006:286-290.
27. Torre D, Tambini R. Acyclovir for treatment of infectious mononucleosis: a meta-analysis. *Scand J Infect Dis.* 1999 31:543-547.
28. Straus SE. The chronic mononucleosis syndrome. *J Infect Dis.* 1988;157:405-412.
29. Maeda A, Wakiguchi H, Yokoyama W, et al. Persistently high Epstein-Barr virus (EBV) loads in peripheral blood lymphocytes from patients with chronic active EBV infection. *J Infect Dis.* 1999;179:1012-1015.
30. Glade PR. General features of infectious mononucleosis. In: Glade PR, ed. Proceedings of Symposium, New York, 1972. Philadelphia: JB Lippincott Company; 1973: 1-18.
31. Finch SC. Clinical symptoms and signs of infectious mononucleosis. In: Carter RL, Penman HG, eds. *Infectious Mononucleosis.* Oxford, England: Blackwell Scientific Publications; 1969:19-46.
32. Leach CT, Sumaya CV. Epstein-Barr virus. In: Feigin RD, Cherry JD, Demmler GJ, Kaplan SL, eds. *Textbook of Pediatric Infectious Diseases.* 5th ed. Philadelphia: Elsevier Saunders; 2004:1932-1956.

SECTION 18

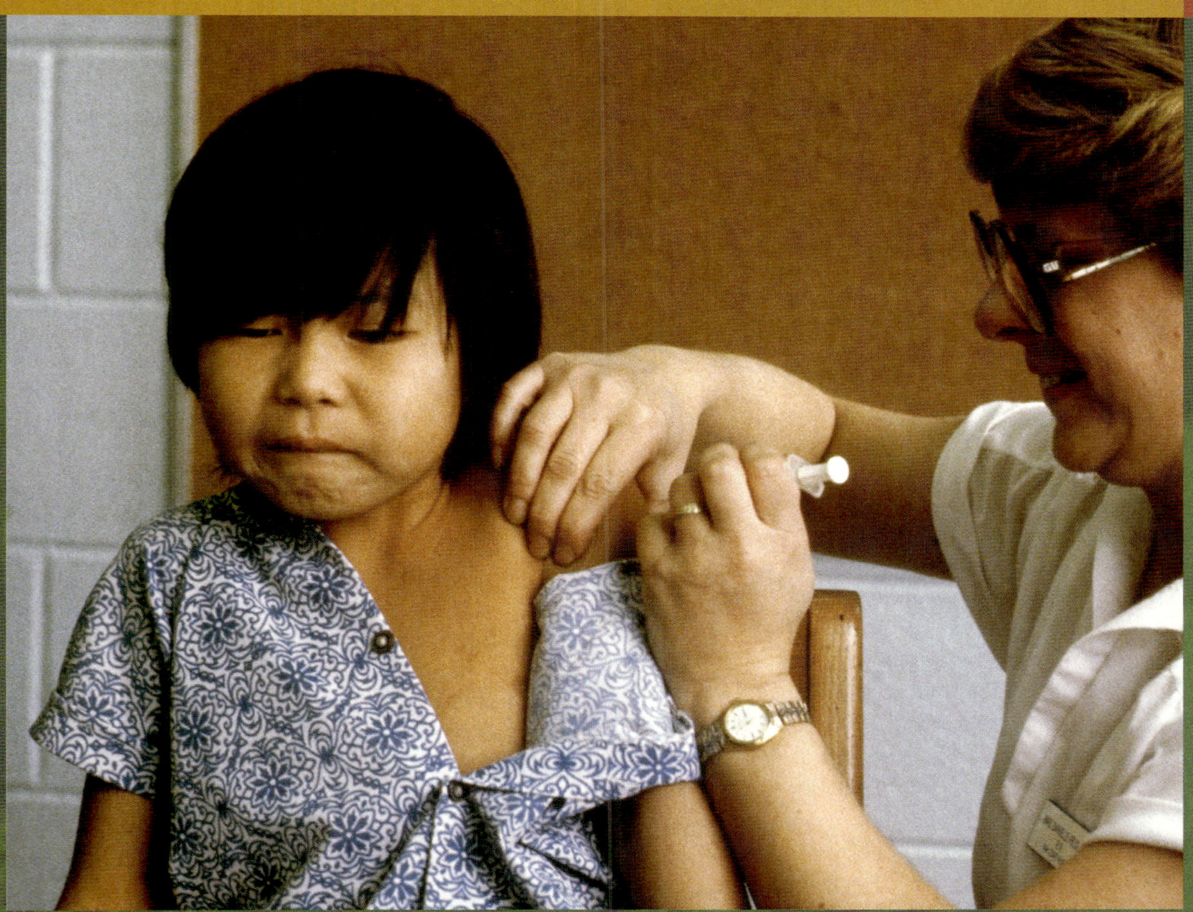

Travel-Related Infections

CHAPTER 64

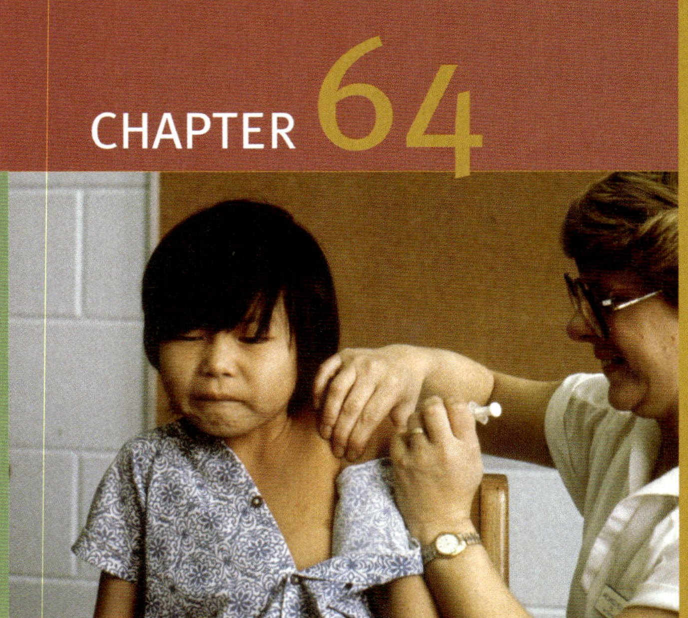

Pretravel Preparation

John C. Christenson

INTRODUCTION

A family of five with children of 2, 4, and 6 years of age is planning a trip to Costa Rica. They will visit the jungle for a bird-watching trip. They wonder if they need medications to prevent malaria.

A similar family is planning to visit relatives in Nigeria during the dry season in March. What vaccines and medications do they need?

Clinicians caring for children are frequently asked these questions. Children visiting developing countries are at risk of travel-related illnesses such as malaria and diarrheal diseases. Accidents and injuries may also occur. To help prevent these, clinicians must know how to find the needed information and provide appropriate medical advice. Others may choose to refer the child and family to a travel medicine clinic. For some communities, travel clinics are too distant for routine referrals, thus the clinician is called upon to provide the needed services.

EPIDEMIOLOGY

Approximately 1 billion passengers travel by air every year. Of these, over 50 million will visit a developing country.[1,2] While children only account for 4% of this group, approximately 25% of travel-related hospitalizations are in children. In one study, 40% of pediatric travelers to the tropics or subtropics experienced traveler's diarrhea.[3] As a consequence, close to 20% required bed confinement. In another study, imported febrile illnesses, such as malaria, represented 1% of hospital admissions.[4] At one pediatric travel clinic, children frequently traveled to high-risk regions, such as Africa, Latin America, and Southeast Asia.[5] Unfortunately many pediatric-age travelers (and/or their parents) do not comply with effective preventive measures.[6] Many of these travelers needed prophylaxis against malaria and vaccinations to protect against hepatitis A and typhoid fever.

While there is great comfort in visiting friends and relatives abroad, studies have shown that these travelers are at the highest risk of acquiring an infection. Of travelers visiting developing countries, 25–40% do so to visit friends and relatives (VFRs).[7] Only 16% of VFRs who were originally immigrants sought pretravel medical advice. In addition, VFRs were frequently prescribed inappropriate prophylaxis or none at all, had longer stays, and spent time in high-risk areas.[8]

Traveling for international adoption also poses specific risks for accompanying children. Adopted children may have gastrointestinal parasites and other enteric pathogens; may have scabies; or be a chronic carrier for hepatitis B. They may transmit pertussis or measles to the adopting family. The adopting family needs to be counseled pretravel and receive the necessary vaccines and prophylactic medications.[9]

TRAVEL ASSESSMENT AND ADVICE

Children are traveling for diverse reasons; to study abroad, with parents on international adoption trips, for adventurous exploration, missionary and humanitarian work, to visit family and relatives, and for ecologic projects. While most travel for short periods of time, others may be relocating because of parental work. Not all parents realize the importance of planning ahead to keep their families healthy. Because certain vaccines and medications need to be given days or weeks before travel, and because not all clinicians provide travel advice, appointments with a travel medicine specialist should be made at least 1 month before travel.

To successfully advise families about their travel health needs, it is important to know exactly where and when they are going. Some infections may be acquired only in certain countries or regions within countries. Clinicians planning to counsel travelers need to have up-to-date information on disease activity. Epidemics of meningococcal disease, hepatitis A, SARS, poliomyelitis, and measles have occurred recently. These may force changes in travel plans or immunization needs. Up-to-date country-specific information can be obtained from various sources such as the Travelers' Health Sections of the Centers for Disease Control and Prevention (www.cdc.gov/health) and the World Health Organization (www.who.int/ith). In addition, the International Association for Medical Assistance to Travelers (www.iamat.org) offers detailed advice to travelers, and Shoreland (www.shoreland.com) offers Travax®, an online subscription service with medical travel information for physicians. While containing useful information, travel books may not have the latest up-to-date information on disease activity.

Because of unfamiliarity with travel medicine, reimbursement issues for travel visits, and lack of specific vaccines, many clinicians refer their patients (and families) to travel medicine clinics. A list of these appears on Web sites of the International Society of Travel Medicine (www.istm.org) and the American Society of Tropical Medicine and Hygiene (www.astmh.org). Unfortunately, some families get inappropriate travel advice from peers, friends, relatives, neighbors, and at times medical providers. Inadequate information may also come from travel brochures or travel agents.

Before travel, a health assessment of the whole family is important. Is anyone taking medications? Are there any allergies? Immunization records need to be reviewed. Is everyone up-to-date? Proper travel advice will result from a careful assessment of travel plans and individual needs. Appropriate measures include provision of vaccines and prophylactic medications, risk-reducing/disease prevention education, and frequently medications for self-treatment.

A concise summary of advice frequently given to travelers appears in Table 64–1.

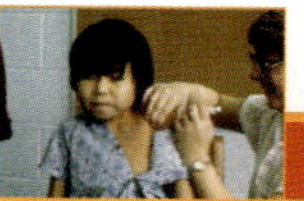

Table 64–1.

General Travel Recommendations

- Prevent high altitude illness: acclimatization is important. Acetazolamide can be used as prophylaxis. Information source: www.high-altitude-medicine.com/ams/html.
- Waterfalls, rivers, streams (rafting, kayaking) in the tropics: high risk for leptospirosis. Doxycycline could be used as prophylaxis in children older than 8 y.
- Avoid cutaneous larva migrans, other parasitic infections (hookworms): do not walk barefoot on ground or dry sand. Use a towel at the beach or lay in the turf.
- Avoid swimming in freshwater in the tropics: prevent schistosomiasis, intestinal parasitic infections, traveler's diarrhea and hepatitis. Chlorinated pools are fine.
- Be careful crossing streets: watch out for bikes and motorcycles; and vehicle on the left lane.
- Safety and injury prevention: use car seats, seat belts. Sit in the back seats. Never leave children unattended. Childproof all rooms.
- Pack a first aid kit. Keep all prescription medications in their original containers. Place in carry-on hand luggage.
- Bring photocopies of passports and birth certificates (especially for US-born children of expatriates): makes replacement easier if original passport is lost or stolen.
- Avoid boredorm: bring cards, books, games, and snacks.
- Best seats for children on planes: bulk head (more leg space). Bassinettes may be available.
- Ear discomfort: provide child with something to drink or eat during ascent and descent.
- Get medical and evacuation insurance (InternationalSOS, Medex, Travelex, Diner's Club, others).
- During long flights: get out of your seat and walk: Avoid "economy-class" thrombosis.
- Protect against sun exposure.

IMMUNIZATIONS

Travel immunizations are categorized as *required, recommended,* or *routine. Routine* vaccinations and boosters against measles, mumps, rubella, polioviruses, varicella, pertussis, influenza, and diphtheria should normally be given at appropriate ages. However, sometimes travel plans require that they be administered on an accelerated schedule. If necessary, first doses, doses within a series, and boosters can all be administered early. For example, young infants can receive the first doses of most routine vaccines as early as 6 weeks of age. Infants can receive a measles vaccine as early as 6 months for travel to high-risk areas. The American Academy of Pediatrics Redbook® is an excellent resource for this information.[10] Frequently administered travel vaccines appear in Table 64–2.

Currently, only two vaccines generally fall into the *required* category. Yellow fever vaccination is the only vaccine that requires documentation on an official certificate of vaccination. Countries with endemic and/or epidemic yellow fever may require proof for entry. The vaccine must have been administered at least 10 days before intended entry, and an official stamp must appear on the certificate.[11] Only authorized practitioners and clinics are allowed to administer yellow fever vaccine and issue this official certificate. Children younger than 4 months should never receive yellow fever vaccine because of the risk of developing postvaccination encephalitis. Children older than 9 months can

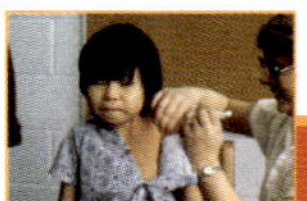

Table 64–2.

Travel Vaccinations

Vaccine	Formulation	Route and Dose	Schedule	Indications	Comment
Hepatitis A	Pediatric: Havrix® (GlaxoSmithKline); 720 EU VAQTA® (Merck); 25 U	IM; 0.5 mL	Primary series: 2 doses, 6–18 mo apart Booster: currently not recommended	Children ≥1 y old	Inactivated vaccine. Lifelong protection is likely
	Adult: Havrix® (GlaxoSmithKline); 1440 EU VAQTA® (Merck); 50 U	IM; 1.0 mL	Primary series: 2 doses, 6–18 mo apart Booster: currently not recommended	Adults ≥19 y old	Inactivated vaccine. Lifelong protection is likely
Hepatitis A and B	Twinrix® (GlaxoSmithKline)	IM; 1.0 mL	Primary series: 3 doses at 0, 1, and 6 mo Accelerated schedule: 0, 7, and 21 d; fourth dose 12 mo later Boosters: not needed	Adults ≥18 y old	Inactivated vaccine. Lifelong protection is likely. Accelerated schedule is as effective
Immunoglobulin, human	Injectable	IM	Travel <3 mo duration: 0.02 mL/kg body weight. Travel >3 mo duration: 0.06 mL/kg body weight every 4–6 mo	Infants <1 y of age	Passive immunizations against hepatitis A. Will require delay of measles and varicella vaccinations (at least 3 mo)
Japanese encephalitis virus	Inactivated	SC; 1.0 mL	Primary series: 3 doses at days 0, 7, and 30. Booster: 1 dose at 24 mo interval	Travel to high-risk areas; prolonged stays	Allergic reactions can be life-threatening. Persons need to be observed for 30 min after each dose and the series must be completed ≥10 d before departure
Meningococcal	Quadrivalent: A, C, Y, W135	SC; 0.5 mL	Primary series: single dose Booster: 5 y in persons ≥4 y old; 2–3 y in children 2–4 y old	≥2 y old	Required for entry to Saudi Arabia during the Hajj
Meningococcal conjugate	Quadrivalent: A, C, Y, W135	IM; 0.5 mL	Primary series: single dose Booster: unknown	Not previously vaccinated ≥11–12 y old	Required for entry to Saudi Arabia during the Hajj
Rabies	Inactivated	IM; 1.0 mL	Preexposure series: 3 doses at days 0, 7, and 21 or 28. Booster: depends on risk category and serological testing. Postexposure: rabies immune globulin; day 0; vaccines at days 0, 3, 7, 14, and 28		Consider for young travelers planning prolonged stays; especially away from large urban centers with adequate medical care systems and airport
Typhoid fever	Live-attenuated Ty21a1	Oral	1 capsule every-other-day for 4 doses. Boosters: every 5 y	Persons ≥6 y old	If series sequence not completed, all 4 doses need to be repeated. Contraindicated in immunocompromised hosts. Cannot be taken with hot beverage.

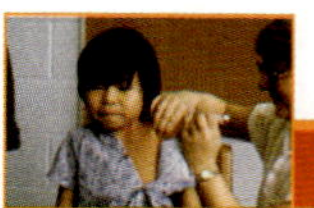

Table 64–2. (continued)

Travel Vaccinations

Vaccine	Formulation	Route and Dose	Schedule	Indications	Comment
					Person must not be taking antibiotics
	Injectable Polysaccharide Vi antigen	IM; 0.5 mL	Primary series: one dose. Booster: every 2 y	Persons ≥2 y old	Inactivated vaccine
Yellow fever	Live injectable	SC; 0.5 mL	Primary series: one dose. Dose must be given at least 10 d before arrival to risk area. Booster: every 10 y.	≥9 mo old.	Contraindicated in immunocompromised hosts. Avoid in pregnancy, unless high-risk travel cannot be avoided. Contraindicated in infants <4 mo of age. Avoid in persons with thymus disorders. Caution in persons ≥60 y old (high risk for vaccine-related infection). Requires official certificate of vaccination

be vaccinated safely. For children between the ages of 6 and 9 months, the risk of acquiring the disease must be greater than the potential side effects of the vaccine. Travel to yellow fever endemic regions should be postponed if at all possible for children in these younger age groups.[11]

The quadrivalent meningococcal vaccine (A, C, Y, W135) is required by Saudi Arabia for all visitors making the Hajj pilgrimage to Mecca and Medina. Polio vaccination has also been required in recent years.

Most other vaccines fall in the *recommended* category. Since the incidence of hepatitis A is high in the developing world, travelers should receive the safe and highly protective hepatitis A vaccine. Passively transferred maternal antibodies blunt the immune response to hepatitis A vaccination in children younger than 1 year. This is especially so in infants younger than 6 months born from seropositive mothers.[12] Passive immunization with gamma globulin can also prevent hepatitis A infection but it is generally reserved for infants younger than 1 year of age.

Typhoid fever results from the consumption of contaminated water or food as well as by intimate contact with documented *Salmonella typhi* carriers. Vaccination is recommended for even short-term travel to high-risk areas in the Indian Subcontinent, Asia, Africa, and Latin America; and for travelers planning to stay for extended periods of time in most areas of the developing world.[13] Injectable and oral vaccine formulations are available. The live-attenuated Ty21a oral vaccine (Vivotif Berna) is recommended for travelers older than 6 years. This formulation has fewer side effects and confers longer protection than the injectable capsular polysaccharide vaccine (Typhium Vi), which can be given to travelers as young as 2 years of age.[14]

Because of a high incidence of invasive meningococcal disease, travelers to Sub-Saharan Africa are advised to receive the meningococcal vaccine. While this vaccination is generally recommended for children older than 2 years, it can confer protection in younger patients against some serogroups, especially serogroup A.[15] The quadrivalent conjugate vaccine is routinely recommended for children and adults at 11–55 years of age. It confers higher antibody titers and longer duration of protection.[16]

Rabies vaccination is recommended for travelers visiting remote areas of the developing world where access to prompt postexposure administration of rabies immunoglobulin and vaccine is less likely. Travelers, especially children, planning extended stay abroad (usually to rural areas) may need Japanese encephalitis virus or tick-borne encephalitis vaccines.

While no vaccine or toxoid is 100% effective or safe, those described above are generally well tolerated with minimal side effects, such as fever, injection site pain, and redness. In most cases, severe side effects are not observed when appropriately administered. Live vaccines such as measles–mumps–rubella, yellow fever, oral typhoid, and varicella should never be administered to immunocompromised travelers.

INSECT BITE PROTECTION

The most effective way of preventing malaria and other mosquito-borne diseases such as dengue fever, chikungunya, yellow fever, and Japanese encephalitis virus is to avoid mosquito bites. This is achievable through the proper use of protective clothing (permethrin-treated long-sleeved shirts and blouses and long pants; closed shoes, and hats) and effective insect repellents; avoidance of outdoor activities during peak mosquito biting times, and by sleeping in dwellings with door and window screens or air conditioning; and/or by using permethrin-impregnated bed nets while sleeping. Dark colored clothing, floral fragrances such as those in perfumed soaps, lotions, hair care products, and deodorants may attract mosquitoes. When possible, these should be avoided.

There are many insect repellents on the market, and the choice of which one to use can be confusing to parents. *N,N*-diethyl-3-methylbenzamide, formerly known as *N,N*-diethyl-m-toluamide (DEET), is the most effective insect repellent available. Products with ≥30% DEET can be used safely in children, but higher concentrations are not necessary.[17] Products containing 20–30% DEET protect an individual for 4–5 hours,[18] while products with lower concentrations protect for shorter periods.[17] Products with microencapsulated DEET (such as UltraThon®) may provide protection for even longer periods of time. The use of higher concentrations of DEET does not correlate with increased toxicity, but inappropriate use does. While wristbands are popular among some travelers, protection is measured in seconds or minutes. Natural products, such as those containing citronella, confer limited protection and are not recommended for protection in the tropics.

Recently, a new insect repellent, 7–15% picaridin (KBR 3023), was released in the Unites States. In clinical trials, picaridin was found to be as effective as DEET, but at a concentration of 20%.[19,20]

Because of potential absorption through mucosal membranes, insect repellents containing DEET should not be applied to the faces of young children. In addition, they should not be applied to the hands of young children since they tend to bring them to their mouths. Once the family returns indoors, the insect repellent can be washed off if the area is screened, air conditioned, or they are under bednets.

While malaria-transmitting mosquitoes usually bite between dusk and dawn, other disease-transmitting mosquitoes are diurnal biters, so insect repellents and proper clothing may be needed during the day as well. The application of permethrin to clothing also reduces bites. Permethrin 0.5% on clothing will last an average of 2 weeks. Parents can purchase permethrin at most recreational outdoor stores or via the Internet. Insect repellents and permethrin-impregnated clothing will also minimize bites by ticks, flies, and other insects. Inspection of children's clothing and skin after returning from outdoors is important to minimize tick exposures. Permethrin-impregnated bednets are also protective.

MALARIA

The risk of infection and type of malaria in the developing world varies from country to country. Before providing advice, clinicians should familiarize themselves with the worldwide distribution of chloroquine-susceptible and chloroquine-resistant *Plasmodium falciparum* and other species. Since resistance is not a problem in Central America, chloroquine can be used there. Most malaria-endemic areas of Africa, Asia, and South America have chloroquine-resistant *P. falciparum*. For these areas, mefloquine, doxycycline, primaquine, or atovaquone-proguanil are used. Parts of Southeast Asia have strains of *P. falciparum* that are mefloquine-resistant.

The choice of antimalarial medication is also influenced by duration of travel, cost, and ease of administration. Most travelers prefer not to take medications every day. Others dislike the idea of taking medications for 4 weeks after returning home. Some travelers will only need intermittent protection against malaria since they are traveling in and out of malaria regions. Doxycycline is the cheapest option. While inexpensive, travelers must be aware of the potential for photosensitivity reactions and yeast superinfection.

Certain antimalarial agents cannot be used in certain patient populations. For example, while chloroquine is safe in pregnancy, doxycycline and atovaquone-proguanil should be avoided; but mefloquine can be given safely after the first trimester. Doxycycline is also contraindicated in children under the age of 8 years.

Since suspensions or elixir formulations of these medications are not available in the United States, and are not palatable, the pharmacist needs to compound these in ways that children will find acceptable. Grinding down tablets and dividing them in portions according to body weight is desirable. The contents in a little sachet-envelope or small gel capsule can then be poured onto food or mixed with chocolate syrup. To minimize gastrointestinal discomfort, all antimalarial medications should always be taken with meals. To avoid "pill

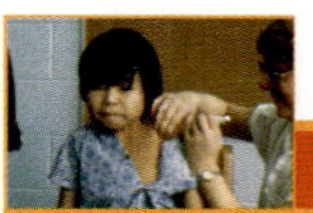

Table 64–3.

Summary of Antimalarial Prophylaxis Regimens

Medication	Adult Dose	Pediatric Dose	Comments
Chloroquine	500 mg salt (300 mg base) tablet. One tablet weekly	8.3 mg/kg salt (5.0 mg/kg base) weekly	Start at least 1 wk before arrival at risk site. Continue for 4 wk after leaving malaria region.
Doxycycline	100 mg tablet. One tablet daily.	≥8 y old: 2 mg/kg daily. Maximum dosage, 100 mg/d.	Start 1–2 d before arrival in malaria region. Continue for 4 wk after departure.
Mefloquine (Lariam®)	250 mg salt (228 mg base) tablet. One tablet weekly.	Dose given weekly. ≤9 kg: 5 mg/kg salt 10–19 kg: 1/4 tablet 20–30 kg: 1/2 tablet 31–45 kg: 3/4 tablet >45 kg: 1 tablet	Start at least 2 wk before arrival at risk site. Continue for 4 wk after leaving malaria region.
Atovaquone-proguanil (Malarone®)	250/100 mg adult tablet. One tablet daily	62.5/25 mg pediatric tablet. 5–8 kg: 1/2 tablet once daily. >8–10 kg: 3/4 tablet once daily. >10–20 kg: 1 tablet once daily. >20–30 kg: 2 tablets once daily. >30–40 kg: 3 tablets once daily. >40 kg: 1 adult tablet once daily	Start 1–2 d before arrival in malaria region. Take for 7 d after departure.
Primaquine	26.3 mg salt (15 mg base). Two tablets once daily; for 14 d	0.8 mg/g of salt form (0.5 mg/kg of base) once daily; for 14 d	Terminal prophylaxis. Must have G6 PD level prior to administration.

esophagitis," medications should be taken while awake, upright, and with sufficient fluids.

To maximize effectiveness, antimalarial prophylaxis medications need to be started before entering an endemic region. Chloroquine needs to be started at least 1 week prior to arrival, mefloquine at least 1–2 weeks. Doxycycline and atovaquone-proguanil can be started 24–48 hours prior.[16,21,22] Dosage information appears on Table 64–3.

Travelers need to be alerted regarding potential side effects. Because medications may require discontinuation, alternate prophylaxis should be discussed before travel. A different medication may be needed that may not be available in the destination country. Some travelers are concerned about the potential of neuropsychiatric disturbances with mefloquine. This medication is contraindicated in people with seizure disorders and in those suffering from anxiety and depression. It is also contraindicated in people with cardiac conduction abnormalities. While most side effects such as nausea and upset stomach are minor, less common ones may be more disturbing. Among these are strange vivid dreams, insomnia, dizziness, weakness, anxiety, and agitation. Children generally tolerate antimalarial medications better than adults.[23] However, approximately 10% of children experience difficulties with mefloquine such as vivid dreams, diarrhea, vomiting, changes in sleep patterns, headaches, and even hallucinations. About 23% of children taking chloroquine experience nausea, headaches, vomiting or changes in sleep. But, while 5–8% of adults will discontinue these agents because of side effects, only 1% of children will do so. Atovaquone-proguanil (Malarone®) has the least potential for side effects.

Despite taking appropriate antimalarial prophylaxis during travel malaria may still manifest itself weeks to months after returning from an endemic area. Families spending extended periods of time in an endemic area where *Plasmodium vivax* and *Plasmodium ovale* are present may need to receive terminal prophylaxis. This is intended to eliminate the hypnozoite stage of the parasite in the liver. This is achieved by taking primaquine for a period of 14 days. A glucose-6-phosphate dehydrogenase level should be checked before administering primaquine because it may cause severe hemolysis in individuals who are glucose-6-phosphate dehydrogenase deficient.

The goal of antimalarial prophylaxis is to rapidly clear infections and reduce mortality and morbidity caused by the malaria parasite. Because no regimen is 100% effective it is important that families be educated about methods of bite prevention and the need to seek care immediately if someone develops a febrile illness during or after a trip to an endemic area. Malaria is discussed further in Chapter 66 (Malaria) and Chapter 65 (Fever in the returned traveler).

TRAVELER'S DIARRHEA

Traveler's diarrhea is a common problem among visitors to the developing world. A study by Pitzinger and associates showed a 60% attack rate in children younger than 2 years of age.[3] Travelers to Northern Africa, India, and Latin America were the most affected. Approximately 19% of affected travelers were confined to bed, with 15% requiring treatment by a physician and approximately 1% requiring hospitalization.

Approximately 80% of traveler's diarrhea is caused by bacterial pathogens such as enterotoxigenic *Escherichia coli*, *Campylobacter jejuni*, nontyphoidal *Salmonella*, and *Shigella*. Traveler's diarrhea may also be caused by noroviruses (Norwalklike viruses), rotavirus, and parasites such as *Giardia lamblia* or *Entamoeba histolytica*.

Traveler's diarrhea can be prevented by avoiding contaminated food and beverages. Tap water or products prepared with it, such as ice, should be avoided. Travelers should avoid foods that are not boiled, cooked, or peeled. Pasteurized milk products, bottled water (especially carbonated), and sodas are usually safe. Proper hand hygiene before eating is particularly important in children.

If diarrhea occurs, parents need to be prepared to prevent or treat dehydration with oral fluids. Powdered oral rehydration salts can be purchased before the trip but are also available in most countries. Undiluted fruit juices, sport drinks, or soda are not appropriate rehydration solutions. They contain large amounts of sugar, which may worsen the diarrhea. With certain enteric infections, vomiting can be a problem and some younger children may require IV rehydration. However, most children can tolerate small amounts of fluids by mouth. By using a spoon or dropper to give 1–5 mL/min, rehydration can be achieved. Rehydrating a seriously dehydrated child can require 1–1½ ounces of fluid per pound of weight over a 2–4-hour period.

Since most cases of traveler's diarrhea are caused by bacteria, antimicrobial therapy can be used to reduce the duration and severity (Table 64–4). Fluoroquinolones, such as ciprofloxacin and levofloxacin are commonly recommended for use in adults. However not all clinicians are comfortable using these in children. Much has been published in the literature about the risks of arthropathies and tendinopathies with fluoroquinolones but a review of existing data has shown the agents to be effective and safely tolerated by children.[24] An equally effective agent is azithromycin. This antimicrobial agent is now considered by many to be the preferred agent for children.[25] In Thailand where fluoroquinolone-resistant *Campylobacter* is a common cause of traveler's diarrhea, azithromycin is clearly useful. Trimethoprim-sulfamethoxazole is no longer recommended because of widespread resistance.[26]

While antidiarrheal medications, such as loperamide and bismuth subsalicylate, are frequently used by adults, loperamide should not be used in young children because of the risk of paralytic ileus, severe vomiting, and drowsiness. However, bismuth subsalicylate has been shown to be safe and efficacious when used in children. Concern over the use of salicylate-containing antidiarrheal drugs and Reye syndrome does exist, but up to this moment there is no clear evidence to support the association.

In the developed world, empiric antibiotics are generally not prescribed for children with diarrhea. The association of antibiotic use, hemolytic uremic syndrome (HUS) and diarrhea caused by enterohemorrhagic *E. coli* is well known. Fortunately, effective treatment of enteric infections in the developing world has not led to an increase in HUS. HUS-associated enterohemorrhagic *E. coli* strains are rare outside developed countries. It is still wise to counsel parents that if a child develops bloody diarrhea, fever and abdominal pain, prompt medical evaluation is necessary.

Table 64–4.

Antibiotics Commonly Prescribed for Self-Treatment of Diarrheal Illness

Medication	Adult Dose	Pediatric Dose
Ciprofloxacin*	1000 mg single daily dose; 1–3 d	10–15 mg/kg/dose twice daily; 1–3 d
Levofloxacin*	500 mg daily; 1–3 d	10 mg/kg once daily; 1–3 d
Azithromycin	1000 mg single daily dose; 1–3 d	10 mg/kg single daily dose; 1–3 d
Rifaximin	200 mg three times daily†	Not available

**Not currently approved by the Food and Drug Administration for use in children but clinical studies supporting safety and efficacy have been published and dosing guidelines are available.*

†Children ≥12 y of age and adults.

Probiotics, such as *Lactobacillus* GG, have been used to treat antibiotic-associated and rotavirus-associated diarrhea with some success. However, there is insufficient data at this time to support their routine use in the prevention or treatment of traveler's diarrhea.

A newly approved nonabsorbable semisynthetic derivative of rifampin, rifaximin, has been shown to be effective in treating traveler's diarrhea. Unfortunately, rifaximin is not recommended for the treatment of invasive intestinal bacterial pathogens such as *Shigella*, *Salmonella*, or *Campylobacter*.[27,28] While routinely it is not recommended, chemoprophylaxis has been shown to reduce the occurrence of traveler's diarrhea and possibly postinfectious irritable bowel syndrome.[28] Studies in children are still lacking.

ADDITIONAL TRAVEL PROBLEMS

Acute respiratory tract infections such as those caused by influenza virus are common among travelers, especially those traveling within the Northern Hemisphere during the period of December through February; and those visiting friends or relatives, and staying longer than 30 days.[29] Infections by parainfluenza virus, adenovirus, human metapneumovirus, coronaviruses, and rhinoviruses have also been documented.[30]

Young infants are frequently flown around the world to visit family. For years, many have expressed concerns over young infants suffering from inflight hypoxia and sudden infant death syndrome during long flights. There is no clear evidence to support this concern. While pretravel fitness-to-fly assessments appear reasonable for young expremature infants with history of lung disease; healthy-term infants appear physiologically capable for travel.[31,32]

ILLNESS AFTER TRAVEL

Fever, skin conditions, and diarrhea are among the most common problems afflicting returned travelers.[33] A brief discussion of these and when it is necessary to seek medical attention should be discussed before travel. An initial evaluation for these problems require a complete assessment of travel history, countries and regions visited, duration of travel, activities while in country, vaccination history, use of prophylactic and therapeutic medications, and compliance with preventive measures. In returned travelers from the tropics, determining an incubation period greatly influences diagnostic and therapeutic considerations. An onset of fever >3 weeks after return generally eliminates dengue fever, yellow fever, and rickettsias as potential etiologic causes. Common skin problems of pediatric travelers are scabies, fungal dermatosis, and parasitic infections. Among the latter, cutaneous larva migrans or creeping eruption, a pruritic serpentiginous skin condition commonly caused by the larval migration of *Ancylostoma braziliense*; and myiasis, resulting from the tissue invasion of the fly larvae, are frequently reported.

Returned travelers may complain of acute or prolonged diarrhea. Causes of acute disease are usually identified through stool cultures and examination for ova and parasites (plus antigen assays). The detection of less common parasites as *Cyclospora cayetanensis* may require special stains. Giardiasis, tropical sprue, and other parasitic infections may cause chronic problems in some travelers.

Tuberculosis and anemia are usually observed only in returned travelers who have spent extended periods of time abroad. Short-term travelers do not require routine screening. Clinicians can consult with specialists in infectious diseases, and tropical and travel medicine when evaluating pediatric travelers with the above problems. Fever in the returned traveler is discussed further in Chapter 65.

REFERENCES

1. Ryan ET, Kain KC. Health advice and immunizations for travelers. *N Engl J Med.* 2000;342:1716-1725.
2. Cossar JH, Reid D, Fallon RJ, et al. A cumulative review of studies on travelers, their experience of illness and the implications of these findings. *J Infect.* 1990;21:27-42.
3. Pitzinger B, Steffen R, Tschopp A. Incidence and clinical features of traveler's diarrhea in infants and children. *Pediatr Infect Dis J.* 1991;10:719-723.
4. Riordan FAI, Tarlow MJ. Imported infections in East Birmingham children. *Postgrad Med J.* 1998;74:36-37.
5. Christenson JC, Fischer PR, Hale DC, Derrick D. Pediatric travel consultation in an integrated clinic. *J Travel Med.* 2001;8:1-5.
6. Klein JL, Millman GC. Prospective, hospital based study of fever in children in the United Kingdom who had recently spent time in the tropics. *BMJ.* 1998;316:1425-1426.
7. Leder K, Tong S, Weld L, et al. Illness in travelers visiting friends and relatives: a review of the GeoSentinel Surveillance Network. *Clin Infect Dis.* 2006;43:1185-1193.
8. Bacaner N, Stauffer B, Boulware DR, Walker PF, Keystone JS. Travel medicine considerations for North American immigrants visiting friends and relatives. *JAMA.* 2004; 291:2856-2864.
9. Barnett ED, Chen LH. Prevention of travel-related infectious diseases in families of internationally adopted children. *Pediatr Clin N Am.* 2005;52:1271-1786.
10. American Academy of Pediatrics. In: Pickering LK, Baker CJ, Long SS, McMillan JA, eds. *Red Book 2006 Report of the Committee on Infectious Diseases.* 27th ed. Elk Grove, IL: American Academy of Pediatrics; 2006.
11. Barnett ED. Yellow fever: epidemiology and prevention. *Clin Infect Dis.* 2007;44:850-856.
12. Bell BP, Negus S, Fiore AE, et al. Immunogenicity of an inactivated hepatitis A vaccine in infants and young children. *Pediatr Infect Dis J.* 2007;26:116-122.

13. Steinberg EB, Bishop R, Dempsey AF, et al. Typhoid fever in travelers: Who should be targeted for prevention? *Clin Infect Dis.* 2004;39:186-191.
14. Basnyat B, Maskey AP, Zimmerman MD, Murdoch DR. Enteric (typhoid) fever in travelers. *Clin Infect Dis.* 2005; 41:1467-1472.
15. Memish ZA. Meningococcal disease and travel. *Clin Infect Dis.* 2002;34:84-90.
16. Hill DR, Ericsson CD, Pearson RD, et al. The practice of travel medicine: guidelines by the Infectious Diseases Society of America. *Clin Infect Dis.* 2006;43:499-539.
17. Fradin MS. Mosquitoes and mosquito repellents: a clinician's guide. *Ann Intern Med.* 1998;128:931-940.
18. Fradin MS, Day JF. Comparative efficacy of insect repellents against mosquito bites. *N Engl J Med.* 2002;347:13-18.
19. Costantini C, Badolo A, Ilboudo-Sanogo E. Field evaluation of the efficacy and persistente of insect repellents DEET, IR3535, and KBR 3023 against *Anopheles gambiae* complex and other Afrotropical vector mosquitoes. *Trans R Soc Trop Med Hyg.* 2004;98:644-652.
20. Badolo A, Ilboudo-Sanogo E, Ouédraogo AP, Costantini C. Evaluation of the sensitivity of *Aedes aegypti* and *Anopheles gambiae* complex mosquitoes to two insect repellents: DEET and KBR 3023. *Trop Med Int Health.* 2004;9:330-334.
21. Fischer PR, Bialek R. Prevention of malaria in children. *Clin Infect Dis.* 2002;34:493-498.
22. Baggild AK, Parise ME, Lewis LS, Kain KC. Atovaquone-proguanil: Report from the CDC expert meeting on malaria chemoprophylaxis (II). *Am J Trop Med Hyg.* 2007; 76:208-223.
23. Albright TA, Binns HJ, Katz BZ. Side effects of and compliance with malaria prophylaxis in children. *J Travel Med.* 2002;9:289-292.
24. Alghashan AA, Nahata MC. Clinical use of fluoroquinolones in children. *Ann Pharmacother.* 2000;34: 347-359.
25. Stauffer WM, Konop RJ, Kamat D. Traveling with infants and young children. Part III: traveler's diarrhea. *J Travel Med.* 2002;9:141-150.
26. Tribble DR, Sanders JW, Pang LW, et al. Traveler's diarrhea in Thailand. Randomized, double-blind trial comparing single-dose and 3-day azithromycin-based regimens with a 3-day levofloxacin regimen. *Clin Infect Dis.* 2007;44: 338-346.
27. Taylor DN, Bourgeois AL, Ericsson CD, et al. A randomized, double-blind, multicenter study of rifaximin compared with placebo and with ciprofloxacin in the treatment of traveler's diarrhea. *Am J Trop Med Hyg.* 2006;74: 1060-1066.
28. Adachi JA, DuPont HL. Rifaximin: a novel nonabsorbed rifamycin for gastrointestinal disorders. *Clin Infect Dis.* 2006;42:541-547.
29. Leder K, Sundararajan V, Weld L, et al. Respiratory tract infections in travelers: a review of the GeoSentinel Surveillance Network. *Clin Infect Dis.* 2003;36:399-406.
30. Luna L, Paming M, Grywna K, Pfefferle S, Drosten C. Spectrum of viruses and atypical bacteria in intercontinental air travelers with symptoms of acute respiratory infection. *J Infect Dis.* 2007;195:675-679.
31. Udomittipong K, Stick SM, Verheggen M, et al. Pre-flight testing of preterm infants with neonatal lung disease: a retrospective review. *Thorax.* 2006;61:343-347.
32. Ryan ET, Wilson ME, Kain KC. Illness after international travel. *N Engl J Med.* 2002;347:505-516.
33. Milner AD. Effects of 15% oxygen on breathing patterns and oxygenation in infants. *BMJ.* 1998;316:873-874.

CHAPTER 65

Fever in the Returned Traveler

Matthew B. Laurens, Julia Hutter, and Miriam K. Laufer

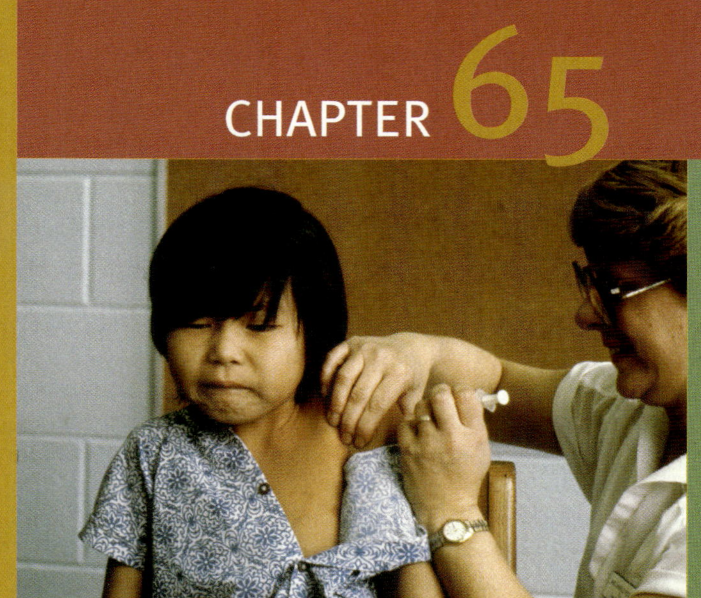

DEFINITIONS AND EPIDEMIOLOGY

More than 50 million people travel to the tropics and the developing world every year and are exposed to diseases that are not commonly seen in the United States and other developed countries. Even though child travelers represent only a small fraction of this number, they constitute about a quarter of all travel-related hospital admissions.[1] Management of sick children after international travel is complicated: febrile illness caused by common, universally transmitted infections such as respiratory and gastrointestinal viruses is extremely common in this population, yet children are also vulnerable to tropical infections acquired during the travel. Although pediatric data are lacking, the etiology of fever among returned travelers is generally equally distributed among the tropical diseases, commonly acquired infections (those found both in developed and developing countries) and illnesses of unknown etiology. Thus, a complete evaluation requires elements that are not usually included in a general pediatric review: assessment of travel vaccinations and prophylaxis, specific destination and exposure history, and probable incubation period. The most common tropical diseases in the returning traveler are malaria, traveler's diarrhea, dengue, rickettsiosis, and typhoid fever.

Resources available to assist in this evaluation include the Centers for Disease Control (CDC) travel Web site (http://www.cdc.gov/travel), the CDC's publication entitled *Health Information for International Travel* also known as The Yellow Book (http://www.cdc.gov/travel/yb/) and the World Health Organization Web site with information on the health risks by country (http://www.who.int/countries/en/). Physician-staffed travel medicine clinics are also a good source of support when evaluating illness in returned travelers.

CLINICAL PRESENTATION

Evaluation of Fever After Travel

Pretravel vaccination

Immunization records, and especially-travel specific immunization records that are often recorded on an International Certificate of Vaccination, may help to guide the evaluation. Some immunizations are highly effective and patients who have been vaccinated are at almost no risk for disease. These infections include hepatitis A and yellow fever. Other vaccines provide incomplete protection. The typhoid fever vaccinations (live and inactivated) have 50–80% efficacy against *Salmonella typhi* and offer no or limited protection against *Salmonella paratyphi*, an increasingly common cause of typhoid fever. The polysaccharide and conjugate *Neisseria meningitidis* vaccines only prevent infection with serotypes A, C, Y, and W-135.

Medication during travel

For patients who attended a travel clinic prior to travel, antimalarial medication may have been prescribed. Compliance with antimalarial prophylaxis is often poor because of the requirement for prolonged administration and real or perceived side effects. In the United States, approximately 20% of cases of malaria among travelers occured in individuals who reported taking appropriate prophylaxis.[2]

Self-treatment for traveler's diarrhea while abroad is generally recommended. For returned travelers, it is possible that febrile illnesses were partially treated by short courses of therapy with azithromycin, fluoroquinolones, or antifolates. These medications may alter the typical presentation or interfere with diagnosis of bacterial and parasitic infections, including typhoid fever and malaria.

Detailed travel history

The precise locations visited should be elicited with specific questions about the itinerary. Developing countries have variable distributions of disease risk, as indicated in Table 65–1. Within countries, the distribution of disease is not uniform, so country level information may not be sufficient to determine risk of some diseases. The resources listed above provide detailed description of the prevalence of diseases within countries, when available. Specific descriptions of travel conditions including the type of accommodation and rural versus urban areas should be elicited. Those staying with family members or in open-air lodges may have more exposures to mosquitoes compared to those staying in air-conditioned hotels. Rural areas may have a higher risk for malaria than urban areas depending on the country visited. In contrast, dengue is more frequently transmitted in urban settings. Also important to ask is the weather pattern of the area visited as mosquito-borne pathogens are more likely to occur during the rainy season when compared to dry months whereas endemic meningococcal meningitis spreads during the dry season. Occasionally, the mode of transportation used may be important, as some diseases have been linked to outbreaks on airplanes and cruise ships.

Exposure history

Specific potentially infectious contacts should be elicited, including exposure to animals, animal bites or freshwater lakes and ponds that may harbor schistosomes or leptospires. Other important factors in assessing risk of disease are foods eaten and where these foods were prepared, type of water consumed and its source, and history of mosquito and/or tick bites. For adolescents and young adults, a history of sexual contact, types of sexual activity and protective measures used should be obtained. Tattooing, body piercing, and intravenous drug use are also potential sources of infection for adolescent travelers. Although it is helpful to identify exposures to individuals with known infections, such as tuberculosis or meningitis, this level of detail is often not available as travelers come into contact with many individuals they do not know well during travel and diagnostic capacity may be limited. Another important aspect is to inquire about the health of others who traveled together with the child. Family members typically accompany pediatric travelers and the trip may have been part of a commercial or informal group tour. Others in the group might have shared the same exposure and developed a similar illness.

Incubation period

The estimated incubation period may assist in determining the cause of a child's fever. This period is a range from the first to the last possible encounter with the putative exposure. In general, incubation periods can be considered short (<1 wk), occurring almost immediately after exposure or moderate in duration, in which case some delay between exposure and clinical manifestation of disease is common. Some of the diseases cause a chronic or relapsing illness that may present with a remote history of international travel. Table 65–2 lists likely incubation periods for infectious causes of fever in the returned traveler.

Physical examination

Many of the travel-related infections discussed below present with fever without any distinguishing physical findings. They may be associated with nonspecific symptoms and laboratory abnormalities such as anemia, jaundice, hepatosplenomegaly, or lymphadenopathy. Table 65–3 lists some of the physical findings that may help to direct the subsequent evaluation of a travel-related illness.

DIFFERENTIAL DIAGNOSIS

The differential diagnosis for fever in the returned traveler must include both travel-related and cosmopolitan illnesses. The detailed discussion below will focus on illnesses associated with travel. Table 65–4 contains a list of common and uncommon travel-related causes of fever.

DIAGNOSIS

The initial evaluation should focus on identifying critical infections and gathering baseline data. The acute, life-threatening infection in this context is likely to be malaria. If exposure to malaria is possible based on the travel history, a thick and thin smear for malaria should be obtained. If the results are negative but there is clinical suspicion of malaria, the smears can be repeated at least three times every 12 hours. Blood cultures should be drawn preferably before antibiotic therapy is started. Identification and sensitivity testing of organisms may be crucial because of the widespread antimicrobial resistance. If a patient presents during the acute phase of infection, a serum sample should be stored for later comparison of serologic titers for diagnosis.

General screening laboratory tests rarely provide a definitive diagnosis but may offer support of a particular etiology and establish a baseline to follow in ill patients. A blood count with differential can be helpful. Neutrophil predominance is often seen in bacterial infections, including leptospirosis and enteric fever; lymphocytosis is more common in viral or rickettsial infection, while eosinophilia typically occurs in acute schistosomiasis or with other helminthic infections. Leukopenia is typically seen in dengue fever and can be seen in enteric fever. Thrombocytopenia is characteristic of dengue and

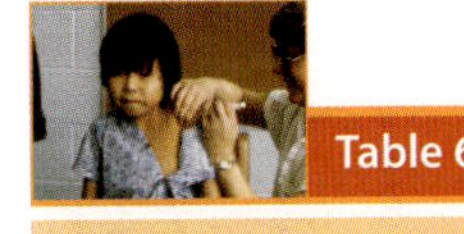

Table 65–1.

The Distribution of Diseases by Specific Regions

Key Region	Malaria	Dengue	Hepatitis A	Rickettsiae	Typhoid Fever	Leptospirosis	Amebiasis	Schistosomiasis	Trypanosomiasis	Tb	Yellow Fever
North Africa	S	S	W	W	S, H	S	W	S, H		W, H	
Central, E, W Africa	W, H	S, H	W	W	S, H	W, H	S	W, H	S, H	W, H	S, H
Southern Africa	S, H	S	S, H	W, H	S	S	S	S, H	S	W, H	
Mexico, Central America, Caribbean	S	S, H	W, H	S	S, H	W, H	W	S	S	S, H	L
South America	S, H	S, H	W	S	S, H	W, H	W	S	S	S, H	S, H
East Asia	S	S, H	W, H	W	S	W	S	S		W	
Southeast Asia	W	W, H	W, H	W, H	W	W, H	S	W		W	
South Asia	W, H	S, H	W	W, H	W, H	W, H	W	L		W	
Middle East	W, H	S, H	W	S	S	S	W	S		W	

L, local transmission documented but rare; S, sporadic, focal, or seasonal transmission in region; W, widespread transmission; H, epidemic activity or high-risk infection in some areas; Blank, no reported cases (does not necessarily mean there is no risk).

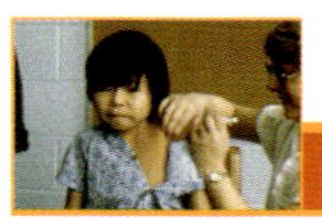

Table 65–2.

Incubation Periods of Travel-Related Infections

Short (<1 wk)	Moderate Duration (<1 mo)	Chronic or Relapsing Illness
Enteric bacterial and viral infections	Malaria	Malaria (*P. vivax and P. ovale*)
Pneumonia	Hepatitis A	Hepatitis B, C
Influenza and parainfluenza	Typhoid fever	Schistosomiasis
Dengue and other arboviral infections	Rickettsia	Amebiasis (colonic or hepatic)
Meningococcal infections	Leptospirosis	Lymphatic filariasis
Yellow fever and other viral hemorrhagic fevers	Amebiasis (colonic or hepatic)	Tuberculosis
Plague	Anthrax	Leishmaniasis
	Acute schistosomiasis (Katayama fever)	Chagas disease
	Brucellosis	Tick-borne or louse-borne relapsing fever
	HIV-acute retroviral syndrome	HIV
	Rabies	Meliodosis
	Brucellosis	
	Measles	
	African sleeping sickness (African trypanosomiasis)	
	Chagas disease (American trypanosomiasis)	
	Tick-borne or louse-borne relapsing fever	
	Hantavirus	
	Meliodosis	

malaria. Elevated hematocrit may be a sign of impending deterioration in a patient with dengue. Hepatic transaminases will be very high in viral hepatitis although mild elevation is common in most systemic infections inlcuding typhoid fever, rickettsial infections, malaria and schistosomiasis. Elevated bilirubin occurs in viral hepatitis, leptospirosis, and malaria. Renal dysfunction may be seen in leptospirosis and in some cases of malaria. Urine or stool microscopy may reveal schistosoma eggs.

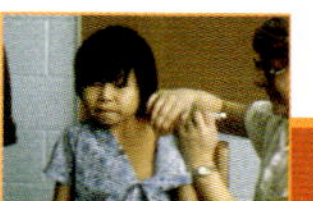

Table 65–3.

Physical Findings Associated with Travel-Related Illness

Organ System	Finding	Potential Diagnoses
Vital signs	Pulse-temperature dissociation	Typhoid fever, rickettsial disease
Skin	Maculopapular rash	Dengue fever, leptospirosis, rickettsial disease, acute HIV infection, hepatitis B
	Pink macules (rose spots)	Typhoid fever
	Necrotic ulcer (eschar)	Rickettsial diseases, Buruli ulcer
	Petechiae (or other evidence of bleeding)	Dengue fever, meningococcemia
	Jaundice	Hepatitis, leptospirosis, malaria
Eyes	Conjunctivitis	Leptospirosis
Lungs	Inspiratory crackles or wheezes	Tuberculosis, pulmonary leptospirosis
	Pleural effusion	DHF
Abdomen	Splenomegaly	Malaria, visceral leishmaniasis, typhoid fever, brucellosis
	Tenderness	Typhoid fever
Lymph nodes	Disseminated lymphadenopathy	Leptospirosis, tuberculosis, acute HIV infection, visceral leishmaniasis, brucellosis, tularemia
	Localized lymphadenopathy	Rickettsial infection extrapulmonary tuberculosis, trypanosomiasis, filariasis, plague

HIV, human immunodeficiency virus.

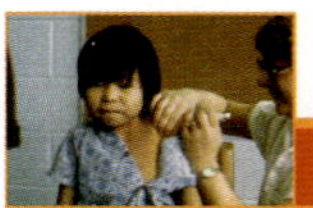

Table 65–4.

Specific Infectious Causes of Illness Among Febrile Returned Travelers, in Order of Decreasing Frequency

Illness	Prevalence (%)	Diagnostic Test	Treatment
Malaria	21	Thick and thin blood films. May need to repeat if negative	Quinidine plus either doxycycline or clindamycin, atovaquone-proguanil or mefloquine If *P. vivax* or *P. ovale* is confirmed, may use chloroquine and should administer primaquine* to treat the liver stage infection
Dengue	6	Serologic diagnosis	Supportive care: - Fluid support and resuscitation - Monitor for bleeding - Blood product transfusion if needed
Rickettsial infection	2	Serological diagnosis PCR where available	Doxycycline
Typhoid fever	2	Blood or bone marrow aspirate culture	Ceftriaxone or a fluoroquinolone for empiric therapy until susceptibility profile is known
Leptospirosis	Rare	Serology (rapid testing is available) with confirmatory culture, PCR, or MAT	Penicillin, doxycycline, cefotaxime, ceftriaxone, or azithromycin
Acute schistosomiasis (Katayama fever)	Rare	Concentrated stool and/or filtered urine examination Serological testing	Severe acute disease: Praziquantel and corticosteroids Mild-moderate acute disease: timing of therapy is controversial, consult tropical infectious disease specialist
Amebic liver abscess	Rare	Serology plus CT scan of liver	Metronidazole or tinidazole After treatment, administer paromomycin, iodoquinol, or diloxanide furoate to eliminate intestinal colonization

**Should only be administered after ascertaining normal G6PD levels.*

CT, computed tomography; MAT, microscopic agglutination test; PCR, polymerase chain reaction.

Adapted from Wilson ME, Weld LH, Boggild A, et al. Fever in returned travelers: Results from the geosentinel surveillance network. Clin Infect Dis. 2007;44(12):1560–1568.

Further evaluation should be tailored around history and clinical presentation. Table 65–5 lists specific syndromes and suggested laboratory evaluation.

INITIAL MANAGEMENT

A tiered approach to the initial management of this population of patients should focus on controlling potential life-threatening illnesses, followed by assessment for the most likely causes, then finally consideration of less common causes, if the initial evaluation is negative. An algorithm is shown in Figure 65–1. If exposure to malaria is possible and laboratory capabilities do not permit immediate, reliable readings of the malaria blood smear, empiric therapy should be considered. In the child traveler, frequent causes of fever such as pneumonia, urinary tract infection, and bacteremia should be evaluated and empiric therapy prescribed according to standard guidelines. If the first battery of tests does not yield a definite diagnosis or the patient appears very ill, consultation with an infectious disease specialist experienced in tropical medicine should be considered.

Infection control should be reviewed urgently in cases of sick patients who have traveled abroad, as international contagious diseases may have a different clinical presentation than the usual triggers for isolation procedures in hospitals in developed countries. Isolation should be instituted immediately in cases suspicious of viral hemorrhagic fever, tuberculosis, or any unusual respiratory condition. Respiratory symptoms in the context of recent intensive exposure to birds should prompt immediate isolation and evaluation for avian influenza. Consider contacting local public health authorities if you suspect a potentially contagious source.

DIAGNOSIS AND MANAGEMENT OF SPECIFIC INFECTIONS

Malaria

Malaria is caused by four human *Plasmodium* species: *falciparum*, *vivax*, *ovale*, and *malariae*. *P. falciparum* is the most common infecting species and causes a potentially lethal form of the disease. More than 1000 cases of

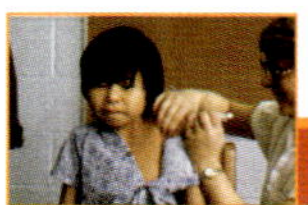

Table 65–5.

Evaluation for Fever in Returned Travelers who have Localizing Signs or Symptoms

Diarrhea	Stool examination for ova and parasites ■ Include antigen detection assays for *Giardia*, *Cryptosporidium*, *Entameba histolytica*, and special staining for *Cryptosporidium*, *Cyclspora*, and *microsporidium* as indicated. ■ Multiple O and P specimens may be needed to detect *Strongyloides* as a result of the intermittent shedding of eggs Stool culture is most useful if antibiotics were not administered
Lower respiratory tract	Acute: ■ Chest radiograph, assessment for viral respiratory pathogens ■ Legionella antigen, bacterial and fungal sputum, and blood culture; if clinically indicated ■ Evaluation for disseminated helminth infection: schistosomiasis, strongyloidiasis, hookworm, ascariasis Prolonged: ■ Tuberculosis screening and sputum microscopy ■ HIV testing ■ Testing for histoplasmosis or coccidiomycosis (if exposure is suspected)
Central nervous system symptoms	■ Imaging of central nervous system for increased intracranial pressure prior to LP, cerebral edema, ischemic lesion, parasitic lesions, abscess ■ CSF culture and direct examination for organisms (bacteria, parasites) ■ Serology for leptospirosis, dengue, rickettsiae, rabies
Petechiae or hemorrhage	■ Blood culture ■ Serological tests for viruses (Ebola, Lassa, Marburg, yellow fever), serology for rickettsia, leptospirosis and dengue, coagulation panel
Eosinophilia	■ Stool examination for ova and parasites ■ As indicated based on exposure: serology for schistosomiasis, strongyloiasis, examination of blood smears or skin snips for microfilariae
Adenopathy	■ Blood culture ■ Serology for leptospirosis, HIV, Epstein-Barr virus and cytomegalovirus, bartonella, toxoplasma, tularemia, and rickettsiae ■ Tuberculin skin testing ■ Culture and stain body fluids or tissues for: acid fast bacilli, leishmaniasis, trypanosomiasis (depending on region)

HIV, human immunodeficiency virus; O and P, ova and parasites.

malaria occur in the United States every year, almost all are imported cases.[2] Malaria parasites are transmitted to the human by the bite of *Anopheles* mosquitoes. After injection into the blood stream by the mosquito, the parasites immediately enter the liver and replicated there. In *falciparum* malaria, the parasites exit the liver after 1–2 weeks and begin the blood stage of infection, which causes disease. As the parasites replicate in red blood cells, rupture and infect new cells, the typical signs and symptoms of fever, chills and anemia develop. Respiratory and gastrointestinal complaints may also be associated with malaria. The time from initial infection to clinical illness may be prolonged in patients who received antimalarial prophylaxis, treatment with antibiotics with antimalarial properties or preexisting immunity. *P. vivax* and *P. ovale* have the unique ability to persist for long periods of time in the liver as hypnozoites. Blood stage infection that causes malaria illness can develop months to years after exposure. In the absence of treatment of the liver stage of the disease (typically with primaquine), disease can recur even after effective treatment of the blood-stage parasites. The diagnosis and management of malaria is discussed in Chapter 66.

Dengue

Dengue virus is the most important arboviral infection among travelers.[3] It is transmitted by the *Aedes aegypti* mosquito and typically presents as a nonspecific, self-limited febrile illness, but secondary infection (infection with a new serotype) can cause the severe manifestations of dengue hemorrhagic fever (DHF) and dengue shock syndrome (DSS).

Dengue is responsible for 11–33% of fevers among children in Southeast Asia.[4,5] Although the incidence of dengue in Latin America is similar to Southeast Asia, the disease is more evenly distributed among the adults and children in both the Americas. Dengue is the

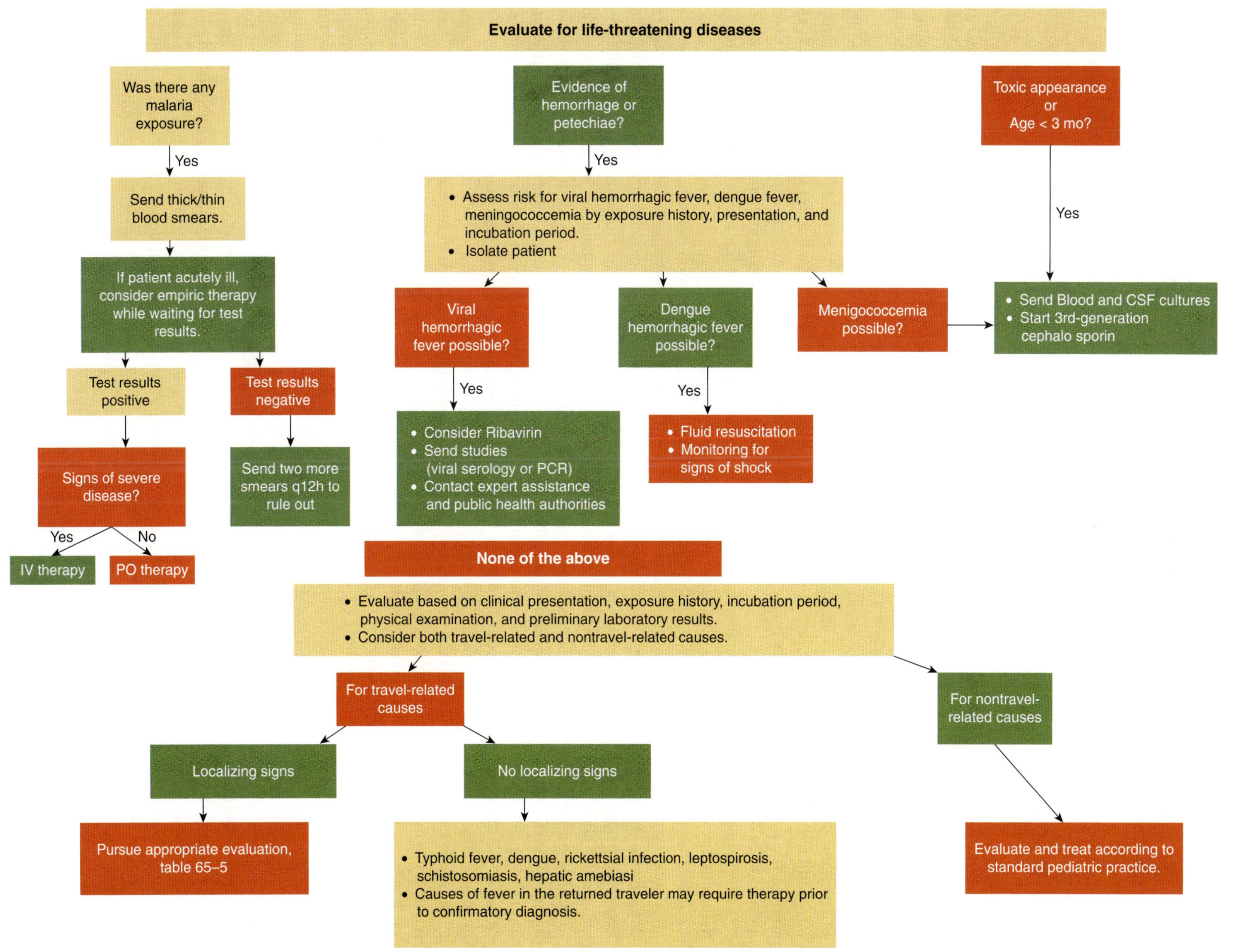

Evaluate for life-threatening diseases
Was there any malaria exposure?
Yes
Send thick/thin blood smears.
If patient acutely ill, consider empiric therapy while waiting for test results.
Test results positive
Test results negative
Signs of severe disease?
Yes
No
IV therapy
PO therapy
Send two more smears q12h to rule out
Evidence of hemorrhage or petechiae?
Yes
• Assess risk for viral hemorrhagic fever, dengue fever, meningococcemia by exposure history, presentation, and incubation period.
• Isolate patient
Viral hemorrhagic fever possible?
Yes
• Consider Ribavirin
• Send studies (viral serology or PCR)
• Contact expert assistance and public health authorities
Dengue hemorrhagic fever possible?
Yes
• Fluid resuscitation
• Monitoring for signs of shock
Menigococcemia possible?
Toxic appearance or Age < 3 mo?
Yes
• Send Blood and CSF cultures
• Start 3rd-generation cephalo sporin
None of the above
• Evaluate based on clinical presentation, exposure history, incubation period, physical examination, and preliminary laboratory results.
• Consider both travel-related and nontravel-related causes.
For travel-related causes
Localizing signs
Pursue appropriate evaluation, table 65–5
No localizing signs
• Typhoid fever, dengue, rickettsial infection, leptospirosis, schistosomiasis, hepatic amebiasi
• Causes of fever in the returned traveler may require therapy prior to confirmatory diagnosis.
For nontravel-related causes
Evaluate and treat according to standard pediatric practice.

FIGURE 65–1 ■ Algorithm for management of febrile returned traveler.

leading cause of systemic febrile illness among travelers returning from Southeast Asia, the Caribbean, and Central America.[6] Dengue occurs in most other regions of the world but is extremely rare in travelers to Africa.

Symptomatic dengue infection is classified into three syndromes: dengue fever, DHF, and DSS. The typical presentation of dengue fever includes fever, severe headache, myalgias, and arthralgias. The pain is so severe that it is often referred to as "break-bone fever." Rash may appear after the onset of fever. A typical finding that occurs in approximately 50% of patients with dengue fever is a positive tourniquet test. The test is performed by inflating a blood pressure cuff halfway between the systolic and diastolic blood pressures for approximately 5 minutes. After release, the number of petechiae in a 2.5 × 2.5 cm patch is counted. Greater than 20 petechiae indicates a positive test. The fever may have a "saddleback pattern" in which a second episode of fever and symptoms develop after an initial resolution. Mild mucosal bleeding may occur, but rarely is the amount life threatening. Fatigue may linger for up to 6 months after dengue infection.

DHF and DSS occur almost exclusively in individuals who have previous infection with a heterologous strain of one of the four dengue serotypes. DHF and DSS are clinical syndromes with World Health Organization-defined case definitions that have been called into question recently and may undergo revision.[7] In general, the criteria for DHF are: fever for 2–7 days, hemorrhage, thrombocytopenia (<100,000 platelets/mm^3) and hemoconcentration (>20% rise in hematocrit over baseline), or evidence of increased capillary permeability (pleural effusion, ascites, low serum protein). The tourniquet test is almost always positive. The severe presentation of DSS usually occurs after the thrombocytopenia and plasma leakage. It is characterized by a rapid, weak pulse with narrowed pulse pressure or hypotension with cool extremities and restlessness.[8]

The diagnosis of dengue is most frequently made by comparing paired serological titers. A specimen should be obtained within the first 5 days of symptoms. This acute-phase sample can be used for virus isolation and detection of IgG and IgM. In dengue, IgM frequently rises later in the course of illness so early diagnosis is often difficult. A convalescent phase specimen should be obtained at least 1 week after the onset of symptoms. The testing is done by the CDC and the specimens can be sent directly or through the state laboratory. In dengue-endemic countries, rapid tests are often used, but none are available in the United States.

The treatment of dengue is symptomatic with an emphasis on fluid resuscitation. In patients with dengue fever, a rising hematocrit is often the first sign of impending DHF/DSS and increased fluid administration may avert severe disease. In patients who develop shock, a fluid bolus of 25 cc/kg over 2 hours followed by maintenance plus replacement fluids is associated with excellent survival. Colloid and crystalloid are equally effective in most patients but colloid is preferred in the most severe cases.[9,10] Antipyretics that interfere with coagulation, such as aspirin and nonsteroidal anti-inflammatory drugs, should be avoided in cases of dengue because of the increased risk of hemorrhage.

Rickettsial Infections

Rickettsial infections present with an influenza-like febrile illness often associated with rash and an eschar at the site of inoculation. Because these infections are difficult to diagnose, rickettsial illnesses are under-recognized.[11] Clinical suspicion and obtaining appropriate specimens for diagnosis are therefore essential.

Rickettsial infections are usually transmitted by arthropod vectors such as ticks, lice, fleas, and mites. Most travelers with rickettsial infections do not recall an arthropod bite.[12] Outdoor activities during travel including camping, hiking and safari excursions in areas of known transmission increase the risk of exposure to these infections.

The most common rickettsial infection in travelers is African tick bite fever. The disease occurs as a result of the infection with *Rickettsia africae* carried by ticks in sub-Saharan Africa. The ticks that carry the infection usually feed on cattle but also on large animals found in game parks. Other rickettsial infections occasionally found in travelers include Mediterranean spotted fever, murine typhus and scrub typhus, caused by *R. conorii*, *R. typhi*, and *Orientia tsutsugamushi*, respectively.[13]

The incubation period is around 1–2 weeks. Common symptoms include fever, myalgia, headache, and rash. An eschar at the site of the original insect bite with regional lymphadenophathy is a characteristic finding. Infections often cause leukopenia, thrombocytopenia, and elevated liver enzymes. The ticks that carry African tick bite fever attack aggressively, and it is common for infected individuals to have several eschars representing multiple bites after exposure. There are no life-threatening complications of African tick bite fever and no fatalities have been reported.[14] Complications have rarely been reported with Mediterranean spotted fever and murine typhus, but untreated scrub typhus can lead to multiorgan failure and death.

The mainstay of diagnosis is serological testing. Indirect immunofluorescence assay and enzyme immunoassay are the recommended and commercially available techniques with the highest sensitivity and specificity for rickettsial infection. Low or moderate levels of antibodies during the initial phase of the illness may represent previous exposure to rickettsial infection, and cross-reactivity of antibodies between different rickettsial species may occur. Definitive diagnosis can only be made with the detection of a fourfold rise in IgG titers between acute and convalescent specimens over a 2–3-week period. High IgM titers may aid in the confirmation of acute or recent infection. These serological assays often cannot distinguish the specific species causing infection. Further testing at reference laboratories may be required, if speciation is needed. Polymerase chain reaction (PCR) assays of whole blood or tissue yield rapid results, but are currently only available in reference and research laboratories. Diagnosis can also be made through immunohistologic detection by indirect immunofluorescence assay staining of tissue samples. Shell vial culture of the organisms for species diagnosis is potentially hazardous and should only be done by specialized laboratories.

Treatment must be initiated based on clinical suspicion because of the delay in obtaining confirmatory laboratory results. It is most effective if initiated within the first week of illness. Doxycycline 2 mg/kg (100 mg maximum) administered twice a day is given orally or intravenously. The duration of therapy is usually 5–14 days depending on the severity of illness and the response to therapy. Treatment should continue for 3 days after defervescence.[15] Even though doxycycline may cause dental staining in children younger than 8 years, the risk of a short course of therapy is justified in the face of this potentially life-threatening disease. Chloramphenicol is effective in treating most forms of rickettsiosis. Although this medication is rarely used in the United States, it is frequently administered for a variety of illnesses in developing countries. Third-generation cephalosporins are active against scrub typhus and ciprofloxacin is an effective alternative to treat Mediterranean spotted fever.

Almost all rickettsial infections respond rapidly to doxycycline. If treatment is initiated based on clinical suspicion and there is no response after 48 hours, the diagnosis of rickettsial infection should be reconsidered.

Leptospirosis

Leptospirosis is a disease caused by the pathogenic spirochete *Leptospira* species found in urine and feces of wild and domestic animals. It is endemic in tropical and subtropical climates where outbreaks may be seasonally related to increased rainfall and warmer weather. Exposure can occur through direct contact with animals or their excretions, contact with infected freshwater or after flooding in urban or rural areas where infected animals live. Transmission occurs when mucous membranes or compromised skin contact contaminated water, soil, or vegetation. After hematogenous dissemination, the pathogen can invade a wide variety of tissues. Disease is caused by both direct infection and the host immune response.

Most cases of leptospirosis are subclinical and do not come to medical attention. Recognized cases of systemic leptospirosis classically present with biphasic illness, although this might not be appreciated by the patient. The initial, acute presentation is characterized by a febrile illness with headache, myalgia, and prostration. Conjunctival suffusion and muscle tenderness are characteristic findings during this stage. The acute, septicemic phase is followed by the immune phase where antibody is produced and organisms are excreted in urine. During this stage of the illness, most patients recover and develop immunity to further infection, but a minority may progress to severe leptospirosis. In cases of severe disease, aseptic meningitis and anterior uveitis can develop. Spontaneous pulmonary hemorrhage syndrome associated with leptospirosis is increasing in frequency and is associated with a 50% mortality rate.[16] The classical form of severe disease is icteric leptospirosis, known as Weil's disease, with jaundice, renal failure, and hemorrhage. The characteristic laboratory finding is elevated bilirubin out of proportion to liver transaminases. As a result of a similar clinical presentation and geographic distribution, leptospirosis is often confused with dengue fever.[17]

Microscopic agglutination test (MAT) is most commonly employed to make a diagnosis. Rapid tests are available from the CDC, but should always be confirmed by either a culture of blood or other body fluids, a positive PCR of blood or serum, or demonstration of seroconversion based on the MAT performed on samples obtained 2 weeks apart.[18] Blood culture specimens should be obtained early in the course of illness as leptospiremia begins before symptom onset and ends 1 week after illness onset. After the second week of illness, the organisms are excreted in urine, so a urine culture may be diagnostic. Urinary excretion may persist for several weeks. Special medium for blood and body fluid cultures is available commercially, but growth may take up to 13 weeks.[19]

The treatment of leptospirosis requires early antibiotic therapy, monitoring and supportive care. Penicillin, doxycycline, cefotaxime, ceftriaxone, and azithromycin are effective therapies. Although penicillin has been considered the treatment of choice for severe disease, trials in Thailand found that cephalosporins and doxycycline are as effective as penicillin in the treatment of severe disease and have the advantage of also treating rickettsial infections that may either be clinically indistinguishable at first or occur concurrently.[20,21] Ceftriaxone allows for once-daily dosing and does not require adjustment in renal failure. Jarisch-Herxheimer reaction can occur with the initiation of beta-lactam therapy.

Typhoid Fever

Typhoid fever, also known as enteric fever, is most commonly caused by infection with *S. typhi* and less often, but with increasing frequency, *S. paratyphi.* The vast majority of cases in the United States are travel related. *S. typhi* and *S. paratyhpi* only infect humans and are transmitted through the fecal–oral route with an infectious dose of 10^3 to 10^6 organisms.[22] Common sources for infection are water and food contaminated by infected individuals. Chronic carriers are asymptomatic and the carrier state can be prolonged. The highest incidence of disease is found in South Asia, followed by Southeast Asia and travel-associated infection occurs in a similar distribution.[6]

When *S. typhi* is ingested, the low gastric pH serves as a key barrier in preventing further passage. Surviving organisms then enter the small intestine to adhere to and penetrate mucosal cells. After invasion, the bacteria travel through intestinal lymph nodes and can invade bone marrow, liver, and spleen. Salmonella organisms multiply in mononuclear cells and then cause clinically apparent disease when large numbers of organisms enter the general circulation.

The incubation period for typhoid fever is approximately 7–14 days. The onset of generalized nonspecific symptoms, such as fever, malaise, and headache usually correlates with the release of the organism into the bloodstream. Fever rises in a "stepladder" pattern to 39–40°C by the second week of illness, when patients often start to appear toxic and have sustained fever. Diarrhea is more common in children, while constipation occurs more frequently in adults. Other common symptoms are nausea, vomiting, and abdominal cramping. Because of the widespread use of suboptimal selection or dose of antibiotics, presentation and course of illness may be atypical.

Frequent physical examination findings are hepatomegaly, splenomegaly and abdominal tenderness. The pathognomonic rose spots, blanching erythematous macular lesions approximately 2–4 mm in diameter, are seen in about a third of cases. Relative bradycardia in relation to the amount of fever is considered a characteristic sign of typhoid fever, but only occurs in about a quarter of cases. Hematologic evaluation may show early leukocytosis or leukopenia, anemia, thrombocytopenia, and clotting abnormalities. Commonly, liver enzymes are moderately elevated. Pyuria, proteinuria, and casts may be seen on urine analysis. EKG may show nonspecific ST-wave and T-wave abnormalities.

Complicated disease occurs in approximately 10% of cases in endemic areas. The most common complications are intestinal perforation and hemorrhage. Encephalopathy with altered mental status and intermittent confusion, delirium, or coma is associated with a high case fatality rate. Extraintestinal infections are rare but the organism can cause meningitis, pneumonia, myocarditis, hepatitis and splenic and liver abscesses.[23] The incidence of complicated disease and case fatality for typhoid fever is very low in the United States where adequate access to diagnosis and therapy is available. In the developing world, poorly or untreated cases of complicated disease carry a fatality rate of 30–50%.[24,25]

Following illness, 45% of children younger than 5 years excrete Salmonella for 12 weeks or more, compared to 5% of older children and adults.[26] Approximately 1–5% of patients become chronic carriers harboring Salmonella in the gallbladder or rarely in the genitourinary system for more than 1 year.[27]

Cultures of blood or bone marrow positive for *S. typhi* or *S. paratyphi* are diagnostic. Stool cultures are useful in identifying excretion and chronic carriage, but are not diagnostic for enteric fever. The sensitivity of blood cultures ranges from 30% to 90%. The highest yield results from large volume blood cultures obtained early in the course of illness. Bone marrow cultures have much higher sensitivity (85–90%) and remain positive after antibiotic treatment is initiated.[28] Although bone marrow aspirate is an invasive procedure, it should be considered in patients in whom there is a high suspicion for typhoid fever and blood cultures are negative. Isolation of an organism for susceptibility testing is especially important in patients returning from South and Southeast Asia where highly resistant *S. typhi* strains circulate.

The classic serologic test for *S. typhi*, the Widal test, has low sensitivity and specificity. Newer serologic rapid test kits and nucleic acid identification are being developed but are not yet commercially avaible.[29]

Treatment is complicated by widespread plasmid-mediated multidrug resistance to traditional first choice antibiotics such as chloramphenicol, ampicillin, and trimethoprim-sulfamethoxazole. Fluoroquinolones are preferred because they achieve high intracellular concentration and are excreted in the biliary system, where Salmonellae often cause chronic infection that leads to the persistent carrier state. The risk of administering a relatively short course of fluoroquinolones to young children is generally outweighed by the excellent efficacy of the drug and the ability to administer the medication orally. Ofloxacin or ciprofloxacin (15 mg/kg) is recommended for 5–7 days for uncomplicated disease and 10–14 days for complicated disease. Intravenous third-generation cephalosporins are also effective and there is increasing evidence that azithromycin may be an effective oral alternative.[27,30]

In some areas of South and Southeast Asia, chromosomally acquired resistance to fluoroquinolones—the current first choice treatment—has become prevalent over the last decade.[31] Assessment of fluoroquinolone clinical susceptibility should be based on both fluoroquinolone (such as ciprofloxacin or ofloxacin) and quinolone (nalidixic acid) disk testing. Nalidixic acid-resistance based on in vitro testing, even when the fluoroquinolone MIC falls within the susceptible range, is a predictor of poor clinical response to fluoroquinolones.[32] Therefore, infections should be treated as if they are fluoroquinolone resistant if they are resistant to nalixidic acid.

First line therapy for fluoroquinolone-resistant typhoid fever is a third-generation cephalosporin such as ceftriaxone (75 mg/kg for 10–14 days) or cefotaxime (80 mg for 10–14 days). Azithromycin (10 mg/kg for 7 days) is another option.[27,33] Hospitalization for parenteral antibiotic therapy is recommended for infants, patients who cannot tolerate oral medication, or anyone suspected of having complicated disease such as intestinal perforation or hemorrhage, shock, or encephalopathy. Hospitalization for intravenous antibiotics should be considered for all patients until the susceptibility pattern of the infecting organism is identified. Dexamethasone should be considered in patients with altered mental status or shock.

Diarrhea

Traveler's diarrhea is the leading cause of illness among returned travelers. The most common causes are: *Escherichia coli*, *Campylobacter jejuni*, *Shigella* spp., and *Salmonella* spp. Typical traveler's diarrhea may present with low-grade fever but fever is rarely a prominent complaint. This should be distinguished from dysentery which is a febrile illness with blood and mucus in the stool. Dysentery is typically caused by *Shigella* and *E. coli.* Other causes of inflammatory enteritis associated with fever that can occur after travel include *Campylobacter,* amebic dysentery, schistosomiasis, trichinosis, cholera, and typhoid fever. Most parasitic infections such as *Cryptosporidium*, *Cyclospora*, and microsporidium cause persistent diarrhea without systemic symptoms.

Prior to travel, patients are advised to carry a course of antibiotics to treat traveler's diarrhea while abroad. In cases of diarrhea in returned travelers, a bacterial stool culture may demonstrate the infecting organism. It is therefore appropriate to obtain a microbiological specimen and then begin an empiric course of antibiotics. The standard treatment for traveler's diarrhea is cirpofloxacin for 1–3 days. In children, azithromycin is another option. In cases of persistent diarrhea, stool can be examined for ova and parasites as described in Table 65–5.

Hepatitis

With the recent introduction of hepatitis A into the pediatric vaccination schedule and widespread practice of pretravel immunization, this infection is found infrequently in travelers. Evaluation of hepatitis should therefore include febrile syndromes that present with hepatitis, such as typhoid fever, rickettsial infections, leptospirosis, malaria, and schistosomiasis. For the minority of patients who have not been vaccinated for hepatitis A or B, serologic testing should be obtained. Acute infection with hepatitis C is unlikely in the absence of significant exposures such as blood transfusion, injection drug use, body piercing, and unprotected intercourse. Travelers to South Asia and North Africa may be at risk for infection with hepatitis E, but infections usually occur in outbreaks and infection in children is rare.

REFERENCES

1. Cossar JH, Reid D, Fallon RJ, et al. A cumulative review of studies on travellers, their experience of illness and the implications of these findings. *J Infect.* 1990;21(1):27-42.
2. Skarbinski J, James EM, Causer LM, et al. Malaria surveillance–United States, 2004. *MMWR Surveill Summ.* 2006; 55(4):23-37.
3. Wilder-Smith A, Schwartz E. Dengue in travelers. *N Engl J Med.* 2005;353(9):924-932.
4. Anderson KB, Chunsuttiwat S, Nisalak A, et al. Burden of symptomatic dengue infection in children at primary school in thailand: a prospective study. *Lancet.* 2007; 369(9571):1452-1459.
5. Phuong HL, De Vries PJ, Nga TT, et al. Dengue as a cause of acute undifferentiated fever in Vietnam. *BMC Infect Dis.* 2006;6:123.
6. Freedman DO, Weld LH, Kozarsky PE, et al. Spectrum of disease and relation to place of exposure among ill returned travelers. *N Engl J Med.* 2006;354(2):119-130.
7. Deen JL, Harris E, Wills B, et al. The WHO dengue classification and case definitions: time for a reassessment. *Lancet.* 2006;368(9530):170-173.
8. World Health Organization. *Dengue Haemorrhagic Fever: Diagnosis, Treatment, Prevention and Control.* 2nd ed. Geneva, Switzerland: World Health Organization; 1997.
9. Ngo NT, Cao XT, Kneen R, et al. Acute management of dengue shock syndrome: a randomized double-blind comparison of 4 intravenous fluid regimens in the first hour. *Clin Infect Dis.* 2001;32(2):204-213.
10. Wills BA, Nguyen MD, Ha TL, et al. Comparison of three fluid solutions for resuscitation in dengue shock syndrome. *N Engl J Med.* 2005;353(9):877-889.
11. Raeber PA, Winteler S, Paget J. Fever in the returned traveller: remember rickettsial diseases. *Lancet.* 1994; 344(8918):331.
12. Jelinek T, Loscher T. Clinical features and epidemiology of tick typhus in travelers. *J Travel Med.* 2001;8(2):57-59.
13. Jensenius M, Fournier PE, Raoult D. Rickettsioses and the international traveler. *Clin Infect Dis.* 2004;39(10): 1493-1499.
14. Jensenius M, Fournier PE, Kelly P, Myrvang B, Raoult D. African tick bite fever. *Lancet Infect Dis.* 2003;3(9):557-564.
15. American Academy of Pediatrics. Rickettsial diseases & endemic typhus. In: Pickering LK, Baker CJ, Long SS, Mcmillan JA, eds. *Red Book: 2006 Report of the Committee on Infectious Diseases.* 27th ed. Elk Grove Village, IL: American Academy of Pediatrics; 2006:567-569,706-707.
16. Mcbride AJ, Athanazio DA, Reis MG, Ko AI. Leptospirosis. *Curr Opin Infect Dis.* 2005;18(5):376-386.

17. Vinetz JM. Leptospirosis. *Curr Opin Infect Dis.* 2001;14(5): 527-538.
18. Human leptospirosis: guidance for diagnosis, surveillance, and control. Geneva, Switzerland: World Health Organization/International Leptospirosis Society; 2003. http://www.who.int/csr/don/en/WHO_CDS_CSR_EPH_2002.23.pdf. Accessed August 12, 2008.
19. Levett PN. Leptospirosis. *Clin Microbiol Rev.* 2001;14(2): 296-326.
20. Panaphut T, Domrongkitchaiporn S, Vibhagool A, Thinkamrop B, Susaengrat W. Ceftriaxone compared with sodium penicillin G for treatment of severe leptospirosis. *Clin Infect Dis.* 2003;36(12):1507-1513.
21. Suputtamongkol Y, Niwattayakul K, Suttinont C, et al. An open, randomized, controlled trial of penicillin, doxycycline, and cefotaxime for patients with severe leptospirosis. *Clin Infect Dis.* 2004;39(10):1417-1424.
22. Hornick RB, Greisman SE, Woodward TE, Dupont HL, Dawkins AT, Snyder MJ. Typhoid fever: pathogenesis and immunologic control. 2. *N Engl J Med.* 1970;283(14): 739-746.
23. Huang DB, Dupont HL. Problem Pathogens: extra-intestinal complications of *Salmonella enterica* serotype typhi infection. *Lancet Infect Dis.* 2005;5(6):341-348.
24. Rogerson SJ, Spooner VJ, Smith TA, Richens J. Hydrocortisone in chloramphenicol-treated severe typhoid fever in Papua New Guinea. *Trans R Soc Trop Med Hyg.* 1991; 85(1):113-116.
25. Punjabi NH, Hoffman SL, Edman DC, et al. Treatment of severe typhoid fever in children with high dose dexamethasone. *Pediatr Infect Dis J.* 1988;7(8):598-600.
26. American Academy of Pediatrics. Salmonella infections. In: Pickering LK, Baker CJ, Long SS, Mcmillan JA, eds. *Red Book: 2006 Report of the Committee on Infectious Diseases.* 27th ed. Elk Grove Village, IL: American Academy of Pediatrics; 2006:579-584.
27. World Health Organization. Background document. In: Ivanoff B, Chaignat CL, eds. *The Diagnosis, Treatment and Prevention of Typhoid Fever.* Geneva, Switzerland: World Health Organization; 2003.
28. Bhan MK, Bahl R, Bhatnagar S. Typhoid And Paratyphoid Fever. *Lancet.* 2005;366(9487):749-762.
29. Kawano RL, Leano SA, Agdamag DM. Comparison of serological test kits for diagnosis of typhoid fever in the Philippines. *J Clin Microbiol.* 2007;45(1):246-247.
30. Frenck RW, Jr., Nakhla I, Sultan Y, et al. Azithromycin versus ceftriaxone for the treatment of uncomplicated typhoid fever in children. *Clin Infect Dis.* 2000;31(5): 1134-1138.
31. Threlfall EJ, Ward LR, Skinner JA, Smith HR, Lacey S. Ciprofloxacin-resistant *Salmonella typhi* and treatment failure. *Lancet.* 1999;353(9164):1590-1591.
32. Wain J, Hoa NT, Chinh NT, et al. Quinolone-resistant *Salmonella typhi* in Viet Nam: molecular basis of resistance and clinical response to treatment. *Clin Infect Dis.* 1997; 25(6):1404-1410.
33. Parry CM, Ho VA, Phuong Lt, et al. Randomized controlled comparison of ofloxacin, azithromycin, and an ofloxacin-azithromycin combination for treatment of multidrug-resistant and nalidixic acid-resistant typhoid fever. *Antimicrob Agents Chemother.* 2007;51(3):819-825.

CHAPTER 66

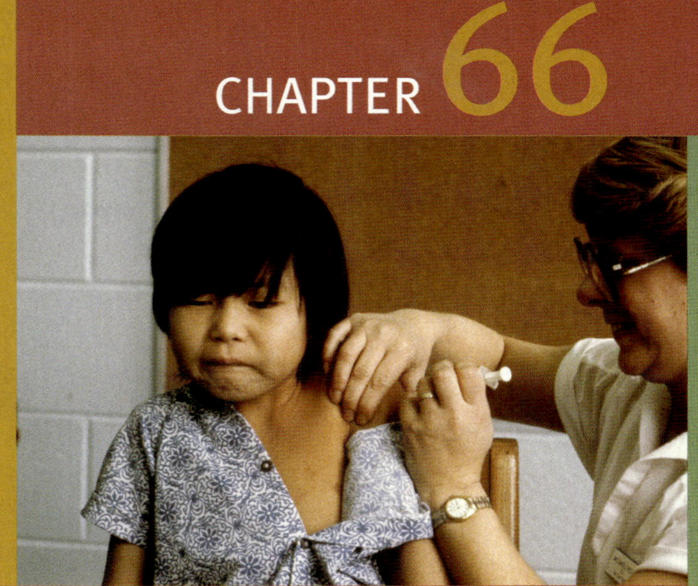

Malaria

Nadia A. Sam-Agudu and Chandy C. John

DEFINITIONS AND EPIDEMIOLOGY

Malaria is a leading cause of childhood morbidity and mortality worldwide. The burden of this disease is largely borne by children in sub-Saharan Africa. Approximately 60% of clinical cases, and more than 75% of the greater than 1 million annual deaths from malaria occur in this region, mostly in children younger than 5 years.[1,2] According to a survey, one in five childhood deaths in sub-Saharan Africa is caused by malaria.[3] In the United States, local malaria transmission, which was once endemic, has been extremely rare since the 1950s.[4] However, American physicians continue to encounter patients with malaria, mostly immigrants, refugees, returned travelers, and military personnel, who acquired their infections in endemic areas. An average of 1200 malaria cases and 13 related deaths occur in the United States every year.[4] Most of the cases are imported, most are caused by *Plasmodium falciparum*, and most are acquired in Africa.[4]

Malaria is a parasitic infectious disease that has been in existence for centuries. The name "malaria" is of Italian origin, meaning "bad air," reflecting the belief in medieval times that it was caused by exposure to foul air in swamps and marshes. This is true to some extent, because the mosquito vector breeds well in warm, humid environments. As a result, the disease is highly prevalent in tropical and subtropical areas, including sub-Saharan Africa, the Indian subcontinent, South-East Asia, and South America (Figure 66–1). Malaria is caused by the parasitic protozoan *Plasmodium,* among which there are approximately 120 species that infect mammals. Human malaria is caused by four *Plasmodium* species: *P. falciparum*, *Plasmodium vivax*, *Plasmodium ovale*, and *Plasmodium malariae. P. falciparum* is prevalent in the tropics and subtropics, specifically in sub-Saharan Africa, the Indian subcontinent, South-East Asia, and the Western Pacific.[5] It accounts for the majority of all human *Plasmodium* infections worldwide. *P. vivax* is commonly found in Asia, South America, parts of Europe, North Africa the Middle East, and the Western Pacific, particularly in Papua New Guinea.[5] It is rarely found in sub-Saharan Africa, and is virtually nonexistent in West Africa. *P. malariae* occurs sporadically in all malaria endemic areas, but is largely restricted to sub-Saharan Africa and the Western Pacific.[6] *P. ovale* is the rarest of all 4 species, and is found mainly in West Africa and the Western Pacific.[6] The definitive vector is the female *Anopheles* mosquito, which requires a blood meal in order to lay eggs.

PATHOGENESIS

The life cycle of *Plasmodium* takes place in both the human host and mosquito vector (Figure 66–2): (1) The female *Anopheles* mosquito takes a blood meal, during which it injects sporozoites (human infective stage) into the human host. The sporozoites pass through the bloodstream into the liver, (2) where, during the liver stage, they mature into schizonts, which rupture and release merozoites. Some *P. vivax* and *P. ovale* sporozoites remain dormant in the liver as hypnozoites, which may release merozoites into the bloodstream weeks, months, or even years later, causing relapses. After merozoites are released from the liver, (3) they invade red blood cells (RBCs), and during the blood stage, mature into trophozoites (ring-form), (4) in the RBCs, trophozoites multiply asexually into schizonts that rupture and release merozoites, which in turn infect more RBCs. As merozoites leave the RBC, the latter is ruptured and destroyed. As thousands of merozoites leave and rupture

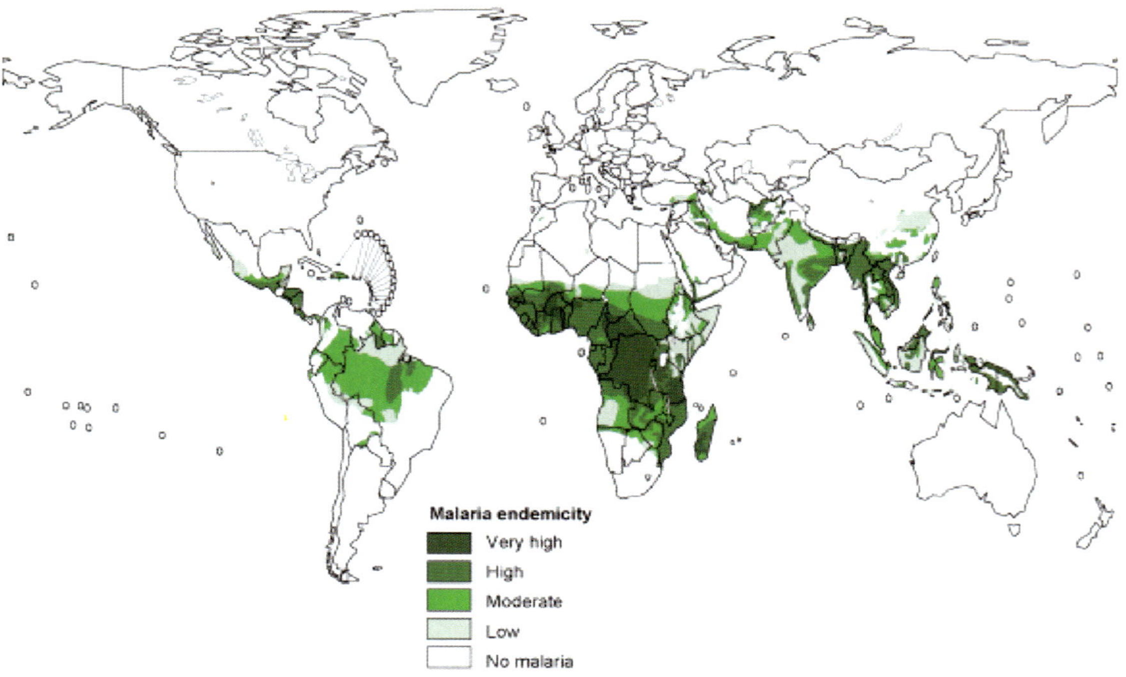

FIGURE 66–1 ■ Global malaria risk distribution. (*With permission from the World Health Organization.*)

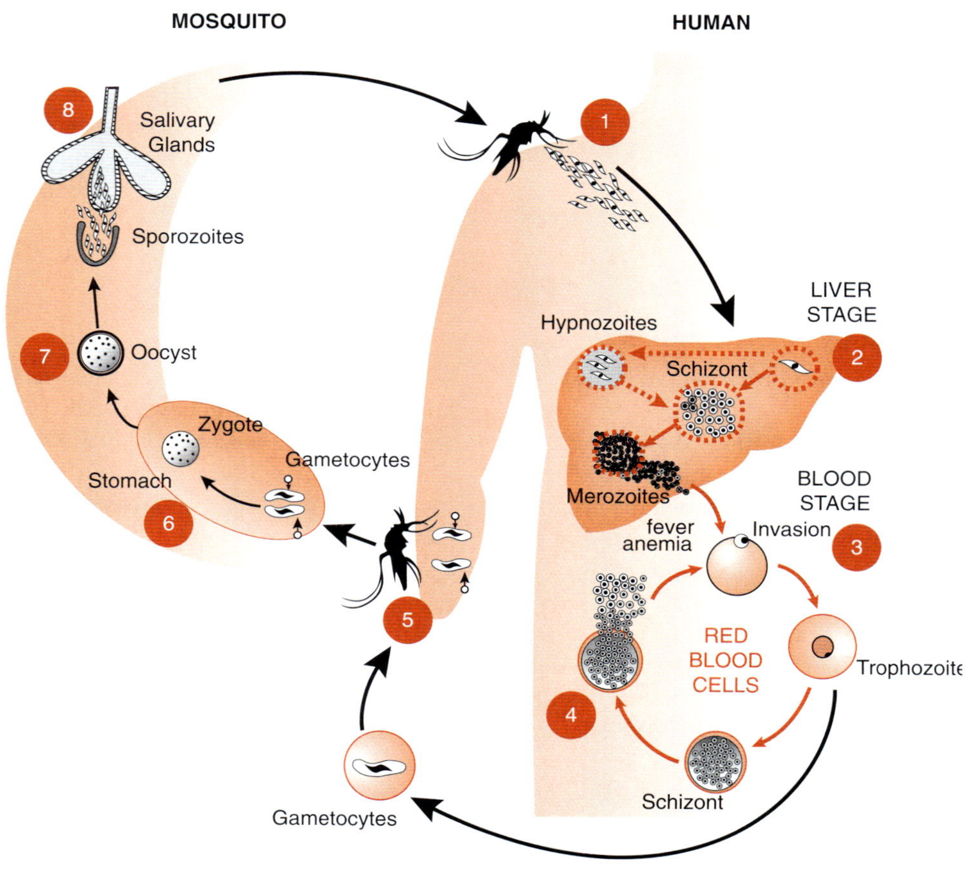

FIGURE 66–2 ■ *Plasmodium* life cycle. (*Courtesy of Adrian Akyeampong.*)

RBCs, the host becomes progressively anemic. In addition, schizont rupture and merozoite release from RBCs have been associated with a systemic proinflammatory cytokine response, in particular tumor necrosis factor-alpha (TNF-α), interleukin-1, and interferon-gamma (IFN-γ), which in turn elevate core temperature and cause fever,[7,8] (5) a small proportion of trophozoites develop into the gametocyte (sexual stage), the form that is infective to the mosquito. Both male and female gametocytes are ingested by an *Anopheles* mosquito during a blood meal from the infected human host, (6) they combine to form zygotes in the mosquito stomach (sexual reproduction), (7) zygotes then invade the mosquito midgut wall and develop into oocysts which mature, rupture and release sporozoites, and (8) the sporozoites migrate to the mosquito salivary glands and are injected into the next human host during a blood meal, thus continuing the cycle.

CLINICAL PRESENTATION

Blood-stage malaria parasites are responsible for the clinical manifestations of infection. The incubation period (from sporozoite inoculation to symptoms) may be as short as a few days to a week (*P. falciparum*), as long as months (*P. vivax*, *P. ovale*), or even years (*P. malariae*). The average range, however, is between 8 and 20 days.[9,10] Clinical manifestations may commence with a brief flu-like prodrome of headache and malaise, myalgias and arthralgias, mild diarrhea, and low-grade fever. This is typically followed by intermittent episodes of high fever, coincident with the release of merozoites from RBCs. Depending on the species, merozoite release occurs at fairly specific intervals. For *P. falciparum*, *P. vivax* and *P. ovale*, this typically occurs every 48 hours and for *P. malariae*, every 72 hours. However, in practice, temperature spikes may be irregular, and may not necessarily be diagnostic of any particular species. This clinical syndrome of mild-to-moderate symptoms without signs of severity or vital organ dysfunction is termed uncomplicated malaria.[11] This is how most children who have acquired malaria elsewhere will present in clinics in the Western world. However, without prompt and/or appropriate treatment at this point, the risk of complications may rise, and the child may develop severe disease (see *P. falciparum* in section "Species Variation" and also see section "Other Complications").

History and Physical

A child with uncomplicated malaria will present as one with an acute febrile illness, often with no localizing signs. Most of the time, there will be history of recent travel to an endemic area, although there are rare reports of local US transmission.[4] Ninety-eight percent of US returned travelers with *P. falciparum* malaria experience their first symptoms within 3 months of arrival.[4] They most likely will present with or will have a history of fever, and may have associated chills, headache, cough, tachypnea, nausea, vomiting, diarrhea, anorexia, or fatigue/weakness. Vital signs may show tachypnea and/or tachycardia (caused by fever and/or anemia), blood pressure is usually normal. Rarely, hypotension is seen with malaria ("algid malaria"). In many cases, this may be caused by concurrent bacteremia and sepsis.[10] Jaundice is not typical in young children,[12] but if present, may reflect an underlying hematologic disorder such as sickle cell disease, thalassemia, or glucose-6-phosphate dehydrogenase (G6PD) deficiency. Jaundice is also seen in more severe disease. Splenomegaly and/or hepatomegaly may be present, depending on the duration or severity of illness. Skin examination may reveal pallor, especially in the palms, soles, and conjunctivae of dark-skinned children. Skin rashes are not typically present in malaria manifestations.

The majority of children with uncomplicated malaria (no signs of severe disease or vital organ dysfunction) will respond to oral antimalarial chemotherapy, but for reasons that are not entirely clear, a proportion may progress to severe/complicated malaria.[10] Neurologically, the child may have had or may be having seizures, but hypoglycemia and dehydration should be ruled out before a diagnosis of cerebral malaria is entertained (see *P. falciparum* in section "Species Variation"). If cerebral malaria is also ruled out, a diagnosis of febrile seizures should be considered. Seizures are common in children with malaria who are admitted to hospitals in developing countries, but they are generally not associated with significantly increased mortality or other adverse outcomes in the absence of impaired consciousness.[13] Table 66–1 lists the signs and symptoms of malaria in children.

Species Variation

P. falciparum

P. falciparum produces the most severe forms of malarial infection. Severe malaria in children in endemic areas depends on age and level of transmission. In these regions, infection and clinical symptoms in infants younger than 6 months are rare and/or mild, possibly as a result of passive immunity from transferred maternal antibodies. Children in endemic areas of high transmission are generally susceptible to severe disease between 6 months and 6 years of age[13–15]; in low transmission areas, the incidence of severe disease may continue to young adulthood and beyond.[15,16]

Severe malaria may manifest as one or all of three overlapping syndromes: cerebral malaria, severe malarial anemia, and respiratory distress.[12,17] *P. falciparum* is responsible for the overwhelming majority of severe malaria cases. Unlike the other three species, *P. falciparum* infects RBCs of all ages, resulting in higher levels of

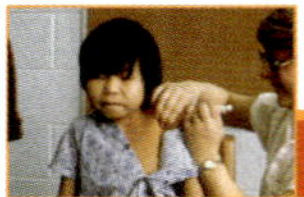

Table 66–1.

Signs and Symptoms Associated with Malaria in Children

Age Group	Uncomplicated Malaria	Severe Malaria
Congenital/newborn	Fever Irritability Lethargy Poor feeding Jaundice Hepatosplenomegaly Anemia Thrombocytopenia	NA
Infants/children younger than 5 y	Fever Cough Diarrhea Headache Chills/Rigors Vomiting Hepatosplenomegaly Anemia Thrombocytopenia	Respiratory distress/acidosis Severe anemia* Hypoglycemia‡ Multiple seizures Impaired consciousness Prostration Severe thrombocytopenia†
Adolescents/older children	Fever Headache Chills/Rigors Vomiting Hepatosplenomegaly Anemia Jaundice Thrombocytopenia	Impaired consciousness Multiple seizures Prostration Severe anemia* Severe thrombocytopenia† Hypoglycemia‡ Respiratory distress/acidosis Pulmonary edema Jaundice Renal impairment

*<5 g/dL
†<20,000/µL
‡<40 mg/dL
NA, not applicable.

parasitemia, severe anemia, and poorer prognosis. In contrast, *P. vivax* and *P. ovale* infect young RBCs, and *P. malariae* infects more mature RBCs.

P. falciparum is the only human species that causes cerebral malaria, a serious complication of infection that has significant morbidity and mortality (Figure 66–3). The World Health Organization defines cerebral malaria as the presence of *P. falciparum* asexual parasitemia and coma, with no other cause of coma identified.[12] The peak incidence of CM by age varies according to transmission level and geographic area, with younger children (age 1–10 years) typically affected in sub-Saharan Africa[14,15,18] and other children and young adults often affected in southeast Asia and Papua New Guinea.[10,12] Mortality from cerebral malaria is estimated at between 15% and 40% in endemic areas.[19,20] Ten to twenty percent of cerebral malaria survivors will suffer acute neurological sequelae such as ataxia, hemiparesis, and cortical blindness, most of which resolve over time.[20–22] A significant proportion may have seizures/epilepsy, and >20% show long-term cognitive impairment after cerebral malaria.[23] The histopathological hallmark of cerebral malaria is the engorgement of cerebral blood microvessels with parasitized and non-parasitized RBCs.[16,18] This results in mechanical obstruction and presumably cerebral hypoxia. In addition, the presence of parasite antigens triggers cytokine production, particularly IFN-γ and TNF-α.[14] In relatively lower concentrations, TNF-α and IFN-γ inhibit growth of malaria parasites, however, excessive production of these proinflammatory cytokines may be deleterious to the host.[7,8,24] Proinflammatory cytokine excess may worsen hypoxia and hypoglycemia, and promote sequestration,[18,24] thereby contributing to the development and progression of cerebral malaria.

A child with cerebral malaria will present with a febrile illness and coma while living in or after traveling to an endemic area. They may have anorexia and vomiting, and neurologically may exhibit seizures, coma, and/or brainstem abnormalities.[16] Duration of symptoms preceding the coma may be brief, typically 1 or 2 days. The Blantyre Coma Scale (Table 66–2) is a

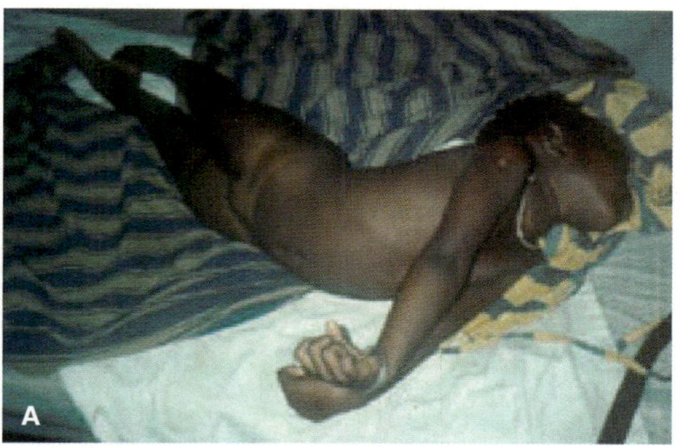

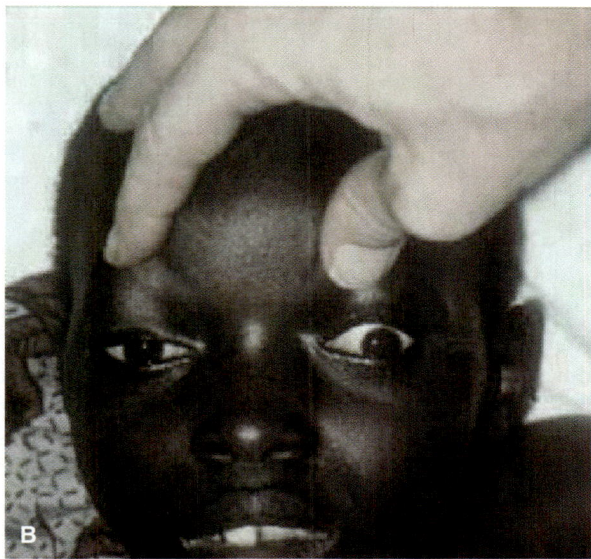

FIGURE 66–3 ■ **(A)** Gambian child with cerebral malaria (note severe extensor posturing); **(B)** Dysconjugate gaze in comatose Gambian child with cerebral malaria. (*With permission from the World Health Organization.*)

Table 66–2.

The Blantyre Coma Scale for Children*

Assessment	Score
A. Best motor response	
Nonspecific or no response	0
Withdraws limb from pain	1
Localizes painful stimulus	2
B. Best verbal response	
None	0
Moan or inappropriate cry	1
Appropriate cry	2
C. Eye movements	
Does not follow a moving object	0
Does follow a moving object	1
Total	(0–5)

**Children with cerebral malaria will have a score of* <*3.*

modified form of the Glasgow Coma Scale that was developed to objectively assess neurological status in children younger than 5 years. A Blantyre coma score of less than 3 denotes a state of unarousable coma and is required for a diagnosis of cerebral malaria.[10,12] Once coma is confirmed, and there is evidence of asexual forms of *P. falciparum* on blood smear (Figure 66–4), antimalarial and supportive treatment should not be delayed. Obtaining a lumbar puncture for cerebrospinal fluid (CSF) analysis will depend on how stable the patient is for the procedure. Unless there are signs of increased intracranial pressure, indicating that a lumbar puncture is unsafe, CSF should be obtained to rule out meningitis or encephalitis as a cause of coma. If there are signs of increased intracranial pressure, lumbar puncture should be deferred, and consideration given to empiric therapy

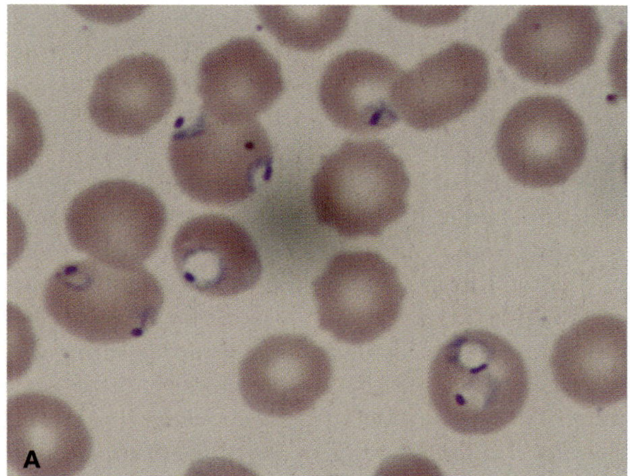

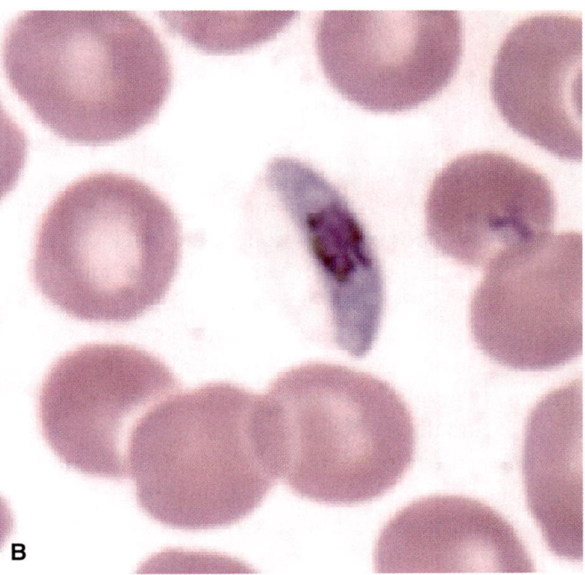

FIGURE 66–4 ■ **(A)** Giemsa-stained thin blood smear showing *P. falciparum* ring trophozoites (note that some RBCs are multiply infected); **(B)** Typical "banana"-shaped *P. falciparum* gametocyte on thin blood smear. (*With permission from the Centers for Disease Control and Prevention.*)

for meningitis until CSF can be obtained. Children with cerebral malaria should have normal CSF values (<5 leukocytes/μL, no erythrocytes, normal protein and glucose level).[10,25] However, patients with hypoglycemia may have low or undetectable glucose levels in the CSF. *Plasmodium* forms are not seen on CSF staining, since these organisms sequester in the cerebral microvasculature. If the CSF examination points to another diagnosis, such as bacterial meningitis, further investigation and appropriate management should be initiated. A number of children present with *P. falciparum* parasitemia and impaired consciousness, but do not meet the strict definition of cerebral malaria (*P. falciparum* parasitemia plus coma). These children have increased mortality,[13] and likely have a slightly less severe manifestation of the same pathophysiologic process as children with cerebral malaria. They should be evaluated and treated in the same way as children with strictly defined cerebral malaria.

Severe malarial anemia is defined as *P. falciparum* asexual parasitemia associated with a hemoglobin concentration of <5 g/dL or a hematocrit of <15%.[12] Severe malarial anemia affects many more children than cerebral malaria; however, the mortality rate of severe malarial anemia is much lower than that of cerebral malaria. The peak incidence of severe malarial anemia is in children younger than 3 years.[17] The severity of anemia roughly correlates with the level of parasitemia, but there is great individual variation. Children with severe malarial anemia may develop respiratory distress as a result of metabolic acidosis from reduced oxygen-carrying capacity and supply. Severe malarial anemia may occur alone or in combination with other complications of falciparum malaria. The presence of severe anemia in association with *P. falciparum* parasitemia does not necessarily mean that the latter is the only cause of the former. Particularly in children at risk, or in developing countries, other causes for anemia, such as nutritional/vitamin deficiencies, should be ruled out if possible.

Respiratory distress is more common in children than adults, and is usually secondary to metabolic acidosis from poor perfusion rather than to pulmonary edema.[10,12,25] Children may be tachypneic or have a low respiratory rate. If they have severe metabolic acidosis, they may exhibit Kussmaul's respirations. Respiratory distress is a poor prognostic sign of severe malaria in children,[26,27] and the acid/base status and volume status of all children with respiratory distress should be evaluated immediately. Since children with pneumonia may present similarly, correlations should be made with clinical presentation and appropriate lab tests (including chest radiograph) in order to arrive at a correct diagnosis.

P. vivax

P. vivax (Figure 66–5) is a relatively infrequent cause of mortality, altough in some areas of Oceania, mortality from *P. vivax* rivals that from *P. falciparum*.[28–30] It is a major cause of morbidity in areas where it is common (Indian subcontinent, southeast Asia, Oceania, South America). It is one of two human *Plasmodium* strains (the other being *P. ovale*) responsible for "relapsing" malaria infection. After liver invasion, *P. vivax* sporozoites may develop into either tissue schizonts or hypnozoites, which are responsible for clinical relapses. The hypnozoites remain dormant in the liver while tissue schizonts develop and continue the cycle, mounting a primary attack. The *P vivax* asexual blood stage cycle is typically "tertian," that is, merozoite release from RBCs occurs every 48 hours, or every third day (the first day is counted as day one). After a certain period, typically within weeks to months of the initial attack, the latent hypnozoites activate, develop into tissue schizonts, and reestablish the blood stage cycle, causing clinical symptoms. It is imperative, therefore, that any patient diagnosed with *P. ovale* or *P. vivax* infection be treated not only for the initial attack, but also for the hypnozoites that lie dormant in the liver.

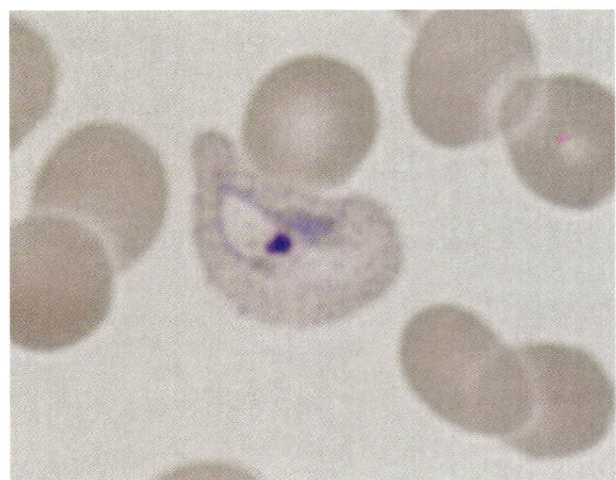

FIGURE 66–5 ■ Large, ameboid trophozoite of *P. vivax* on thin blood smear (note the fine stippling caused by Schuffner's dots, and enlargement and distortion of the RBC). (*With permission from Dr. Jon Rosenblatt, Mayo Clinic Laboratories.*)

P. ovale

P. ovale infection occurs in West Africa, the Phillipines, Indonesia, and Papua New Guinea. The clinical course and fever pattern for *P. ovale* is similar to that of *P. vivax* infection; however, clinical symptoms are milder, and there is less likelihood of relapse.[10]

P. malariae

P. malariae infection (Figure 66–6) has patchy distribution in tropical and subtropical regions worldwide. In comparison to the other three human *Plasmodium* species, it exhibits slow development in both the human and mosquito hosts. Infection with *P. malariae* is the mildest but also the most chronic, and may persist in the

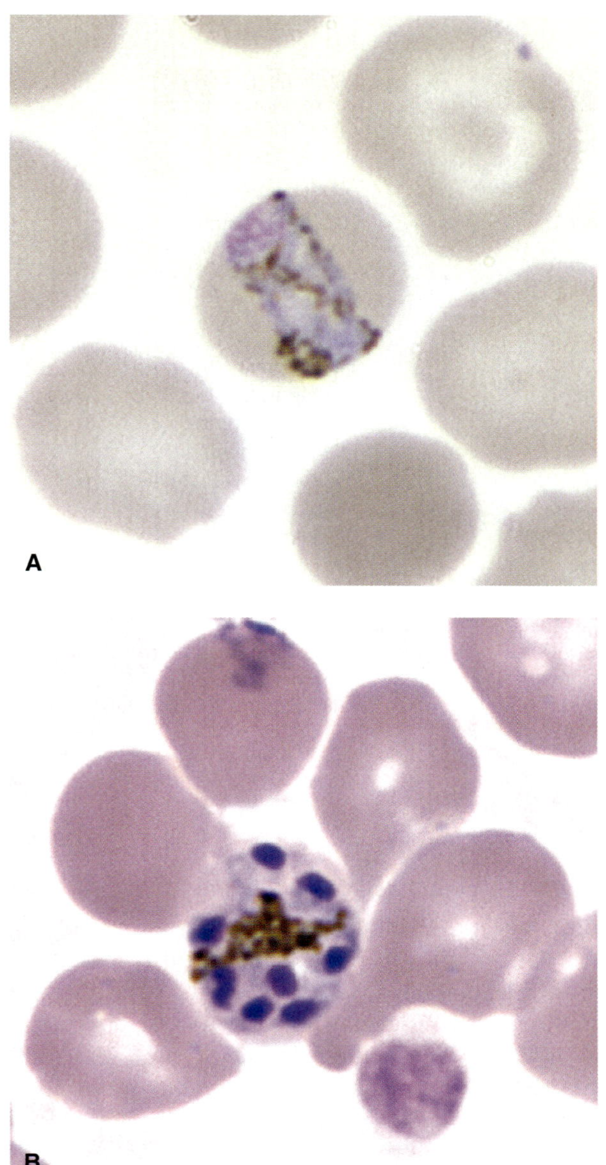

FIGURE 66–6 ■ (A) Characteristic "band" trophozoite of *P. malariae* on thin blood smear (note intact shape and size of the RBC); **(B)** *P. malariae* schizont. (*With permission from the Centers for Disease Control and Prevention.*)

human host for many years. It appears that this chronicity is not caused by hypnozoites, but rather, recrudescence of the initial attack from small numbers of blood stage forms that have persisted in internal organs.[10] As such, patients can present with *P. malariae*-related illness long after they have left endemic areas where they first acquired the infection. Even though *P. malariae* infection is generally mild, it can cause a chronic nephrotic syndrome which has a poor prognosis.[6,10]

P. knowlesi

There is now evidence that *P. knowlesi*, a *Plasmodium* species that usually infects monkeys, has crossed over to cause malaria in humans in southeast Asia, notably in Malaysia[31]. *P. knowlesi* is now considered a fifth human malaria species. It is not clear at this point if *P. knowlesi* preferentially infects a subset of red cells, but it multiplies rapidly and can cause very high levels of parasitemia. Morphologically, it can be confused with *P. malariae* on microscopic examination.

P. knowlesi malaria, because of its rapid life cycle, can cause high level parasitemia, severe seizures and rapidly lead to death[32]. Since *P. knowlesi* can be mistaken for *P. malariae* on microscopy, it should be considered in any severely ill patient with malaria acquired in southeast Asia, particularly in patients who are thought to have *P. malariae* infection on microscopy but have high-level parasitemia, as high-level parasitemia with *P. malariae* infection is unusual. PCR testing at a reference lab is currently the only way to identify *P. knowlesi* infection. Cloroquine plus sulfadoxine-pyrimethamine should be used to treat *P. knowlesi* infections[31,32]; quinine is an alternative in severely ill patients.

Mixed infections

It is not uncommon for patients to present with concurrent infections from two or more *Plasmodium* species. Mixed infections are common in endemic malarious areas. The most common types of mixed infections are *P. falciparum/P. vivax* in subtropical regions, and *P. falciparum/P. malariae* in tropical Africa,[10] however, *P. falciparum/P. ovale* is particularly common in West Africa.

Other Complications

Additional complications, generally caused by *P. falciparum*, are listed below; other species will be mentioned, if they are more likely to cause a particular complication.

Convulsions/seizures

Seizures are quite common in children with mild or severe malaria, and children are more likely than adults to have seizures with malarial infection.[12,18] Fifty to eighty percent of children with cerebral malaria have seizures.[10,12] In a recent study, close to 40% of all children admitted with malaria in a malaria endemic area experienced seizures.[13] However, in children with malaria, seizures may also occur as a result of profound hypoglycemia, dehydration, or fever, and may be generalized, focal, single, or multiple in nature.[12]

Hypoglycemia

Children are more likely than adults to develop hypoglycemia. It is especially common in children younger than 3 years, those with seizures, high levels of

Table 66–3.

Differential Diagnosis of Malaria Symptomatology

Children Age Group	Common	Uncommon
Newborn/Infant	Viral syndrome	TORCH infections
	Influenza	Viral hepatitis
	Otitis media	Meningitis
	Bacteremia/sepsis	
	Pneumonia	
Young child	Influenza	Bacteremia
	Gastroenteritis	Hepatitis B, C, E
	Pneumonia	Aseptic meningitis
	Dengue fever	Bacterial meningitis
	Yellow fever	Salmonella infection
	Hepatitis A	Leptospirosis
	Acute hemolysis*	Rickettsial infection
Adolescent/older child	Influenza	Hepatitis B, C, E
	Gastroenteritis	Aseptic meningitis
	Yellow fever	Bacterial meningitis
	Dengue fever	Salmonella infection
	Hepatitis A	Leptospirosis
	Acute hemolysis*	Rickettsial infection

*May be because of G6PD deficiency, sickle cell anemia, and drugs.
TORCH: **T**oxoplasma, **R**ubella, **C**ytomegalovirus, **H**erpes Simplex Virus.

parasitemia, or in deep coma.[12] The manifestations of hypoglycemia are similar to those of cerebral malaria, and it is critically important to treat the former as soon as possible in order to establish or rule out cerebral malaria. In some cases, treatment of hypoglycemia reverses neurological symptoms that may have been ascribed to cerebral malaria. Note that quinine can induce or worsen hypoglycemia, so blood glucose levels should be closely monitored during its use.

Acute renal failure

Acute renal failure is more common in older children and adults, and is characterized by elevated serum creatinine and blood urea, and oliguria or anuria caused by acute tubular necrosis.[12,33,34] The incidence of acute renal failure in falciparum malaria is between 1% and 4%; it may reach up to 60% in patients with severe malaria.[32] It is usually reversible with appropriate treatment. Blackwater fever is a rarer form of acute renal failure associated with *P. falciparum* malaria, and results from severe intravascular hemolysis and hemoglobinuria.[33] Patients present with flank pain, vomiting, severe anemia and oliguria with passage of dark, cola-colored urine, hence the name "blackwater." G6PD deficiency should be excluded in patients with hemoglobinuria, since antimalarial and other oxidant drugs (notably primaquine) can trigger hemolysis in such individuals, even without malarial infection.[12]

Hyperreactive malarial splenomegaly

Also known as tropical splenomegaly syndrome, hyperreactive malarial splenomegaly (HMS) is defined as gross splenomegaly (>10 cm below the costal margin) in a long-term resident of a malarious area, presence of antimalarial antibodies, elevated serum IgM, and clinical and immunological response to antimalarial treatment.[35,36] HMS occurs in areas of intense malaria transmission, and is more common in young and middle-aged adults.[36,37] Although the exact mechanism is unclear, there is thought to be an exaggerated polyclonal B lymphocyte stimulation in response to chronic and repeated exposure to any of the 4 human malaria parasites.[10,36,37] As a result, high levels of antimalarial antibodies are produced, and there is accompanying immune complex deposition in the liver and spleen. Patients present with a grossly enlarged spleen, often with hepatomegaly, abdominal pain, anemia, cachexia, and hypersplenism (normochromic, normocytic anemia, thrombocytopenia, leucopenia, and reticulocytosis).[36–38] There may be no evidence for acute malarial infection on blood smear. In some cases, patients develop massive hemolysis and/or overwhelming infection, which increases mortality. The backbone of treatment is long-term administration of chloroquine, proguanil, or sulfadoxine-pyrimethamine,[35,36] with most patients achieving significant reduction in spleen size. In general, chloroquine has been the drug of choice; repeated

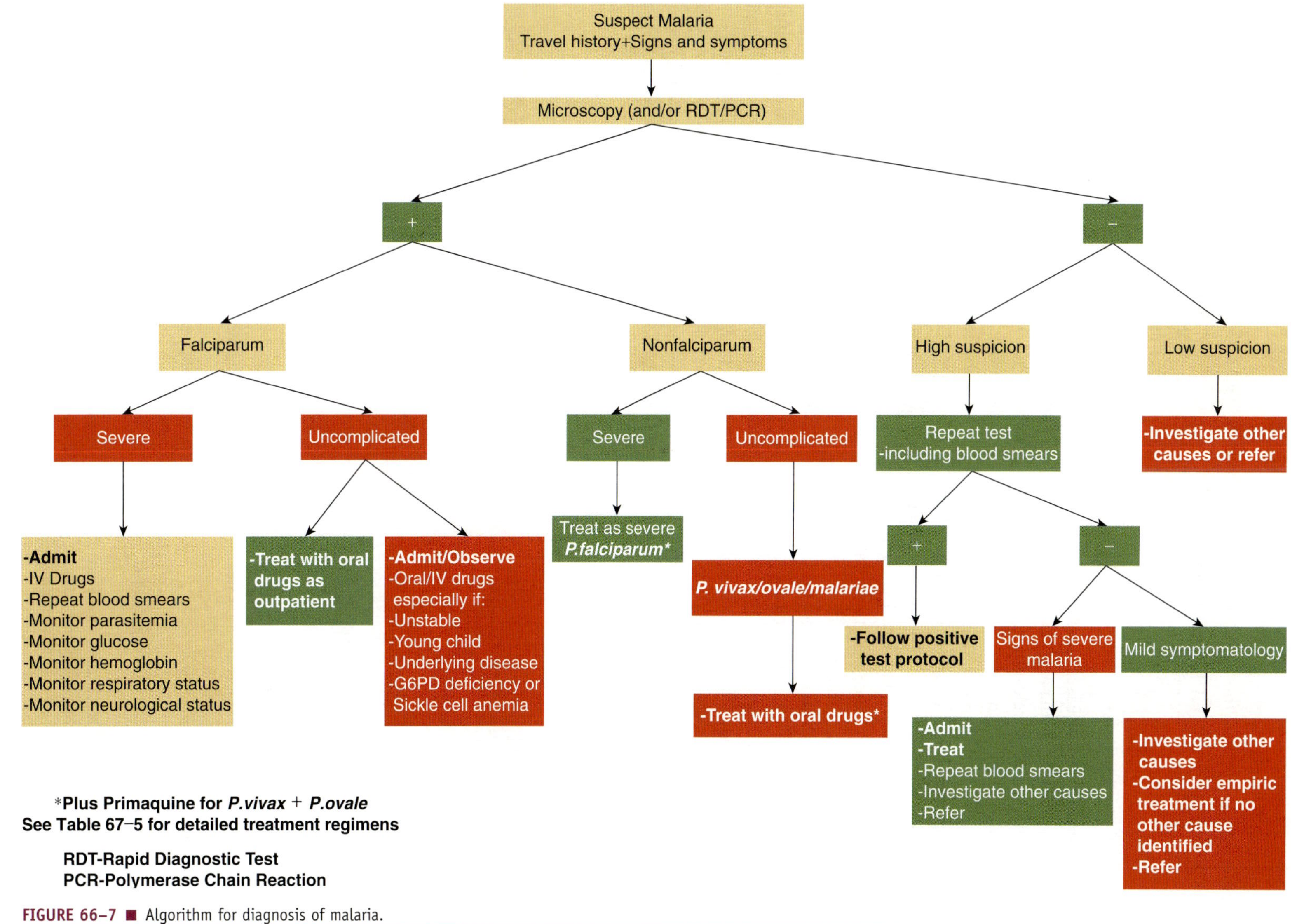

FIGURE 66–7 ■ Algorithm for diagnosis of malaria.

treatment with sulfadoxine-pyrimethamine is generally avoided because of the increased risk of Stevens-Johnson syndrome with prolonged therapy. The treatment course is several months to up to a year, or until splenomegaly has adequately improved.

Congenital malaria infection

As with other infectious diseases such as rubella, cytomegalovirus, and varicella, malaria can be transmitted transplacentally to the developing fetus from the mother. In endemic areas, up to 1 in 4 babies born to infected mothers are parasitemic, but many of these children are asymptomatic and clear parasitemia without treatment.[39] *P. falciparum* and *P. vivax* are most often implicated in pregnancy-related and congenital malaria. Malaria may cause or exacerbate maternal anemia, which may lead to placental insufficiency. As a result, infants with congenital malaria can also present with low birth weight because of intrauterine growth retardation.[12] Symptomatic infants usually present at 2–8 weeks of life, and may have fever, poor oral intake, lethargy, anemia, and hepatosplenomegaly.[12,39] Cerebral malaria, and the organ dysfunction of severe malaria is rare in infants.[12,16]

DIFFERENTIAL DIAGNOSIS

The signs and symptoms of malaria are protean, and do not particularly distinguish it from other diagnoses. This is a problem, especially in endemic areas where many other infectious diseases and febrile illnesses also exist. However, the *collective* array of signs and symptoms, acuity of illness should raise the suspicion of malaria in the majority of cases. In the United States, malaria should be considered in any child returning from travel in a malarious area with fever and/or splenomegaly. Conditions that may present similarly to malaria are listed in Table 66–3.

DIAGNOSIS

The diagnosis of acute malaria can be straightforward if the right tests are done at the appropriate times. The gold standard for clinical diagnosis is light microscopy of thin and thick Giemsa-stained blood smears to identify parasites. Thick blood smears are best for establishing the presence of *Plasmodium* parasites; thin smears aid in species identification. Blood samples should be collected and sent to the laboratory as soon as possible, since it can take several hours to prepare, dry, and examine the thick

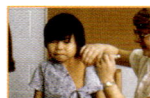

Table 66–4.

Diagnostic Tests for Malaria

Test	When to Order: Uncomplicated Malaria	When to Order: Severe Malaria	Comments
Thick, thin blood smears	Immediately	Immediately, every 6–24 h	From finger, toe, or heel
Polymerase chain reaction/RDT	Immediately	Immediately	In addition to blood smears if severe disease
Total serum IgM	NA	NA	For diagnosis of HMS; not helpful in acute malaria
Supportive tests			
Fingerstick glucose	Not usually indicated	Immediately, monitor closely	Rapidly identify and treat hypoglycemia
Complete blood count	Routine	Immediately, monitor closely	Identify anemia and thrombocytopenia
Electrolyte panel	Not usually indicated	Immediately, monitor closely	Identify hypoglycemia and renal impairment
Blood gases	Not usually indicated	Immediately, monitor closely	Identify acidosis
Bilirubin	Not usually indicated	Immediately	
Lumbar puncture	Not usually indicated	If cerebral malaria suspected, and patient stable	Should not delay treatment
Imaging			
Chest xray	Not usually indicated	Immediately, if respiratory distress and lung examination findings	Rule out pneumonia Rule out pulmonary edema

RDT, rapid diagnostic test; IgM, immnoglobulin; HMS, Hyperreactive malarial splenomegaly; NA, not applicable.

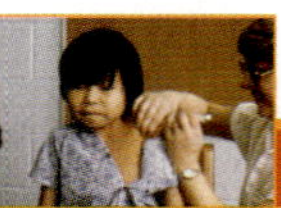

Table 66–5.

Drug Treatments for Malaria

Drug	Adult Dosage	Pediatric Dosage**
I. Uncomplicated malaria		
A. *P. ovale, P. malariae* and chloroquine-sensitive *P. vivax* and *P. falciparum*		
Chloroquine phosphate* (PO)[a]	1 g (600 mg base) at 0h; then 500 mg (300 mg base) at 6h, 24h, & 48h	10 mg base/kg (max. 600 mg base) at 0h; then 5 mg base/kg at 6h, 24h, & 48h
Hydroxychloroquine (PO)	800mg (620 mg base) at 0h; then 400mg (310 mg base) at 6h, 24h, & 48h	10mg base/kg at 0h; then 5 mg base/kg at 6h, 24h, & 48h
B. Chloroquine-resistant *P. vivax*[¶]		
Quinine sulfate* (PO)	650 mg salt 3 times daily × 3–7d[‡]	30 mg salt/kg/d in 3 doses × 3–7d[‡]
+ doxycycline^ (PO)	100 mg twice daily × 7d	4 mg salt/kg/d in 2 doses × 7d
Mefloquine (PO)	750 mg × 1, then 500mg 12 hrs later	15 mg/kg × 1, then 10mg/kg 12 hrs later
C. Relapse prevention: *P. vivax* & *P. ovale* only[§]		
Primaquine phosphate (PO)	30 mg base orally once daily × 14d	0.5 mg base/kg orally once daily × 14d
D. Chloroquine-resistant *P. falciparum*[†]		
Quinine sulphate* (PO)	650 mg salt 3 times daily × 3–7d[‡]	30 mg/kg/d in 3 doses × 3–7d[‡]
+ doxycycline^ (PO)	100mg twice daily × 7d	4.4 mg/kg/d in 2 doses × 7d
or + tetracycline^ (PO)	250mg 4 times daily × 7d	25 mg/kg/d in 4 doses × 7d
or + clindamycin (PO)	20mg/kg/d in 3 doses × 7d	20 mg/kg/d in 3 doses × 7d
Atovaquone/proguanil (Malarone)* (PO)	Adult tab: 250mg atovaquone/100mg proguanil 2 adult tabs twice daily × 3d, or 4 adult tabs once daily × 3d	Pediatric tab: 62.5 mg atovaquone/25mg proguanil <5kg: not indicated 5–8 kg: 2 ped tabs once daily × 3d >8–10kg: 3 ped tabs once daily × 3d >10–20kg: 1 adult tab once daily × 3d >20–30kg: 2 adult tabs once daily × 3d >30–40kg: 3 adult tabs once daily × 3d >40kg: use adult dosing
Mefloquine PO	750 mg salt × 1, then 500mg 6–12 hrs later	15 mg salt/kg × 1, then 10mg/kg 6–12 hrs later
II. Severe malaria (due to any species, regardless of region or resistance pattern)		
Quinidine gluconate* (IV)	10 mg salt/kg loading dose (max. 600 mg) in normal saline over 1–2 hrs, then 0.02 mg salt/kg/min until oral therapy (as in I.D) can be started	10 mg salt/kg loading dose (max. 600 mg) in normal saline over 1–2 hrs, then 0.02 mg salt/kg/min until oral therapy (as in I. D) can be started
+ Tetracycline OR Doxycycline OR Clindamycin	Dosage as in I.D	
Quinine dihydrochloride(IV)	20 mg/kg loading dose in 5% dextrose over 4 hrs, then 10 mg/kg over 2-4 hrs q8h (max.1800 mg/d) until oral therapy (as in I.D) can be started	20 mg/kg loading dose in 5% dextrose over 4 hrs, then 10 mg/kg over 2-4 hrs q8h (max.1800 mg/d) until oral therapy (as in I.D) can be started
+ Tetracycline OR Doxycycline OR Clindamycin	Dosage as in I. D	Dosage as in I.D

Data sources: CDC, JAMA 2007; The Medical Letter, 2004.
* *Drug of choice*
** *Maximum for all pediatric dosages is the adult dosage.*
[¶] *Infections acquired in Papua New Guinea and Indonesia*
[‡] *Treat for 7d if infection acquired in Southeast Asia; 3d if elsewhere*
^ *Do not use in children < 8yrs old*
[§] *Concurrent with regular treatment. Check for G6PD defiiciency before dosing.*
[†] *See Figure 8*
[††] *Please see text for treatment of P. knowlesi infection.*
[a] *Abbreviations: PO = orally, IV = intravenously.*

smears. If the initial blood smear is negative, and malaria is still suspected, blood smears should be repeated at 6-, 12- or 24-hour intervals for 48–72 hours[10,40] in order to increase sensitivity. Even after malaria is diagnosed, blood smears should be sent at similar intervals in order to monitor parasite density (percentage of infected RBCs on a thin film), as a measure of response to therapy. If malaria is strongly suspected, the patient is severely ill, and/or laboratory diagnosis is not possible, appropriate antimalarial therapy should be initiated, pending referral of the patient or the availability of blood smear results. The algorithm in Figure 66–7 provides a guide for diagnosis and management of malaria. Table 66–4 lists the most important tests and when to order them. Immunity or partial immunity plays an important role in the host's susceptibility to severe disease.[7,8,25] A child older than 6 years, and who has a prior history of malaria infection, and has recently (<2 years prior) lived in a malarious area may be at least partially immune.[25] Outpatient management may be appropriate for a child with this profile who has no evidence of malaria complications and does not appear acutely ill.

Several rapid diagnostic tests (RDTs) based on parasite antigen detection by immunochromatography for all four human *Plasmodium* spp. have been developed. In general, the overall sensitivities of these tests are better for *P. falciparum* than for the other 3 strains, and the best RDTs have a sensitivity and specificity that approaches that of microscopy.[41–43] RDTs also require less user training and take less time to provide a result. In June 2007, the U.S. Food and Drug Administration (FDA) approved the first RDT for use in hospitals and commercial laboratories in the United States.[44] Molecular diagnosis by polymerase chain reaction is available, and is more accurate than light microscopy, however, it is expensive and requires a specialized laboratory.[44] Serology (detection of antimalaria antibodies) does not detect current infection; it only indicates past exposure if positive.[44] Serology is only otherwise useful for diagnosing suspected hyperreactive malarial splenomegaly in a patient.

TREATMENT

As a result of the limited availability, malaria treatment in the United States currently does not include artemisinin and its derivatives. Artemisinin is derived from the herb *Artemisia annua,* which has been used in Chinese medicine for centuries. Artemisinin and its derivatives (artesunate, artemether, artemotil, dihydroartemisinin) produce rapid parasite clearance and symptom resolution, and are the World Health Organization's backbone for falciparum malaria treatment worldwide.[11] The Centers for Disease Control and Prevention is working to make intravenous artesunate available in the United States under an Investigational New Drug protocol in 2007.[40] It is critical

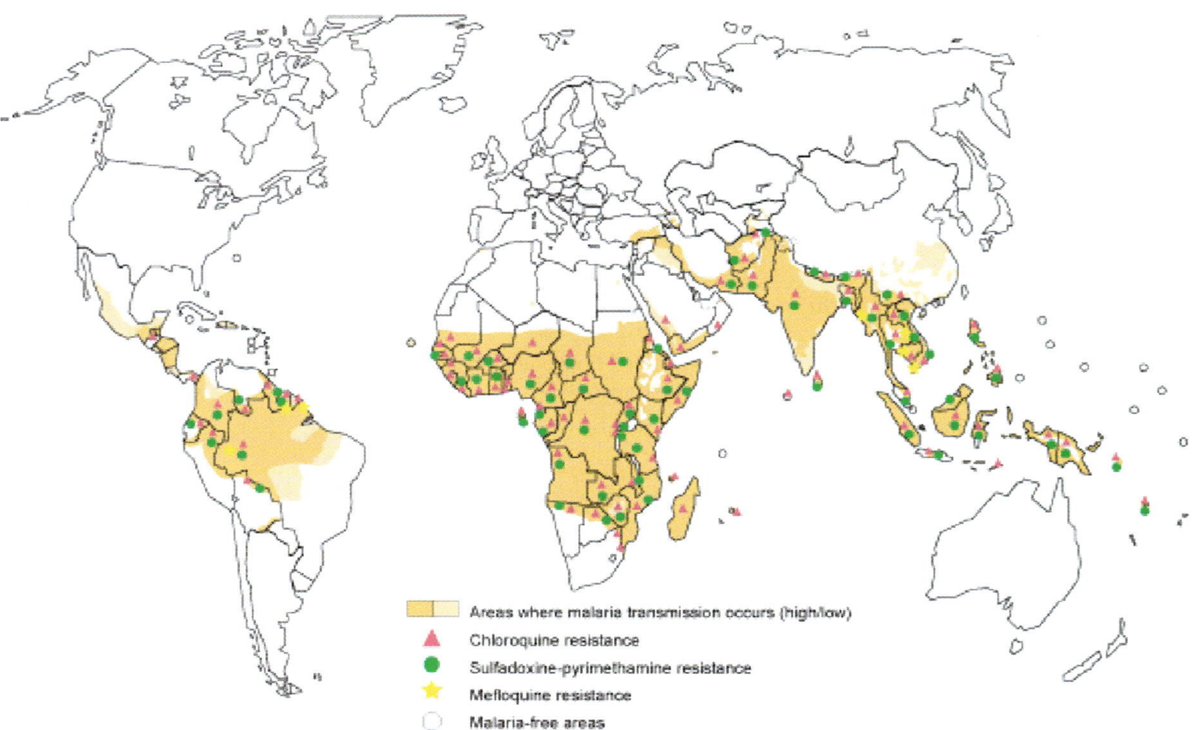

FIGURE 66–8 ■ Worldwide distribution of *P. falciparum* drug resistance, up to 2004. (*With permission from the World Health Organization*).

to differentiate between severe and uncomplicated malaria, as treatment regimens for these two conditions differ. The hallmarks of severe malaria are outlined in Table 66–1, but these criteria were developed for children in malaria endemic countries. In general, any ill-appearing child requiring hospitalization should be considered to have severe malaria and should receive treatment with intravenous antibiotics. Table 66–5 provides a list of drug combinations and doses for both adults/older children and young children. Figure 66–8 represents the drug-resistant *P. falciparum* regions in the world.

WHEN TO REFER

Given that malaria is no longer endemic in the United States, general practitioners today are much less comfortable with diagnosing and treating malaria. Depending on location of their practice, and the population of immigrants/refugees there, physicians may rarely, if ever, see a case of malaria. Therefore, the threshold for referring a patient to a specialist should be much lower for malaria than for infectious diseases commonly encountered in the United States. A specialist should be one that is trained in pediatric infectious diseases, clinical tropical medicine or both. If the patient is not able to be transferred, a telephone consultation should be done with a specialist. Blood smear slides may also be sent to a reference laboratory, for examination by experienced personnel. In general, infants, pregnant women, and patients with underlying hematologic or immunologic disease should be referred for subspecialty evaluation. In addition, any patient who has signs and symptoms of complicated malaria should also be referred. If a practitioner has any level of discomfort with managing a patient with suspected malaria, they should refer that patient to a specialist, after providing appropriate initial care.

MALARIA PROPHYLAXIS

Malarial infection in US travelers is largely preventable. Travelers should have thorough counseling and appropriate chemoprophylaxis (depending on age, medical history, drug sensitivities, and destination). Recommended drugs and doses for malaria prophylaxis are provided in Chapter 64. In addition to prophylaxis, travelers should be advised to take protective measures, as no prophylaxis is 100% effective. The Centers for Disease Control and Prevention Yellow Book[45] provides practical information that can guide practitioners in counseling travelers about a variety of conditions, including malaria. Currently, there is no malaria vaccine, and so prevention is limited largely to chemoprophylaxis for travelers, and intermittent preventive treatment, bednets, and indoor residual spraying for residents in endemic areas. However, intensive research in malaria vaccine development continues, as success in this field could have a significant impact on morbidity and mortality in children worldwide.

REFERENCES

1. Snow RW, Craig M, Deichmann U, Marsh K. Estimating mortality, morbidity and disability due to malaria among Africa's non-pregnant population. *Bull World Health Organ.* 1999;77(8):624-640.
2. Snow RW, Guerra CA, Noor AM, Myint HY, Hay SI. The global distribution of clinical episodes of *Plasmodium* falciparum malaria. *Nature.* 2005;434(7030):214-217.
3. Rowe AK, Rowe SY, Snow RW, et al. The burden of malaria mortality among African children in the year 2000. *Int J Epidemiol.* 2006;35(3):691-704.
4. Skarbinski J, James EM, Causer LM, et al. Malaria Surveillance–United States, 2004. *MMWR Surveill Summ.* 2006; 55(4):23-37.
5. World Malaria Report 2005, Malaria burden. 2005. http://www.rollbackmalaria.org/. Accessed March 18, 2007.
6. Mueller I, Zimmerman PA, Reeder JC. *Plasmodium malariae* and *Plasmodium ovale*—the 'bashful' malaria parasites. *Trends Parasitol.* 2007;23(6):278-283.
7. Miller LH, Baruch DI, Marsh K, Doumbo OK. The pathogenic basis of malaria. *Nature.* 2002;415(6872):673-679.
8. Stevenson MM, Riley EM. Innate immunity to malaria. *Nat Rev.* 2004;4(3):169-180.
9. Seear MD. The child with an acute fever-malaria. *Manual of Tropical Pediatrics.* 1st ed. Cambridge: Cambridge University Press; 2000:58-68.
10. Warrell D, Gilles H, eds. *Essential Malariology.* 4th ed. London: Arnold; 2002.
11. Guidelines for the Treatment of Malaria. 2006. http://www.who.int/malaria/docs/treatmentguidelines2006.pdf. Accessed May 30, 2007.
12. World Health Organization, Communicable diseases cluster. Severe falciparum malaria. *Trans R Soc Trop Med Hyg.* 2000;94(suppl 1):S1-S90.
13. Idro R, Ndiritu M, Ogutu B, et al. Burden, features, and outcome of neurological involvement in acute falciparum malaria in Kenyan children. *J Am Med Assoc.* 2007; 297(20):2232-2240.
14. Hunt NH, Golenser J, Chan-Ling T, et al. Immunopathogenesis of cerebral malaria. *Int J Parasitol.* 2006;36(5): 569-582.
15. Reyburn H, Mbatia R, Drakeley C, et al. Association of transmission intensity and age with clinical manifestations and case fatality of severe *Plasmodium falciparum* malaria. *J Am Med Assoc.* 2005;293(12):1461-1470.
16. Idro R, Jenkins NE, Newton CR. Pathogenesis, clinical features, and neurological outcome of cerebral malaria. *Lancet Neurol.* 2005;4(12):827-840.
17. World Health Organization, Child Health Epidemiology Reference Group. Estimates of the Burden of Malaria Morbidity in Africa in Children Under the Age of Five Years; 2005 April. http://www.who.int/child_adolescent_health/documents/pdfs/cherg_malaria_morbidity.pdf. Accessed April 15, 2007.

18. Newton CR, Hien TT, White N. Cerebral Malaria. *J Neurol Neurosurg Psychiatry*. 2000;69(4):433-441.
19. Newton CR, Taylor TE, Whitten RO. Pathophysiology of fatal falciparum malaria in African children. *Am J Trop Med Hyg*. 1998;58(5):673-683.
20. Murphy SC, Breman JG. Gaps in the childhood malaria burden in Africa: cerebral malaria, neurological sequelae, anemia, respiratory distress, hypoglycemia, and complications of pregnancy. *Am J Trop Med Hyg*. 2001; 64(suppl 1–2):57-67.
21. Newton CR, Krishna S. Severe falciparum malaria in children: current understanding of pathophysiology and supportive treatment. *Pharmacol The*. 1998;79(1):1-53.
22. Carter JA, Ross AJ, Neville BG, et al. Developmental impairments following severe falciparum malaria in children. *Trop Med Int Health*. 2005;10(1):3-10.
23. Boivin MJ, Bangirana P, Byarugaba J, et al. Cognitive impairment after cerebral malaria in children: a prospective study. *Pediatrics*. 2007;119(2):E360-E366.
24. Clark IA, Budd AC, Alleva LM, Cowden WB. Human malarial disease: a consequence of inflammatory cytokine release. *Malar J*. 2006;5:85.
25. Stauffer W, Fischer PR. Diagnosis and treatment of malaria in children. *Clin Infect Dis*. 2003;37(10):1340-1348.
26. Marsh K, Forster D, Waruiru C, et al. Indicators of life-threatening malaria in African children. *N Engl J Med*. 1995;332(21):1399-1404.
27. English M, Waruiru C, Amukoye E, et al. Deep breathing in children with severe malaria: indicator of metabolic acidosis and poor outcome. *Am J Trop Med Hyg*. 1996; 55(5):521-524.
28. Ozen M, Gungor S, Atambay M, Daldal NN. Cerebral malaria owing to *Plasmodium vivax*: case Report. *Ann Trop Paediatr*. 2006;26(2):141-144.
29. Kochar DK, Saxena V, Singh N, Kochar SK, Kumar SV, Das A. *Plasmodium vivax* malaria. *Emerg Infect Dis*. 2005; 11(1):132-134.
30. Mohapatra MK, Padhiary KN, Mishra DP, Sethy G. Atypical manifestations of *Plasmodium vivax* malaria. *Indian J Malariol*. 2002;39(1-2):18-25.
31. Cox-Singh J, Davis TM, Lee, KS, et al. Plasmodium knowlesi malaria in humans is widely distributed and potentially life threatening. *Clin Infect Dis*. 2008;46:165-171.
32. Singh B, L Kim Sung Matusop A, et al. A large focus of naturally acquired Plasmodium knowlesi infections in human beings. *Lancet* 2004;363:1017-1024.
33. World Health Organization. Management of Severe Malaria: A Practical Handbook. http://www.who.int/malaria/docs/hbsm_tochtm#intro. Accessed May 31, 2007.
34. Eiam-Ong S. Malarial nephropathy. *Semin Nephrol*. 2003;23(1):21-33.
35. Singh RK. Hyperreactive malarial splenomegaly in expatriates. *Travel Med Infect Dis*. 2007;5(1):24-29.
36. Fakunle YM. Tropical splenomegaly. Part 1: Tropical Africa. *Clin Haematol*. 1981;10(3):963-975.
37. Sigueira-Batista R, Quintas LE. Tropical splenomegaly syndrome: a review from Brazil. *East Afr Med J*. 1994; 71(12):771-772.
38. Bedu-Addo G, Bates I. Causes of massive tropical splenomegaly in Ghana. *Lancet*. 2002;360(9331):449-454.
39. Fischer PR. Congenital malaria: an African survey. *Clin Pediatr*. 1997;36(7):411-413.
40. Griffith KS, Lewis LS, Mali S, Parise ME. Treatment of malaria in the United States: a systematic review. *J Am Med Assoc*. 2007;297(20):2264-2277.
41. Moody A. Rapid Diagnostic Tests for malaria parasites. *Clin Microbiol Rev*. 2002;15(1):66-78.
42. Palmer CJ, Bonilla JA, Bruckner DA, et al. Multicenter study to evaluate the optimal test for rapid diagnosis of malaria in U.S. Hospitals. *J Clin Microbiol*. 2003;41(11): 5178-5182.
43. Richter J, Harms G, Müller-Stöver I, Göbels K, Häussinger D. Performance of an immunochromatographic test for the rapid diagnosis of malaria. *Parasitol Res*. 2004;92(6): 518-519.
44. Centers for Disease Control and Prevention. Malaria: diagnosis and treatment. 2007. http://www.cdc.gov/malaria/diagnosis_treatment/diagnosis.htm. Accessed July 12, 2007.
45. Centers for Disease Control and Prevention. *Yellow Book: Health Information for International Travel 2008. Prevention of Specific Infectious Diseases—Malaria.* Atlanta: US Department of Health and Human Services, Public Health Service, 2007. http://wwwn.cdc.gov/travel/contentyellowbook.aspx.

CHAPTER 67

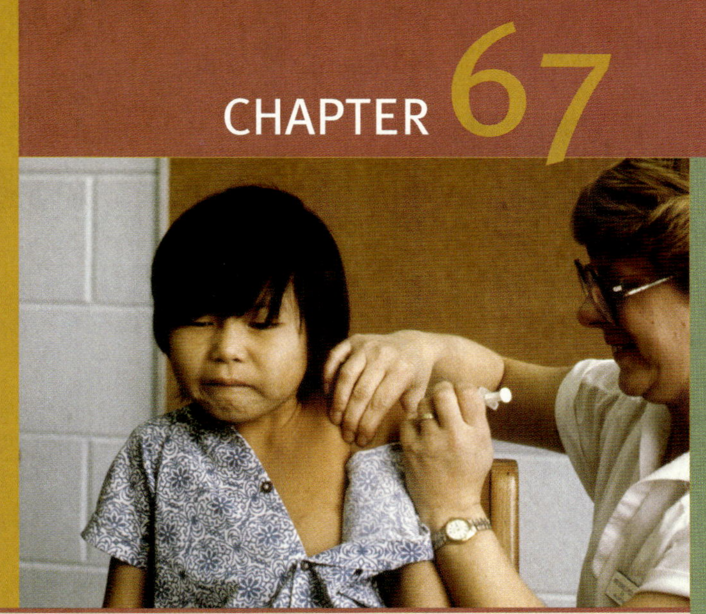

Intestinal Parasites

Nisha Manickam and Michael Cappello

Infections caused by intestinal parasites represent major causes of global morbidity, including malnutrition, diarrhea with dehydration, and anemia. For example, nearly 2 billion people, mostly in resource-poor countries, are infected with one or more of the soil-transmitted nematodes, while cestodes and trematodes are common food-borne infections worldwide. Intestinal protozoa are important causes of diarrhea in travelers, as well as immigrants, refugees, and international adoptees. With the increased global mobility of persons and populations, physicians in the United States are encountering parasitic diseases with increased frequency, requiring familiarity with their clinical features and management. This chapter will focus on the four major classes of intestinal parasite: nematodes, trematodes, cestodes, and protozoa.

NEMATODES (TABLE 67–1)

Nematodes are unsegemented roundworms belonging to the phylum Nematoda. Many species are found worldwide, but most favor tropical climates. In general, nematodes are cylindrical in shape with tapered ends. They vary greatly in size from up to 40 cm in length (*Ascaris lumbricoides*) to less than 1 cm (*Strongyloides stercoralis, Enterobius vermicularis,* and hookworm species). The common finding in this group of worms is the antigenically inert outer layer called the cuticle, which serves as a barrier of protection from host antibodies and digestive enzymes.[1,2] Nematodes have separate adult male and female genders, with females typically larger in size.

Ascaris lumbricoides

Epidemiology

A. lumbricoides is the most prevalent of nematode infections, with an estimated 1.4 billion persons infected worldwide. Of those, only a portion have signs of clinical disease, with an estimated 20,000 deaths yearly due to complications of ascariasis.[3] Infection occurs in both tropical and temperate climates,[2] and in both rural and urban environments,[4] typically where adequate moisture and poor sanitation are found. In the United States, the majority of infected individuals are immigrants from endemic areas.[3]

Pathogenesis

Infection occurs when individuals ingest eggs, often contained in food contaminated with human fecal material, which hatch in the small intestine. The first-stage larvae penetrate the intestinal mucosa, enter venous circulation, and travel to the lungs. They then access the alveolar space and migrate up the trachea where they are swallowed, thus returning to the small intestine. During tissue migration, the larvae undergo a series of molts, eventually maturing into adults in the small intestine. Adult females release eggs that are eventually excreted in feces.

Clinical presentation

A hallmark of *Ascaris* infection occurs 5–6 days after egg ingestion, just as the larvae travel to the lungs. Termed Loeffler's syndrome, patients often experience wheezing, dyspnea, cough, and fever lasting 10–12 days. Dense pulmonary infiltrates on chest X-ray and moderate

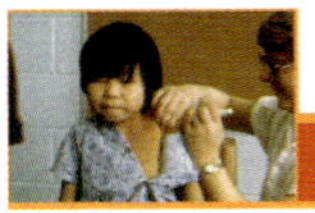

Table 67–1.

Nematodes

Organism	Epidemiology	Clinical Caveats
Ascaris lumbricoides	■ Highest prevalence occurs in tropical and subtropical regions, especially in areas with inadequate sanitation. ■ In the United States, transmission has occurred in rural areas of the southeastern states.	■ May cause Loffler's syndrome (pulmonary infiltrates, cough, wheezing, dyspnea, and fever) with peripheral eosinophilia during the migration of larvae through lung tissue. ■ Treatment may trigger movement of the adult intestinal worms and can lead to intestinal obstruction.
Strongyloides species	■ Tropical and subtropical areas including the southeastern US. ■ More frequently found in rural areas, institutional settings, among World War II and Vietnam war veterans, and lower socioeconomic groups.	■ Hyperinfection may occur in persons undergoing chemotherapy or taking systemic corticosteroids—therefore persons from endemic areas should be screened prior to therapy.
Hookworm (*Necator americanus* and *Ancylostoma duodenale*)	■ Worldwide distribution, mostly in areas with moist, warm climate.	■ Heavily infected children may have growth stunting, cognitive delays, iron deficiency anemia, hypoalbuminemia, and eosinophilia.
Enterobius vermicularis (pinworm)	■ The most common helminth infection in the United States (an estimated 40 million persons infected). ■ Worldwide distribution, with infections more frequent in young children and among persons living in crowded conditions. ■ More common in temperate than tropical countries.	■ Common in children in daycare settings, pinworm is diagnosed best using the scotch-tape test.
Trichuris trichiura	■ Worldwide distribution, favoring tropical areas, especially those with poor sanitation practices. ■ Also found in the southern US. ■ More common among children than adults.	■ Heavy infections can mimic inflammatory bowel disease, with hemorrhagic colitis known as *Trichuris* dysentery. ■ Rectal prolapse can also develop.

eosinophilia (up to 40%) may also be noted. Light to moderate infections may be asymptomatic, although common symptoms include abdominal pain, nausea, anorexia, and diarrhea or constipation. In contrast, those with heavy chronic infections may experience intestinal obstruction, nutritional deficiencies, and cognitive delays.[2] Adult worms may also migrate to the bile duct and pancreatic duct, leading to ascending cholangitis, acute pancreatitis, or obstructive jaundice.[5]

Diagnosis

The diagnosis of *A. lumbricoides* infection requires identification of characteristic eggs, larvae, or adult worms. When adult worms are producing eggs in the small intestine, light microscopy can be used to identify eggs in the feces. Fertilized eggs are either round or ovoid in shape and measure 60–75 μm in diameter, while unfertilized eggs are elongated and measure up to 90 μm in diameter (Figure 67–1).[6] Adult worms may also be passed in stool or exit via the mouth or nares. Adult female worms range in size from 20 to 35 cm in length

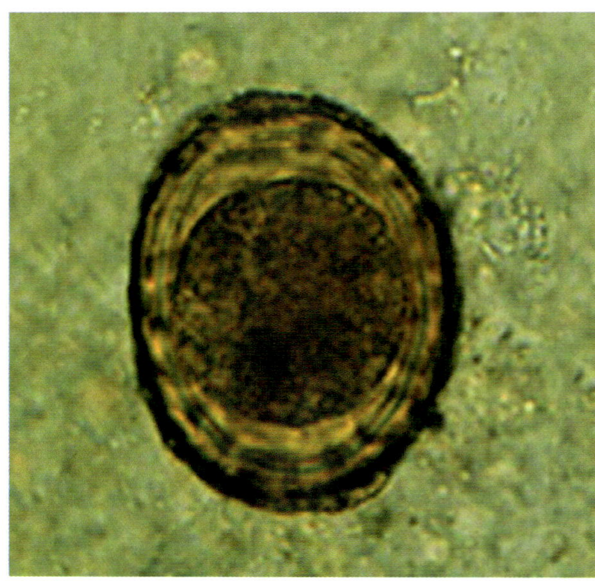

FIGURE 67–1 ■ *Ascaris lumbricoides* egg. The unicellular stage shown here would be detected in a stool specimen. (*Courtesy of the Centers for Disease Control.*[6])

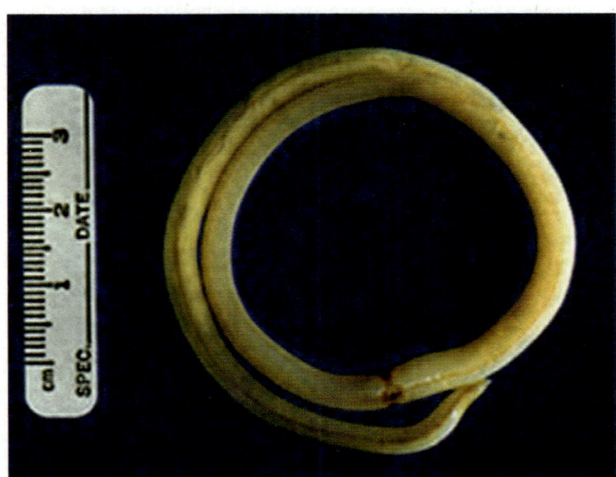

FIGURE 67–2 ■ Adult female *Ascaris lumbricoides*. (*Courtesy of the Centers for Disease Control.*[6])

and 3–6 mm in diameter, while males are slightly smaller.[7] The worms are pink in color and tapered at both ends (Figure 67–2). In individuals with Loeffler's syndrome, larvae can occasionally be detected in sputum or bronchoalveolar lavage fluid.

Imaging studies, including abdominal radiographs, ultrasound, and computed tomography (CT) can also establish a diagnosis in heavily infected individuals. On radiographs, large collections of worms can produce a "whirlpool" effect as they contrast with bowel gas.[8] Barium is occasionally ingested by the worms, allowing for visualization of the alimentary canal. Ultrasound can detect biliary or pancreatic migration of worms and endoscopic retrograde cholangiopancreatography(ERCP) can aid in removal. CT of the abdomen with oral contrast often reveals cylindrical filling defects within the intestinal lumen. The GI tract of the *Ascaris* worms can occasionally be seen as a slender thread of contrast within the filling defects.[9]

Treatment

For *A. lumbricoides*, the treatments of choice are the benzimidazole anthelminthics, albendazole and mebendazole. Ivermectin and nitazoxanide are also active against *A. lumbricoides* and can be considered alternative agents (Table 67–5).[10] Treatment may trigger active movement of the worms, leading to obstruction or extraintestinal migration.

Strongyloides Species

Epidemiology

Human infection with *Strongyloides* is usually caused by *S. stercoralis,* which is endemic to the tropics and subtropics, including parts of the southeastern United States and Appalachia. By contrast, *Strongyloides fuelleborni* is found in the South Pacific, mainly Papua New Guinea, and parts of Africa. It is estimated that 56 million people are infected with *S. stercoralis.*[11] In the United States, those at highest risk for strongyloidiasis include veterans of World War II and Vietnam, immigrants and refugees from endemic areas, as well as those seropositive for human T-lymphocyte lymphotropic virus type I.[12]

Pathogenesis

Third-stage free-living larvae penetrate the host skin and gain access to the bloodstream. Once in the venous circulation, their migration is similar to *A. lumbricoides,* first traveling to the lungs then migrating to the trachea and ultimately into the small intestine. It is here that the larvae become fully mature adults and embed into the intestinal epithelium. The females shed eggs into the gut, which develop into first-stage larvae that are excreted in feces (Figure 67–3).

Strongyloides species are unique among nematodes in that they can complete their entire life cycle outside the host (free living cycle) or multiply within a single host (autoinfective cycle). In autoinfection, larvae develop into the infectious stage within the gut and

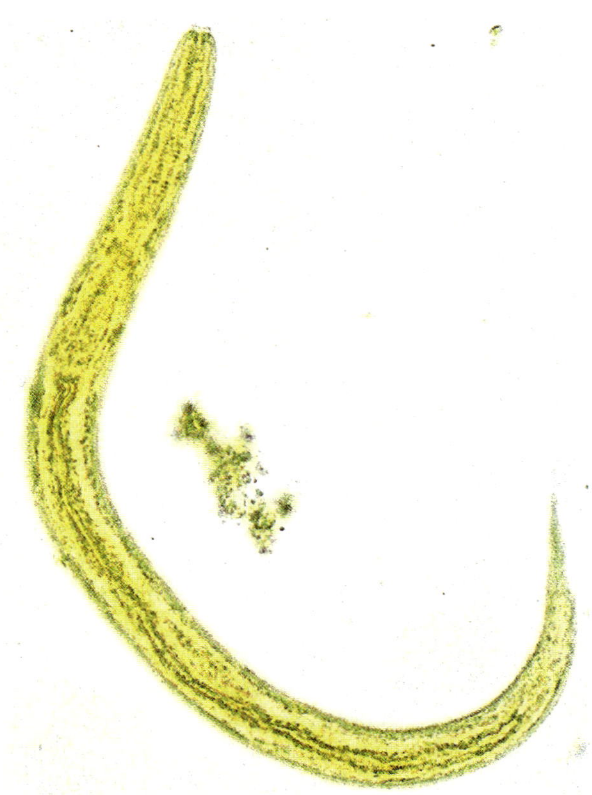

FIGURE 67–3 ■ Iodine-stained first-stage larvae of *Strongyloides stercoralis* as would be detected in stool. (*Courtesy of Ash and Orihel.*[7])

penetrate the colonic mucosa or perianal skin. Thus, persons can have chronic infections lasting for decades after leaving an endemic area.

Clinical presentation

Acute infection is characterized by "larva currens," a serpiginous urticarial rash at the site of skin penetration.[13] Migrating larvae in the lung can occasionally induce dyspnea, dry cough, and wheezing. Loeffler's syndrome, characterized by cough, interstitial infiltrates, and eosinophilia, may develop in those with moderate to severe infection, although less commonly than with *Ascaris* infection. Intestinal symptoms are usually absent in immunocompetent individuals; however, severe, prolonged infections in children can lead to chronic diarrhea, vomiting, weight loss, abdominal distention, malnutrition and lethargy.[8] In chronic infection, larva currens is often seen in the perianal area representing autoinfection. In Papua New Guinea, an infantile form of strongyloidiasis (due to *S. fuelleborni*), called "swollen belly syndrome," is characterized by abdominal distention, diarrhea, failure to thrive, protein malnutrition, and hypoalbuminemia.[14]

A feature of *S. stercoralis* infection is the phenomenon of hyperinfection or disseminated infection. This occurs when a person's cell-mediated immune response is deficient, often due to the administration of immunosuppressives, such as glucocorticoids. Disseminated infection usually involves the bowel (paralytic ileus), central nervous system (CNS) (meningitis, brain abscess), and the lungs (pneumonitis), and may be complicated by secondary bacterial infection and septicemia.[15] For this reason, persons from endemic areas about to undergo chemotherapy or long-term steroid therapy are usually screened for evidence of *S. stercoralis* infection.

Diagnosis

S. stercoralis is unique among intestinal nematodes in that eggs passed by adult female worms develop into larvae within the gut and are excreted in the feces. Although light microscopy may be used to identify larvae, the sensitivity is poor. Multiple samples will increase the detection rate, from 10% with one specimen up to 50% with three.[8] Occasionally, the use of a string test or duodenojejunal aspiration can be used to detect larvae.[16] With this method, the patient swallows a weighted gelatin capsule attached to a string with the free end taped to the patients' cheek or neck. After approximately 4 hours, the string is removed and examined for evidence of parasites under light microscopy. In disseminated infection, examination of sputum or lung tissue may also reveal larvae. Peripheral eosinophilia is often found in persons with chronic strongyloidiasis, but may be absent in hyperinfection.[17]

Serology can aid in the diagnosis of *S. stercoralis* infection, especially in those with asymptomatic eosinophilia.[18,19] However, antibodies persist for years after treatment, thereby limiting the use of serologic tests for distinguishing past from current infection.

Treatment

The drug of choice for strongyloidiasis is ivermectin (Table 67–5). Alternatives include albendazole and thiabendazole.[10] In the setting of disseminated infection, it is important to evaluate patients for evidence of concomitant bacterial infection, as well as taper steroids or immunosuppressives as tolerated.[20]

Hookworm Species (*Ancylostoma duodenale* and *Necator americanus*)

Epidemiology

The hookworm species *A. duodenale* and *N. americanus* are estimated to infect 740 million people worldwide,[5,21] and infection was once endemic in the southeastern United States.[22] Other species *Ancylostoma ceylanicum* and the dog hookworm *Ancylostoma caninum* less commonly cause intestinal disease. Hookworms primarily infect persons in rural areas and may be associated with farming certain crops (mulberry leaves, sweet potatoes, tea,[23] and coffee).

Pathogenesis

The life cycle of hookworms begins when third-stage larvae in the soil contact and penetrate human skin, enter the venous circulation, and are carried to the lungs. After migrating up the trachea, the worms are swallowed and ultimately reach the small intestine. Adult hookworms attach to the intestinal mucosa, lacerating mucosal vessels and ingesting blood (Figure 67–4A and B). The adults mate in the gut, and females release eggs that are excreted in feces (usually appearing within 6–8 weeks after infection).[24]

Clinical presentation

Acute infection may cause ground itch, characterized by pruritus and rash, at the site of skin penetration.[2] Migration of larvae through the lungs can produce a pneumonitis similar to that seen with *A. lumbricoides*, although usually less severe. Intestinal disease is usually manifested by nonspecific abdominal pain. Heavy worm burdens, however, may be associated with epigastric pain, nausea, exertional dyspnea, headache, and fatigue. Ingestion of large numbers of *A. duodenale* larvae may be associated with a condition called Wakana disease, which is characterized by eosinophilia, nausea, vomiting, and dyspnea.[24]

Chronic infection may lead to anemia, malnutrition, and growth delay, and can be associated with

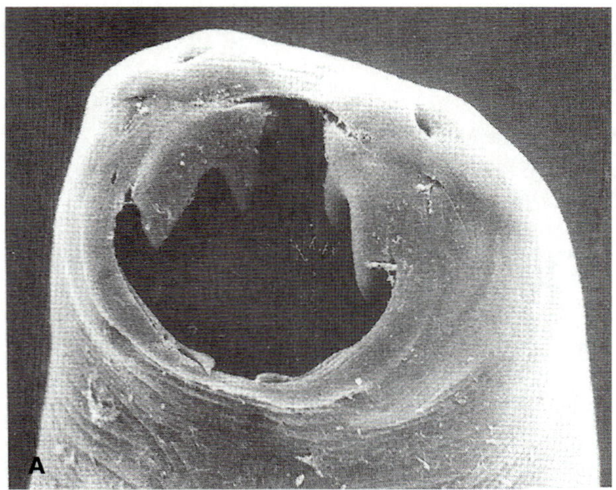

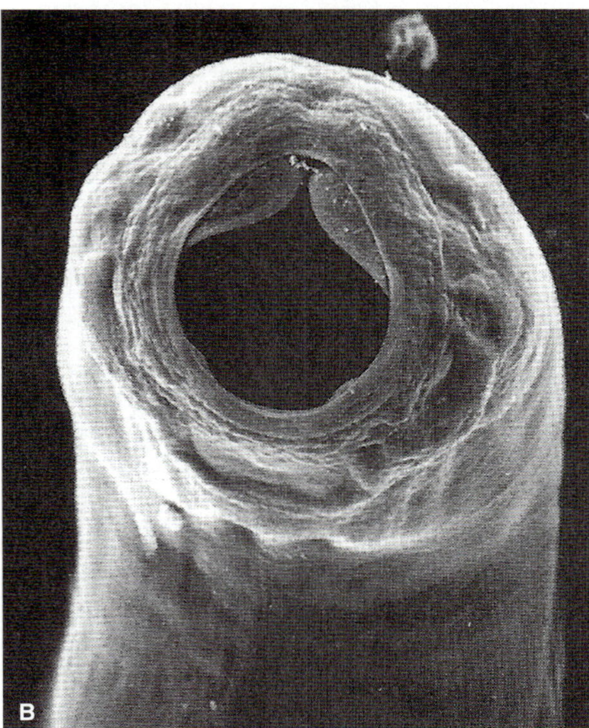

FIGURES 67–4 ■ Stereoscans of two adult hookworms **(A)** *Necator americanus* and **(B)** *Ancylostoma duodenale* revealing cutting plates and teeth, respectively. (*Courtesy of Muller, Worms and Human Disease.*[2])

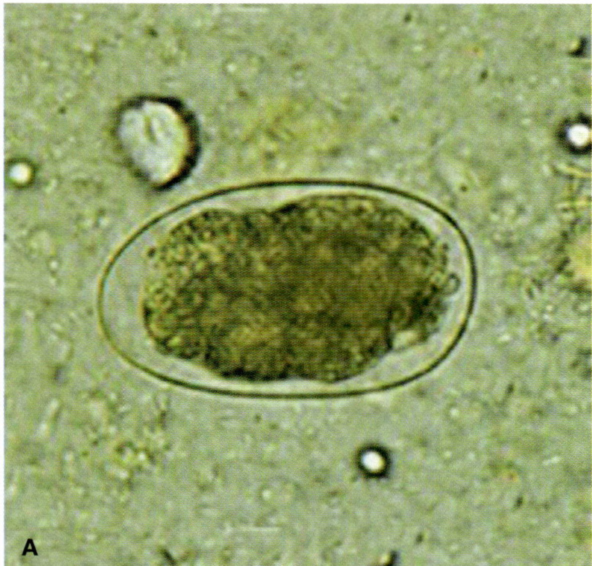

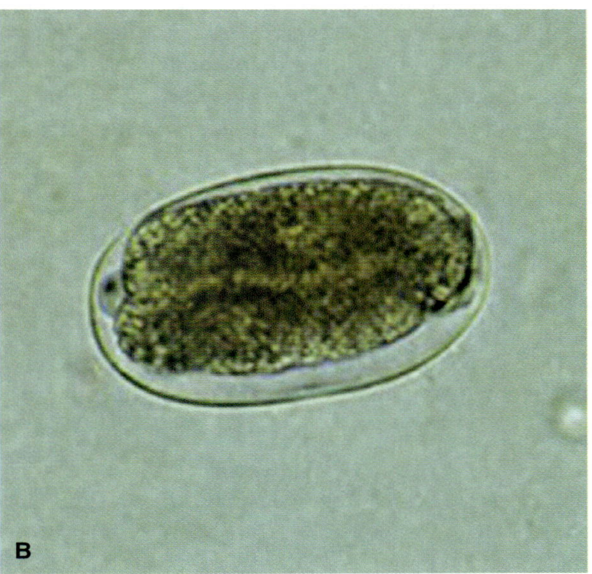

FIGURES 67–5 ■ Eggs of two hookworm species **(A)** *Ancylostoma duodenale* and **(B)** *Necator americanus* revealing similar morphology. (*Courtesy of the Centers for Disease Control.*[6])

cognitive delay. It is estimated that each adult hookworm can feed on up to 0.2 mL of blood per day, resulting in iron-deficiency anemia and hypoproteinemia.[4] A form of neonatal disease, similar to that caused by *S. fuelleborni*, is characterized by melena, abdominal distention, hypotension, and severe anemia.[25,26]

Diagnosis

Identification of eggs in fecal samples is the mainstay of diagnosis. The eggs are 50–75 μm in length by 35–45 μm in width, with a thin shell and oval or ellipsoid shape (Figure 67–5A and B).[6] Heavily infected persons also have iron-deficiency anemia, hypoalbuminemia, and mild eosinophilia.

Treatment

Hookworm infection is generally treated with albendazole or mebendazole, with pyrantel pamoate a suitable alternative (Table 67–5). .Nitazoxanide may also have activity,[27] although data are limited. Eradication programs in endemic countries have relied on targeted chemotherapy of children, which results in short-term improvements in blood hemoglobin levels and nutritional status.[24] However, high rates of reinfection and potential emergence of anthelminthic resistance may limit the long-term benefit of current control measures.[26]

Enterobius vermicularis

Epidemiology

E. vermicularis (pinworm) is the most common nematode infection in developed countries, mainly affecting preschool children. Infection occurs through fecal–oral contamination, ingestion of fomites (airborne eggs), and/or retroinfection.[28]

Pathogenesis

Once pinworms eggs are ingested, they hatch and release larvae in the small intestine. Here they undergo several molts until they mature into adults and eventually reach the colon (usually a 5-week process). Female adult pinworms migrate out of the intestine at night and deposit eggs on the perianal skin. Each female can produce as many as 11,000 eggs per day,[29] which become infectious within hours.

Clinical presentation

Pruritus ani, caused by the inflammatory response directed at eggs deposited on the perianal skin, may lead to secondary cellulitis and subcutaneous abscess formation.[30] Aberrant migration of the adult worms may result in endometritis, salpingitis, and rarely appendicitis.[28,31]

Diagnosis

Since eggs are deposited in the perianal area instead of in the feces, they are not detected using standard microscopy for ova and parasites. For this reason, it is recommended that a piece of clear adhesive tape be looped over a tongue depressor so that the adhesive surface is on the outside. The tape is then pressed against the perianal skin in several places and attached to a glass slide, which is examined under light microscopy for the presence of eggs. The optimal time for this test is early morning before bathing. Pinworm eggs are ovoid and measure 50–60 μm in length by 20–30 μm in width (Figure 67–6).[6] Adult worms may reach 1 cm in length and are distinguished by bilateral cuticular ridges termed alae.[2]

Treatment

E. vermicularis infection is treated with mebendazole, albendazole, or pyrantel pamoate (Table 67–5).[10] A second treatment after 2 weeks is recommended to eradicate developing larvae, as these anthelminthics are not ovicidal. Recurrent disease is common, most often due to reinfection from an infected close contact.

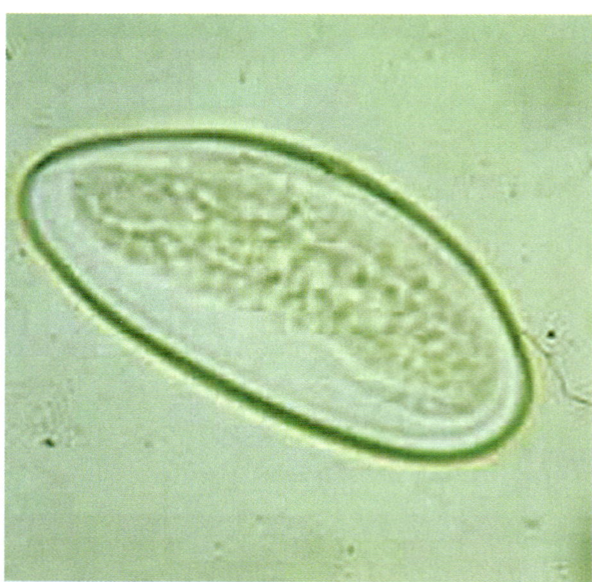

FIGURE 67–6 ■ Egg of *Enterobius vermicularis* (pinworm). (*Courtesy of the Centers for Disease Control.*[6])

Trichuris trichiura

Epidemiology

Also known as the whipworm, infections with *T. trichiura* occur in most parts of the tropics, similar to *A. lumbricoides* and hookworm. The estimated number of people infected worldwide is 795 million.[21]

Pathogenesis

The life cycle is similar to that of *E. vermicularis* in that infectious eggs are swallowed and hatch in the small intestine. Larvae undergo several molts until they mature into adults and eventually reside in the colon. The adult whipworms, which can reach 5 cm in length, embed into the colonic mucosa where the males and females mate. Here the females excrete up to 20,000 eggs per day in the stool, taking at least 2–3 months from infection before egg production starts.[2] Unlike *E. vermicularis* eggs, which become infectious soon after deposition, the eggs of *T. trichiura* only become infectious after 15–30 days.[6]

Clinical presentation

Light infections are usually asymptomatic. Heavy infections can lead to a severe inflammatory colitis known as *Trichuris* dysentery,[32] characterized by melena and mucus in the stool. Mucosal edema also may develop, leading to rectal prolapse (Figure 67–7). Chronic infections can lead to a colitis that mimics inflammatory bowel disease and may be associated with growth delay and cognitive deficits.[33]

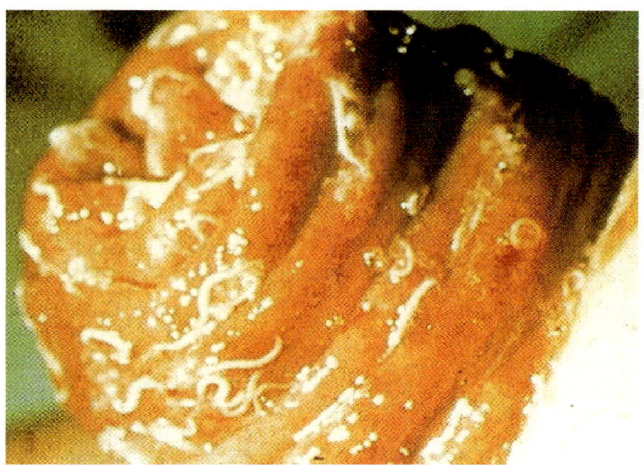

FIGURE 67–7 ■ Rectal prolapse with numerous visible adult worms of *Trichuris trichiura*. (*Courtesy of Sun.*[8])

Diagnosis

Light microscopy is most commonly used to detect characteristic eggs in the feces. The eggs are oval in shape (sometimes referred to as "barrel shaped"), and have a three-layer eggshell as well as transparent bipolar mucoid plugs (Figure 67–8). They usually measure 50–54 × 22–23 μm.[6]

Treatment

The drug of choice for *T. trichiura* infection is mebendazole (500 mg in a single dose for light infections; 100 mg bid × 3 days for heavy infections). Alternative drugs are albendazole and ivermectin (Table 67–5). Of note, *T. trichiura* is resistant to pyrantel pamoate.[10]

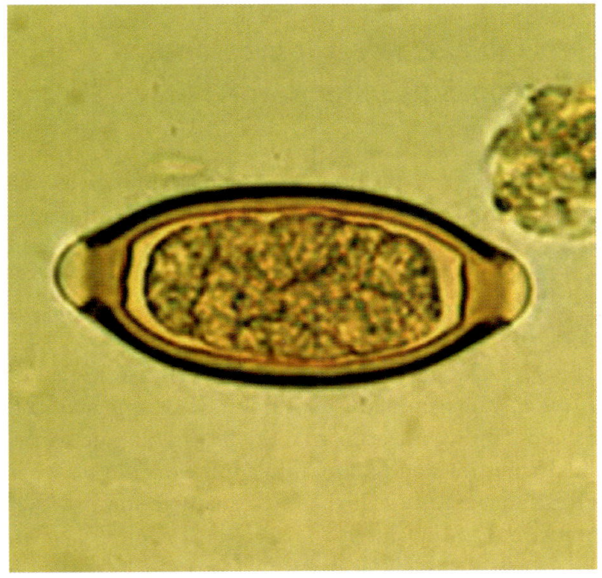

FIGURE 67–8 ■ Unembryonated egg, as seen in stool, of *Trichuris trichiura*. Note the barrel shape with polar prominences, referred to as "polar plugs." (*Courtesy of the Centers for Disease Control.*[6])

PREVENTION OF NEMATODES

Education, targeted chemotherapy, and improved sanitation efforts (building of proper latrines) helped to reduce the burden of intestinal nematode infections in the United States.[22] In resource poor countries, mass deworming may reduce nutritional deficiencies and growth stunting, although this strategy confers only short-term benefit due to high rates of reinfection. For travelers to endemic areas, education about transmission is important. Wearing proper footwear and proper cooking of food and filtering (or boiling) of drinking water may reduce the risk of transmission. Although currently in development, no vaccines are yet available for human soil-transmitted nematode infections.

TREMATODES (TABLE 67–2)

Trematodes, also known as flukes, belong to the phylum Platyhelminthes and are characteristically flat and leaf-like. An estimated 50 million people are infected with intestinal flukes in North Africa, the Middle East, and East and Southeast Asia.[34] Many trematodes are hermaphrodites, with both male and female reproductive organs in a single worm. Each trematode has two suckers, an anterior oral sucker that connects to the alimentary canal, and a posterior ventral sucker that attaches the worm to the host (Figure 67–9).[2] These worms have no true intestine, as the alimentary canal ends in a blind pouch. Liquid waste is therefore expelled through specialized excretory cells known as flame cells, and insoluble waste must be regurgitated through the apical sucker.[4] Unique to trematodes is the requirement of the snail as an intermediate host. The major intestinal flukes are *Fasciolopsis buski, Heterophyes heterophyes,* and *Metagonimus yokogawai.*

Fasciolopsis buski

Epidemiology

Found predominantly in the Far East, *F. buski* is endemic in the Yangtze basin provinces of China and parts of Southeast Asia and India where both pigs and water plants are farmed.[2]

Pathogenesis

When human feces containing eggs contaminate a body of water, the eggs embryonate and hatch, releasing larvae called miracidium. The miracidium infect specific freshwater snails and develop into cercariae, which are shed and encyst on plants. Here, the larvae develop into metacercaria. When raw or undercooked plants (watercress, bamboo shoots, and water chestnuts) containing these metacercaria are consumed by humans, the larvae migrate to the small intestine and mature into adult

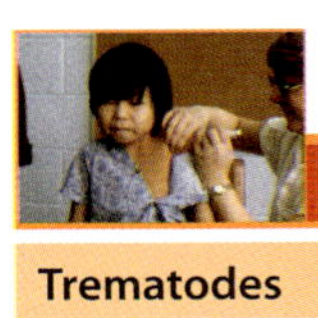

Table 67–2.

Trematodes

Organism	Epidemiology	Clinical Caveats
Fasciolopsis buski	■ Predominantly in the Asia (endemic in the Yangtze basin provinces of China) and parts of Southeast Asia and India where both pigs and water plants are farmed. ■ Related to consumption of undercooked plants such as watercress, bamboo shoots and water chestnuts.	■ Heavy infections can lead to intestinal ulceration, microabscesses, and obstruction.
Heterophyes heterophyes *Metagonimus yokogawai*	■ Endemic in most parts of Asia, Egypt, and the Middle East. ■ Most common fluke in the Far East, but also found in Siberia, Manchuria, the Balkan states, Israel, and Spain.	■ Eggs can migrate to the heart (causing valvular damage) and brain. ■ Related to consumption of raw or undercooked fish in endemic areas. ■ Symptoms usually include diarrhea and abdominal pain. ■ Like *H. heterophyes*, migration of eggs to the heart and brain has been reported.

flukes. The larvae take approximately four months to fully mature at which time they can produce up to 28,000 eggs per fluke per day.[2]

Clinical presentation

Clinical symptoms result from the attachment of the flukes to the intestinal mucosa causing inflammation, ulceration, and microabscesses. Heavy worm burdens (>500 adult worms) can produce significant symptoms, such as diarrhea, constipation, abdominal pains, nausea, and vomiting. Heavy infections with *F. buski* can also lead to intestinal obstruction or a protein-losing enteropathy.[34]

Diagnosis

Recovery of characteristic eggs in the stool is the key to diagnosis. The eggs may be best demonstrated after concentrating stool, especially in the case of light infections.

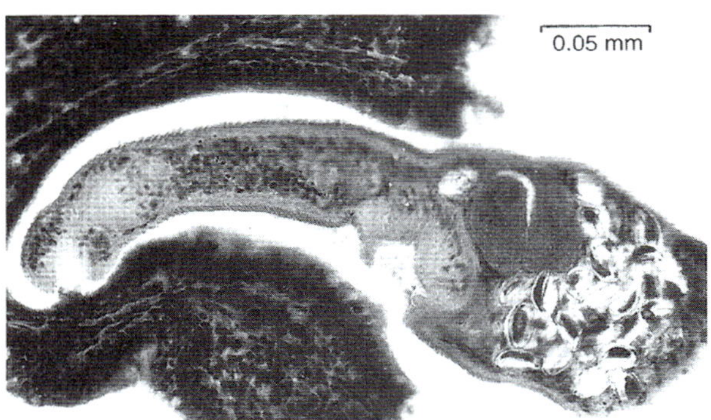

FIGURE 67–9 ■ Adult *Heterophyes heterophyes* fluke attached to intestinal mucosa. (*Courtesy of Muller.*[2])

F. buski has larger eggs than the other intestinal flukes and measures 130–140 by 80–85 μm in size (Figure 67–10A).[2] The eggs are operculated and are unembryonated when deposited. The adult flukes, if recovered, reach up to 7.5 cm in length and 2.5 cm in width, and are easily recognized when compared to other *Fasciola* species because of the absence of a cephalic cone (Figure 67–10B).[35]

Treatment

The preferred treatment for *F. buski* is praziquantel (Table 67–5).[10]

Heterophyes heterophyes and *Metagonimus yokogawai*

Epidemiology

H. heterophyes can be found in most parts of Asia, as well as in North Africa and the Middle East. *M. yokogawai* represents the most common intestinal fluke in the Far East, but has also been found in Spain, Israel, and Serbia.[2]

Pathogenesis

The life cycles of these species are very similar to that of *F. buski*. When humans consume raw or undercooked fish containing metacercaria, the larvae migrate to the small intestine and mature into adult worms. The types of fish that transmit disease are usually found in either brackish or fresh water.[34]

Clinical presentation

The smaller flukes (*H. heterophyes and M. yokogawai*) can penetrate the intestinal mucosa, eliciting a granulomatous

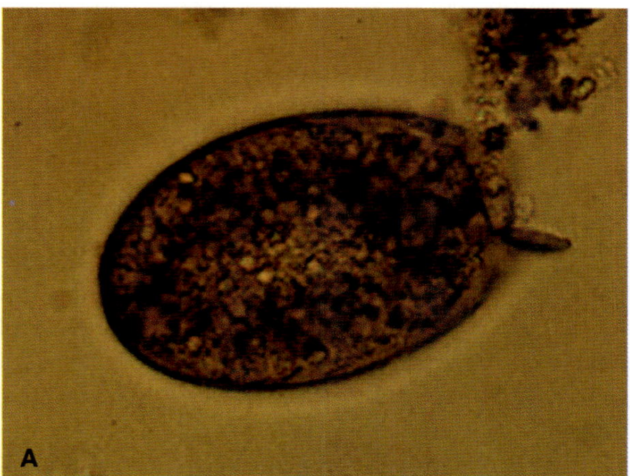

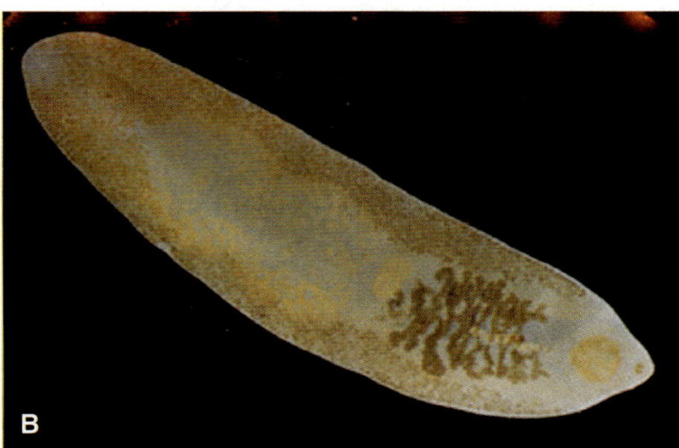

FIGURE 67–10 ■ The **(A)** egg and **(B)** adult fluke of *Fasciolopsis buski*. (*Courtesy of the Centers for Disease Control.*[6])

response. They may occasionally migrate to ectopic sites, such as the heart and brain via the bloodstream and lymphatics. Symptoms include abdominal pain, intermittent diarrhea, anorexia, and nausea.[34]

Diagnosis

The eggs of *H. heterophyes* and *M. yokogawai* are much smaller in size than *F. buski*. Treatment may result in expulsion of the adult worms, allowing for a definitive diagnosis. The adult worms of *H. heterophyes* and *M. yokogawai* are 1–1.7 mm in length by 0.3–0.4 mm in width and 1–2.5 mm in length by 0.4–0.75 mm in width, respectively (Figure 67–11A and B).[6]

Treatment

Similar to *F. buski*, the preferred treatment is Praziquantel (Table 67–5).[10]

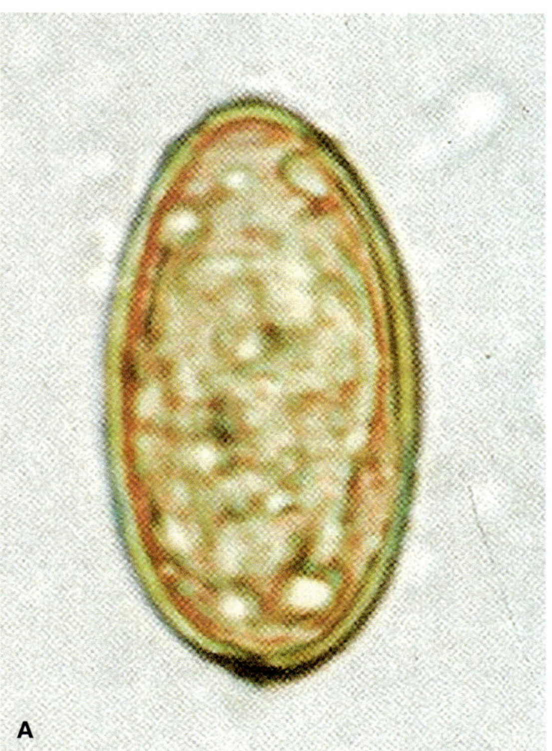

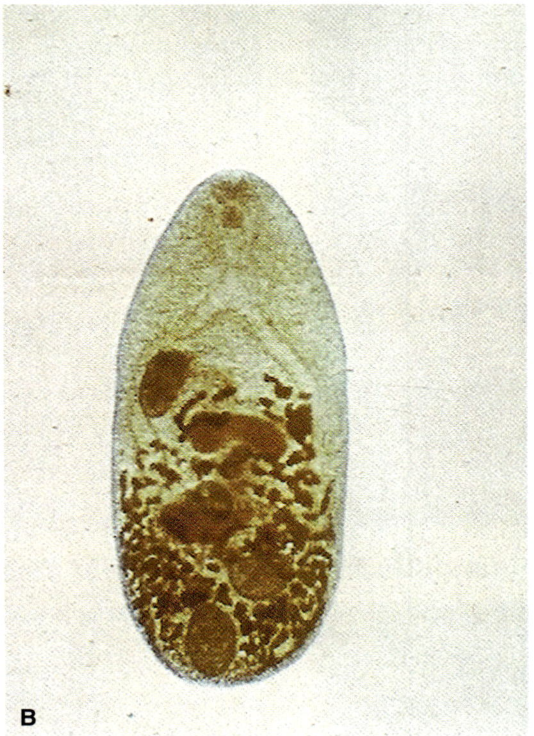

FIGURE 67–11 ■ The **(A)** egg and **(B)** adult fluke of *Metagonimus yokogawai*. (*Courtesy of Yamaguchi.*[62])

PREVENTION OF TREMATODES

Properly cooking plants (such as bamboo shoots and watercress) may help to prevent infection. The practice of eating raw fish in endemic areas should also be discouraged. Ultimately, improving sanitary conditions in endemic areas to prevent fecal contamination in water sources where plants and fish live is the most effective long-term control strategy.

CESTODES (TABLE 67–3)

Cestodes, belonging to the phylum Platyhelminthes, are also commonly known as tapeworms because of their flat, ribbon-shaped appearance. The tapeworm morphology consists of a scolex, which attaches to the host's intestinal mucosa via suckers or sucking grooves, and/or hooks. Just posterior to the scolex is the neck, which gives rise to the growth of proglottids. The tapeworm grows distally in a process known as strobilation; thus the further away from the neck region, the proglottids become successfully more mature and then gravid. Once they fill with eggs, the proglottid becomes detached and is excreted in the stool. Similar to flukes, tapeworms are hermaphroditic, as each proglottid contains both ovaries and testes. There are four major groups of cestodes, but only those in the orders Cyclophylidea (*Taenia saginata, Taenia solium, Hymenolepis nana)* and Pseudophylidea (*Diphylobothrium latum)* are important intestinal pathogens.

Taenia saginata and *Taenia solium*

Epidemiology

T. saginata, the beef tapeworm, is endemic to Europe, Africa and South America because of the customary practice of consuming undercooked beef. *T. solium,* related to pork consumption, is common in Mexico, Central and South America, parts of Africa and Southeast Asia.[2] Infection with the larval stages of *T. solium,* called cysticercosis, is a major cause of seizures in resource-poor countries.

Pathogenesis

The life cycles of *T. saginata* and *T. solium* are quite similar. When either cattle or pigs consume feed contaminated with human feces containing *Taenia* eggs, the eggs hatch in the intestine and travel via the bloodstream and lymphatics to somatic tissues. Here, they develop into the larval forms (cysticerci). When humans ingest undercooked beef or pork containing cysticerci, the larvae are released from the cyst and attach to the intestinal epithelium via the scolex. Here the tapeworms grow distally, reaching lengths of 2–4 m for *T. solium* (800–900 proglottids) and 5–25 m for *T. saginata* (1000–2000 proglottids).[8] Maturation into the adult form takes 6–8 weeks for *T. solium* and 10–12 weeks for *T. saginata,* at which time proglottids may be shed.[36] If untreated, tapeworms can survive for up to 25 years for *T. solium,* and 10 years for *T. saginata.*[8]

If humans ingest *T. solium* eggs directly via fecal–oral contamination, the eggs hatch and invade the circulatory system and disseminate to somatic tissues. Neurocysticercosis is the term that refers to CNS invasion by the larvae.

Table 67–3.

Cestodes

Organism	Epidemiology	Clinical Caveats
Taenia saginata	■ Worldwide distribution—endemic in Europe, Africa and South America where there are customary practices of eating undercooked beef.	■ Most people become aware of infection during passage of proglottids in stool. ■ *T. saginata* are usually expelled as single proglottids and may even crawl out of the anus.
Taenia solium	■ Worldwide distribution—common in Mexico, Central and South America, parts of Africa and Southeast Asia. Related to the consumption of undercooked pork.	■ *T. solium* proglottids are expelled in chains of 5-6 proglottids. These tapeworms can live up to 25 years if left untreated. ■ Neurocysticercosis follows ingestion of eggs (fecal–oral transmission), not from eating pork.
Hymenolepis nana	■ Most common tapeworm infection in humans with a worldwide distribution (although more common in temperate areas).	■ When children are infected, many experts recommend treating the whole family, as person-to-person spread has been documented.
Diphylobothrium latum	■ Endemic in Japan and Northern Europe. Can also be found in Asia, Uganda, Chile, North America and the former Soviet Union. In the United States, cases have been reported after consumption of imported fish from endemic areas.	■ Related to consumption of raw or undercooked infected fish. ■ Chronic infection can lead to macrocytic anemia from vitamin B12 deficiency.

Clinical presentation

Intestinal taeniasis is usually asymptomatic. Occasionally infected individuals experience vague symptoms, including abdominal pain, nausea, diarrhea, and appetite changes. Many become aware of infection only after the passage of tapeworm segments in the stool.[36]

Diagnosis

Demonstration of eggs or gravid proglottid segments in the feces is necessary for the diagnosis of intestinal taeniasis. For *T. solium* and *T. saginata,* the eggs are morphologically indistinguishable, described as brown and spherical, measuring 31–43 μm in diameter (Figure 67–12). [6] The gravid proglottid segments allow for distinction between species. *T. solium* proglottids are usually expelled passively in chains of five or six segments while that of *T. saginata* are expelled as single proglottids and may even crawl out of the anus. The uterine branches and testicular follicles in each segment also differ; *T. solium* have fewer uterine branches (5–10) and testicular follicles (150–200) while that of *T. saginata* have 15–30 branches and 300–400 testicular follicles (Figure 67–13A and B).[8]

Occasionally, the scolex will be passed in the stool and will allow for differentiation between species. The scolex of *T. solium* has a rostellum with a double row of hooklets (22–32) and four suckers. In contrast, *T. saginata* has an unarmed rostellum (the absence of hooklets) (Figure 67–14A and B).[37]

Fecal coproantigen detection assays have been developed to detect *Taenia*-specific antigens in human specimens.[38] This is a sensitive and specific test, although not widely available. Serology is useful for the diagnosis of *T. solium* infection in the setting of cysticercosis, especially neurocysticercosis, although its role in diagnosing intestinal disease is less certain.

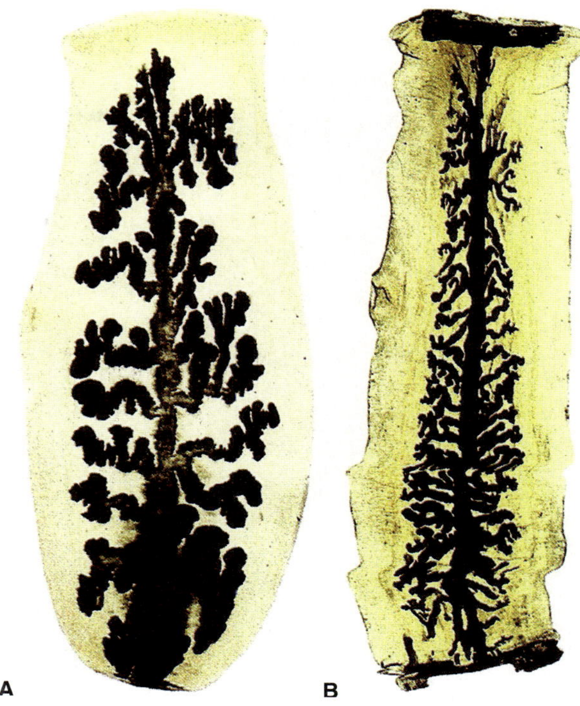

FIGURES 67–13 ■ To identify *Taenia* species, India ink can be injected into the uterus via the lateral genital pore of proglottids passed in stool. The number of branches corresponds to the type of species, i.e., **(A)** *Taenia solium* has 13 or fewer branches and **(B)** *Taenia saginata* usually has 15 or more. (*Courtesy of Ash and Orihel.*[7])

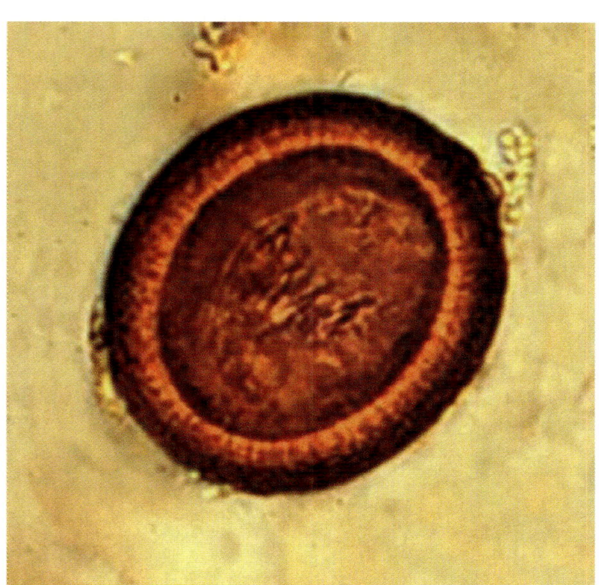

FIGURE 67–12 ■ The eggs of *Taenia saginata and Taenia solium* tapeworms are indistinguishable by light microscopy. (*Courtesy of the Centers for Disease Control.*[6])

Treatment

The mainstay of treatment for intestinal taeniasis is praziquantel (Table 67–5).[10] One to three months after therapy, patients should be examined for evidence of eggs in the stool to document cure.

Hymenolepis nana

Epidemiology

H. nana, also known as the dwarf tapeworm, is the most common tapeworm to infect humans, and has a global distribution.[39]

Pathogenesis

H. nana does not require an intermediate host. Rather, humans ingest eggs (via fecal–oral contamination) that hatch in the small intestine releasing a larval form called the oncosphere. This penetrates the intestinal mucosa and matures into cysticercoid larva in the lymphatics of the intestinal villi. The cysticercoid then migrates back into the intestinal lumen, where it attaches via its scolex and grows distally as it matures, eventually achieving

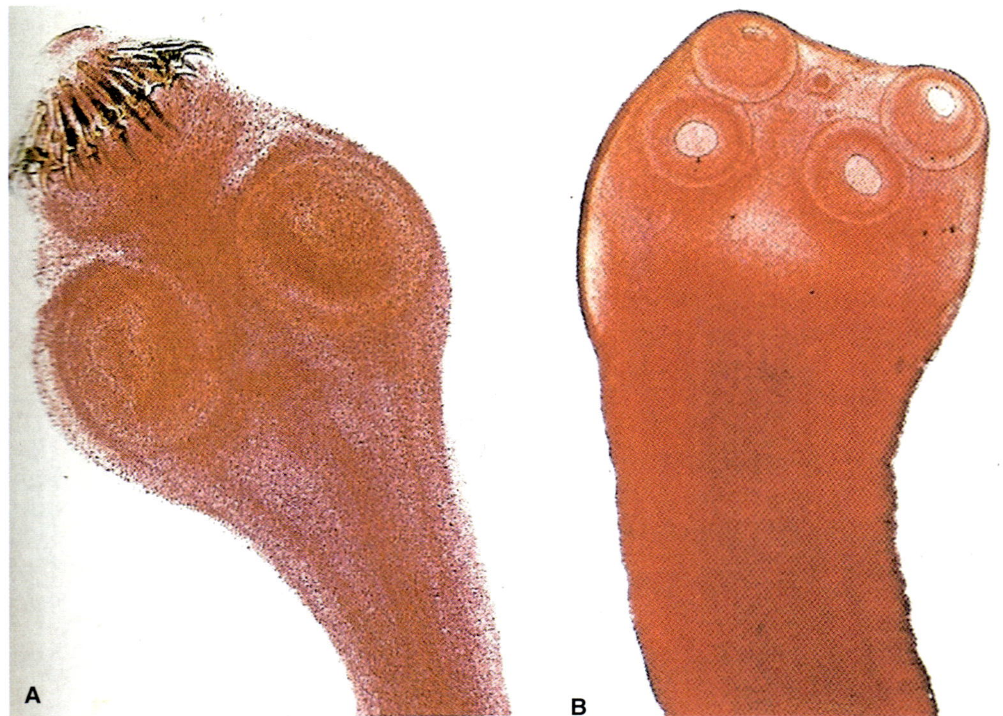

FIGURES 67–14 ■ The scolex of **(A)** *Taenia solium* revealing a spherical shape with a double row of hooklets and **(B)** *Taenia saginata* with a square head and four suckers. (*Courtesy of Yamaguchi.*[62])

lengths of 2–4 cm.[36] It takes 3–4 weeks from the start of infection before eggs appear in the stool.[39] This entire life cycle can be completed in a single host, unlike the other intestinal tapeworms.

Clinical presentation

While most cases are asymptomatic, heavy infection with *H. nana* (>1000 worms) can cause intestinal inflammation with diarrhea, abdominal pain, anorexia, and pruritus ani.[36,39]

Diagnosis

As noted above, *H. nana* adult worms are much smaller in size than other tapeworms, and contain up to 200 proglottids.[2] The scolex has four suckers and hooklets. The diagnosis is usually made by demonstration of eggs in feces. The eggs measure 30–55 μm in diameter and can be spherical or oval shaped with a two-layered shell (Figure 67–15).[6]

Treatment

The treatment of choice is praziquantel (Table 67–5). One to three months after therapy, patients should be rechecked for evidence of eggs in the stool to document cure.[10]

Similar to *E. vermicularis* (pinworms), when children are infected with *H. nana,* many experts recommend screening and treating family members, since person-to-person spread has been documented.

Diphylobothrium latum

Epidemiology

D. latum, the fish tapeworm, is endemic in Japan and Northern Europe where consumption of raw fish is common.[8] An estimated 20 million people are infected

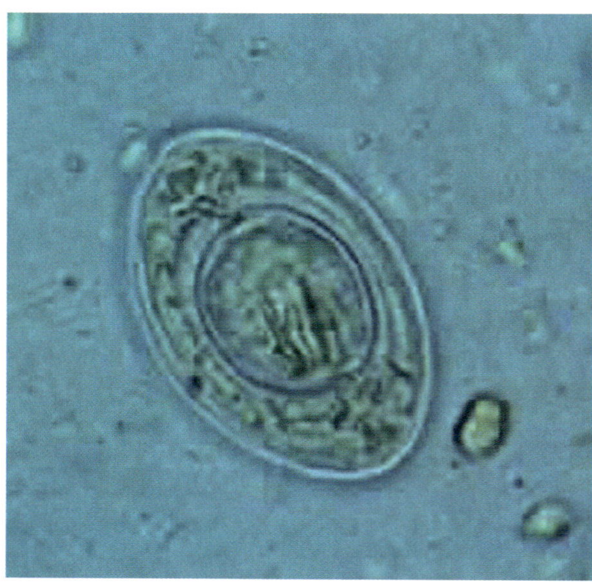

FIGURE 67–15 ■ Egg of *Hymenolepis nana.* (*Courtesy of the Centers for Disease Control.*[6])

worldwide.[2] Infection has been reported after the consumption of sushi[40] and in the United States after sampling raw gefilte fish.[8]

Pathogenesis

The life cycle of *D. latum* requires two intermediate hosts prior to human infection. When eggs from human feces contaminate water, the eggs hatch and form coracidium (a larval form). When ingested by a small freshwater crustacean, termed a copepod, the next larval stage, called the procercoid, develops. If a fish ingests the infected copepod, the procercoid invades the stomach wall of the fish and disseminates to the muscle tissue, where it matures to a plerocercoid larvae. When humans ingest raw or undercooked infected fish, the plerocercoid larvae matures into adult form and can grow to 15 m in length[39] with 3000–4000 proglottid segments (Figure 67–17A and B).[8]

Clinical presentation

Most infected individuals are asymptomatic, however, some may experience nonspecific symptoms such as abdominal pain, weight loss, vomiting, and anorexia. Chronic infection can lead to macrocytic anemia from vitamin B12 deficiency.[2] Although up to 40% of patients may have subclinical vitamin B12 deficiency, only 2% develop anemia.[8]

Diagnosis

Diagnosis of *D. latum* requires the detection of eggs or proglottid segments in feces, which usually appear one month after consumption of infected fish. The eggs are released from a uterine pore and measure 55 by 60 μm and have both an operculum and a small knob (Figure 67–16).[8] If passed in the stool, the scolex of *D. latum* has a spoon shape and contains bothria (grooves) that allow attachment to the intestinal wall. Unlike the *Taenia* species, there are no suckers or hooklets.[8]

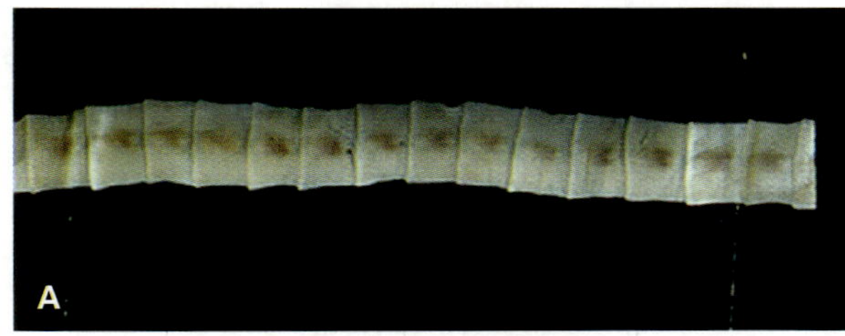

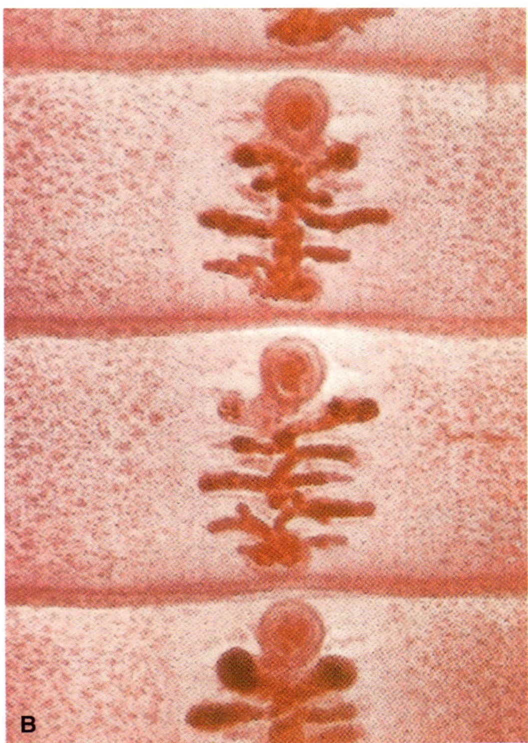

FIGURES 67–17 ■ Section of proglottid segments of *Diphylobothrium latum*. **(A)** Reveals that the proglottid segments are of greater width than height, with a centrally positioned genital pore. **(B)** Shows a close-up of the gravid proglottid segments. The center of each segment has a coiled uterus which is sometimes described as a "rosette." (*Courtesy of the Centers for Disease Control and Yamaguchi.*[6,62])

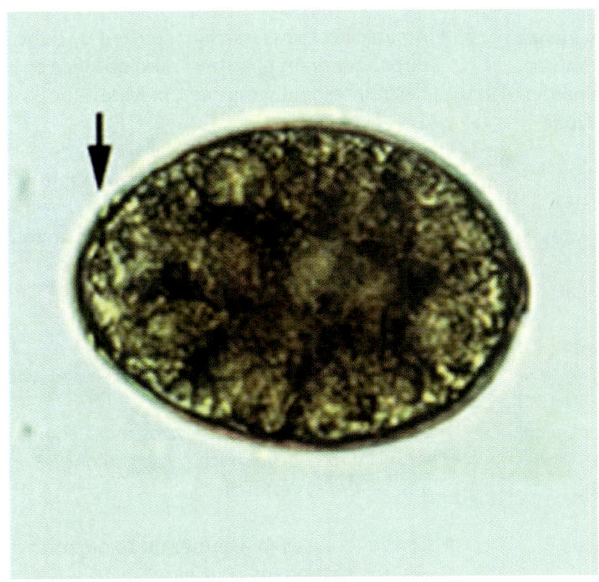

FIGURE 67–16 ■ Unembryonated egg of *Diphylobothrium latum*. Arrow points toward operculum. (*Courtesy of the Centers for Disease Control.*[6])

Treatment

The recommended treatment is praziquantel (Table 67–5). As with other tapeworms, a repeat stool specimen should be examined 1 to 3 months after treatment to document cure.

PREVENTION OF CESTODES

Prevention of tapeworm infections requires education and safe eating practices. Thoroughly cooking beef, pork and fish will kill cysticerci and plerocercoids, thereby preventing infection. Prevention of *H. nana* infection requires adequate sanitation.

PROTOZOA (Table 67–4)

Intestinal protozoa are unicellular organisms spread via ingestion of contaminated food and water. The most common intestinal protozoa are *Giardia lamblia* and *Entamoeba histolytica* (known as amebiasis), both of which cause disease worldwide. Other species cause significant disease primarily in those who are immunocompromised, including *Cryptosporidium parvum*, *Cyclospora cayetanensis*, and *Isospora belli*. The pathogenic potential of two other protozoa, *Blastocystis hominis* and *Dientamoeba fragilis*, is controversial.

Giardia lamblia

Epidemiology

In the United States, *G. lamblia* remains a common cause of waterborne diarrhea, with numerous outbreaks recorded. The prevalence in developed countries is estimated at 2–5% while that in developing countries may be as high as 20–30%.[41] Those at highest risk appear to be infants and young children (especially those in day care centers, where person-to-person transmission can occur), immunocompromised individuals (especially those with common variable immunodeficiency and X-linked agammaglobulinemia), and travelers to high prevalence areas (accounting for 5% of traveler's diarrhea).[42] Contaminated water serves as the most common source of human infection in the United States, with waterborne outbreaks occurring in mountainous areas as well as swimming pools after a fecal accident. There is also reason to believe that mammals (both wild and domestic) serve as reservoirs for this organism. Transmission may also occur through sexual activity as a result of oroanal contact.[41]

Pathogenesis

After ingestion of as few as 10–100 *Giardia* cysts, the organisms excyst in the small intestine and release two trophozoites, which embed within the crypts. Here the

Table 67–4.

Protozoa

Organism	Epidemiology	Clinical Caveats
Giardia lamblia	■ Worldwide distribution, although more prevalent in warm climates. In the United States, outbreaks have been related to contaminated water sources. Young children, immunocompromised persons, and travelers to endemic areas are at highest risk.	■ Chronic infection is characterized by steatorrhea, weight loss, secondary lactase deficiency, vitamin A and B12 deficiency, and hypoalbuminemia.
Entamoeba histolytica	■ Worldwide distribution—with higher incidence in developing countries where food and water sources may be subject to fecal contamination. In the United States, high-risk groups include travelers and recent immigrants.	■ Amebic liver abscess, characterized by right upper quadrant pain, fever, and absence of gastrointestinal symptoms, may develop.
Cryptosporidium parvum	■ Worldwide distribution. ■ Immunocompromised persons, especially those with AIDS have higher infection rates.	■ Usually self-limited in immunocompetant persons. ■ Characterized by watery diarrhea, abdominal pain and cramping, and occasionally fever.
Cyclospora cayetanensis	■ Most common in tropical and subtropical areas. ■ Food-borne outbreaks have been linked to contaminated imported foods such as raspberries and basil.	■ Abdominal cramps, nonbloody watery diarrhea can last up to 6 weeks in immunocompetant persons. ■ Humans are the only known reservoir.
Isospora belli	■ Worldwide distribution—especially in tropical and subtropical areas. ■ More common in immunocompromised persons.	■ Symptoms are similar to *Cyclospora*. Persons with HIV may have much more prolonged and severe symptoms.
Blastocystis hominis and *Dientamoeba fragilis*	■ Worldwide distribution. Occurs in all ages.	■ Controversial as to whether these organisms are true pathogens of disease. ■ Some experts advocate treating symptomatic persons if no other cause has been found.

trophozoites multiply by binary fission and encyst. After being excreted in feces, cysts may contaminate water sources and infect animals, which serve as a reservoir for human infection.[41] *Giardia* cysts survive for months in cool, moist conditions, and are relatively resistant to chlorination.[42,43]

Clinical presentation

Some individuals who harbor *G. lamblia* may be asymptomatic, serving as a reservoir for infection of others. Symptoms of infection include acute diarrhea, especially in travelers, who may also experience weight loss, abdominal discomfort, and flatulence beginning within 7 days of cyst ingestion. Chronic giardiasis occurs in 30–50% of infected persons, and is characterized by steatorrhea, weight loss, secondary lactase deficiency, Vitamin A and B12 deficiency, and even hypoalbuminemia.[41] In young children with chronic infection, nutritional deficiencies can lead to delays in growth and development.

Diagnosis

Stool examination for trophozoites and cysts should be performed using light microscopy. Trophozoites are more commonly found in watery stools, and cysts are more commonly found in formed specimens.[6] At least three specimens should be submitted and occasionally the stool must be concentrated to confirm the diagnosis. The cysts are round or oval and measure 8–12 μm in length (Figure 67–18A). The trophozoites are pear-shaped and measure 9–20 μm in length with two large nuclei and one large central karyosome (Figure 67–18B and C).[6]

Currently, fecal antigen detection and serology are both commercially available to help aid in diagnosis.[43] Fecal antigen testing has reported sensitivities of

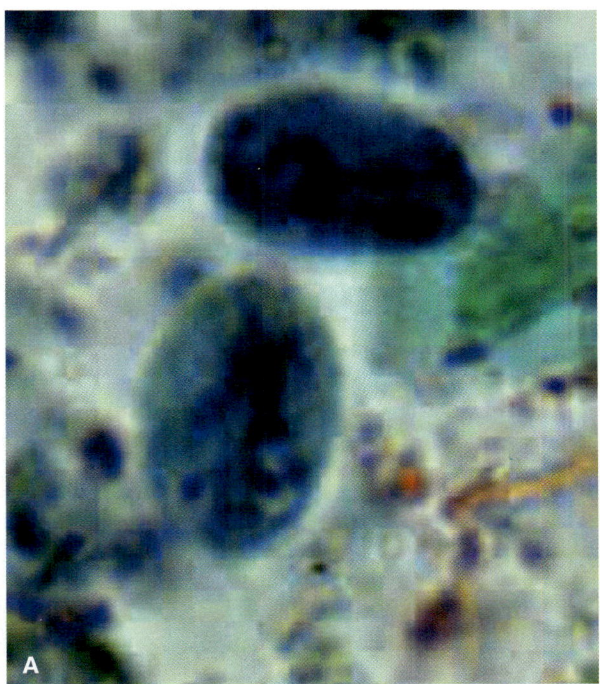

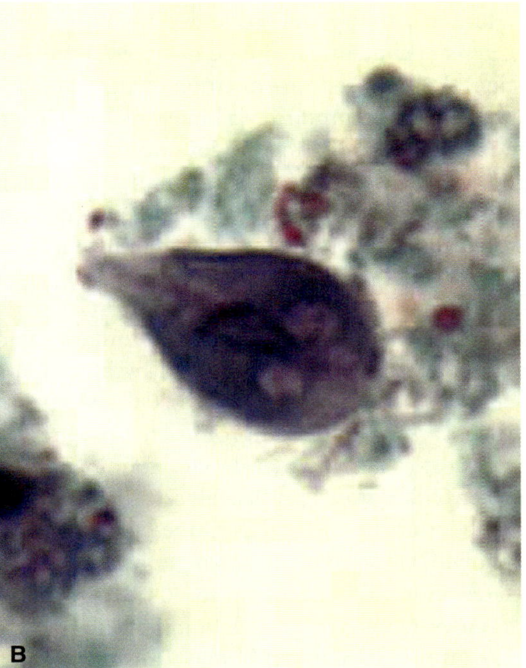

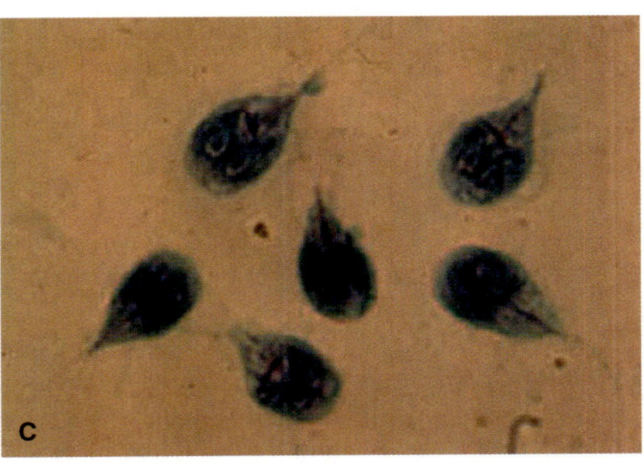

FIGURES 67–18 ■ **(A)** Cysts of *Giardia lamblia* viewed after staining with iron-hematoxylin. Trophozoites of *Giardia lamblia* in **(B)** trichrome stain and **(C)** culture. (*Courtesy of the Centers for Disease Control.*[6])

87–100%.[41] Serology, on the other hand, is not helpful in distinguishing past from present infection.

Treatment

The drugs of choice are metronidazole, nitazoxanide, and tinidazole (Table 67–5). Alternatives include paromomycin and furazolidone.[10]

Entamoeba histolytica

Epidemiology

The prevalence of *E. histolytica* is highest in developing countries, where water and food are subject to fecal contamination. In the United States, the majority of disease is found among immigrants from Mexico, Central America, South American, Asia, and the Pacific Islands.[44] Travelers to endemic areas are also at risk.

Pathogenesis

The life cycle of *E. histolytica* is similar to that of *G. lamblia*. Humans, thought to be the primary reservoir, ingest cysts in contaminated food or water. In the small intestine, they excyst to form trophozoites, which are highly motile and reproduce via binary fission. Here the trophozoites may lead to the development of flask-shaped ulcers and mucosal thickening mimicking inflammatory bowel disease. To complete the life cycle, the trophozoites encyst and are passed in the feces.

Clinical presentation

Many infected individuals are asymptomatic. Some develop amebic colitis, characterized by bloody diarrhea, abdominal pain, and tenderness. Others, especially those who are immunocompromised,[45] pregnant, or receiving corticosteroids, may develop fulminant colitis, with fever, leukocytosis, profuse bloody diarrhea, widespread abdominal pain, and peritoneal signs. Many of these individuals develop intestinal perforation, with an associated mortality rate of up to 40%.[44] Amebomas, which represent annular granulation tissue in the colon that can mimic carcinoma,[46] may cause obstructive symptoms.

A common extraintestinal manifestation is *amebic* liver abscess, which occurs in the absence of gastrointestinal symptoms and is characterized by fever, right upper quadrant pain, and tenderness.[44]

Diagnosis

Light microscopy, perhaps the most commonly used method of diagnosing amebiasis, does not differentiate *E. histolytica* from other commensal organisms, such as *Entamoeba dispar*. The trophozoites are 15–20 μm in size (range of 10–60 μm) and have a single nucleus with granular cytoplasm (Figure 67–19A). The cysts usually measure 12–15 μm and have four nuclei (Figure 67–19B).[6] Commercially available enzyme-linked immunosorbent assay (ELISA) can identify specific *E. histolytica* antigens in the stool.[47,48] These are more sensitive than microscopy and can distinguish *E. histolytica* from *E. dispar*.

In the setting of liver abscess, serology is highly sensitive (>94%) and specific (>95%).[44] Currently, the Centers for Disease Control (CDC) offers *E. histolytica* antibody detection via enzyme immunoassay (EIA).

Treatment

To limit the spread of disease, even asymptomatic carriers should be treated. The drugs of choice vary depending on the severity and location of disease (Table 67–5). Individuals with symptomatic disease should be treated with a luminal agent, such as paromomycin or iodoquinol, after primary treatment is given to eradicate colonization. Amebic liver abscess can usually be treated with metronidazole, although surgical intervention is occasionally necessary.[44]

Cryptosporidium parvum

Epidemiology

C. parvum is prevalent worldwide, with an estimated 20% of children in the United States seropositive. In developing countries, studies reveal up to a 90% seroprevalence in young children.[49] Higher infection rates are seen in immunocompromised individuals, particularly in persons with acquired immunodeficiency syndrome (AIDS).[50] Some reasons for its widespread prevalence include chlorine resistance, a small infectious dose, and possible zoonotic transmission. In the United States, a 1993 outbreak of *C. parvum* in Wisconsin was traced to contamination of the public water source.[51]

Pathogenesis

Infection with *C. parvum* begins with the ingestion of oocysts. Once in the GI tract, the oocysts excyst and release sporozoites, which attach to intestinal epithelial cells. Sporozoites undergo asexual reproduction and release merozoites, which either infect new epithelial cells or mature into gametocytes. Gametocytes undergo sexual reproduction, and when fertilized, form thin and thick walled cysts. The thin walled cysts autoinfect the host, while thick walled cysts are released in the feces.[50]

Clinical presentation

Persons with *C. parvum* infection range from being asymptomatic to having profuse watery diarrhea with extraintestinal infection. In immunocompetent persons, the incubation period of 7–10 days is followed by abdominal pain and cramping, watery diarrhea with mucous (without hematochezia), weight loss, and occasionally fever and vomiting.[50] Children in developing

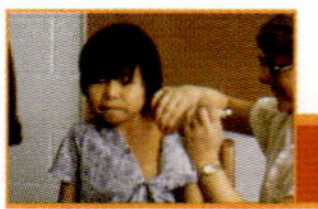

Table 67–5.

Medications for Treatment of Intestinal Parasites

Parasite	Treatment	Adult Dose	Pediatric Dose
Nematodes			
Ascaris lumbricoides	Albendazole	400 mg once	400 mg once
	Mebendazole	100 mg BID × 3 d or 500 mg once	100 mg BID × 3 d or 500 mg once
	Ivermectin	150–200 μg/kg once	150–200 μg/kg once
	Alternative:		
	Nitazoxanide	500 mg × 3 d	1–3 y: 100 mg BID × 3 d 4–11 y: 200 mg BID × 3 d
Enterobius vermicularis	Pyrantel pamoate	11 mg/kg once (max 1g); repeat in 2 wk	11 mg/kg once (max 1g); repeat in 2 wk
	Mebendazole	100 mg once; repeat in 2 wk	100 mg once; repeat in 2 wk
	Albendazole	400 mg once; repeat in 2 wk	400 mg once; repeat in 2 wk
	Alternative:		
	Nitazoxanide	500 mg × 3 d	1–3 y: 100 mg BID × 3 d 4–11 y: 200 mg BID × 3 d
Trichuris trichiura	Mebendazole	100 mg BID × 3 d or 500 mg once	100 mg BID × 3 d or 500 mg once
	Alternatives:		
	Albendazole	400 mg × 3 d	400 mg × 3 d
	Ivermectin	200 μg/kg daily × 3 d	200 μg/kg daily × 3 d
	Nitazoxanide	500 mg × 3 d	1–3 y: 100 mg BID × 3 d 4–11 y: 200 mg BID × 3 d
Strongyloides stercoralis	Ivermectin	200 μg/kg/d × 2 d	200 μg/kg/d × 2 d
	Alternatives:		
	Albendazole	400 mg BID × 7 d	400 mg BID × 7 d
	Thiabendazole	50 mg/kg/d in 2 doses × 2 d (max 3g/d)	50 mg/kg/d in 2 doses × 2 d (max 3g/d)
	Nitazoxanide	500 mg × 3 d	1–3 y: 100 mg BID × 3 d 4–11 y: 200 mg BID × 3 d
Hookworm sp. *Ancylostoma duodenale,* *Necator americanus*	Albendazole	400 mg once	400 mg once
	Mebendazole	100 mg BID × 3 d or 500 mg once	100 mg BID × 3 d or 500 mg once
	Pyrantel Pamoate	11 mg/kg (max 1 g) × 3 d	11 mg/kg (max 1 g) × 3 d
	Alternative:		
	Nitazoxanide	500 mg x 3 d	1–3 y: 100 mg BID × 3 d 4–11 y: 200 mg BID × 3 d
Trematodes			
Fasciolopsis buski	Praziquantel	75 mg/kg/d in 3 doses × 1 d	75 mg/kg/d in 3 doses × 1 d
	Alternative:		
	Nitazoxanide	500 mg × 3 d	1–3 y: 100 mg BID × 3 d 4–11 y: 200 mg BID × 3 d
Metagonimus yokogawai	Praziquantel	75 mg/kg/d in 3 doses × 1 d	75 mg/kg/d in 3 doses × 1 d
Heterophyes heterophyes	Praziquantel	75 mg/kg/d in 3 doses × 1 d	75 mg/kg/d in 3 doses × 1 d
Cestodes			
Taenia solium (Intestinal infection)	Praziquantel	5–10 mg/kg once	5–10 mg/kg once
	Alternative:		
	Niclosamide	2 g once	50 mg/kg once

(*continued*)

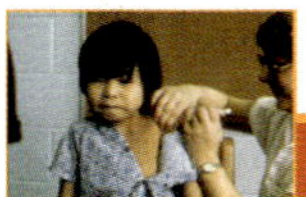

Table 67–5. (continued)

Medications for Treatment of Intestinal Parasites

Parasite	Treatment	Adult Dose	Pediatric Dose
Taenia saginata	Praziquantel	5–10 mg/kg once	5–10 mg/kg once
	Alternative:		
	Niclosamide	2 g once	50 mg/kg once
	Nitazoxanide	500 mg × 3 d	1–3 y: 100 mg BID × 3 d 4–11 yrs: 200 mg BID × 3 d
Diphylobothrium latum	Praziquantel	5–10 mg/kg once	5–10 mg/kg once
	Alternative:		
	Niclosamide	2 g once	50 mg/kg once
Hymenolepis nana	Praziquantel	25 mg/kg once	25 mg/kg once
	Alternative:		
	Nitazoxanide	500 mg × 3 d	1–3 y: 100 mg BID × 3 d 4–11 y: 200 mg BID × 3 d
Protozoa			
Entamoeba histolytica	*Asymptomatic:*		
	Iodoquinol	650 mg TID × 20 d	30–40 mg/kg/d (max 2g) in 3 doses × 20 d
	Paromomycin	25–35 mg/kg/d in 3 doses × 7 d	25–35 mg/kg/d in 3 doses × 7 d
	Mild to moderate intestinal disease:		
	Metronidazole	750 mg TID × 7–10 d	35–50 mg/kg/d in 3 doses × 7–10 d
	Tinidazole	2 g once daily × 5d	50 mg/kg/d (max 2g) in 1 dose × 3 d
	Severe intestinal and extraintestinal disease:		
	Metronidazole	750 mg TID × 7–10 d	35–50 mg/kg/d in 3 doses × 7–10 d
	Tinidazole	2 g once daily × 5 d	50 mg/kg/d (max 2g) × 5 d
	Alternative:		
	Nitazoxanide	500 mg × 3 d	1–3 y: 100 mg BID × 3 d 4–11 y: 200 mg BID × 3 d
Giardia lamblia	Metronidazole	250 mg TID × 5 d	15 mg/kg/d in 3 doses × 5 d
	Nitazoxanide	500 mg BID × 3 d	1–3 y: 100 mg q12 h × 3 d 4–11 y: 200 mg q12 h × 3 d
	Tinidazole	2 g once	50 mg/kg once (max 2g)
	Alternatives:		
	Paromomycin	25–35 mg/kg/d in 3 doses × 7 d	25–35 mg/kg/d in 3 doses × 7 d
	Furazolidone	100 mg QID × 7–10 d	6 mg/kg/d in 4 doses × 7–10 d
Isospora belli	Trimethoprim-sulfmethoxazole	TMP 160mg/ SMX 800 mg (1 DS tab) BID × 10 d	TMP 5 mg/kg, SMX 25 mg/kg BID × 10 d
	Alternative:		
	Nitazoxanide	500 mg × 3 d	1–3 y: 100 mg BID × 3 d 4–11 y: 200 mg BID × 3 d
Cryptosporidium Non-HIV infected	Nitazoxanide	500 mg BID × 3 d	1–3 y: 100 mg BID × 3 d 4–11 y: 200 mg BID × 3 d
Cyclospora cayetanensis	Trimethoprim-sulfmethoxazole	TMP 160mg/ SMX 800 mg (1 DS tab) BID × 7–10 d	TMP 5 mg/kg, SMX 25 mg/kg BID × 7–10 d
	Alternative:		
	Nitazoxanide	500 mg × 3 d	1–3 y: 100 mg BID × 3 d 4–11 y: 200 mg BID × 3 d

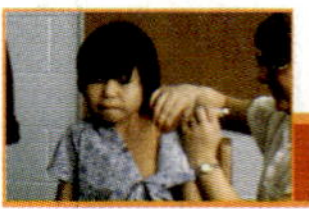

Table 67–5. (continued)

Medications for Treatment of Intestinal Parasites

Parasite	Treatment	Adult Dose	Pediatric Dose
Dientamoeba fragilis	Iodoquinol	650 mg TID × 20d	3–40 mg/kg/d (max 2 g) in 3 doses × 20d
	Paromomycin	25–35 mg/kg/d in 3 doses × 7d	25–35 mg/kg/d in 3 doses × 7 d
	Tetracycline	500 mg QID × 10d	40 mg/kg/d (max 2 g) in 4 doses × 10d
	Metronidazole	500-750 mg TID × 10d	20–40 mg/kg/d in 3 doses × 10 d
Blastocystis hominis	Metronidazole	750 mg TID × 10d	
	Iodoquinol	650 mg TID × 20d	
	Trimethoprim-sulfmethoxazole	1 DS tab BID × 7d	
	Alternative:		
	Nitazoxanide	500 mg × 3d	1–3 y: 100 mg BID × 3 d 4–11 y: 200 mg BID × 3 d

Modified from Drugs for parasitic infections. Med Lett Drugs Ther 2004;46(1189):1–12.

countries may develop chronic infection, leading to malnutrition and growth delay.

In persons with AIDS or other immunocompromised conditions, infection may be more severe. Those with low CD4 counts (<50/mm^3) may have profuse (up to 2 L per day) and watery diarrhea. These patients are less likely to spontaneously clear the infection, and may have extraintestinal disease, such as biliary infection.[50]

Diagnosis

The diagnosis of cryptosporidiosis is usually made by demonstration of oocysts in stool using light microscopy

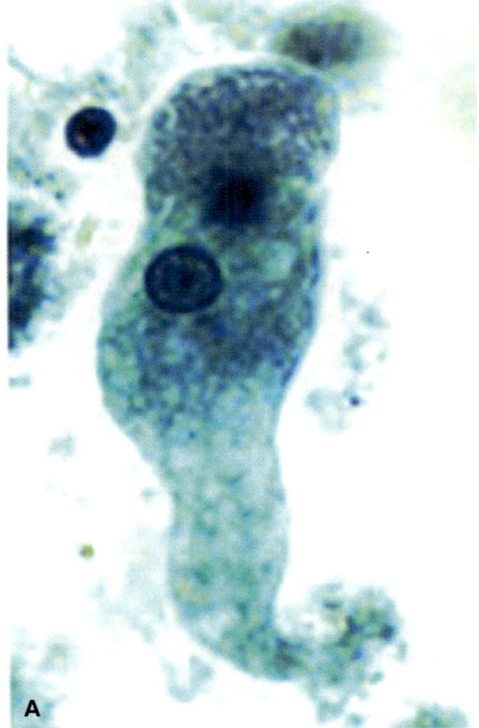

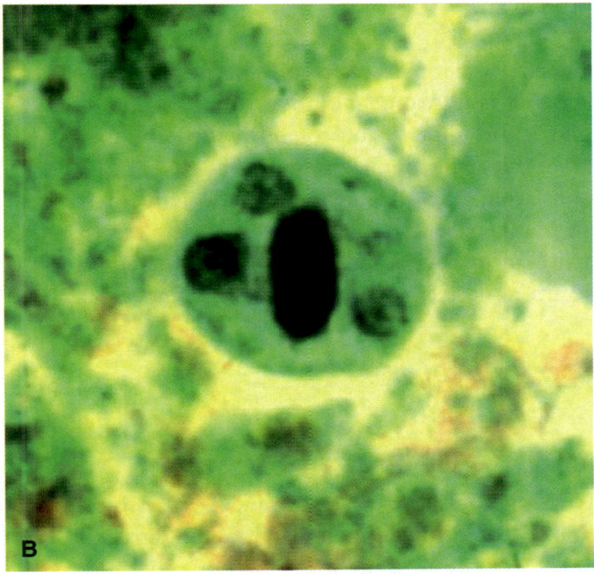

FIGURE 67–19 ■ (A) Trophozoite of *Entamoeba histolytica* revealing a single nucleus and centrally placed karyosome with a ground glass-appearing cytoplasm. **(B)** Cyst of *Entamoeba histolytica* stained with trichrome showing four visible nuclei. Courtesy of the Centers for Disease Control.[6]

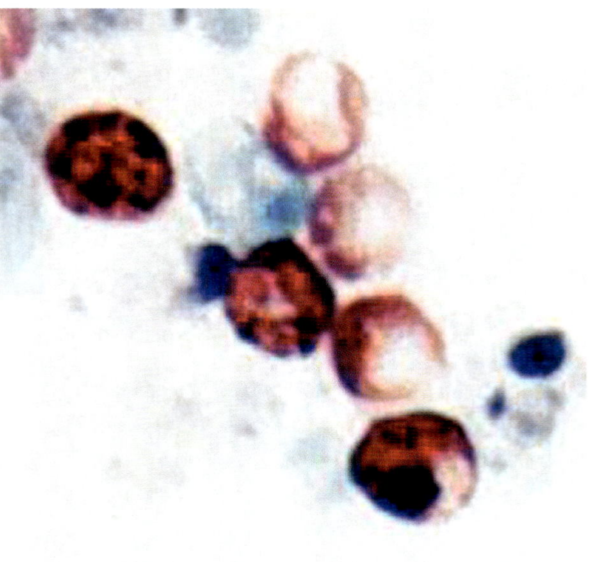

FIGURE 67–20 ■ Oocyst of *Cryptosporidium parvum* stained with a modified acid-fast method. Courtesy of the Centers for Disease Control.[6]

and modified acid-fast staining. Of note, clinical laboratories do not routinely perform this test, and one must therefore request examination specifically for *C. parvum.*[49] The oocysts are 4–6 μm in size and round with no visible nuclei (Figure 67–20).[52] Direct fluorescent antibody tests, specific fecal antigen tests, and polymerase chain reaction (PCR) techniques with high sensitivities and specificities are also available.[49,50] Serology is available, but because of the widespread prevalence of antibodies to *C. parvum,* a positive result is not diagnostic of current infection.

Treatment

In immunocompetent persons, cryptosporidiosis is usually self-limited, and treatment is not required. Malnourished children or adults with prolonged shedding may benefit from therapy with nitazoxanide (Table 67–5).[53,54] For persons with AIDS, therapy with nitazoxanide may also confer some benefit, but recent evidence shows that highly active antiretroviral therapy (HAART) therapy is most effective at decreasing the duration of illness.[49]

Cyclospora cayetanensis and *Isospora belli*

Epidemiology

Humans are the only known reservoirs for *C. cayetanensis,* unlike *I. belli,* which can infect both humans and animals. These spore-forming protozoa typically cause disease in tropical and subtropical regions.[55] *C. cayetanensis* can also be found in developed countries, mainly in persons who have traveled to an endemic area or by consumption of contaminated food from an endemic area. In human immunodeficiency virus (HIV)-infected patients with CD4 T-cell counts less than 200/mm^3, persistent infections are being increasingly identified.[56]

In the United States, several large outbreaks of *C. cayetanensis* have been reported related to consumption of contaminated raspberries imported from Guatemala, as well as basil grown in the United States and Mexico.[15] Waterborne transmission has also been documented.[57,58]

Pathogenesis

Oocysts released in the feces of persons infected with either *C. cayetanensis* or *I. belli* are unsporulated and require several weeks to become infectious. Humans ingest the infectious oocysts, which enter the small intestine epithelium and replicate intracellularly. Newly formed oocysts rupture the epithelial cells and are shed in human feces to complete the transmission cycle.[56]

Clinical presentation

In immunocompetent individuals, infection with either *Cyclospora* or *Isospora* can lead to abdominal cramps and watery, nonbloody diarrhea lasting for up to 6 weeks. Accompanying symptoms include nausea, vomiting, muscle aches, fatigue, and low-grade fever. In highly endemic areas, asymptomatic as well as relapsing–remitting infections occur.[55] In immunocompromised individuals, including those with HIV infection, the clinical course can be more severe and prolonged.

Diagnosis

The diagnosis is best accomplished by examination of the stool by light microscopy. Often more than one sample is needed (preferably three), and if the sample cannot be examined promptly, the stool should be refrigerated or placed in a preservative. Several diagnostic techniques are available, including wet mounts using differential interference contrast or UV fluorescence microscopy. Special stains, such as modified acid-fast and safranin, may also be used. *C. cayetanensis* is round and measures 8–10 μm in diameter (Figure 67–21), while *I. belli* cysts are larger and ellipsoidal in shape, measuring 25–30 μm (Figure 67–22).[6]

Treatment

The treatment of choice for both infections is trimethoprim/sulfamethoxazole. Refer to the Table 67–5 for details.

Blastocystis hominis and *Dientamoeba fragilis*

Epidemiology

The degree to which these two protozoa cause intestinal disease remains controversial. Both share a worldwide

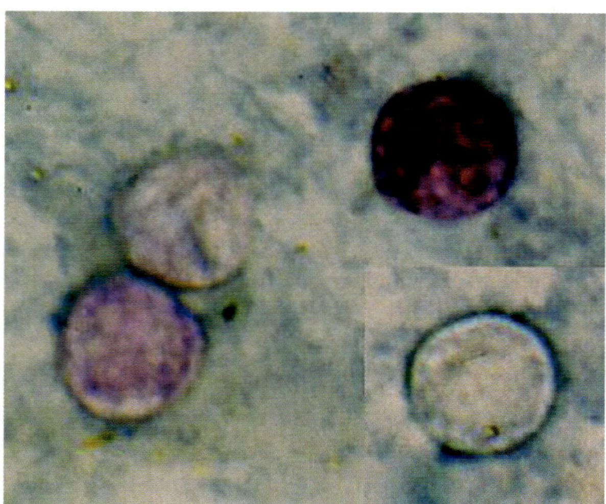

FIGURE 67–21 ■ Oocyst of *Cyclospora cayetanensis* from feces preserved with 10% formalin stained with a modified acid-fast method. Courtesy of the Centers for Disease Control.[6]

distribution and occur in all ages. Prevalence studies have shown that these organisms are common in both developed and resource-poor countries, and in symptomatic as well as healthy asymptomatic individuals. Up to 15% of stool samples in the United States are positive for *B. hominis* compared to reported rates of 30–50% in developing countries.[59] Surveillance for *D. fragilis* suggests that it occurs less commonly in the United States than *B. hominis.*[60]

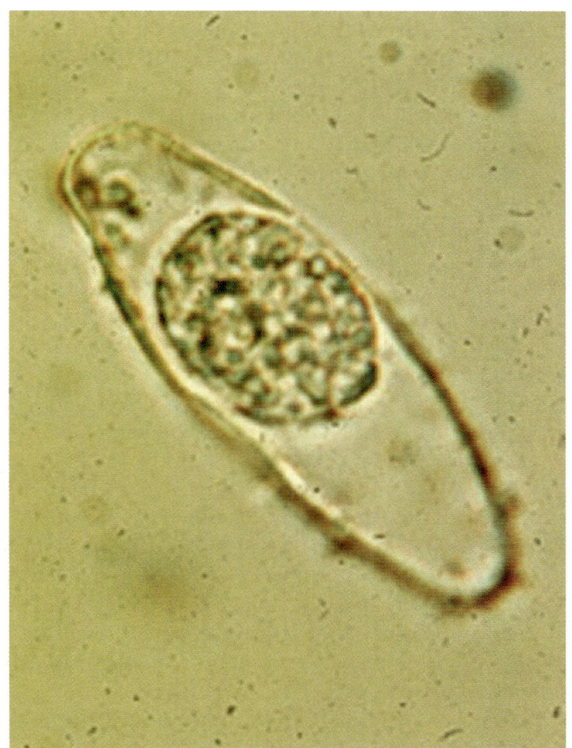

FIGURE 67–22 ■ Immature oocyst of *Isospora belli* containing one sporoblast. Courtesy of the Centers for Disease Control.[6]

Pathogenesis

The life cycles and mechanisms of pathogenesis for these two protozoa remain poorly understood. In the case of *B. hominis,* four forms of the protozoa have been described: vacuolar, granular, ameboid, and cystic. However, the phenotype most involved in transmission has not yet been defined. For *D. fragilis,* a cyst form has not been identified, and so it is unclear how this pathogen survives in the environment, as well as the acidity of the stomach if the route of transmission is fecal–oral.

Clinical presentation

Much of the known spectrum of illness associated with carriage of these organisms comes from case reports, rather than well-controlled clinical studies. Symptoms of nausea, anorexia, abdominal pain, vomiting, fatigue, and watery diarrhea have been reported, although many individuals who harbor these organisms are asymptomatic.[52,59,60] One difficulty in defining the pathogenicity of *B. hominis* and *D. fragilis* is that excretion of these organisms often coincides with excretion of other established intestinal pathogens.

Diagnosis

B. hominis usually measures between 5 and 40 μm and lacks a cell wall. A stained smear of unconcentrated stool (usually with hematoxylin or trichrome stain) is the preferred method of diagnosis.[59] The size of *D. fragilis* also varies widely.[60] They have a rounded appearance on wet mount and as the name suggests, they are binucleate and rapidly degenerate after excretion in the feces. Similar to *B. hominis,* permanently stained smears of stool are the preferred method of diagnosis.

Treatment

There are no consensus guidelines for treatment of *Blastocystis* or *Dientamoeba.* In the absence of symptoms, treatment is not warranted. However, if a patient has symptoms and no other pathogens have been identified, treatment with antiparasitic agents (Table 67–5) may be considered. Case reports and small placebo-controlled trials suggest that treatment may improve symptoms in some individuals.[59–61]

PREVENTION OF PROTOZOAN INFECTIONS

Similar to other intestinal parasites, precautions to prevent fecal–oral contamination will potentially reduce transmission of intestinal protozoa. For travelers, bottled, filtered, or boiled water should be used for drinking and brushing teeth. Consumption of ice and raw fruits and vegetables should be avoided.

REFERENCES

1. Bungiro RD, Cappello, M. Helminth infections. *Encyclopedia of Gastroenterology*. Amsterdam: Elsevier; 2004.
2. Muller R. *Worms and Human Disease*. 2nd ed. Walling ford, Oxon, UK: CABI Publishing; 2002.
3. Khuroo MS. Ascariasis. *Gastroenterol Clin North Am.* 1996;25(3):553-577.
4. Jones BF, Cappello, M. Nematodes. *Encyclopedia of Gastroenterology*. Amsterdam: Elsevier; 2004.
5. Bethony J, Brooker S, Albonico M, et al. Soil-transmitted helminth infections: Ascariasis, trichuriasis, and hookworm. *Lancet.* 2006;367(9521):1521-32.
6. DPDx—Laboratory identification of parasites of public concern. Centers for Disease Control and Prevention.
7. Ash L, Orihel, T. *Atlas of Human Parasitology*. 3rd ed. Chicago, IL: American Society of Clinical Pathologists; 1990.
8. Sun T. *Parasitic Disorders: Pathology, Diagnosis, And Management*. 2nd ed. Baltimore: Williams & Wilkins; 1999.
9. Beitia AO, Haller JO, Kantor A. CT findings in pediatric gastrointestinal ascariasis. *Comput Med Imaging Graph.* 1997;21(1):47-49.
10. Drugs for parasitic infections. *Med Lett Drugs Ther.* 2004; 46(1189):1-12.
11. Zaha O, Hirata T, Kinjo F, Saito A. Strongyloidiasis—Progress in diagnosis and treatment. *Intern Med.* 2000; 39(9):695-700.
12. Cappello M, Hotez, P. Intestinal nematodes. In: Sarah S, Long MD, eds. *Long, Pickering and Prober's Principles and Practice of Pediatric Infectious Diseases*. 2nd ed. Philadelphia, PA: Churchill Livingstone; 2003.
13. Gill GV, Welch E, Bailey JW, Bell DR, Beeching NJ. Chronic *Strongyloides stercoralis* infection in former British Far East prisoners of war. *QJM.* 2004;97(12): 789-95.
14. Ashford RW, Barnish G, Viney ME. *Strongyloides fuelleborni kellyi*: infection and disease in Papua New Guinea. *Parasitol Today.* 1992;8(9):314-8.
15. Lewthwaite P, Gill GV, Hart CA, Beeching NJ. Gastrointestinal parasites in the immunocompromised. *Curr Opin Infect Dis.* 2005;18(5):427-435.
16. Jones JE. String test for diagnosing giardiasis. *Am Fam Physician.* 1986;34(2):123-126.
17. Vadlamudi RS, Chi DS, Krishnaswamy G. Intestinal strongyloidiasis and hyperinfection syndrome. *Clin Mol Allergy.* 2006;4:8.
18. Genta RM. Predictive value of an enzyme-linked immunosorbent assay (ELISA) for the serodiagnosis of strongyloidiasis. *Am J Clin Pathol.* 1988;89(3):391-394.
19. van Doorn HR, Koelewijn R, Hofwegen H, et al. Use of enzyme-linked immunosorbent assay and dipstick assay for detection of *Strongyloides stercoralis* infection in humans. *J Clin Microbiol.* 2007;45(2):438-442.
20. Simpson WG, Gerhardstein DC, Thompson JR. Disseminated *Strongyloides stercoralis* infection. *South Med J.* 1993;86(7):821-825.
21. de Silva NR, Brooker S, Hotez PJ, Montresor A, Engels D, Savioli L. Soil-transmitted helminth infections: updating the global picture. *Trends Parasitol.* 2003;19(12):547-551.
22. Boccaccio M. Ground itch and dew poison; the Rockefeller Sanitary Commission 1909-14. *J Hist Med Allied Sci.* 1972;27(1):30-53.
23. Traub RJ, Robertson ID, Irwin P, Mencke N, Andrew Thompson RC. The prevalence, intensities and risk factors associated with geohelminth infection in tea-growing communities of Assam, India. *Trop Med Int Health.* 2004;9(6):688-701.
24. Hotez PJ, Brooker S, Bethony JM, Bottazzi ME, Loukas A, Xiao S. Hookworm infection. *N Engl J Med.* 2004;351(8): 799-807.
25. Yu SH, Jiang ZX, Xu LQ. Infantile hookworm disease in China. A review. *Acta Trop.* 1995;59(4):265-270.
26. Bundy DA, de Silva NR. Can we deworm this wormy world? *Br Med Bull.* 1998;54(2):421-432.
27. Diaz E, Mondragon J, Ramirez E, Bernal R. Epidemiology and control of intestinal parasites with nitazoxanide in children in Mexico. *Am J Trop Med Hyg.* 2003;68(4):384-385.
28. Cook GC. Enterobius vermicularis infection. *Gut.* 1994; 35(9):1159-1162.
29. Grencis RK, Cooper ES. Enterobius, trichuris, capillaria, and hookworm including ancylostoma caninum. *Gastroenterol Clin North Am.* 1996;25(3):579-597.
30. Mattia AR. Perianal mass and recurrent cellulitis due to *Enterobius vermicularis. Am J Trop Med Hyg.* 1992;47(6): 811-815.
31. Arca MJ, Gates RL, Groner JI, Hammond S, Caniano DA. Clinical manifestations of appendiceal pinworms in children: an institutional experience and a review of the literature. *Pediatr Surg Int.* 2004;20(5):372-375.
32. Jung RC, Beaver PC. Clinical observations on *Trichocephalus trichiurus* (whipworm) infestation in children. *Pediatrics.* 1951;8(4):548-557.
33. Ezeamama AE, Friedman JF, Acosta LP, et al. Helminth infection and cognitive impairment among Filipino children. *Am J Trop Med Hyg.* 2005;72(5):540-548.
34. Liu LX, Harinasuta KT. Liver and intestinal flukes. *Gastroenterol Clin North Am.* 1996;25(3):627-636.
35. Roberts L, Janovy, J. Gerald D. *Schmidt & Larry S. Roberts' Foundations of Parasitology*. 7th ed. New York, NY: McGraw-Hill; 2005.
36. Held M, Cappello, M. Cestodes. *Encyclopedia of Gastroenterology*. Amsterdam: Elsevier; 2004.
37. Flisser A, Viniegra AE, Aguilar-Vega L, Garza-Rodriguez A, Maravilla P, Avila G. Portrait of human tapeworms. *J Parasitol.* 2004;90(4):914-916.
38. Allan JC, Craig PS. Coproantigens in taeniasis and echinococcosis. *Parasitol* Int. 2006;55 (suppl):S75-S80.
39. Schantz PM. Tapeworms (cestodiasis). *Gastroenterol Clin North Am.* 1996;25(3):637-653.
40. Stadlbauer V, Haberl R, Langner C, Krejs GJ, Eherer A. Annoying vacation souvenir: fish tapeworm (*Diphyllobothrium* sp.) infestation in an Austrian fisherman. *Wien Klin Wochenschr.* 2005;117(21-22):776-779.
41. Farthing MJ. Giardiasis. *Gastroenterol Clin North Am.* 1996;25(3):493-515.
42. Katz DE, Taylor DN. Parasitic infections of the gastrointestinal tract. *Gastroenterol Clin North Am.* 2001;30(3): 797-815, x.

43. Ali SA, Hill DR. Giardia intestinalis. *Curr Opin Infect Dis.* 2003;16(5):453-460.
44. Stanley SL, Jr. Amoebiasis. *Lancet.* 2003;361(9362): 1025-1034.
45. Bowley DM, Loveland J, Omar T, Pitcher GJ. Human immunodeficiency virus infection and amebiasis. *Pediatr Infect Dis J.* 2006;25(12):1192-1193.
46. Haque R, Huston CD, Hughes M, Houpt E, Petri WA, Jr. Amebiasis. *N Engl J Med.* 2003;348(16):1565-1573.
47. Leo M, Haque R, Kabir M, et al. Evaluation of *Entamoeba histolytica* antigen and antibody point-of-care tests for the rapid diagnosis of amebiasis. *J Clin Microbiol.* 2006; 44(12):4569-4571.
48. Haque R, Mollah NU, Ali IK, et al. Diagnosis of amebic liver abscess and intestinal infection with the TechLab Entamoeba histolytica II antigen detection and antibody tests. *J Clin Microbiol.* 2000;38(9):3235-3239.
49. Kosek M, Alcantara C, Lima AA, Guerrant RL. Cryptosporidiosis: an update. *Lancet Infect Dis.* 2001;1(4): 262-269.
50. Chen XM, Keithly JS, Paya CV, LaRusso NF. Cryptosporidiosis. *N Engl J Med.* 2002;346(22):1723-1731.
51. Franzen C, Muller A. Cryptosporidia and microsporidia—Waterborne diseases in the immunocompromised host. *Diagn Microbiol Infect Dis.* 1999;34(3):245-262.
52. Stark D, van Hal S, Marriott D, Ellis J, Harkness J. Irritable bowel syndrome: a review on the role of intestinal protozoa and the importance of their detection and diagnosis. *Int J Parasitol.* 2007;37(1):11-20.
53. Abubakar I, Aliyu SH, Arumugam C, Hunter PR, Usman NK. Prevention and treatment of cryptosporidiosis in immunocompromised patients. *Cochrane Database Syst Rev.* 2007(1):CD004932.
54. Ochoa TJ, White AC, Jr. Nitazoxanide for treatment of intestinal parasites in children. *Pediatr Infect Dis J.* 2005;24(7):641-642.
55. Mansfield LS, Gajadhar AA. *Cyclospora cayetanensis*, a food- and waterborne coccidian parasite. *Vet Parasitol* 2004;126(1-2):73-90.
56. Petri WA, Jr. Protozoan parasites that infect the gastrointestinal tract. *Curr Opin Gastroenterol.* 2000;16(1):18-23.
57. Herwaldt BL. *Cyclospora cayetanensis*: A review, focusing on the outbreaks of cyclosporiasis in the 1990s. *Clin Infect Dis.* 2000;31(4):1040-1057.
58. Davis AN, Haque R, Petri WA, Jr. Update on protozoan parasites of the intestine. *Curr Opin Gastroenterol.* 2002;18(1):10-14.
59. Sohail MR, Fischer PR. *Blastocystis hominis* and travelers. *Travel Med Infect Dis.* 2005;3(1):33-38.
60. Johnson EH, Windsor JJ, Clark CG. Emerging from obscurity: biological, clinical, and diagnostic aspects of *Dientamoeba fragilis. Clin Microbiol Rev.* 2004;17(3):553-570, table of contents.
61. Stark D, Beebe N, Marriott D, Ellis J, Harkness J. *Dientamoeba fragilis* as a cause of travelers' diarrhea: report of seven cases. *J Travel Med.* 2007;14(1):72-73.
62. Yamaguchi T. *Clinical Parasitology.* London: Wolfe Medical Publications, Ltd; 1981.

CHAPTER 68

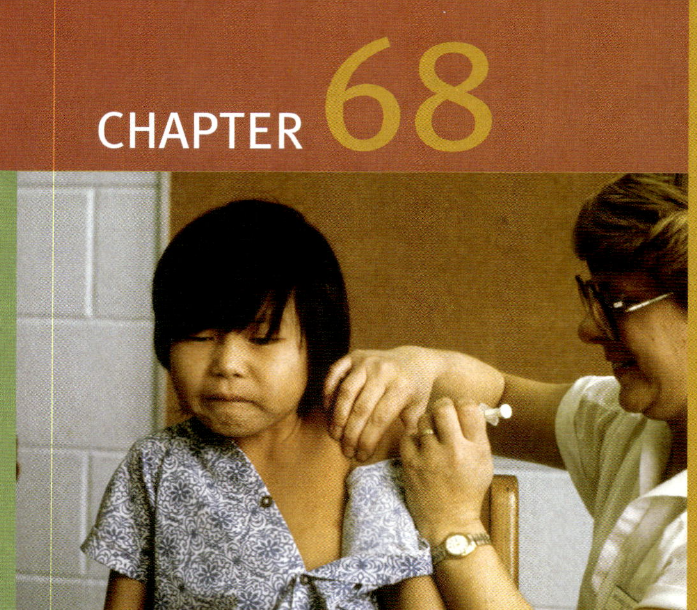

International Adoption and Infectious Diseases

Laurie C. Miller and Emma Jacobs

DEFINITIONS AND EPIDEMIOLOGY

Since 1986, more than 320,000 children have been adopted by American families from other countries. More than 20,000 children have arrived annually in each of the last 5 years, most commonly from China, Guatemala, Russia, and South Korea[1] (Figure 68–1). Infectious diseases are one of the most common and immediate medical concerns among newly arrived international adoptees.[2–6] The recent increase in adoptions from Africa (especially Ethiopia and Liberia) has broadened the range of infectious disease concerns among new arrivals. Infectious diseases in new adoptees affect not only the child, but may also present risks to family members and the community.[7]

Pediatricians play an important role in the care of internationally adopted children, especially in relation to infectious diseases. Pediatricians are often asked to interpret information about prior infectious diseases in preadoptive medical records given to prospective adoptive families and to provide health advice to families who travel to receive their children. Pediatricians must evaluate newly arrived adoptees for infectious diseases, and remain aware of the possibility of latent or "missed" infections that may manifest months or even years later. The physician must also assess the validity of vaccine records from various birth countries. This chapter will review these topics. Infectious disease risks to families and communities will be highlighted, and some of the diagnostic dilemmas specific to international adoptees will be considered. Detailed discussions of the specific diseases mentioned in this chapter are found in other sections of this book.

Preadoptive Screening for Infectious Diseases in the Child's Country of Origin

Nearly all children undergo testing for hepatitis B, HIV, and syphilis ("RW" in Russia or Kazakhstan, "TRUST" in China) prior to placement in international adoptions. However, the results may be outdated or inaccurate (performed in an inadequate laboratory, see *HIV* below). Prospective parents often ask the pediatrician for advice about repeating these tests in country before they agree to accept the child. This is rarely advisable, because laboratory accuracy and sterile phlebotomy equipment cannot be guaranteed. Furthermore, negative test results do not preclude later infection. In some countries (Ethiopia, Nepal, some regions of Russia and Kazakhstan), specialized laboratories offer polymerase chain reaction (PCR) tests for hepatitis B, hepatitis C, or HIV. These results can be reassuring in cases where maternal antibodies are suspected, but parents must be cautioned that valid test results are not guaranteed.

International Adoption and Travel Medicine

Most adoptive parents travel to receive their children; many countries require multiple trips or prolonged in-country residence in order to complete legal adoption requirements. A travel medicine consultation may help parents prepare for travel-related illnesses (e.g., diarrhea, malaria), as well as infectious diseases potentially transmitted by their new child. Travelling adults should have updated vaccinations for polio, tetanus, measles,

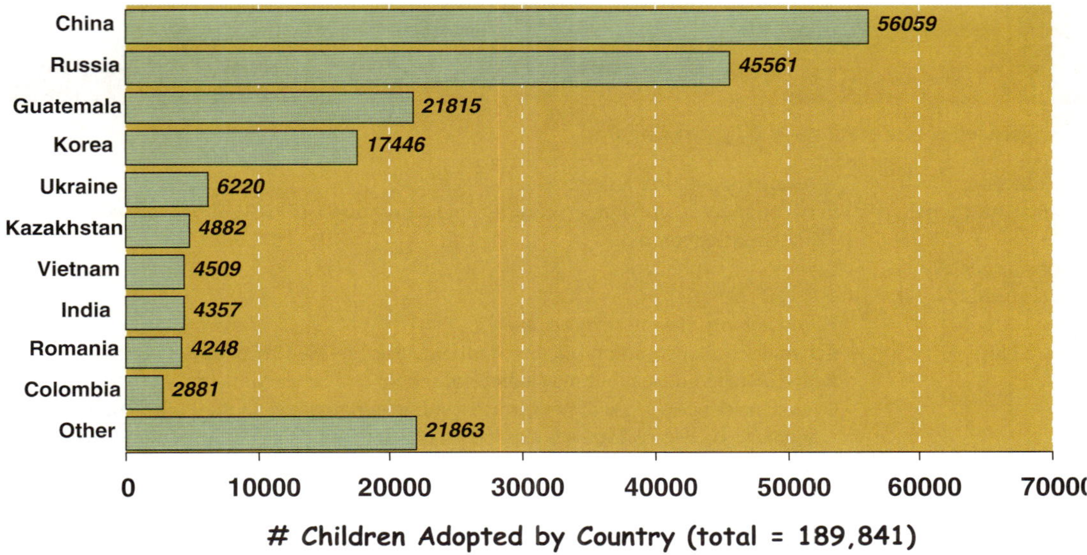

FIGURE 68–1 ■ International adoptions by the US families: 1997–2006.

mumps, rubella vaccination (MMR), varicella, influenza, hepatitis A and B. Depending on the destination, vaccines against typhoid, yellow fever, meningococcus, or Japanese encephalitis may be recommended.[7,8] Child travelers may also need destination-specific vaccinations.[9–11] In addition, all children awaiting a new sibling should be updated on vaccines, whether or not they are travelling. For prolonged stays in some destinations, vaccination against rabies and tuberculosis (Bacille Calmette-Guerin [BCG]) may be advisable.[11] Several Web sites contain up-to-date health recommendations for specific destinations.[12,13] Travelling children should be carefully supervised for unfamiliar risks related to sanitation, water, street dogs, and traffic.[11,14,15]

Prospective parents frequently request advice about medications to bring on their trip for their newly adopted child. Most acute illnesses can be satisfactorily managed by the child's local physicians in the birth country, using locally available medications. Sterile needles and syringes are available in pharmacies in many countries without prescriptions. A few medications and supplies may be useful for illnesses during travel[16] (Table 68–1). It is advisable for parents to arrange in advance of travel for needed communication with physicians at home (e.g., via e-mail).

Common Infectious Diseases in Internationally Adopted Children

The infectious diseases of internationally adopted children reflect endemic diseases in their birth countries, as well as the conditions in which the children reside prior to adoption (Table 68–2). Orphanages, like other congregate settings, increase the risks of respiratory, gastrointestinal, and skin infections. Hygiene practices may be suboptimal, and children often have increased susceptibility to infections caused by malnutrition or concurrent medical problems. "Exotic" infectious diseases are relatively uncommon, in part reflecting the limited exposure of most children to the world outside of their orphanages.

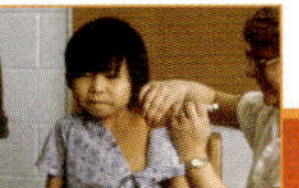

Table 68–1.

Basic Supplies to Consider for Travel (adjust as appropriate for child's age and location)
Adhesive plasters
Alcohol wipes
Amoxicillin
Antibacterial gel
Antibiotic ointment
Antihistamine
Antipyretics
Azithromycin (or cefixime)
Cold/cough preparation
Diaper rash cream
Dosage syringe
Insect repellent
Nasal aspirator
Pedialyte
Permethrin (Elimite)
Sunscreen
Sodium sulamyd optic drops
Thermometer

Adapted from Borchers DA. Adoption Medical Travel Guide. www.adoptivefamilies.com/pdf/travelmed.pdf. Accessed August 27, 2008.

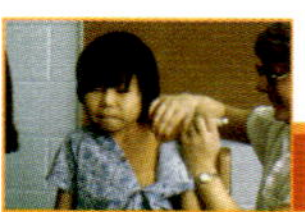

Table 68–2.

Infectious Diseases of Internationally Adopted Children

Respiratory infections	Very common in orphanages
Gastrointestinal infections	Very common in orphanages; parasitic infections found in ~50% of new arrivals. Enteric bacterial infections uncommon
Skin infections (especially impetigo, scabies)	Common in orphanages
Dental caries	Very common; may be severe
Tuberculosis	Active disease uncommon but latent tuberculosis in ~10–15% of all new arrivals
Hepatitis A	Active disease unusual but may infect household and other contacts
Hepatitis B	Overall incidence ~3–5% of new arrivals who tested negative in their birth countries. Incidence seems to be decreasing with expanding use of hepatitis B vaccine and improved testing in birth countries to identify infected children
Hepatitis C	Rare although history of maternal antibodies common
HIV	Very rare although increase expected as adoptions of younger infants from endemic areas increase
Syphilis	History of treated congenital syphilis in ~10–15% of children from Russia; rare from other countries. Untreated syphilis very rare
Vaccine-preventable diseases	Measles, varicella, pertussis, mumps, rubella reported in new arrivals and family members[6,17] diseases
"Exotic" diseases	Very rare although malaria becoming more common with increase in adoptions from Africa

Adapted from Miller LC. International adoption: infectious diseases issues. CID. 2005;40:286–293; Miller LC. The Handbook of International Adoption Medicine. New York: Oxford University Press; 2005.

CLINICAL PRESENTATION AND DIAGNOSIS

Screening Newly Arrived Internationally Adopted Children for Infectious Diseases

Standard screening tests are recommended for all newly arrived internationally adopted children (Table 68–3). Tests should be done even if recent results from the child's country of origin are available because of uncertain validity of tests performed in an unknown laboratory. Because of the potentially long incubation periods of some infections, repeat testing for HIV, hepatitis B, hepatitis C, and tuberculosis is recommended 6 (or more) months after the child arrives in the United States.

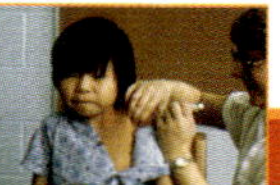

Table 68–3.

Recommended Screening Tests for New Arrivals[2,5,15]

Infectious disease screening

Hepatitis A IgM and IgG
Hepatitis B surface antigen, surface antibody, core antibody*
Hepatitis C*
HIV ELISA (also consider PCR, if <6 months of age)*
Mantoux test*
RPR
Stool for ova and parasites, giardia antigen (repeat later if symptoms warrant)
Titers to verify immunity from administered vaccines (see text)

Other screening tests

CBC
Lead*
Urinalysis
T4, TSH
AST, ALT, Bilirubin, Alkaline phosphatase
Calcium, phosphorus
Vision and hearing screening
Developmental testing

Additional tests to consider based on clinical findings, country of origin and age of the child

H. pylori stool antigen
Malaria smear
Stool cultures for bacterial pathogens
Newborn screen to State Board of Health (usually includes hemoglobin electrophoresis)
G-6-PD screen
Sickle cell screen

**Repeat 6 (or more) months after arrival in the United States.*

Infectious Diseases After Arrival in the United States

Human immunodeficiency virus infection (HIV)

Many internationally adopted children come from countries with high rates of HIV infection. To date, however, very few adoptees have arrived in the United States with this disease.[2] In seven studies describing a total of 1089 children adopted to the United States, Australia, and France, no child with HIV infection was identified, although three had transient antibodies to HIV.[18–24] An informal multicenter survey of 7299 adopted children evaluated in 17 international adoption clinics between 1990 and 2002 found only 12 infected children (0.16%, from Panama, Russia, Cambodia, Romania, and Vietnam).[25] The actual proportion of HIV-infected children is likely somewhat less, as this survey included only children who were evaluated in specialized clinics. The reason for the low rate of infection may reflect accurate preadoptive testing in the birth countries (thus only seronegative children are placed) and low risk of acquisition in orphanages or foster care. However, a recent outbreak of HIV in orphanages in Kazakhstan highlights the risks of exposure.[26] Serologic testing (ELISA) for both HIV-1 and HIV-2 is recommended for all children at arrival in the United States, and again 6 (or more) months after arrival.[4] Some[27] but not all[15] experts recommend PCR testing for HIV DNA for new arrivals younger than 6 months of age at arrival.

Hepatitis B

International adoption and other types of immigration are now the most common sources of children in the United States with hepatitis B infection.[28] In a recent survey by the Centers for Disease Control and Prevention, adoptees from China, Bulgaria, Russia, Phillipines, Ukraine, and Vietnam accounted for 32% of young children reported with hepatitis B infection.[29] Worldwide, about 2 billion people—one-third of the world's population—have present or past evidence of infection with hepatitis B. Nearly 75% of infected people reside in Asia.[30] The 350–375 million with chronic infection have approximately 15–25% risk of dying from hepatitis B virus-related liver disease, including end-stage cirrhosis and hepatocellular carcinoma.[31,32] The four serotypes (adw, ayw, adr, and ayr) and seven genotypes (A to G) of the hepatitis B virus show distinct geographic distributions; these relate to clinical outcomes and responses to drug treatments.[31,33,34] Universal hepatitis B vaccination of newborns was established in only 54% of countries worldwide as of 2000, representing approximately one-third of the global birth cohort.[35] By 2003, 72% of "high prevalence" nations had universal infant vaccine programs.[32]

Hepatitis B screening is nearly universal for children prior to placements in international adoptions. With few exceptions (sibling groups, identified special needs), only seronegative children are considered eligible for adoption. Despite negative serological tests in the country of origin, consistently about 3–5% of new arrivals have hepatitis B infection.[18–24,36] Some series report slightly higher rates of 5–7%.[6,37] The discrepancy between test results in the birth country and those obtained after arrival has been attributed to inaccurate laboratories or infection acquired after testing was completed. Children awaiting international adoption often receive multiple injections; infection rates in some orphanages have been high (35% or more in some orphanages in Romania in the early 1990s[7,38]). Unfortunately, reuse or improper disposal of needles remains a widespread practice in many parts of the world.[39] A recent World Health Organization study found that nearly one-third of injections in developing countries were administered using unsterile equipment; in parts of the Middle East and Asia, this figure rose to 75%.[40]

Because of these risks, prospective adoptive families must be counseled on the risks of household transmission of hepatitis B[41–45,46] and preferably be fully immunized before travelling to receive their new child. Adoption of a child with hepatitis B is well recognized as a source of infection within the family, with transmission rates as high as 64%.[45] In a recent study of 124 unvaccinated Dutch expatriates residing in Nigeria, nearly 10% of the adults and 13% of children acquired hepatitis B infection.[47] Risk of hepatitis B infection was associated with adoption of a Nigerian child and the duration of time the child had resided with the family. Extended family and community members are also at risk of acquiring infection. For example, nearly all unvaccinated parents of 31 hepatitis B-infected international adoptees in Belgium as well as a teacher, grandfather, and teenage family friend became infected, although few individuals reported blood or body fluid contact with the infected child.[7]

A history of vaccination in the adopted child does not insure absence of hepatitis B infection. Only approximately 70% of children who received 3 doses of hepatitis B vaccine in their birth countries had detectable antibody,[37,48] while 13% of previously vaccinated adoptees had hepatitis B core antibody, reflecting prior infection.[37]

Because of these risks, vaccination of family members prior to adoptive placement is urgently recommended. Although most families have adequate time to receive hepatitis B vaccine using the conventional schedule (0, 1, 6 months), occasional families may need an accelerated schedule. Three vaccine doses administered over 3–4 weeks (at 0, 7, and 21 days) induces immunity in more than 75% of adults by 2 months and in 90% by 1 year; a fourth dose (administered 12 months later) for long-term immunity is usually suggested.[40] If needed, this schedule is also successful in inducing immunity in children.[49] Immunity appears to be long-lasting (at least 10 years) for most individuals. High-risk individuals (family members of infected children) should be tested for antibody titers at intervals and offered booster shots if the titer falls below 10 mIU/mL.[31]

Newly adopted children should be tested at arrival and again 6 months later (HBsAg, core Ab, and sAb).[2,6,15] The "hepatitis panel" (HBsAg, IgM core Ab) offered by some commercial laboratories is inadequate. Documentation of surface antibody status is useful to assess the need for additional hepatitis B vaccination (although its presence in infants may reflect maternal antibody and not denote long-lasting immunity). Children found to have HBsAg should undergo additional testing, including liver function tests (ALT, AST, bilirubin, alkaline phosphatase, albumin), HBeAg, HBeAb, α-fetoprotein, and quantitative viral HBV DNA by PCR, and be immunized against hepatitis A (if not immune). Isolated HB core Ab may indicate that the individual is recovering from acute HBV infection, distantly immune with nondetectable levels of HBsAb, has a false-positive core Ab (IgG or polyclonal core Ab may represent maternal antibody in infants), or has a false-negative HBsAg (actually a carrier). These individuals should be retested for liver transaminases, HBsAg and HBsAb (and HBV DNA by PCR) within 1–2 months. Liver ultrasound and consultation with a gastroenterologist are recommended for children with elevated transaminases and/or persistent HBsAg.

Many international adoptees acquire hepatitis B via vertical transmission. A recent study of perinatally infected children of varying ethnic groups found that ~30% develop anti-HBe during ~10 years of follow-up, while <5% clear hepatitis B sAg during this period .[50, 51]

Rare circumstances associated with hepatitis B infection, including infection with viral mutants (altered S gene protein, resulting in "surface antigen negative disease") or superinfections with >1 genotype have not yet been reported in international adoptees. However, some have speculated that early malnutrition may promote severe disease expression.[52]

Hepatitis C

Hepatitis C infection is rare among international adoptees (~1%).[5] However, the presence of hepatitis C antibodies is noted on many medical reports of prospective adoptees from Russia (most other countries do not screen for this infection). These usually represent maternal antibodies; some of these mothers likely acquired hepatitis C infection via injection drug use (thus indicating a possible adverse prenatal exposure for the child). Results of RNA PCR testing in Russian specialty laboratories may be offered for some of these children; results should be interpreted with caution, as reliability of these tests may be uncertain even under the best conditions. Qualitative PCR tests in the first 6 months of life have relatively poor sensitivity in identifying infection.[53] Even between 9 and 15 months of age, infected children may have negative PCR tests as a result of fluctuations in viremia or technical issues related to the assay.

As with hepatitis B, long-term carriage of hepatitis C increases the risk of hepatocellular carcinoma (~1.9–6.7% of patients after 20 years of disease[54]). Acquisition of infection via vertical transmission may reduce the risks of long-term carriage[55] although this is controversial.[56] Ethnic differences contribute to the development of hepatocellular carcinoma, with Asians, Hispanics, Native Americans, and Pacific Islanders noted to have the highest incidence.[54] Coinfection with hepatitis B or HIV also increases the morbidity of HCV infection.

All newly adopted children should be screened for hepatitis C. Because false-negative tests may occur early after infection, children should be retested 6 or more months after arrival.[57] Infected children should be referred to a hepatologist for consideration of drug treatment (e.g., pegylated interferon-ribavirin or other combinations) and ongoing management.

Hepatitis A

Screening for hepatitis A in new arrivals has not routinely been recommended. However, one report has highlighted the risks of hepatitis A not only in new arrivals and their household contacts, but also non-household contacts (e.g., short-term visitors to the child's home).[57A] Among the 27 cases of hepatitis A reported in this outbreak, 19% were adoptees, 7% were unvaccinated travelers, 48% were non-traveling contacts of the adoptees, and 26% were non-traveling contacts of the adoptees. Thus, hepatitis A screening should now be considered routinely in new arrivals.

Tuberculosis

International adoptees have multiple risk factors for infection with *Mycobacterium tuberculosis*, including birth in countries with high prevalence of tuberculosis, poor access to health care, residence in institutions where caregivers may not be screened for tuberculosis infection, young age, and malnutrition. Fortunately, few children arrive with active disease. In those with active disease, extrapulmonary (especially lymphadenitis Figure 68–2) is more usual than pulmonary disease. Latent tuberculosis, however, is relatively common. Most series report latent tuberculosis infection (positive tuberculin skin test [TST], no clinical disease) in approximately

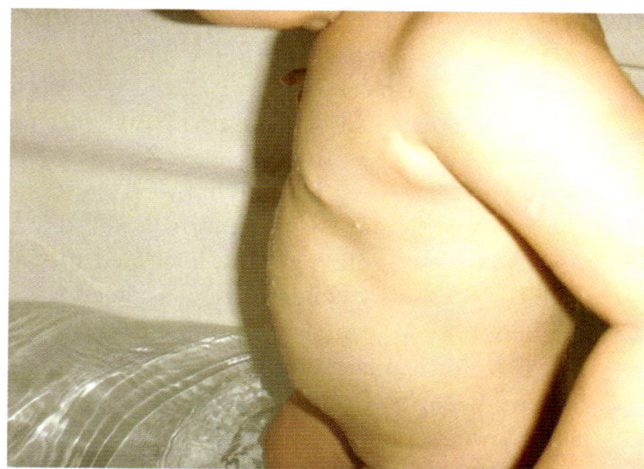

FIGURE 68–2 ■ Axillary lymphadenopathy in a child with tuberculosis.

5–20% of new arrivals.[5] Children from Russia and Ukraine appear to be at higher risk for this infection.[24,37] In a recent report of internationally adopted children in Italy, 30% of non-BCG vaccinated children had latent tuberculosis infection.[37] It is vital to recognize that latent disease may activate, especially in young children, creating a public health hazard. An outbreak of tuberculosis affecting 56 people in a small town in North Dakota was traced to a child adopted from the Marshall Islands.[58]

TSTs should be placed on all internationally adopted children after arrival and again 6 months later. There are many potential pitfalls in diagnosis. False-negative TSTs may result if the test is placed within 4–6 weeks of live virus vaccine administration (for example, MMR or varicella), if the child is malnourished, very young, immunosuppressed, has a concurrent viral or bacterial infection, or was recently exposed to tuberculosis.[4] False-positives most commonly result from prior BCG vaccination or infection with nontuberculous mycobacteria.

Most international adoptees receive BCG vaccination in their birth countries. When properly administered, the BCG vaccine leaves a small scar over the deltoid muscle. Cross-reactivity between purified protein derivative and BCG usually wanes by 6–12 months of age[59–61] when the vaccine is given in early infancy. TST is recommended for newly arrived adoptees regardless of the child's BCG status[15,62]; results are interpreted *without* consideration of prior BCG vaccination. Reactions ≥10 mm are considered positive. In these children, chest radiographs should be obtained, along with careful physical examination for signs of tuberculosis disease. If these investigations are negative, then the child is considered to have latent infection and prophylactic treatment with isoniazid for 9 months is recommended. Reactions in the 5–9-mm range warrant careful evaluation and follow-up, some experts recommend chest radiographs and consideration of prophylactic treatment as recent exposure cannot be excluded.[6,63] Because of the prevalence of multiple-drug resistant tuberculosis in many of the countries of origin of international adoptees, consultation with an infectious disease specialist should be obtained in any child with suspicion of active disease.

A new class of diagnostic tests, interferon-γ release assays, has recently been developed to improve specificity and sensitivity over the century-old TST. To date, these tests have not been adequately studied in children, especially among high-risk populations, and their utility in the diagnosis of latent TB infection is not yet well understood.[64–66] A recent report suggests this test is less sensitive than TST.[67] However, such tests may aid in diagnosis in the future and may be especially valuable in BCG-vaccinated children. These tests are discussed further in Chapter 36.

Some clinicians have recommended chest radiographs for all new arrivals as a means to identify children with tuberculosis infection. A recent survey of approximately 1600 international adoptees in the Netherlands found that routine chest radiography yielded new information in only 2% of cases. Furthermore, false-positive results (findings with no clinical significance) occurred in more than 3% of children. Therefore, routine chest radiography rarely modifies management but may result in additional and unnecessary testing of children with false-positive results.[68]

Intestinal parasites

Approximately 25% of newly arrived international adoptees have intestinal parasites. The prevalence varies depending on country of origin—infections are common in children from Eastern Europe, South Asia, and Africa but rare in children from South Korea.[4,19,20,22–24,36,69,70] *Giardia intestinalis* is the parasite most frequently identified; 8% of international adoptees in Sweden had this infection, with risk per 100,000 children ranging from 0 to 50,000.[71] Some children have persistent or difficult-to-treat infections. Options for eradication include repeating treatment with metronidazole (longer duration or higher dose), or administering alternative agents such as furazolidone, tinidazole, quinacrine, albendazole, or nitazoxanide.[5] Other parasites are often found, including *Entamoeba histolytica, Dientamoeba fragilis, Ascaris lumbricoides, Trichuris trichuria,* Hookworms, *Hymenolepsis nana, Strongyloides stercoralis,* and others. Some children have multiple parasites. Organisms such as *Blastocystis hominis, Entamoeba coli, Entamoeba hartmanni, Entamoeba polecki, Entamoeba dispar, Cryptosporidium, Microsporidium, Cyclospora, Isospora, Iodamoeba buetschlii,* and *Endolimax nana* are usually considered nonpathogens and do not require treatment.

Symptoms of infestation include diarrhea, flatulence, odoriferous stools, abdominal pain, failure to thrive, and anemia. However many children are asymptomatic.[4] Impaired neuropsychiatric function (unrelated to anemia) has been attributed to parasitic infection, with improved cognition after treatment.[72–75]

All newly arrived children should be screened for intestinal parasites. Three samples are recommended to improve detection rate[4]; immunoassay of giardia antigen alone is inadequate. Follow-up samples should be obtained after treatment to verify eradication and to screen for additional parasites. Parasites are sometimes missed in initial stool screening; retesting is advisable if later symptoms appear.[2] A recent survey of intestinal parasites in immigrant children included serologic tests for *Strongyloides* (positive in 1%, equivocal in 10%) and *Schistosoma* (positive in 2%).[76]

Only some parasites induce eosinophilia (especially hookworm, *Strongyloides, Ascaris,* and *Toxocara*).

Children with unexplained eosinophilia after initial stool screening should be reevaluated, and less common parasitic causes of eosinophilia considered (filariasis, schistosomiasis, cutaneous larva migrans).[77] Specific serological testing is available for schistosomiasis, strongyloidiasis, filariasis, echinococcosis, and toxocariasis. Even mild eosinophilia may indicate a pathogenic parasite: evaluation of Southeast Asian immigrants with eosinophilia and negative stool examinations eventually revealed a pathogenic parasite in 95%, most commonly hookworm, *Strongyloides*, or *E. histolytica*.[78] In children with persistent eosinophilia and no obvious diagnosis, empirical treatment with a broad-spectrum antihelminthic is reasonable.[77] Options include mebendazole, pyrantel, or albendazole,[79] although the first two are not effective for strongyloidiasis, tapeworm, or schistosomiasis. Other explanations should be sought if the eosinophil count does not return to normal.[79] Current treatment guidelines for parasites are available in the Red Book[15] and other sources.[80,81]

Bacterial enteric pathogens and Helicobacter pylori

Bacterial enteropathogens (*Salmonella, Shigella, Enteropathogenic E. coli*, or *Campylobacter)* are relatively uncommon in newly arrived adoptees, but children with diarrhea, flatulence, and abdominal pain should be tested for these infections and treatment given to prevent disease transmission.

Some children arriving from orphanages are infected with *H. pylori*.[82] This organism can cause diarrhea, growth faltering, anemia, dyspepsia, and malnutrition.[83] Stool antigen testing for *H. pylori* in young children is both sensitive and specific.[83,84] Some strains acquired in the developing world are resistant to usual drug therapies (e.g., amoxicillin and clarithromycin).[85]

Syphilis

Most—but not all—internationally adopted children are screened for congenital syphilis in their birth countries.[5] Medical records provided at the time of adoption indicate that approximately 15% of children adopted from Russia have a history of congenital syphilis. Details of treatment are rarely provided, however, these children virtually all have negative rapid plasma reagin (RPR) tests on arrival in the United States. Characteristic dental malformations are sometimes seen even when adequate treatment has been provided. Other medical or neurologic complications have not yet been reported in this group of children. Rarely, children arrive with unrecognized, untreated congenital syphilis, or even more uncommonly, with syphilis resulting from sexual abuse. Thus, all children should be tested upon arrival with a nonspecific treponemal test, such as RPR. If this is negative and the child is asymptomatic (and sexual abuse is not suspected), then no additional testing is needed. Children with prior treated congenital syphilis should have careful clinical evaluation and follow-up RPR testing at 1, 2, 4, 6, and 12 months of age. Ophthalmologic and audiologic evaluations should be obtained, as well as screening for neurologic and developmental disorders.[5,6]

Children with positive RPR tests or physical findings consistent with syphilis should have confirmatory treponemal tests (MHA-TP or FTA-ABS), lumbar puncture (if there is consideration of neurosyphilis[86]), dark-field examination of body fluids (such as nasal discharge), long-bone X-rays, as well as vision and hearing tests. After successful treatment, nontreponemal antibody titers become nonreactive over time, while treponemal tests remain positive for life.[6] Detailed recommendations for management of children with positive screening serology on arrival may be found in the Red Book.[15]

Skin infections

Skin infections such as scabies, pediculosis, ringworm, impetigo, and molluscum contagiosum are relatively common in new arrivals, and may spread readily within the new household. Scabies should be suspected in almost any pruritic rash appearing within several weeks of arrival; response to treatment is often diagnostic.

Malaria and unusual infections

As the number of adoptions from Africa has increased (>3000 in past 10 years), concerns about malaria and other tropical diseases has risen. Splenomegaly, anemia, and thrombocytopenia at arrival should prompt consideration of malaria. Some experts suggest routine malaria screens (thick and thin blood smears) for any child adopted from an endemic area. Maps showing malaria risks are readily available online.[13,30,87,88] In a survey of Liberian children immigrating to Minnesota, 65% had positive malaria smears, one-third were completely asymptomatic, and one-third had splenomegaly only.[78] Children from India and South Asia may also be at risk for this infection.[36]

The global epidemic of SARS (severe acute respiratory syndrome) in 2003 serves as a vivid reminder of the potential role of newly arrived adoptees as vectors for transmissible diseases. Although none was laboratory-confirmed, 17 adoptees from China and their family members were investigated as "suspect" or "probable" cases.

Other tropical diseases remain rare (e.g., tungiasis,[89] leprosy,[36] gnathostomiasis[90]). Several cases of *Pneumocystis jiroveci* (formerly *P. carinii*) pneumonia[5,91,92] and one case of fatal measles-related subacute sclerosing panencephalitis have been reported.[93]

Recently, international adoptees were found to be a source for methicillin-resistant *Staphlyococcus aureus*.[94]

PREVENTION

Management of immunizations is a major concern for physicians caring for newly arrived international adoptees. Deficiencies in vaccine records and reduced immunogenicity of vaccines administered in other countries have been widely recognized (Table 68–4). Lack of protective antibody titers in children with seemingly adequate vaccination records may result from provision of nonimmunogenic vaccines to orphanages, improper storage or administration of vaccines, incorrect documentation of administered immunizations, or impaired response to vaccines caused by malnutrition, illness, or stress. As a result of these deficiencies, there have been several reports of transmission of vaccine-preventable diseases (measles,[17] pertussis[6]) to adoptive families, travellers, and community members. Notably, vaccine requirements for entry into the United States are waived for international adoptees. Adopting parents must agree to complete their child's needed vaccines after arrival in the United States.

Specific updated recommendations for management of vaccines in new arrivals are available online[15,102] (Table 68–5). Exceptions to these recommendations include vaccine records from South Korea, Guatemalan foster care (where children receive vaccines in private medical clinics), and probably also India[27] and Colombia.[78] A recent cost-analysis suggests that presumptive immunization rather than prevaccination serotesting of young international adoptees and other immigrant children improves the percentage of protected patients and saves costs.[103] However, availability of combination vaccines and the desire of many parents to avoid unnecessary needle sticks were not included in the analysis.

Table 68–4.

Immunizations in Internationally Adopted Children

Countries of Origin	N	Comments
		Vaccine Records
Many countries[69]	128	Deficient in 37%
Russia[18]	32	Age appropriate according to the US schedule: 16% DPT, 53% polio, 84% measles
Many countries[101]	~160	Age appropriate according to the US schedule: 100% DTP, 99% polio, 100% hepatitis B, 79% measles, 96% mumps, 92% rubella (see also below)
		Protective Vaccine Titers
China, Russia, other E. European countries[95]	26	≥ 3 DTP vaccines: 35% had protective immunity to tetanus and diphtheria (only 12% of former orphanage residents were immune)
Many countries[96]	4	≥ 3 vaccines: 100% lacked immunity to ≥1 serotype polio
Many countries[97]	51	≥ 2 DTP or hepatitis B vaccines: protective immunity for diphtheria 100%, tetanus 80%, hepatitis B 67%
Many countries[98]	70	Protective titers: ≥3 polio vaccines, 65%; ≥3 DTP vaccines, 61–88%; measles 90%
Mostly China[99]	133	≥3 DTP and polio vaccines: ~60% had protective immunity to tetanus, diphtheria, polio
Many countries[48]	504*	9% age-appropriate (according to the US schedule) for DTP, polio, hepatitis B, and MMR; 67% current for ≥1 series
Guatemala[100]	103†	28% age-appropriate (according to the US schedule) for DTP, polio, hepatitis B, MMR
Predominantly Eastern Europe[37]	88	≥3 vaccines: protective immunity for polio 38%, diphtheria 96%, tetanus 91%, hepatitis B 69%; ≥1 vaccine: measles 62%, mumps 56%, rubella 86%
Many countries[101]	~160	≥2 vaccines: protective immunity for diphtheria 99%, tetanus 88%, polio 95%, hepatitis B 82%. ≥1 vaccine: measles 92%, mumps 67%, rubella 92%

**178 Records available.*
†56 Records available.
DTP, diphtheria, tetanus and pertussis vaccination; MMR, measles, mumps and rubella vaccination.

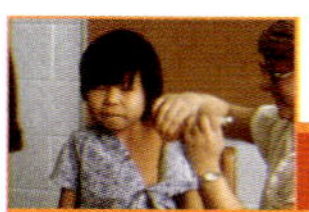

Table 68–5.

Vaccine Management for Internationally Adopted Children

	Recommended Approach	Alternative Approach
Hepatitis B	Test for HbsAg, sAb, core Ab before immunizing ■ If sAb positive, complete series for total of 3 vaccines to provide long-term protection ■ If core Ab positive, give 1 dose vaccine and retest in 1 month	Begin series at time tests obtained; management pending test results
Polio	For children with ≥3 doses, measure neutralizing antibody to types 1, 2, and 3. If antibody present to all 3 serotypes, continue age-appropriate schedule. If antibody absent, repeat series	Give single dose IPV and then measure neutralizing antibodies to types 1, 2, and 3
DTaP	Continue age-appropriate schedule. If severe local reaction, test for antibody to tetanus and diphtheria (*Note*: DTaP needed to protect children <7 y against pertussis)	■ Test for antibodies to tetanus and diphtheria before immunizing ■ Administer single dose of DTaP, then test in 1 month and continue schedule for children with ≥3 doses ■ Repeat all doses
MMR	Age-appropriate administration	■ Test for measles antibody; if present give single dose MMR to children >1 y ■ Test for all 3 antibodies; immunize appropriately for children >1 y (single antigen preparations may be difficult to obtain)
Varicella	■ Serologic testing, followed by age-appropriate administration if seronegative ■ Age-appropriate administration	Typical scarring may not be accepted by schools, day care, etc. as evidence of immunity

Barnett ED. Immunizations and infectious disease screening for internationally adopted children. Pediatr Clin North Am. 2005;52:1287–1309; Stauffer WM, Kamat D, Walker PF. Screening of international immigrants, refugees, and adoptees. Prim Care Clin Office Pract. 2002;29:870-905; Atkinson WL, Pickering LK, Schwartz B, Weniger BG, Iskander JK, Watson JC. General Recommendations on Immunization: Recommendations of the Advisory Committee on Immunization Practices (ACIP) and the American Academy of Family Physicians (AAFP). Vol. 2004, 2002.

REFERENCES

1. Immigrant visas issued to orphans coming to the U.S. http://travel.state.gov/adopt.html. Accessed August 27, 2008.
2. Miller LC. International adoption: infectious diseases issues. *CID*. 2005;40:286-293.
3. Murray TS, Groth E, Weitzman C, Cappello M. Epidemiology and management of infectious diseases in international adoptees. *Clin Microbiol Rev*. 2005;18: 510-520.
4. Staat MA. Infectious disease issues in internationally adopted children. *Pediatr Infect Dis J*. 2002;21:257-258.
5. Miller LC. *The Handbook of International Adoption Medicine*. New York: Oxford University Press; 2005.
6. Barnett ED. Immunizations and infectious disease screening for internationally adopted children. *Pediatr Clin North Am*. 2005;52:1287-1309.
7. Chen LH, Barnett ED, Wilson ME. Preventing infectious diseases during and after international adoption. *Ann Intern Med*. 2003;139:371-378.
8. Wilson ME, Kimble J. Posttravel hepatitis A: probable acquisition from an asymptomatic adopted child. *Clin Infect Dis*. 2001;33:1083-1085.
9. Mackell SM. Vaccinations for the pediatric traveler. *CID*. 2003;37:1508-1516.
10. Christenson JC. Preparing children for travel to tropical and developing regions. *Pediatr Ann*. 2004;33:676-684.
11. Maloney S, Weinberg M. Prevention of infectious diseases among international pediatric travelers: considerations for clinicians. *Semin Pediatr Infect Dis*. 2004;15: 137-149.
12. Centers for Disease Control and Prevention. *The Yellow Book. Health information for international travel*. http://www.cdc.gov/travel/contentyellowbook.aspx. Accessed August 27, 2008.
13. World Health Organization. International travel and health. http://www.who.int/ith/. Accessed, 2004.
14. Hostetter MK. Epidemiology of travel-related morbidity and mortality in children. *Pediatr Rev*. 1999;20:228-233.
15. American Academy of Pediatrics. In: Pickering LK, Baker CJ, Long SS, McMillan JA, eds. *2006 Red Book: Report of the Committee on Infectious Diseases*. Elk Grove Village, IL: American Academy of Pediatrics; 2006.
16. Borchers DA. Adoption Medical Travel Guide. http://Adoptivefamilies.com/pdf/travelmed.pdf. Accessed August 27, 2008.

17. Measles among adults associated with adoption of children in China. *MMWR.* 2007;56:144-146.
18. Albers LH, Johnson DE, Hostetter MK, Iverson S, Miller LC. Health of children adopted from the former Soviet Union and Eastern Europe. Comparison with preadoptive medical records. *JAMA.* 1997;278:922-924.
19. Hostetter MK, Iverson S, Thomas W, McKenzie D, Dole K, Johnson DE. Medical evaluation of internationally adopted children. *N Engl J Med.* 1991;325:479-485.
20. Johnson DE, Miller LC, Iverson S, et al. The health of children adopted from Romania. *JAMA.* 1992;268: 3446-3451.
21. Bureau JJ, Maurage C, Bremond M, Despert F, Rolland JC. Children of foreign origin adopted in France. Analysis of 68 cases during 12 years at the University Hospital Center of Tours. *Arch Pediatr.* 1999;6:1053-1058.
22. Miller LC, Kiernan MT, Mathers MI, Klein-Gitelman M. Developmental and nutritional status of internationally adopted children. *Arch Pediatr Adolesc Med.* 1995;149:40-44.
23. Miller LC, Hendrie NW. Health of children adopted from China. *Pediatrics.* 2000;105:E76.
24. Saiman L, Aronson J, Zhou J, et al. Prevalence of infectious diseases among internationally adopted children. *Pediatrics.* 2001;108:608-612.
25. Aronson J. *HIV in Internationally Adopted Children.* Washington, DC: Joint Council for International Children's Services; 2002.
26. Trial scrutinizes infant HIV outbreak in Kazakhastan. National Public Radio. www.npr.org/templates/story/story.php?storyid=E954147. Accessed August 28, 2008.
27. Hostetter M. Infectious diseases in internationally adopted children: findings in children from China, Russia, and Eastern Europe. *Adv Pediatr Infect Dis.* 1999;14:147-161.
28. Elisofon SA, Jonas MM. Hepatitis B and C in children: current treatments and future strategies. *Clin Liver Dis.* 2006;10:133-148.
29. Shepard C, Finelli L, Bell B, Miller J. Acute hepatitis B among children and adolescents – United States 1990-2002. *MMWR.* 2004;53:1015-1018.
30. Centers for disease control and prevention. Hepatitis, viral, type B. http://www.cdc.gov/travel/yellowbookch4-hepb.aspx. Accessed August 28, 2008.
31. Kao JH, Chen DS. Global control of hepatitis B infection. *Lancet.* 2002;2:395-403.
32. Blumberg BS. The curiosities of hepatitis B virus. *Proc Am Thorac Soc.* 2006;3:14-20.
33. Kao JH, Chen PJ, Lai MY, Chen DS. Hepatitis B genotypes correlate with clinical outcomes in patients with chronic hepatitis B. *Gastroenterology.* 2000;118: 554-559.
34. Snitbhan R, Scott RM, Bancroft WH, Top FH, Jr., Chiewsilp D. Subtypes of hepatitis B surface antigen in Southeast Asia. *J Infect Dis.* 1975;131:708-711.
35. Alter MJ. Epidemiology and prevention of hepatitis B. *Semin Liver Dis.* 2003;23:39-46.
36. Smith-Garcia T, Brown JS. The health of children adopted from India. *J Community Health.* 1989;14: 227-241.
37. Vivano E, Cataldo F, Accomando S, Firenze A, Valenti RM, Romano N. Immunization status of internationally adopted children in Italy. *Vaccine.* 2006;24:4138-4143.
38. Hoksbergen R, van Dijkum C, Stoutjesdijk F. Experiences of Dutch families who parent an adopted Romanian child. *J Devel Behav Pediatr.* 2002;23:403-410.
39. Murakami H, Kobayashi JM, Zhu X, Li Y, Wakai S, Chiba Y. Risk of transmission of hepatitis B virus through childhood immunization in northwestern China. *Soc Sci Med.* 2003;57:1821-1832.
40. Keystone JS. Travel-related hepatitis B: risk factors and prevention using an accelerated vaccination schedule. *Am J Med.* 2005;118:63S-68S.
41. Vernon TM, Wright RA, Kohler PF, Merrill DA. Hepatitis A and B in the family unit. Nonparenteral transmission by asymptomatic children. *JAMA.* 1976;235: 2829-2831.
42. Nordenfelt E, Dahlquist E. HBsAg positive adopted children as a cause of intrafamilial spread of hepatitis B. *Scand J Infect Dis.* 1978;10:161-163.
43. Friede A, Harris JR, Kobayashi JM, Shaw FE, Jr., Shoemaker-Nawas PC, Kane MA. Transmission of hepatitis B virus from adopted Asian children to their American families. *Am J Public Health.* 1988;78:26-29.
44. Christenson B. Epidemiological aspects of the transmission of hepatitis B by HBsAg-positive adopted children. *Scand J Infect Dis.* 1986;18:105-109.
45. Sokal EM, Van Collie O, Buts JP. Horizontal transmission of hepatitis B from children to adoptive parents. *Arch Dis Child.* 1995;72:191.
46. Doganci T, Uysal G, Kir T, Barkirtas A, Kuyucu N, Doganci L. Horizontal transmission of hepatitis B virus in children with chronic hepatitis. *World J Gastroenterol.* 2005;11:418-420.
47. Cobelens FGJ, van Schothorst HJ, Wertheim-Van Dillen PME, Ligthelm RJ, Paul-Steenstra IS, van Thiel PPAM. Epidemiology of hepatitis B infection among expatriates in Nigeria. *CID.* 2004;38:370-376.
48. Schulte J, Maloney S, Aronson J, Gabriel PS, Zhou J, Saiman L. Evaluating acceptability and completeness of overseas immunization records of internationally adopted children. *Pediatrics.* 2002;109:e22.
49. Bosnak M, Dikici B, Bosnak V, Haspolat K. Accelerated hepatitis B vaccination schedule in childhood. *Pediatr Int.* 2002;44:663-665.
50. Boxall EH, Sira J, Standish RA, et al. Natural history of hepatitis B in perinatally infected carriers. *Arch Dis Child Fetal Neonatal Ed.* 2004;89:F456-F460.
51. Choulot JJ, Guerin B. Chronic carriage of hepatitis B virus and adoption. *Med Mal Infect.* 2005;35:S132-S133.
52. Zwiener RJ, Fielman BA, Squires RH, Jr. Chronic hepatitis B in adopted Romanian children. *J Pediatr.* 1992;121: 572-574.
53. European Paediatric Hepatitis C Virus Network; Polywka S, Pembrey L, Tovo P-A, Newell M-L. Accuracy of HCV-RNA PCR tests for diagnosis or exclusion of vertically acquired HCV infection. *Med Virol.* 2005;78: 305-310.
54. El-Serag HB, Mason AC. Rising incidence of hepatocellular carcinoma in the United States. *N Engl J Med.* 1999;340:745-750.
55. Jonas MM. Hepatitis C infection in children. *N Engl J Med.* 1999;341:912-913.
56. Rerksuppaphol S, Hardikar W, Dore GJ. Long-term outcome of vertically acquired and post-transfusion hepatitis C infection in children. *J Gastroenterol Hepatol.* 2004;19:1357-1362.

57. Maggiore G, Caprai S, Cerino A, Silini E, Mondelli MU. Antibody-negative chronic hepatitis C virus infection in immunocompetent children. *J Pediatr.* 1998;132: 1048-1050.

57A. Fischer GE, Teshale EH, Miller C, Schumann C, Winter K, Elson F, et al. Hepatitis A among international adoptees and their contacts. *Clin Infect Dis.* 2008 Sep 15;47(6):812-4.

58. Curtis A, Ridzon R, Vogel R, et al. Extensive transmission of Mycobacterium tuberculosis from a child. *N Engl J Med.* 1999;341:1491-1495.

59. Lifschitz M. The value of the tuberculin skin test as a screening test for tuberculosis among BCG-vaccinated children. *Pediatrics.* 1965;36:624-627.

60. Hizel K, Maral I, Karakus R, Aktas F. The influence of BCG immunisation on tuberculin reactivity and booster effect in adults in a country with a high prevalence of tuberculosis. *Clin Microbiol Infect.* 2004;10:980-983.

61. Menzies D. What does tuberculin reactivity after bacille Calmette-Guérin vaccination tell us? *Clin Infect Dis.* 2000;31(suppl 3):S71-S74.

62. Pediatric Tuberculosis Collaborative Group. Targeted tuberculin skin testing and treatment of latent tuberculosis infection in children and adults. *Pediatrics.* 2004;114:1175-1201.

63. Mandalakas AM, Starke JR. Tuberculosis screening in immigrant children. *Pediatr Infect Dis J.* 2004;23:71-72.

64. Mazurek GH, Jereb J, LoBue P, Iademarco MF, Metchock B, Vernon A. Guidelines for using the Quantiferon-TB Gold Test for detecting Mycobacterium tuberculosis infection, United States. *MMWR.* 2005;54: 49-55.

65. Pai M, Kalantri S, Dheda K. New tools and emerging technologies for the diagnosis of tuberculosis: part 1. Latent tuberculosis. *Expert Rev Mol Diagn.* 2006; 6: 413-422.

66. Tsiouris SJ, Austin J, Toro P, et al. Results of a tuberculosis-specific IFN-gamma assay in children at high risk for tuberculosis infection. *Int J Tuberc Lung Dis.* 2006;10:939-941.

67. Hill PC, Brookes RH, Adetifa IMO, et al. Comparison of enzyme-linked immunospot assay and tuberculin skin test in healthy children exposed to Mycobacterium tuberculosis. *Pediatrics.* 2006;117:1542-1548.

68. Bakker J, Horsthuis K, Cobelens FGJ, Beek FJA, Schulpen TW. Value of routine chest radiography in the medical screening of internationally adopted children. *Acta Paediatrica.* 2005;94:366-368.

69. Jenista JA, Chapman D. Medical problems of foreign-born adopted children. *Am J Dis Child.* 1987;141: 298-302.

70. Aronson J. Medical evaluation and infectious considerations on arrival. *Pediatr Ann.* 2000;29:218-223.

71. Ekdahl K, Andersson Y. Imported giardiasis: impact of international travel, immigration, and adoption. *Am J Trop Med Hyg.* 2005;72:825-830.

72. Boivin MJ, Giordani B. Improvements in cognitive performance for schoolchildren in Zaire, Africa, following an iron supplement and treatment for intestinal parasites. *J Pediatr Psychol.* 1993;18:249-264.

73. Guerrant DI, Moore SR, Lima AA, Patrick PD, Schorling JB, Guerrant RL. Association of early childhood diarrhea and cryptosporidiosis with impaired physical fitness and cognitive function four–seven years later in a poor urban community in northeast Brazil. *Am J Trop Med Hyg.* 1999;61:707-713.

74. Nokes C, Grantham-McGregor SM, Sawyer AW, Cooper ES, Bundy DA. Parasitic helminth infection and cognitive function in school children. *Proc R Soc Lond B Biol Sci.* 1992;247:77-81.

75. Nokes C, McGarvey ST, Shiue L, et al. Evidence for an improvement in cognitive function following treatment of Schistosoma japonicum infection in Chinese primary schoolchildren. *Am J Trop Med Hyg.* 1999;60:556-565.

76. Rice JE, Skull SA, Pearce C, Mulholland N, Davie G, Carapetis JR. Screening for intestinal parasites in recently arrived children from East Africa. *J Paediatr Child Health.* 2003;39:456-459.

77. Schulte C, Krebs B, Jelinek T, Nothdurft HD, von Sonnenburg F, Loscher T. Diagnostic significance of blood eosinophilia in returning travelers. *Clin Infect Dis.* 2002;34:407-411.

78. Stauffer WM, Kamat D, Walker PF. Screening of international immigrants, refugees, and adoptees. *Prim Care Clin Office Pract.* 2002;29:870-905.

79. Looke DFM, Robson JMB. Infections in the returned traveller. *Med J Aust.* 2002;177:212-219.

80. Drugs for parasitic infections. *Med Letter.* 2002;XX:1-12. Available at www.medletter.com Accessed August 28, 2008.

81. Moon TD, Oberhelman RA. Antiparasitic therapy in children. *Pediatr Clin North Am.* 2005;52:917-948.

82. Miller LC, Kelly N, Tannemaat M, Grand RJ. Serologic prevalence of antibodies to *Helicobacter pylori* in internationally adopted children. *Helicobacter.* 2003;8: 173-178.

83. Frenck RW, Fathy HM, Sherif M, et al. Sensitivity and specificity of various tests for the diagnosis of *Helicobacter pylori* in Egyptian children. *Pediatrics.* 2006;118: 1195-1202.

84. Dondi E, Rapa A, Boldorinie R, Fonio P, Zanetta S, Oderda G. High accuracy of noninvasive tests to diagnose *Helicobacter pylori* infection in very young children. *J Pediatr.* 2006;149:817-821.

85. Houben MH, Van Der Beek D, Hensen EF, Craen AJ, Rauws EA, Tytgat GN. A systematic review of *Helicobacter pylori* eradication therapy-the impact of antimicrobial resistance on eradication rates. *Aliment Pharmacol Ther.* 1999;13:1047-1055.

86. Michelow IC, Wendel GD, Norgard MV, et al. Central nervous system infection in congenital syphilis. *N Engl J Med.* 2002;346:1792-1798.

87. Centers for Disease Control and Prevention. *Health Information for the International Traveller, 2005-2006.* Atlanta: US Department of Health and Human Services, Public Health Service; 2005. http://www.cdc.gov/travel/default.aspx. Accessed August 28, 2008.

88. World Health Organization. World Malaria Report, 2005. http://www.rbm.who.int/wmr2005/html/map1.htm. Accessed August 28, 2008.

89. Fein H, Naseem S, Witte DP, Garcia VF, Lucky A, Staat MA. Tungiasis in North America: a report of 2 cases in internationally adopted children. *J Pediatr.* 2001;139: 744-746.

90. Olivan-Gonzalvo G. Gnathostomiasis tras un viaje a China para realizar una adopcion internacional. *Med Clin (Barc)*. 2006;126:757-759.
91. Redman JC. *Pneumocystis carinii* pneumonia in an adopted Vietnamese infant. A case of fulminant disease with recovery. *JAMA*. 1974;230:1561-1563.
92. Giebink GS, Sholler L, Keenan TP, Franciosis RA, Quie PG. *Pneumocystis carinii* pneumonia in two Vietnamese refugee infants. *Pediatrics*. 1976;58:115-118.
93. Bonthius DJ, Stanek N, Grose C. Subacute sclerosing panencephalitis, a measles complication, in an internationally adopted child. *Emerg Infect Dis*. 2000;6: 377-381.
94. Radtke A, Jacobsen T, Bergh K. Internationally adopted children as a source for MRSA. *Eurosurveillance*. 2005; 10:051020.
95. Hostetter MK, Johnson DJ. Immunization status of adoptees from China, Russia, and Eastern Europe (abstract). *Pediatr Res*. 1998;43:147A.
96. Miller LC. Internationally adopted children–immunization status. *Pediatrics*. 1999;103:1078.
97. Staat MA, Daniels D. Immunization verification in internationally adopted children. *Pediatr Res*. 2001;49: 468A.
98. Miller LC, Comfort K, Kelly N. Immunization status of internationally adopted children. *Pediatrics*. 2001;108: 1050-1051.
99. Schulpen TW, van Seventer AH, Rumke HC, van Loon AM. Immunisation status of children adopted from China. *Lancet*. 2001;358:2131-2132.
100. Miller LC, Chan W, Comfort K, Tirella L. Health of children adopted from Guatemala: comparison of orphanage and foster care. *Pediatrics*. 2005;115:e710-e717.
101. Crouch B, Lee PJ, Alonso M, Lane D, Chen JJ, Krilov LR. *Reliability of Immunization Records in Internationally Adopted Children*. Atlanta, GA: American Academy of Pediatrics; 2006.
102. Atkinson WL, Pickering LK, Schwartz B, Weniger BG, Iskander JK, Watson JC. General recommendations on immunization: recommendations of the Advisory Committee on Immunization Practices (ACIP) and the American Academy of Family Physicians (AAFP). Vol. 2004, 2002.
103. Cohen AL, Vennstra D. Economic analysis of prevaccination serotesting compared with presumptive immunization for polio, diphtheria, and tetanus in internationally adopted and immigrant infants. *Pediatrics*. 2006;117: 1650-1655.

SECTION 19

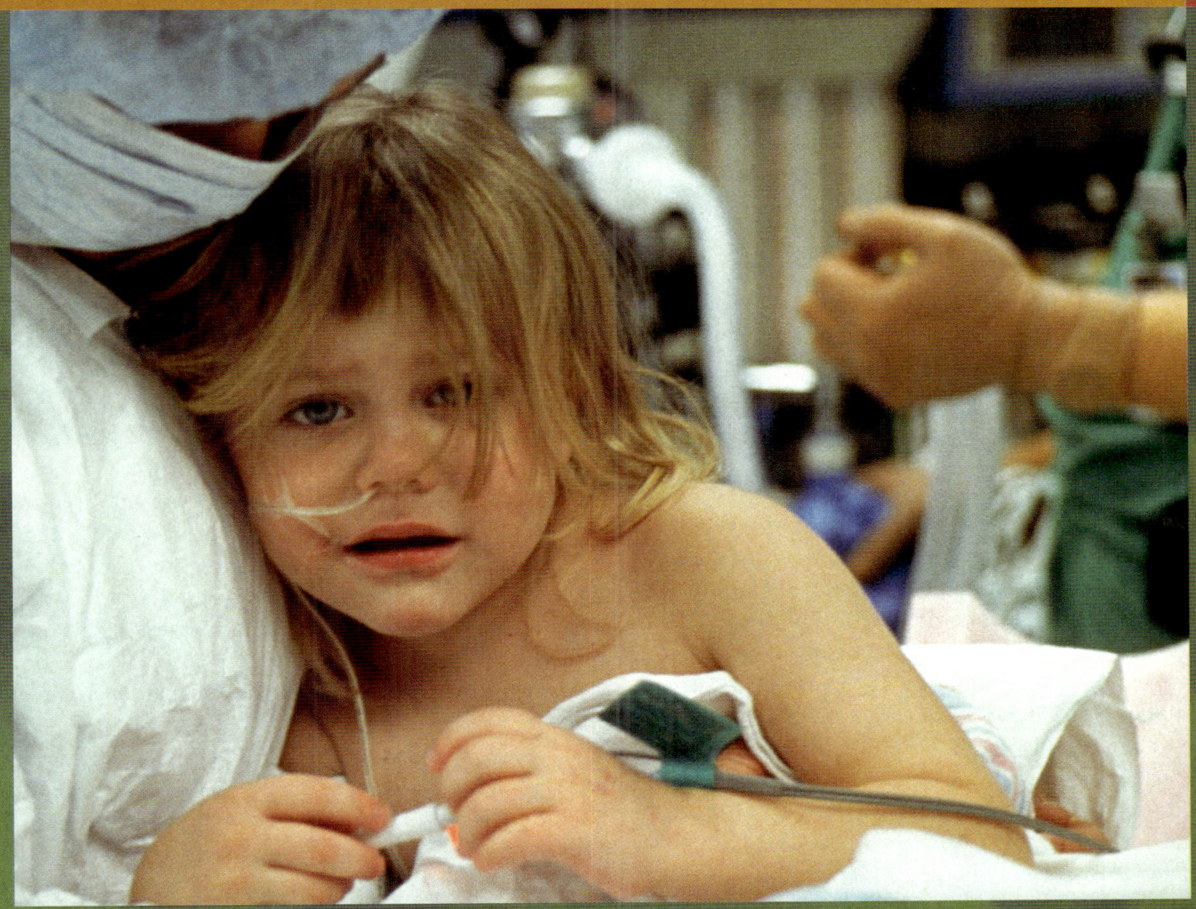

Health-Care Acquired Infections

CHAPTER 69

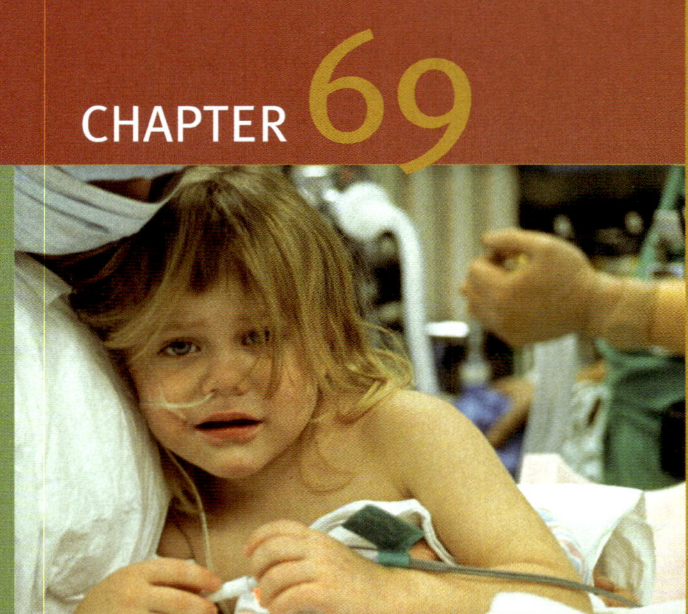

Surgical Site Infections

Peter Mattei

DEFINITIONS AND EPIDEMIOLOGY

Surgical site infections (SSI) are infections that occur in tissues or organs that a surgeon has incised or come into contact with during the course of a surgical procedure or operation. Despite advances in the understanding of risk factors, pathogenesis, and prophylaxis, SSI are still a significant source of morbidity for children who undergo operative procedures. Estimated to occur in 2–6% of children who undergo an operation, SSI in some studies account for up to early one quarter of all nosocomial infections in this age group.[1–7] For the individual, an SSI can mean prolongation of the hospital stay, additional surgical interventions, the risk of further complications and, most importantly, unnecessary pain and anxiety. For society, the treatment of these largely preventable complications substantially increases the overall cost of health care, as the cost of treatment for each patient with an SSI increases by an average of approximately 36%.[8]

It should be noted that nearly all of the studies regarding the microbiology, pathogenesis, prevention, and treatment of SSI have been conducted in adults. Because of the present dearth of studies involving children, we have no choice but to apply the same principles used in adults, with modifications where clinical experience and good judgment dictate.

In the past, subjective terms such as "postoperative wound infection" or "wound abscess" were commonly used to describe SSI and, unless defined very clearly by the author who used them, it was often difficult to understand exactly which disease processes were being discussed. In 1970, the Centers for Disease Control and Prevention (CDC) established the National Nosocomial Infections Surveillance (NNIS) System (now the National Healthcare Safety Network [NHSN]), which eventually helped to more precisely define the various types of SSI.[9] (Table 69–1 and Figure 69–1). The use of these definitions has allowed more accurate comparisons between studies and, perhaps more importantly, has provided a basis for standardization of the criteria used in surveillance programs throughout the United States. These programs and subsequent studies that resulted have provided an abundance of useful data over the past 15–20 years and have helped to enhance our understanding of the risk factors and pathogenesis of SSI.

Several factors are used to define SSI, including the timing of the infection relative to the creation of the incision, the extent of local tissue or organ involvement, and the clinical signs that are suggestive or diagnostic of an actual infection. The question of timing is based on the idea that after a certain period of time, an infection can no longer be presumed to be causally related to the surgical event. The CDC defines an SSI as an infection that occurs within 30 days of an operative procedure, or up to 1 year from the time of surgery if an implant (a "nonhuman-derived implantable foreign body") is placed permanently in a patient at the time of surgery. Although inevitably somewhat arbitrary, this is a consensus based on our current understanding of wound healing and empiric evidence derived from decades of cumulative clinical practice.

Surgical site infections are further described as superficial incisional infections, deep incisional infections, and organ/space infections. Superficial incisional infections include tissue infections (cellulitis) and organized purulent infections (abscess) that involve the skin and subcutaneous fat down to but not including the level of the muscle fascia. Deep incisional infections are those that involve one or more layers of muscle or fascia down to the structure that defines the underlying

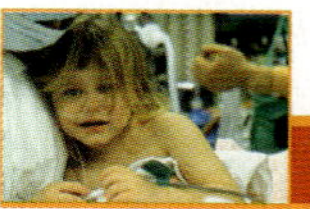

Table 69–1.

Criteria for Defining Surgical Site Infections (SSI)[9]

Type of SSI	Timing	Anatomic Location	Clinical Criteria	Comments
Superficial incisional	<30 d*	Skin and/or subcutaneous tissues	At least one of the following: ■ Purulent drainage from superficial incision ■ Positive wound culture ■ Signs of infection[†] *and* wound is opened by surgeon[‡] ■ Diagnosis of superficial incisional SSI made by surgeon	Do not report: stitch abscess, or circumcision, episiotomy, or burn infections
Deep incisional	<30 d*	Fascia and/or muscle	At least one of the following: ■ Purulent drainage from deep incision ■ Signs of infection and wound is opened by surgeon or wound dehisces[‡] ■ Abscess or infection noted on examination, at reoperation, or by medical imaging ■ Diagnosis of deep incisional SSI made by surgeon	Report infections that involve both superficial and deep tissues as deep incisional SSI
Organ/Space	<30 d*	Organ or space that was opened during surgery	At least one of the following: ■ Percutaneous aspiration of pus from organ/space ■ Positive organ/space fluid culture ■ Abscess or infection noted on examination, at reoperation, or by medical imaging ■ Diagnosis of organ/space SSI made by surgeon	Report organ/space infections that drain through the incision as deep incisional SSI

**Up to 1 year if an implant is placed.*
[†]Pain or tenderness, localized swelling, redness or heat.
[‡]Unless wound cultures are negative.

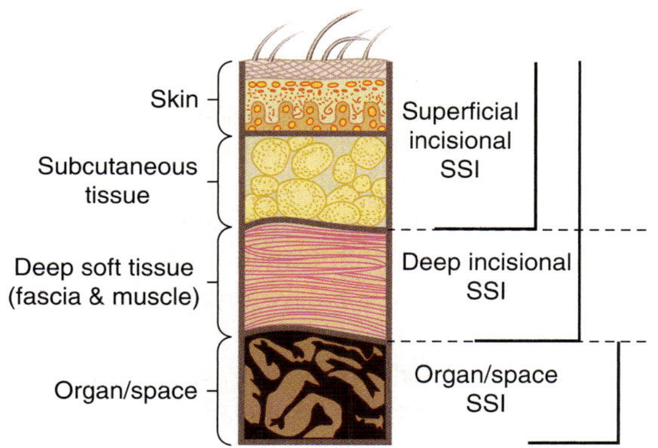

FIGURE 69–1 ■ Cross-section of abdominal wall depicting Centers for Disease Control and Prevention classifications of surgical site infection.

organ space (e.g., peritoneum, pleura, periosteum, or dura). Organ/space infections include infections that involve the underlying body cavity or an organ within that space (Table 69–2).

The NNIS also defines SSI on the basis of specific clinical criteria: (1) the presence of purulent material either draining from the wound or identified by surgical or radiographic means; (2) a positive wound culture; (3) clinical signs or symptoms suggestive of an infection in a wound that has been deliberately opened; or (4) the clinical judgment of a surgeon or attending physician that an infection is present. The criteria therefore vary somewhat depending on the depth of tissues involved and the clinical circumstances. Nevertheless, this practical and reproducible paradigm is used extensively as the standard for defining surgical site infections in the United States and increasingly throughout the world.

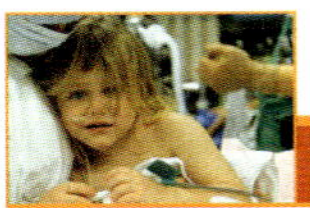

Table 69–2.

Organ/Space Infections[10]

Osteomyelitis
Breast abscess or mastitis
Myocarditis or pericarditis
Disk space
Ear or mastoid
Endometritis
Endocarditis
Eye, other than conjunctivitis
Gastrointestinal tract
Intra-abdominal
Intracranial, brain abscess or dura
Joint or bursa
Lung, upper or lower respiratory tract
Mediastinitis
Meningitis or ventriculitis
Oral cavity (mouth, tongue, or gums)
Spinal abscess
Sinusitis
Arterial or venous infection
Vaginal cuff

Not all infections that occur after a surgical procedure are reportable as SSI. Important exceptions include stitch abscess, which is the result of a very small, localized infection or inflammatory reaction to suture material in the skin, and circumcision, episiotomy, and burn infections, which are not classified as operative procedures by the NNIS.[10]

MICROBIOLOGY

The organisms most commonly isolated from infected surgical sites have been remarkably consistent over the past several decades, with *Staphylococcus aureus*, coagulase-negative staphylococci, *Enterococcus* spp., and *Escherichia coli* being the most common.[11,12] The distribution of less common isolates usually reflect the proximity of the surgical wound to organs or body sites that are known to be colonized or contaminated with certain microbes. Incisions of the head and neck, for example, are more likely to become infected with nose and mouth flora (*Eikenella corrodens, Morraxella catarrhalis,* and *Peptostreptoccus* spp.) while after colorectal surgery, incisions are more likely to become infected with *Enterobacteriaceae* and *Bacteroides* spp. Another recent trend is an increase in infections caused by antimicrobial-resistant organisms, especially methicillin-resistant *S. aureus* (MRSA)[13,14] and *Candida albicans.*[15] The increase in infections due to MRSA is a reflection of the well-documented increase in community-acquired soft-tissue infections caused by this virulent pathogen, the emergence of which is thought to be due to the widespread (and perhaps indiscriminate) use of broad-spectrum antibiotics. Finally, implants such as indwelling central venous catheters may become infected with common skin flora such as *Staphylococcus epidermidis.* Under normal circumstances, these organisms are fairly innocuous but in the presence of a foreign body their virulence is clearly enhanced.

Occasionally, a very unusual organism is isolated from a surgical site infection. When these occur in two or more patients in the form of a local outbreak, it is important to recognize and eliminate the source of contamination and to identify others who might be at risk. Examples include a cluster of postoperative Aspergillus infections that were traced to a contaminated air-handling system in a single operating theater in Texas,[16] and an outbreak of *Pseudomonas aeruginosa* sternal wound infections traced to a surgeon with onychomycosis.[17] These miniepidemics underscore the importance of systematic and honest reporting of SSI data and the usefulness of ongoing hospital infection control procedures.

PATHOGENESIS

The likelihood of developing a surgical site infection depends on a combination of microbial features and host factors.[18–20] The combination of an adequate number of microorganisms of sufficient virulence and a susceptible host under the appropriate local wound conditions is necessary and sufficient to produce a surgical site infection. Certain local factors are known to increase the incidence of infection, in particular the presence of a foreign body such as suture material or a drain.[21] Likewise, the risk of infection is higher if the host is immunocompromised. The augmented virulence of particular pathogens has been attributed to their ability to evade local host defenses, usually by the secretion of toxins or local tissue proteases. For example, some strains of coagulase-negative staphylococci produce an extracellular polysaccharide (slime) that create an effective barrier against host defenses and antimicrobial agents,[22] while some Bacteroides species secrete short chain fatty acids, which impair neutrophil function, and a procoagulant, which inhibits bacterial clearance.[23]

The vast majority of SSI are caused by microorganisms that are part of the patient's skin flora or that colonize the mucosa of a hollow organ that is close to the wound or is violated during the operation.[24] Pathogens may also be introduced by contaminated surgical instruments, operating room personnel, or frank contamination with stool, secretions, or pus. Although it is assumed that most infections are caused by organisms that are introduced into the wound at the time of the operation, there are clearly some cases in which the contamination occurs in the perioperative period. For example, there are published reports of clusters of infections caused by contaminated surgical bandages[25] and contaminated tap water.[26] In addition, it is standard surgical practice is to take special precautions when incisions are located near a colostomy or near the anus, where significant postoperative wound contamination is to be expected. Nevertheless, SSI are generally thought to be due to microorganisms that are present before the patient leaves the operating theater.

Host factors that are important in the development of an SSI include systemic factors as well as wound factors that create a local environment conducive to the growth of microorganisms. Patients who are immunodeficient or who are administered drugs that compromise the immune system such as corticosteroids have a higher incidence of SSI and are more susceptible to opportunistic pathogens.[27] Conditions associated with poor microvascular blood flow or diminished oxygen delivery such as diabetes mellitus, shock, or nicotine abuse may also increase the risk of infection.[9] It was often taught in the past that occlusive surgical dressings should be avoided and that the dressing should be removed on the second postsurgical day to avoid wound infection, however it has since been shown that occlusive dressings pose no risk for infection and may in fact decrease the risk of SSI.[28]

RISK FACTORS

Risk factor assessment for SSI are complicated by the fact that practical risk factors that a clinician or surgeon might use to identify patients at increased risk do not necessarily satisfy the criteria that an epidemiologist would use to define a risk factor in the strictest sense, namely a factor that is an independent predictor of infection based on rigorous multivariate analysis. Nevertheless, in adults, there are numerous local and systemic factors that have been identified as risk factors for the development of SSI. These serve as the basis for preventative measures, many of which have become the standard of patient care in developed countries. Unfortunately, there are still very little data available regarding risk factor assessment in children.

One of the most important and reliable instruments for the assessment of infection risk is the operative wound classification system as defined by the National Research Council (Table 69–3). It is a practical estimate of the degree of contamination of the surgical wound and historically has correlated consistently with the incidence of postoperative wound infection.[29,30] There are four classes: clean, clean contaminated, contaminated, and dirty-infected. Clean wounds result from incisions that are made through intact, uninfected skin, in which the gastrointestinal, respiratory, or genitourinary tract has not been entered,

Table 69–3.

Wound Classification[59]

Wound Class	Definition	Example	Antibiotic Prophylaxis
Clean	■ Elective incision through healthy skin with no inflammation ■ Incision primarily closed or closed over closed-suction drain ■ No break in aseptic technique ■ GI, respiratory or GU tract not entered	Hernia repair	Not indicated*
Clean-contaminated	■ GI, respiratory or GU tract entered with no infection present ■ Incision closed with passive drain ■ Minor break in aseptic technique	Cholecystectomy Appendectomy	Indicated
Contaminated	■ Open fresh traumatic wound ■ Incisions through noninfected inflamed skin ■ Gross GI tract spillage ■ Biliary tract or GU tract entered with infected bile or urine present ■ Major break in aseptic technique	Hemicolectomy	Indicated
Dirty-Infected	■ Old traumatic wound with devitalized tissue, FB, or feces present ■ Incision through infected skin or soft tissues ■ Perforated viscus	Perforated viscus	N/A†

**Recommended when an implant is placed.*
†Requires directed therapy for treatment of infection.

and there has been no break in aseptic technique. Clean-contaminated wounds are those that are associated with entry into the gastrointestinal, respiratory, or genitourinary tract in the absence of infection, or those in which there is more than a minor break in aseptic technique. Wounds that are closed with a passive drain in place and nonperforated appendectomy incisions are also considered to be clean-contaminated. Contaminated wounds are those that are the result of a recent traumatic injury, those in which the incised skin is inflamed but not infected, and those in which there has been a major break in aseptic technique. Incisions exposed to gross gastrointestinal tract spillage or infected bile or urine are also considered contaminated. Dirty-infected wounds are those resulting from neglected traumatic wounds and contain devitalized tissue, foreign material, or fecal matter, and those in which the incised skin is infected. These are technically not at risk for getting infected but are considered already infected. All current wound surveillance programs utilize this wound classification system and documentation of the wound classification is required by major hospital accreditation organizations and most standard operating room protocols.

In addition to the degree of wound contamination, various host factors, mechanical factors, and interventions that increase the risk of SSI have been identified. Host factors include the following: (1) Blood glucose—patients with poorly controlled diabetes are known to be at higher risk for SSI, those with an elevated HgA1c level going into surgery,[31] and those with elevated blood glucose levels (>200 mg/dL) in the postoperative period[32,33] are at higher risk for postoperative infectious complications. (2) Smoking—some studies have confirmed that smokers have a higher risk of SSI[34] but whether this risk can be lessened by having patients abstain from smoking for a period of time prior to their operation is unclear, though overall complication rates are probably lower.[35] (3) Immunosuppressive drugs—patients who take exogenous corticosteroids are thought to be at higher risk of developing SSI, but the data are somewhat equivocal. (4) Nutritional status—patients with severe protein malnutrition appear to have an increased risk of SSI, but it has been difficult to prove that improving nutrition by either the enteral or parenteral route preoperatively can decrease the risk. However, improving nutrition before a major operation has benefits well beyond the risk of SSI and current surgical strategies routinely incorporate nutritional therapy. Furthermore, in terms of lowering the risk of SSI (and most other complications), enteral nutrition has been shown to be clearly superior to parenteral nutrition.[36] (5) Hospital factors—prolonged hospital stay,[37] perioperative blood transfusions,[34] and preoperative colonization with *S. aureus*[38] have all been associated with an increased risk of developing SSI, but whether these are independently associated with an increased risk is yet to be determined. (6) Procedural factors—prolonged operative time, poor oxygen delivery, and hypothermia.[37] Prolonged operative time is the only factor that appears to correlate independently with an increased risk for SSI.[9,39]

Based on epidemiologic data from numerous multivariate analyses, the NNIS developed a risk index score that is supposed to identify patients who are at the highest risk for SSI. For any given operation, the score is generated by counting the number of the following risk factors present: (1) American Society of Anesthesiology (ASA) preoperative assessment score of 3, 4, or 5; (2) the operative incision is classified as either contaminated or dirty-infected; and (3) the operation takes longer than expected by a certain factor than expected.[30] Although the NNIS risk index score is able to predict SSI risk much better than standard wound classification systems and appears to be applicable to many different types of surgical procedures, its usefulness is largely limited to assessment of adults and may not be an accurate predictor of risk in children.[40]

PREVENTION

Surgical delivery systems and personnel work under the assumption that nearly all SSI are preventable. Preventing SSI involves eliminating or minimizing known risk factors, including both host and environmental factors. Modern surgical practice includes standardized procedures specifically designed to prevent SSI (Table 69–4). As these procedures are based on a large amount of data accumulated over many years as well as many ongoing studies, one can expect changes as practices evolve in response to new information. Likewise, the practices described are based on studies that included predominantly adults and therefore require certain modifications when applied to children.

Environmental Interventions

Modern operating theater systems are designed to control environmental infectious risk factors and are aimed principally at the reduction of the number of microorganisms that come into contact with the surgical wound. First and foremost is the concept of aseptic technique. Most surgical instruments can be sterilized in an autoclave, which uses superheated steam under pressure to kill organisms and destroy spores. Optical equipment and electrical appliances are damaged by autoclaves and need to be sterilized ethylene oxide gas or peracetic acid. All drapery and consumable materials such as gauze sponges and suture material are also sterilized. Modern operation theaters have ventilation systems that create positive pressure within the room and fresh filtered air

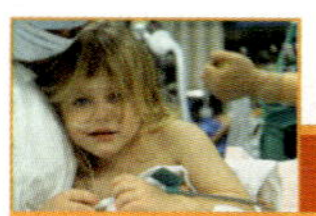

Table 69–4.

Surgical Practice Standards Designed to Prevent SSI

A. Environmental factors
  1. Aseptic technique
    a. Sterilization of instruments
    b. Proper air handling in the operating theater
    c. Concept of the "sterile field"
    d. Decontamination of surgical personnel
    e. Antiseptic skin preparation
  2. Proper surgical technique
    a. Avoiding contamination of the sterile field
    b. Careful handling of tissue
    c. Removing foreign material from the wound
    d. Maintaining blood perfusion and oxygenation
    e. Using closed-suction drainage techniques
    f. Wound closure techniques
  3. Wound care
    a. Sterile dressings
    b. Avoiding postoperative contamination
B. Host factors
  1. Systemic processes
    a. Blood glucose control
    b. Avoidance of nicotine
    c. Minimizing immunosuppressive drugs
    d. Maintaining adequate nutrition
    e. Control of other infections
    f. (Supplemental oxygen)
    g. (Elimination of colonizing pathogens)
  2. Perioperative adjuncts
    a. Prophylactic antibiotics
    b. Hair removal, no shaving
    c. Avoiding hypothermia
    d. (Supplemental oxygen)
    e. (Bowel preparation)
C. Institutional factors
  1. SSI surveillance
    a. Inpatient surveillance
    b. Postdischarge surveillance
  2. Outcomes monitoring
  3. Modification of practice standards

is brought in using laminar flow technology to prevent air turbulence. Surgical personnel are required to apply an antiseptic on their hands and forearms and to wear surgical caps, surgical scrub garments, sterile gowns, surgical masks, and sterile gloves. A methodical and almost ritualized behavior is displayed by all personnel to prevent contamination of the surgical field, which includes a complete covering of the patient and operating table with sterile drapes and towels and meticulous attention to potential contamination.

Local Skin Preparation

The skin of the patient is prepared with an antiseptic solution, typically applied in concentric circles starting at the incision site and working outward. Betadine (povidone–iodine) is the traditional and still the most widely used operative antiseptic. It has a broad spectrum of activity, including gram-positive and gram-negative bacteria, *Mycobacterium tuberculosis*, fungi, and viruses, is easy to apply, is relatively inexpensive, and well-tolerated by most individuals.[41] Isopropyl (or ethyl) alcohol (70% v/v in water) has a similar spectrum of activity, is easy to apply and dries completely; it is also inexpensive and generally well-tolerated. However the use of alcohol is limited, and in some cases prohibited, due to its flammability. Patient fires have been reported when the alcohol has not been allowed to dry completely before electrocautery is used during surgery. Recently there has been a trend toward the use of chlorhexidine gluconate as a substitute for betadine, especially for skin antisepsis prior to central venous access.[42] It is usually supplied in an isopropyl alcohol base and has a broad spectrum of activity and has the advantage of being effective after a single application. It is currently more expensive than betadine, may cause a skin rash in susceptible individuals, and must be allowed to dry completely before starting the operation because of the risk of fire from the alcohol component. In practice, there is no perceptible difference in the incidence of infection regardless of which of the commonly used antiseptics is used. Furthermore, a recent large meta-analysis of available studies failed to show a significant advantage of one antiseptic over another.[43]

Prior to application of antiseptics, the skin of the patient may need to be prepared in other ways. Excessive hair is usually removed prior to making an incision. It is best to clip the hair close to the skin rather than using a shaving razor, which has been shown to increase the risk of SSI,[44] and hair should be removed as close to the time of surgery to avoid the creation of folliculitis. Showering with an antiseptic soap the night before a scheduled operation was formerly a time-honored ritual but has been shown to have no effect on the incidence of SSI.[45] Similarly, mechanical bowel preparation with cathartics and oral antibiotics was the inviolable rule before elective colorectal surgery for decades but has been shown not only to be ineffective in preventing SSI but may actually increase the risk of anastomotic leak and organ-space infection.[46,47]

Antibiotic prophylaxis

One of the most important interventions in the prevention of SSI is the use of prophylactic antibiotics.[48–52] It might seem obvious that the administration of antibiotics to patients felt to be at high risk of SSI would prevent infection, and for the most part this is true. However, there are limitations to the effectiveness of prophylactic antibiotics and there are risks involved as well. Current recommendations are summarized in Table 69–5. Patients with infected wounds are treated with appropriate

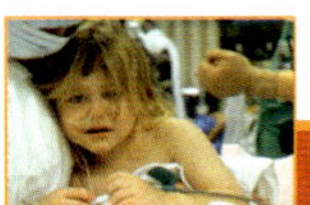

Table 69–5.

Antibiotic Prophylaxis Recommendations[9,51,52]

Wound Class	Likely Pathogens	Recommended Antibiotic Regimen
Clean	*S. aureus*, coagulase-negative staphylococci Less common: gram-negative rods noncardiac thoracic: also *Streptococcus pneumoniae*	■ None, *or* ■ Cefazolin or Cefuroxime, *plus* ■ Vancomycin or Clindamycin, if β-lactam allergic
Clean-contaminated	Gram-negative rodsLess common: *S. aureus*, coagulase-negative staphylococci	■ Cefazolin, Cefuroxime, Cefoxitin, or Cefotetan, *plus* ■ Vancomycin or Clindamycin, if β-lactam allergic
Contaminated	Gram-negative rods, enterococcus, anaerobes	■ Cefazolin plus Metronidazole, or Cefoxitin or Cefotetan OR ■ Clindamycin or Metronidazole plus Gentamicin or Ciprofloxacin

General principles:
1. Antibiotics should be administered within 60 minutes of incision.
2. Antibiotics should be redosed intraoperatively every 3–4 hours (every 2–3 hours for antibiotics with a short half-life, e.g., cefoxitin or every 6–8 hours for antibiotics with a long half-life, e.g., Vancomycin and Metronidazole).
3. Antibiotics chosen should cover most likely pathogens.
4. A single preoperative dose is usually sufficient, though antibiotics may be continued for up to 24 hours postoperatively under some circumstances.

antibiotics and are technically not given "prophylactic" antibiotics. For clean wounds, it is difficult to show a benefit from antimicrobial prophylaxis and the risks, including anaphylaxis and the generation of resistant organisms, may outweigh any small potential benefit. The exception is a clean operation that involves the placement of an implant, such as a heart valve or bone endoprosthesis, or in certain parts of the body, such as the heart, brain, or bone, in which case even a single infection can have deleterious consequences. Although generally not indicated or recommended in most cases, it is nevertheless common practice in some centers to use prophylactic antibiotics routinely in all clean cases because of a perceived decrease in the albeit small number of SSI that are seen in these patients.

The greatest benefit of antimicrobial prophylaxis is for clean-contaminated and contaminated wounds. The choice of antibiotic should reflect the most likely organisms to be encountered and therefore should cover aerobic gram-positive organisms. Coverage for gram-negative bacteria and/or anaerobes should be provided for operations involving exposure to the aerodigestive tract or bowel flora. For prophylaxis to be effective, there should be adequate tissue levels of the antibiotic at the time the incision is made. Antibiotics should therefore be given within 60 minutes prior to the start of the operation, rather than at the time of incision (too late) or "on call" to the operating room (too soon), as was customary in the past. Nearly every study has shown that a single preoperative dose of an appropriate antibiotic is effective in decreasing the incidence of SSI. There are very little data to support the use of antibiotics for the first 24 hours and no data to support their use for more than 1 day after an operation.[48,49]

Intraoperative Interventions

In addition to efforts designed to minimize contamination of the surgical wound, surgeons have long been taught that careful management of the wound during an operation can lower the risk of SSI. First and foremost is gentle handling of tissues. Infections are more likely to develop in wounds in which the skin edges are devascularized and in the presence of devitalized tissue. Wound edges are grasped carefully with noncrushing forceps or skin hooks and only when necessary. Prior to skin closure, the wound is irrigated with sterile normal saline to wash away necrotic debris. Efforts should be made to avoid maneuvers that may decrease the blood supply and delivery of oxygen to the operative field, including unnecessary or poorly designed tissue flaps and the application of dressings that create pressure on the wound or generate a tourniquet effect.

Wound Closure and Postoperative Care

Wound closure is also an important concept in the prevention of SSI. An incision that is infected or grossly contaminated may be treated with one of several techniques. Wounds may be closed with the placement of drains to prevent an infected fluid collection from forming. Closed-suction drains (e.g., Jackson–Pratt or Hemovac drains) decrease the risk of infections while passive drains (e.g., Penrose drains) that are brought out through the incision are not recommended as they have been shown to increase the risk of SSI.[9,53] Finally, in the case of dirty or frankly infected wounds, it is recommended that the wound not be closed at all, and instead is left open and lightly packed with moistened sterile gauze. Options then include (1) delayed primary closure, in which the surgical dressing is left undisturbed for 2–3 days after which the wound edges are brought together primarily in sterile fashion and (2) wound closure by secondary intention, in which the dressings are changed two to three times daily using sterile technique and the wound is allowed to granulate and heal over the course of 2 to several weeks. Some wounds of intermediate risk for SSI pose something of a dilemma regarding the decision to use closed or open wound management. For example, adults who undergo colostomy closure or appendectomy for perforated appendicitis have historically been treated with open wound management due to an expected 50% or greater risk of wound infection, while pediatric surgeons generally utilize primary closure for such wounds because the true incidence of SSI in these circumstances appears to be much lower.[54]

Although most SSI are thought to be caused by intraoperative wound contamination, some may be due to postoperative contamination or the use of surgical dressings that create a local environment conducive to the growth of microorganisms. Wounds that are near the anus or a colostomy should be protected from fecal effluent with barrier dressings or left open to heal by secondary intention. In rare cases, complex wound closures of the buttocks or perianal region are protected by temporary fecal diversion. For most other incisions, it was long felt that a surgical dressing should be placed sterilely in the operating room and then removed after a few days to allow the wound to "breathe." The patient was asked to keep it dry for at least a week. Over the past 10–15 years, these recommendations have all but vanished. Modern dressings are usually "occlusive," not permitting tissue fluid to escape and protecting the wound from exogenous pathogens, and are not removed for 7–14 days, with no increase in the incidence of wound infection. Most popular dressings are also transparent (Tegaderm, Dermabond) allowing clinicians to monitor the wound for signs of infection.

OTHER CONSIDERATIONS

In general, control of host factors that increase the risk of SSI is less of a concern for surgeons who deal primarily with children. Nevertheless, there are circumstances in which it becomes important. Children who are malnourished may benefit from a period of supplemental nutrition, preferably by the enteral route, as parenteral nutrition may increase the risk of infection. Infections present in other parts of the body should be treated aggressively, as there is a correlation between other infections and SSI.[34] Patients who take immunosuppressive medications are usually not able to discontinue them, but the dose of some, such as corticosteroids, can sometimes safely be lowered during the perioperative period. Children with diabetes should have their blood glucose levels monitored frequently and maintained within a narrow range, with insulin administration if necessary, both during the operation and for the first 2–3 days postoperatively. Although the administration of supplemental oxygen via nasal cannula has recently been shown to decrease the incidence of SSI in older patients who undergo colorectal surgery,[55] it will need to be investigated more thoroughly in children before its use can be recommended.

At the institutional level, the most effective means of lowering the incidence of SSI is to establish a system of prospective wound surveillance, with honest reporting of outcomes and modification of practices to reflect new data and changes in practice standards.[56] Aseptic technique should be monitored and violators (re)educated. Wounds are systematically classified according to their degree of contamination and prophylactic antibiotics should be administered according to current standards. Specific cases of SSI should be discussed at regular morbidity and mortality conferences and worrisome trends should be investigated thoroughly with the help of infection control personnel. Inpatients and outpatients with surgical incisions should be surveyed periodically for the presence of infection in the form of systematic audits. Staff should be frequently instructed as to current standards of practice and informed of the results of audits in the form of both positive and instructive feedback. There is a recent trend for the federal government and some private insurers to refuse payment for the treatment of "preventable" nosocomial infections including SSI,[57,58] increasing the visibility of the issue and the importance of careful monitoring and reporting practices.

CLINICAL PRESENTATION

The clinical picture of a surgical wound infection usually follows a more-or-less typical pattern, with predictable variation depending on the type of organism involved[59] (Table 69–6). Most bacterial wound infections become clinically apparent between the fourth and seventh postoperative day (by convention the date of the operation is day zero). Early symptoms include worsening pain and increased swelling. On examination, there is usually erythema, induration of surrounding tissues, and tenderness; the area may be palpably warm. The wound may also be fluctuant, suggesting the presence of liquid beneath the surface; however in children a subcutaneous abscess is most often tense and very tender. In rare cases, especially if there is a significant

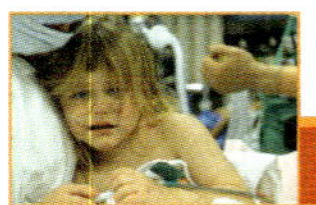

Table 69–6.

Typical Clinical Presentation of Superficial Incision Surgical Site Infections[59]

POD	Class of Organism	Local Findings	Systemic Signs
1–2	Polymicrobial Group A streptococcus *C. perfringens*	Dramatic: wound erysipelas, extreme tenderness, crepitus	Severe: fever, toxemia
3–6	Gram-positive cocci	Significant: erythema, induration, tenderness, copious pus	Minor: low-grade fever, irritability
7–14	Gram-negative rods	Subtle: mild cellulitis, thin foul-smelling drainage	Significant: fever, tachycardia
7–30	Fungus, atypical	Few local signs, scant drainage	Indolent: low-grade fever, malaise

deep component there may be spreading cellulitis or true lymphangitic streaking away from the wound.

The timing of the development of a wound infection can give clues as to the likely organism. Wound infections that develop within the first 24 to 48 hours of an operation are very rare and usually due to infection with *Streptococcus pyogenes* (group A Streptococcus). The presentation is often impressive, with sharply demarcated edema and lymphangitis (wound erysipelas) that spreads rapidly, exquisite tenderness and scant, watery drainage. Patients are typically febrile and toxic-appearing. Gram-positive infections are more likely to present within 3–6 days of an operation. They are heralded by sometimes dramatic local findings of a wound infection while systemic signs of illness are relatively minor. Gram-negative wound infections are usually more subtle in presentation, typically arising in the second postoperative week, and are more likely to cause generalized symptoms despite relatively minor signs of a local wound infection.

DIAGNOSIS AND MANAGEMENT

Most wound infections are easily diagnosed on the basis of history and physical examination. Ultrasound can be useful in some cases to identify a subcutaneous abscess if the physical findings are ambiguous or to exclude the diagnosis before opening a wound unnecessarily. The presence of a deep wound SSI or an organ/space infection is generally confirmed by computed tomography (CT) scan or magnetic resonance imaging (MRI), although ultrasound is sometimes useful, especially in infants and small children.

Unless the physical findings are quite minor, in which case there may be a decision to treat with antibiotics for a wound cellulitis or to simply observe, wounds that are suspected of being infected should be aspirated or opened at the bedside. If pus is encountered, specimens should be sent for Gram stain and culture with sensitivities, and the wound should be adequately drained. It is usually necessary to open the entire length of the wound and to break up loculations of pus. The wound is then allowed to heal by secondary intention. This usually entails packing the wound lightly with saline-moistened gauze, which is changed two to four times daily for 2 weeks or more. However, in some cases, it may be possible to achieve adequate drainage of the entire wound, with or without the use of a passive drain, and to minimize the extent of the wound that is opened.

Deep infections are treated with antibiotics alone if the collection is smaller than approximately 5 cm in diameter, or by image-guided percutaneous aspiration and drainage if the abscess is large and safely accessible. Organ or space infections may require operative intervention if the deep space abscess drains spontaneously through the incision (a "necessitating" infection).

Opening an infected wound can generally be performed at the bedside with minimal discomfort, but requires a great deal of patience, compassion, and skill. The skin edges of an infected wound that is less than 2 weeks old can usually be separated with minimal traction and the release of pus under pressure can provide significant symptomatic relief. Nevertheless, the procedure is rarely completely painless and there is always a great deal of anxiety on the part of the patient and their family members. One hopes that the image of the brusque and busy surgeon ripping open a wound quickly and without warning and then leaving a tearful patient and horrified onlookers in his or her wake is a thing of the past. Though the act of opening a wound takes seconds, in some cases, the entire procedure can take more than 20 minutes. Patients should be given an analgesic and, if necessary, an anxiolytic. It is not uncommon for children to have the procedure done with moderate sedation or even general anesthesia. All equipment, disposables, and culture supplies should be prepared in advance and close at hand. Local anesthetic is generally unnecessary and may not be effective in the presence of acute infection. A gentle separation of the incision can usually be made painlessly if made exactly in the previous incision, which as a rule is insensate. An attempt should be made to break up loculations gently with an examining finger, but vigorous probing with instruments, especially to "test the fascia," is painful, dangerous, and usually unnecessary. The wound should be packed gently with saline-moistened sterile gauze and covered with a clean, dry dressing.

Purulent drainage from a wound should be sent for Gram stain, culture, and sensitivities, even if the most likely organisms are known. Although drainage alone may be sufficient to treat some postoperative wound infections, antibiotics are usually considered an important component of therapy. Patients with systemic toxicity or significant cellulitis should be treated in hospital with broad-spectrum intravenous antibiotics until systemic signs of infection have resolved. Provided the family is reliable and close follow-up is arranged, outpatients with no signs of systemic illness, only minor cellulitis, and a wound that has been adequately drained can usually be treated safely with oral antibiotics and dressing changes at home. Broad-spectrum antibiotics are administered empirically and then the regimen is tailored to the organisms that grow in culture. Initial therapy should especially include coverage against gram-positive organisms, which are the most commonly seen. Coverage against gram-negative organisms and anaerobes should be included if the gastrointestinal tract was opened during the operation. A typical intravenous regimen would include a first-generation cephalosporin such as cefazolin, or for penicillin-allergic patients, clindamycin. Clindamycin is increasingly being used as first-line therapy due to the recent increase in the prevalence of community-acquired MRSA infections. For uncomplicated wound infections that occur after bowel surgery, options include cefazolin and metronidazole, ampicillin/sulbactam alone, or, in penicillin-allergic patients, clindamycin and gentamicin. Organ/space infections that develop after bowel surgery, such as intra-abdominal abscesses, are traditionally treated with "triple antibiotics" (ampicillin or vancomycin, gentamicin, and metronidazole or clindamycin) though many surgeons use ampicillin/sulbactam and gentamicin with excellent results. Some believe that monotherapy with a broad-spectrum antibiotic such as piperacillin/tazobactam is as effective as traditional triple-antibiotic therapy without the risks associated with aminoglycoside administration.[60] Therapy for infections that occur in other types of surgical incisions is based on the organisms most likely to be involved. For example, wounds of the head and neck are more likely to be caused by oral flora and therefore penicillin or clindamycin are ideal choices. Nevertheless, antibiotic choices should be based on culture results in addition to clinical judgment.

Necrotizing Infections

Although exceedingly rare, few surgical site infections are as serious or as terrifying as those that result in tissue necrosis. They can present in the form of necrotizing fasciitis or, less commonly, necrotizing cellulitis. Necrotizing SSI is usually a polymicrobial infection that includes aerobic and anaerobic bacteria and is more common in patients with diabetes and peripheral vascular disease.[61] Less commonly, a necrotizing soft tissue infection can result from infection with a single predominant organism such as group A Streptococcus, *Clostridium perfringens* or *Vibrio vulnificus.* The characteristic soft tissue necrosis is due to microvascular thrombosis that is induced by a procoagulant exotoxin secreted by the microorganisms involved.[62]

These infections are rapidly progressive and potentially lethal unless recognized early and treated aggressively. Necrotizing infections present acutely, often within the first 24–48 hours after surgery. Local signs include edema and erythema of the wound edges, which can spread very quickly, and a watery discharge ("dishwater" discharge) may be seen coming from the wound. The edema often striking and has a raised edge noting an abrupt change to more normal appearing skin ("wound erysipelas"). There is typically extreme pain and exquisite tenderness at and near the incision, although anesthesia of the surrounding skin may also occur. Crepitus may be noted due to gas generated within the tissues. Systemic signs of illness are nearly always apparent, including fever and malaise, and can rapidly progress to overt toxicity and shock. The diagnosis must therefore be confirmed very quickly (within 4–6 hours). In the proper clinical setting, the diagnosis may be made on the basis of physical findings only. In less obvious cases, it may be necessary to perform X-rays to identify gas in the soft tissues, MRI to identify necrotic tissue, or wound exploration with fascia inspection and/or biopsy.

Treatment includes intravenous antibiotics and immediate radical surgical excision of all necrotic tissue. Although monotherapy with broad-spectrum antibiotics like imipenem/cilastin or piperacillin/tazobactam may be effective, multidrug regimens are the mainstay of current therapy. This may include high-dose penicillin or clindamycin and either a fluoroquinolone (in older children and adults) or aminoglycoside (in younger children). Vancomycin may be added if MRSA is suspected and antifungal drugs may be added if a fungal infection is thought to be involved. Antibiotics should be started even before the diagnosis is confirmed with certainty.

Surgical debridement is performed in the operating room under general anesthesia. All necrotic tissue is excised sharply and wound, which may be gigantic, is left open. The wound is inspected several times a day and debrided again if there are signs of further necrosis. After successful therapy, wound management usually requires skin grafts or soft-tissue flaps for closure. Hyperbaric oxygen therapy is advocated by some as a therapeutic adjunct but it is not a substitute for aggressive surgical debridement.[63]

A particularly devastating form of postoperative necrotizing soft-tissue infection is necrotizing fasciitis that involves the perineum and pelvic fascia (Fournier's gangrene), which has been reported after inguinal hernia repair and circumcision.[64,65] Even in the case of successful management, wound management can be extremely challenging and usually results in significant disfigurement and functional impairment. As with all necrotizing infections, early recognition and immediate aggressive medical and surgical management is the key to patient survival.

PEARLS/SPECIAL SITUATIONS

- Surgical site infections are classified as superficial incisional infections, deep incisional infections, and organ/space infections.
- Postoperative occlusive dressings pose no risk for infection and may in fact decrease the risk of surgical site infection.
- Necrotizing surgical site infections present acutely, often within the first 24–48 hours after surgery. Characteristic features may include "dishwater" discharge, wound erysipelas, and crepitus.

REFERENCES

1. Ford-Jones EL, Mindorff CM, Langley JM, et al. Epidemiologic study of 4684 hospital-acquired infections in pediatric patients. *Pediatr Infect Dis J.* 1989;8(10):668-675.
2. Horwitz JR, Chwals WJ, Doski JJ, et al. Pediatric wound infections: a prospective multicenter study. *Ann Surg.* 1998;227(4):553-558.
3. Upperman JS, Sheridan RL, Marshall J. Pediatric surgical site and soft tissue infections. *Pediatr Crit Care Med.* 2005; 6(3 suppl):S36-S41.
4. Bhattacharyya N, Kosloske AM. Postoperative wound infection in pediatric surgical patients: a study of 676 infants and children. *J Pediatr Surg.* 1990;25(1):125-129.
5. Bhattacharyya N, Kosloske AM, Macarthur C. Nosocomial infection in pediatric surgical patients: a study of 608 infants and children. *J Pediatr Surg.* 1993;28(3):338-343; discussion 343-344.
6. Davenport M, Doig CM. Wound infection in pediatric surgery: a study in 1094 neonates. *J Pediatr Surg.* 1993; 28(1):26-30.
7. Sharma LK, Sharma PK. Postoperative wound infection in a pediatric surgical service. *J Pediatr Surg.* 1986;21(10):889-891.
8. Sparling KW, Ryckman FC, Schoettker PJ, et al. Financial impact of failing to prevent surgical site infections. *Qual Manag Health Care.* 2007;16(3):219-225.
9. Mangram AJ, Horan TC, Pearson ML, et al. Guideline for prevention of surgical site infection, 1999. Hospital Infection Control Practices Advisory Committee. *Infect Control Hosp Epidemiol.* 1999;20(4):250-278; quiz 279-280.
10. Horan TC, Gaynes RP. Surveillance of nosocomial infections. In: Mayhall CG, ed. *Hospital Epidemiology and Infection Control.* Philadelphia: Lippincott Williams & Wilkins; 2004:1659-1702.
11. Weiss CA, III, Statz CL, Dahms RA, et al. Six years of surgical wound infection surveillance at a tertiary care center: review of the microbiologic and epidemiological aspects of 20,007 wounds. *Arch Surg.* 1999;134(10): 1041-1048.
12. Brook I. Microbiology and management of post-surgical wounds infection in children. *Pediatr Rehabil.* 2002;5(3): 171-176.
13. Olesevich M, Kennedy A. Emergence of community-acquired methicillin-resistant *Staphylococcus aureus* soft tissue infections. *J Pediatr Surg.* 2007;42(5):765-768.
14. Simor AE, Ofner-Agostini M, Bryce E, et al. The evolution of methicillin-resistant *Staphylococcus aureus* in Canadian hospitals: 5 years of national surveillance. *Can Med Assoc J.* 2001; 165(1):21-26.
15. Jarvis WR, Martone WJ. Predominant pathogens in hospital infections. *J Antimicrob Chemother.* 1992;29 (suppl A):19-24.
16. Lutz BD, Jin J, Rinaldi MG, et al. Outbreak of invasive Aspergillus infection in surgical patients, associated with a contaminated air-handling system. *Clin Infect Dis.* 2003;37(6):786-793.
17. Mermel LA, McKay M, Dempsey J, Parenteau S. Pseudomonas surgical-site infections linked to a healthcare worker with onychomycosis. *Infect Control Hosp Epidemiol.* 2003;24(10):749-752.
18. Hansis M. Pathophysiology of infection—a theoretical approach. Injury 1996;27 (suppl 3):SC5-SC8.
19. Bowler PG. Wound pathophysiology, infection and therapeutic options. *Ann Med.* 2002;34(6):419-427.
20. Barie PS, Eachempati SR. Surgical site infections. *Surg Clin North Am.* 2005;85(6):1115-1135, viii-ix.
21. Leaper DJ. Risk factors for surgical infection. *J Hosp Infect.* 1995;30 (suppl):127-139.
22. Gotz F. Staphylococcus and biofilms. *Mol Microbiol.* 2002;43(6):1367-1378.
23. Rotstein OD. Interactions between leukocytes and anaerobic bacteria in polymicrobial surgical infections. *Clin Infect Dis.* 1993;16 (suppl 4):S190-S194.
24. Gastmeier P, Brandt C, Sohr D, Ruden H. [Responsibility of surgeons for surgical site infections. *Chirurg.* 2006;77(6): 506-511.
25. Pearson RD, Valenti WM, Steigbigel RT. Clostridium perfringens wound infection associated with elastic bandages. *Jama.* 1980;244(10):1128-1130.
26. Lowry PW, Blankenship RJ, Gridley W, et al. A cluster of legionella sternal-wound infections due to postoperative topical exposure to contaminated tap water. *N Engl J Med.* 1991;324(2):109-113.

27. Casanova JF, Herruzo R, Diez J. Risk factors for surgical site infection in children. *Infect Control Hosp Epidemiol.* 2006;27(7):709-715.
28. Hutchinson JJ, McGuckin M. Occlusive dressings: a microbiologic and clinical review. *Am J Infect Control.* 1990;18(4):257-268.
29. Gaynes RP, Culver DH, Horan TC, et al. Surgical site infection (SSI) rates in the United States, 1992-1998: the National Nosocomial Infections Surveillance System basic SSI risk index. *Clin Infect Dis.* 2001;33 (suppl 2): S69-S77.
30. Culver DH, Horan TC, Gaynes RP, et al. Surgical wound infection rates by wound class, operative procedure, and patient risk index. National Nosocomial Infections Surveillance System. *Am J Med.* 1991;91(3B):152S-157S.
31. Dronge AS, Perkal MF, Kancir S, et al. Long-term glycemic control and postoperative infectious complications. *Arch Surg.* 2006;141(4):375-380; discussion 380.
32. Latham R, Lancaster AD, Covington JF, et al. The association of diabetes and glucose control with surgical-site infections among cardiothoracic surgery patients. *Infect Control Hosp Epidemiol.* 2001;22(10):607-612.
33. Guvener M, Pasaoglu I, Demircin M, Oc M. Perioperative hyperglycemia is a strong correlate of postoperative infection in type II diabetic patients after coronary artery bypass grafting. *Endocr J.* 2002;49(5):531-537.
34. Cheadle WG. Risk factors for surgical site infection. *Surg Infect* (Larchmt). 2006;7 (suppl 1):S7-S11.
35. Theadom A, Cropley M. Effects of preoperative smoking cessation on the incidence and risk of intraoperative and postoperative complications in adult smokers: a systematic review. *Tob Control.* 2006;15(5):352-358.
36. Mazaki T, Ebisawa K. Enteral versus parenteral nutrition after gastrointestinal surgery: a systematic review and meta-analysis of randomized controlled trials in the English literature. *J Gastrointest Surg.* 2008;12(4):739-755.
37. Lauwers S, de Smet F. Surgical site infections. *Acta Clin Belg.* 1998;53(5):303-310.
38. Perl TM. Prevention of Staphylococcus aureus infections among surgical patients: beyond traditional perioperative prophylaxis. *Surgery.* 2003;134(5 suppl):S10-S17.
39. Muilwijk J, van den Hof S, Wille JC. Associations between surgical site infection risk and hospital operation volume and surgeon operation volume among hospitals in the Dutch nosocomial infection surveillance network. *Infect Control Hosp Epidemiol.* 2007;28(5): 557-563.
40. Kagen J, Bilker WB, Lautenbach E, et al. Risk adjustment for surgical site infection after median sternotomy in children. *Infect Control Hosp Epidemiol.* 2007;28(4): 398-405.
41. Fleischer W, Reimer K. Povidone-iodine in antisepsis-state of the art. *Dermatology.* 1997;195 (suppl 2):3-9.
42. Chaiyakunapruk N, Veenstra DL, Lipsky BA, Saint S. Chlorhexidine compared with povidone–iodine solution for vascular catheter-site care: a meta-analysis. *Ann Intern Med.* 2002;136(11):792-801.
43. Edwards PS, Lipp A, Holmes A. Preoperative skin antiseptics for preventing surgical wound infections after clean surgery. *Cochrane Database Syst Rev.* 2004(3): CD003949.
44. Tanner J, Moncaster K, Woodings D. Preoperative hair removal: a systematic review. *J Perioper Pract.* 2007;17(3): 118-121, 124-132.
45. Webster J, Osborne S. Meta-analysis of preoperative antiseptic bathing in the prevention of surgical site infection. *Br J Surg.* 2006;93(11):1335-1341.
46. Wille-Jorgensen P, Guenaga KF, Matos D, Castro AA. Preoperative mechanical bowel cleansing or not? An updated meta-analysis. *Colorectal Dis.* 2005;7(4):304-310.
47. Guenaga KF, Matos D, Castro AA, et al. Mechanical bowel preparation for elective colorectal surgery. *Cochrane Database Syst Rev.* 2005(1):CD001544.
48. Ichikawa S, Ishihara M, Okazaki T, et al. Prospective study of antibiotic protocols for managing surgical site infections in children. *J Pediatr Surg.* 2007;42(6):1002-1007; discussion 1007.
49. Andersen BR, Kallehave FL, Andersen HK. Antibiotics versus placebo for prevention of postoperative infection after appendicectomy. *Cochrane Database Syst Rev.* 2005(3):CD001439.
50. Ein SH, Sandler A. Wound infection prophylaxis in pediatric acute appendicitis: a 26-year prospective study. *J Pediatr Surg.* 2006;41(3):538-541.
51. Hedrick TL, Smith PW, Gazoni LM, Sawyer RG. The appropriate use of antibiotics in surgery: a review of surgical infections. *Curr Probl Surg.* 2007;44(10):635-675.
52. Bratzler DW, Houck PM. Antimicrobial prophylaxis for surgery: an advisory statement from the National Surgical Infection Prevention Project. *Am J Surg.* 2005;189(4):395-404.
53. Raves JJ, Slifkin M, Diamond DL. A bacteriologic study comparing closed suction and simple conduit drainage. *Am J Surg.* 1984;148(5):618-620.
54. Henry MC, Moss RL. Primary versus delayed wound closure in complicated appendicitis: an international systematic review and meta-analysis. *Pediatr Surg Int.* 2005; 21(8):625-630.
55. Chura JC, Boyd A, Argenta PA. Surgical site infections and supplemental perioperative oxygen in colorectal surgery patients: a systematic review. *Surg Infect* (Larchmt). 2007; 8(4):455-461.
56. Jarvis WR. Benchmarking for prevention: the Centers for Disease Control and Prevention's National Nosocomial Infections Surveillance (NNIS) system experience. *Infection.* 2003;31 (suppl 2):44-48.
57. Hedrick TL, Anastacio MM, Sawyer RG. Prevention of surgical site infections. *Expert Rev Anti Infect Ther.* 2006; 4(2):223-233.
58. Sipkoff M. Hospitals asked to account for errors on their watch. CMS and states may stop paying for specific hospital-acquired conditions. Will health plans follow suit? *Manag Care.* 2007;16(7):30, 35-37.
59. Mollitt DL. Surgical infections. In: Ziegler MM, Azizkhan RG, Weber TR, eds. *Operative Pediatric Surgery.* New York: McGraw-Hill Professional; 2003:161-177.
60. Results of the North American trial of piperacillin/tazobactam compared with clindamycin and gentamicin in the treatment of severe intra-abdominal infections. Investigators of the Piperacillin/Tazobactam Intra-abdominal Infection Study Group. *Eur J Surg.* (suppl.) 1994(573):61-66.

61. Cainzos M, Gonzalez-Rodriguez FJ. Necrotizing soft tissue infections. *Curr Opin Crit Care.* 2007;13(4):433-439.
62. Flores-Diaz M, Alape-Giron A. Role of Clostridium perfringens phospholipase C in the pathogenesis of gas gangrene. *Toxicon.* 2003;42(8):979-986.
63. Jallali N, Withey S, Butler PE. Hyperbaric oxygen as adjuvant therapy in the management of necrotizing fasciitis. *Am J Surg.* 2005;189(4):462-466.
64. Ameh EA, Dauda MM, Sabiu L, et al. Fournier's gangrene in neonates and infants. *Eur J Pediatr Surg.* 2004;14(6): 418-421.
65. Eke N. Fournier's gangrene: A review of 1726 cases. *Br J Surg.* 2000;87(6):718-728.

CHAPTER 70

Cerebrospinal Fluid Shunt Infections

Jessica K. Hart and Samir S. Shah

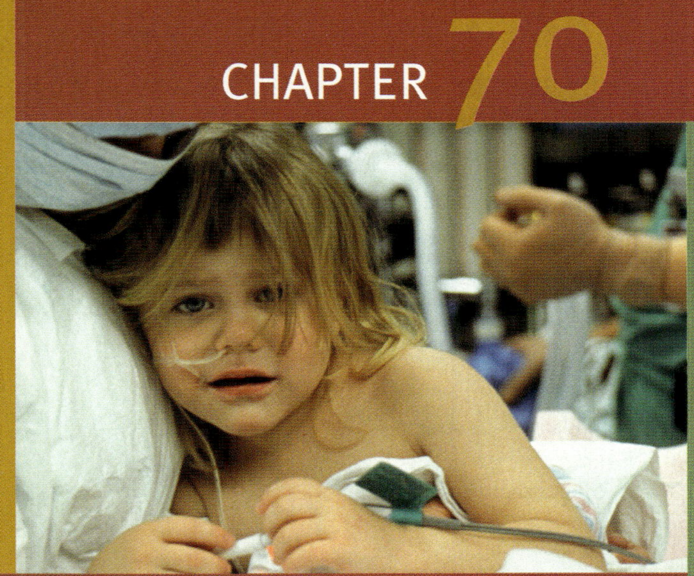

DEFINITIONS AND EPIDEMIOLOGY

Cerebrospinal fluid (CSF), or ventricular, shunts are the predominant mode of therapy for children with hydrocephalus. Common causes of hydrocephalus in children include myelomeningocele, meningocele, obstructive or communicating hydrocephalus, intraventricular hemorrhage, congenital cyst, and central nervous system tumors.[1] The majority of shunts are inserted in the perinatal period. The shunts divert CSF away from the ventricles, preventing increases in intracranial pressure that lead to neurologic sequelae. The typical CSF shunt has a proximal portion that enters the CSF space, an intermediate reservoir that lies outside the skull but underneath the skin, and a distal portion that terminates in either the peritoneal (ventriculoperioteal [VP] shunt), vascular (ventriculoatrial shunt; VA shunt), or pleural space (Figure 70–1).

Infection develops in 5–15% of all CSF shunts;[2,3] most infections occur within 6 months of shunt placement.[3,4] Factors associated with CSF shunt infections include premature birth, young age, neuroendoscope use during shunt insertion, prior shunt infection, and hospital stay more than 3 days at the time of shunt insertion.[1,5–7] Insertion of a VP shunt in a premature neonate (age <3 months) has been associated with a nearly five-fold increase in the risk of shunt infection. Patients younger than 1 year at the time of shunt placement also have a substantially higher risk of shunt infection than those older than 1 year at the time of shunt placement.[8,9] Insertion of a shunt after a previous shunt infection is associated with a four-fold increase in the risk of shunt infection.

The etiologic agents associated with CSF shunt infections are shown in Table 70–1.[10] Staphylococcal species, especially coagulase-negative *Staphylococcus* and *Staphylococcus aureus,* account for almost two-thirds of all shunt infections.[7,11] The remaining infections are produced by a wide variety of organisms, including gram-negative bacilli. Among 92 patients with VP shunts, prior *S. aureus* shunt infection (OR, 5.9; 95% CI: 1.4–25.9) independently increased the odds that *S. aureus* was the causal pathogen.[5] Gram-negative organisms (e.g., *Escherichia coli, Klebsiella pneumoniae, Pseudomonas aeruginosa*) tend to have a delayed onset, suggesting inoculation after surgery.[1,10] *Propionibacterium acnes* has been isolated more often in recent series of VP shunt infections; this bacterium generally causes low-grade, indolent

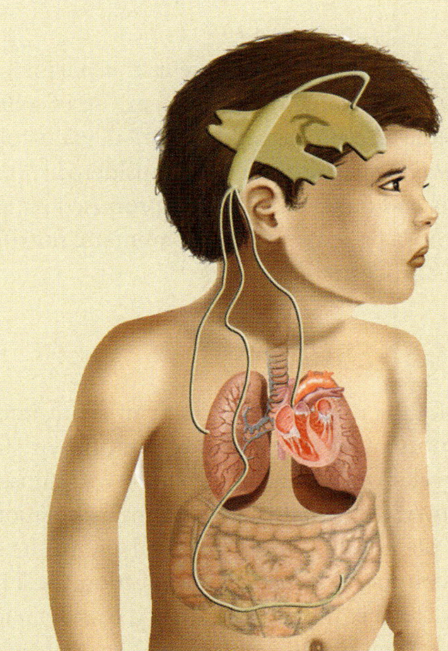

FIGURE 70–1 ■ Types of CSF shunts.

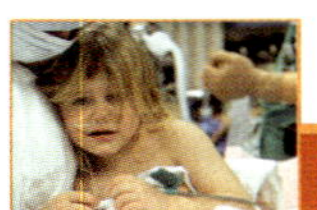

Table 70–1.

Etiology of CSF Shunt Infections

Common	
Coagulase-negative staphylococci	
S. aureus	
Enteric Gram-negative bacilli*	
Less common	
P. acnes	
Viridans group streptococci	
Rare	
Other streptococci†	
Enterococcus spp.	
Candida spp.	
Corynebacterium spp.	

*Usually *E. coli, Klebsiella* spp., *P. aeruginosa*, and *Proteus* species.
†Usually group B *Streptococcus, Streptococcus pyogenes*, or *Streptococcus pneumoniae*.

infections.[12] The apparent increase in *P. acnes* infection is probably a result of the more frequent use of anaerobic culture media and prolonged (up to 7 days) incubation times. *Candida* species should be considered in premature infants and other immunocompromised patients as well as in those patients receiving parenteral nutrition or prolonged corticosteroid therapy.[13]

PATHOGENESIS

There are four common mechanisms of shunt infection: (1) local inoculation of bacteria at the time of surgery, (2) skin breakdown overlying the shunt with subsequent bacterial entry, (3) hematogenous shunt inoculation, and (4) retrograde infection from the distal end of the shunt. The most common mechanism of infection, local inoculation of bacteria at the time of surgery, usually manifests within several weeks of the operation. Bacterial entry following breakdown of skin overlying the shunt may occur if the incision fails to properly heal or if the patient disrupts the healing process by scratching the open wound; gram-positive bacteria are more likely in this scenario. Children, who are relatively immobile, such as those with severe neurologic disability, may develop an overlying decubitus ulcer, which permits bacteria direct access to the shunt. Rarely, accessing the shunt by needle puncture introduces colonizing skin bacteria into the shunt system. Children with shunts in their vascular system (e.g., ventriculoatrial shunts) are continually at risk of infection from bacteremia with retrograde spread to the ventricles. Finally, retrograde infection from the distal end of the shunt as a consequence of viscus (e.g., bowel, gallbladder) perforation may lead to distal catheter contamination; gram-negative bacteria are most commonly isolated in the context of bowel perforation.

CLINICAL PRESENTATION

History and Physical

The patient with a ventricular shunt requires a review of the symptoms and signs associated with increased intracranial pressure and central nervous system infection. Historical information obtained from the patients or their caregivers should include indications for shunt placement, postoperative course, and history of shunt infection or malfunction (Table 70–2).

In infants, the physical examination should include a measurement of head circumference and assessment of size and softness of the anterior fontanelle. The skull and scalp should be palpated and inspected for signs of fluid accumulation or soft tissue infection such as erythema and tenderness to palpation. Characteristics of the burr hole(s) should be noted and all incision sites on the skull, neck, chest, and abdomen should be inspected. Attention should be directed toward swelling and fluctuance, which may represent CSF or a purulent fluid collection.

The extracranial portions of the shunt system should be examined to assess for shunt patency (see Box 70–1). Digital compression of the valve is an integral part of shunt examination. Shunt pumping is easy to

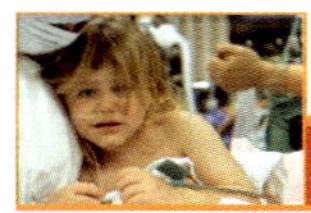

Table 70–2.

Pertinent History and Physical Examination

Important medical history	
Indications for insertion	
Dates of insertion and revision	
Type of valve and reservoir	
Medications and allergies	
History of prior shunt infections: organisms and therapy	
History of shunt malfunction: cause and correction	
Important elements of the physical examination	
Head, Eye, Ear, Nose, Throat	Head Circumference
	Characteristics of fontanelles and position of sutures in infants
	Burr holes: size, number, location, and features (soft, tense, tender)
	Scalp infections
Neurologic	Papilledema, optic atrophy
	Extraocular motor function
	Mental status: alertness, orientation
Neck	Tenderness
	Meningismus
Abdomen	Tenderness
	Ascites
	Masses
	Surgical incision site
Catheter	Position of reservoir, valve, catheter tip
	Palpate catheter connections

Box 70-1 Shunt Assessment

There are many types of devices and shunt systems available. The essential elements of any shunt system include the proximal and distal catheters, a valve, and a reservoir. The valve allows unidirectional flow, incorporates a pumping chamber, and regulates the pressure at which flow will occur by responding to the pressure difference across it. The reservoir is usually located between the two valves. The proximal valve allows flow from the ventricles to the reservoir, while the distal valve allows flow from the reservoir to the distal portion of the catheter.

Step 1 - Compress the proximal bubble: This ensures filling of the distal bubble for the next step, and empties the chamber to test proximal blockage later.

Step 2 - Assess the distal catheter: While still compressing proximally, place a finger over the distal bubble and compress it. This will assess CSF flow through the distal catheter. Normally, there is no resistance to emptying of the fluid through the valve into the abdominal cavity. Undue pressure suggests a distal tube blockage, disconnection, or insufficient tube length resulting from growth of the child.

Step 3 - Assess the proximal catheter: Release the proximal bubble. Now the negative pressure in this bubble should suck fluid into it from the ventricular cavity, usually within 1 second. Any longer delay in filling often suggests a proximal blockage; however, if the shunt has been pumped several times in the previous hours, it may fill slowly because the proximal tip is sitting against the choriod plexus. Since there is no proximal valve, when the distal bubble is compressed, the proximal bubble can be repeatedly depressed to measure resistance to filling of the proximal shunt without draining excessive fluid from above.[41]

perform, does not require special equipment, and can support the diagnosis of overt shunt malfunction. See Box 70–1 for a step-by-step approach to shunt assessment.

A complete neurological examination should also be performed, including cranial nerve assessment and fundoscopy to detect papilledema and optic atrophy (which suggest elevated intracranial pressure). The neck should be palpated to detect cervical and posterior auricular adenopathy which may occur with infections of the shunt insertion site.

Signs and Symptoms of Proximal Shunt Infection

The clinical features of CSF shunt infection depend on the mechanism of infection, the causative pathogen, and the type of shunt. The most common clinical symptoms are fever, headache, nausea, and lethargy (Table 70–3).[2,7] Shunt infection is the cause for shunt malfunction in 3–8% of cases.[14] Table 70–4 presents common signs and symptoms associated with CSF shunt malfunction.[14]

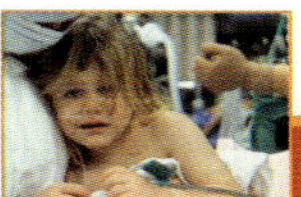

Table 70–3.

Clinical Features Associated with CSF Shunt Infection

Clinical Features
Systemic signs of infection
Fever
Headache
Malaise
Nausea
Vomiting
Irritability
Lethargy or altered mental status
Seizures
Meningismus
Paresis
Focal signs of infection
Pain at distal site (i.e., peritoneum) or wound
Purulent drainage from wound site
Inflammation (erythema, warmth, swelling) along subcutaneous course of the shunt
Signs of shunt malfunction*

**See Table 70– 4.*

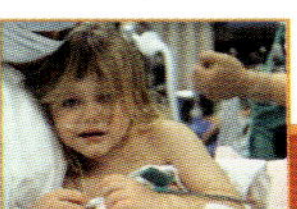

Table 70–4.

Signs and Symptoms Associated with CSF Shunt Malfunction

Underdrainage of CSF (Hydrocephalus)	
Infants	Macrocephaly
	Diastatis of sutures
	Bulging fontanelles
	Seizures
	Respiratory distress
Children	Constant headache
	Irritability
	Poor feeding
	Regression of developmental milestones
All ages	Headache
	Shunt site swelling
	Lethargy
	Vomiting
	Ataxia
	Fever
	Papilledema
	Optic atrophy
	Diplopia
	Abdominal pain or mass
	Bradycardia
Overdrainage of CSF	
Infants	Skull deformities: Rapid decline in head circumference, deep sunken fontanelles, overriding parietal bones
Children	Intracranial hypotension:
	Hypotension
	Headaches that resolve with recumbency
All ages	Slit-ventricle syndrome: Lethargy, postural headaches, nausea, vomiting, altered mental status

Signs of meningitis such as meningismus and photophobia are less common because infected CSF from the ventricles does not easily communicate with CSF in the subarachnoid space. Children with infections caused by indolent organisms such as *P. acnes* may have an insidious course with few overt symptoms. Additionally, children with gram-negative organisms have been described as "well appearing" although half have mild alterations of mental status.[15]

Infections of the external surface are less frequent and usually present with signs of local soft tissue inflammation such as focal swelling, pain, erythema, and purulent drainage from the incision site. Surface shunt infection is usually a complication of surgery because of the direct inoculation of the insertion site at the time of placement.

Signs and Symptoms of Distal Shunt Infection

Signs and symptoms of *distal* shunt infection depend on the location of the shunt tip and whether the internal lumen or the external surface is infected. Intraluminal infection of a ventriculoatrial shunt can result in bacteremia and systemic signs of toxicity, including fever, chills, and tachycardia. Rarely, compression of the reservoir or catheter track of an infected VA shunt can lead to intermittent bacteremia accompanied by fever and chills; this phenomenon has been referred to as the "shampoo clue" by some authors since some cases of VA shunt infection were suspected after inadvertent manipulation of the catheter track during hair washing caused fever and rigors.[16] Severe sepsis or septic shock is uncommon. Intraluminal infection of a ventriculoperitoneal shunt usually produces signs of focal infection.

Other complications of CSF shunts are summarized in Table 70–5.[17–19] Abdominal peritoneal pseudocysts develop as a consequence of clinical or subclinical infections that cause an inflammatory reaction around the catheter tip (Figure 70–2). The pseudocysts may grow quite large since the CSF encased within the pseudocyst cannot be resorbed by the peritoneal cavity. Pseudocysts complicate VP shunt placement in 0.7–4.5% of cases; usually as a late complication, occurring >12 months after initial shunt placement.[17,20,21] Small pseudocysts are more likely than large cysts to be associated with infection, presumably because pseudocysts associated with infection cause symptoms earlier than noninfected pseudocysts. Among patients with abdominal pseudocysts, the abdominal symptoms (Table 70–5) precede central nervous system complaints such as lethargy, headache, and visual disturbances by several days or weeks.

If shunt infection goes untreated for extended periods, immunologic sequelae, such as shunt nephritis can occur. Nephritis in the context of VA shunt infection is caused by deposition of antibody–antigen complexes in the renal glomeruli. "Shunt nephritis," which can be difficult to distinguish from bacterial endocarditis, occurs in 5–15% of VA shunt infections.

DIFFERENTIAL DIAGNOSIS

Shunt infection may occur with or without shunt malfunction. The differential diagnosis should focus on distinguishing shunt-related complications from other causes of headache or altered mental status. In addition to shunt-related infection, other acute infectious causes of headache include meningoencephalitis, brain abscess, sinusitis, orbital disease, and cranial neuralgias (e.g., herpes zoster). Other causes include stroke, subarachnoid hemorrhage, hypoglycemia, hypertension, collagen vascular disease, and migraine headaches.

DIAGNOSIS

Diagnosis of a CSF shunt infection requires either isolation of a pathogen from ventricular fluid, lumbar CSF,

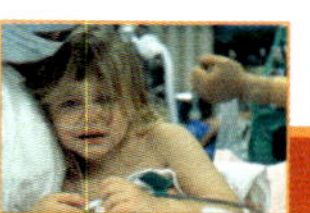

Table 70–5.

Potential Complications of CSF Shunts

Complication	Most Common Signs and Symptoms
Perforated viscus by direct catheter erosion	Abdominal tenderness, rebound tenderness, guarding
Bowel obstruction, ileus, or volvulus	Abdominal pain, fullness, distention; vomiting; failure to pass gas or stool
Ascites (usually in the context of a concurrent illness such as cirrhosis or congestive heart failure)	Abdominal discomfort, fluid wave, dullness to percussion
Abdominal pseudocyst	Abdominal discomfort and distention, nausea, vomiting, presence of an abdominal mass
Pneumocephalus	Headache, altered mental state
Nephritis	Hematuria, proteinuria, edema, hypertension, renal insufficiency or failure

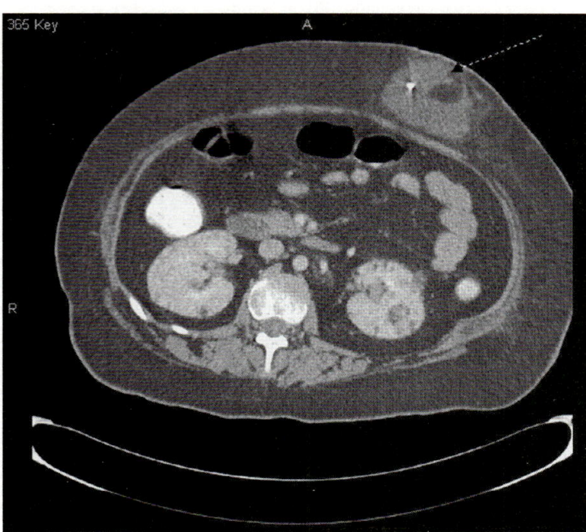

FIGURE 70–2 ■ CT of the abdomen reveals that the distal portion of the ventriculo-peritoneal catheter (the bright white area) is lodged in the subcutaneous tissues resulting in a collection of CSF in the subcutaneous tissues (arrow).

or blood (for VA shunts) or the presence of CSF pleocytosis (usually defined as >50 white blood cells/mm^3 in the context of a CSF shunt) in combination with either shunt malfunction or one or more of the signs or symptoms listed in Table 70–3.

CSF Studies

The CSF should be sent for cell count, glucose, protein, Gram stain, and aerobic and anaerobic bacterial culture (Table 70–6).[22,23] A CSF fungal culture should also be performed in premature infants and in children with other immunocompromising conditions.[13] A mild CSF pleocytosis, low CSF glucose level (hypoglycoracchia), and elevated CSF protein are usually present in cases of ventricular infection. CSF white blood cell counts typically range from 100 to 2500/mm^3 in VP shunt infections although normal CSF parameters (including CSF white blood cell count) have been reported in 17–35% of children with VP shunt infections.[4,10,22] CSF pleocytosis alone is not diagnostic of infection. Mild to moderate pleocytosis (20–500 white blood cells/mm^3) also occurs as a consequence of postsurgical or foreign body (i.e., shunt)-associated inflammation. Furthermore, infections caused by indolent organisms such as *P. acnes* may fail to induce a vigorous inflammatory response.

The types of white blood cells present in the CSF also facilitate the diagnosis of infection. McClinton et al.[24] found that the presence of >10% CSF neutrophils had a specificity of 99% for shunt infection (i.e., almost all patients without shunt infection had very few CSF neutrophils). Furthermore, the positive predictive value of >10% CSF neutrophils was 93% (i.e., almost all patients

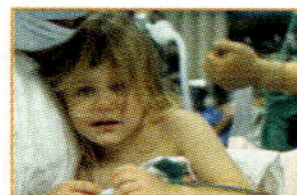

Table 70–6.

Diagnostic Tests for Patients with A CSF Shunt and Suspected Infection

Step 1: Detect shunt malfunction

1. Assess shunt patency (Box 70-1)
2. Shunt series (radiographs of skull, neck, chest, and abdomen)
3. CT or magnetic resonance imaging to diagnose ventriculitis, intracranial abscess, and empyema and identify changes that suggest elevated intracranial pressure

Step 2: Detect infection

1. Blood cultures (especially if ventriculoatrial shunt)
2. Shunt "tap"
   - Gram stain
   - Aerobic and anaerobic culture
   - Cell count and differential
   - Glucose, protein
3. Urinalysis, serum C3 and C4 complement in patients with a ventriculoatrial shunt to diagnose shunt nephritis

with >10% CSF neutrophils had a shunt infection).[24] CSF eosinophilia (>5% of total CSF white blood cell count) has also been associated with both shunt infection and malfunction but may also occur in response to intrathecal antibiotics or as a reaction to the shunt catheter.[24]

Ideally, fluid from the *reservoir* should be obtained by percutaneous aspiration under sterile conditions. Shunt drainage should be performed by a neurosurgeon or a clinician with experience in performing this procedure. The potential complications of draining CSF directly from the shunt include bleeding at the puncture site, CSF leakage, mechanical damage to the valve, and introduction of infection. In addition, draining CSF too rapidly may cause intraventricular or subdural bleeding. Bacteria are identified by Gram stain of CSF obtained from the reservoir in up to 80% of cases although the likelihood of a positive Gram stain depends on the causative organism. *S. aureus* and aerobic gram-negative rods such as *E. coli* typically have positive Gram stain results while *P. acnes*, coagulase-negative staphylcoccci, and viridans group streptococci are positive in <40% of cases.[10] Therefore, a negative Gram stain does not exclude the diagnosis of shunt infection. Although most bacteria causing shunt infections grow within 48–72 hours, cultures should be held for 5–7 days since fastidious organisms such as *P. acnes* may take longer to grow. Contamination and true infection cannot be readily differentiated when bacteria are identified by culture in the context of normal CSF parameters. In such cases, infection should be strongly considered and shunt aspiration should be repeated; a positive culture with the same bacteria usually indicates true infection.

Isolation of bacteria from CSF obtained by *lumbar puncture* suggests CSF shunt infection in the appropriate context. However, children requiring a CSF shunt often have impaired CSF flow. As a consequence, the ventricular fluid may have little or no communication with the lumbar spinal fluid and CSF obtained by lumbar puncture may not suggest infection despite the presence of ventriculitis.

Other Laboratory Studies

Blood should be routinely obtained for culture from patients evaluated for suspected shunt infection. While a negative peripheral blood culture does not rule out a shunt infection, a positive blood culture often influences the choice of antimicrobial therapy. Among patients with confirmed VP shunt infection, blood cultures are positive in 20–30% of cases.[4,10] Peripheral cultures are more likely to be positive in patients with VA shunt infection where blood cultures are positive in 90% of cases.[1,7] Laboratory manifestations of shunt nephritis include anemia, azotemia, hypocomplementemia, as well as hematuria and proteinuria.

Neuroimaging

Neuroimaging studies including X-rays of the skull, neck, chest, and abdomen (the "shunt series") and computed tomography (CT) should be performed as part of the routine evaluation of a child with a suspected CSF shunt infection. Neuroimaging studies may provide evidence of shunt malfunction that accompanies some cases of infection. Specific abnormalities that can be visualized on the shunt series include disconnection of the distal catheter, retraction of the distal catheter tip, and discontinuity near the proximal shunt bulb. Routine performance of shunt series has a low overall yield but on rare occasions detects abnormalities that are missed by CT.[25] Both CT and MRI of the head will detect increased ventricular size; this finding may reflect either increased intracranial pressure or hydrocephalous *ex vacuo*, a condition where the increased ventricle size reflects shrinkage of brain parenchyma rather than an increase in the intracranial pressure. Ventriculitis and meningitis can be visualized on CT and MRI as enhancement of the ventricular ependymal lining or cerebral cortical sulci.[26] In rare cases, subdural empyema or brain abscess may be the first indication of shunt infection. Radiologic imaging of other areas should be considered depending on the location of the distal catheter tip. CT or ultrasound of the abdomen may identify abdominal peritoneal pseudocysts at the distal portion of a VP shunt (Figure 70–2). Some free fluid in the peritoneal cavities is normal but larger amounts should raise concern for infection. Chest radiography detects pleural effusions associated with ventriculopleural shunt infection.

MANAGEMENT

The child with a ventricular shunt infection should be managed in consultation with neurosurgical and Infectious Diseases specialists. Success rates with various treatment strategies are as follows:

- Intravenous antibiotics without shunt removal, <25%;
- Intravenous and intraventricular antibiotics without shunt removal, 40%;
- Intravenous antibiotics with shunt removal and immediate replacement, 75%; and
- Intravenous antibiotics with shunt removal and delayed replacement, >90%.[11,27]

Therefore, optimal management of a CSF shunt infection includes intravenous antibiotics and removal of all components of the infected shunt with placement of a temporary external ventricular drain until the CSF is sterile.[4,8,11,27,28] The external ventricular drain facilitates resolution of the ventriculitis and permits continued monitoring of CSF parameters. Infection complicates fewer than 5% of closed external drainage systems; routine changing of the drainage catheter does not appear to reduce the infection rate.

In cases of distal shunt infection, some neurosurgeons prefer to externalize only the distal portion of the shunt. This strategy still maintains CSF flow and still offers the ability to perform frequent ventricular fluid sampling without subjecting the patient to a more extensive surgical procedure. However, early infection of the proximal portion of the shunt may be obscured by antibiotic treatment and become active after discontinuation of therapy and reinsertion of the distal portion of the shunt.

TREATMENT

Until an organism is isolated, patients should be treated with empiric antibiotic therapy that covers the range of potentially causative pathogens.[28] Reasonable options include vancomycin in combination with ceftazidime, cefepime, or meropenem. Linezolid was successfully used to treat a woman with *Staphylococcus epidermidis* VP shunt infection and a history of Stevens-Johnson syndrome attributed to prior vancomycin therapy.[29] Quinupristin–dalfopristin has also been reported to successfully cure patients with CSF shunt infections caused by coagulase-negative staphylococci.

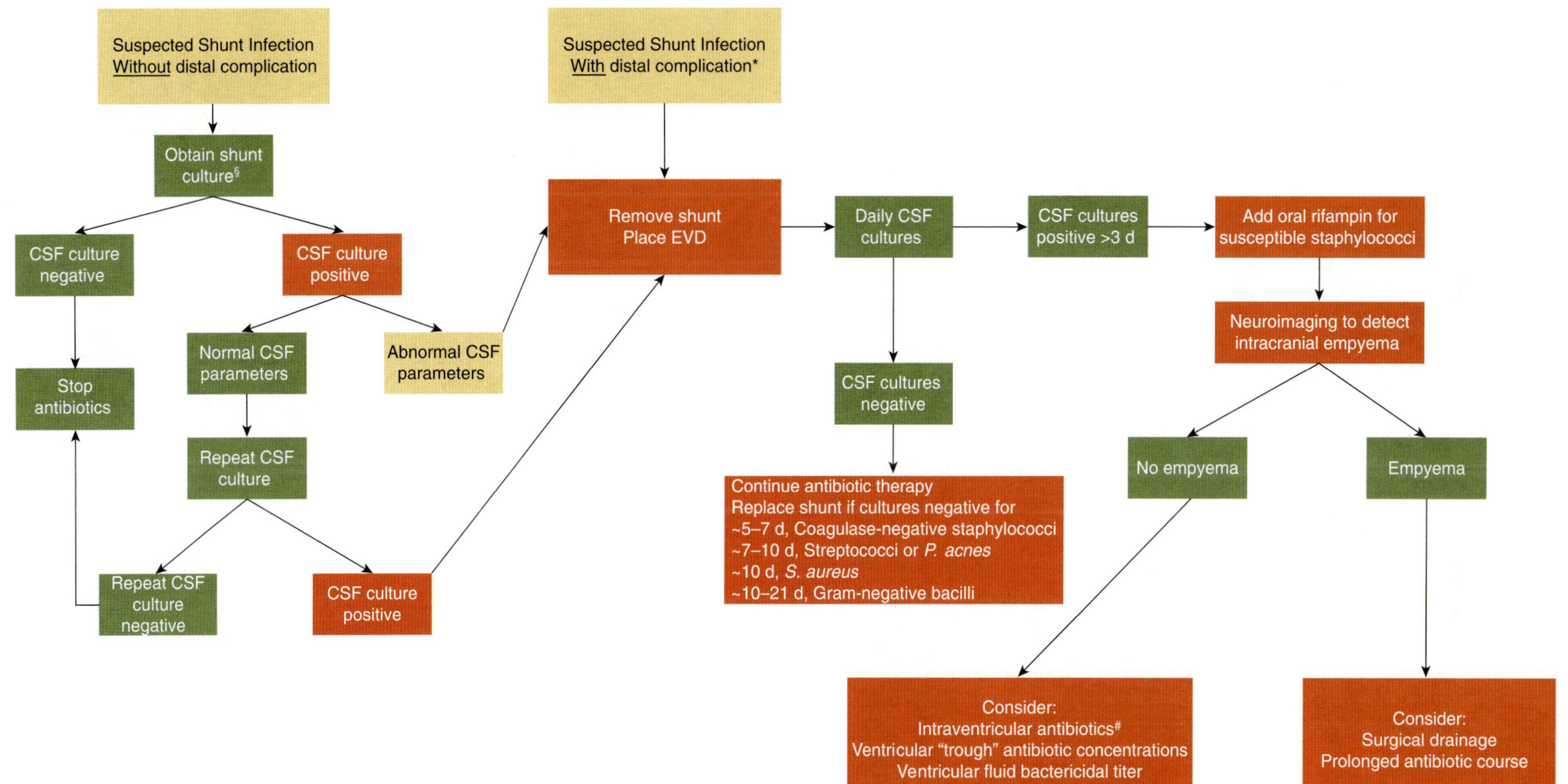

FIGURE 70–3 ■ Algorithm for management of suspected CSF shunt infection.

*Begin empiric therapy with vancomycin in combination with either ceftazidime, meropenem, or cefepime

§Begin empiric therapy if patient is clinically ill or if CSF parameters (e.g., cell count, glucose, protein, or Gram stain) are abnormal, otherwise may begin empiric therapy if culture is positive.

#Depending on organism isolated, consider vancomycin, gentamicin, tobramycin, or amikacin. Some authors have used polymyxin B or colistin for Gram-negative bacteria resistant to commonly used antibiotic agents. Intraventricular administration is not an U.S. Food and Drug Administration-approved indication for any of the listed antibiotics.

Situations that may warrant additional measures include cases of delayed ventricular fluid sterilization (>3 days) and cases where the patient cannot safely undergo surgical catheter removal. First, intraventricular antibiotic administration should be considered. No antibiotic has been approved by the U.S. Food and Drug Administration for intraventricular use. However, commonly used intraventicular antibiotics include vancomycin, gentamicin, tobramycin, and amikacin.[30–32] Polymixin B and colistin have also been administered directly into the ventricles to treat ventricular infections caused by gram-negative bacteria resistant to many commonly used antibiotics.[33–36] Penicillin and cephalosporins should *not* be instilled directly into the ventricles since intraventricular administration of these antibiotics has been associated with increased neurotoxicity, including seizures. Second, rifampin has excellent CSF penetration and should be administered orally (in addition to an intravenous antistaphylococcal agent such as vancomycin) when the infection is caused by susceptible staphylococci.[37,38] Third, neuroimaging should be performed to diagnose an intracranial abscess or empyema. Magnetic resonance imaging is preferred because of its higher sensitivity but contrast-enhanced CT is sufficient in many cases. Finally, either the trough ventricular antibiotic concentration or the ventricular fluid bactericidal titer should be measured to assess the adequacy of antibiotic therapy. No standardized values exist but many experts agree that the trough antibiotic concentration should exceed the minimum inhibitory concentration of the organism by 10-fold or more; lower values indicate suboptimal ventricular fluid antibiotic concentrations. Bactericidal titer measurements may not be readily available since they are technically difficult and time-consuming to perform; if no turbidity is observed after 24 hours of growth, reflecting failure of bacteria to grow at a dilution of 1:8 or higher (i.e., more dilute), then the ventricular antibiotic concentrations are probably sufficient.[11]

Management strategies are summarized in Figure 70–3. Duration of antibiotic therapy varies depending on the causative organism, the time to CSF sterilization, the extent of CSF inflammation, and the patient's clinical response. However, few studies have rigorously analyzed the relationship of duration of therapy to clinical outcome. In general, coagulase-negative staphylococcal infections can be treated for 5–7 days after the first negative culture. Other bacteria should be treated for longer periods *after* CSF sterization: 7–10 days for streptococci and *P. acnes;* 10 days for *S. aureus*; and 10–21 days for gram-negative rods. The isolation of bacteria in the absence of CSF pleocytosis suggests colonization of the shunt catheter; in this situation, some experts recommend a shorter course of therapy than discussed above. While some authors[39] recommend a 3-day period off antimicrobial therapy to verify clearing of infection prior to shunt reimplantation, such a strategy does not appear to benefit the patient.[40] Patients with a complicated course or suppurative complications such as brain abscess or intracranial empyema may require longer therapy. Additional therapy is not typically required once the shunt has been replaced. If the shunt was not initially removed, therapy should be continued for an even longer period of time than mentioned above, although the optimal duration in such cases is not known.

COURSE AND PROGNOSIS

The mortality associated with ventricular shunt infections is low. Potential morbidity includes new or more frequent seizures and worsening neurologic impairment. Infections caused by *S. aureus* and *Candida* species have a substantially higher rate of recurrence despite adequate therapy than infections caused by other organisms.

PEARLS AND SPECIAL SITUATIONS

- Laboratory findings of anemia, azotemia, hematuria, and proteinuria suggest shunt nephritis in a child with a ventriculoatrial shunt.
- Impaired CSF flow can lead to normal CSF findings despite the presence of ventriculitis in specimens obtained by lumbar puncture.

REFERENCES

1. Naradzay JF, Browne BJ, Rolnick MA, Doherty RJ. Cerebral ventricular shunts. *J Emerg Med.* 1999;17(2):311-322.
2. Kontny U, Hofling B, Gutjahr P, Voth D, Schwarz M, Schmitt HJ. CSF shunt infections in children. *Infection.* 1993;21(2):89-92.
3. Mancao M, Miller C, Cochrane B, Hoff C, Sauter K, Weber E. Cerebrospinal fluid shunt infections in infants and children in Mobile, Alabama. *Acta Paediatr.* 1998;87(6):667-670.
4. Ronan A, Hogg GG, Klug GL. Cerebrospinal fluid shunt infections in children. *Pediatr Infect Dis J.* 1995;14(9):782-786.
5. McGirt MJ, Zaas A, Fuchs HE, George TM, Kaye K, Sexton DJ. Risk factors for pediatric ventriculoperitoneal shunt infection and predictors of infectious pathogens. *Clin Infect Dis.* 2003;36(7):858-862.
6. Dallacasa P, Dappozzo A, Galassi E, Sandri F, Cocchi G, Masi M. Cerebrospinal fluid shunt infections in infants. *Childs Nerv Syst.* 1995;11(11):643-648.
7. Morris A, Low DE. Nosocomial bacterial meningitis, including central nervous system shunt infections. *Infect Dis Clin North Am.* 1999;13(3):735-750.
8. Wang KW, Chang WN, Shih TY, et al. Infection of cerebrospinal fluid shunts: causative pathogens, clinical features, and outcomes. *Jpn J Infect Dis.* 2004;57(2):44-48.

9. Pople IK, Bayston R, Hayward RD. Infection of cerebrospinal fluid shunts in infants: a study of etiological factors. *J Neurosurg.* 1992;77(1):29-36.
10. Odio C, McCracken GH, Jr., Nelson JD. CSF shunt infections in pediatrics. A seven-year experience. *Am J Dis Child.* 1984;138(12):1103-1108.
11. Yogev R. Cerebrospinal fluid shunt infections: a personal view. *Pediatr Infect Dis.* 1985;4(2):113-118.
12. Thompson TP, Albright AL. *Propionibacterium acnes* infections of cerebrospinal fluid shunts. *Childs Nerv Syst.* 1998;14(8):378-380.
13. Chiou CC, Wong TT, Lin HH, et al. Fungal infection of ventriculoperitoneal shunts in children. *Clin Infect Dis.* 1994;19(6):1049-1053.
14. Kim TY, Stewart G, Voth M, Moynihan JA, Brown L. Signs and symptoms of cerebrospinal fluid shunt malfunction in the pediatric emergency department. *Pediatr Emerg Care* 2006;22(1):28-34.
15. Stamos JK, Kaufman BA, Yogev R. Ventriculoperitoneal shunt infections with Gram-negative bacteria. *Neurosurgery.* 1993;33(5):858-862.
16. Apsner R, Winkler S, Schneeweiss B, Horl WH. The shampoo clue: two cases of infection of a ventriculoatrial shunt. *Clin Infect Dis.* 2000;31(6):1518-1519.
17. Anderson CM, Sorrells DL, Kerby JD. Intraabdominal pseudocysts as a complication of ventriculoperitoneal shunts. *J Am Coll Surg.* 2003;196(2):297-300.
18. Browd SR, Gottfried ON, Ragel BT, Kestle JR. Failure of cerebrospinal fluid shunts: part II: Overdrainage, loculation, and abdominal complications. *Pediatr Neurol.* 2006; 34(3):171-176.
19. Ugarriza LF, Cabezudo JM, Lorenzana LM, Porras LF, Garcia-Yague LM. Delayed pneumocephalus in shunted patients. Report of three cases and review of the literature. *Br J Neurosurg.* 2001;15(2):161-167.
20. Grosfeld JL, Cooney DR, Smith J, Campbell RL. Intraabdominal complications following ventriculoperitoneal shunt procedures. *Pediatrics.* 1974;54(6):791-796.
21. Rush DS, Walsh JW, Belin RP, Pulito AR. Ventricular sepsis and abdominally related complications in children with cerebrospinal fluid shunts. *Surgery.* 1985;97(4):420-427.
22. Myers MG, Schoenbaum SC. Shunt fluid aspiration: an adjunct in the diagnosis of cerebrospinal fluid shunt infection. *Am J Dis Child.* 1975;129(2):220-222.
23. Noetzel MJ, Baker RP. Shunt fluid examination: Risks and benefits in the evaluation of shunt malfunction and infection. *J Neurosurg.* 1984;61(2):328-332.
24. McClinton D, Carraccio C, Englander R. Predictors of ventriculoperitoneal shunt pathology. *Pediatr Infect Dis J.* 2001;20(6):593-597.
25. Zorc JJ, Krugman SD, Ogborn J, Benson J. Radiographic evaluation for suspected cerebrospinal fluid shunt obstruction. *Pediatr Emerg Care.* 2002;18(5):337-340.
26. Goeser CD, McLeary MS, Young LW. Diagnostic imaging of ventriculoperitoneal shunt malfunctions and complications. *Radiographics.* 1998;18(3):635-651.
27. Schreffler RT, Schreffler AJ, Wittler RR. Treatment of cerebrospinal fluid shunt infections: a decision analysis. *Pediatr Infect Dis J.* 2002;21(7):632-636.
28. Anderson EJ, Yogev R. A rational approach to the management of ventricular shunt infections. *Pediatr Infect Dis J.* 2005;24(6):557-558.
29. Gill CJ, Murphy MA, Hamer DH. Treatment of *Staphylococcus epidermidis* ventriculo-peritoneal shunt infection with linezolid. *J Infect.* 2002;45(2):129-132.
30. Hirsch BE, Amodio M, Einzig AI, Halevy R, Soeiro R. Instillation of vancomycin into a cerebrospinal fluid reservoir to clear infection: pharmacokinetic considerations. *J Infect Dis.* 1991;163(1):197-200.
31. Pickering LK, Ericsson CD, Ruiz-Palacios G, Blevins J, Miner ME. Intraventricular and parenteral gentamicin therapy for ventriculitis in children. *Am J Dis Child.* 1978;132(5):480-483.
32. Laborada G, Cruz F, Nesin M. Serial cytokine profiles in shunt-related ventriculitis treated with intraventricular vancomycin. *Chemotherapy.* 2005;51(6):363-365.
33. Bukhary Z, Mahmood W, Al-Khani A, Al-Abdely HM. Treatment of nosocomial meningitis due to a multidrug resistant Acinetobacter baumannii with intraventricular colistin. *Saudi Med J.* 2005;26(4):656-658.
34. Clifford HE, Stewart GT. Intraventricular administration of a new derivative of polymyxin B in meningitis due to Ps. pyocyanea. *Lancet.* 1961;2:177-180.
35. Fernandez-Viladrich P, Corbella X, Corral L, Tubau F, Mateu A. Successful treatment of ventriculitis due to carbapenem-resistant Acinetobacter baumannii with intraventricular colistin sulfomethate sodium. *Clin Infect Dis.* 1999;28(4):916-917.
36. Ng J, Gosbell IB, Kelly JA, Boyle MJ, Ferguson JK. Cure of multiresistant Acinetobacter baumannii central nervous system infections with intraventricular or intrathecal colistin: case series and literature review. *J Antimicrob Chemother.* 2006;58:1078-1081.
37. Archer GL, Tenenbaum MJ, Haywood HB, III. Rifampin therapy of *Staphylococcus epidermidis.* Use in infections from indwelling artificial devices. *JAMA.* 1978;240(8): 751-753.
38. Ring JC, Cates KL, Belani KK, Gaston TL, Sveum RJ, Marker SC. Rifampin for CSF shunt infections caused by coagulase-negative staphylococci. *J Pediatr.* 1979;95(2):317-319.
39. Tunkel AR, Kaufman B. Cerebrospinal fluid shunt infections. In: Mandell GL, Bennett J, Dolin R, eds. *Principles and Practice of Infectious Diseases.* 6th ed. Philadelphia, PA: Elsevier; 2005:1126-1132.
40. Wang KC, Lee HJ, Sung JN, Cho BK. Cerebrospinal fluid shunt infection in children: efficiency of management protocol, rate of persistent shunt colonization, and significance of 'off-antibiotics' trial. *Childs Nerv Syst.* 1999; 15(1):38-43; discussion -4.
41. Fleisher G, Ludwig, S, Henretig, FM, Silverman, BK, Ruddy, RM. *Textbook of Pediatric Emergency Medicine.* 5th ed. Philadelphia, PA: Lippincott Williams & Wilkins; 2005.

CHAPTER 71

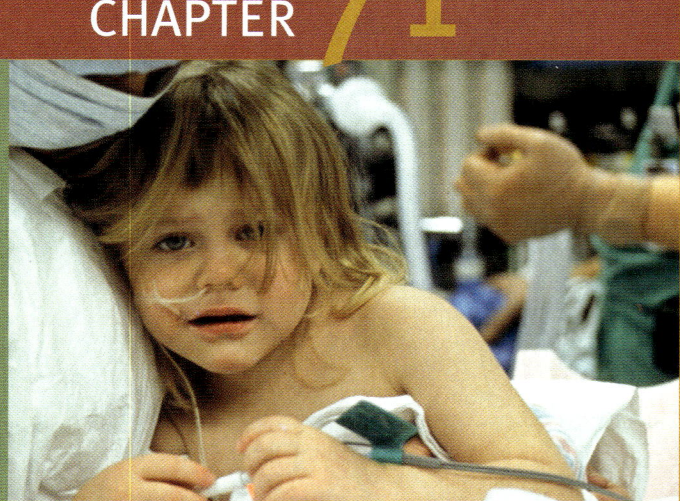

Catheter-Associated Infections

Kristina Bryant and Matthew M. Zahn

DEFINITIONS AND EPIDEMIOLOGY

Each year, more than 5 million central venous catheters are inserted in patients in the United States. Types of catheters are listed in Table 71–1. A substantial proportion of these are used in children for delivery of intravenous fluids, total parenteral nutrition, antibiotics, and chemotherapy. Infectious complications occur in 5–26% of all patients with central venous catheters. According to data reported to the National Nosocomial Infection Surveillance System (NNIS) between 1992 and 2003, the pooled mean catheter-associated bloodstream infection (CA-BSI) rate in pediatric intensive care unit patients was 7.3/1000 catheter days.[1] Rates in neonatal intensive care units (NICUs) ranged from 3.7/1000 catheter days in infants with birth weights >2500 g to 10.6/1000 catheter days in infants with birth weights <1000 g. In addition to patient factors such as immunosuppression and prematurity, longer duration of catheter use,[2] use of multiple central lines,[3] dialysis,[2] extracorporeal membrane oxygenation therapy,[2] total parenteral nutrition,[4] mechanical ventilation,[5] and receipt of packed red blood cell transfusion[6] are all associated with increased risk of infection. In premature infants, duration of intravenous lipid use has been associated with coagulase-negative staphylococci (CoNS) bacteremia and fungemia.[7]

Types of catheter-associated infection are listed in Table 71–2. Various definitions have been proposed for central venous catheter-associated bloodstream infection (CVC-BSI), including catheter-related BSI (CR-BSI) and catheter-associated BSI. CR-BSI—a BSI attributable to the catheter—is often difficult to diagnose in children because obtaining a peripheral culture is not always

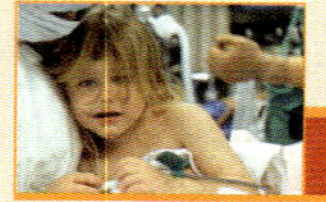

Table 71–1.

Types of Central Catheters

Catheter Type	Insertion Site	Comments
Nontunneled CVC	Subclavian, jugular, femoral veins	For short-term intravenous therapy, typically less than 21 d
Tunneled CVC	Subclavian, jugular, and femoral veins	Broviac, Hickman, Groshong; can remain in place for months to years
Totally Implantable	Subclavian or internal jugular	"Infusaport" or "port"; can remain in place for months to years
Percutaneously inserted central catheter (PICC)	Peripheral vein in the arm, leg or scalp; terminates in central vein	Commonly used for outpatient therapy; can remain in place for weeks to months
Umbilical	Umbilical artery or vein	Used in neonates Umbilical artery catheters should not be used >5 d Umbilical venous catheters can be used up to 14 d

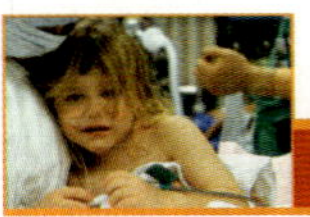

Table 71–2.

Types of Central Catheter-Related Infection

Local infection (in the absence of concomitant bloodstream infection)	
Exit site infection	Erythema or induration within 2 cm of the the catheter exit site
Tunnel infection	Tenderness, erythema, or induration within 2 cm of the subcutaneous tract of a tunneled catheter
Pocket infection	Purulent fluid in the subcutaneous pocket of a totaled implanted vascular catheter with or without spontaneous drainage or skin necrosis
CVC-BSI	
CR-BSI	Catheter-tip culture yields ≤15 colony-forming units of the same organism as is grown from a peripheral blood sample *or* Positive CVC and peripheral culture *and* 1. Quantitative blood culture from CVC has 5–10-fold greater colony-forming units count than peripheral culture *or* 2. CVC culture turns positive more than 2 h prior to peripheral culture
CA-BSI	Recognized pathogen cultured from 1 or more blood cultures *and* 1. Central venous catheter in use in the 48-h period before the development of infection 2. Pathogen cultured from the blood not related to infection at another site

feasible and catheters are often not removed for diagnostic purposes because of the difficulty of inserting another catheter. Therefore, CA-BSI—a BSI in the context of a catheter—is a practical definition used in many children's hospitals. This definition is also used for nosocomial infection surveillance.

Totally implantable devices are associated with the lowest rates of infection, followed by tunneled central venous catheters and percutaneously inserted central catheters. Catheter location is also important. The highest rates of infection are associated with jugular catheters, followed by femoral and subclavian catheters.

Staphylococcus aureus and gram-negative bacilli cause most catheter insertion or exit site infections. Etiologic agents associated with CVC-BSI are listed in Table 71–3.[8] The relative frequency of each pathogen varies by patient population. In NICU patients, CoNS account for approximately 50% of CVC-BSI; enterococci are also common pathogens.[4] In pediatric intensive care units, CoNS are likewise common (37.7%), followed by gram-negative bacteria (25%), enterococci, and *Candida* species.[9] *Pseudomonas aeruginosa* and viridans streptococci are also important considerations in patients with febrile neutropenia. In patients with short gut syndrome, enteric gram-negative bacilli and yeast predominate, probably because of translocation of bacteria from the gastrointestinal tract and subsequent seeding of the catheter.[10,11]

Few studies have described the epidemiology of patients who develop catheter-related infections in home care settings. Overall, gram-negative bacilli appear to cause a disproportionate number of infections acquired in home care, particularly in the context of a polymicrobial infection. CoNS, *Pseudomonas*, and *Acinetobacter* species were identified most often in one study of pediatric oncology patients receiving home infusion therapy.[12] Among children with cancer, gram-negative bacteria accounted for 44% of CVC-BSIs acquired in home care but only 18% of those acquired in the hospital setting.[13] In another study of pediatric patients receiving intravenous antistaphylococcal therapy at home for osteomyelitis, *P. aeruginosa* and enteric bacilli accounted for nearly all of the infections; one-third of infections were polymicrobial.[14] More recently, children with BSI caused by *Stenotrophomonas maltophilia* were four times

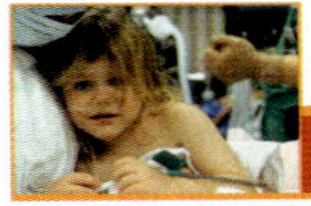

Table 71–3.

Etiology of CVC-BSI

Common
Coagulase-negative staphylococci
Enterococci
S. aureus
Candida albicans

Less common
Enteric gram-negative bacilli
Klebsiella species
Escherichia coli
Enterobacter species
Pseudomonas species
Non-*albicans Candida* species

Rare
Rapidly-growing mycobacteria†
Anaerobic bacteria
Malassezia furfur

†*Especially mycobacterium fortuitum, mycobacterium abscesses, mycobacterium chelonae.*

more likely to acquire their infection in home care than those with BSIs caused by other gram-negative rods.[15]

PATHOGENESIS

The pathogenesis of catheter-related infection varies by catheter type. Most infections of nontunneled catheters are related to migration of skin flora at the catheter exit site down the extraluminal surface of the catheter, probably by capillary action.[16,17] By contrast, infection of tunneled catheters most often results from colonization of the catheter hub during catheter use, with subsequent intraluminal colonization of the catheter and dissemination to the blood.[18] Catheter colonization is common and does not always result in CVC-BSI; the risk of infection appears to be related to the number of organisms present.[19] Hematogenous seeding of catheters as a result of infection at another site (i.e., the abdomen or the lungs) occasionally occurs and contaminated infusates are rare causes of CVC-BSI.[20]

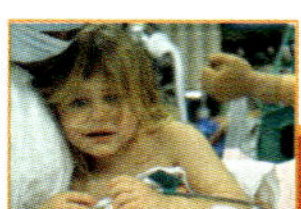

Table 71–5.

Signs and Symptoms of Catheter-Associated Infection

Systemic
Fever
Hypothermia
Malaise
Hypotension
Delayed capillary refill
Apnea
Feeding intolerance
Cardiac murmur (if endocarditis is present)

Local
Erythema at catheter exit site or over tunnel tract
Drainage from catheter exit site
Fluctuence or induration overlying totally implanted catheter or tunnel tract
Malfunction of catheter

CLINICAL PRESENTATION

History and Physical

The patient's past medical history should be documented, with particular emphasis given to factors that may place the patient at risk for specific infections or indicate a potential offending pathogen (Table 71–4). Patients with CVC-BSI can have a broad spectrum of symptoms (Table 71–5). Systemic symptoms of CVC-BSI generally include fever, and fever is often the only sign of disease. Any patient with a central line and fever must be considered to potentially have a CVC-BSI. Patients can present with sepsis, and a patient's hemodynamic status should always be noted, including capillary refill and blood pressure. Alternatively, patients with catheter infection can present with minimal outward signs of disease. Symptoms in the neonate in particular can be insidious and include apnea, feeding intolerance, temperature regulation problems, increased oxygen requirement, and lethargy. GI symptoms such as abdominal distension can occasionally occur.[21] Catheter malfunction can be an early sign of infection.

Symptoms may vary by organism causing infection, but overlap occurs. CoNS classically causes relatively mild clinical symptoms, although neonates with CVC-BSI may manifest with sepsis syndrome. Gram-negative and fungal CVC-BSIs are more likely to present with severe systemic symptoms. Symptoms associated with a CVC-BSI often become more prominent with manipulation of the line, such as during flushing or pushing medications. Clinical findings overall can be unreliable: Findings with good sensitivity have poor specificity (e.g., fever), and those with good specificity have poor sensitivity (e.g., catheter site findings).

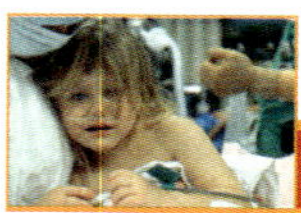

Table 71–4.

Pertinent Medical History

Type of catheter
Indications for catheter placement
Date of catheter placement
Symptoms that may indicate alternate source of fever (e.g., upper respiratory tract symptoms, diarrhea, rash, etc.)
Underlying illnesses
Previous culture history
Current antibiotic regimen

Local Catheter Infection Signs

The physical examination of any patient with suspected CVC-associated infection includes an examination of the catheter site. Dressings should be removed to allow for adequate evaluation of the exit site. Local infections generally present with some combination of erythema, induration, tenderness, and/or drainage around the catheter site (Figures 71–1 and 71–2). Local infection may be confused with simple soft tissue inflammation. Local signs may be absent in neutropenic patients with catheter site infections because of an inability to mount an inflammatory response. CVC-BSI often presents without any local signs of infection.

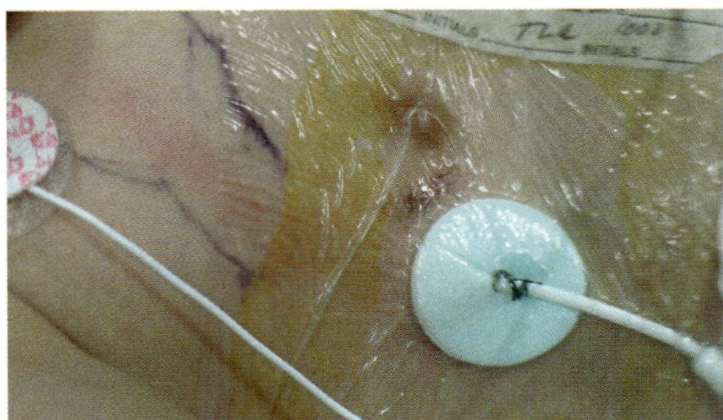

FIGURE 71–1 ■ Linear erythema seen with a tunnel infection.

Other Physical Examination Findings

Thorough, repeated evaluations for other potential infectious etiologies that can cause fever and systemic symptoms should be performed in all patients with suspected CVC-BSI, especially those with positive blood cultures. A thorough evaluation for endocarditis must always be performed, especially in the setting of repeatedly positive blood cultures. This includes cardiac examination to search for new murmurs and a search for evidence of embolic disease such as pulmonary lesions, splinter hemorrhages in the nail beds, Osler nodes (red-purple, tender, raised), and Janeway lesions (hemorrhagic, nontender, flat).

DIAGNOSIS

Catheter site infection is a clinical diagnosis. Cultures of the local catheter site, especially when purulent drainage is present, may help guide antimicrobial therapy. CVC-BSI infection is definitively diagnosed by isolation of a pathogen by blood culture in the appropriate clinical setting. When CVC-BSI is suspected, blood cultures should be obtained whenever possible both from the CVC and a peripheral vein (Table 71–6). At least 1 mL of blood should be drawn for culture in young children. Up to 30 mL may be obtained in older adolescents and adults. The sensitivity of blood cultures increase with the volume of blood drawn.[22]

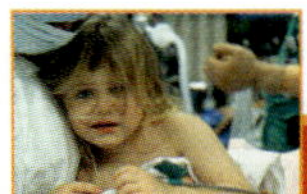

Table 71–6.

Diagnostic Evaluation of Suspected CVC-Infection

Quantitative blood culture from each lumen of catheter (at least 1 mL)
Quantitative blood culture from peripheral vein (at least 1 mL)
Gram stain and culture of exudate at catheter exit site (if present)
Semiquantitative or quantitative culture of catheter tip (if catheter is removed)
Complete blood count

Optional tests

- CRP test
- Serum electrolytes
- Echocardiogram, if endocarditis suspected
- Doppler ultrasound, if thrombophlebitis is suspected

Exclude infection at other sites

- Chest radiograph to evaluate pneumonia, if tachypnea or hypoxia is present
- Abdominal radiograph, if abdominal distention or feeding intolerance
- Urinalysis and urine culture

A positive blood culture drawn from an in-dwelling catheter can represent true CVC-BSI, catheter-colonization or simple contaminant. Distinguishing infection caused by common skin flora, such as CoNS, from other infections can be challenging, A positive peripheral blood culture in conjunction with a positive catheter culture is stronger evidence of catheter-related disease than catheter culture alone. Standard laboratory criteria for diagnosing a CVC-BSI are listed in Table 71–2. When both peripheral and catheter cultures of equal volume have been drawn, quantitative culture methods can also distinguish true infection from contaminated culture. When a CVC culture turns positive more than 2 hours before a peripheral culture, a CVC-BSI is likely.[23] CVC-BSI is also likely when a comparison of quantitative cultures yields a CVC-to-peripheral ratio of 5:1 or more. If the catheter is removed, catheter tip cultures are useful in confirming catheter-related infection. Isolation of identical organisms from the central catheter tip and peripheral blood culture is strong evidence of CVC-BSI. Prior antibiotic exposure, however, often leads to a negative result.

Adjunctive laboratory tests include a complete blood count. The white blood cell count may be significantly high or low. Thrombocytopenia is often

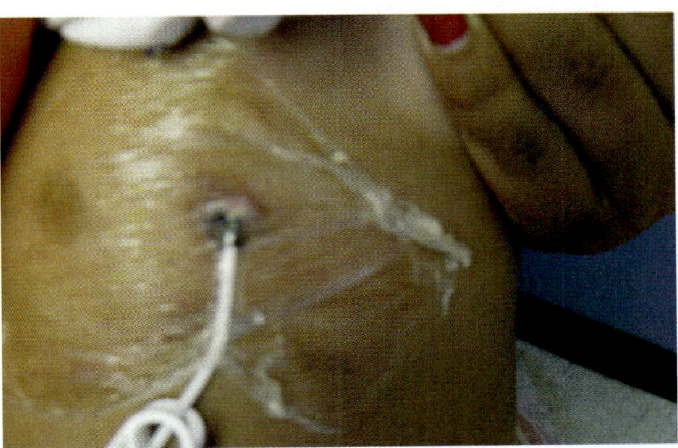

FIGURE 71–2 ■ Erythema, induration and purulent drainage in a patient with a catheter exit site infection.

present in the face of systemic fungal disease.[24] A C-reactive protein test (CRP) may be helpful in assessing the likelihood of BSI in children with CVCs. CRP has been used to guide empiric therapy in febrile children but specific cutoff values for the diagnosis of CVC-BSI have not yet been determined. Cultures from other potential sites of infection, such as endotracheal tubes or foley catheters, should also be obtained.

Management of Suspected CVC Infection

An approach to the management of suspected CVC-BSI is outlined in Figure 71–3. Those with mild illness can undergo initial evaluation, including blood culture, without initiation of empiric antibiotic therapy. More seriously ill children must have empiric antibiotic therapy begun immediately. Typical empiric regimens include antimicrobials active against gram-positive and gram-negative bacteria. Because of the prevalence of methicillin-resistant *S. aureus* and CoNS at many centers, vancomycin is appropriate for gram-positive coverage. An aminoglycoside (gentamicin, tobramycin, amikacin) or a beta-lactam with antipseudomonal activity (ceftazidime, cefepime, piperacillin-tazobactam or meropenam) are options for gram-negative coverage. In severely ill patients or those at risk for multidrug resistant gram-negative infections, empiric gram-negative coverage with both an aminoglycoside and a beta-lactam should be considered.

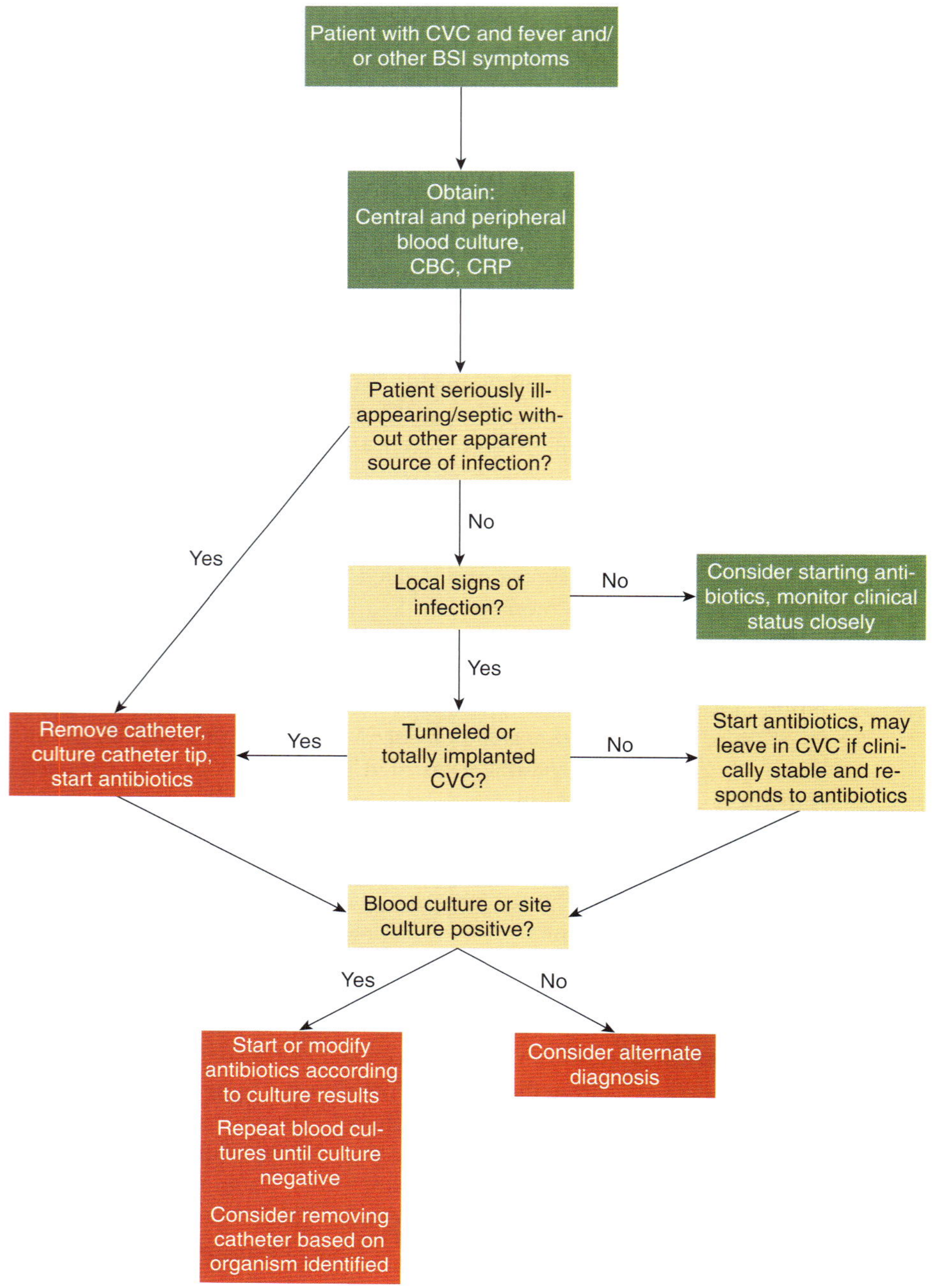

FIGURE 71–3 ■ Management of the child with suspected CVC-associated infection.

Because the sites for venous access are often limited in children, immediate catheter removal is not always feasible. Catheter exit site infections are sometimes successfully treated with systemic and local antibiotics without catheter removal. In contrast, pocket or tunnel infections necessitate catheter removal. If the patient appears septic, consideration should be given to catheter removal without awaiting confirmatory culture results. When a culture yields a preliminary positive result, a repeat blood culture should be obtained. Persistently positive blood cultures despite effective antimicrobial therapy should prompt CVC removal and a search for metastatic infections such as endocarditis, meningitis, osteomyelitis or septic thrombosis.

DIFFERENTIAL DIAGNOSIS

The differential diagnosis for fever in a patient with a central venous catheter is broad and varies among different at-risk patient groups. In an otherwise healthy outpatient with an indwelling catheter, the likelihood of CVC-associated BSI is high.[25] In an ICU setting, the development of fever in a patient with a central venous catheter heralds a catheter-related infection in only 12% of patients.[26] Careful evaluation for other sources of fever, including catheter-associated urinary tract infection, ventilator-associated pneumonia, and nosocomial viral infection, is indicated. A positive blood culture alone does not confirm catheter-associated infection; other sources of infection must be excluded. For example, the source of gram-negative bacteremia in a NICU patient may be an intra-abdominal process such as necrotizing enterocolitis rather than infection attributable to the catheter.

TREATMENT

Definitive therapy of CVC-BSI is based on the type of infection, the antimicrobial susceptibility pattern of the organism, and the presence of metastatic infections. The optimal duration of therapy for children with uncomplicated CVC-associated infection has not been defined, but recommendations have been extrapolated from adult treatment guidelines.[22] In general, tunnel and pocket infections are treated with 10–14 days of systemic antibiotic therapy in addition to catheter removal. Shorter courses may be effective for exit site infections, especially when the catheter is removed.

The treatment of CVC-associated BSI is summarized in Table 71–7. Treatment of *S. aureus*, fungi, or mycobacteria requires catheter removal, as does persistent bacteremia with any organism. Most uncomplicated cases of CVC-BSI are treated with 10–14 days of antibiotic therapy. A shorter course of therapy (5–7 days) is appropriate for CoNS when the catheter is removed. A longer course of therapy (21 days) is recommended by some experts for *S. aureus* BSI. An echocardiogram should be performed when *S. aureus* is isolated from serial (2 or more) blood cultures, or in any child with congenital heart disease and *S. aureus* BSI. Although routine catheter removal is not necessary for most cases of CVC-BSI caused by enteric gram-negative organisms, delayed catheter removal in neonates with either *S. aureus* or gram-negative rod infection is associated with infection related-complications, including osteomyelitis, meningitis, vital organ abscess, and death.[27]

Fungal infections are treated for at least 14 days after blood cultures are negative. Ophthalmologic examination should be routinely performed in children with candidemia to detect retinitis; this examination may be performed 1–2 weeks after negative cultures because dissemination may occur at any point during active candidemia. When blood cultures are persistently positive for *Candida* species, an ultrasound of the liver and spleen should be performed to evaluate for hepatosplenic candidiasis, as well as echocardiogram to evaluate for endocarditis.

Antibiotic Lock Therapy

Antibiotic lock therapy entails flushing a mixture of anticoagulant and antibiotic into a catheter and allowing the solution to dwell for a period of time. Treatment of CVC-BSI with lock therapy with or without concurrent systemic antibiotics can be effective in instances of hard-to-clear infection when maintaining the catheter is vital. Antibiotic lock therapy has also been effective as prophylaxis, lowering rates of infection in patients with underlying illness, such as short gut syndrome, that place them at increased risk of repeated CVC-BSIs.[28] Some caveats exist: Tunnel or pocket infections are unlikely to respond,[29] and treatment of CoNS has been more effective than treating *S. aureus* or pseudomonal infection. Vancomycin has been most comprehensively studied in lock preparations,[30,31] although multiple other antibiotics have been used,[32] including amphotericin B to treat fungal disease.[33] Duration of therapy in many successful studies has been 2 weeks.[22] Appropriate concentrations of antibiotic solutions and dwell times are still being established.[33] The specific indications for antibiotic lock therapy remain to be defined.

In general, complicated CVC infections should be managed in conjunction with appropriate pediatric subspecialists (Table 71–8). Infectious disease consultation may be helpful (1) when the infection is caused by an unusual or multidrug resistant organism or (2) when the symptoms of sepsis persist, regardless of appropriate antimicrobial therapy and catheter removal. Endocarditis may require consultation with a cardiologist or cardiovascular surgeon. The infection control team should

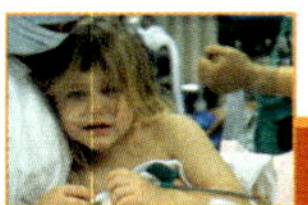

Table 71–7.

Treatment of CVC-BSI

Organism	Antimicrobial Agent	Duration	Routine Catheter Removal
Coagulase-negative staphylococcus	Vancomycin 15 mg/kg/dose every 6 h	10–14 d*	No
Methicillin-susceptible *S. aureus*	Oxacillin 50 mg/kg/dose every 6 h	14 d†	Yes
Methicillin-resistant *S. aureus*	Vancomycin 15 mg/kg/dose every 6 h	14 d†	Yes
Enteric gram-negative bacilli	Cefepime 50 mg/kg/dose every 8–12 h‡ *or* Meropenem 20 mg/kg/dose every 8 h	10–14 d	No
Enterococci	Ampicillin 50 mg/kg/dose every 6 h (susceptible isolates) *or* Vancomycin15 mg/kg/dose every 6 h Add gentamicin, if endocarditis is present	10–14 d	No
P. aeruginosa	Cefepime or meropenem with an aminoglycoside	10–14 d	Yes
C. albicans, *C. parapsilosis*, *C. lusitaniae* *C. glabrata* *C. kruzei*	Fluconazole 6 mg/kg every 24 h Amphotericin B 1 mg/kg every 24 hours *or* Caspofungin 70 mg/m^2 as a loading dose, followed by 50 mg/m^2 every 24 h§	14 d after the first negative culture	Yes

**5–7 Days is sufficient, if CVC is removed.*
†Some experts recommend 21-day course.
‡Every 8-h dosing is recommended for febrile neutropenia.
§Hepatic insufficiency requires dose adjustment.

be notified if a contaminated infusate is suspected as the source of a CVC-BSI.

PREVENTION

Most catheter-associated infections are preventable. Measures proven to decrease rates of catheter-related infection are outlined in Table 71–9.[28] Concurrent implementation of these measures as part of a "bundle" or comprehensive prevention program leads to greater reductions in infection rates than does implementation of any single measure.[34] Scheduled replacement of catheters as a method to decrease infections is not recommended and is associated with a higher rate of mechanical complications.

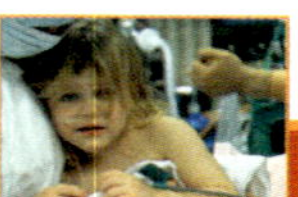

Table 71–8.

When to Refer to a Subspecialist

Bloodstream infection complicated by endocarditis, meningitis, osteomyelitis, or septic thrombosis
Persistently positive blood cultures despite appropriate antimicrobial therapy and catheter removal
Infection with rare or multidrug-resistant organism
Persistent fever, hypotension, or other signs of sepsis despite negative blood cultures

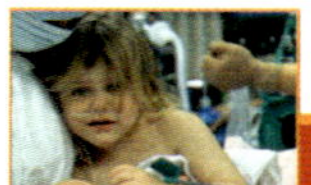

Table 71–9.

Strategies to Prevent CVC-BSI

Education of personnel who will insert and maintain catheters
Hand hygiene before catheter insertion or manipulation of the hub
Skin antisepsis with 2% chlorhexidine gluconate at insertion and at dressing change
Full sterile barrier precautions at the time of catheter insertion
Removal of catheter when no longer necessary

Modification to these practices or additional measures may be required in specific patient populations. For instance, chlorhexidine gluconate is currently labeled for use in infants ≥2 months of age, although some experts advocate its use in younger infants with birth weights ≥1500 grams. Limitation of intravenous lipid use in NICU patients may reduce the risk for the development of CoNS bacteremia or fungemia. In adults, femoral catheters are associated with higher infection rates and should be avoided when possible.[35] Insufficient data exist to recommend against femoral catheterization in children.[36]

Additional preventive measures include the use of antimicrobial/antiseptic impregnated catheters. Catheters coated with chlorhexidine/silver sulfadiazine or minocycline/rifampin have been shown to reduce the risk of CVC infection in adults.[37,38] The additional cost of these catheters justify their use if other measures fail to decrease CVC-BSI.[28] Use of a chlorhexidine-impregnated sponge (Biopatch™) at the insertion site of short-term CVC reduces catheter-colonization and CR-BSI in adults.[39] Data in pediatric patients are limited. A study involving 705 neonates demonstrated decreased catheter tip colonization in infants randomized to Biopatch™ use but no difference in BSI rates.[40] Contact dermatitis was noted in some extremely low birth weight infants.

PEARLS

- Obtain at least 1 mL of blood for culture in infants
- Symptoms associated with a CVC-BSI often become more prominent with flushing of the line
- Catheter removal is essential in the treatment of CVC-BSI caused by *S. aureus* and *Candida* species

REFERENCES

1. National Nosocomial Infections Surveillance (NNIS) System Report, data summary from January 1992 through June 2003, issued August 2003. *Am J Infect Control.* 2003; 31(8):481-498.
2. Odetola FO, Moler FW, Dechert RE, VanDerElzen K, Chenoweth C. Nosocomial catheter-related bloodstream infections in a pediatric intensive care unit: Risk and rates associated with various intravascular technologies. *Pediatr Crit Care Med.* 2003;4(4):432-436.
3. Almuneef MA, Memish ZA, Balkhy HH, Hijazi O, Cunningham G, Francis C. Rate, risk factors and outcomes of catheter-related bloodstream infection in a paediatric intensive care unit in Saudi Arabia. *J Hosp Infect.* 2006; 62(2):207-213.
4. Sohn AH, Garrett DO, Sinkowitz-Cochran RL, et al. Prevalence of nosocomial infections in neonatal intensive care unit patients: Results from the first national point-prevalence survey. *J Pediatr.* 2001;139(6):821-827.
5. Grohskopf LA, Sinkowitz-Cochran RL, Garrett DO, et al. A national point-prevalence survey of pediatric intensive care unit-acquired infections in the United States. *J Pediatr.* 2002;140(4):432-438.
6. Elward AM, Fraser VJ. Risk factors for nosocomial primary bloodstream infection in pediatric intensive care unit patients: a 2-year prospective cohort study. *Infect Control Hosp Epidemiol.* 2006;27(6):553-560.
7. Avila-Figueroa C, Goldmann DA, Richardson DK, Gray JE, Ferrari A, Freeman J. Intravenous lipid emulsions are the major determinant of coagulase-negative staphylococcal bacteremia in very low birth weight newborns. *Pediatr Infect Dis J.* 1998;17(1):10-17.
8. Wisplinghoff H, Seifert H, Tallent SM, Bischoff T, Wenzel RP, Edmond MB. Nosocomial bloodstream infections in pediatric patients in United States hospitals: epidemiology, clinical features and susceptibilities. *Pediatr Infect Dis J.* 2003;22(8):686-691.
9. Richards MJ, Edwards JR, Culver DH, Gaynes RP. Nosocomial infections in pediatric intensive care units in the United States. National Nosocomial Infections Surveillance System. *Pediatrics.* 1999;103(4):e39.
10. Kurkchubasche AG, Smith SD, Rowe MI. Catheter sepsis in short-bowel syndrome. *Arch Surg.* 1992;127(1):21-24.
11. Weber TR. Enteral feeding increases sepsis in infants with short bowel syndrome. *J Pediatr Surg.* 1995;30(7): 1086-1088; discussion 8-9.
12. Kellerman S, Shay DK, Howard J, et al. Bloodstream infections in home infusion patients: the influence of race and needleless intravascular access devices. *J Pediatr.* 1996; 129(5):711-717.
13. Shah SS, Manning ML, Leahy E, Magnusson M, Rheingold SR, Bell LM. Central venous catheter-associated bloodstream infections in pediatric oncology home care. *Infect Control Hosp Epidemiol.* 2002;23(2):99-101.
14. Ruebner R, Keren R, Coffin S, Chu J, Horn D, Zaoutis TE. Complications of central venous catheters used for the treatment of acute hematogenous osteomyelitis. *Pediatrics.* 2006;117(4):1210-1215.
15. Kagen J, Zaoutis TE, McGowan KL, Luan X, Shah SS. Bloodstream Infection Caused by *Stenotrophomonas maltophilia* in Children. *Pediatr Infect Dis J.* 2007;26(6): 508-512.
16. Cooper GL, Schiller AL, Hopkins CC. Possible role of capillary action in pathogenesis of experimental catheter-associated dermal tunnel infections. *J Clin Microbiol.* 1988;26(1):8-12.
17. Safdar N, Maki DG. The pathogenesis of catheter-related bloodstream infection with noncuffed short-term central venous catheters. *Intensive Care Med.* 2004;30(1):62-67.
18. Linares J, Sitges-Serra A, Garau J, Perez JL, Martin R. Pathogenesis of catheter sepsis: a prospective study with quantitative and semiquantitative cultures of catheter hub and segments. *J Clin Microbiol.* 1985;21(3):357-360.
19. Sherertz RJ, Raad, II, Belani A, et al. Three-year experience with sonicated vascular catheter cultures in a clinical microbiology laboratory. *J Clin Microbiol.* 1990;28(1): 76-82.
20. Held MR, Begier EM, Beardsley DS, et al. Life-threatening sepsis caused by Burkholderia cepacia from contaminated intravenous flush solutions prepared by a compounding pharmacy in another state. *Pediatrics.* 2006;118(1): e212-e215.

21. Maayan-Metzger A, Linder N, Marom D, Vishne T, Ashkenazi S, Sirota L. Clinical and laboratory impact of coagulase-negative staphylococci bacteremia in preterm infants. *Acta Paediatr.* 2000;89(6):690-693.
22. Mermel LA, Farr BM, Sherertz RJ, et al. Guidelines for the management of intravascular catheter-related infections. *Clin Infect Dis.* 2001;32(9):1249-1272.
23. Raad I, Hanna HA, Alakech B, Chatzinikolaou I, Johnson MM, Tarrand J. Differential time to positivity: a useful method for diagnosing catheter-related bloodstream infections. *Ann Intern Med.* 2004;140(1):18-25.
24. Benjamin DK, Jr., Ross K, McKinney RE, Jr., Benjamin DK, Auten R, Fisher RG. When to suspect fungal infection in neonates: a clinical comparison of *Candida albicans* and *Candida parapsilosis* fungemia with coagulase-negative staphylococcal bacteremia. *Pediatrics.* 2000;106(4):712-718.
25. Farr BM. Nosocomial infections related to use of intravascular devices inserted for short-term vascular access. In: Mayhall CG, ed. *Hospital Epidemiology and Infection Control.* Philadelphia, PA: Lippincott Williams & Wilkins; 2004:232-240.
26. Quilici N, Audibert G, Conroy MC, et al. Differential quantitative blood cultures in the diagnosis of catheter-related sepsis in intensive care units. *Clin Infect Dis.* 1997;25(5):1066-1070.
27. Benjamin DK, Jr., Miller W, Garges H, et al. Bacteremia, central catheters, and neonates: when to pull the line. *Pediatrics.* 2001;107(6):1272-1276.
28. O'Grady NP, Alexander M, Dellinger EP, et al. Guidelines for the prevention of intravascular catheter-related infections. *Pediatrics.* 2002;110(5):e51.
29. Dugdale DC, Ramsey PG. *Staphylococcus aureus* bacteremia in patients with Hickman catheters. *Am J Med.* 1990;89(2):137-141.
30. Safdar N, Maki DG. Use of vancomycin-containing lock or flush solutions for prevention of bloodstream infection associated with central venous access devices: a meta-analysis of prospective, randomized trials. *Clin Infect Dis.* 2006;43(4):474-484.
31. Garland JS, Alex CP, Henrickson KJ, McAuliffe TL, Maki DG. A vancomycin-heparin lock solution for prevention of nosocomial bloodstream infection in critically ill neonates with peripherally inserted central venous catheters: A prospective, randomized trial. *Pediatrics.* 2005;116(2):e198-e205.
32. Messing B, Peitra-Cohen S, Debure A, Beliah M, Bernier JJ. Antibiotic-lock technique: A new approach to optimal therapy for catheter-related sepsis in home-parenteral nutrition patients. *JPENJ Parenter Enteral Nutr.* 1988;12(2):185-189.
33. Anthony TU, Rubin LG. Stability of antibiotics used for antibiotic-lock treatment of infections of implantable venous devices (ports). *Antimicrob Agents Chemother.* 1999;43(8):2074-2076.
34. Pronovost P, Needham D, Berenholtz S, et al. An intervention to decrease catheter-related bloodstream infections in the ICU. *N Engl J Med.* 2006;355(26):2725-2732.
35. Merrer J, De Jonghe B, Golliot F, et al. Complications of femoral and subclavian venous catheterization in critically ill patients: A randomized controlled trial. *JAMA.* 2001;286(6):700-707.
36. Venkataraman ST, Thompson AE, Orr RA. Femoral vascular catheterization in critically ill infants and children. *Clin Pediatr (Phila).* 1997;36(6):311-319.
37. Darouiche RO, Raad, II, Heard SO, et al. A comparison of two antimicrobial-impregnated central venous catheters. Catheter Study Group. *N Engl J Med.* 1999;340(1):1-8.
38. Veenstra DL, Saint S, Saha S, Lumley T, Sullivan SD. Efficacy of antiseptic-impregnated central venous catheters in preventing catheter-related bloodstream infection: A meta-analysis. *JAMA.* 1999;281(3):261-267.
39. Maki DG, Mermel LA, Kluger DM, et al. The efficacy of a chlorhexidine-impregnated sponge (Biopatch) for the prevention of intravascular catheter-related infection: A prospective randomized controlled multicenter study (Abstract 1430). In: 40th Interscience Conference on Antimicrobial Agents and Chemotherapy; September 17-20, 2000 Toronto, Canada.
40. Garland JS, Alex CP, Mueller CD, et al. A randomized trial comparing povidone-iodine to a chlorhexidine gluconate-impregnated dressing for prevention of central venous catheter infections in neonates. *Pediatrics.* 2001;107(6):1431-1436.

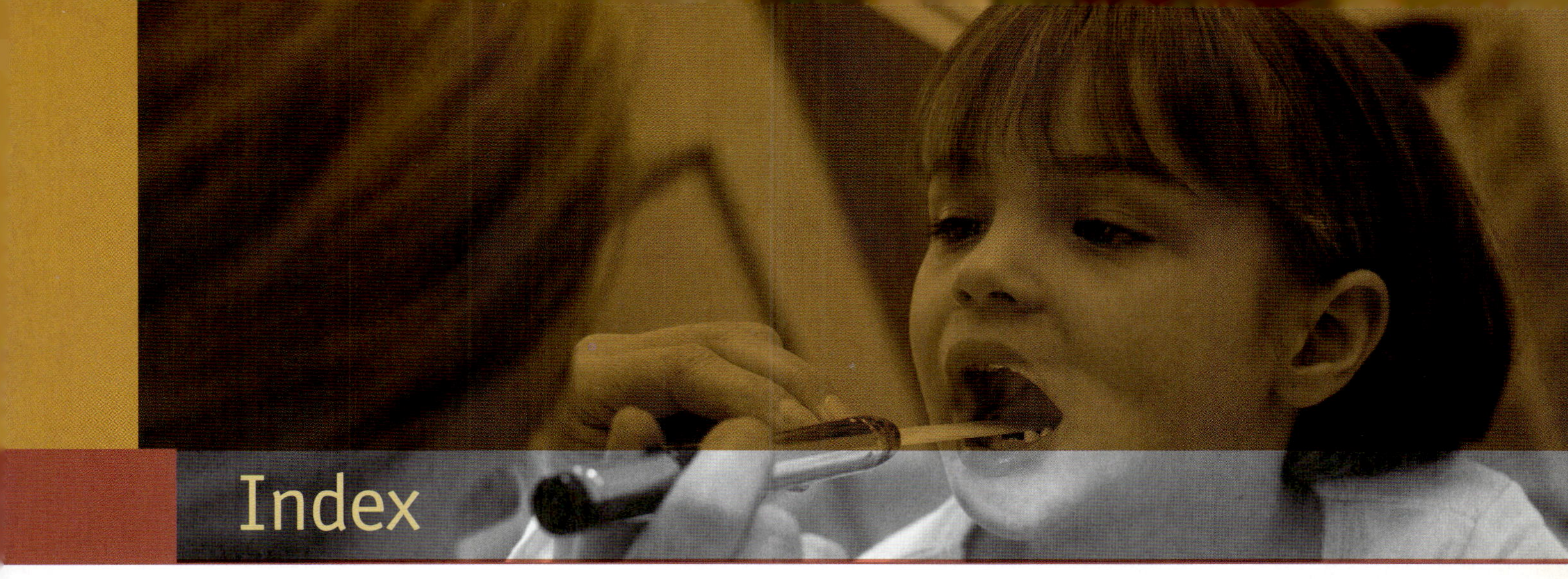

Index